| Water-Soluble Vitamins | | | | | | | Minerals | | | | | |
Ascorbic Acid (mg)	Folacin[6] (µg)	Niacin[7] (mg)	Riboflavin (mg)	Thiamin (mg)	Vitamin B_6 (mg)	Vitamin B_{12} (µg)	Calcium (mg)	Phosphorus (mg)	Iodine (µg)	Iron (mg)	Magnesium (mg)	Zinc (mg)
35	50	5	0.4	0.3	0.3	0.3	360	240	35	10	60	3
35	50	8	0.6	0.5	0.4	0.3	540	400	45	15	70	5
40	100	9	0.8	0.7	0.6	1.0	800	800	60	15	150	10
40	200	12	1.1	0.9	0.9	1.5	800	800	80	10	200	10
40	300	16	1.2	1.2	1.2	2.0	800	800	110	10	250	10
45	400	18	1.5	1.4	1.6	3.0	1200	1200	130	18	350	15
45	400	20	1.8	1.5	1.8	3.0	1200	1200	150	18	400	15
45	400	20	1.8	1.5	2.0	3.0	800	800	140	10	350	15
45	400	18	1.6	1.4	2.0	3.0	800	800	130	10	350	15
45	400	16	1.5	1.2	2.0	3.0	800	800	110	10	350	15
45	400	16	1.3	1.2	1.6	3.0	1200	1200	115	18	300	15
45	400	14	1.4	1.1	2.0	3.0	1200	1200	115	18	300	15
45	400	14	1.4	1.1	2.0	3.0	800	800	100	18	300	15
45	400	13	1.2	1.0	2.0	3.0	800	800	100	18	300	15
45	400	12	1.1	1.0	2.0	3.0	800	800	80	10	300	15
60	800	+2	+0.3	+0.3	2.5	4.0	1200	1200	125	18+[8]	450	20
60	600	+4	+0.5	+0.3	2.5	4.0	1200	1200	150	18	450	25

[5]Total vitamin E activity, estimated to be 80 per cent as α-tocopherol and 20 per cent other tocopherols. See text for variation in allowances.

[6]The folacin allowances refer to dietary sources as determined by *Lactobacillus casei* assay. Pure forms of folacin may be effective in doses less than one-fourth of the RDA.

[7]Although allowances are expressed as niacin, it is recognized that on the average 1 mg of niacin is derived from each 60 mg of dietary tryptophan.

[8]This increased requirement cannot be met by ordinary diets; therefore, the use of supplemental iron is recommended.

Normal and Therapeutic Nutrition

Corinne H. Robinson M.S., R.D. Nutrition Consultant and

Professor of Nutrition Emeritus. Formerly, Head, Department of Nutrition and Food, Drexel University, and Instructor, Normal and Therapeutic Nutrition, School of Nursing, Thomas Jefferson University, Philadelphia

with the assistance of
Marilyn R. Lawler M.S., R.D. Chief Therapeutic Dietitian, Yale–New Haven Hospital, and

Instructor, Normal and Therapeutic Nutrition, Division of Nursing Education, Southern Connecticut State College, New Haven

14th edition

Normal and Therapeutic Nutrition

MACMILLAN PUBLISHING CO., INC.
New York
COLLIER MACMILLAN PUBLISHERS
London

Earlier editions: *Dietetics for Nurses* by Fairfax T. Proudfit copyright 1918, 1922, 1924, 1927 by Macmillan Publishing Co., Inc., copyright renewed 1946, 1950, 1952, 1955 by Fairfax T. Proudfit; *Nutrition and Diet Therapy* by Fairfax T. Proudfit copyright 1930, 1934, 1938, 1942 by Macmillan Publishing Co., Inc., copyright renewed 1958 by Fairfax T. Proudfit, 1962, 1966 by The First National Bank of Memphis; *Nutrition and Diet Therapy* by Fairfax T. Proudfit and Corinne H. Robinson copyright 1946, 1950, 1955 by Macmillan Publishing Co., Inc.; *Normal and Therapeutic Nutrition* by Fairfax T. Proudfit and Corinne H. Robinson © 1961 by Macmillan Publishing Co., Inc.; *Proudfit-Robinson's Normal and Therapeutic Nutrition* by Corinne H. Robinson © copyright 1967 by Macmillan Publishing Co., Inc.

Macmillan Publishing Co., Inc.
866 Third Avenue, New York, New York 10022

Collier-Macmillan Canada, Ltd., Toronto, Ontario

Library of Congress catalog card number: 74—169980

Printing: 5 6 7 8 9 10 11   Year: 4 5 6 7 8 9

The photographs appearing on the title pages for each unit were supplied by the following organizations and are used by permission:

Units I and XV, Medical College of Virginia, Health Sciences Division, Virginia Commonwealth University, Richmond
Unit II, College of Home Economics, Drexel University, Philadelphia
Unit III, World Health Organization
Units IV and VII, Division of Nutrition, Pennsylvania Department of Health
Unit V, U.S. Department of Agriculture
Unit VI, *Minneapolis Sunday Tribune*
Units VIII, XIII, and XIV, School of Nursing, College of Allied Health Sciences, Thomas Jefferson University, Philadelphia
Units IX, X, XI, XII, Yale—New Haven Hospital, New Haven

To the memory of my husband

Howard West Robinson

Preface to the Fourteenth Edition

Good nutrition for people of all ages, for health maintenance as well as restoration of health, is an economic, political, and humanitarian concern. Unfortunately, millions of people in North America experience some degree of malnutrition as a result of ignorance or poverty, or both. Consumers do not find it easy to evaluate the nutritive quality of the numerous new foods that constantly appear in the market or to separate fact from misinformation; those whose health is impaired are especially susceptible to half-truths and false claims. By providing nutritional services and extending nutrition education, nutritionists and dietitians, nurses and physicians, home economists, dental hygienists and dentists, and other health workers have an unparalleled opportunity to work toward the improvement of the nutritional status of the population. They must be prepared to correlate their particular skills in a team effort toward meeting the increased demands for first-rate nutritional care.

Normal and Therapeutic Nutrition is intended especially for students of nursing and dietetics. It will also serve as a useful reference for the practicing dietitian, nutritionist, nurse, physician, dentist, and home economist. The text aims to assist the student to realize three broad objectives: (1) the development of a good background in the science of nutrition that can be used as a basis for decisions in the dietary planning for any age group in health and in illness; (2) the acquisition of practical knowledge concerning the selection of foods according to nutritive values and costs, the care and preparation of foods so that nutritive values are retained, and the psychologic and cultural factors that govern the acceptance of foods; and (3) the ability to apply techniques of education and dietary counseling so that the principles of normal and therapeutic nutrition can be interpreted to the layman in terms that are appropriate for his living environment.

The overall organization in two parts, "Normal Nutrition" and "Therapeutic Nutrition," remains the same as in the preceding edition. The placement of content in Parts One and Two has been carefully correlated in order to maintain a unified approach, keep repetition to a minimum, and permit flexibility in course planning. For example, Part One could be used in a single broad-fields course that includes chemistry, physiology, and nutrition; or, instead of separate courses in normal and therapeutic nutrition, Parts One and Two can be used simultaneously in a single course in clinical nutrition.

To accomplish the aims of the text, the content has been revised and expanded in two important ways, namely, in the discussions pertaining to the science of nutrition, and in the emphasis placed upon nutrition education and dietary counseling.

The increased emphasis upon nutritional science is particularly evident in Units I and II. "Introduction to the Study of the Nutritive Processes" (Chapter 2) has been rewritten to include current concepts of cell structure and function, a brief review of digestive processes, a discussion of the several mechanisms by which nutrients are absorbed, and the metabolic interrelationships that exist. The discussion of the functions and metabolism of all of the nutrients has been expanded (Chapters 4 through 12). Chemical formulas for many of the nutrients, some key reactions, and new diagrams of several metabolic pathways are illustrated. Mineral elements are now discussed in two chapters. The first of these (Chapter 8) includes a discussion of mineral elements in general, calcium, phosphorus, magnesium, sulfur, iron, and other trace elements. "Fluid and Electrolyte Balance" (Chapter 9) describes the role of sodium, potassium, chlorine, and water, and the physiologic and biochemical mechanisms that regulate fluid and acid-base balance. More detail has also been included in Chapter 12, "The Water-Soluble Vitamins," for those vitamins for which allowances were first set in 1968 by the Food and Nutrition Board. Revised summary tables of the minerals and vitamins appear at the ends of Chapters 9, 10, and 12.

Education for normal nutrition as well as the specialized requirements in illness has been emphasized throughout the text. In order to accomplish this the content of Unit VII, "Nutrition and Public Health," has been expanded to two chapters. In the first of these chapters the national and international problems of nutrition are considered, with particular emphasis upon the factors of poverty and ignorance. On the basis of these problems, the role of public and private agencies in providing nutritional services and the methods by which nutrition education is extended are discussed in Chapter 26, "Nutrition Education and Services Through Community Action." The rehabilitation of the patient insofar as nutritional care is concerned and the dietary counseling of the patient and his family are discussed in Chapter 28, "Coordinated Nutritional Services for Patients."

Gray-tint areas in the text identify specific guidelines for nutrition education. A section entitled "Points for Emphasis in Nutrition Education," appearing at the close of the chapters in Unit II, presents a summary of important concepts pertaining to the nutrients that can be used as a basis for education of the layman. Likewise, guidelines for counseling are provided for the major therapeutic dietary regimens described in Part Two.

Many chapters of the text have been largely rewritten in order to report the applications of current research. The recommendations of the Committee on Maternal and Infant Nutrition of the National Research Council are taken into account in the discussion of diet in pregnancy (Chapter 21). A number of new dietary regimens are fully described in the chapters of Part

Two. A new chapter, "Malabsorption Syndrome," has been added to Unit X, "Diet in Disturbances of the Gastrointestinal Tract." It brings together in one place the descriptions of a number of conditions with related symptomatology, and includes a full description of the Medium-Chain Triglyceride Diet, Lactose-Restricted Diet, Sucrose-Restricted Diet, and Gluten-Restricted Diet. The dietary management in five types of hyperlipidemia is described in Chapter 42, "Hyperlipidemia and Atherosclerosis." The rationale and details of the Controlled Protein, Potassium, and Sodium Diet for renal failure with and without dialysis are discussed in Chapter 44, "Diet in Diseases of the Kidney."

Particular attention has been given to learning aids for the student. The two-column format, new to this edition, lends itself to ease in reading. A glossary of over 500 frequently used terms is included for the first time. Each table, chart, line drawing, and photograph has been selected to supplement the written text and to emphasize some aspect of nutritional science and its application. Problems and review questions are intended to aid in the formulation of appropriate attitudes in nutritional practice as well as the correlation of materials studied. References for further study, at the end of each chapter, include representative writings from the current literature as well as older, classic works in nutrition.

The Appendix includes seven tables pertaining to the nutritive values of foods, height and weight tables for children and adults, and tables of normal constituents of the blood and urine. Table A-1, "Nutritive Values of the Edible Part of Foods," containing 615 food listings, is the 1970 revision prepared by the Consumer and Food Services of the U.S. Department of Agriculture. Table A-2 has been expanded to include values for folacin, pantothenic acid, and vitamins E, B_6, and B_{12} as well as for sodium, potassium, magnesium, and phosphorus.

Many people have contributed in numerous ways to this edition. The assistance of Miss Marilyn R. Lawler, Chief Therapeutic Dietitian, Yale–New Haven Hospital, is gratefully acknowledged for the revision of Unit X, "Diet in Disturbances of the Gastrointestinal Tract" (Chapters 34 to 37), and Unit XI, "Dietary

Modifications for Surgical Conditions" (Chapter 38), and for the extension of Table A-2 to include vitamin values. Appreciation is expressed to the staff of the Consumer and Food Economics Research Division of the U.S. Department of Agriculture for information pertaining to the nutritive values of foods, food consumption data, and food economics; to Mrs. Marjorie C. Zukel for materials on fat-controlled diets; and to Miss Dorothy Youland for information pertaining to nutritional activities of public health agencies. Many individuals, companies, and agencies generously gave permission to quote from published articles and to use photographs from their files.

Many photographs were taken expressly for this edition. Sincere appreciation is expressed to the following individuals and organizations who supplied them: Miss Marilyn R. Lawler, Chief Therapeutic Dietitian, Mr. Albert P. Freije, Director of Special Services, and Dr. Doris Johnson, Director of Dietetics, Yale–New Haven Hospital, New Haven; Miss Margaret C. McClean, Instructor in Nutrition, and Miss Doris E. Bowman, Director, School of Nursing, Thomas Jefferson University, Philadelphia; Miss Natalie Scardamaglia, Dietitian, and Mr. Eugene Cole, Director, Allied Services for the Handicapped, Scranton; Miss Isabelle G. A. Wozniczak, Patient Coordinator, and Dr. Robert Warner, Medical Director, Children's Rehabilitation Center, Buffalo; Miss Sophia M. Podgorski, Director, Division of Nutrition, Pennsylvania Department of Health, Harrisburg; Miss Erna Behrend and Miss Betty Moore, Nutritionists, Medical College of Virginia, Richmond; and Miss Elizabeth C. Doherty, Acting Director, Dietetic Technician Program, Pittsburgh. Appreciation is also expressed to the students, patients, nurses, and dietitians whose photographs are included.

My husband, Howard W. Robinson, contributed a great deal to each of six editions of this text. He encouraged me with his interest and enthusiasm and sustained me with his patience. His advice was generous and thoughtful, not only on matters pertaining to physiologic chemistry but often to the precise wording for expressing an idea. His death occurred during the preparation of this edition, thus bringing to a close a collaboration of more than a quarter century.

I am deeply grateful to the staff of The Macmillan Company for their cooperation, courtesy, and careful attention to every detail, and especially to Miss Joan C. Zulch, Medical Editor, who seems never at a loss for new ideas and who skillfully guides the book from its inception to its completion.

CORINNE H. ROBINSON

Contents

Part One Normal Nutrition

Part Two   Therapeutic Nutrition

Appendices

Part One
Normal Nutrition

Unit I

Introduction to the Study of Nutrition

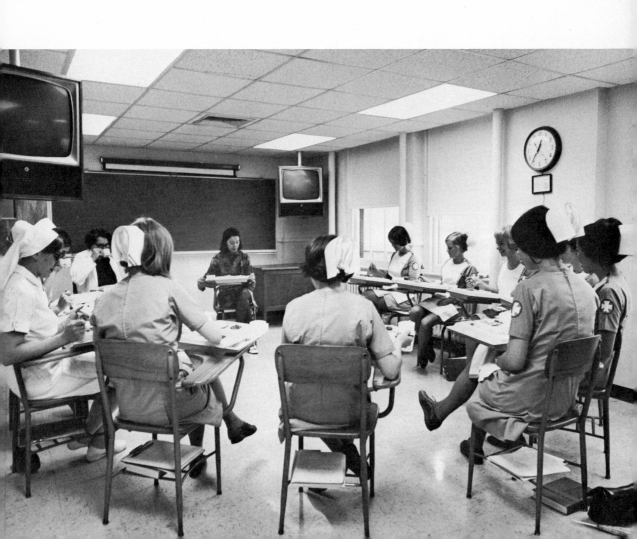

1 Food and Its Relation to Health

THE MEANINGS OF FOOD, NUTRITION, AND NUTRITIONAL CARE

What does food mean to you? Food—menu—diet—hunger—nutrition—malnutrition. What images do these words bring to your mind? Are they oriented to your senses? To your social enjoyment? To your concerns about your own well-being? To your emotions? Do they raise questions about the quality of life for your fellow human beings? When you sit down to your next meal you will have definite ideas—positive or negative—about that meal and the specific foods that are served to you.

By your eyes you will delight in the texture variations and color combinations of the food, the artistic touch of a garnish, and the beautiful table appointments; or perhaps you may be repelled because the food lacks color and is carelessly served. By your nose you will enjoy the tantalizing odors of meat or of freshly baked rolls, or the fragrance of fully ripened fruit; or possibly the odor of grease which has been too hot or of vegetables which have been cooked too long may bring about anorexia and even nausea. By your sense of taste you will experience countless flavors—the salty, sweet, bitter, and sour and their variations; you will feel the textures of smooth or fibrous, crisp or soft, creamy or oily, moist or dry foods.

But your senses alone do not describe what your next meal, or any meal, means to you. Is the meal merely a way of staying alive and keeping in health; an opportunity for fellowship with your family and friends; a way to celebrate an event; an occasion for stimulating conversation; a means of satisfying your feelings when you are hurt and depressed; a display of prestige by which you show that you can afford certain foods others cannot; a token of security and love; a means of asserting your independence; a cause of concern because some foods might make you ill; an occasion of self-denial; something you enjoy leisurely; taken for granted as your right; a precious gift from God for which you are thankful? What other feelings are evoked by the food you eat?

Next to the air you breathe and the water you drink, food has been basic to your existence. In fact, food has been the primary concern of man in his physical environment throughout all recorded history. By food, or its lack, the destinies of men are greatly influenced. Man must eat to live, and what he eats will affect in a high degree his ability to keep well, to work, to be happy, and to live long.

You bring to the study of nutrition your lifetime experience with food which may serve you well in further improving your nutrition and the nutrition of your fellowmen. But it may also be that you have many incorrect ideas and such strong feelings about food that it will take much patience and perseverance on your part to change your attitudes and motivations. As you enter upon this study it is well for you to examine carefully your present feelings about food, as well as your current knowledge of nutrition, so that you can build upon what is good in your dietary pattern and correct that which is undesirable. (See Figures 1–1 and 1–2.)

Definitions. *Health* as defined by the World Health Organization of the United Nations is the "state of complete physical, mental and social well-being and not merely the absence of disease or infirmity."*

Nutrition is "the science of foods, the nutri-

* *World Health Organization—What It Is, What It Does, How It Works.* Leaflet, Geneva, Switzerland, 1956.

4

ents and other substances therein; their action, interaction, and balance in relationship to health and disease; the processes by which the organism ingests, digests, absorbs, transports, and utilizes nutrients and disposes of their end products. In addition, nutrition must be concerned with social, economic, cultural, and psychological implications of food and eating."[†]

† Robinson, W. D.: "Nutrition in Medical Education," in *Proceedings Western Hemisphere Nutrition Congress*—1965. American Medical Association, Chicago, 1966, p. 206.

Figure 1–1. An abundant food supply for an affluent society. For most people in the United States the cultural, emotional, social, and physiologic needs for food can be easily satisfied from a choice of 10,000 or more items available in the supermarket. Even in an affluent society there are people of low income who cannot satisfy their needs from this abundance. (Courtesy, U.S. Department of Agriculture.)

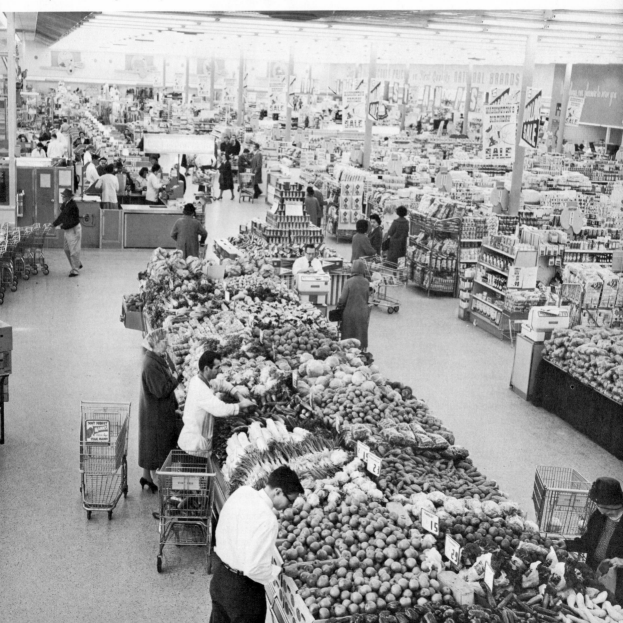

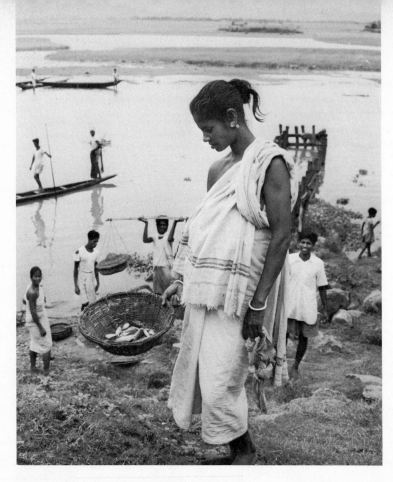

Figure 1–2. Poverty, hunger, and malnutrition are the fate of more than half of the world's population. Even when food is scarce, it has meanings to people in terms of social customs, religious beliefs, and psychologic satisfactions as well as nutritional needs. (Courtesy, P. N. Sharma and World Health Organization.)

Nutrients are the constituents in food that must be supplied to the body in suitable amounts. These include water, proteins and the amino acids of which they are composed, fats and fatty acids, carbohydrates, minerals, and vitamins.

Nutritional status is the condition of health of the individual as influenced by the utilization of the nutrients. It can be determined only by the correlation of information obtained through a careful medical and dietary history, a thorough physical examination, and appropriate laboratory investigations.

Nutritional care is "the application of the science and art of human nutrition in helping people select and obtain food for the primary purpose of nourishing their bodies in health or in disease throughout the life cycle. This participation may be in single or combined functions: in feeding groups involving food selection and management; in extending knowledge of food and nutrition principles; in teaching these principles for application according to particular situations; and in dietary counseling."[*]

Good nutrition and malnutrition. *Good, adequate,* and *optimum* are terms applied to that quality of nutrition in which the essential nutrients in correct amounts and balance are utilized to promote the highest level of physical and mental health throughout the entire life cycle. The student will be able to develop a more comprehensive description of the attributes of good nutrition through the study of the specific functions of each nutrient and the physical and biochemical measures that characterize the adequacy of supply and utilization.

Malnutrition is an impairment of health resulting from a deficiency, excess, or imbalance of nutrients. It includes *undernutrition,* which

[*] Committee on Goals of Education for Dietetics, Dietetic Internship Council: "Goals of the Lifetime Education of the Dietitian," *J. Am. Diet Assoc.,* **54**:92, 1969.

refers to a deficiency of calories and/or one or more essential nutrients, and *overnutrition,* which is an excess of one or more nutrients and usually of calories.

Good nutrition: a multidisciplinary effort. The achievement of good nutrition requires (1) application of agricultural science and technology to produce sufficient amounts of plant and animal foods of high nutritive value; (2) processing of foods for maximum retention of nutritive values; (3) adequate storage, transportation, and marketing facilities to make foods available at times and places where needed; (4) appropriate governmental controls to ensure the wholesomeness and nutritive quality of the food supply; (5) economic conditions that make it possible to procure the necessary foods at a cost within the reach of all; (6) educational programs in nutrition within the schools and at the community level; and (7) efficient use of food within the home, public eating place, and institution.

The perspective of nutrition held by each of the specialists who help to assure an adequate food supply obviously would be quite different. The combined efforts in the scientific disciplines related to food and nutrition and in food production and technology to supply food for the nation and the world ultimately concern each and every individual so that he may enjoy the benefits of good nutrition—health, happiness, efficiency, and longevity. The final decisions on food consumption are made individually, even though the selection may have been determined by others. In every walk of life the individual has a vital stake in the quality and quantity of food that is available to him and can benefit by increased knowledge of the principles of nutrition and their application to his daily living.

DIETARY TRENDS IN THE UNITED STATES

Changes in patterns of living. The population of the United States has shifted from rural to urban centers; but even on the farm most families now purchase much more of their food than was customary half a century ago. Americans have the benefits of many labor-saving devices in their occupations and in their homes. They work fewer hours in a week, so that the way in which they spend their leisure may be decisive in determining their food needs. Leisure, to many people, means little activity—riding rather than walking, watching television rather than leading an active outdoor life, and so on.

Greater numbers of married women are working away from home than ever before, which means that there is less time for food preparation, more expensive ready-prepared foods are used, and shopping is less frequent. Husbands, as well as wives, are shopping for and preparing foods; sometimes children, especially teen-agers, may be given too much freedom in their food choices thus resulting in poor nutrition. Marriages occur at an earlier age with pregnancy often presenting an additional stress on the young woman who has not fully matured and who may have been the victim of poor dietary practices.

The average American family of today has a higher income and is spending more of it for food. With this higher income, more meals are eaten in restaurants. More workers are receiving meals at their place of work rather than carrying lunches, and more children are participating in school lunch programs. The family eats fewer meals together, and in far too many families some meals may be skipped by one or more persons. Breakfast is an often neglected meal, although some families have found that this is the one time of the day when they can plan to be together.

The scientific and technologic advances reach into every aspect of daily life, including the quantity, quality, variety, and attractiveness of the foods we eat. Frozen foods including complete meals, baked foods of all kinds, and mixes for almost every part of the meal are commonplace items in the supermarkets. The number of brands and the variety are so great that the shopper finds it difficult indeed to make wise selections.

Dietary adequacy. Since 1936 the U.S. Department of Agriculture has conducted five comprehensive surveys of food consumption in the United States. The most recent survey, covering the four seasons from spring 1965 through winter 1966, included 15,000 households of one or more persons.[1] The households were selected from urban, rural nonfarm, and farm families in four regions—Northeast, North Central, South, and West—in such a manner that the results of the survey would be representative of practices throughout the United States. Trained interviewers obtained information on family characteristics, the quantities of food purchased, the expenditures for food purchased, practices with respect to the use of certain foods, the number of meals eaten away from home, and the expenditure for food eaten away from home. In addition, the actual amounts of foods consumed by selected individuals were also determined.

The adequacy of the diets was evaluated according to the Recommended Dietary Allowances (RDA) described fully in Chapter 3. This standard describes the desirable levels of nutrient intakes for various age categories and provides a margin of safety for most individuals. In the U.S. Department of Agriculture survey a *good* diet was one that provided the nutrients at levels equal to or in excess of the RDA. A diet was rated *poor* if it provided less than two thirds of the RDA for one or more nutrients. When diets provide less than two thirds of the RDA for a prolonged period of time, it is expected that some individuals may show some signs of deficiency.

In the decade following the 1955 survey the following changes in food selection occurred: (1) less milk and milk products, flour and cereal foods, vegetables, and fruits; and (2) more meat, fish, and poultry, baked foods, and snack foods such as soft drinks, pretzels, and doughnuts. These changes resulted in a decline in the quality of diets from 1955 to 1965. Only 50 per cent of the diets were rated good in 1965 whereas in 1955 this rating was given to 60 per cent of all diets. Poor diets accounted for 20 per cent of all diets in 1965 and 15 per cent in 1955. (See Figure 1–3.)

The nutrients most frequently supplied at low levels in 1965 as well as in 1955 were calcium, ascorbic acid, and vitamin A. For each of these the incidence of poor intakes was higher in 1965. These changes in food consumption and their adverse effect on the nutritive value of diets suggest important points to be emphasized in nutrition education.

NUTRITIONAL PROBLEMS IN THE UNITED STATES

Increasing awareness of malnutrition. Although the 1965 household survey of food consumption indicated that only half the diets could be rated as good, it provided no measure of the nutritional status of the population. Because of the prevailing high level of affluence in the United States people have come to believe that hunger, and its sequel malnutrition, do not exist except as a consequence of disease—at least to any appreciable degree. Even many physicians, nurses, and nutritionists have assumed that "It can't happen here."

The shocking facts of the widespread existence of malnutrition in the United States have been brought to the attention of the public by many

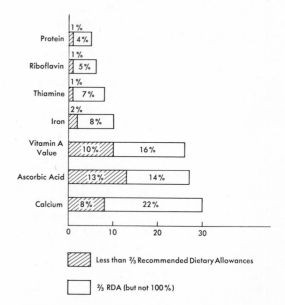

Figure 1–3. Calcium, vitamin A, and ascorbic acid are the nutrients most frequently supplied at levels below the Recommended Dietary Allowances, according to data from the household dietary survey of 1965. (Courtesy, Agricultural Research Service, U.S. Department of Agriculture.)

means in recent years, including a television documentary, the publication of *Hunger, U.S.A.*,[2] and the concerns of citizen groups for the quality of life in the city ghettos and in some rural regions. The picture of malnutrition has surely been overdrawn by some and has been lightly brushed over by others. Nevertheless, the awakening to the fact that many Americans, especially among the 30 million poor, were malnourished led to the investigations of the Senate Poverty Committee in 1967, the hearings of the Select Committee on Nutrition and Human Needs of the U.S. Senate in 1968–1969, and the White House Conference on Food, Nutrition, and Health in December 1969. These investigations and conferences have resulted in significant legislation pertaining to new programs for assistance and for education, as well as a greater acceptance of responsibility on the part of professional and lay groups.

Nutritional status in the United States. Regional studies coordinated by the U.S. Department of Agriculture on the nutritional status of people of various ages, ethnic origin, and geographic areas have shown the existence of malnutrition in vulnerable segments of the population.[3] For the most part these studies have been conducted on people of middle income and have not been fully representative of the nation as a whole.

In 1967 the first comprehensive National Nutrition Survey was initiated by the Nutrition Program of the Public Health Service.[4] The survey was made on about 70,000 people living in low-income areas of 10 states, including Massachusetts, New York, West Virginia, South Carolina, Michigan, Louisiana, Kentucky, Texas, Washington, and California. In these low-income areas one half the families had incomes below $3000 and 80 per cent of the total families had incomes under $5000. All age groups were represented in the sample.

The information developed during the survey included (1) socioeconomic data: number in family, educational level, income, environment; (2) dietary evaluation: sources of food, preparation facilities, food and nutrient intake, and food attitudes; (3) physical examination: hair, eyes, skin, lips, anthropometric measurements, bone

x-rays; (4) laboratory analyses of blood and urine: hemoglobin, hematocrit, serum proteins, vitamin A, carotene, and ascorbic acid; urinary creatinine, thiamine, and riboflavin; and (5) dental examinations: decayed, filled, and missing teeth; condition of gums; ability to bite and chew.

In the hearings before the Senate Committee on Nutrition and Human Needs, Drs. Schaefer and Johnson, on the basis of this survey, stated that there was an "alarming prevalence" of characteristics of the malnourished. All the signs usually seen in the malnourished of Central America, Africa, and Asia were also seen in the people examined in the United States. The fact that these people enjoyed better health than those in other countries was attributed to a more sanitary supply of water, milk, and other foods, adequate disposal of wastes, and generally better hygienic conditions. Only preliminary results of the survey have been published at the time of this writing; these partial findings are summarized below. (See also Figure 1–4.)

1. *Anemia:* there was frequent occurrence in all age categories; one third of all children under six years had unacceptable hemoglobin levels.

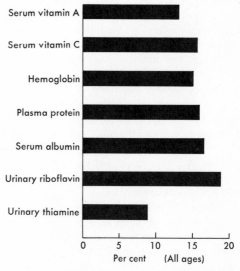

Figure 1–4. Laboratory findings of the National Nutrition Survey: percentage of population with less than adequate levels. (Courtesy, Drs. A. E. Schaefer and O. C. Johnson. Reprinted from *Nutrition Today*, 4:6 [Spring], 1969, by permission.)

2. Dental problems: for each 100 persons 90 needed fillings or extractions; 45 had some degree of periodontal disease and 20 had severe periodontal disease; 18 of every 100 persons over 10 years of age had trouble or pain in biting and chewing.

3. Retarded growth: height was considerably below average in children from one to three years; bone development was retarded.

4. Vitamin A deficiency: low serum vitamin A levels were seen in about one third of all children under six years. Eight cases of Bitot's spots on the conjunctiva were reported.

5. Endemic goiter: about 5 per cent of the population had enlarged thyroid, owing to lack of iodine.

6. Vitamin C deficiency: low serum vitamin C levels were found in 12 to 16 per cent of the various age groups; scorbutic gums were present in 1 person of every 25.

7. Vitamin D deficiency: this was observed in 4 per cent of children under six years; 18 cases of rickets were diagnosed.

8. Protein malnutrition: low serum proteins were found in one of every six persons of all ages. Four to five per cent of children had winged scapula and pot belly indicating protein malnutrition. Seven cases of severe protein-calorie malnutrition (kwashiorkor and marasmus) were diagnosed in preschool children.

Although the initial survey was confined to low-income areas, there is no reason to believe that the conditions described above would be absent in people of ample income. In fact, anemia and dental problems are known to be widely prevalent, and the other deficiencies probably exist to a varying degree. Many of the problems of malnutrition that particularly affect people of middle- and upper-income levels are those of nutritional excesses.

1. Obesity is estimated to be present in every fifth person over 30 years of age, with a higher frequency in women than in men. Overweight is present in increasing numbers of children and young adults.

2. Atherosclerosis, hypertension, cardiovascular disease, and other degenerative diseases have a complex etiology. Excessive calorie intake, high

intake of saturated fats, and a high proportion of simple sugars are among the more important aspects of these problems.

All the conditions enumerated above will be discussed in some detail throughout the various chapters of this text.

GLOBAL PROBLEMS IN NUTRITION

Scope of malnutrition. Most of the world's people today, as always, are engaged in a struggle for food. In relatively few countries, such as the United States, Canada, and western European countries, is food abundant and of great variety. More than half the world's people are caught in a relentless sequence of ignorance, poverty, malnutrition, disease, and early death. There are no completely reliable statistics on either morbidity or mortality from malnutrition, but one estimate places the daily death toll from malnutrition at 10,000.[5]

The world's population increases by approximately 180 to 200 thousand persons each day, so that the expansion of food production to keep pace with, and to move ahead of, this population growth must assume staggering proportions. The world production of agricultural, fishery, and forest products has increased greatly during the last few years. Even developing countries have realized substantially greater yields of the staple cereals. Nevertheless, in many countries the population increase has been even greater than that in food production so that the net amount of food available per capita is actually decreased.

Protein-calorie malnutrition is the single greatest world problem in nutrition. In its severe forms, kwashiorkor and marasmus, it affects millions of preschool children. In fact, in some countries, three children may be dead before the first one gets to school. Those children who do survive are physically and mentally retarded—perhaps irreversibly so.

Anemia—especially in mothers and young children—vitamin A deficiency, and riboflavin deficiency are especially frequent. Rickets, scurvy, pellagra, beriberi, and endemic goiter occur in severe forms in some parts of the world.

The characteristics of these deficiencies will be described in the chapters related to the specific nutrients involved.

Responsibility for world nutrition. No thinking man or woman can afford to avoid the fact that so many of the world's people simply do not have enough to eat, nor can he, even in his own self-interest, evade the responsibility for alleviating hunger. In chronic starvation lie the frustration, tension, and envy of masses of people who will ultimately resort to violence.

World peace cannot be guaranteed by supplying adequate food alone, but one road to world peace is surely through a better-fed world population. Beyond this, charity and brotherhood are at the root of Christianity and indeed of all ethical systems, and to practice them should be on the conscience of mankind.

A number of groups under the United Nations are directly concerned with global problems of nutrition, namely the Food and Agriculture Organization (FAO); World Health Organization (WHO); United Nations Children's Fund (UNICEF); United Nations Educational, Scientific and Cultural Organization (UNESCO).

The challenge of the future is forcefully emphasized by B. R. Sen, Director-General, Food and Agriculture Organization, in his closing remarks to the foreword of the *State of Food and Agriculture, 1965:*

It is abundantly clear that the next 35 years to the end of the century will be a most critical period in human history. As we stand at this watershed looking into the future, there is much that has been accomplished during the two decades of FAO's existence which can give us cause for hope. There has been a breakthrough in world awareness of the dimensions of hunger and malnutrition. Man's right to food has come to be universally recognized as one of his fundamental rights. Agriculture has gained in status in the economy of developing countries. Food surpluses have become available for the relief of malnutrition and for assisting the economic growth of food-deficient nations. FAO has attracted the dedication and moral commitment of countless people all over the world in the attainment of its cherished objectives. All of these are no mean achievement. I earnestly hope that in this next phase of FAO's history more and more attention will be

given to the human factor in economic and social progress, since the ultimate goal of our endeavor as well as the instrument for achieving it is Man.*

Some Goals in the Study of Nutrition

At the beginning of any study it is well for the student to take time to determine the goals that he should set for himself. These will not be the same for all individuals because students begin the study with quite differing backgrounds of knowledge and experience, and because their professional interests are likely to vary widely. Moreover, it must be anticipated that the goals will, in fact, change as the study progresses and the student becomes more aware of the field. Worthwhile goals are not fully achieved within the space of a few months but should provide the basis for an ongoing lifetime program of education. The discussion that follows will give the student some background for setting up his own goals with reference to personal and family nutrition, and toward a professional career in the health sciences.

Personal and family nutrition. Regardless of one's future professional career, the first goals in the study of nutrition should be directed to oneself. Physical and mental health are essential assets to meet the exciting, and sometimes arduous, requirements of one's life work. Those who expect to help other people achieve better health through nutrition must be enthusiastic and living examples of the benefits of the application of nutrition knowledge.

Nutrition education applied to the individual also reaches the family. This is especially important for young men and women as they establish their own families. Within the family the wife and mother is the principal decision-maker for the family's food. She plans the menus, selects the foods, and prepares them. Although she makes every effort to please her husband, her

* Sen, B. R.: Foreword in *The State of Food and Agriculture 1965, review of the second postwar decade.* Food and Agriculture Organization of the United Nations, Rome, 1965, p. 4.

influence also molds many of his habits. The food habits of children are formed by the prevailing attitudes and practices within the home.

Professional goals. Professional people in any discipline related to health are engaged in activities related to education, prevention, and therapy. Of these, education of the population promises long-range benefits to the greatest numbers. Teachers, nurses, nutritionists, home economists, dietitians, and physicians assume varying responsibilities for individual and group education. The elementary and secondary schools afford the best opportunity for helping the child to establish attitudes and practices concerning food selection which will lead him to a more healthful, productive life. The role of teaching nutrition in the classroom belongs not only to the home economics teacher but also to the elementary teacher of the various grades. The school nurse and physician have many opportunities to note defects in health which suggest the need for improved nutrition; they can influence children in changing food habits, provide guidance to mothers, help to plan meaningful experiences in the classroom, and lend their support to the school food service program. The school lunch is part of the educational program in that each meal becomes a laboratory experience which demonstrates that good nutrition and good food are, in fact, partners. The athletic

program can be an effective adjunct to nutrition education, when the nutrition practices recommended by coaches are based upon the facts of nutrition science.

Voluntary and governmental agencies together with industry are accepting responsibility for nutrition programs with limitless boundaries. The researcher in nutrition and food sciences is equally at home in the laboratories of a food company, a university, a hospital, or in the public health field. (See Figure 1–5.) Nutritionists, dietitians, and home economists, depending upon their education and particular interests, are the experts who interpret a product for a company; develop new uses for a food; advise mothers and children concerning their diets in a clinic; serve as consultants to a public health team; supervise food service in a college dormitory, industrial cafeteria, or hospital; assist individuals and groups in dietary selection; and teach in nursing schools, colleges, and universities.

Today's nurse is an educator as well as a therapist. Her concern is for the maintenance as well as the restoration of health. Traditionally, the nurse has been associated with patient care, and indeed this continues to be a central concern of nursing. The interpretation of this role, however, has been considerably extended in recent years to the concept of continuity of care. The nurse in the hospital soon learns that she cannot

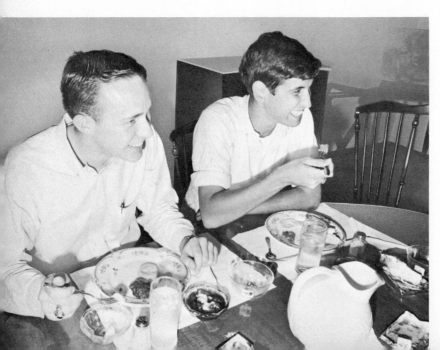

Figure 1–5. These premedical students are shown participating in research by eating carefully controlled diets to determine the effects of carbohydrates on metabolism. (Courtesy, U.S. Department of Agriculture.)

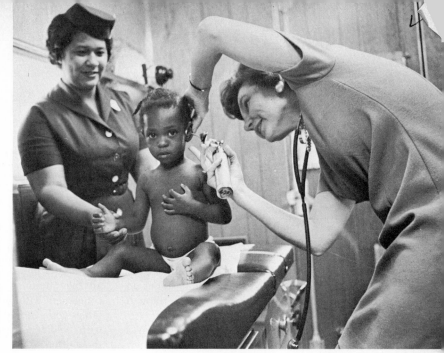

Figure 1–6. Public health nurses help families through clinic services and education to maintain good health. The nutritional status and health are determined by a physician's examination. Extra food is part of the free health care at this public clinic. (Courtesy, Larry Rana and U.S. Department of Agriculture.)

limit her concern for the patient to the bedside, but that she also has some responsibility for effecting the smooth transition of the patient from the hospital to his home. To implement continuity of care, she knows that with respect to nutritional needs the patient may require instruction in the proper choice of foods in the market, assistance in planning for the best use of his food money, and practical suggestions for food preparation with meager facilities, or in the face of physical handicaps. Some of the assistance required by the patient may be provided by the nurse, but more often a team effort—nurse, dietitian, social worker—is needed. (See also Chapters 27 and 28.)

In the community the nurse is often the coordinator of services. The public health nurse encounters a legion of problems and needs related to nutrition: perhaps she needs to show one mother how to prepare an infant formula; another person needs to know how to budget her limited income so that she can buy enough milk; another needs actual instruction in food preparation for an ill member of the family; another has been given a diet that does not fit in with the religious practices of the family; or a pregnant woman may need to know what foods she must eat and how to provide for them in her budget. (See Figure 1–6.)

Objectives for the student. To achieve the personal and professional goals the student should consider the following more specific aims in his study of nutrition.

1. Acquire the proper attitude and convictions relative to the importance of nutrition in regulating one's own health, that of the family, and that of individuals of the community.

2. Gain an appreciation of the kinds of health problems arising from poor nutrition that exist in his own community, the nation, and throughout the world.

3. Acquire knowledge concerning the science of nutrition:

    a. Functions, digestion, absorption, and metabolism of proteins, fats, carbohydrates, minerals, and vitamins.

    b. The interrelationship of nutrients.

    c. The nutritive requirements of individuals and the variations that may be imposed by activity, climate, stage of life cycle, and disease.

4. Gain appreciation and understanding of the meanings that food has for people and how these are related to economic, psychologic, and cultural factors.

5. Develop the ability to interpret the principles of nutrition in the selection of an adequate diet:

a. By knowing the food sources of the nutrients.

b. By applying consumer information to the planning of meals and the selection of food for quality and economy.

6. Develop awareness of opportunities for improving nutrition through the education of individuals.

7. Develop the ability to counsel people on an individual or group basis by adapting nutrition information to specific health, socioeconomic, and cultural needs.

8. Know where to look for reliable sources of information and how to evaluate publications on food and nutrition and the claims made through product advertising.

9. Become familiar with agencies concerned with nutrition and health in order to utilize their services and contribute to their functioning.

Some guidelines for nutrition study. It is often said that one can judge a workman by the way in which he uses his tools. This is also true of the use a student makes of the study tools available to him. First, one must become acquainted with a tool and gain some practice in using it before it becomes comfortable to use. With your text, for example, look through the table of contents to learn something of the topics that are covered and the sequence of their presentation. Then browse through the book to become aware of the kinds of study aids that are provided.

Terminology in any study is basic to understanding and the time used in developing the ability to use nutrition terms with accuracy and ease is well spent. Terms especially related to nutrition are, for the most part, defined at the point of their first use. Those terms that are used frequently throughout the text have also been listed in the Glossary in the Appendix.

Nutrition is related to other sciences, especially biochemistry and physiology (see Figure 1–7), and it should be studied in the context of these sciences. If you have already completed courses in the biologic sciences, the discussion in this text pertaining to the metabolism of the nutrients will help to correlate the earlier studies with nutritive processes as well as reinforcing the learning. If you do not yet have a background in the biologic sciences, you may find the study of metabolism to be a little difficult at this point. Then it is recommended that you read the discussion on metabolism to gain an overall perspective, but that you defer detailed study to a subsequent time.

Many tables, diagrams, charts, and photographs have been carefully selected to emphasize and to summarize important points made in the discussion. If you study these you will find that they reinforce the reading of the text itself. The tables of food composition in the Appendix contain a gold mine of information. Perhaps half of all the questions people will pose to you are concerned with nutritive values, and in these tables you can find the answers. But to use them with confidence means that you must consult them often.

Review questions at the end of each chapter will help you to focus on the important points that have been made. The suggested problems are examples of situations that may be encountered in making applications of the principles of nutrition. You will soon learn to find answers to problems that come within your own daily experiences.

Any student of nutrition should be aware of the current issues before the public. You will find that your interest will be deeper if you try to relate your course of study to some of the reporting in newspapers and magazines, for example. Try to evaluate what you read in the popular publications with what you learn in your study.

Additional references have been included for each chapter to enable you to read more exten-

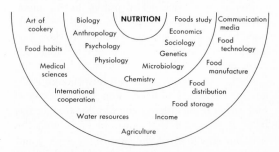

Figure 1–7. Good nutrition for everyone is dependent upon the application of the principles of many sciences and the coordination of many disciplines.

sively on selected topics, to familiarize you with reliable publications in nutrition, to foster the habit of consulting the literature, and perhaps even to provide the starting point for a term paper you may wish to develop. The references included are at a reading level comparable to this text.

PROBLEMS AND REVIEW

1. What is your understanding of the following terms: nutrition, malnutrition, foodstuff, nutrient, health, food, nutritional care?
2. Industrial and economic developments have been a powerful factor in the changing of our food habits. List several of these which have had an influence on our dietary habits within your lifetime.
3. Within your experience give an example of a situation in which the community has fostered better nutrition.
4. Select an article related to food from the daily newspaper or a popular magazine and discuss its merits.
5. In what ways is a knowledge of the following sciences helpful in the study of nutrition: bacteriology, chemistry, sociology, psychology?
6. What is the difference between a dietary survey and a nutritional status study?
7. *Problem*. Start a list of resources for the study of nutrition and dietetics. Add to this list as you continue in your study. Include only those books and journals which you have examined. Include the names of official and voluntary agencies in your own community and at state, federal, and international levels as you become familiar with the work they do in the area of nutrition.
8. *Problem*. Compile a list of characteristics which describe a person who is in good nutritional status. How do you measure up with this?
9. *Problem*. Review the suggested objectives for study in this chapter. Then prepare a statement in your own words which best describes the goals you think are most important. Limit your statement to 300 words; be concise but exact.

CITED REFERENCES

1. *Dietary Levels of Households in the United States, Spring 1965*. ARS 62–17, U.S. Department of Agriculture, Washington, D.C., 1968.
2. *Hunger, U.S.A*. Citizen Board of Inquiry into Hunger and Malnutrition in the United States, Washington, D.C., 1968.
3. Morgan, A. F., ed.: *Nutritional Status U.S.A*. California Agricultural Experiment Station, Bull. 769, Berkeley, 1959.
4. Schaefer, A. E., and Johnson, O. C.: "Are We Well Fed? The Search for the Answer," *Nutr. Today*, 4(No. 1):2–11, 1969.
5. "Fortified Foods: the Next Revolution," *Chem. Eng. News*, 48:36–43, Aug. 10, 1970.

ADDITIONAL REFERENCES

Adelson, S. F.: "Changes in Diets of Households, 1955 to 1965. Implications for Nutrition Education Today," *J. Home Econ.*, 60:448–55, 1968.
Berg, A.: "Priority of Nutrition in National Development," *Nutr. Rev.*, 28:199–204, 1970.
Briggs, G. M.: "Editorial: Hunger and Malnutrition," *J. Nutr. Educ.*, 1:4–6, Winter 1970.
Coffey, J. D.: "World Food Supply and Population Explosion," *J. Am. Diet. Assoc.*, 52:43–48, 1968.

Goldsmith, G. A.: "More Food for More People," *Am. J. Public Health,* **59**:694–704, 1969.

Harper, A. E.: "Nutrition: Where Are We? Where Are We Going?" *Am. J. Clin. Nutr.,* **22**:87–98, 1969.

King, C. G.: "America's Role in World Nutrition," *Bordens Rev. Nutr. Res.,* **30**:2–9, 1969.

Lamont-Havers, R. W.: "Trends in Human Nutrition Research," *J. Am. Diet. Assoc.,* **52**:300–303, 1968.

Mayer, J.: "A Report on the White House Conference on Food, Nutrition and Health, December 2–4, 1969," *Nutr. Rev.,* **27**:247–51, 1969.

Mehrens, G. L.: "Anticipating the Year 2000," *J. Am. Diet. Assoc.,* **52**:467–70, 1968.

Pyke, M.: "Scientific Technology and the Mercenary Society," *J. Nutr. Educ.,* **1**:20–22, Winter 1970.

Stare, F. J.: "Nutritional Improvement and World Health Potential," *J. Am. Diet. Assoc.,* **57**:107–10, 1970.

Todhunter, E. N.: "The Evolution of Nutrition Concepts—Perspectives and New Horizons," *J. Am. Diet. Assoc.,* **46**:120–28, 1965.

"White House Conference on Food, Nutrition and Health. Recommendations of Panels on Nutrition Teaching and Education," *J. Nutr. Educ.,* **1**:24–39, Winter 1970.

2 Introduction to the Study of the Nutritive Processes: Digestion, Absorption, and Metabolism

Some understanding of the metabolic processes that take place in the body is important to the study of nutrition. The purposes of this chapter are to present an overview of the nutritive processes that will be discussed in somewhat more detail in the chapters to follow on normal and therapeutic nutrition, and to review briefly some aspects of digestion, absorption, and metabolism as a framework for the study of nutrition. Many details have intentionally been omitted, for it is assumed that students who are using this text have already completed courses in physiology and chemistry. The student who desires further review or greater depth of study may consult one of the standard texts of physiology and chemistry, some of which have been listed at the end of this chapter.

The processes of metabolism are so complex that it is impossible to tell the story exactly as it happens. For the sake of simplicity, single aspects are usually described in more or less detail; for example, one can trace the digestion, absorption, and intermediary metabolism of a given carbohydrate, or of any other nutrient, more or less independently of any other. This can give a misleading impression to the student inasmuch as the multitude of metabolic events occur simultaneously within the cells. Each metabolic event is affected by other events that preceded it or occurred at the same moment in time. The utilization of any nutrient is interrelated with that of many others. The story of metabolism is an unending one that invites the interest and continuing research by physiologists, histologists, cytologists, microbiologists, biochemists, nutritionists, and others.

Composition of the body. Water accounts for roughly two thirds of the body weight and is distributed in all tissues. About three fourths of the water is in the *intracellular* compartment (fluid within the cells), and one fourth is in the *extracellular* compartment, which includes the blood circulation, the lymph, and the interstitial fluids which bathe all cells. Tissues vary considerably in their water content, with bones, teeth, and adipose tissue, for example, containing appreciably less than muscle and nervous tissue.

Proteins and fats each account for about 18 per cent of body weight, with considerable variations depending upon the amount of fat deposition. The percentage of fat in the newborn infant is relatively low, but in the obese adult the percentage of fat may exceed that of protein by a wide margin.

Only about three fourths of a pound of carbohydrate is present in the body. This is chiefly in the form of fuel storage, with only a small amount being involved in the structure of the tissues.

The predominating chemical elements in the body are oxygen, 65 per cent; carbon, 18 per cent; hydrogen, 10 per cent; and nitrogen, 3 per cent. Together they represent about 96 per cent of body weight. The remaining 4 per cent is made up of the mineral elements, of which calcium and phosphorus account for three fourths.

Many of the most important body constituents are organic compounds present in such small amounts that they have no significant effect on the total body weight. Among these are the vitamins, hormones, and enzymes.

Cells as functioning units. The human body may be studied at various levels of organization: the organism as a whole; organs and tissues; cells that make up the organs and tissues; and structural components within cells. Nutritional processes of the organism as a whole are the sum total of the physical and chemical activities that take place within the cell and the relationships that exist between the cells and the surrounding environment.

The simplest living organism consists of a single cell such as a bacterium or yeast cell that is capable of respiration, ingestion, digestion, absorption, circulation, synthesis of new materials, breakdown of materials for energy, response to the environment, excretion, and reproduction. Survival of the cell is dependent upon a favorable external environment. The cells of complex organisms such as those in the human being carry out these multiple activities but cannot exist independently; they function through intricate coordination with other cells. Cells are so tiny that they can be seen only with a light microscope. Many structures within cells have been identified by means of the electron microscope that permits magnification of 100,000 times or more. Cells are of infinite variety in size, shape, and specialized functions. They also possess some structures and functions in common so that it is possible to diagram and describe a so-called typical cell. (See Figure 2–1.)

Figure 2–1. Diagram of a cell as it would appear under an electron microscope.

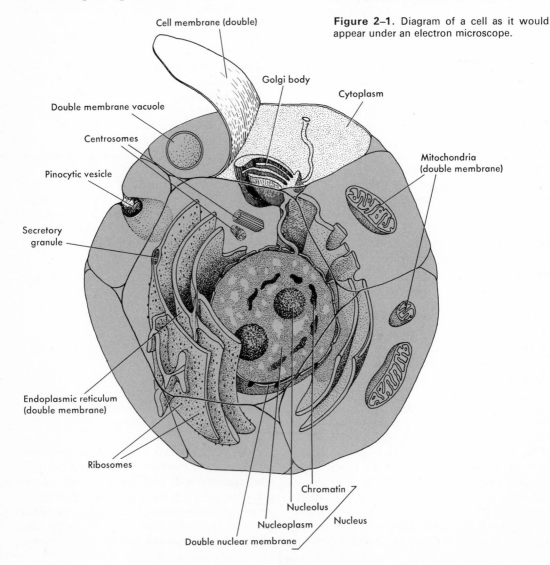

Cell membrane (double)

Golgi body

Cytoplasm

Double membrane vacuole

Centrosomes

Pinocytic vesicle

Mitochondria (double membrane)

Secretory granule

Endoplasmic reticulum (double membrane)

Ribosomes

Chromatin

Nucleolus

Nucleus

Nucleoplasm

Double nuclear membrane

The *cell membrane* surrounds the protoplasm, maintains the constancy of the internal environment, and establishes dynamic equilibrium with the external environment by its highly selective ability to regulate the kinds and amounts of materials that enter and leave the cell.

The *nucleus* of the cell is the storehouse for deoxyribonucleic acid (DNA), the genetic plan for the construction of proteins that enable new cells to have the characteristics of the parent cell.

The *cytoplasmic matrix* is the continuous phase extending from the cell membrane throughout the cell and surrounding the *organelles* or living structures as well as certain lifeless materials known as *inclusions*. The organelles include the mitochondria, lysosomes, and endoplasmic reticulum.

Mitochondria are rod-shaped or round structures that vary in size and shape depending upon their activity. Within the mitochondria are hundreds to thousands of oxidative enzymes that are responsible for carrying on the reactions that yield the high-energy compound adenosine triphosphate (ATP). ATP supplies the energy needed by the cell to carry on its activities.

Lysosomes are membranes, or bags, that contain digestive enzymes. When the membrane bursts, the cell itself is digested, this being normal as worn-out cells are replaced by new. Lysosomes also release amino acids from proteins and are able to engulf bacteria and other substances. The phagocytic activity is a special property of the white blood cells.

The *endoplasmic reticulum* is the system of channels that allows flow of materials to and from the various parts of the cell as well as to the extracellular environment. The endoplasmic reticulum is associated with several special structures that vary considerably according to the type of cell. *Ribosomes* are the site of protein synthesis according to the genetic information supplied by the nucleus. They are abundant in cells where protein synthesis is great, but are lacking in some cells, such as red blood cells, where protein synthesis does not take place. The *Golgi complex* appears as flattened bags and is well developed in secretory cells. It stores and concentrates enzymes and secretes them on demand.

The nature of enzymes. All living tissues, plant and animal, produce thousands of enzymes without which the myriad chemical reactions could not take place. Enzymes are organic catalysts of a protein nature which remarkably increase the rate of reactions without becoming a part of the reaction products. When protein is denatured (as by heating), the enzyme activity is lost. A small amount of enzyme will accomplish a chemical change on a great deal of substance, sometimes as much as 4,000,000 times its own weight. Enzymes, like all organic materials, are gradually used up, and therefore they must be continuously synthesized by the living cell.

Some enzymes are simple proteins, whereas others consist of a protein and another grouping which is loosely or firmly bound to the protein molecule. In an enzyme system the protein molecule is called the *apoenzyme;* its attached grouping is called the *prosthetic group.* For many enzyme systems the prosthetic group is comprised of *coenzymes,* which are organic compounds, including several of the vitamins. The same *coenzyme,* it should be noted, may be used in different enzyme systems; it is the protein molecule that gives an enzyme its particular specificity. Some enzymes may require the presence of a *cofactor* (e.g., a mineral element) for their proper functioning.

Some enzymes are produced in an inactive form known as *proenzyme* or *zymogen* and require some other substance to activate them. For example:

$$\text{Trypsinogen} \xrightarrow[\text{(activator)}]{\text{enterokinase}} \text{Trypsin}$$
(proenzyme or zymogen)   (active enzyme)

$$\text{Protein} + \text{water} \xrightarrow{\text{trypsin}} \text{Proteoses, peptones,}$$
(substrate)   polypeptides

Most enzymes participate in only one chemical reaction on a single substance, although some act on a class of compounds. Thus, a single cell contains hundreds to thousands of enzymes that are responsible for as many different actions. An enzyme, such as *lactase,* will split only the sugar lactose; it has no action on the sugar sucrose, or on any other sugar, protein, or fat. The enzyme which converts the amino acid phenylalanine to another amino acid, tyrosine, cannot be replaced by any other enzyme; if it is missing, the congenital condition known as *phenylketonuria* exists.

Enzymes are classified broadly by the functions they perform. Among the many important functions are hydrolysis, oxidation, dehydrogenation, and transfer of chemical groupings; thus, hydrolases, oxidases, dehydrogenases, and transferases.

Enzymes are inactivated but not destroyed at freezing temperatures; they are destroyed at the temperatures at which proteins coagulate. Enzyme activity is affected by the pH (hydrogen ion concentration) of the medium. Pepsin, which digests proteins in the stomach, is one of the few enzymes active in the very acid reaction of the stomach whereas the enzymes found in the intestines are active at a somewhat alkaline pH.

Metabolism. The series of processes necessary for the building of cells and tissues and their continuous functioning is known as *metabolism*. This broad term implies the coordination of a number of processes:

1. Ingestion, or the intake of food.

2. Digestion, which prepares foods for their use by the body.

3. Absorption of nutrients from the gastrointestinal tract into the circulation.

4. Transportation of nutrients by the circulatory system to the sites for their use, and of wastes to the points of excretion.

5. Respiration, which supplies oxygen to the tissues for the oxidation of food, and which removes waste carbon dioxide. The circulatory system is again responsible for transportation of these gases.

6. Use of materials: oxidation to create heat and energy; incorporation into new cells and tissues.

7. Excretion of wastes: undigested food wastes and certain body wastes from the bowel; carbon dioxide by the lungs; nitrogenous, mineral salt, and other wastes from metabolism by the kidneys and by the skin.

Numerous physical and chemical methods have been developed for measuring the metabolic changes that occur with variations in nutrition. Analyses of blood, urine, and somewhat less frequently, of feces for various constituents are utilized in nutrition research. Part of the study of nutrition is concerned with a knowledge of such changes and an interpretation of their significance in assessing the quality of nutrition.

Functions of food. "You are what you eat" is, in a sense, true inasmuch as food supplies the nutrients needed as a source of energy for activity of the body, and as structural materials for every cell of the body. In the latter capacity, not only do the nutrients furnish the materials that give the body its structure and proportions, but they are used for the synthesis of the numerous regulatory substances that are essential to life.

The nutrients that supply energy include carbohydrates, fats, and proteins. In forming body structures, water, proteins, fats, carbohydrates, and minerals all participate. All nutrients—water, amino acids, fatty acids, sugars, mineral elements, and vitamins—are involved in the innumerable regulatory activities.

DIGESTION

Purposes. Only a few substances contained in foods are suitable for use by the body without change, namely, water, simple sugars, and some mineral salts and vitamins. *Digestion* includes the mechanical and chemical processes whereby complex food materials are hydrolyzed to forms that are suitable in size and composition for absorption into the mucosal wall and for utilization by the body. The nutrients that are absorbed include amino acids, fatty acids, glycerol, simple sugars, minerals, and vitamins.

In addition to its hydrolytic activities the gastrointestinal tract controls the amounts of certain substances that will be absorbed, for example, calcium and iron; prevents the absorption of unwanted molecules; synthesizes enzymes and hormones that are required for the digestive process; eliminates the wastes remaining from the digestion of food as well as certain endogenous wastes; and renews its own structure every 24 to 48 hours.

The digestive organs. The gastrointestinal tract is a tube about 25 to 30 feet long in the adult and includes the mouth, esophagus, stomach, small intestine (duodenum, jejunum, and ileum), and large intestine (cecum, colon, rectum, and anal canal). The liver and pancreas, although situated apart from the tract itself, are important for the secretions that they contribute to the digestive process. (See Figure 2–2.)

The structure of the walls of the gastrointestinal tract is grossly similar throughout but is adapted in its detail for the particular functions of a given organ. The wall consists of four layers: a mucosal lining; circular muscle fibers; longitudinal muscle fibers; and an outer covering known as the serosa. (See Figure 2–3.)

Muscular controls are in effect at several points along the tract to permit the influx of food to the next site for digestion and, under normal conditions, to prevent the backward flow of food (regurgitation). These are the cardiac opening from the esophagus to the stomach; the pyloric sphincter at the gastric-duodenal juncture; and the ileocecal valve, which permits the passage of material from the ileum into the large intestine.

Controls for activity of the digestive tract. The secretion of digestive juices and the motor activity of the tract, and hence the speed and completeness of digestion, are regulated by nervous, chemical, and physical factors.

Everyone is familiar with the fact that the thought, sight, or smell of foods creates the desire for food and increases the flow of saliva and gastric juices. On the other hand, an unpleasant environment or worry and fear may depress the secretion of digestive juices and thus delay digestion. Strong emotions such as anger often increase gastric secretion, but sometimes depress it. The autonomic nervous system exercises continuous control of the secretory and motor activity throughout the entire tract. The pressure of food against the mucosal surfaces and specific characteristics of foods serve as stimuli to the nerves.

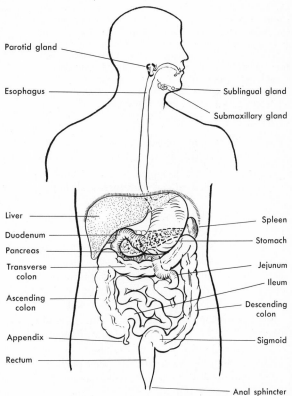

Figure 2–2. The digestive tract.

Parotid gland

Esophagus

Sublingual gland

Submaxillary gland

Liver

Spleen

Duodenum

Stomach

Pancreas

Transverse colon

Jejunum

Ileum

Ascending colon

Descending colon

Appendix

Sigmoid

Rectum

Anal sphincter

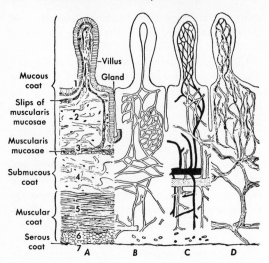

Figure 2–3. Diagram of a cross section of small intestine. *A* shows coats of intestinal wall and tissues of coats: (*1*) columnar epithelium, (*2*) areolar connective tissue, (*3*) muscularis mucosae, (*4*) areolar connective tissue, (*5*) circular layer of smooth muscle, (*6*) longitudinal layer of smooth muscle, (*7*) areolar connective tissue and endothelium. *B* shows arrangement of central lacteal, lymph nodes, and lymph tubes. *C* shows blood supply; arteries and capillaries *black,* veins *stippled. D* shows nerve fibers, the submucous plexus lying in the submucosa, the myenteric plexus lying between the circular and longitudinal layers of the muscular coat. (Courtesy, Miller, M. A., and Leavell, L. C.: *Kimber-Gray-Stackpole's Anatomy and Physiology*, 16th ed. The Macmillan Company, New York, 1972.)

Hormones are the chemical messengers produced at a given site as a result of stimulation by specific foods. Table 2–1 presents a summary of the hormones that affect secretory and motor activity.

Mechanical digestion. Rhythmic coordinated muscle activity causes foods to be reduced to minute particles and intimately mixed with digestive juices so as to facilitate movement throughout the tract, and to provide for maximum exposure to the hydrolyzing enzymes and contact with the absorbing surfaces of the mucosal wall.

By mastication solid foods are cut, ground, mixed with saliva, and prepared for swallowing. Within seconds rhythmic contractions of the muscles of the esophagus force the food particles into the fundus of the stomach, which serves as a reservoir. Each addition of food expands the stomach walls just enough to hold the contents and pushes the mass preceding it forward toward the central part of the organ. Because there is little motor or secretory activity in the fundus, food may remain there for an hour or more, thus allowing salivary digestion of carbohydrates to continue for awhile. Small, regular contractions in the middle region of the stomach gradually increase in rate and intensity. The food is mixed with gastric juice, broken up further, and finally reduced to a thin, souplike consistency called *chyme.*

The pyloric valve opens from time to time to permit small amounts of chyme to enter the duodenum. The rhythmic movements of the intestine are known as *peristalsis.* In the small intestine the circular muscle fibers have a constricting and squeezing action so that the chyme is constantly mixed with the digestive enzymes and given maximum exposure to the absorbing surfaces. This motion of the circular muscles is referred to as segmentation. As the longitudinal muscle fibers contract, a wavelike motion is produced that gradually moves the food mass forward. The muscular activity of the tract also serves as a stimulus to the secretion of the digestive juices and increases the blood supply to the digestive organs.

Motility through the tract. The rate at which foods move through the digestive tract depends upon the consistency, composition, and amount of food eaten. Liquids begin to leave the stomach from 15 minutes to ½ hour after ingestion, a fact that explains why liquid diets do not have great satiety value. Carbohydrates, when eaten alone, leave the stomach more rapidly than do proteins. Fats check the secretion of gastric juices and retard peristaltic activity so that their presence in the diet delays the emptying of the stomach. Normally, the stomach empties in four to six hours. A small meal should pass from the stomach in one to four hours.

The unabsorbed food residue from the small intestine begins to pass through the ileocecal valve into the large intestine in from 2 to 5½ hours, but 9 hours or more from the time of eating may be required for the last of a large meal to pass this point. The length of time required to eliminate food residues as feces varies

Table 2–1. Hormones That Regulate Secretory and Motor Activity of the Digestive Tract

Hormone	Where Produced	Stimulus to Secretion	Action
Gastrin	Pyloric and duodenal mucosa	Food in the stomach, especially proteins, caffeine, spices, alcohol	Stimulates flow of gastric juice
Enterogastrone	Duodenum	Acid chyme, fats	Inhibits secretion of gastric juice; reduces motility
Cholecystokinin	Duodenum	Fat in duodenum	Contraction of gallbladder and flow of bile to duodenum
Secretin	Duodenum	Acid chyme; polypeptides	Secretion of thin, alkaline, enzyme-poor pancreatic juice
Pancreozymin	Duodenum; jejunum	Acid chyme; polypeptides	Secretion of thick, enzyme-rich pancreatic juice
Enterocrinin	Upper small intestine	Chyme	Secretion by glands of intestinal mucosa

widely; a range of 20 to 36 hours after the consumption of the meal is typical.

Chemical digestion. A complex mixture of substances is presented to the various sites of the tract for hydrolysis. Depending upon the location, these include food materials in various stages of hydrolysis, secretions of digestive fluids containing enzymes and hormones, cellular materials from the desquamating mucosa, bile, bacteria, and various products of metabolism within the body that have entered the tract.

A large volume of digestive juices is produced daily by the secretory cells of the digestive tract and by the pancreas and liver. These juices are 98 to 99 per cent water and contain varying proportions of inorganic and organic compounds. One of the organic compounds of importance is mucin, a glycoprotein that lends the slippery quality to mucus and thus facilitates the smooth movement of food throughout the tract. Mucus also furnishes a protective coating to the gastric and duodenal mucosa against the corrosive action of hydrochloric acid. Except for bile, the digestive juices contain enzymes that are appropriate for a particular stage of hydrolysis. Most of the hydrolytic activity on foodstuffs occurs in the small intestine. The final stages of hydrolysis for some nutrients, for example, the disaccharides, occurs within the mucosal cell itself and not in the lumen. Table 2–2 presents a summary of the digestive juices, their components, and the results of enzyme activity.

Functions of the large intestine. The secretions within the large intestine contain much mucus and are alkaline in nature but contain no hydrolytic enzymes. Almost all the nutrients have been absorbed before the food residues enter the large intestine. The cecum fills slowly, and the peristaltic waves that carry the mass toward the rectum together with antiperistaltic waves that force it back spread the digested materials over the walls of the large intestine so that considerable amounts of water are absorbed.

Bacteria of various types are established in the colon shortly after birth and are of three types: (1) fermentative, (2) putrefactive, and (3) *Escherichia coli*. Much fermentation of carbohydrate residues and putrefaction of protein residues occurs in the large intestine. Under normal conditions these reactions cause no trouble.

Foods that are fibrous increase the bulk of the feces and also stimulate the muscular contractions that promote normal evacuation. Feces contain not only the residues of food digestion but also dead and live bacteria, residues from the digestive juices, debris from cellular desquamation, and some endogenous metabolic wastes.

Table 2–2. Digestive Juices and Their Actions

Site of Secretion	Stimuli to Secretion	Daily Volume and pH	Important Constituents	Action

Mouth: saliva
Salivary glands
  Submaxillary
  Sublingual
  Parotid
	Psychic: thought, sight, smell, taste
	Mechanical: presence of food in mouth
	Chemical: contact of sugar, salt, spices, etc., on taste buds
		1000–1500 ml
		pH 5.9–6.8
			Mucin
			*Amylase** (ptyalin)
				Lubrication
				Cooked starch → dextrins, maltose
				Enzyme activity in the mouth is not important

Stomach: gastric juice Parietal cells	Psychic: as above Mechanical: contact with mucosa; distention Hormonal: gastrin increases flow; enterogastrone inhibits	1500–2500 ml pH 2.0–2.5	HCl	Pepsinogen → pepsin Bactericidal Reduces ferric iron to ferrous iron
Chief cells			*Pepsinogen* *Pepsin*	Inactive form of pepsin Proteins → proteoses, peptones, polypeptides
Columnar epithelium			Mucin *?Lipase* *?Rennin* (infants only) Intrinsic factor	Lubrication; protects gastric and duodenal lining Emulsified fats → fatty acids + glycerol (action is negligible) Casein → paracasein Enables absorption of vitamin B_{12}
Liver: bile	Cholecystokinin contracts gallbladder and releases bile to duodenum	500–1100 ml pH 6.9–8.6	Bile salts Bile acids Bile pigments Cholesterol Mucin	Neutralizes acid chyme Emulsifies fats for action of lipase Facilitates absorption of fats and fat-soluble vitamins

Organ	Hormonal/nervous control	Amount, pH	Constituent*	Action
Pancreas: pancreatic juice	Secretin	600–800 ml pH 7–8	Thin, watery, alkaline, enzyme-poor juice	Neutralizes acid chyme
	Pancreozymin		*Amylase*	Starch → dextrins, maltose
			Chymotrypsinogen	Inactive form of enzyme
			Chymotrypsin	Proteins → proteoses, peptones, polypeptides
			Trypsinogen	Inactive enzyme
			Trypsin	Proteins → proteoses, peptones, polypeptides
			Peptidase	Polypeptides → smaller peptides, amino acids
			Lipase	Fats → monoglycerides, fatty acids, glycerol
Small intestine: Intestinal juice (succus entericus)	Enterocrinin	2000–3000 ml pH 7–8	*Enterokinase*	Trypsinogen → trypsin
	Presence of food in small intestine		*Peptidases*	Polypeptides → amino acids
			Nucleinase	Nucleic acid → nucleotides
			Nucleotidase	Nucleotides → nucleosides + phosphoric acid
			Lecithinase	Lecithin → diglycerides + choline phosphate
Within mucosal cells			*Sucrase* (invertase)	Sucrose → glucose + fructose
			Maltase	Maltose → glucose + glucose
			Lactase	Lactose → glucose + galactose

*Constituents in italics are enzymes.

ABSORPTION

The nature of absorption. The process whereby nutrients are moved from the intestinal lumen into the blood or lymph circulation is known as absorption and results in a net gain of nutrients to the body. It is an active process in that substances are moved into the body against forces that would normally cause a flow in the opposite direction. It is also a selective process by which some materials, such as glucose, are transported in their entirety across the cell; others, for example, calcium and iron, are absorbed only according to body need; and still others, such as intact proteins, are held back.

Absorption requires that the nutrient penetrate the cell wall, cross the cell, exit from the cell into the lamina propria, and cross the epithelium of the blood or lymph vessels. In some instances absorption includes a metabolic change within the cell before it is transferred to the circulation. The absorption of specific nutrients will be discussed in Unit II.

Sites and rates of absorption. Absorption appears to take place primarily from the duodenum and jejunum.[1] A notable exception is vitamin B_{12}, which has a specific absorption site in the lower ileum. Bile is reabsorbed from the distal part of the intestine. Most, if not all, substances that are proximally absorbed can also be absorbed by the ileum; thus, those substances that escaped absorption proximally are absorbed distally.

Normally, 98 per cent of the carbohydrate, 95 per cent of the fat, and 92 per cent of the protein in the diet is hydrolyzed and the end products are absorbed. These percentages are sometimes referred to as *coefficients of digestibility*. Malabsorption can occur under a variety of circumstances: a reduction in the number of functioning villi; an increase in motility so that the time of exposure to absorptive surfaces is inadequate; a lack of specific enzymes or of bile; an interference by insoluble compounds; and removal of part of the intestine by surgery.

The absorptive surface. The small intestine provides an absorbing surface that is probably 600 times as great as its external surface area.[2]

This is possible because of the arrangement of the mucosal wall in numerous folds, the 4 to 5 million villi that constitute the mucosal lining, and the 500 to 600 microvilli that form the "brush border" of each epithelial cell of the villus.

Villi are visible by a light microscope. They are tiny finger-like projections of the mucosa and consist of a single layer of epithelial cells resting on the lamina propria, which is a bed of supporting connective tissue supplied by arterial and venous blood vessels and lacteals or lymph channels. (See Figure 2–3.)

Microvilli can be seen only by means of an electron microscope. They elaborate some of the hydrolytic enzymes, and the final stages for hydrolysis of some substances such as disaccharides are completed here and not in the lumen of the intestine.

Mechanisms for absorption. Four mechanisms have been postulated to explain absorption, although it must be emphasized that the pores, carriers, and pumps that are hypothesized have not been seen.[2]

1. *Simple diffusion through pores or channels.* Substances of very low molecular weight (probably 100 or less), such as water and some electrolytes, appear to move freely across the membrane from the side of higher concentration to the side of lower concentration. This mechanism would operate in the direction of the circulation after meals when the concentration of these small molecules in the intestinal lumen is higher than that in the blood and lymph. Being a two-way channel, this mechanism is effective in maintaining osmotic equilibrium. The molecular size of most nutrients is too great for diffusion by pores.

2. *Carrier-facilitated passive diffusion.* Water-soluble nutrients cannot penetrate the lipid-rich membrane of the cell. Therefore, they are attached to "carriers" or "ferries" that facilitate crossing the cell membrane. This is known as *facilitated diffusion*. In passive diffusion the nutrients move downhill, that is, from an area of higher concentration to one of lower concentration; no energy is required for this mechanism. When the concentration of nutrients in the circulation is equal to or exceeds that in the

lumen, nutrients can no longer passively diffuse. They would remain in the intestinal tract until excreted in the feces, representing a large wastage of essential nutrients.

3. *Active transport.* The absorption of most nutrients is probably accounted for by active transport. As in passive diffusion, carriers are necessary for the penetration of the cell membrane. Active transport involves the uphill pumping of nutrients from the lumen into the circulation; that is, the nutrient is moved from a site of lower concentration to one of higher concentration. Energy is required for active transport and is supplied by ATP from the metabolism of glucose within the cell. Sodium plays an essential role in the active transport of water, sugars, and amino acids.[3] The metabolic energy required for the operation of the sodium pump also serves for the transport of these other nutrients, thus serving as an energy-saving device.

4. *Pinocytosis.* In some instances the cell appears to "drink up" or surround a substance and to extrude it into the interior of the cell. Some fats appear to be absorbed by this process. Occasionally, intact proteins may be absorbed in this fashion, helping to explain the incidence of allergy.

INTERMEDIARY METABOLISM

Intermediary metabolism refers to the physical and chemical changes that take place in the internal environment. As pointed out earlier, these changes are the sum total of the activities occurring within each and every cell. The nutrients diffuse from arterial capillary blood into the interstitial fluids surrounding the cells and thence are absorbed by processes such as those described in the preceding section. Likewise, the cells dispose of waste materials to the interstitial fluid and in turn to the venous circulation.

Anabolism refers to those processes by which new substances are synthesized from simpler compounds: for example, enzymes, hormones, and tissue proteins from amino acids, glycogen from glucose, and fats from fatty acids. *Catabolism* refers to the breakdown of complex substances to simpler compounds: for example, the oxidation of glucose to yield energy, carbon dioxide, and water, and the breakdown of fats to glycerol and fatty acids.

The enzyme systems of a given cell determine the specific functioning of that cell. A compound—for example, glucose—that is to be utilized by the cell is attacked by one enzyme after another in assembly-line fashion until the desired end product has been achieved. If a single enzyme in the cell is missing, there is a breakdown in the assembly line and all sorts of problems arise. During the last 25 years a better understanding of enzyme activities has led to the identification, and in some cases effective treatment, of the so-called inborn errors of metabolism seen in far too many infants. The condition *galactosemia* results from the lack of a specific enzyme needed for using galactose; *phenylketonuria*, likewise, results from an enzyme defect that leads to failure to utilize the amino acid phenylalanine.

The metabolic pool. The term *metabolic pool* is often used to refer to the total supply of a given nutrient that is momentarily available for metabolic purposes. For example, the metabolic pool of amino acids at any given moment would include all the amino acids available from dietary sources plus those available from cellular breakdown. From this mixture of amino acids the cells have available the appropriate ones for synthesizing a new protein. The metabolic pool should not be thought of as having specific physical boundaries from which materials may be drawn, but rather as constituting the environment for the cells and the tissues.

Dynamic equilibrium. Cellular materials are constantly being broken down and equally rapidly synthesized. The rate of cellular turnover is exceedingly high, being especially so in the most active organs such as the intestinal wall and the liver. In spite of the remarkable rate of turnover, the body tends to maintain a state of equilibrium, often referred to as *dynamic equilibrium*, or *homeostasis*. The maintenance of equilibrium is governed by an adequate supply of nutrients, a normal complement of enzyme systems, and by the secretion of hormones that regulate metabolic rates.

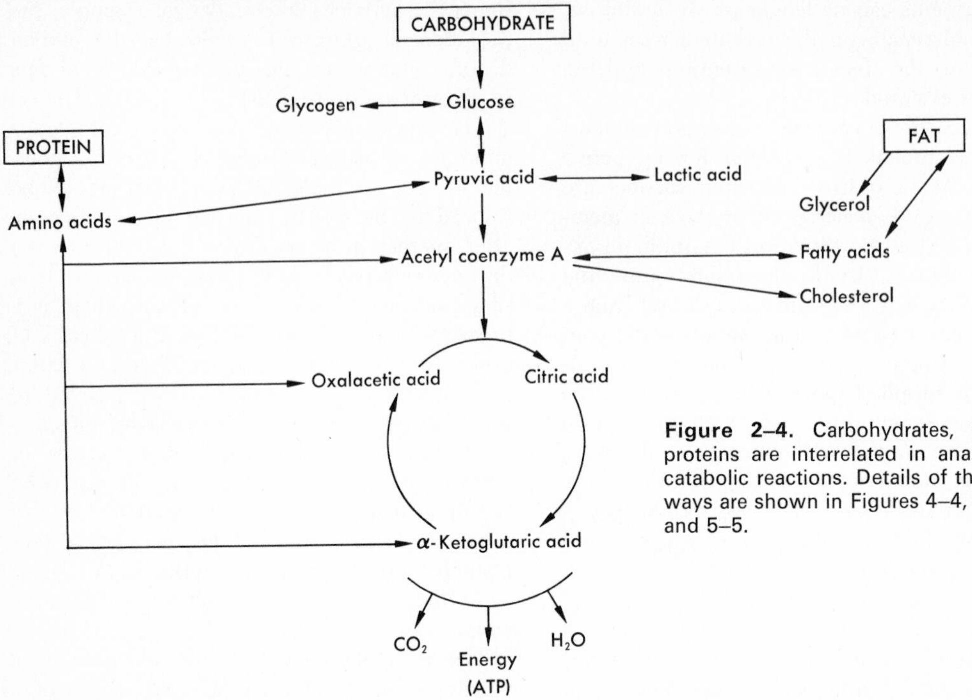

Figure 2–4. Carbohydrates, fats, and proteins are interrelated in anabolic and catabolic reactions. Details of these pathways are shown in Figures 4–4, 4–7, 5–3, and 5–5.

Common pathways. Carbohydrate, fat, and protein are metabolized in an interdependent fashion. Glucose, fatty acids, and amino acids can enter the common pathway that yields energy. Glucose can be metabolized to fatty acids and cholesterol, and some oxidative products of glucose can combine with amino groups to form amino acids. Amino acids are potential sources of both glucose and fatty acids; and so on.

Not only are these major nutrients intertwined in their utilization, but they are dependent upon the correct concentrations of electrolytes and vitamins for making these changes take place. Figure 2–4 is a simplified diagram showing how the metabolism of protein, fat, and carbohydrate is interrelated. Further details of the metabolic pathways are presented in Unit II.

PROBLEMS AND REVIEW

1. What is meant by the following terms: digestion; coefficient of digestibility; peristalsis; segmentation?
2. An enzyme is a catalyst produced by living cells. Name five characteristics of enzymes.
3. In what way does the chewing of food aid digestion in the stomach?
4. It is important that foods be attractively served. How does this facilitate good digestion?
5. Pepsin is a proteolytic enzyme which is secreted by the gastric mucosa as a proenzyme, pepsinogen. How is the pepsinogen activated? What is the substrate on which pepsin acts?
6. Many pediatricians permit children to have foods such as fruit and bread or crackers between meals but advise against the use of milk for such feedings. Why would milk be more likely to interfere with the appetite for the following meal?
7. In what ways would a deficient secretion of hydrochloric acid interfere with digestion?
8. *Problem.* A meal consisted of 25 gm protein, 35 gm fat, and 50 gm carbohydrate. Using

the coefficients of digestibility typical of American diets, calculate the amounts that would be actually absorbed.

9. What conditions are necessary so that the tissues can maintain homeostasis?
10. Explain what is meant by passive diffusion; active transport; carrier-mediated transport.

CITED REFERENCES

1. Booth C. C.: "Sites of Absorption in the Small Intestine," *Fed. Proc.,* **26**:1583–88, 1967.
2. Ingelfinger, F. J.: "Gastrointestinal Absorption," *Nutr. Today,* **2**:2–10, March 1967.
3. Curran, P. F.: "Ion Transport in Intestine and Its Coupling to Other Transport Processes," *Fed. Proc.,* **24**:993–99, 1965.

ADDITIONAL REFERENCES

Asimov, I.: *The Chemicals of Life.* The New American Library of World Literature, New York, 1962.

Crane, R. K.: "A Perspective of Digestive-Absorptive Function," *Am. J. Clin. Nutr.,* **22**:242–49, 1969.

Grollman, S.: *The Human Body: Its Structure and Function,* 2nd ed. The Macmillan Company, New York, 1969.

Guyton, A. C.: *Textbook of Medical Physiology,* 3rd ed. W. B. Saunders Company, Philadelphia, 1966.

McMillan T. J.: "Your Basic Food Needs: Nutrients for Growth," in *Food for Us All—Yearbook of Agriculture 1969.* U.S. Department of Agriculture, Washington, D.C., pp. 254–59.

Miller, M. A., and Leavell, L. C.: *Kimber-Gray-Stackpole's Anatomy and Physiology,* 16th ed. The Macmillan Company, New York, 1972.

Nasset, E. S.: "Role of Digestive System in Protein Metabolism," *Fed. Proc.,* **24**:953–58, 1965.

Neurath, H.: "Protein-Digesting Enzymes," *Sci. Am.,* **211**:68–79, Dec. 1964.

Review: "Exercise and Gastrointestinal Absorption in Human Beings," *Nutr. Rev.,* **26**:167–68, 1968.

————: "Fat Absorption Physiology and Biochemistry," *Nutr. Rev.,* **26**:168–70, 1968.

————: "Time Response of Jejunal Sucrase and Maltase Activity in Man," *Nutr. Rev.,* **27**:259–61, 1969.

Spencer, R. P.: "Intestinal Absorption of Amino Acids. Current Concepts," *Am. J. Clin. Nutr.,* **22**:292–99, 1969.

Williams, R. J.: "We Abnormal Normals," *Nutr. Today,* **2**:19–23, Dec. 1967.

3 Dietary Guides and Their Uses

RECOMMENDED DIETARY ALLOWANCES

Development of dietary allowances. Man has always been concerned about the kinds and amounts of foods that would keep him physically fit. Nevertheless, significant progress in identifying the nutrients needed by the body and the amounts required under varying circumstances has come about principally in this century as a result of thousands of investigations in research laboratories. Periodically, summaries of such research have been made in order to recommend the levels of intake desirable for various categories of the population. The first national effort in the United States came about late in 1940 when the Food and Nutrition Board of the National Research Council was organized to guide the government in its nutrition program. One of the first activities of this Board was the careful review of research on human requirements for the various nutrients. This led to the publication of the Recommended Dietary Allowances in 1943. The Board has evaluated new research from time to time and has published seven revisions of the standards.

The 1973 Recommended Dietary Allowances are listed in Table 3–1. They assume a "reference" man and woman weighing 70 and 58 kg, respectively, 23 to 50 years of age, and living in a temperate climate. Adjustments are made for age, for body size, for change in environment, and for change in activity.

The bulletin published by the Food and Nutrition Board[1] gives a full description of the bases used to establish these recommendations and also includes a discussion of the needs for other nutrients such as fat, carbohydrate, water, and many minerals and vitamins not listed in the table. When diets are planned to meet the recommended levels set forth in the table, it is safe to assume that the body's needs for the nutrients not listed will also be met. The allowances for specific nutrients, and factors that modify the needs, are discussed in more detail in the chapters of Unit II.

The bulletin prepared for each revision of the RDA has described the purposes, interpretation, and intended uses of the dietary allowances. These are summarized in the paragraphs that follow.

Interpretation. It is important to recognize the bases that have been used in the development of the dietary allowances. The stated levels of nutrients for each age-sex category are value judgments set by the Food and Nutrition Board, composed of a committee of nutritional scientists. They are based upon available knowledge, and revisions are made at five-year intervals to incorporate newer knowledge.

The allowances have been derived by applying statistical analyses to the available data on the requirements of different individuals. The use of the word "allowance" rather than "requirement" should be especially noted. The allowances are designed to take care of "practically all of the healthy people in the United States." Thus, they are neither minimum requirements nor average needs. Let us take a hypothetical example: Suppose ten adults who have been subjects in research studies were found to have satisfactory calcium balances with the following calcium intakes; 425, 540, 570, 590, 600, 610, 630, 735, and 795 mg. The average requirement for the group is 609 mg, but this level of intake would not be enough for the three persons whose balances were satisfactory at higher levels of intake. But if the allowance is set at 800 mg,

Table 3-1. Food and Nutrition Board, National Academy of Sciences—National Research Council Recommended Daily Dietary Allowances,[1] Revised 1973

Designed for the maintenance of good nutrition of practically all healthy people in the U.S.A.

	(years) From up to	Weight (kg)	Weight (lbs)	Height (cm)	Height (in)	Energy (kcal)[2]	Protein (g)	Fat-Soluble Vitamins					Water-Soluble Vitamins							Minerals					
								Vitamin A Activity (RE)[3]	Vitamin A Activity (IU)	Vitamin D (IU)	Vitamin E Activity[5] (IU)	Ascorbic Acid (mg)	Folacin[6] (μg)	Niacin[7] (mg)	Riboflavin (mg)	Thiamin (mg)	Vitamin B6 (mg)	Vitamin B12 (μg)	Calcium (mg)	Phosphorus (mg)	Iodine (μg)	Iron (mg)	Magnesium (mg)	Zinc (mg)
Infants	0.0–0.5	6	14	60	24	kg×117	kg×2.2	420[4]	1,400	400	4	35	50	5	0.4	0.3	0.3	0.3	360	240	35	10	60	3
	0.5–1.0	9	20	71	28	kg×108	kg×2.0	400	2,000	400	5	35	50	8	0.6	0.5	0.4	0.3	540	400	45	15	70	5
Children	1–3	13	28	86	34	1300	23	400	2,000	400	7	40	100	9	0.8	0.7	0.6	1.0	800	800	60	15	150	10
	4–6	20	44	110	44	1800	30	500	2,500	400	9	40	200	12	1.1	0.9	0.9	1.5	800	800	80	10	200	10
	7–10	30	66	135	54	2400	36	700	3,300	400	10	40	300	16	1.2	1.2	1.2	2.0	800	800	110	10	250	10
Males	11–14	44	97	158	63	2800	44	1,000	5,000	400	12	45	400	18	1.5	1.4	1.6	3.0	1200	1200	130	18	350	15
	15–18	61	134	172	69	3000	54	1,000	5,000	400	15	45	400	20	1.8	1.5	1.8	3.0	1200	1200	150	18	400	15
	19–22	67	147	172	69	3000	54	1,000	5,000	400	15	45	400	20	1.8	1.5	2.0	3.0	800	800	140	10	350	15
	23–50	70	154	172	69	2700	56	1,000	5,000		15	45	400	18	1.6	1.4	2.0	3.0	800	800	130	10	350	15
	51+	70	154	172	69	2400	56	1,000	5,000		15	45	400	16	1.5	1.2	2.0	3.0	800	800	110	10	350	15
Females	11–14	44	97	155	62	2400	44	800	4,000	400	10	45	400	16	1.3	1.2	1.6	3.0	1200	1200	115	18	300	15
	15–18	54	119	162	65	2100	48	800	4,000	400	11	45	400	14	1.4	1.1	2.0	3.0	1200	1200	115	18	300	15
	19–22	58	128	162	65	2100	46	800	4,000	400	12	45	400	14	1.4	1.1	2.0	3.0	800	800	100	18	300	15
	23–50	58	128	162	65	2000	46	800	4,000		12	45	400	13	1.2	1.0	2.0	3.0	800	800	100	18	300	15
	51+	58	128	162	65	1800	46	800	4,000		12	45	400	12	1.1	1.0	2.0	3.0	800	800	80	10	300	15
Pregnant						+300	+30	1,000	5,000	400	15	60	800	+2	+0.3	+0.3	2.5	4.0	1200	1200	125	18+[8]	450	20
Lactating						+500	+20	1,200	6,000	400	15	60	600	+4	+0.5	+0.3	2.5	4.0	1200	1200	150	18	450	25

[1] The allowances are intended to provide for individual variations among most normal persons as they live in the United States under usual environmental stresses. Diets should be based on a variety of common foods in order to provide other nutrients for which human requirements have been less well defined. See text for more-detailed discussion of allowances and of nutrients not tabulated.

[2] Kilojoules (KJ) = 4.2 × kcal.

[3] Retinol equivalents.

[4] Assumed to be all as retinol in milk during the first six months of life. All subsequent intakes are assumed to be one-half as retinol and one-half as β-carotene when calculated from international units. As retinol equivalents, three-fourths are as retinol and one-fourth as β-carotene.

[5] Total vitamin E activity, estimated to be 80 percent as α-tocopherol and 20 percent other tocopherols. See text for variation in allowances.

[6] The folacin allowances refer to dietary sources as determined by Lactobacillus casei assay. Pure forms of folacin may be effective in doses less than one-fourth of the RDA.

[7] Although allowances are expressed as niacin, it is recognized that on the average 1 mg of niacin is derived from each 60 mg of dietary tryptophan.

[8] This increased requirement cannot be met by ordinary diets; therefore, the use of supplemental iron is recommended.

there is a generous margin of safety for 8 of the 10 persons and the level is just above the requirements of the remaining two.

Except for calories the allowances provide a margin of safety for most people; that is, the allowances are sufficiently higher than the average needs so that almost all of the population is covered. The margin differs for each nutrient because of variations in body storage and individual needs, and because some nutrients (vitamins A and D) may be toxic when taken in excessive amounts. The allowances may not meet the needs of those persons who have been depleted because of illness or injury or from long periods of inadequate food intake. Because the allowances are generous, they could be temporarily reduced in emergency situations such as a disaster when there is a limited food supply.

Uses. The allowances should be used to encourage the development of good food habits that will result in the best possible health, and, by contrast, the prevention of disease. Except for iron, the allowances can be fully met for all age categories by the food supplies currently available in the United States.

The allowances are useful for planning the food supplies that should be available to the population, and for planning diets for groups of individuals, for example in a hospital or other institution. They are also used in dietary surveys to show how actual intakes of nutrients compare with these standards, so that recommendations can be made for the improvement of food patterns as well as production and distribution of food supplies.

In the practice of dietetics the allowances are frequently used to determine the adequacy of a given diet, whether it be the food intake of an individual or the nutritive quality of a proposed diet. When the nutrient intake of a healthy individual is equal to, or exceeds, the recommended allowances, it is highly likely that the diet is meeting the needs of that person in terms of his full potential for growth or productivity. On the other hand, if a diet fails to provide the RDA, it must not necessarily be classified as "poor," nor must it be assumed that malnutrition will occur. Because of the margin of safety, it should be obvious that some persons can, in fact, ingest a diet that does not meet the recommended allowances and yet remain in good nutritional health. A determination of nutritional status can be made only when clinical signs, biochemical data, and dietary intake are correlated. Since it is not practical to determine which individuals have requirements higher than average, it is generally good practice for each person to aim to achieve the recommended allowances in his intake.

Dietary guides in other countries. Dietary allowances have been established for the populations of many countries. In addition, the World Health Organization and the Food and Agriculture Organization of the United Nations have adopted recommendations for allowances for many nutrients. The aim of the various standards is essentially to provide a level of nutrition that maintains good health for substantially all of the population.[2] The allowances are not minimum requirements, nor are they average needs.

The allowances in various countries differ because they are intended for the population of a given environment—for example, climate, occupation and activity, dietary practices—and therefore they are not interchangeable. For example, more calories would be allowed for men and women in a country where considerable physical activity is involved in daily work than in a country where work is mechanized and activity is sedentary. The increased calorie allowances in turn necessitate increased allowances of some of the B complex vitamins such as thiamine. The allowances in the various countries also differ because of varying interpretations of data by committees who set up the allowances.[2] As research becomes more extensive these differences are narrowing somewhat. A comparison of allowances set up for men and women by four groups is shown in Table 3–2.

Labeling. The Food and Drug Administration has recently published extensive regulations for food labeling, including nutritional information. The labels for many processed foods will state the caloric, protein, fat, and carbohydrate values per serving, and will also list the percentages of U.S. Recommended Daily Allowances (U.S.RDA)

Table 3-2. Dietary Allowances for Adults by Four Standards

	United States† 1973	Food and Agriculture Organization*†	Canada† 1964*	United Kingdom† 1969*
Body weight, kg	70-58	65	72-57	65-56
Calories	2700-2000	3200-2300	2850-2400	3000-2500
Protein, gm	56-46	46-39	50-39	87-73
Calcium, mg	800	400-500‡	500	800
Iron, mg	10-18		6-10	12
Vitamin A, I.U.	5000-4000	750 mcg	3700	5000
R.E.	1000-800	(retinol)		
Thiamine, mg	1.4-1.0	1.3-0.9	0.9-0.7	1.2-1.0
Riboflavin, mg	1.6-1.2	1.8-1.3	1.4-1.2	1.8-1.5
Niacin, mg equiv	18-13	21.1-15.2	9-7	12-10
Ascorbic acid, mg	45		30	20

Recommended Dietary Allowances, 7th ed. Food and Nutrition Board, National Research Council–National Academy of Sciences, Washington, D.C., 1968, pp. 68–69.

†The first figure in each column refers to men, and the second to women Where the allowance for men and women is the same, only one figure is given.

‡This allowance for calcium represents a range for men and women.

of important minerals and vitamins. The U.S. RDA replaces the Minimum Daily Requirements (MDR) used in labeling for many years. There are three tables of U.S.RDA: for adults and children over 4 years; for infants and children under 4 years; and for pregnant and lactating women. Although the basis for the U.S.RDA is the table of Recommended Dietary Allowances (Table 3–1), the U.S.RDA is more limited and is intended to be used only as a standard for nutritional labeling. The two tables must not be used interchangeably.

A DAILY FOOD GUIDE

Foods as sources of nutrients. All foods provide for the energy needs of the body. In addition, most foods furnish nutrients needed for tissue structure and for regulatory functions. No single food meets all these needs. Even a food like milk, which is generally considered to be the most nearly perfect food, does not contain all the food constituents in optimum amounts. Milk is an excellent source of protein for tissue building, it provides more calcium than any other food for bone and tooth formation,

and it gives the most abundant supply of riboflavin. In other minerals and vitamins, too, milk is relatively rich. However, its ascorbic acid content is low, so that the need for citrus fruits or other vitamin-C-rich food becomes readily apparent. Milk is also deficient in iron; thus, the place of egg, meats, green leafy vegetables, and fruits becomes evident. One could continue in this manner to evaluate each food. A variety of foods becomes one of the best guarantees that a diet will be adequate.

Four food groups. A standard such as the Recommended Dietary Allowances is of practical value only when it is interpreted into a selection of foods to meet the recommended levels. This may be accomplished through dietary calculations as described in the next section of this chapter. However, simple guides for the general public are essential, and these have been developed by nutrition committees of government agencies and others.

One of these guides, "A Daily Food Guide" (Table 3–3 and Figure 3–1), provides a foundation for a day's meals and includes food choices which permit flexibility for seasonal, regional, and budgetary considerations. The specific nutrient contributions made by foods in each of the Four Food Groups will be discussed in the chap-

Table 3–3. A Daily Food Guide*

Milk Group (8-ounce cups)
   2 to 3 cups for children under 9 years
   3 or more cups for children 9 to 12 years
   4 cups or more for teen-agers
   2 cups or more for adults
   3 cups or more for pregnant women
   4 cups or more for nursing mothers

Meat Group
   2 or more servings. Count as one serving:
      2 to 3 ounces lean, cooked beef, veal, pork, lamb, poultry, fish—without bone
      2 eggs
      1 cup cooked dry beans, dry peas, lentils
      4 tablespoons peanut butter

Vegetable-Fruit Group (½ cup serving, or 1 piece fruit, etc.)
   4 or more servings per day, including:
      1 serving of citrus fruit, or other fruit or vegetable as a good source of vitamin C, or 2 servings
      of a fair source
      1 serving, at least every other day, of a dark-green or deep-yellow vegetable for vitamin A
      2 or more servings of other vegetables and fruits, including potatoes

Bread-Cereals Group
   4 or more servings daily (whole grain, enriched, or restored). Count as one serving:
      1 slice bread
      1 ounce ready-to-eat cereal
      ½ to ¾ cup cooked cereal, corn meal, grits, macaroni, noodles, rice, or spaghetti

*"A Daily Food Guide" in *Consumers All* Yearbook of Agriculture, 1965, U.S. Department of Agriculture, Washington, D.C., 1965, p. 394.

ters on the nutrients in Unit II. See also Table 13–2, page 205, for calculation of the nutritive contributions of the Four Food Groups.

The basic diet. The minimum number of servings for the adult of each of the Four Food Groups will be used as a basis for dietary planning throughout this text. The protein, mineral, except for iron, and vitamin needs are substantially met by this plan (see Table 13–2), and the caloric levels are approximately sufficient for basal energy requirements. The size of each portion will obviously need to be modified for preschool and school children and for teenagers to provide the correct amounts of the various nutrients.

To fully meet the energy needs, additional foods may be selected from the fats and sweets or from one or more of the four groups. The nutrient intake will remain essentially at the level calculated for the basic diet if additional energy is provided chiefly from fats and sweets, but

the further selection of foods from one or more of the four groups will substantially increase the nutritive value of the diet.

COMPOSITION OF FOODS

Factors affecting food composition. The nutritive values of foods are determined, for the most part, by chemical methods. In some instances, such as the evaluation of protein quality or of digestibility, or the determination of vitamin D, animal feeding (bioassay) is used. Certain of the B vitamins and some of the amino acids are best determined by observing the reproduction, or selected metabolic processes, of microorganisms (microbiologic assay).

The values for nutrients in tables of food composition are customarily expressed as averages of analyses of food samples. For some nutrients numerous analyses have been made, but

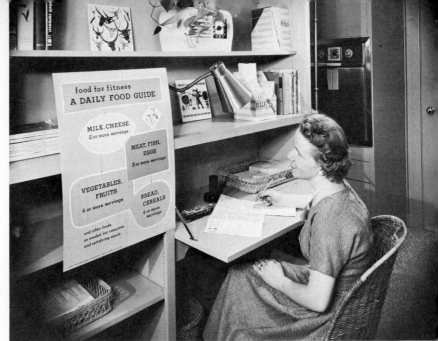

Figure 3–1. Selecting foods from the Four Food Groups of the Daily Food Guide helps to ensure nutritious meals. (Courtesy, U.S. Department of Agriculture.)

for other nutrients the number of determinations has been much more limited. Obviously, the actual nutritive value of a food may be expected to vary more or less widely from the average. Some of the more important factors which account for variation in food composition are discussed briefly below.

The nature of the soil might be expected to produce variations in the composition of foods. At the present time, the only correlation that has been fully established is that a low-iodine content of the soil is reflected in a low-iodine content of foods. The quantity of vitamins, or of other nutrients, has been found to be largely independent of the soil composition. Contrary to certain cultists who criticize the use of chemical fertilizers and who emphasize so-called organic farming, Maynard[3] presented evidence that soils that are chemically fertilized are highly productive of foods of good nutritive value.

The variety of plant and the climate are important determinants of nutritive value. The latter cannot be controlled, but much progress has been made in developing plant varieties that have superior nutritive qualities. For example, strains of corn and wheat are helping to improve the food supply in many of the developing countries.

The conditions of storage—length of time, temperature, light—are known to modify the nutritive value of foods. Some nutrients such as ascorbic acid are rapidly lost when the temperature is high or when foods are bruised. Other nutrients may be lost to a varying degree but not quite so readily as ascorbic acid.

Divergent procedures in food preparation are major factors that affect the nutritive value of a food as it is consumed. Losses in food preparation may be brought about through solubility of the nutrient in water, or through destruction of the nutrient. The latter is increased with high temperature and is also dependent upon the pH of the medium in which it is cooked. The amount of peelings removed, the size of pieces subjected to cooking, the temperature used, the length of time for cooking, the amount of water used, the length of time food is held after cooking—as on a steam table—are but a few of the many variables which may result in wide differences between two foods that were identical at the start of the cooking procedure.

Processing techniques may enhance or interfere with the nutritive value of foods. Dehydration, canning, and freezing yield foods of high nutritive value, but each, in certain ways, modifies somewhat the nutrient contribution of a given food. No doubt this list could be lengthened, but it should suffice to emphasize to the student that a given value for a nutrient in a table of food composition represents an approximation and not a precise value.

Tables of food composition. In view of the foregoing discussion, one might be tempted to ask what useful purposes can be served by referring to a table of nutritive values. First, tables of food composition serve as a basis for comparing one food with another; for example, an examination of the calcium content of many foods leads one to the conclusion that milk is clearly the best source. Although every medium-sized orange could not be expected to yield exactly the same number of milligrams of ascorbic acid, the tables do give information on the relative magnitude of ascorbic acid in orange as compared with apple, for example. Second, tables of food composition make it possible to calculate the nutritive values of any diet and to compare these values with a given standard. Third, with the information on nutritive values, one can plan diets that meet requirements for specific needs—for example, a high-protein diet or a sodium-restricted diet. Finally, the tables provide a ready reference to answer numerous questions concerning the nutritive value of foods; they are useful in counteracting misinformation about nutritive values.

The several tables of food values in the Appendix have been derived from compilations made from time to time, chiefly by investigators in the U.S. Department of Agriculture. Just as the purchase of food involves certain units of measure such as ounces, pounds, pints, quarts, so the amount of nutrients in a food is expressed in certain units—grams (gm), milligrams (mg), sometimes micrograms (mcg), and international units (I.U.). In Table A–1 of the Appendix the nutritive values are expressed for the edible part of household portions of food, thus making it simple to determine the contribution of full or fractional portions of food. Other tables give the nutritive values for 100-gm edible portion of food.

Dietary Evaluation

Purposes of dietary evaluation. A dietary evaluation may be qualitative—that is, through questioning of the subject it may be established that certain foods are, or are not, being included; recommendations for dietary improvement can often be made on such a basis without the necessity for detailed calculations. Nurses and dietitians make such evaluations prior to counseling patients regarding a dietary modification. Such qualitative evaluations are also useful as a starting point for nutrition education for the lay public.

The discussion that follows is concerned with dietary calculations since the student and professional person must be able to use tables of food composition with facility. Most tools that are useful in carrying out one's work entail the development of skill on the part of the user. At first a tool may seem cumbersome and awkward; in fact, it may seem to impede progress rather than help to move things forward. So it is with a table of food composition—one of the most valuable of tools in the application of nutritional science. The beginning student often looks upon dietary calculations as being both time consuming and tedious. However, if long-range goals are kept in mind, the time spent in learning to use tables with confidence will be rewarding. Among the outcomes from experience in dietary calculations are the following:

1. A greater consciousness of food habits and their relation to nutrition and health.

2. Familiarity with tables of food composition and the kinds of information they provide.

3. Facility in using food tables whether to calculate a complete dietary or to seek specific answers concerning nutritive values of a single food.

4. Knowledge concerning the important sources of each of the nutrients.

5. Ability to make recommendations for the improvement of dietaries based upon the calculation of dietary intakes.

6. Appreciation of the importance of keeping orderly and accurate records of dietary intake so that any calculations may be as reliable as possible.

7. The habits of preparing neat and concise reports which have been carefully checked for their accuracy so that coworkers may use the information with complete confidence.

Table 3–4. Nutritive Value of a Breakfast

Food	Household Measure	Weight gm	Energy calories	Protein gm	Fat gm	Carbohydrate gm	Minerals Ca mg	Fe mg	A I.U.	Vitamins Thiamine mg	Riboflavin mg	Niacin mg	Ascorbic Acid mg
Prunes, cooked	3	45	49	tr	tr	13	10	0.8	310	0.01	0.03	0.4	tr
Scrambled eggs	2	128	220	14	16	2	102	2.2	1380	0.10	0.36	tr	0
Bacon, cooked	2 strips	15	90	5	8	1	2	0.5	0	0.08	0.05	0.8	—
Toast, enriched	1 1/2 slices	33	105	3	2	20	31	0.9	tr	0.09	0.08	0.9	tr
Butter	2 pats	14	100	tr	12	tr	3	0	470	—	—	—	0
Coffee													
Cream, light	1 tablespoon	15	30	1	3	1	15	tr	130	tr	0.02	tr	tr
Total			594	23	41	37	163	4.4	2290	0.28	0.54	2.1	tr
Recommended Dietary Allowances													
Woman, 23–50 years			2000	46			800	18	4000	1.0	1.2	13	45
Per cent of RDA			30	50			20	24	57	28	45	15	0

Calculation of the nutritive value of a diet. The method described below may be applied to the diet for a day, for one meal, or for a recipe. It may be used for the calculation of a single nutrient such as protein or for all nutrients listed in a given table. Study these steps carefully before you begin your calculations. See sample calculation of a breakfast, Table 3–4.

1. Study the arrangement of Table A–1, noting especially the units of measure for each nutrient.

2. Keep an accurate record, in household measures, of the foods eaten at each meal. Record the information directly after each meal if at all possible; do not rely on the memory. Include any foods or beverages taken between meals. Specify the exact kinds of foods eaten. Note these descriptive terms: *scrambled* eggs; *cooked* prunes; *light* cream; *enriched* toast; *fried* beef liver. These descriptions enable anyone who is making the evaluation to select the correct items from the table of food composition.

3. If the evaluation is for an entire day, list the total amount, in household measures, for the same foods eaten at different meals. For example: one slice enriched bread at breakfast, ¾ slice at lunch, and ½ slice at dinner would be recorded on the calculation sheet as 2¼ slices.

4. Calculate the nutritive values for each food of the diet or recipe by multiplying the values for the stated portion in Table A–1 by the amounts actually eaten. For example, if three cooked prunes are eaten, all nutritive values shown in the table would be multiplied by ⅙, since the values are given for 17 to 18 prunes.

5. When recording the results of your calculations, use only as many decimal places as appear in the original table. For example, 11.3 gm fat is recorded as 11 gm fat; but 11.5 gm fat would be recorded as 12 gm. A calculated value for thiamine of 0.074 mg would be recorded as 0.07 mg since the table lists only two decimal places for thiamine.

6. Check each of your calculations to be sure it is correct before entering the result on the final calculation sheet.

7. Record all data so that numbers are legible and digits and decimal points are aligned.

8. Total the amount of each nutrient contained in the entire diet or recipe.

9. Compare the actual totals of the diet with the Recommended Dietary Allowances of the individual for whom the evaluation was made. If there are wide deviations between the two, it is especially important to look for possible errors in calculations, misplacement of decimal points, or mistakes in additions.

10. Calculate for each of the nutrients the percentage of the Recommended Dietary Allowances provided by the diet.

11. Summarize the study by listing ways in which the diet can be improved.

PROBLEMS AND REVIEW

1. List the Recommended Allowances for yourself. If a dietary calculation indicated that you were getting less than these allowances in one or more respects, how should you interpret this?

2. State the characteristics of the reference woman. How do you differ?

3. List five reasons why two oranges may differ in ascorbic acid content.

4. Two students had hamburger for lunch, each raw hamburger weighing 4 ounces. One student received more calories in her hamburger than did the other. Explain.

5. Examine the tables in the Appendix to become familiar with the information they provide.

6. *Problem.* Using Table A-1, list five fresh fruits that are the most outstanding sources of vitamin A. In your community, which of these, if any, are not practical for dietary planning?

7. *Problem.* Use Table A-1 to find answers to the following questions:
   a. A woman asks whether whole-wheat bread is more nutritious than enriched white bread.
   b. A teen-ager wants to know if potatoes are more fattening than ice cream.
   c. A mother asks if she can substitute tomato juice for orange juice in her child's diet.
   d. A man asks if beefsteak is richer in protein than Swiss cheese.

8. *Problem.* Keep a careful record of your own food intake for three days. See page 37 for directions.

   a. Score your diet according to the Daily Food Guide. What food group, if any, requires more emphasis in order to improve your diet?

   b. Select one of the three days that is most typical of your usual practice. Calculate the nutritive values using Table A-1. Compare your intake with your recommended allowances.

   c. Keep this evaluation for reference as you study the nutrients in Unit II.

CITED REFERENCES

1. Food and Nutrition Board: *Recommended Dietary Allowances,* 8th ed., National Research Council–National Academy of Sciences, Washington, D.C., 1973.
2. Patwardhan, V. A.: "Dietary Allowances—An International Point of View," *J. Am. Diet. Assoc.,* **56:**191–94, 1970.
3. Maynard, L. A.: "Effect of Fertilizers on the Nutritional Value of Foods," *J.A.M.A.,* **161:**1478, 1961.

ADDITIONAL REFERENCES

"A Daily Food Guide," in *Consumers All—Yearbook of Agriculture 1965.* U.S. Department of Agriculture, Washington, D.C., 1965, p. 394.

"Dietary Standards for Canada," *Can. Bull. Nutr.,* **6:** No. 1, 1964.

Goldsmith, G. A.: "Interests and Activities of the Food and Nutrition Board," *J. Am. Diet. Assoc.,* **52:**37–42, 1968.

Gormican, A.: "Inorganic Elements in Foods Used in Hospital Menus," *J. Am. Diet. Assoc.,* **56:**397–403, 1970.

Hollingsworth, D. F.: "Recommended Intakes of Nutrients for the United Kingdom," *J. Am. Diet. Assoc.,* **56:**200–202, 1970.

Miller, D. F., and Voris, L.: "Chronologic Changes in the Recommended Dietary Allowances," *J. Am. Diet. Assoc.,* **54:**109–117, 1969.

Sabry, Z. I.: "The Canadian Dietary Standard," *J. Am. Diet. Assoc.,* **56:**195–99, 1970.

Sebrell, W. H., Jr.: "The New Recommended Dietary Allowances," *Nutr. Rev.,* **26:**355–57, 1968.

Standal, B. R., *et al.:* "Fatty Acids, Cholesterol, and Proximate Analyses of Some Ready-to-Eat Foods," *J. Am. Diet. Assoc.,* **56:**392–96, 1970.

Todhunter, E. N.: "Food Composition Tables in the U.S.A.," *J. Am. Diet. Assoc.,* **37:**209–14, 1960.

Watt, B. K.: "Concepts in Developing a Food Composition Table," *J. Am. Diet. Assoc.,* **40:**297–300, 1962.

Watt, B. K.: "Nutritive Values of Foods and Use of Tables Listing Them," in *Food for Us All—Yearbook of Agriculture 1969.* U.S. Department of Agriculture, Washington, D.C., pp. 315–18.

Unit II

The Nutrients: Their Characteristics, Functions, Metabolism, Food Sources, Daily Allowances

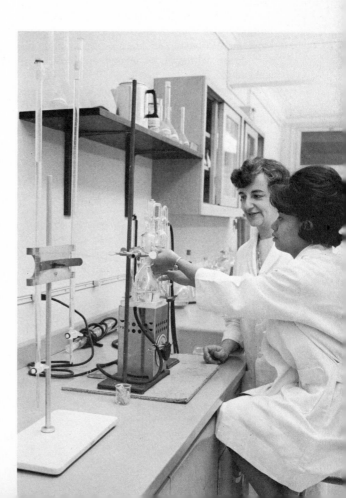

4 Proteins and Amino Acids

Importance of protein. In 1838 a Dutch chemist, Mulder, described certain organic material which is "unquestionably the most important of all known substances in the organic kingdom. Without it no life appears possible on our planet. Through its means the chief phenomena of life are produced."* Berzelius, a contemporary of Mulder, suggested that this complex nitrogen-bearing substance be called *protein* from the Greek word meaning to "take the first place."[1]

Proteins is now retained as a group name to designate the principal nitrogenous constituents of the protoplasm of all plant and animal tissues; they are necessary for tissue synthesis and in the regulation of certain body functions. To say that proteins are more important than are other nutrients is not appropriate, however, for we shall see in the study of nutrition that an inadequate dietary supply or an interference with the utilization of any nutrient can have serious consequences.

One of the most crucial problems facing mankind with its expanding population is an adequate supply of foods that furnish the necessary quantity and quality of protein. Protein-calorie malnutrition, a broad term that encompasses kwashiorkor and marasmus together with milder stages of these diseases, is the major nutritional problem of the developing countries of the world. Literally millions of infants and young children are victims of these diseases in Asia, Africa, Central America, the West Indies, and South America. Many of the children who survive are unable to achieve their full physical growth and development. Even more serious is the threat that the most severely malnourished may be retarded in their mental development and that this retardation may be irreversible.

In the United States there is an abundance of protein of good quality but even so some people do not get enough, either because of ignorance concerning the selection of a good diet or because of lack of money to purchase protein foods, which are generally the most expensive items of the diet. Occasionally, an infant is seen with severe protein-calorie malnutrition. The number of children who may have milder protein deficiencies and who are therefore increasingly susceptible to infections is not known.

A full understanding of the role of proteins in body functions, of daily requirements, and of food sources to meet these needs is essential for the planning of adequate diets for the healthy in all stages of the life cycle and also for therapeutic modifications for the ill. Moderate to severe protein deficiencies are often encountered during illness because of inadequate intake or faulty absorption or metabolism.

COMPOSITION, STRUCTURE, AND CLASSIFICATION

Composition. Proteins are extremely complex nitrogenous organic compounds in which amino acids are the units of structure. They contain the elements carbon, hydrogen, oxygen, nitrogen, and, with few exceptions, sulfur. Most proteins also contain phosphorus, and some specialized proteins contain very small amounts of iron, copper, and other inorganic elements.

The presence of nitrogen distinguishes protein from carbohydrate and fat. Proteins con-

---

*Mulder, G. J.: *The Chemistry of Animal and Vegetable Physiology*. Quoted in Mendel, L. B.: *Nutrition: The Chemistry of Life*. Yale University Press, New Haven, Conn., 1923, p. 16.

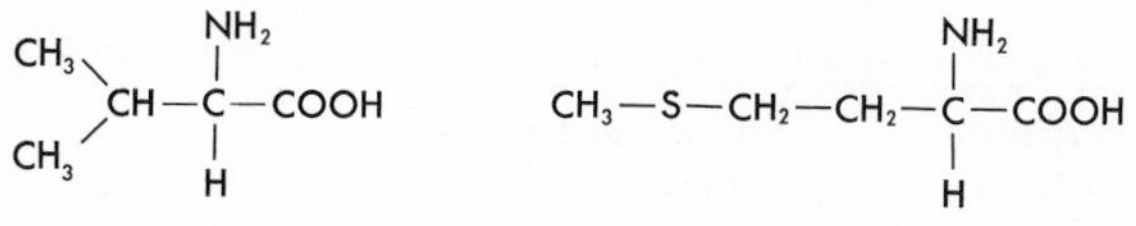

Figure 4–1. Amino acids with different groupings attached to the carbon that holds the amino group.

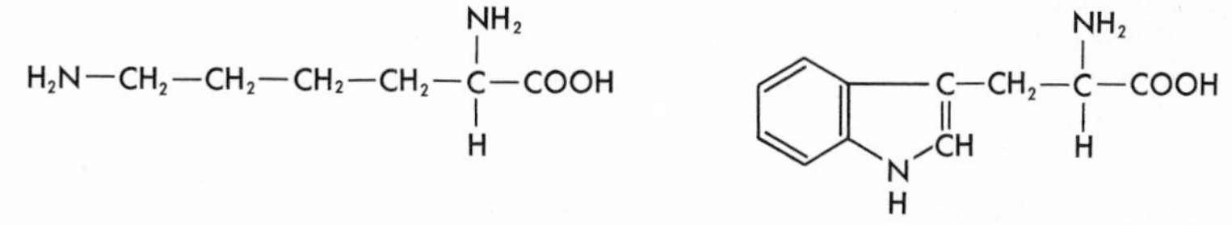

Valine   Methionine

Lysine   Tryptophan

tain an average of 16 per cent nitrogen and have a molecular weight that varies from 13,000 or less to many millions. These large molecules form *colloidal* solutions that do not readily diffuse through membranes.

Structure. Twenty-two amino acids are widely distributed in proteins, and small amounts of four or five additional amino acids have been isolated from one or more proteins. Some amino acids—ornithine and citrulline—are important intermediates in metabolism but are not constituents of intact proteins. See page 54.

All the amino acids obtained by hydrolysis from native proteins are α-amino acids; that is, the amino group (NH_2) is attached to the carbon adjacent to the carboxyl group ($COOH$). The amino acids, except glycine, are optically active and are of the L-configuration; not all amino acids of the D-configuration are utilized in the body.

The structure of an amino acid may be represented thus:

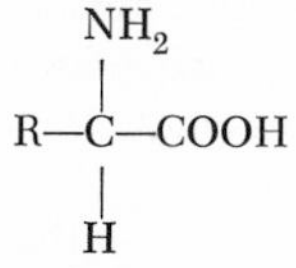

$$R—\overset{\overset{\displaystyle NH_2}{|}}{\underset{\underset{\displaystyle H}{|}}{C}}—COOH$$

By varying the grouping (R) which is attached to the carbon containing the amino group, many different amino acids are possible. Examples of variations in the R grouping are shown in Figure 4–1. (See also Table 4–1.)

Proteins consist of chains of amino acids joined to each other by the peptide linkage; that is, the amino group of one amino acid is linked to the carboxyl group of another amino acid by the removal of water. (See Figure 4–2.) Thus, two amino acids form a dipeptide, three amino acids form a tripeptide, and so on. Proteins consist of hundreds of such linkages.

Specificity of protein. The nature of a protein is first determined by the sequence in which the amino acids are linked and also by the amounts of each amino acid present. For example, tripeptides containing these sequences would differ from each other:

Glycine—Tryptophan—Methionine
Tryptophan—Glycine—Methionine
Glycine—Tryptophan—Valine

Some polypeptide chains might be relatively short; some might be open chains, whereas others might be closed or cyclic chains. Moreover, the nature of the protein is determined by the manner in which the polypeptide chains are bound together to form the protein molecule. *Fibrous* proteins consist of long polypeptide chains bound together in more or less parallel fashion; these are characteristic of proteins of muscle

Figure 4–2. Peptide linkage (CONH). The carboxyl group of one amino acid is linked to the amino group of another amino acid by the removal of water. Proteins consist of long chains of amino acids thus linked.

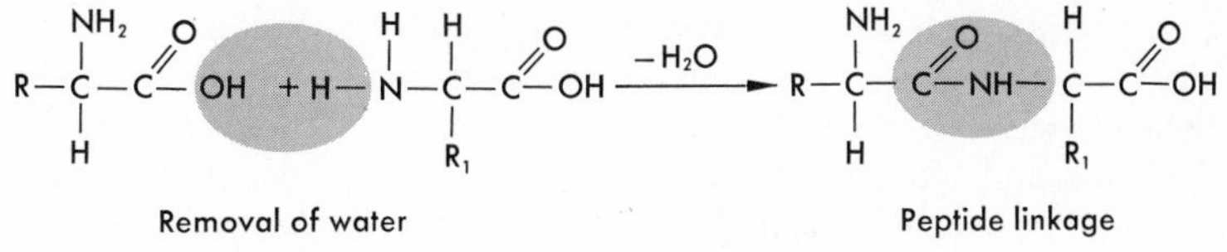

Removal of water   Peptide linkage

Table 4–1. Classification of Amino Acids

Classification	Essential Amino Acids	Nonessential Amino Acids
Neutral—one amino and one carboxyl group		
Aliphatic	Threonine	Glycine
	Valine	Alanine
	Leucine	Serine
	Isoleucine	
Aromatic—contains benzene ring	Phenylalanine	Tyrosine*
Heterocyclic	Tryptophan	Proline
		Hydroxyproline
	Histidine (children)	
Sulfur-containing	Methionine	Cystine*
		Cysteine
Basic—two amino and one carboxyl group	Lysine	Arginine*
		Hydroxylysine
Acid—one amino and two carboxyl groups		Aspartic acid
		Glutamic acid

*These amino acids are classed as semiessential See text (page 45).

fibers, hair, and collagen. *Globular* proteins are round to ellipsoidal; these include hemoglobin, insulin, and albumins and globulins.

In view of the number of amino acids and the innumerable ways and proportions by which they may be combined, it should not be surprising that proteins are so numerous and so highly specific. Each species synthesizes protein that is characteristic. Moreover, each species also synthesizes for its manifold functions proteins that are tailored to these specific needs. Thus, serum albumin, insulin, hemoglobin, keratin, collagen, and myosin have specific structures and functions; they are not interchangeable.

Classification. Proteins may be classified on the basis of their physical and chemical properties or their nutritional qualities.

Physical-chemical properties. Each of the three groups within this classification may be subdivided into a number of classes according to solubility.

1. Simple proteins upon hydrolysis by acids, alkalies, or enzymes yield only amino acids or their derivatives. Examples of this group are albumins and globulins found within all body cells and in the blood serum; keratin, collagen,

and elastin in supportive tissues of the body and in hair and nails; globin in hemoglobin and myoglobin; and zein in corn, gliadin and glutenin in wheat, legumin in peas, and lactalbumin and lactoglobulin in milk.

2. Conjugated proteins are composed of simple proteins combined with a nonprotein substance. This group includes lipoproteins, the vehicles for the transport of fats in the blood; nucleoproteins, the proteins of the cell nuclei; phosphoproteins, such as casein in milk and ovovitellin in eggs; metalloproteins, such as the enzymes that contain mineral elements; mucoproteins, found in connective tissues, mucin, and gonadotropic hormones; chromoproteins, such as hemoglobin and visual purple; and flavoproteins, which are enzymes that contain the vitamin riboflavin.

3. Derived proteins are substances resulting from the decomposition of simple and conjugated proteins. These include rearrangements within the molecule without breaking the peptide bond, such as that occurring with coagulation, and also substances formed by hydrolysis of the protein to smaller fragments referred to as proteoses, peptones, and peptides.

Essential and nonessential amino acids. The importance of the amino acid composition of proteins was shown by Osborne and Mendel in 1915, who observed that rats failed to grow or even survive if some amino acids were omitted from the diet, but that the elimination of other amino acids had no such harmful effects. (See Figure 4–3.) Later work by others, especially by Dr. William C. Rose,[2] established that this was also true for human beings. Thus, amino acids came to be classified as *essential* and *nonessential*. Strictly speaking, all the amino acids are essential units for the synthesis of the protein molecule. However, the body can manufacture many amino acids if it has an adequate nitrogen source, but it cannot produce certain others in adequate amounts to meet body needs. Those amino acids which cannot be synthesized in sufficient amounts by the body and which must be provided in the diet are essential. The human adult requires eight essential amino acids, and growing children require nine or perhaps ten. Arginine is classified as semiessential since growth is retarded if it is not available. The presence of cystine and tyrosine in the diet will reduce the requirement for methionine and phenylalanine, respectively; hence, they are also classed as semiessential. The student should learn to recognize the names of the essential amino acids since they are being referred to more and more frequently in writings on protein nutrition. (See Table 4–1.)

Figure 4–3. Effect of protein quality. These rats of the same age were fed a bread diet. The two rats on the right received bread to which lysine, the limiting amino acid in grains, had been added. This improvement of the protein quality led to the greater gain. (Courtesy, E. I. DuPont de Nemours and Company, Inc.)

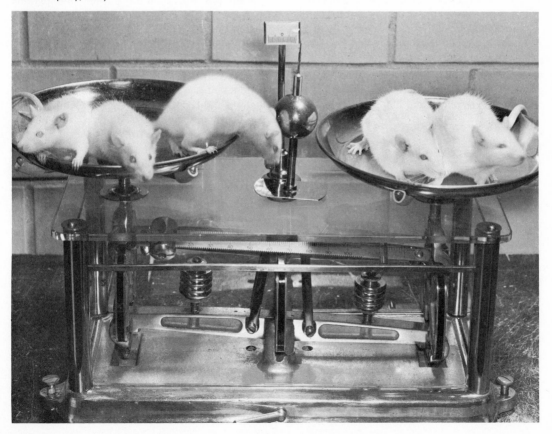

Complete and incomplete proteins. Depending upon their ability to maintain life and promote growth, proteins have long been classified as *complete, partially complete,* and *totally incomplete.* A complete protein contains enough of the essential amino acids to maintain body tissues and to promote a normal rate of growth. Such proteins are sometimes referred to as having a *high biologic value.* Egg, milk, and meat (including poultry and fish) proteins are all complete but not necessarily identical in quality. Wheat germ and dried yeast have a biologic value approaching that of animal sources.

Partially complete proteins will maintain life, but they lack sufficient amounts of some of the amino acids necessary for growth. Gliadin, which is one of a number of proteins found in wheat, is a notable example of proteins of this class. Adults under no physiologic stress can maintain satisfactory nutrition for indefinite periods when consuming sufficient amounts of protein from certain cereals or legumes.

Totally incomplete proteins are incapable of replacing or building new tissue, and hence cannot support life, let alone promote growth. Zein, one of the proteins found in corn, and gelatin are classic examples of proteins which are incapable of even permitting life to continue.

FUNCTIONS

Maintenance and growth. Proteins constitute the chief solid matter of muscles, organs, and endocrine glands. They are major constituents of the matrix of bones and teeth; skin, nails, and hair; and blood cells and serum. In fact, every living cell and all body fluids, except bile and urine, contain protein. The first need for amino acids, then, is to supply the materials for the building and the continuous replacement of the cell proteins throughout life.

Regulation of body processes. Body proteins have highly specialized functions in the regulation of body processes. For example, hemoglobin, an iron-bearing protein that is the chief constituent of the red blood cells, performs a vital role in carrying oxygen to the tissues. The plasma proteins are of fundamental importance in the regulation of osmotic pressure and in the maintenance of water balance. The blood proteins. have a role in the maintenance of the normal slightly alkaline reaction of the blood. The body's resistance to disease is maintained in part by antibodies which are protein in nature.

Enzymes which are specific catalysts for metabolic processes are protein in nature. Governing the metabolic reactions are hormones, many of which are protein in nature—insulin, epinephrine, and thyroid hormone, to name but a few.

Amino acids also have specific functions in metabolism. Tryptophan serves as a precursor for niacin, one of the B-complex vitamins; methionine supplies labile methyl groups for the synthesis of choline, a compound that helps to prevent storage of fat in the liver; glycine contributes to the formation of the porphyrin ring in the hemoglobin molecule and is also an important constituent of the purines and pyrimidines in nucleic acid.

Energy. Proteins are a potential source of energy, each gram of protein yielding on the average 4 calories. The energy needs of the body take priority over other needs, and if the diet does not furnish sufficient calories from carbohydrate and fat, the protein of the diet as well as tissue proteins will be catabolized for energy. When amino acids are used for energy they are then lost for synthetic purposes. Conversely, when amino acids are incorporated into the protein molecule they are not furnishing energy until such time as the tissue proteins are again being catabolized.

DIGESTION AND ABSORPTION

Digestion. The purposes of digestion are to hydrolyze proteins to amino acids so that they can be absorbed and to destroy the biologic specificity of the proteins by such hydrolysis. (See also Chapter 2.) In addition to the foods ingested, the mixture to be digested includes a sizable amount of protein that is constantly being released from the worn-out cells of the mucosa and of the digestive enzymes themselves.[3] The endogenous and exogenous sources of the amino acids are indistinguishable and present a mixture for absorption that differs from that provided by the diet alone.

Saliva contains no proteolytic enzyme, and thus the only action in the mouth is an increase in the surface area of the food mass as a result of the chewing of food. Most of the hydrolysis of protein occurs in the stomach, duodenum, and jejunum. A given enzyme is capable of splitting only specific linkages; it does not attack each and every linkage. Pepsinogen, produced in the stomach, is activated by hydrochloric acid. Pepsin brings about cleavage of the peptide chain at points where phenylalanine or tyrosine provides an amino group.[4] Such splitting of the chain results in shorter fragments often referred to as proteoses.

Trypsinogen, one of the inactive proteases produced by the pancreas, is activated to trypsin by enterokinase, an enzyme produced in the intestinal wall. At a pH of 8 to 9, trypsin splits peptide linkages at points where lysine or arginine provide the carboxyl group.[4] Chymotrypsinogen, another inactive pancreatic enzyme, is activated by trypsin. Chymotrypsin attacks the peptide chain at linkages in which the carboxyl group is provided by phenylalanine, tyrosine, methionine, or tryptophan. Thus, with cleavage at these specific points, the protein molecule will have been split into many smaller fragments.

Peptidases split off amino acids at the terminal linkages. Carboxypeptidases split off the amino acids next to a terminal carboxyl group, and amino peptidases attack the linkages next to the terminal amino group. The mucosal epithelium contains peptidases, and dipeptide hydrolysis probably occurs at the membrane surfaces.

Effect of protein denaturation. Proteolytic enzymes not only bring about the splitting of the peptide linkages but they also split the cross-links that connect the peptide chains. During moderate heating of proteins some of the cross-linkages are split, thereby facilitating digestion. On the other hand, excessive heating results in the formation of linkages that are resistant to the digestive enzymes. As a consequence the amino acids so linked may not be available at a rate that is necessary for incorporation into new proteins.

One resistant linkage is that of lysine with carbohydrate as a result of high heat, usually prolonged. The brown crust of bread contains less available lysine than does the white crumb; toasting of bread results in small losses. If breakfast cereals are processed at high temperatures, they are also subject to such losses. The American diet provides an abundance of essential amino acids, and the reduced availability of lysine, as described above, is not of any significance. These changes may be important when relatively low-protein diets of poor quality are consumed.

Effect of enzyme inhibitors. Some foods such as navy beans and soybeans contain substances that inhibit activity of enzymes such as trypsin. Consequently, the utilization of the proteins of these foods is less efficient. Heating inactivates these inhibitors, thereby improving the digestibility of the protein.

Absorption. Amino acids are absorbed from the proximal intestine into the portal circulation. The rates of absorption are regulated by complex mechanisms not fully understood. These rates are dependent upon (1) the total load of amino acids released through digestion, (2) the proportions of the various amino acids present in the mixture to be absorbed, (3) the availability of carriers to ferry the amino acids into the mucosal cells, and (4) the uptake of amino acids by tissues. Within the intestinal lumen the concentration of free amino acids is at no time great. Apparently, the liberation of amino acids through digestion is coordinated with the rate of absorption. As a consequence, there is a minimal loss of amino acids in the feces. The rate of absorption also appears to be controlled by the levels existing in the blood. Amino acids are rapidly removed from the circulation, and the concentration in the blood at any given time is relatively low.

Active transport and specific carriers. Amino acids are absorbed by active transport, but some diffusion of amino acids also occurs. The amino acids are in competition for the carriers, some amino acids being absorbed much more rapidly than others. In one study an essential amino acid mixture in amounts usually present in a protein meal was administered into the jejunum of normal adults, and the rates of absorption were measured.[5] Methionine, leucine, isoleucine, and valine had the highest rates of absorption, and these were two to three times as rapid as that for threonine, which was the lowest. Whether these same rates would apply to a protein meal fed intact is not known. If they do, as is strongly suspected, a protein that might contain an excess of a rapidly absorbed amino acid such as leucine would be less effective than a more balanced protein inasmuch as carriers would be less available for the amino acids with the lower rates of absorption.

On the average, 92 per cent of the amino acids present in the typical American diet are released through digestion and absorbed. Proteins that are well balanced in their amino acid composition, as in milk, eggs, and meat, show even higher rates of absorption. Most plant proteins have excesses of some amino acids and deficiencies of others, and the percentage of amino acids absorbed is somewhat less. In part this results from the competition of amino acids for carriers to transport them across the mucosal cells, and in part it may be explained by link-

ages resistant to digestion as explained above. A point of practical importance in dietary planning is that some protein of good quality should be present in each meal so that the available mixture of amino acids at any given time is optimum in quality as well as quantity.

METABOLISM

Strictly speaking, the metabolism of proteins is the metabolism of the amino acids. Each cell within the body utilizes the available amino acids to synthesize all the numerous proteins required for its own functions and also makes use of amino acids to furnish energy. In addition, some specialized cells, such as those of the liver, also synthesize proteins and nonprotein nitrogenous substances that are required for the functioning of the body as a whole. Whether the fate of an amino acid, at any given moment, is that of anabolism or catabolism is determined by a number of interrelated factors. (See Figure 4–4.)

Methods for study of protein metabolism.

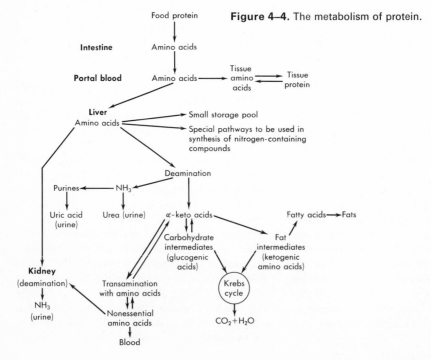

Figure 4–4. The metabolism of protein.

Numerous techniques are available to the biochemist and nutritionist for the study of protein metabolism. Hundreds of investigators since the nineteenth century have assayed the quality of proteins from single foods and food mixtures and have measured the requirements for proteins or amino acids under varying dietary and physiologic conditions by means of *nitrogen balance* studies. These studies on infants, children, and adults as well as on experimental animals—especially rats—have included measurements of the dietary intake of protein or amino acids and of the excretion of nitrogen in the urine and feces. The nitrogen balance technique requires continuous supervision of subjects for weeks or even months so that precise controls of dietary intake and 24-hour quantitative collections of urine and feces are assured. A metabolic ward staffed by technically skilled personnel is the best insurance that the controls are adequate. The method is time consuming, tedious, and expensive. By nitrogen balance only the total nitrogen metabolism of the body is measured, without information on what is happening in specific tissues.

The biochemist in a clinical laboratory or conducting research in protein metabolism makes use of many methods that supplement or take the place of nitrogen balance studies. These include the determination of the concentration in the blood of the protein fractions, amino acids, and nonprotein nitrogenous constituents—total nonprotein nitrogen, urea nitrogen, creatinine, and uric acid. Tracers are often used to study the fate of an amino acid including its absorption, its incorporation into tissues, its pathway through intermediate substances, or its excretion in the urine.

A study of the nitrogenous constituents in the urine opens another door to a better understanding of the metabolism of protein. From such measurements it is possible to determine the level of nitrogen catabolism that is taking place, to detect abnormalities in amino acid metabolism (as in phenylketonuria) or in nonprotein nitrogenous compounds (as in gout), and to evaluate the ability of the kidney to excrete nitrogenous products. (See Tables A–14 and A–15.)

Nitrogen balance. Nitrogen balance studies are based on the fact that protein, on the average, contains 16 per cent nitrogen; thus, 1 gm nitrogen is equivalent to 6.25 gm protein. The balance may be expressed thus:

$$\text{Nitrogen balance} = \text{Nitrogen intake} - \text{nitrogen excretion (urine} + \text{feces} + \text{skin)}$$

Nitrogen excretion. The fecal nitrogen includes that from undigested dietary protein and also nitrogen from undigested endogenous sources. The latter are composed of the undigested protein fractions of desquamated cells of the intestinal mucosa, the used-up enzymes from the digestive juices, and bacterial cells. The daily fecal excretion of nitrogen by the adult is approximately 1 gm, but this varies with the quality of the protein fed, the gastrointestinal motility, and so on. The difference between the amount of nitrogen in the diet and the fecal nitrogen is the amount of nitrogen absorbed and available for tissue use.

More than 90 per cent of the urinary nitrogen results from the deamination of the amino acids in the body and is excreted chiefly as urea with small amounts of ammonia. Nonprotein nitrogenous end products include creatinine, uric acid, and a number of others. When the calorie intake is fully adequate and the protein intake is just sufficient to cover the repletion of body tissues, the urinary nitrogen is at its lowest level. As the protein intake increases above the tissue maintenance requirement the excess amino acids are not stored but are used for energy, thereby increasing the amount of urinary nitrogen. Therefore, in studies of the minimum protein requirement by the nitrogen balance technique it is always necessary to determine the balance at gradually decreasing levels of intake until the point of negative balance is reached. That level just above negative balance that is just sufficient for tissue replacement represents the *minimum* protein requirement under the conditions of the experiment.

Nitrogen is also lost through perspiration and from the desquamated cells of the skin surfaces, the hair, and the nails. Such losses are extremely difficult to measure. A few studies have shown that the average daily losses by the adult male are about 1.4 gm nitrogen. When people live and work at high environmental temperatures so that sweating is profuse, the losses from the skin have been found to be as high as 3.75 gm nitrogen (equivalent to 23 gm protein) in 24 hours.[6]

States of balance. Nitrogen equilibrium is that state of balance when the intake of nitrogen is equal to that which is excreted. A state of equilibrium is normal for the healthy adult. It is established at any level of protein intake that exceeds the minimum requirement, provided that the calorie intake is also adequate.

Positive nitrogen balance is that state in which the intake of nitrogen exceeds the excretion. It indicates that new protein tissues are being synthesized, as in growing children or during pregnancy. Positive nitrogen balance also occurs when tissues depleted of protein during illness or injury are being replenished, or when muscles are being developed, as in athletic training. Positive nitrogen balance should not be interpreted as storage in the usual sense. There is no further addition of protein to already well-nourished cells.

Negative nitrogen balance is that condition in which the excretion of nitrogen exceeds the intake. An individual with a negative nitrogen balance is losing nitrogen from tissues more rapidly than it is being replaced—an undesirable state of affairs. It may occur because (1) the calorie content of the diet is inadequate and therefore tissues are being broken down to supply energy; (2) the quality of the protein is poor and the needs for tissue replacement are not being met; or (3) injury, immobilization, and disease are causing excessive breakdown of tissues.

Dynamic equilibrium. The liver is the key organ in the metabolism of protein. It selectively removes amino acids from the portal circulation for the synthesis of its own proteins and for many of the specialized proteins such as lipoproteins, plasma albumins, globulins, and fibrinogen as well as nonprotein nitrogenous substances such as creatine. The liver is also the principal organ for the synthesis of urea.

Amino acids are transported throughout the body by the systemic circulation and are rapidly removed from the circulation by the various tissue cells. Likewise, amino acids and products of amino acid metabolism are constantly added to the circulation by the tissues. The *amino acid pool* available to the tissues at any given location at any given moment thus includes dietary sources (exogenous) and tissue breakdown (endogenous sources). These sources are indistinguishable. Body proteins are not rigid structures, but there is a continuous taking up and release of amino acids. In the adult the gains and losses are about equal, and the state is known as *dynamic equilibrium.*

The rate of turnover varies widely in body tissues. The intestinal mucosa, for example, renews itself every one to three days—a fantastic rate of repletion! The liver also has a high rate of turnover. Muscle proteins have a much slower rate of turnover, but the size of the muscle mass in the body is so great that the net daily release of amino acids is considerable. The turnover rate of collagen is very slow and that of the brain cells is negligible.

Protein reserves. Although the body does not store protein in the sense that it stores fat, or glycogen, or vitamin A, certain "reserves" are available from practically all body tissues for use in an emergency. Based upon animal studies, about one fourth of the body protein can be depleted and repleted.[7] Thus, the vital functions of the organism may be protected for 30 to 50 days of total starvation or for much longer periods of partial starvation. It should be apparent that the use of these reserves eventually requires restoration of tissues to their normal protein composition.

Anabolism or catabolism? Whether an amino acid is utilized for the synthesis of new proteins or is deaminized and used for energy depends upon a number of factors.

1. The "all-or-none" law. All the amino acids needed for the synthesis of a given protein must be simultaneously present in sufficient amounts. If a single amino acid is missing, the protein cannot be constructed. If a given amino acid is present only to a limited extent, the protein can be formed only as long as the supply of that amino acid lasts. The amino acid in short supply is known as the *limiting amino acid.* If one or more amino acids are missing from the pool, the remaining amino acids are unavailable for later synthesis and will be catabolized for energy.

2. *Adequacy of calorie intake.* For protein synthesis to proceed at an optimum rate, the calorie intake must be sufficient to supply the energy needs. A deficiency of calories necessitates the use of some dietary and tissue proteins for energy.

3. *The nutritional and physiologic state of the individual.* The rate of synthesis is high during growth and in tissue repletion following illness or injury. In the adult synthesis just balances tissue depletion when the calorie intake is adequate.

Protein catabolism is greatly increased immediately following an injury, burns, and immobilization because of illness. It is also increased as a result of fear, anxiety, or anger. For example, unmarried pregnant girls who are worried about their future often have a negative nitrogen balance in spite of diets that appear to be adequate.

4. *Development of specific tissues.* Some tissues may be synthesized even though the overall nitrogen balance might be negative. Thus, the fetus and maternal tissues may be developed at the expense of the mother when her diet is inadequate. Another example of specific tissue development is that of rapidly growing tumors that use amino acids at the expense of normal tissues.

5. *Hormonal controls.* The pituitary growth hormone has an anabolic effect during infancy and childhood, and the estrogens and androgens exert an anabolic effect during preadolescent and adolescent years. By bringing about normal carbohydrate metabolism insulin has an indirect anabolic effect by reducing the breakdown of proteins to supply glucose. Insulin probably facilitates the transport of amino acids into the cell. In normal amounts thyroid hormone also stimulates growth.

Among the hormones that increase the catabolism of body tissues are adrenocortical hormones which stimulate the breakdown of tissue proteins to yield glucose. An excessive production of thyroxine also increases the breakdown of proteins.

Synthesis of proteins. Each cell is capable of synthesizing all the proteins for its own functions but not those of a different type of cell. The specific protein that will be synthesized is governed by the *genetic code,* or amino acid program, that exists within the nucleus of each cell. The synthesis of protein takes place in the cytoplasm of the cell. The model for protein synthesis was established by Watson and Crick in 1962. (See Figure 4–5.)

Within the nucleus of the cell are giant molecules of a substance known as deoxyribonucleic acid (DNA). These molecules consist of two intertwining chains containing 5-carbon sugar (deoxyribose) and phosphate groupings that form a long double-helix molecule. These chains are the backbone of the molecule. Four nitrogenous bases (adenine, guanine, cytosine, and thymine) are joined in pairs and attached by hydrogen bonds to the sugar-phosphate chain to give a firm structure that resembles a spiral staircase. The arrangement of the bases within the molecule designates the specific amino acids that will be used and the sequence of their attachment to one another.

Since the synthesis of the protein takes place in the cytoplasm, the plan must be carried from the DNA molecules in the nucleus. This is the function of *messenger ribonucleic acid* (mRNA). Ribonucleic acid is a compound that resembles DNA except that the 5-carbon sugar is ribose and uracil is substituted for thymine. The information in DNA is copied within the nucleus to mRNA, which then moves to the ribosomes which are the site of synthesis in the cytoplasm.

Amino acids enter the cell by active transport from the metabolic pool. Some of the nonessential amino acids may be synthesized within the cell itself. The amino acids are activated in a reaction that requires the energy-rich compound ATP. Then they form a complex with another type of RNA, known as *transfer RNA;* the transfer RNA is specific for each amino acid. The RNA-amino acid complex is then moved to the messenger RNA where the peptide linkage is formed according to the pattern carried from DNA. When the synthesis has been completed, the protein is set free from the ribosomes to perform its function in the cell, and the transfer

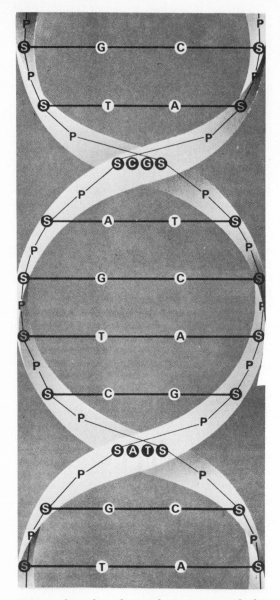

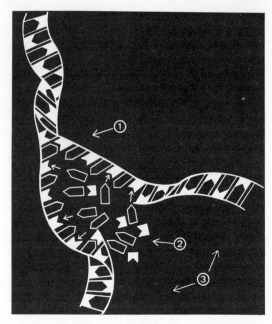

Figure 4–5. (*Left*) The Watson-Crick DNA model. Shown here are only a few of the thousands of turns in the double-helix structure of the molecule. The two outer ribbons are the backbone of the molecule, consisting of the sugar (*S*) deoxyribose and phosphate (*P*). Cross-links between the two ribbons are pairs of bases: adenine (*A*), guanine (*G*), cytosine (*C*), and thymine (*T*). (Courtesy, World Health Organization.)
(*Right*) Shows replication of the molecule. The two chains of the DNA molecule are "unzipped" at (*1*); sugars, phosphates, and bases move about in the nucleus (*2*) and attach to form two new double-helix arrangements (*3*). (Courtesy, World Health Organization.)

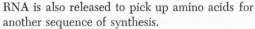

RNA is also released to pick up amino acids for another sequence of synthesis.

The daily synthesis of protein in the adult has been estimated to be about 1.3 gm per kilogram, or about 91 gm for the 70-kg man.[8] Almost all the amino acids for this daily replacement are supplied by tissue proteins that have been broken down, supplemented with amino acids from dietary sources.

Synthesis of nonessential amino acids. The materials for the formation of the nonessential amino acids are keto acids such as pyruvic and α-ketoglutaric acid formed in the metabolism of carbohydrates (see page 70) and ammonia that is released through deamination of amino acids. The synthesis involves a process known as *transamination* in which enzymes known as *transaminases* and pyridoxal phosphate, a coenzyme containing vitamin B_6, are involved. By this mechanism a new amino acid is formed without the appearance of ammonia in the free state. Glutamic acid often serves as a donor of nitrogen in this reaction. The general reaction is as follows:

$$R_1CHNH_2COOH + R_2COCOOH \rightleftarrows$$
    Amino acid$_1$ Keto acid$_2$
$$R_2CHNH_2COOH + R_1COCOOH$$
          Amino acid$_2$ Keto acid$_1$

Catabolism. When amino acids are used for energy, the amino group is removed and a keto acid remains. Most of the deamination of amino acids occurs in the liver, but some also occurs in the kidney. Ammonia is liberated from the amino acids by oxidative enzymes according to the following general reaction:

$$RCHNH_2COOH + \tfrac{1}{2}\,O_2 \rightarrow RCOCOOH + NH_3$$
  Amino acid   Keto acid Ammonia

The two fractions resulting from the deamination of the amino acids are disposed of in the following ways.

Keto acids. The keto acids enter the common pathway for energy metabolism at various points of the cycle depending upon the amino acids from which they were derived. There they may be completely oxidized to yield energy, carbon dioxide, and water. The common pathway for the release of energy is described in Chapter 5 (page 71). (See also Figure 4–6.)

Instead of being used immediately for energy, keto acids may be synthesized to glycogen or fat. Some of the amino acids—accounting for about 58 per cent of the protein molecule—are said to be *glucogenic,* whereas other amino acids—slightly less than half of the protein molecule—are potentially *ketogenic.* These distinctions are not fully valid, however. For example, from Figure 4–6 it may be noted that a number of amino acids are converted to pyru-

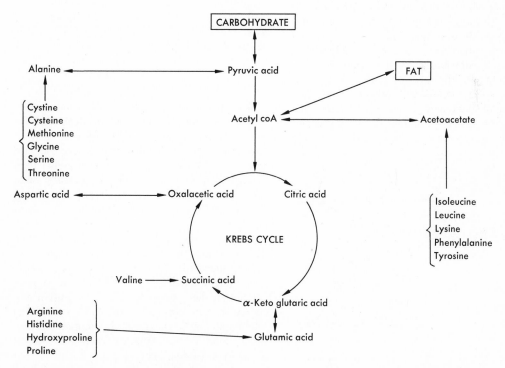

Figure 4–6. Amino acids enter the pathways common to carbohydrate and fat metabolism. Most amino acids are glucogenic; some are ketogenic; and a few may be either ketogenic or glucogenic.

vic acid, which, in turn, can form glucose or can combine with coenzyme A and proceed to form fatty acids.

Disposal of ammonia. Most of the ammonia released through deamination is synthesized to urea. A small amount of ammonia may be used in the formation of new amino acids or purines, pyrimidines, creatine, and other important nonprotein nitrogenous substances. The transfer of amino groups by transamination has been described on page 52.

The liver is the primary organ for the synthesis of urea. This is an essential mechanism for the disposal of ammonia, which is highly toxic if it enters the systemic circulation. When the function of the liver is seriously impaired, ammonia enters the circulation and produces harmful effects on the central nervous system.

The Krebs-Henseleit cycle is a mechanism that explains the formation of urea. (See Figure 4–7.) This is an energy-requiring process. The ammonia combines with carbon dioxide (available from oxidation in the Krebs cycle) and ATP to form a carbamyl phosphate. This compound combines with ornithine—an amino acid—to initiate the urea cycle. A second molecule of ammonia is contributed to the cycle from aspartic acid. In the presence of arginase, an enzyme, and magnesium, arginine yields one molecule of urea and of ornithine. Thus, one turn of the cycle has effected the release of ammonia in the form of urea and is able to recycle again.

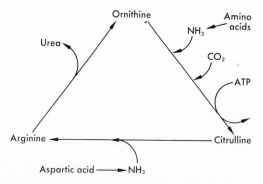

Figure 4–7. The Krebs-Henseleit cycle. A mechanism for disposing of ammonia by urea synthesis.

The excretion of urea and other nitrogenous products in the urine entails an obligatory excretion of fluid as well. In the absence of sufficient fluid the work of the kidney will be increased.

DIETARY PROTEIN ALLOWANCES

The daily protein allowances may be stated in terms of the amounts of protein or of the amounts of essential amino acids and nitrogen.

Recommended protein allowance. The protein allowance for adults recommended by the Food and Nutrition Board is 56 gm for the 70-kg man and 46 gm for the 58-kg woman.[9] On the basis of desirable body weight the allowance is 0.8 gm per kilogram, or 0.4 gm per pound. With this information the allowance for adults of any given size is easily calculated.

Research studies have shown that the average healthy adult consuming a protein-free diet that is adequate in calories loses nitrogen from his body proportional to the amount of his functioning protoplasm as expressed by his basal metabolic rate. This is about 20 mg protein per kilocalorie of basal metabolism. For a woman weighing 58 kilograms with a metabolic rate of 1400 kcal, 28 gm of ideal protein $\dfrac{(1400 \times 20)}{1000}$ would replace this loss. The protein allowance would be correspondingly increased or decreased for greater or lesser body weight. An additional allowance of about 30 per cent is necessary to take care of some persons who have higher than average requirements. Such an increase takes care of almost all of the adult population and also provides a "margin of safety" for most persons.

Dietary proteins are not all capable of producing 1 gm tissue protein for each gram of protein ingested. The protein efficiency of a diet containing animal foods is higher than a pure vegetarian diet (see page 57). The protein efficiency is also lowered if the calorie intake is inadequate or if the meal distribution of protein is poor. Typical American diets are assumed to have a protein efficiency of about 70 per cent. From these considerations it should be apparent that the recommended allowances are not *requirements* or minimum levels of intake. Therefore, diets that contain less protein than the allowances cannot be equated with protein deficiency.

Allowances for growth. The allowances for infants are based upon human milk as the source of protein. The allowance decreases from 2.2 gm per kilogram during the first six months to 2.0 gm per kilogram for the second half year. For children from 1 to 10 years the daily allowances range from 23 to 36 gm. On the basis of body weight, these are equivalent to 1.8 to 1.2 gm per kilogram, the higher level being given during the second and third years and gradually decreasing with age.

An additional 30 gm protein per day during pregnancy will take care of the growth of the fetus and of the maternal tissues. During lactation, an increase in the protein allowance of 20 gm is satisfactory for the production of an upper limit of 1200 ml milk. These allowances take into account the variability of individual needs and the efficiency of protein.

Essential amino acid requirements. Dr. Rose[10,11] has determined the quantitative requirements of the essential amino acids for healthy young men by feeding a controlled diet which included a mixture of pure amino acids flavored with lemon juice and sugar, and wafers made of cornstarch, sucrose, centrifuged butterfat, corn oil, and vitamins. Similar studies have been reported for young women and for infants.[12,13] The minimum requirements on the basis of these studies are summarized in Table 4–2; they suffice only when the diet provides enough nitrogen for the synthesis of the nonessential amino acids so that the essential amino acids will not be used for this purpose. On a weight basis, it will be noted that the infant requirements are several times as high—a fact that one would expect in view of the high rate of tissue synthesis during infancy.

Table 4–2. Minimum Essential Amino Acid Requirements Compared with Amino Acids in the United States per Capita Food Supply*

Essential Amino Acid	Minimal Requirements			U.S. per Capita Food Supply† gm
	Infants mg per kg	Men gm per day	Women gm per day	
Histidine	32			
Isoleucine	90	0.70	0.45	5.2
Leucine	120	1.10	0.62	8.0
Lysine	90	0.80	0.50	6.1
Methionine				
In absence of cystine		1.10		
In presence of 15 mg cystine per kg	85			
In presence of 50 mg cystine per kg	65			
In presence of 200 mg cystine			0.35	
In presence of 810 mg cystine		0.20		
Phenylalanine				4.6
In absence of tyrosine		1.10		
In presence of 175 mg tyrosine per kg	90			
In presence of 1100 mg tyrosine		0.30		
In presence of 900 mg tyrosine			0.22	
Threonine	60	0.50	0.30	3.9
Tryptophan	30	0.25	0.16	1.2
Valine	93	0.80	0.65	5.5

*Table arranged from data summarized by: Williams, H. H.: "Amino Acid Requirements," *J. Am. Diet. Assoc.,* **35**: 929, 1959.

†Phipard, E. F.: "Protein and Amino Acids in Diets," *Nutr. Committee News,* U.S. Department of Agriculture, Washington, D.C., May 1959.

Reference protein. The protein requirement was described a number of years ago by a nutrition committee of the Food and Agriculture Organization in terms of a reference pattern of amino acids. This pattern was based upon the kinds and amounts of amino acids required by healthy human beings to meet obligatory nitrogen losses in urine, feces, and skin. The *reference protein* was one which would produce 1 gm of tissue for each gram consumed; thus, it would have a biologic value of 100. Other individual foods or diets could thus be compared with this reference protein to measure their biologic values. After a series of investigations, it was found that the amino acid patterns in human milk and whole eggs corresponded most closely to the pattern required by humans. Therefore, in 1965 the joint FAO/WHO committee recommended that these proteins be used as a reference pattern.[14]

FOOD SOURCES

Protein content of foods and dietaries. The average protein composition of common foods is shown in Table 4–3. The protein concentration is high in dry milk, meat, fish, poultry, cheese, and nuts; intermediate in eggs, legumes, flours and cereals, and liquid milk; and low in most fruits and vegetables. One pint of liquid milk furnishes more than one fourth of the recommended daily allowance for most categories. Breads and cereals supply an appreciable amount of protein by virtue of the amounts that are consumed in a day. Legumes make a relatively small contribution in the United States because they are not eaten with frequency. In some countries of the world legumes are a major source of proteins.

In the United States the food supply available

Table 4–3. Average Protein Content of Foods in Four Food Groups*

Food	Average Serving	Protein gm	Protein Quality Limiting Amino Acids
Milk Group			
Milk, whole or skim	1 cup	9	Complete
Nonfat dry milk	7/8 ounce (3–5 tablespoons)	9	Complete
Cottage cheese	2 ounces	10	Complete
American cheese	1 ounce	7	Complete
Ice cream	1/8 quart	3	Complete
Meat Group			
Meat, fish, poultry	3 ounces, cooked	15–25	Complete; higher protein for lean cuts
Egg	1 whole	6	Complete
Dried beans or peas	1/2 cup cooked	7–8	Incomplete; methionine
Peanut butter	1 tablespoon	4	Incomplete; several amino acids borderline
Vegetable-Fruit Group			
Vegetables	1/2 cup	1–3	Incomplete
Fruits	1/2 cup	1–2	Incomplete
Bread-Cereals Group			
Breakfast cereals, wheat	1/2 cup cooked 3/4 cup dry	2–3	Incomplete; lysine
Bread, wheat	1 slice	2–3	Incomplete; lysine
Macaroni, noodles, spaghetti	1/2 cup cooked	2	Incomplete; lysine
Rice	1/2 cup cooked	2	Incomplete; lysine and threonine
Cornmeal and cereals	1/2 cup cooked	2	Incomplete, lysine and tryptophan

*These values represent approximate group averages. For specific food items, consult Table A–1, in the Appendix.

for consumption furnishes 99 gm protein per capita daily. The percentages supplied by each food group are: meat, fish, poultry, 41; eggs, 6; legumes and nuts, 5; milk and milk products, 23; fruits and vegetables, 7; and flour and cereal products, 18.[15]

The protein contribution made by the recommended number of servings from the Four Food Groups is shown in Figure 4–8. Inasmuch as some of the foods added to this basic list for calories usually would contain some protein, the daily intake would be sufficient to meet the needs of healthy people of all ages.

Supplementation of plant foods. The biologic value of a protein is a measure of the proportion of absorbed nitrogen that is retained and is directly proportional to the essential amino acid composition of foods. A general rule of thumb used in planning diets for adults in the United States is to allow at least one third of the protein from complete protein foods. For children and during repletion of proteins following illness, from one half to two thirds of the protein from complete protein sources is recommended.

The amino acid composition of foods may be calculated from values listed in Table A–5. Plant foods usually contain insufficient quantities of one or more of these four essential amino acids: lysine, threonine, tryptophan, and methionine. Also, they may contain poor balances of other amino acids so that excesses of some interfere with the utilization of those that are more limiting. In spite of these shortcomings, the chief source of protein in diets for most of the world's people is from plants. Even in the United States and other countries that have much available animal protein, plant proteins help to stretch the supply of expensive protein foods. How can this be done?

1. When an appreciable amount of plant proteins is fed with a small amount of animal proteins, the quality of the mixture is as effective as if only animal protein had been fed. For example, cereal foods are usually low in lysine, but milk supplies ample amounts of the missing lysine. Thus, macaroni and cheese, cereal and milk, or bread and milk are supplementary. Likewise, a relatively small amount of meat, egg, or cheese in a rice, noodle, or macaroni casserole is an effective combination. For the best use of the protein foods, some complete protein should be included in each of the meals of the day, rather than allotting all of it to one meal.

2. Plant foods may supplement one another since they are not all deficient in the same amino acids. For example, corn and dry beans are not satisfactory if either is the sole source of protein. When eaten together, as in countries of Central America, the biologic value of the protein is significantly improved. Hardinge and his associates[16] found that legumes, whole grains, nuts, and vegetables provided a satisfactory combination of amino acids for a group of pure vegetarians. One of the tremendously

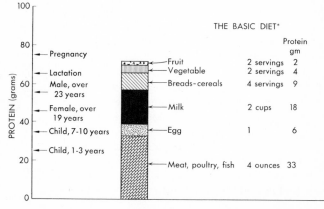

Figure 4–8. The Four Food Groups of the Basic Diet meet the recommended allowances for protein. The addition of 1 cup of milk will fulfill increased needs during pregnancy. Note the high proportion of complete protein furnished by the milk and meat groups. See Table 13–2 for complete calculation.

important areas of nutrition research today is directed toward the development of mixtures of plant proteins whereby the limiting amino acid of one food is provided by another. *Incaparina* was the first such mixture to be used successfully in infant and child feeding.[17] Many other such mixtures have been developed and are being tested throughout the developing countries of the world. (See also Chapter 26.)

3. Some essential amino acids—lysine and methionine—can now be produced at costs sufficiently low that it is economical to add them to foods in which they are deficient. Such additions must be made with caution since the possibility exists that an imbalance of amino acids could be created in low-protein diets, thereby depressing growth.[18] Wheat fortified with lysine is now being tested in selected areas of India.

PROTEIN DEFICIENCY

Because the protein intake in the United States is high, and because the quality is exceptionally good, one would not expect to see many individuals exhibiting the clinical symptoms of severe deficiency. A reduced protein intake over an extended period of time leads eventually to depletion of the tissue reserves and then to the lowering of blood protein levels. The speed with which the deficiency develops depends upon the quality and quantity of the protein intake, the caloric intake, the age of the individual and other factors. According to Youmans,[19] edema (known as "nutritional edema" as distinct from edema of circulatory origin) is the first clinical sign; this is dependent upon posture and becomes more marked in the legs at the end of the day. As the condition becomes more severe, edema becomes more generalized.

Protein deficiency is sometimes seen among pregnant women from low-economic groups ignorant of the essentials of a good diet. Miscarriage, premature birth, and anemia are frequent in these women. Other vulnerable groups are the elderly who have too little income to secure food, insufficient understanding of the importance of diet, lack of incentive to eat, or poor health; and the chronically ill who have

poor appetites but increased protein requirements. Although symptoms of protein deficiency may not be detectable, the stress of an infection or surgery on such an individual may result in delayed convalescence or poor wound healing.

Protein-calorie malnutrition. *Kwashiorkor* occurs in children shortly after weaning, usually between ages one and four years, and is characterized by growth failure, edema, skin lesions, and changes in hair color. The liver is extensively infiltrated with fat. The principal dietary defect is a lack of protein in the foods available to the child when he is weaned. (See Figure 4–9.)

Marasmus is usually seen at a somewhat earlier age than kwashiorkor and is caused by a deficiency of both protein and calories. Growth failure is even more severe than in kwashiorkor, but edema is usually absent.

One of the most serious problems associated with protein-calorie malnutrition is the possi-

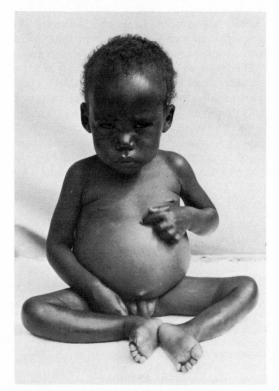

Figure 4–9. Child suffering from kwashiorkor—Africa. (Courtesy, M. Autret and the Food and Agriculture Organization.)

bility that mental development may be permanently impaired. The protein deficiencies constitute the major nutritional problem in the world today and will be discussed more extensively in Chapter 25.

SOME POINTS FOR EMPHASIS IN NUTRITION EDUCATION

1. Proteins are made up of building units called amino acids. They are required by people of all ages to replace tissues that are constantly being broken down. Children and pregnant and lactating women need additional protein for synthesis of new proteins.

2. Proteins, like carbohydrates and fats, contribute calories to the diet. If too few calories are included in the diet, protein will be used for energy. Then it cannot also be used for building tissues.

3. Muscular work does not increase the requirement for protein.

4. Some amino acids, called essential, must be supplied in the diet because the body cannot make them.

5. Animal protein foods, except gelatin, are complete because they contain balanced proportions of the essential amino acids. Include some good-quality protein at each meal.

6. About one sixth of the day's allowance for protein for the adult will be supplied by 1 ounce meat, fish, or poultry, or 1 cup milk, or 1 egg, or 1 ounce cheese.

7. Proteins from plant foods are incomplete but they are useful in reducing the amount of expensive animal proteins that are needed. Breads, cereals, dry beans and peas, and peanut butter when combined with small amounts of eggs, cheese, meat, fish, and poultry give just as good an assortment of amino acids as a large amount of animal foods.

8. Incomplete protein foods should be combined in the same meal with complete protein foods. The protein should be distributed in each of the meals of the day, rather than largely at one meal.

PROBLEMS AND REVIEW

1. Describe the synthesis of tissue proteins. Under what circumstances would synthesis be accelerated?
2. Name four ways in which proteins are used in the regulation of body functions.
3. Explain why proteins are considered to be a wasteful source of energy.
4. *Problem.* Prepare an outline or diagram which shows the steps in the digestion of protein.
5. What is meant by an essential amino acid; complete protein; high biologic value; supplementary value of protein?
6. What is meant by positive nitrogen balance; negative nitrogen balance; nitrogen equilibrium? When does each condition occur?
7. How can you explain the fact that a person on a low-protein, high-calorie diet is less likely to go into negative nitrogen balance than one who is on a low-calorie diet of the same protein level?
8. How can you explain the fact that some vegetarians maintain good protein nutrition while others do not?
9. *Problem.* Plan a diet for a woman which provides **46** gm of protein, of which not more than one third is in the form of animal protein. What foods are especially important in such a diet plan?
10. What happens to protein which is eaten in excess of body requirements? Why is it important to provide a margin of safety in planning for the daily protein allowance?
11. What foods would you include in your own diet to ensure an adequate protein intake? How would you modify this plan for a growing child?

12. *Problem.* A diet contains 3000 calories and 150 gm of protein. What percentage of the calories is supplied by protein?

13. *Problem.* One pint of milk supplies 18 gm of protein. What amounts of these foods would be required to replace the protein of the milk: buttermilk; nonfat dry milk; evaporated milk; ice cream; Cheddar cheese; eggs; halibut; beef liver; sirloin steak; peanut butter; oatmeal? How does the quality of protein in the various foods listed above compare?

14. *Problem.* On the basis of current market prices, calculate the cost for the amounts of foods which were needed to replace the protein of 1 pint milk (problem 13). What conclusions can you draw from this calculation?

15. A friend asks you whether she should buy lysine-enriched bread in preference to the usual enriched loaf of bread. How would you reply?

16. What are the effects of insufficient protein in the diet?

CITED REFERENCES

1. Vickery, H. B.: "The Origin of the Word Protein," *Yale J. Biol. Med.*, **22**:387–93, 1950.
2. Rose, W. C., *et al.*: "Further Experiments on the Role of Amino Acids in Human Nutrition," *J. Biol. Chem.*, **148**:457–58, 1943.
3. Nasset, E. S.: "Role of the Digestive Tract in the Utilization of Protein and Amino Acids," *J.A.M.A.*, **164**:172–77, 1957.
4. Albanese, A. A., and Orto, L. A.: "The Proteins and Amino acids," in Wohl, M. G., and Goodhart, R. S.: *Modern Nutrition in Health and Disease*, 4th ed. Lea & Febiger, Philadelphia, 1968, p. 99.
5. Adibi, S. A., and Gray, S. J.: "Intestinal Absorption of Essential Amino Acids in Man," *Gastroenterology*, **52**:837–45, 1967.
6. Consolazio, C. F.: "Comparisons of Nitrogen, Calcium, and Iodine Excretion in Arm and Total Body Sweat," *Am. J. Clin. Nutr.*, **18**:443–48, 1966.
7. Allison, J. B., and Wannamacher, R. N., Jr.: "The Concept and Significance of Labile and Over-All Protein Reserves of the Body," *Am. J. Clin. Nutr.*, **16**:445–52, 1965.
8. Sprinson, D. B., and Rittenberg, D.: "The Rate of Interaction of the Amino Acids of the Diet with Tissue Proteins," *J. Biol. Chem.*, **180**:715–26, 1949.
9. Food and Nutrition Board: *Recommended Dietary Allowances*, 8th ed. National Academy of Sciences–National Research Council, Washington, D.C., 1973.
10. Staff Report: "Rose Reports Human Amino Acid Requirements," *Chem. Eng. News*, **27**:1364, 1949.
11. Rose, W. C., *et al.*: "The Amino Acid Requirements of Man. XV. The Valine Requirements: Summary and Final Observations," *J. Biol. Chem.*, **217**:987–95, 1955.
12. Leverton, R. M., *et al.*: "The Quantitative Amino Acid Requirements of Young Women," *J. Nutr.*, **58**:59, 83, 219, 341, 355, 1956.
13. Holt, L. E., and Snyderman, S. E.: "The Amino Acid Requirements of Children," in Cole, W. H., ed.: *Some Aspects of Amino Acid Supplementation*. Rutgers University Press, New Brunswick, N.J., 1956, pp. 60–68.
14. FAO/WHO Expert Group: *Protein Requirements*. Tech. Rep. 301, World Health Organization, Geneva, 1965.
15. "Nutritional Review," *National Food Situation*. U.S. Department of Agriculture, Washington, D.C., Nov. 1969, pp. 28–30.
16. Hardinge, M. G., *et al.*: "Nutritional Studies of Vegetarians. V. Proteins and Essential Amino Acids," *J. Am. Diet. Assoc.*, **48**:25–28, 1966.
17. Scrimshaw, N. S.: "Progress in Solving World Nutrition Problems," *J. Am. Diet. Assoc.*, **35**:441–48, 1959.
18. Elvehjem, C. A.: "Amino Acid Balance in Nutrition," *J. Am. Diet. Assoc.*, **32**:305–308, 1956.
19. Youmans, J. B.: "The Clinical Detection of Protein Deficiency," *J.A.M.A.*, **128**:439–41, 1945.

ADDITIONAL REFERENCES

Apgar, B. J.: "Mountain Climbing in a Laboratory," in *Science for Better Living—Yearbook of Agriculture 1968*. U.S. Department of Agriculture, Washington, D.C., pp. 307–10.

Ashworth, A., and Harrower, A. D. B.: "Protein Requirements in Tropical Countries: Nitrogen Losses in Sweat and Their Relation to Nitrogen Balance," *Br. J. Nutr.*, 21:833–43, 1967.

Asimov, I.: *The New Intelligent Man's Guide to Science*. Basic Books, Inc., New York, 1965, pp. 487–530; 561–76.

Brown, W.: "Present Knowledge of Protein Nutrition," *Postgrad. Med.*, 41:A109–16, Feb. 1967; A107–12, March 1967; A119–26, April 1967.

Christensen, H. N.: "Amino Acid Transport and Nutrition," *Fed. Proc.*, 22:1110–14, 1963.

Hegsted, D. M.: "Minimum Protein Requirements of Adults," *Am. J. Clin. Nutr.*, 21:352–57, 1968.

Kies, C., *et al.*: "Determination of First Limiting Nitrogenous Factor in Corn Protein for Nitrogen Retention in Human Adults," *J. Nutr.*, 86:350–56, 1965.

————: "Effect of 'Non-specific' Nitrogen Intake on Adequacy of Cereal Proteins for Nitrogen Retention in Human Adults," *J. Nutr.*, 86:357–61, 1965.

Lewis. H. B.: "Fifty Years of Study of the Role of Protein in Nutrition," *J. Am. Diet. Assoc.*, 28:701–706, 1952.

Mitchell, H. S.: "Protein Limitation and Human Growth," *J. Am. Diet. Assoc.*, 44:165–72, 1964.

Review: "Factors Causing Changes in Plasma Amino Acid Patterns," *Nutr. Rev.*, 27:241–44, 1969.

————: "The Influence of Amino Acid Deficiencies on Hepatic Protein Synthesis," *Nutr. Rev.*, 27:233–35, 1969.

————: "Tissue Protein Turnover Rates," *Nutr. Rev.*, 27:181–82, 1969.

Scrimshaw, N. S.: "Nature of Protein Requirements. Way They Can Be Met in Tomorrow's World," *J. Am. Diet. Assoc.*, 54:94–102, 1969.

5 Carbohydrates

Photosynthesis. Carbohydrates are the most abundant organic compounds in the universe. They include the structural parts of plants in the form of cellulose as well as stores of starches and sugars. The sun is the ultimate source of energy for living organisms. By an exceedingly complex process known as photosynthesis the energy of the sun is utilized by chlorophyll, the green coloring matter in leaves, to synthesize carbohydrate from carbon dioxide of the air and water of the soil. This is probably the most important reaction

$$6\ CO_2 + 6\ H_2O + \text{light energy} \rightarrow C_6H_{12}O_6 + 6\ O_2$$
$$\text{chemical}$$
$$\text{energy}$$

for the continuance of life inasmuch as the energy stored in the leaves, stems, roots, and seeds is used in turn by animal species.

Dietary significance. Starches and sugars account for about half of the caloric intake in the United States and up to four fifths of the calories in most Oriental diets. Try to imagine meals that exclude all foods containing starches and sugars such as breads, cakes, cookies, pastries, and puddings; breakfast cereals, macaroni, rice, spaghetti, noodles; fruits and vegetables; jellies, jams, candies, and sweetened beverages. As you think of such a limitation you soon realize how important carbohydrate-rich foods are for the energy, satiety, variety, and palatability they afford the diet.

A liberal use of carbohydrate has a number of distinct advantages. The yield of energy per acre of land is far greater from plant foods than from animal foods because the animal must first convert the energy of the plants it consumes into protein and fat. Cereal grains, legumes, and roots are somewhat less subject to deterioration than are animal foods. For these reasons, carbohydrate-rich foods are less expensive. Generally, as the income decreases, the consumption of carbohydrate foods increases, and that of protein-rich foods decreases. Carbohydrates are sparing of the body economy, for they are easily digested, and also help to conserve tissue proteins. When the dietary selection is made from whole-grain or enriched cereals and breads, rather than refined foods, a bonus of B complex vitamins and iron is added.

Composition. Carbohydrates are simple sugars or polymers such as starch that can be hydrolyzed to simple sugars by the action of digestive enzymes or by heating with dilute acids. Like thousands of organic compounds they contain carbon, hydrogen, and oxygen. Generally, but not always, the hydrogen and oxygen are present in the proportion to form water; hence the term *carbohydrate*. However, many compounds such as acetic acid ($C_2H_4O_2$) and lactic acid ($C_3H_6O_3$) that are not carbohydrate also contain hydrogen and oxygen in the same proportions as water.

CLASSIFICATION, DISTRIBUTION, AND CHARACTERISTICS

Carbohydrates are classified as monosaccharides, or simple sugars, disaccharides, or double sugars, and polysaccharides, which include many molecules of simple sugars.

Monosaccharides. These are compounds that cannot be hydrolyzed to simpler compounds. Although naturally occurring simple sugars may contain 3 to 7 carbon atoms, only the hexoses (6-carbon atoms) are of dietary importance. Pentoses (5-carbon atoms) and a number of derivatives of monosaccharides are of physiologic importance, but they need not be present in the diet.

Glucose, galactose, fructose, and mannose have the same empiric formula, $C_6H_{12}O_6$. They differ in the arrangement of the groupings about the carbon atoms (see Figure 5–1) and are distinctive in their physical properties, such as solubility and sweetness. Glucose, galactose, and mannose possess an aldehyde grouping (CHO) and are known as aldohexoses. Fructose possesses a ketone grouping (CO) and is known as a ketohexose.

Glucose, galactose, and mannose rotate the plane of polarized light to the right (dextrorotatory), whereas fructose rotates the plane to the left (levorotatory). These natural sugars are designated as D-sugars, not because of their plane of rotation, but because the asymmetric carbon atom next to the primary alcohol group has the same orientation as in the triose D-glycerose ($CHO \cdot CHOH \cdot CH_2OH$).

Glucose, also known as dextrose, grape sugar, or corn sugar, is somewhat less sweet than cane sugar and is soluble in hot or cold water. It is found in sweet fruits such as grapes, berries, and oranges and in some vegetables such as sweet corn and carrots. It is prepared commercially as corn syrup or in its crystalline form by the hydrolysis of starch with acids. Glucose is the chief end product of the digestion of the di- and polysaccharides, is the form of carbohydrate circulating in the blood, and is the carbohydrate utilized by the cell for energy.

Fructose (levulose or fruit sugar) is a highly soluble sugar that does not readily crystallize. It is much sweeter than cane sugar and is found in honey, ripe fruits, and some vegetables. It is also a product of the hydrolysis of sucrose.

Galactose is not found free in nature, its only source being from the hydrolysis of lactose. *Mannose* is of limited distribution in foods and of little consequence in nutrition.

Ribose, xylose, and *arabinose* are three pentoses that do not occur free in nature but are constituents of pentosans in fruits and the nucleic acids of meats. Ribose is of great physiologic importance as a constituent of riboflavin, a B complex vitamin, and of ribonucleic acid (RNA) and deoxyribonucleic acid (DNA). It is rapidly synthesized by the body and is not a dietary essential.

Disaccharides. Disaccharides, or double sugars, result when two hexoses are combined with the loss of one molecule of water, the empiric formula being $C_{12}H_{22}O_{11}$. They are water soluble, diffusible, and crystallizable and vary widely in their sweetness. They are split to simple sugars by acid hydrolysis or by digestive enzymes.

Sucrose is the table sugar with which we are familiar and is found in cane or beet sugar, brown sugar, sorghum, molasses, and maple sugar. Many fruits and some vegetables contain small amounts of sucrose.

Lactose, or milk sugar, is produced by mammals and is the only carbohydrate of animal origin of significance in the diet. It is about one

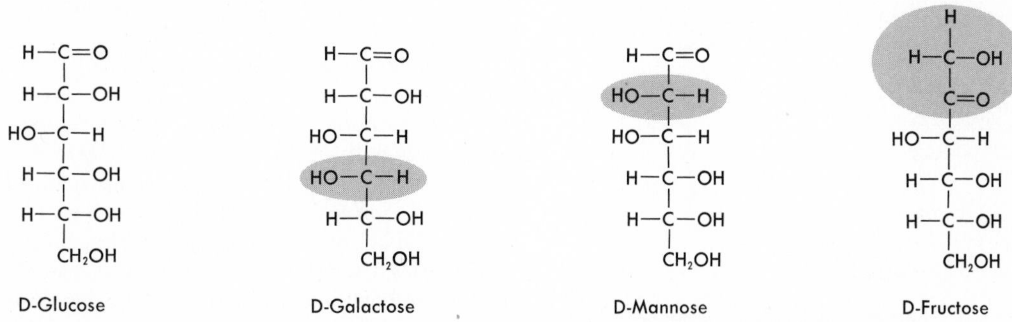

Figure 5–1. These hexoses differ in the arrangement of the groupings about the carbon atoms. The encircled grouping shows how the sugar differs from glucose in its structure. Fructose is a ketose; the others are aldoses.

sixth as sweet as sucrose and dissolves poorly in cold water. The concentration of lactose in milk varies from 2 to 8 per cent, depending upon the species of animal.

Maltose, or malt sugar, does not occur to any appreciable extent in foods. It is an intermediate product in the hydrolysis of starch. Maltose is produced in the malting and fermentation of grains and is present in beer and malted breakfast cereals. It is also used with dextrins as the source of carbohydrate for some infant formulas.

Polysaccharides. Polysaccharides $(C_6H_{10}O_5)_n$, are complex compounds with a relatively high molecular weight. They are amorphous rather than crystalline, are not sweet, are insoluble in water, and are digested with varying degrees of completeness. Starches, dextrins, glycogen, and several indigestible carbohydrates are of nutritional interest.

Starch is the storage form of carbohydrate in the plant and a valuable contributor to the energy content of the diet. It consists of numerous glucose units linked in two types of chains: (1) amylose, comprised of long, straight chains of glucose, and (2) amylopectin, consisting of shorter, branched chains of glucose. (See Figure 5–2.) The starch granules are encased in a cellulose-type wall and are distinctive in size and shape for each source. When starch is cooked in moist heat, the granules absorb water and swell, and the walls of the cell are ruptured, thus permitting more ready access to the digestive enzymes. Amylopectin has colloidal properties so that thickening of a starch-water mixture occurs when heat is applied.

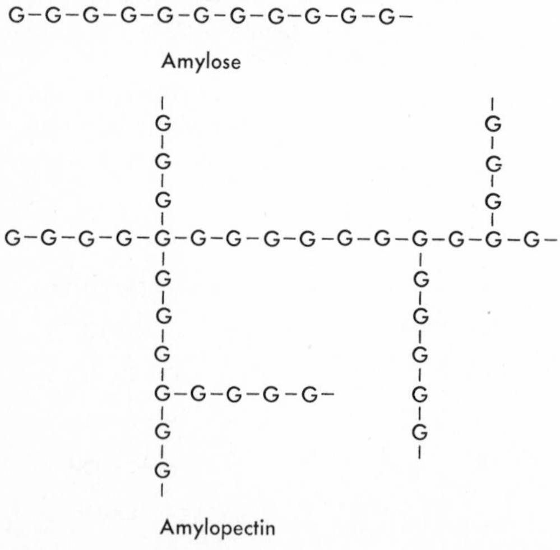

Dextrins are intermediate products in the hydrolysis of starch and consist of shorter chains of glucose units. Some dextrins are produced when flour is browned or bread is toasted.

Glycogen, the so-called "animal starch," is similar in structure to the amylopectin of starch, but contains many more branched chains of glucose. It is rapidly synthesized from glucose in the liver and muscle.

Indigestible polysaccharides. Cellulose is the most abundant organic compound in the world, comprising at least 50 per cent of the carbon in vegetation. Wood and cotton are chiefly cellulose, but the skins of fruits, the coverings of seeds, and the structural parts of edible plants are the only forms of cellulose and hemicellulose with which we are concerned in the study of nutrition. Ruminants are able to utilize cellulose for energy because of the presence of specific enzymes in the rumen, but for man cellulose is an indigestible dietary constituent.

Several indigestible polysaccharides have useful properties in food processing. *Pectins,* found in ripe fruits, have the ability to absorb water and to form gels, a property utilized in making fruit jellies. *Agar* is obtained from seaweed and is useful for its gelling properties. *Carrageen* (Irish moss) and *alginates* from seaweed are often used to enhance the smoothness of foods such as ice cream and evaporated milk.

Carbohydrate derivatives. Sugars react chemically to form sugar alcohols, amino sugars, glycosides, uronic acids, and many complex compounds with lipids and proteins. *Glycerol* is the 3-carbon alcohol that is a component of glycerides. *Sorbitol,* a sugar alcohol, is sweet, is water soluble, and is found in cherries, plums, and berries. About 70 per cent of it can be metabolized without appearing in the blood as glucose, and it has occasionally been suggested as a substitute for sugar in diabetic diets.

G–G–G–G–G–G–G–G–G–G–G–

Amylose

Figure 5–2. The starch molecule is composed of (1) amylose, with straight chains of glucose units, and (2) amylopectin, with branched chains of glucose units.

Ascorbic acid, one of the water-soluble vita-mins, is a hexose derivative that can be syn-thesized by plants and by some animals but not by the human being. Numerous carbohydrate derivatives are constituents of connective, ner-vous, and other tissues and are involved in many metabolic functions. (See below.)

FUNCTIONS

Almost all of the dietary carbohydrate is even-tually utilized to meet the energy needs of the body. A very small fraction of the available car-bohydrate is used for the synthesis of a num-ber of regulatory compounds.

Energy. Each gram of carbohydrate when oxidized yields, on the average, 4 calories. Some carbohydrate in the form of glucose will be used directly to meet immediate tissue energy needs, a small amount will be stored as glycogen in the liver and muscles, and some will be stored as adipose tissue for later conversion to energy. Glucose is the sole form of energy for the brain and nervous tissue and must be available mo-ment by moment for the functioning of these tissues. Any failure to supply glucose, or the oxygen for its oxidation, is rapidly damaging to the brain.

Glycogen is the storage form of carbohydrate in the body. At any given time about 100 gm glycogen can be stored in the liver and is avail-able to replenish the glucose level of the blood. Cardiac, smooth, and skeletal muscles contain about 200 to 250 gm glycogen that is instantly available within the muscle but is not available for regulation of the blood sugar level. Together, muscle and liver glycogen if completely used could meet no more than half the day's energy need.

Protein-sparing action. The body will use carbohydrate preferentially as a source of energy when it is adequately supplied in the diet, thus sparing protein for tissue building. Since meet-ing energy needs of the body takes priority over other functions, any deficiency of calories in the diet will be made up by using adipose and pro-tein tissues.

Regulation of fat metabolism. Some carbohy-drate is necessary in the diet so that the oxida-tion of fats can proceed normally. When carbo-hydrate is severely restricted in the diet, fats will be metabolized faster than the body can take care of the intermediate products. The ac-cumulation of these incompletely oxidized prod-ucts leads to ketosis. Carbohydrate must be al-most completely lacking in the diet for acidosis to occur under normal conditions, but it is common in uncontrolled diabetes mellitus. See page 86.

Role in gastrointestinal function. Several reg-ulatory functions have been attributed to lactose. One of these is the promotion of the growth of desirable bacteria in the small intestine. Some of these bacteria are useful in the synthesis of cer-tain B complex vitamins. Lactose also enhances the absorption of calcium. It is undoubtedly no accident of nature that milk, which is the out-standing source of calcium, is also the only dietary source of lactose.

Cellulose, hemicellulose, and pectins yield no nutrients to the body. These indigestible sub-stances aid in the stimulation of the peristaltic movements of the gastrointestinal tract, and by absorbing water give bulk to the intestinal con-tents.

Carbohydrate in body compounds. Structur-ally, carbohydrate accounts for a very small part of the weight of the body. Nevertheless, mono-saccharides are vitally important constituents of numerous compounds that regulate metabolism. Among these are:

Glucuronic acid, which occurs in the liver and is also a constituent of a number of mucopolysac-charides. Glucuronic acid in the liver combines with toxic chemicals and bacterial by-products and is thus a detoxifying agent.

Hyaluronic acid, a viscous substance that forms the matrix of connective tissue.

Heparin, a mucopolysaccharide, a substance that prevents the clotting of blood.

Chondroitin sulfates found in skin, tendons, carti-lage, bone, and heart valves.

Immunopolysaccharides as part of the body's mecha-nism to resist infections.

Deoxyribonucleic acid (DNA) and ribonucleic acid (RNA), the compounds that possess and transfer the genetic characteristics of the cell.

Galactolipins as constituents of nervous tissue.

Glycosides as components of steroid and adrenal hormones.

DIGESTION AND ABSORPTION

Digestion. The purpose of carbohydrate digestion is to hydrolyze the di- and polysaccharides of the diet to their constituent simple sugars. This is accomplished by enzymes of the digestive juices (see Table 2-2, page 24) and yields these end products:

Starch →Glucose
Sucrose →Glucose + fructose
Maltose→Glucose + glucose
Lactose→Glucose + galactose

Although some hydrolysis of starch to maltose occurs in the mouth by the action of salivary amylase and continues in the stomach until the food mass is acidified, the principal site of digestion of carbohydrate is in the small intestine. Salivary amylase does not act upon raw starch but pancreatic amylase hydrolyzes both raw and cooked starch to dextrins and, in turn, to maltose. Cooked starch is more rapidly hydrolyzed because the cell walls have been ruptured and the enzymes have more ready access to the starch granules.

Disaccharidases are produced within the mucosal cell and are not secreted into the lumen of the intestine.[1] Sucrose, lactose, and maltose are hydrolyzed within the brush border of the epithelial cell.

Fiber. Cellulose and hemicellulose cannot be hydrolyzed by enzymes of the human digestive tract, therefore yield no energy, and are excreted in the feces. Tough fibers including seeds, skins, and structural parts of plant foods are broken into smaller particles, whereas the more tender fibers of young plants may be partially disintegrated by bacterial action within the large intestine. The cooking of foods also softens fibers and partially disintegrates them.

Available carbohydrate. The total carbohydrate values reported in tables of food composition include not only the fully digestible starches and sugars but also nondigestible components such as cellulose, hemicellulose, and pectins. Thus, the amount of carbohydrate actually available to the body is the difference between the total carbohydrate and the amount of fiber that is present. The carbohydrate of refined flours and cereals, sugars, and sweets is completely, or almost completely, digested, whereas that from fibrous vegetables, fruits with seeds, and whole-grain cereals and flours is somewhat less completely digested.

Absorption. Glucose, fructose, and galactose are absorbed into the portal circulation and are carried to the liver. Glucose and galactose can be absorbed by passive diffusion with a carrier as an intermediary as long as the concentration at the luminal surface is greater than that in the circulation. When the concentration in the circulation exceeds that at the luminal surfaces, active transport is required. This is effected by the sodium pump and a mobile carrier system.[1] In other words, the energy that is required to pump sodium out of the cell also serves to transport glucose and galactose. The energy to operate the sodium pump is provided by glucose within the epithelial cell. Active transport undoubtedly accounts for the principal means whereby glucose and galactose are absorbed. Fructose apparently is absorbed only by passive diffusion.

Most absorption occurs from the jejunum. When the concentration of sugar in the intestine is great, the need for carriers to ferry sugars across the epithelial cells may exceed the numbers present; hence, some sugars will move along the tract to carrier sites in the ileum.

The rate of absorption is about equal for galactose and glucose, whereas fructose is absorbed about half as rapidly. Mannose and xylose are poorly absorbed, indicating a high level of selectivity at the absorption sites.

About 97 to 98 per cent of the carbohydrate in diversified American diets is digested and absorbed. The fuel factor of 4 calories per gram is based upon this level of absorption. In countries where plant foods comprise most of the diet so that the unavailable carbohydrate is correspondingly higher, the percentage of carbohydrate absorbed is lower, and the energy value per gram of dietary carbohydrate is somewhat lower.

INTERMEDIARY METABOLISM

Glucose is quantitatively the most important carbohydrate available to the body whether it be by absorption from the diet or by synthesis within the body. Galactose and fructose from the diet or from endogenous sources are rapidly synthesized to glucose in the liver. Therefore, any discussion of carbohydrate metabolism is essentially that of glucose. (See Figure 5–3.)

Glucose metabolism consists of an interrelated series of biochemical reactions that are facilitated by enzymatic activity. Glucose metabolism cannot be completely separated from the metabolism of fats and proteins. On the one hand, proteins and fats are potential sources of glucose, and on the other, glucose can be converted to fatty acids, glycerol, and certain amino acids. A number of points in the sequence of glucose metabolism are also the crossroads for amino acid and fatty acid metabolism, and in some respects one nutrient can substitute for another. For example, a decrease in carbohydrate metabolism is accompanied by an increase in fatty acid

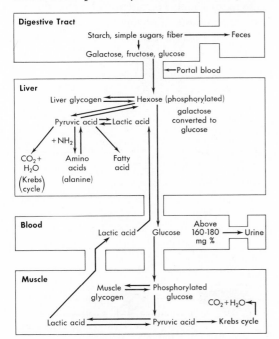

Figure 5–3. Pathways of carbohydrate metabolism.

oxidation. Moreover, trace amounts of certain mineral elements and several of the B complex vitamins are essential for enzyme activity. Thus, the metabolism of the nutrients is interdependent, and the lack of any one of them affects the total metabolism of the organism. For example, when there is a deficiency of any one of the vitamins, the result is a failure of the reaction to take place at the point where that vitamin is essential. Any reactions subsequent to this point, therefore, cannot occur.

The details of these elegant metabolic mechanisms are beyond the scope of this text, but they are well described in a number of texts on biochemistry. Nevertheless, the nurse and nutritionist frequently encounter patients with some defect in carbohydrate metabolism. The following paragraphs will furnish a general understanding of the mechanisms for the regulation of the blood glucose and a broad outline of the anaerobic and aerobic phases of glucose metabolism.

The liver in carbohydrate metabolism. Following absorption from the small intestine, the monosaccharides are carried by the portal vein to the liver. Just as the control tower in an airport regulates the flow of traffic in the air, so the liver exercises the principal control of the pathways that glucose (and other nutrients) shall take. The purposes of the transformations that take place in the liver are to regulate the level of glucose in the blood—not too much and not too little—and to synthesize certain essential compounds from glucose. The chemical changes are facilitated by enzymes that are specific for each reaction. The liver is under the influence of hormones secreted by the pancreas, adrenal, pituitary, and thyroid glands. Inasmuch as the liver is the chief organ for the regulation of glucose metabolism, it is understandable that any disturbance in liver function can have more or less profound effects on carbohydrate metabolism. The paragraphs that follow will help to explain how the liver maintains the regulation of the blood glucose.

The blood glucose. By means of the blood circulation glucose is made continuously available to each and every cell of the body as a source of energy and for the synthesis of a variety of substances. The glucose taken from the circulation by the cells is constantly replaced so that the blood glucose level is maintained within relatively narrow limits. (See Figure 5–4.)

In the fasting state the blood glucose concentration is normally 70 to 90 mg per 100 ml. Shortly after a meal it rises to about 140 to 150 mg per 100 ml, but within a few hours the concentration will have returned to the fasting level. Should the blood sugar level reach 160 to 180 mg per 100 ml some glucose will be excreted in the urine (glucosuria). This level, varying somewhat from one individual to another, is known as the *renal threshold for glucose*. The regulation of the blood sugar level by the liver is so efficient that glucosuria does not normally occur. Occasionally, an individual who has a lower renal threshold for glucose but who has no other abnormalities will excrete some glucose following meals that are especially rich in carbohydrate.

A blood sugar concentration in excess of normal levels is known as *hyperglycemia;* this is characteristic of diabetes mellitus. A glucose concentration below normal levels is known as *hypoglycemia* and may occur in certain abnormalities of liver function, or when insulin is produced in excessive amounts by the pancreas.

Sources of blood glucose. Glucose is available to the circulation (1) from absorbed sugars from the diet; (2) by breakdown of liver glycogen (glycogenolysis); (3) by conversion from glucogenic amino acids and the glycerol of fats (gluconeogenesis); and to a lesser extent (4) by the reconversion of pyruvic and lactic acids formed in the glycolytic pathway. Fatty acids and ketogenic acids do not contribute to the blood glucose nor does muscle glycogen.

Since absorbed sugars are only intermittently available, the liver maintains a constant supply of sugar to the blood by the release of glucose from glycogen. If the glycogen reserves are depleted, protein and fat from body reserves or from dietary sources are used to replenish the glucose of the blood. Amino acids must be deaminized before the remainder of the molecule can enter the pathway of carbohydrate metabolism. Approximately half the amino acids are glucogenic. Only the glycerol fraction of fats, representing about 10 per cent of the total molecule, can be converted to glucose.

Hormones. Several mechanisms under the influence of hormones increase the supply of glucose to the blood. *Thyroid hormone* increases the rate of absorption from the gastrointestinal tract. *Glucagon,* a hormone secreted by the cells of the

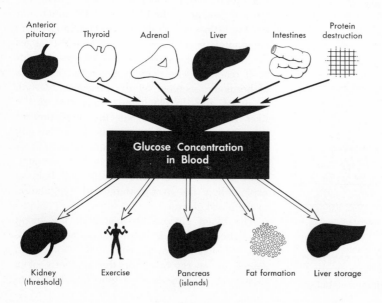

Figure 5–4. Factors influencing the level of blood sugar. (Courtesy, the Lilly Research Laboratories, Indianapolis.)

pancreas, is believed to activate phosphorylase, thus initiating glycogenolysis. *Epinephrine*, produced by the adrenal gland under conditions of stress, increases the rate of glycogen breakdown. *Steroid hormones* accelerate the catabolism of proteins, thus bringing about gluconeogenesis. *Adrenocorticotropic hormone* is antagonistic to the action of insulin and thus prevents the blood sugar level from dropping.

Removal of glucose from the blood. Six pathways are available for the removal of glucose from the blood: (1) the continuous uptake of glucose by every cell in the body and its oxidation for energy; (2) the conversion of glucose to glycogen by the liver (glycogenesis); (3) the synthesis of fats from glucose (lipogenesis); (4) the synthesis of numerous carbohydrate derivatives (see page 65); (5) glycolysis in the red blood cells; and (6) elimination of glucose in the urine when the renal threshold is exceeded.[2]

The amount of glycogen that can be formed is limited, but there is no limit to the amount of fat that is formed. Glycogen reserves are maintained at their maximum level by diets high in carbohydrate. A diet high in protein and relatively low in carbohydrate will result in moderate glycogen reserves, but a diet high in fat and low in carbohydrate and protein will result in poor glycogen reserves.

Insulin. Only one hormone is known to lower the blood sugar. An increase in the concentration of blood glucose stimulates the release of insulin, the hormone produced by the beta cells of the islands of Langerhans. Insulin lowers the blood glucose by several actions: (1) facilitating the synthesis of glycogen in the liver; (2) the active transport of glucose across cell membranes; and (3) the conversion of glucose to fatty acids.

Oxidation of glucose. Glucose is not oxidized in a single explosive reaction to yield energy and the end products, carbon dioxide and water. Rather, numerous intermediate steps, catalyzed by a specific enzyme at each stage, permit the gradual release of energy. (See Figure 5–5.) The catabolism of glucose includes *glycolysis*, an anaerobic phase that terminates with pyruvic acid and lactic acid, and the *citric acid cycle*, an aerobic phase in which carbon dioxide and water are released. A number of the intermediate

products formed in these pathways are the crossroads for carbohydrate, fat, and protein metabolism.

High-energy phosphate compounds. Certain phosphate compounds trap large amounts of energy and are known as high-energy phosphate compounds. Adenosine triphosphate (ATP) is one such compound. It contains three phosphate groupings, two of which are held to the rest of the molecule by high-energy bonds. On demand ATP gives up one of its phosphate groupings to yield a burst of energy for the work of the cell. The energy required to reconvert ADP to ATP is supplied by the metabolism of glucose. In the glycolytic pathway the yield of energy is low, whereas in the citric acid cycle it is about 15 times as great.

Glycolysis. The chemical reactions that constitute glycolysis, also known as the Embden-Meyerhof pathway, are catalyzed by a specific enzyme in each case, some of which require the presence of inorganic phosphate, inorganic ions, NAD (nicotineamide adenine dinucleotide), and NADP (nicotineamide adenine dinucleotide phosphate). The reactions do not require oxygen. Almost all of the glucose catabolized in the body undergoes breakdown through these steps.

Phosphorylation. The entrance of glucose into the cell is facilitated by insulin. Within the cell the first step in glycolysis is the combination of glucose with ATP in the presence of glucokinase and magnesium to form glucose-6-phosphate and ADP. The phosphorylated glucose then proceeds through the glycolytic pathway to pyruvic and lactic acids. Glucose-6-phosphate also leads to the synthesis of glycogen and may, to a lesser extent, proceed through an alternate oxidative pathway known as the *pentose shunt*.

Conversion to trioses. The hexose molecule is split to trioses, which undergo a series of changes until pyruvic acid ($CH_3COCOOH$) is formed. One of the trioses—dihydroxyacetone phosphate —instead of proceeding to pyruvic acid may be sidetracked to form α-glycerophosphate, which furnishes the glycerol molecule for the synthesis of neutral fats. (See page 85.)

Lactic acid. Pyruvic acid can proceed anaerobically to form lactic acid, which is utilized for

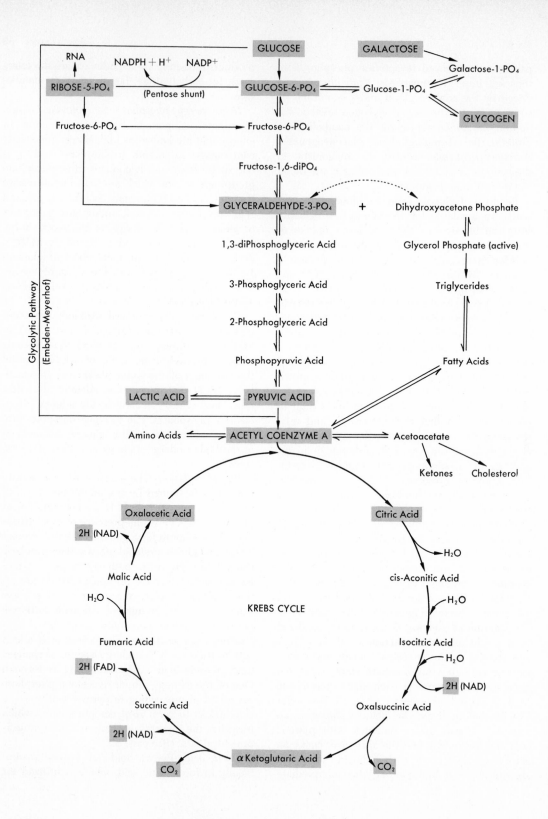

muscle contraction under conditions when the energy need exceeds the supply of oxygen. Under normal conditions only a small amount of lactic acid is formed. About one fifth of the lactic acid produced in the muscle is further oxidized through the citric acid cycle; the rest is resynthesized in the muscle to glycogen or reenters the blood circulation and is synthesized by the liver to glycogen.

The pentose shunt. An aerobic bypass for glycolysis may be utilized especially by the liver and adipose tissue. This is also known as the *hexose monophosphate shunt* or the *oxidative shunt.* Through the reactions occurring in this pathway ribose, which is a constituent of RNA, is synthesized. Also NADPH is produced, which is essential for the synthesis of fatty acids and for the utilization of lactic acid in muscular work.

Aerobic metabolism. Most of the pyruvic acid formed in the glycolytic pathway is decarboxylated to a 2-carbon fragment (acetate). For the complex reactions involved in decarboxylation and the formation of active acetate these are required: NAD, thiamine pyrophosphate, lipoic acid, magnesium, and coenzyme A.

Coenzyme A is a complex molecule of which pantothenic acid, a B complex vitamin is a constituent. Acetyl coenzyme A is derived not only from pyruvic acid but also from the oxidation of fatty acids (see page 85) and from certain amino acids (see page 53). Acetyl coenzyme A is something like the hub of a wheel in that it can proceed in a number of directions—through the citric acid cycle to yield energy or to form a number of new compounds. (See Figure 5–5.)

Citric acid cycle. This is also known as the *tricarboxylic acid* cycle or the Krebs cycle for the man who first formulated the sequence. Through this cycle about 90 per cent of the energy of the body is produced.

The citric acid cycle is initiated by the condensation of oxalacetic acid with acetyl coenzyme A to form citric acid. In one turn of the cycle the 2 carbon atoms from acetyl coenzyme A are oxidized to carbon dioxide and water. The overall reaction is:

$$CH_3COOH + 2\ O_2 \rightarrow 2\ CO_2 + 2\ H_2O$$

One molecule of carbon dioxide is released in the formation of α-ketoglutaric acid and 1 in the formation of succinyl coenzyme A.

The oxidizing agents in this cycle are coenzymes: NAD and FAD (flavin adenine dinucleotide) can exist in the oxidized or reduced form. The oxidized form of these coenzymes oxidizes the reactants in the cycle in steps as indicated. The coenzymes are reduced to $NADPH_2$ and $FADH_2$ and subsequently are reoxidized in reactions in which inorganic phosphorus takes part (oxidative phosphorylation). In this process two molecules of ATP are formed for every molecule of $FADH_2$ oxidized. Thus the coenzymes are regenerated and a small amount can oxidize a large quantity of citric acid cycle acids. For every molecule of acetyl coenzyme A that is oxidized in the cycle 12 ATP molecules are produced.

CARBOHYDRATE IN THE DIET

Dietary allowances. The low-carbohydrate diet of the Eskimos and the high-carbohydrate diets of many Oriental peoples indicate that man can be healthy with wide variations in carbohydrate intake. This wide variation is compatible with health because carbohydrates, fats, and proteins are interchangeable in meeting the energy needs of the body.

Although the minimum requirement for carbohydrate is not known, the Food and Nutrition Board[3] suggests that individuals on a normal diet should include at least 100 gm carbohydrate

Figure 5–5. Glucose is oxidized anaerobically to pyruvic and lactic acids—the Embden-Meyerhof pathway. Glucose may also be oxidized through the pentose shunt. Pyruvic acid is decarboxylated to form acetate. Active acetate condenses with oxalacetic acid, and each turn of the Krebs cycle releases 2 molecules of CO_2 and 8 hydrogen ions and uses up 2 molecules of water.

daily to maintain metabolic processes. Most Americans consume diets that range between 200 and 300 gm carbohydrate.

The exact amount of fiber essential for normal laxation is not known. Cowgill[4] recommended 100 mg fiber per kilogram, or about 5 to 6 gm per day for the adult. As with digestible carbohydrates, individuals apparently can adjust to widely varying levels of fiber in the diet. A recent study[5] showed that vegetarians who had four times as much fiber in the diet as non-vegetarians did not experience any adverse effects on the digestive tract.

Dietary sources. Flour and cereal products furnish about 36 per cent and sugars and sweets about 37 per cent of the carbohydrate in the food supply in the United States. The remainder of the carbohydrate is provided by fruits, vegetables, and dairy products.

The carbohydrate composition of typical foods is shown in Table 5–1. Pure sugars are 100 per cent carbohydrate, and syrups, jellies, and jams contain 65 to 80 per cent. Cereal foods, flours, and crackers contain 65 to 85 per cent carbohydrate on a dry weight basis, chiefly in the form of starch.

Table 5–1. Carbohydrate Content of Some Typical Foods

Food	Per 100 gm of Food gm	Per Serving Portion		
		Measure	Weight gm	Carbo-hydrate gm
*Complex Carbohydrates**				
Bread, all kinds	50–56	1 slice	25	13
Cereals, breakfast, dry	68–84	1 cup wheat flakes	30	24
Crackers, all kinds	67–73	4 saltines	11	8
Flour, all kinds	71–80	2 tablespoons	14	11
Legumes, dry	60–63	1/2 cup navy beans, cooked	95	20
Macaroni, spaghetti, dry	75	1/2 cup cooked	70	16
Nuts	15–20	1/4 cup peanuts	36	7
Pie crust, baked	44	1/6 shell	30	13
Potatoes, white, raw	17	1 boiled	122	18
Rice, dry	80	1/2 cup cooked	105	25
Complex and Simple Carbohydrates (1/2 and 1/2)				
Cake, plain and iced	52–68	1 piece layer, iced	75	45
Cookies	51–80	1 chocolate chip	10	6
Simple Carbohydrates				
Beverages, carbonated	8–12	8 ounces cola	246	24
Candy (without nuts)	75–95	1 ounce milk chocolate	28	16
Fruit, dried	59–69	4 prunes	32	18
Fruit, fresh	6–22	1 apple	150	18
		1 orange	180	16
Fruit, sweetened, canned or frozen	16–28	1/2 cup peaches	128	26
		3 ounces frozen strawberries	85	24
Ice cream	18–21	1/2 cup	67	14
Milk	5	1 cup	244	12
Pudding	16–26	1/2 cup vanilla	128	21
Sugar, all kinds	96–100	1 tablespoon white	11	11
Syrups, molasses, honey	65–82	1 tablespoon molasses	20	13
Vegetables	4–18	1/2 cup green beans	63	4
		1/2 cup peas	80	10

*Foods are grouped according to the predominating type of carbohydrate present.

Fruits and vegetables vary widely in their carbohydrate concentration. Those with a high water content such as spinach, cabbage, other leafy vegetables, and melons contain 6 per cent or less of carbohydrate and are correspondingly low in calories. Potatoes, sweet potatoes, Lima beans, corn, and bananas are somewhat lower in water content and furnish approximately 20 per cent carbohydrate or more. Dried beans and peas and dried fruits have a carbohydrate content in excess of 60 per cent. For convenience in dietary planning, fruits and vegetables have been grouped according to their carbohydrate content. (See Table A–4.)

The degree of ripeness determines the relative proportions of sugars and starches in fruits and vegetables. Green bananas are high in starch and low in sugar, whereas ripe bananas have little starch and consist primarily of sugars. Freshly picked and immature vegetables, on the other hand, for example, sweet corn, tender peas, and young carrots, contain more sugar and less starch than mature vegetables.

Milk is the only animal food contributing to the daily carbohydrate intake. Freshly opened oysters and scallops contain some glycogen, but the amount is of no practical significance. The glycogen in liver is rapidly converted to lactic and pyruvic acids when the animal is slaughtered.

The principal sources of fiber are raw fruits, especially those with skins and seeds, vegetables such as celery, corn, and Lima beans, and whole-grain breads and cereals.

Problems related to carbohydrate consumption. The total amount of carbohydrate available for consumption in the United States is about 100 gm less than it was 60 years ago. (See Figure 5–6.) During this period of time, the consumption of sugars and sweets has gradually increased and that of cereals, breads, and potatoes has substantially decreased.

These changes in the carbohydrate supply reflect a more generous economy, the influence of a more sedentary way of life, and the effects of technology and the marketing system. They may also have some adverse effects on the nutritional status of the individual.

Nutritional adequacy. An excessive intake of sugars, candies, pastries, cakes, and cookies may crowd out essential foods, thus resulting in nutrient deficiencies as well as problems of overweight. The establishment of food habits early in life with respect to the judicious consumption of sweets can scarcely be overemphasized. Although some sweets may be given to children, these foods should not be categorized as the "good food" (in taste) that is "bad" for one, nor should they be used as rewards or bribes to achieve a desired behavior—for example, eating the vegetable on the plate!

Some individuals consume normal amounts of carbohydrate, but their choices are restricted to the sweets and unenriched breads. Others, believing that breads and cereals contribute to overweight, omit the bread-cereal group from their diets. In either instance the intake of B complex vitamins and iron is correspondingly reduced. Four servings of enriched or whole-grain breads and cereals should be included daily before nutritionally inferior carbohydrate foods are added.

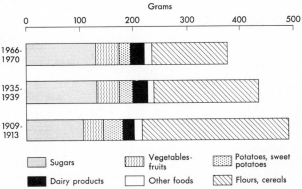

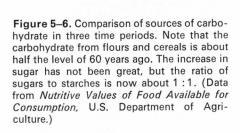

Figure 5–6. Comparison of sources of carbohydrate in three time periods. Note that the carbohydrate from flours and cereals is about half the level of 60 years ago. The increase in sugar has not been great, but the ratio of sugars to starches is now about 1 : 1. (Data from *Nutritive Values of Food Available for Consumption,* U.S. Department of Agriculture.)

Dental caries. The causes of tooth decay are many and complex. Nevertheless, if the consumption of sweets by a child leads to reduced intake of other foods, some defects in tooth structure may be expected if some of the essential nutrients are missing. Any carbohydrates in contact with the tooth surfaces for a period of time provide a favorable medium for the rapid growth of bacteria; sticky candies and other sweets may be especially harmful. Brushing the teeth after eating sweets or, at the very least, rinsing the mouth with water is helpful in removing the carbohydrate residues from the teeth.

Gastrointestinal irritation. An excessive intake of concentrated sweets sometimes leads to irritation of the gastrointestinal mucosa and may, in certain disorders, favor increased fermentation and gas production. Some individuals experience distention, flatulence, and diarrhea after drinking milk because of a deficiency of the enzyme lactase in the intestinal mucosa.

Serum lipids. The shift from the complex carbohydrates to the simpler forms may bring about an elevation in the serum triglycerides.[6-8] This increase in serum triglycerides is believed to increase the incidence of cardiovascular disease. Other research workers have pointed out that these changes are not of the same order of magnitude as those seen with alterations in the amount and nature of fat. (See also Chapter 6.)

SOME POINTS FOR EMPHASIS IN NUTRITION EDUCATION

1. Carbohydrates include sugars, starches, and fiber from plant foods. Milk, which contains lactose, or milk sugar, is the only important animal source of carbohydrate.
2. The principal function of carbohydrate is to furnish energy for the body. In the United States about half of the energy value of the diet is provided by carbohydrate.
3. Equally good nutrition can be maintained on diets that are low in carbohydrate and those that are high in carbohydrate. In certain disease conditions carbohydrates may need to be moderately or severely restricted, whereas in other conditions a high carbohydrate intake is necessary.
4. Only a small amount of carbohydrate is stored in the body in the form of glycogen. If there is an excess of carbohydrate beyond the body's immediate need, it is stored as fat.
5. Wheat, corn, rice, potatoes, sweet potatoes, sugars, and sweets are the important sources of carbohydrate and calories in the American diet because they are used so frequently and appear in so many forms.
6. Weight for weight, fresh fruits and vegetables contain much less carbohydrate than breads and cereals. The fiber of fruits and vegetables is important for helping to maintain normal elimination.
7. Enriched and whole-grain breads and cereals are best buys for low-cost diets. They contribute not only energy but substantial amounts of protein, B complex vitamins, and iron.
8. Sugars and sweets are concentrated sources of energy and are valued for the palatability they give to the diet.
9. Sugars and sweets should not be permitted to replace essential foods needed for proteins, minerals, and vitamins. Unless used with discretion they may contribute to dental caries, especially in children.
10. Dark-brown sugar and molasses contain some minerals, especially iron. The contribution made to the daily intake of minerals is, however, likely to be small.

PROBLEMS AND REVIEW

1. What are the important differences between the three classes of carbohydrates?
2. In the United States about half of the calories are furnished by carbohydrate. Under what circumstances would you expect this proportion to increase?

3. Drinking a glass of fruit juice removes feelings of hunger quickly but for a relatively short period of time. Explain this on the basis of the physiologic and biochemical reactions that have taken place.

4. Even though you eat a diet that is high in carbohydrate the blood glucose will not usually reach the renal threshold. Explain the mechanisms whereby the blood sugar is maintained within such narrow limits.

5. If an individual is not eating, what mechanisms provide for the maintenance of a normal blood sugar?

6. If carbohydrate is eaten in excess of the body's need for energy, what happens to it?

7. Of what practical importance is cellulose in the diet?

8. *Problem.* Calculate the carbohydrate content of 60 gm bread; 120 gm potato; 150 gm orange.

9. *Problem.* Calculate the carbohydrate and caloric content of your diet for one day. What percentage of the calories were derived from carbohydrate? What percentage of your calories were derived from cereal foods and breadstuffs; cakes, pies, and other baked sweets; sugars, candy, carbonated beverages? What improvements could you suggest for the selection of carbohydrates in your diet?

10. *Problem.* Plan a midafternoon and bedtime snack that will furnish 100 gm. carbohydrate. What points should you consider in planning for these snacks?

11. What reasons can you give for reducing the intake of sugars and sweets? What legitimate role do they have in the diet?

CITED REFERENCES

1. Levine, R.: "Role of Carbohydrate in the Diet," in Wohl, M. G., and Goodhart, R. S., eds.: *Modern Nutrition in Health and Disease,* 4th ed. Lea & Febiger, Philadelphia, 1968, p. 157.

2. West, E. S., *et al.*: *Textbook of Biochemistry,* 4th ed. The Macmillan Company, New York, 1966, p. 1039.

3. Food and Nutrition Board: *Recommended Dietary Allowances,* 7th ed. Pub. 1694. National Academy of Sciences–National Research Council, Washington, D.C., 1968, p. 10.

4. Cowgill, G. R., and Anderson, W. E.: "Laxative Effects of Wheat Bran and 'Washed' Bran in Healthy Men. A Comparative Study," *J.A.M.A.,* **98**:1866–75, 1932.

5. Hardinge, M. G., *et al.*: "Nutritional Studies of Vegetarians. III. Dietary Levels of Fiber," *Am. J. Clin. Nutr.,* **6**:523–25, 1958.

6. Yudkin, J.: "Dietary Fat and Dietary Sugar in Relation to Ischaemic Heart Disease and Diabetes," *Lancet,* **2**:4–5, July 4, 1964.

7. Grande, F., *et al.*: "Effects of Carbohydrates of Leguminous Seeds, Wheat and Potatoes on Serum Cholesterol Concentration in Man," *J. Nutr.,* **86**:313–17, 1965.

8. Antar, M. A., *et al.*: "Changes in Retail Market Food Supplies in the United States in the Last Seventy Years in Relation to the Incidence of Coronary Heart Disease, with Special Reference to Dietary Carbohydrates and Essential Fatty Acids," *Am. J. Clin. Nutr.,* **14**:169–78, 1964.

ADDITIONAL REFERENCES

Anderson, J. T.: "Dietary Carbohydrate and Serum Triglycerides," *Am. J. Clin. Nutr.,* **20**:168–75, 1967.

Bibby, B. G.: "Cariogenicity of Foods," *J.A.M.A.,* **177**:316–21, 1961.

Grande, F.: "Dietary Carbohydrates and Serum Cholesterol," *Am. J. Clin. Nutr.* **20**:176–84, 1967.

Groen, J. J.: "Effect of Bread in the Diet on Serum Cholesterol," *Am. J. Clin. Nutr.*, **20**:191–97, 1967.

Hardinge, M. G., *et al.:* "Carbohydrates in Foods," *J. Am. Diet. Assoc.*, **46**:197–204, 1965.

Harper, A.E.: "Carbohydrates," in *Food—the Yearbook of Agriculture 1959*. U.S. Department of Agriculture, Washington, D.C., pp. 88–100.

Review: "The Role of Carbohydrates in the Diet," *Nutr. Rev.*, **22**:102–105, 1964.

Stevens, H. A., and Ohlson, M. A.: "Estimated Intake of Simple and Complex Carbohydrates," *J. Am. Diet. Assoc.*, **48**:294–96, 1966.

Tank, G.: "Recent Advances in Nutrition and Dental Caries," *J.A.M.A.*, **46**:293–97, 1965.

Yudkin, J.: "Evolutionary and Historical Changes in Dietary Carbohydrates," *Am. J. Clin. Nutr.*, **20**:108–15, 1967.

6 Lipids

of substituting special margarines and cooking oils for regular margarines, butter, and solid fats? Are there any disadvantages to such changes? Definitive answers to some of these questions are not yet possible. The informed nurse, dietitian, and physician are people who can look at specific questions with an overall perspective and provide sound guidance to the public.

COMPOSITION, CLASSIFICATION, AND CHARACTERISTICS

Composition. Lipids include fats, oils, and fatlike substances that have a greasy feel and that are insoluble in water but soluble in certain organic solvents such as ether, alcohol, and benzene. Like carbohydrates, fats are organic compounds of carbon, hydrogen, and oxygen, but the resemblance ends there. Fats have a much smaller proportion of oxygen than do carbohydrates and differ importantly in their structure and properties. Some lipids also contain other elements such as phosphorus and nitrogen.

Classification. Lipids are usually classified in three groups.

1. *Simple lipids.* Triglycerides are esters of fatty acids and glycerol. A simple triglyceride is one in which the three fatty acids are the same. A mixed triglyceride is one in which at least two of the fatty acids are different. (See Figure 6–1.) This group accounts for about 98 per cent of fats in foods and over 90 per cent of the total fat in the body.

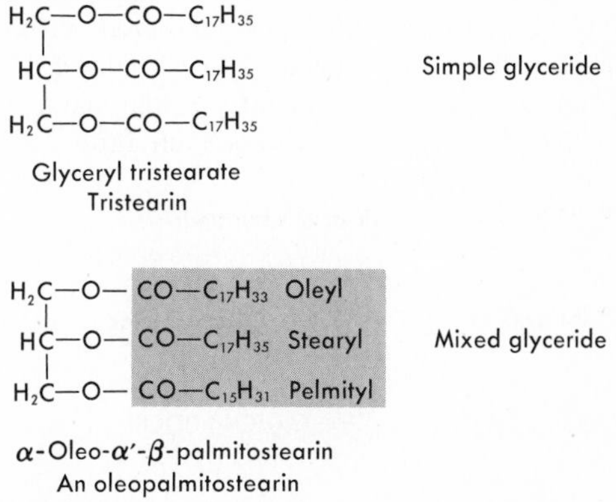

Dietary significance. Fats are prominent constituents of the American diet, supplying as much as two fifths of the total calorie intake. Anyone who has been forced to drastically restrict his intake of fats appreciates how much they contribute to the palatability of the diet whether it be the butter or margarine on bread, sauces for meats and vegetables, dressings on salads, or cakes, cookies, pastries, and other desserts.

Because fats are a concentrated source of energy it is possible to ingest the needed calories without excessively bulky diets. Meals that are moderate in fat content also have greater satiety than those that are low in fat. This results from the longer time that a food mixture containing fat remains in the stomach, thus delaying hunger.

The fat in many foods is also a carrier of fat-soluble vitamins. For example, the elimination of butter or margarine, whole milk, whole-milk cheeses, and egg yolk means that the diet must be planned with especial care to include sufficient vitamin A from other sources.

Many Americans today, on the basis of advertising and research reported by mass media, are raising important questions about the fat content of their diets. They ask: Should we reduce the fat in our diets? Should we omit whole milk and eggs because they are high in saturated fats and in cholesterol? What are the possible benefits

$$H_2C—O—CO—C_{17}H_{35}$$
$$HC—O—CO—C_{17}H_{35} \qquad \text{Simple glyceride}$$
$$H_2C—O—CO—C_{17}H_{35}$$

Glyceryl tristearate
Tristearin

$$H_2C—O—CO—C_{17}H_{33} \; \text{Oleyl}$$
$$HC—O—CO—C_{17}H_{35} \; \text{Stearyl} \qquad \text{Mixed glyceride}$$
$$H_2C—O—CO—C_{15}H_{31} \; \text{Pelmityl}$$

α-Oleo-α'-β-palmitostearin
An oleopalmitostearin

Figure 6–1. A simple and a mixed triglyceride.

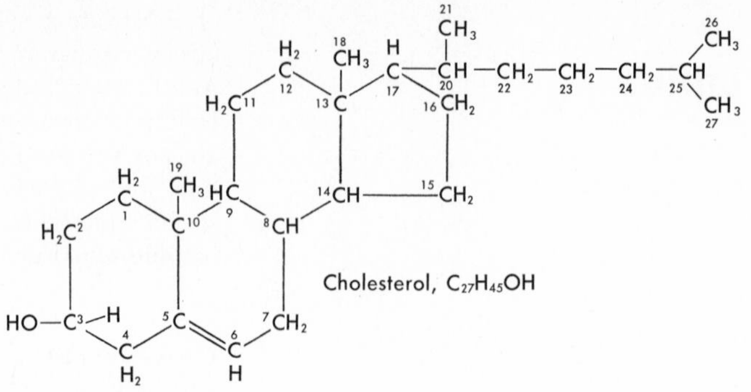

Figure 6–2. (A) In lecithin a phosphate group and choline replace one of the fatty acids of the glyceride. (B) The composite benzene ring structure of cholesterol is typical of the structure of many sterols.

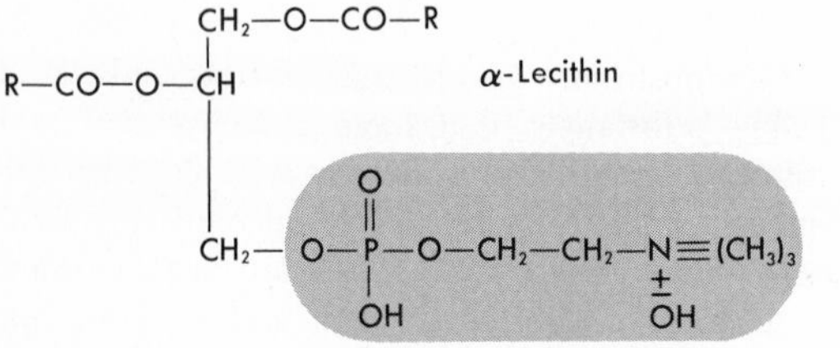

Waxes are esters of fatty acids and long-chain or cyclic alcohols. This group includes the esters of cholesterol, vitamin A, and vitamin D.

2. *Compound lipids.* Upon hydrolysis this group yields other molecules such as phosphoric acid and a nitrogen base in addition to fatty acids and glycerol. (See Figure 6–2.) Among these are phospholipids such as lecithin, cephalin, and sphingomyelin; the cerebrosides that contain a molecule of glucose or galactose; and the lipoproteins.

3. *Derived lipids.* These include fatty acids; alcohols (glycerol and sterols); carotenoids; and the fat-soluble vitamins A, D, E, and K.

Fatty acids. Most fatty acids in foods and in the body are straight, even-numbered carbon chains, containing as few as 4 or as many as 24 carbon atoms. Short-chain fatty acids contain 4 and 6 carbon atoms, medium-chain fatty acids

contain 8 to 12 carbon atoms, and long-chain fatty acids contain more than 12 carbon atoms.

Fatty acids are "saturated" or "unsaturated." A fatty acid in which each of the carbon atoms in the chain has two hydrogen atoms attached to it is saturated:

$$\begin{array}{cc} H & H \\ | & | \\ -C-C-. \\ | & | \\ H & H \end{array}$$

An unsaturated fatty acid is one in which a hydrogen atom is missing from each of two adjoining carbon atoms, thus necessitating a double bond between the two carbon atoms:

$$\begin{array}{cc} H & H \\ | & | \\ -C=C-. \end{array}$$

The formulas for four fatty acids that contain 18 carbon atoms but that differ in their saturation are shown in Figure 6–3.

$CH_3(CH_2)_{16}COOH$ Stearic acid (saturated)

$CH_3(CH_2)_7$ CH=CH $(CH_2)_7COOH$ Oleic acid (monounsaturated)

$CH_3(CH_2)_4$ CH=CH CH_2 CH=CH $(CH_2)_7COOH$ Linoleic acid (2 double bonds; polyunsaturated)

CH_3CH_2 CH=CH CH_2 CH=CH CH_2 CH=CH $(CH_2)_7COOH$ Linolenic acid (3 double bonds; polyunsaturated)

Figure 6–3. These fatty acids contain 18 carbon atoms but differ in the level of saturation.

Unsaturated fatty acids can exist as geometric isomers. In the *cis* form the molecule folds back upon itself at each double bond. In the *trans* form the molecule extends to its maximum length.

cis form   *trans* form

The form in which a fatty acid occurs markedly influences the melting point and other properties of the fat. Food and body fats exist principally in the *cis* form.

Characteristics of fats. The nature of fats—their hardness, melting point, and flavor—is determined by the length of the carbon chain and the level of saturation of the fatty acids as well as the order in which the fatty acids are attached to the glycerol molecule. A tremendous number of fats exists in nature. Each food fat—beef, lamb, chicken, olive oil, for example—has its distinctive flavor and hardness.

Hardness. Fatty acids containing 12 carbon atoms or less and unsaturated fatty acids are liquid at room temperature. Saturated fatty acids containing 14 carbon atoms or more are solid at room temperature. Food and body fats contain mixtures of short- and long-chain fatty acids and of saturated and unsaturated fatty acids. No natural fat is made up completely of either saturated or unsaturated fatty acids.

The distribution of fatty acids in a number of fats is shown in Table 6–1. Oleic, palmitic, and stearic acids predominate in animal fats. These fats are solid at room temperature and are often referred to as "saturated." In general, herbivora have harder fats that carnivora, and land animals have harder fats than aquatic animals. Lamb and beef fat, with their high content of palmitic and stearic acids, are much harder than pork and chicken fat, which contain somewhat more of the

unsaturated fatty acids. Fats from fish have a high proportion of polyunsaturated fatty acids containing 20 to 24 carbon atoms. The proportion of saturated fatty acids is high in milk fat, but this fat is soft because of the presence of many short-chain fatty acids.

Oleic and linoleic acids predominate in vegetable fats, except for coconut oil. Corn, cottonseed, and soybean oils are very rich in linoleic acid, whereas peanut and olive oils are rich in oleic acid and correspondingly lower in linoleic acid. Of the vegetable fats coconut oil is unique in that it is composed largely of lauric acid, which is liquid at room temperature. Coconut oil is classed as a "saturated" fat, and other vegetable fats as "unsaturated." Those fats that have a high proportion of fatty acids with two or more double bonds are referred to as "polyunsaturated."

Hydrogenation. In the presence of a catalyst such as nickel, liquid fats can be changed to solid fats by introducing hydrogen at the double bonds of the carbon chain. In the manufacture of vegetable shortenings and margarines, some, but not all, of the double bonds in the oils are hydrogenated, thereby giving fats that are somewhat soft and plastic. During hydrogenation some of the fatty acids are changed from the *cis* to the *trans* form, but both forms are utilized by the body. Hydrogenation reduces the linoleic acid content of the fat.

Emulsification. Fats are capable of forming emulsions with liquids, a property that is essential for their digestion and absorption. Emulsification of fats is also utilized in the homogenization of milk and in the preparation of mayonnaise.

Saponification refers to the formation of a soap of fatty acid and a cation. In the alkaline medium of the intestine, for example, free fatty acid may combine with calcium to form an insoluble compound that is excreted in the feces. In certain diseases characterized by poor fat absorption—sprue, for example—the loss of calcium in this manner could be significant.

Rancidity. Air at room temperature can induce oxidation of fats, resulting in the changes in odor and flavor commonly known as rancidity. These changes are accelerated upon exposure to light and in the presence of traces of certain minerals.

Table 6–1. Typical Major Fatty Acid Analyses of Some Fats of Animal and Plant Origin*†

				Saturated						Unsaturated				
		Capric	Lauric	Myristic	Palmitic	Stearic	Arachidic	Behemic	Palmitoleic	Oleic	Linoleic	Linolenic	Arachidonic	Other Polyenoic Acids
	4–8	10.0	12.0	14.0	16.0	18.0	20.0	22.0	16.1	18.1	18.2	18.3	20.4	
Animal														
Lard				1.5	27.0	13.5			3.0	43.5	10.5	0.5		
Chicken			2.0	7.0	25.0	6.0			8.0	36.0	14.0			
Egg					25.0	10.0				50.0	10.0	2.0	3.0	
Beef				3.0	29.0	21.0	0.5		3.0	41.0	2.0	0.5	0.5	
Butter	5.5	3.0	3.5	12.0	28.0	13.0			3.0	28.5	1.0			
Human milk		1.5	7.0	8.5	21.0	7.0	1.0		2.5	36.0	7.0	1.0	0.5	
Menhaden				9.0	19.0	5.5			16.0					48.5
Human adipose‡			0.1–2	2–6	21–25	2–8			3–7	39–47	4–25			2–8
Vegetable														
Corn					12.5	2.5	0.5			29.0	55.0	0.5		
Peanut					11.5	3.0	1.5	2.5		53.0	26.0			
Cottonseed				1.0	26.0	3.0			1.0	17.5	51.5			
Soybean					11.5	4.0				24.5	53.0	7.0		
Olive					13.0	2.5			1.0	74.0	9.0	0.5		
Coconut	7.0	6.0	49.5	19.5	8.5	2.0				6.0	1.5			

*Food and Nutrition Board: *Dietary Fat and Human Health*. Pub. 1147, National Academy of Sciences—National Research Council, Washington, D.C., 1966, p. 6.

†Composition is given in weight percentages of the component fatty acids (rounded to nearest 0.5) as determined by gas chromatography. The number of carbon atoms and the number of double bonds is indicated under the common name of the fatty acid. These data were derived from a variety of sources. They are representative determinations rather than averages, and considerable variation is to be expected in individual samples from other sources.

‡Adapted from West, E. S., *et al.: Textbook of Biochemistry*, 4th ed. The Macmillan Company, New York, 1966, p. 134.

They occur more readily in fats that have a high proportion of unsaturated fatty acids. Some fats are naturally protected from rapid oxidation by the presence of antioxidants, one of which is vitamin E. Commercially processed fats and oils are usually protected by the addition of small amounts of antioxidants.

Effect of heat. Excessive heating of fats leads to the breakdown of glycerol, producing a pungent compound (acrolein) which is especially irritating to the gastrointestinal mucosa. Fatty acids are also oxidized by prolonged heating at high temperatures. Under ordinary conditions of home or commercial frying no adverse effects on nutritional properties have been found.

FUNCTIONS

Important source of energy. The primary function of fat is to supply energy, each gram of fat yielding approximately 9 calories when oxidized. This energy is continuously available from the stores in adipose tissue. The high density and low solubility of fats make them an ideal form in which to store energy. In fact, not only fats as such are stored in adipose tissue, but any glucose and amino acids not promptly utilized are also synthesized into fats and stored.

Adipose tissue, which consists principally of triglycerides, is stored in the subcutaneous tissues and in the abdominal cavity. It also surrounds the organs and is laced throughout muscle tissue. Many examples could be cited of individuals who have survived total starvation for 30 or 40 days, or partial starvation for much longer periods of time. Their survival was possible only because of the energy available from the adipose tissues.

Insulation and padding. The subcutaneous layer of fat is an effective insulator and reduces losses of body heat in cold weather. Excessive layers of subcutaneous fat, as in obesity, may interfere with heat loss during warm weather, thus increasing discomfort. The vital organs such as the kidney are protected against physical injury by a padding of fat. Fats and oils also have some value as a lubricant for the gastrointestinal tract.

Essential fatty acids. Linoleic acid is an essential fatty acid; that is, it cannot be synthesized in the body and must be present in the diet. In the body linoleic acid is rapidly converted to arachidonic acid, the physiologically functioning polyunsaturated fatty acid. Young animals that are fed a diet deficient in polyunsaturated fatty acids fail to grow and are afflicted with an eczemalike dermatitis. These conditions are corrected when linoleic acid is added to the diet. Similarly, Hansen[1] found that the inclusion of essential fatty acids in the diet of infants who had eczema led to improvement of the skin and to greater gains in weight. (See Figure 6–4.)

The essential fatty acids are constituents of phospholipids that form cellular membranes and thus appear to have a role in regulating cell permeability and in the transport of lipids in the circulation.

Linolenic acid, another of the polyunsaturated fatty acids, promotes normal growth in animals but it does not cure the dermatitis that occurs from fatty acid deficiency. It is, therefore, not an essential fatty acid and is not a substitute for linoleic acid.

Phospholipids. All cells contain phospholipids, but brain, nervous tissue, and liver are especially rich in them. The phospholipid level in the body is not reduced even in starvation, suggesting the vital role that they must play in metabolism. Phospholipids are powerful emulsifying agents and have an affinity for water. Hence, they are essential to the digestion and absorption of fats and they facilitate the uptake of fatty acids by the cells.

Phospholipids comprise a significant proportion of the blood lipoproteins but their function in lipid transport is not clearly understood. They are manufactured and removed by the liver and apparently do not enter the tissue cells, which readily synthesize their own supply of phospholipid.

Cholesterol. The concentration of cholesterol is high in the liver, the adrenal, the white and gray matter of the brain, and the peripheral nerves. It is present in small amounts in almost all body tissues and constitutes an important fraction of the blood lipoproteins. It is synthesized by the liver to meet body needs regardless

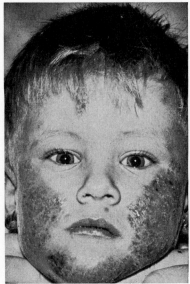
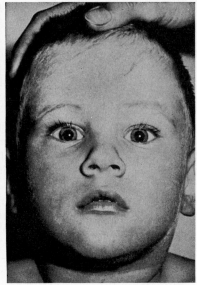

Figure 6–4. Child, 2 1/2 years old, showing (*A*) eczema present since two months of age; (*B*) condition one month after fresh lard was added to the diet. (Courtesy, Dr. A. E. Hansen, Galveston, Texas.)

A   B

of dietary intake. Cholesterol furnishes the nucleus for the synthesis of provitamin D, adrenocortical hormones, steroid sex hormones, and bile salts.

DIGESTION AND ABSORPTION

Digestion. Almost all the fats presented to the digestive tract for hydrolysis are triglycerides. Only a small fraction of dietary fat consists of cholesterol esters and phospholipids. Fats are hydrolyzed primarily in the small intestine. Although gastric lipase may bring about some hydrolysis of finely divided fats from foods such as egg yolk and cream, the action is not important.

As the chyme enters the duodenum, the presence of fat stimulates the intestinal wall to secrete *cholecystokinin,* a hormone that is carried to the gallbladder by the bloodstream. Cholecystokinin stimulates the contraction of the gallbladder, thereby forcing bile into the common duct and thence into the small intestine.

Bile has several important functions in fat digestion and absorption: (1) it stimulates peristalsis; (2) it neutralizes the acid chyme so as to provide the optimum hydrogen ion concentration for enzyme activity; (3) it emulsifies fats, thereby increasing the surface area exposed to enzyme action; and (4) it lowers the surface tension so that intimate contact between the fat droplets and the enzymes is possible.

The triglycerides are hydrolyzed stepwise by lipase; that is, one of the end fatty acids is removed at the time yielding in turn a diglyceride and then a monoglyceride. Only about one fourth to one half of the triglycerides are completely hydrolyzed to glycerol and fatty acids. Phospholipids are hydrolyzed by a number of phospholipases that can attack the several linkages of the molecule. The end products of lipid hydrolysis that are presented for absorption include fatty acids, glycerol, monoglycerides, and probably some diglycerides and triglycerides.

Speed of digestion. Fats reduce the motility of the gastrointestinal tract, and hence any diet containing fat remains in the stomach longer than one that is low in fat. Fats that are liquid at body temperature are hydrolyzed more rapidly than those that are solid at body temperature. Typical mixed diets contain complex mixtures of fats including short- and long-chain as well as saturated and unsaturated fatty acids.

Adults normally experience no difficulty in digesting fats from any source. Infants and young children, as well as some elderly persons, seem to have somewhat better tolerance for the softer, more highly emulsified fats such as those in dairy products. They also may experience some discomfort following meals that are high in fat.

Fried foods are digested somewhat more slowly than foods prepared by other methods of cookery because the food particles coated with fat must be broken up before they can be acted upon by enzymes. Properly fried foods do not normally cause digestive difficulties, even for persons who require therapeutic diets. When the frying temperature is too low, foods absorb excessive amounts of fat, thus lengthening the time required for digestion. On the other hand, if foods are fried at too high a temperature the resulting decomposition products may be irritating to the intestinal mucosa.

Absorption. The free fatty acids, monoglycerides, some diglycerides and triglycerides, and cholesterol are complexed with bile salts to form *micelles,* which are water-soluble microscopic particles that can penetrate the mucosal membrane. Plant sterols are not absorbed, and their presence in the intestine may reduce the amount of cholesterol that is absorbed. At the point of contact of the micelle with the brush border of the epithelial cell, the lipids are apparently released from the complex and enter the cell by mechanisms not fully understood. *Pinocytosis,* that is, engulfing the fat and subsequently releasing it to the interior of the cell, is believed to be one of the operative mechanisms. When the lipids are released from the micelle, new products of hydrolysis of fats can again combine with the bile salts. Eventually the bile salts are absorbed by active transport from the lower ileum. Most of the absorption of fats occurs from the jejunum.

Fatty acids that contain 12 carbon atoms or less are absorbed into the portal circulation without reesterification in the mucosal cell. They are attached to albumin for their transportation, and they may be used within the liver or released to other tissues in the body. The glycerol resulting from fat hydrolysis is also carried by the portal circulation.

Fatty acids that contain 14 carbon atoms or more are resynthesized to new triglycerides within the epithelial cell of the mucosa before they are extruded into the lymph circulation. The new fats are formed by the addition of two fatty acids to a monoglyceride molecule or by esterification of glycerol with three fatty acids. See page 85 for a further description of fat synthesis. Cholesterol is also reesterified within the epithelial cell.

Chylomicrons. In order to penetrate the lipoprotein membrane of the epithelial cell for entrance to the lymph circulation, the newly formed fats are made soluble by surrounding them with a lipoprotein envelope consisting chiefly of phospholipids and a very small amount of protein. These particles are known as *chylomicrons,* having first been identified in chyle (lymph). They are of very low density and give to the lymph a milky appearance.

Completeness of digestion and absorption. Normally about 95 per cent of dietary fats and 80 per cent of dietary cholesterol are absorbed. Mineral oil, which is not a true fat, is not absorbed from the intestine. This fact is mentioned in order to emphasize that mineral oil should never be used in food preparation inasmuch as it may seriously interfere with the absorption of fat-soluble vitamins. When mineral oil is used as a laxative, it should not be taken at mealtime.

A number of factors may reduce the amount of fat that is digested and absorbed. Among these are increased motility so that food is moved along the tract too rapidly for complete enzyme action; disease of the biliary tract so that the secretion of bile is deficient or does not reach the small intestine; disease of the pancreas so that lipase is not secreted; and reduction in the absorbing surfaces as in celiac disease or following surgery on the small intestine. When fat absorption is decreased, large amounts of fat are excreted in the feces (steatorrhea) with a consequent serious loss of calories. (See Chapter 36.)

METABOLISM

The blood is the means of transportation of lipids from one site to another, and the liver and adipose tissues are the specialized organs that control lipid metabolism. The synthesis of new lipids (lipogenesis) and the catabolism of lipids (lipolysis) are continuously taking place. These reactions are catalyzed by specific enzymes under the control of nervous and hormonal mechanisms.

Blood lipids. Since fats are insoluble in water, proteins provide the mechanism for their transport in the aqueous medium of the blood. These protein-lipid complexes are known as *lipoproteins*. The chylomicrons synthesized in the intestinal mucosa (see page 83) are large particles consisting principally of triglycerides. They may give a milky appearance to blood serum shortly after a fat-rich meal, but they are rapidly hydrolyzed by lipoprotein lipase and the released fats are used by the tissues. The blood serum is thus "cleared."

Alpha- and beta-lipoproteins. The greatest concentration of lipids in the blood consists of two classes of lipoproteins. *High-density* or *α-lipoproteins* contain a large proportion of protein, phospholipid, and cholesterol. This class is little affected by changes in diet or by age. *Low-density* or *β-lipoproteins* include a number of groups that vary widely in density and in their proportions of triglycerides, cholesterol, phospholipids, and protein. Those that approach the particle size of chylomicrons consist principally of triglycerides and only small amounts of protein and other lipids. This class is especially elevated in carbohydrate-induced hyperglyceridemia. Another group of β-lipoproteins contains a large proportion of cholesterol and is elevated with increasing age and when diets are rich in saturated fatty acids, and to a lesser extent when diets contain substantial amounts of cholesterol. Patients who have had a myocardial infarction, those who have angina pectoris, and those individuals who are considered to be high risks for cardiovascular disease usually show increased concentrations of the β-lipoprotein group. Other pathologic conditions in which this group is often elevated include diabetes mellitus, nephrosis, hypothyroidism, and xanthomatosis.

Free fatty acids (FFA), also designated as nonesterified fatty acids (NEFA), are the principal source of fatty acids made available to the cells for energy. They enter the circulation as the result of the hydrolysis of triglycerides, chiefly by adipose tissue. The fatty acids are attached rather tightly to plasma albumin and do not circulate in their free state. At the cell surfaces the fatty acid is released with ease from its carrier. The concentration of FFA in the blood at any given time is quite low, but the rate of turnover is so rapid that several thousand calories are transported daily in the circulation in this way. The concentration of free fatty acids is somewhat higher in the circulation during fasting, indicating more rapid release from adipose tissue. It is somewhat lower when carbohydrate is being absorbed, indicating that carbohydrate is being used for energy as well as synthesized to fat. (See Table A–14.)

Adipose tissue and fat metabolism. Like other tissues, adipose tissue is constantly being remolded. It synthesizes, stores, and releases fat. It consists chiefly of triglycerides and is supplied with the enzymes that are required for lipogenesis and lipolysis. Fat synthesis and breakdown take place continuously, but they are in equilibrium when the energy needs of the body are exactly met. If the energy supplied to the body is in excess of the body's needs, lipogenesis exceeds the rate of lipolysis and adipose tissue is stored (weight is gained) regardless of whether calories are derived from fat, carbohydrate, or protein. Insulin is required for the synthesis of fats.

When a calorie deficit exists, the adipose tissue will be catabolized more rapidly than it is being synthesized (weight is lost). The release of fatty acids from adipose tissue is accelerated by the same hormones that increase glucose breakdown: epinephrine, norepinephrine, glucagon, growth hormone, adrenocorticotropic hormone, and thyrotropic hormone.

The liver and fat metabolism. The liver is the key organ in the regulation of fat metabolism. It is able to accomplish the shortening or lengthening of the carbon chain of the fatty acids and to introduce double bonds into fatty acids. For example, a double bond can be introduced into stearic acid to yield oleic acid. On the other hand, a second double bond cannot be introduced into oleic acid to yield linoleic acid. With a dietary supply of linoleic acid, this essential fatty acid can be converted to arachidonic acid by adding a 2-carbon unit and by introducing two additional double bonds.

The liver hydrolyzes the triglycerides brought to it, re-forms new triglycerides, and again releases them to the circulation. It converts FFA to triglycerides and phospholipids and synthesizes lipoproteins. It releases them to the circulation and also removes them from the circulation, thus maintaining control over the blood levels.

The liver is probably the chief regulator of the total body content of cholesterol and of the circulating blood cholesterol. It governs the endogenous synthesis of cholesterol, the removal of cholesterol from the circulation, the production of bile acids from cholesterol, and the excretion of cholesterol and bile acids by way of the bile into the intestine.

Certain *lipotropic* substances must be present to prevent the accumulation of fat in the liver. They include choline, vitamin B_{12}, betaine, and possibly inositol. Methionine, one of the essential amino acids, donates methyl groups for the synthesis of choline and is therefore a lipotropic substance.

Synthesis of fats. Triglycerides are synthesized by the epithelial cells of the intestinal mucosa, by the adipose tissue, and by the liver. In order to synthesize triglycerides a source of α-glycerophosphate is essential. This is furnished by the normal oxidation of glucose that occurs in each of these tissues through the Embden-Meyerhof pathway (see page 69). A second source of α-glycerophosphate is available from the glycerol released from fat hydrolysis in the intestinal mucosa and in the liver.[2] The glycerol so released combines with ATP in the presence of glycerokinase to form α-glycerophosphate. Adipose tissue does not contain glycerokinase and cannot convert glycerol to the active form.

The fatty acids for the triglyceride molecule are available from the hydrolysis of fats and also through synthesis from acetyl coenzyme A derived through the oxidation of fats, glucose, and

some amino acids. The synthesis of fats from acetyl coenzyme A is accomplished essentially by building up the carbon chain by successive additions of 2-carbon fragments. NADPH, a niacin-containing coenzyme, is required for this synthesis. It is made available through the pentose shunt of the glycolytic pathway (see page 71). The synthesis of fatty acids from acetyl coenzyme A is thus seen to be dependent upon normal carbohydrate metabolism and to require insulin. Free fatty acids are not esterified directly with glycerophosphate but must first be converted to fatty acyl coenzyme A. They are then attached stepwise to glycerophosphate to form the triglyceride.

Oxidation of fatty acids. All cells of the body except those of the central nervous system can oxidize fatty acids to yield energy. Beta oxidation is the major pathway for the oxidation of fatty acids. By this process oxidation occurs at the carbon that is beta from the carboxyl group. This requires coenzyme A and is accomplished in five steps, the end result of which is a fatty acid that is two carbons shorter plus a molecule of acetyl coenzyme A:

$$CH_3(CH_2)_{16}COOH + \text{Coenzyme A} \rightarrow$$
Stearic acid

$$CH_3(CH_2)_{14}COOCoA + CH_3COOCoA$$
Palmityl coenzyme A   Acetyl coenzyme A

This sequence is repeated until all of the fatty acid has been broken down to acetyl coenzyme A. Acetyl coenzyme A can enter the Krebs cycle for oxidation to energy, carbon dioxide, and water, or it can be used for the synthesis of new fatty acids, cholesterol, and other compounds. (See Figure 6–5.)

The glycerol made available from the hydrolysis of fatty acids enters the glycolytic pathway by combining with ATP to form glycerophosphate. Thus, it is a potential source of glucose, glycogen, and energy or may be the backbone for the new glyceride molecule.

Ketogenesis. Within the liver two molecules of acetyl coenzyme A can condense to form acetoacetyl coenzyme A, which in turn yields acetoacetic acid, beta-hydroxybutyric acid, and

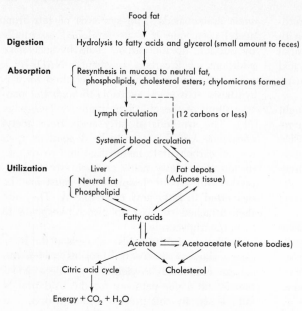

Food fat

Digestion   Hydrolysis to fatty acids and glycerol (small amount to feces)

Absorption   { Resynthesis in mucosa to neutral fat,
phospholipids, cholesterol esters; chylomicrons formed }

Lymph circulation   (12 carbons or less)

Systemic blood circulation

Utilization   Liver   Fat depots
{ Neutral fat   (Adipose tissue)
Phospholipid }

Fatty acids

Acetate ⇌ Acetoacetate (Ketone bodies)

Citric acid cycle   Cholesterol

Energy + CO_2 + H_2O

Figure 6–5. The utilization of fat in the body.

acetone. These compounds are known as *ketone bodies* and the process as *ketogenesis*. The ketone bodies are normally produced in small amounts by the liver. Although the liver does not possess the enzymes necessary for their further oxidation, the tissues utilize them to yield energy. In certain circumstances, such as uncontrolled diabetes mellitus and starvation, carbohydrate metabolism is greatly reduced, and the production of acetyl coenzyme A from fat oxidation is greatly increased. The reduction in carbohydrate metabolism means that the amount of oxalacetate available to combine with acetyl coenzyme A in the Krebs cycle is also reduced. The liver synthesizes vastly increased amounts of the ketones —far beyond the ability of the tissues to oxidize them. The principal effect of the increased production is a disturbance of the acid-base balance. Acetoacetic acid and β-hydroxybutyric acid are fairly strong acids and combine with the available base. They are excreted (ketonuria) and the alkali reserve is reduced. Acetone, being volatile, is excreted by the lungs.

Cholesterol metabolism. The liver and intestine are the chief sites of cholesterol synthesis, but all cells are able to produce some cholesterol. The endogenous production of cholesterol has been variously estimated at 1000 to 2000 mg

daily and is apparently independent of the dietary supply. Acetyl coenzyme A is the direct precursor of cholesterol, and thus any donor of acetyl coenzyme A—fatty acids, glucose, and some amino acids—is a potential source of cholesterol.

The body is unable to break down the cholesterol nucleus, but the liver converts it by enzyme action to bile acids. This is apparently rate limited,[3] and therefore any excess supply may pose problems of disposal. Cholesterol as such and bile acids are constituents of bile, and excretion occurs from the intestine.

As stated in a preceding section, cholesterol is transported in the blood in the lipoproteins. The determination of the cholesterol concentration in blood serum is conveniently made in the laboratory, and any increase in blood levels correlates well with the increase in the concentration of the class of β-lipoproteins that occur in certain pathologic conditions. The serum cholesterol concentration in apparently normal adults may range from 150 to 250 mg per 100 ml, although a level above 200 mg per 100 ml is now considered by some investigators to be undesirable. About three fourths of the serum cholesterol is esterified. The concentration of cholesterol varies considerably and may be increased during periods of emotional stress, physical inactivity, and overeating. A single determination is probably of limited significance.

FAT IN THE DIET

Dietary allowances. The Food and Nutrition Board has not set precise recommendations for either the quantity or type of fat that should be included in the normal diet. The Board has indicated that dietary modifications may be justified for many Americans in order to lower blood serum concentrations of cholesterol and triglyceride, and that such modifications must always give consideration to the calorie and nutrient balances.[4]

People of the Orient consume diets that provide around 10 per cent or less of the calories from fat, whereas Americans derive up to 40 per cent of their calories from fat. These extremes are based on patterns of food consumption that differ tremendously. Neither of them can be described categorically as affording the greatest promise of good health.

Since the calorie value of the diet is derived mainly from fat and carbohydrate, any drastic restriction in the one means that the other must be increased in order to maintain caloric equilibrium. In normal individuals it is debatable whether it is desirable to markedly increase the carbohydrate intake in order to restrict the fat intake, let us say, to 20 to 25 per cent of the calories.

As little as 1 per cent of the calories from linoleic acid is sufficient to prevent symptoms of essential fatty acid deficiency in infants.[4] The Food and Nutrition Board suggests that formulas containing 3 per cent of total calories from linoleic acid may be expected to prevent subclinical deficiencies and to establish some reserves against stress. Essential fatty acid deficiency has not been demonstrated in adults, and the exact requirement for linoleic acid is not known. The average mixed diet is believed to be more than adequate.

Food sources. Oils, lard, hydrogenated shortening, butter, margarine, bacon, and salad dressings are the most concentrated sources of fat.

A small amount of them will contribute importantly to the calorie level of the diet.

So-called "invisible" fats represent about three fifths of the fat in the American diet. These sources include meats, poultry, fish, dairy products (excluding butter), eggs, and baked products. Meats, poultry, and fish vary widely in their fat content. The amount of fat ingested from meat will depend upon the cut that was used, whether fat was carefully trimmed, whether fat drippings were used, and upon the method of preparation. Lean cuts of beef, pork, lamb, and veal differ little in their fat content. Fish is somewhat lower in fat than is meat. Fish that have a colored flesh are somewhat higher in fat than those with white flesh.

All of the fat in the egg is in the yolk, about one third of this being in the form of phospholipid. Whole milk, cream, ice cream, and whole-milk cheeses furnish appreciable amounts of fat. Fruits, vegetables, legumes, cereals, and flours are low in fat. On the other hand, nuts contain an appreciable amount of fat.

Linoleic acid. Corn, cottonseed, and soy oils are good sources of linoleic acid. Some special margarines now available in food markets are processed by adding hydrogenated fat to oils, thereby retaining a greater proportion of linoleic acid. These margarines are much softer than regular margarines. In the labeling of such margarines the words *liquid oil* appear first, followed by a listing of hydrogenated oil and other ingredients. Fish and poultry furnish small amounts of linoleic acid.

Cholesterol. Only animal foods furnish cholesterol. Liver, egg yolk, kidney, brains, sweetbreads and fish roe are rich sources. Much smaller concentrations are found in whole milk, cream, butter, cheese, and meat.

An individual who eats no eggs or organ meats probably ingests not more than 200 mg cholesterol daily; if, in addition, he uses skim milk and substitutes vegetable margarine for butter, the intake will be further reduced to 100 to 150 mg daily. Each egg yolk adds about 275 mg cholesterol. (See Table A–6.)

Fat in the American diet. The fat content of the basic diet pattern is shown in Table 6–2. Note that the basic list of foods supplies approx-

Table 6–2. Fat Content of Basic Diet

| | Measure | Total Fat gm | Fatty Acids | | | Cholesterol mg |
			Saturated gm	Oleic gm	Linoleic gm	
Milk, whole	2 cups	18	10	6	tr	25
Egg	1	6	2	3	tr	275
Meat, fish, poultry, lean	4 ounces	10	4	5	1	120
Vegetables-fruit	4 servings	tr	tr	tr	tr	—
Bread	3 slices	3	tr	1	tr	—
Total fat in basic diet		37	16	15	1	420
Typical Additions of Fat to Basic Diet						
Butter	3 teaspoons	12	6	4	tr	37
French dressing	1 tablespoon	6	1	1	3	—
Corn oil in cooked foods	1 tablespoon	14	1	4	7	—
Cherry pie	1 piece	15	4	7	3	—
Total fat		84	28	31	14	457

imately equal amounts of saturated and oleic acids, a proportion that is quite characteristic of American diets. The choice of additional foods to supply the needed energy requirements affords a wide range of possibilities for modifying the kind as well as the amount of fat that is included. In the example given, the use of salad dressing and corn oil increases the linoleic acid content considerably.

Some important changes have taken place in the consumption of fat in the United States since the beginning of this century. The total amount of fat available for consumption at the present time is 155 gm daily.[5] This represents about 42 per cent of the total calories available. The contributions of each of the food groups to the total fat is as follows:

	Per Cent
Fats and oils including butter	42.3
Meat, poultry, and fish	34.9
Dairy products excluding butter	12.7
Dry beans, peas, nuts, soya flour	3.5
Eggs	3.3
Flour and cereal products	1.4
Coffee and cocoa	1.2
Fruits and vegetables	0.9

The total amount of fat available for consumption and the percentage of calories available from fat have shown a steady increase since the early part of the century. Socioeconomic changes have resulted in a steady decline in the intake of cereal foods, breadstuffs, and potatoes, which are low in fat, and an increase in the intake of meats and fat-rich foods including ice cream, table spreads, and other fats. The use of butter has sharply declined, but this has been replaced by margarine. Hydrogenated shortenings have replaced, to a large extent, shortenings of animal origin. Vegetable oils are used much more widely so that the average intake of linoleic acid is greater than that in earlier decades.

Problems related to fat in the diet. Because fats are so concentrated a source of energy, small quantities rapidly increase the calorie intake. It should be self-evident that the individual who does not exercise moderation in the use of fats can rapidly increase his caloric intake beyond his needs and thus become overweight.

The evidence is strong that a high intake of saturated fats and of cholesterol increases the concentration of blood cholesterol and certain lipoprotein fractions. These elevated levels of blood lipids appear to be highly correlated with the incidence of cardiovascular diseases. A fuller discussion of this important problem is presented in Chapter 42.

Some Points for Emphasis in Nutrition Education

1. Fats are essential constituents of the body, being the principal way in which the body stores energy.

2. Fats are the most concentrated source of energy in the diet and furnish more than twice as many calories, gram for gram, as do carbohydrates and proteins. Consequently, a small volume of fatty food will increase the calorie intake considerably.

3. When an individual consumes a diet that provides more calories than he needs, the excess calories will be stored as fat regardless of the composition of the diet. On the other hand, when an individual consumes a diet that supplies fewer calories than he needs, adipose tissue will furnish the additional needs.

4. A diet that provides 35 per cent of the calories from fat allows a wide latitude of food choice that is acceptable to Americans. Some of the foods chosen should be good sources of vitamin A.

5. Foods fried at the proper temperature may be used in moderation by most people. Preferably they should not be given to very young children.

6. Cholesterol is an essential constituent of body tissues and is required for the regulation of important body functions. It does not need to be in the diet because the liver readily synthesizes it. On the other hand, a modest intake as provided by the recommendations for the Four Food Groups is compatible with good nutrition.

7. A diet that contains a high proportion of saturated fatty acids and of cholesterol is one of many factors that is believed to contribute to cardiovascular disease.

8. In advising Americans about ways to modify their diets without resorting to distorted dietary patterns or faddism, the following guidelines seem appropriate: (a) Include first those basic foods that are essential for protein, minerals, and vitamins. (b) Select fats for food preparation from oils rich in linoleic acid as well as from solid fats. (c) Trim visible fats from meats; use more poultry and fish. (d) Substitute fruits and low-calorie desserts more frequently for high-fat desserts. (e) In choosing foods for additional calories, place emphasis on the maintenance of normal weight.

Problems and Review

1. Prepare an outline that shows the digestion, absorption, and metabolic fate of triglycerides supplied by the diet.
2. Give several reasons why fat is a useful constituent of the diet.
3. What is a hydrogenated fat? Give several examples. How does it compare in nutritional value with the fat from which it was made?
4. What effect will the inclusion of fatty foods such as fried potatoes and pork chops have on the digestion of the meal as a whole?
5. *Problem.* Compare the fat and calorie values of ½ cup ice cream; 1 tablespoon mayonnaise; 1 ounce cream cheese; 2 teaspoons butter; 1 cup milk.
6. *Problem.* Calculate your own fat intake for one day. Which of the foods you ate are good sources of linoleic acid? What percentage of the total calories in your diet was derived from fat?
7. A margarine may be manufactured from 100 per cent vegetable oil but may still be a poor source of linoleic acid. Explain why this might be true.
8. *Problem.* Examine the labels of three or four brands of special types of margarine. What information do they give you about their value as sources of linoleic acid? How do these margarines compare with regular margarines in cost?
9. What is the nutritional significance of linoleic acid? Of cholesterol? Of phospholipids?

10. What points would you emphasize in the selection of fats for good nutrition?
11. A patient tells you that he has not been eating butter, eggs, or whole milk because he read in a magazine that cholesterol causes heart disease. How would you respond to this?

CITED REFERENCES

1. Hansen, A. F.: "Essential Fatty Acids in Infant Feeding," *J. Am. Diet. Assoc.,* **34**:239–41, 1958.
2. Isselbacher, K. J.: "Metabolism and Transport of Lipid by Intestinal Mucosa," *Fed. Proc.,* **24**:16–22, 1965.
3. Connor, W. E., *et al.:* "Cholesterol Balance and Fecal Neutral Steroid and Bile Acid Excretion in Normal Men Fed Dietary Fats of Different Fatty Acid Composition," *J. Clin. Invest.,* **48**:1363–75, 1969.
4. Food and Nutrition Board: *Recommended Dietary Allowances,* 7th ed. Pub. 1694. National Academy of Sciences–National Research Council, Washington, D.C., 1968.
5. Friend, B.: "Nutritional Review," *National Food Situation.* Economic Research Service, U.S. Department of Agriculture, Washington, D.C., Nov. 1970, pp. 21–25.

ADDITIONAL REFERENCES

Bennion, M., and Park, R. L.: "Changes in Frying Fats with Different Foods," *J. Am. Diet. Assoc.,* **52**:308–12, 1968.
Call, D. L., and Sánchez, A. M.: "Trends in Fat Disappearance in the United States (1909–1965)," *J. Nutr.,* 93 (Pt. II); 1–28, 1967.
Council on Foods and Nutrition: "The Regulation of Dietary Fat," *J.A.M.A.,* **181**:411–29, 1962.
Fleischman, A. I., *et al.:* "Studies on Cooking Fats and Oils," *J. Am. Diet. Assoc.,* **42**:394–98, 1963.
Food and Nutrition Board: *Dietary Fat and Human Health.* Pub. 1147. National Academy of Sciences–National Research Council, Washington, D.C., 1966.
Grollman, A.: "A Common-Sense Guide to Cholesterol," *Today's Health,* **44**:3, Aug. 1966.
Hansen, A. E., *et al.:* "Role of Linoleic Acid in Infant Nutrition," *Pediatrics,* **31** (Pt. II): 171–92, 1963.
Hodges, R. E.: "Dietary and Other Factors Which Influence Serum Lipids," *J. Am. Diet. Assoc.,* **52**:198–201, 1968.
Keys, A.: "Blood Lipids in Man—A Brief Review," *J. Am. Diet. Assoc.,* **51**:508–16, 1967.
Mead, J. F.: "Present Knowledge of Fat," *Nutr. Rev.,* **24**:33–35, 1966.
Review: "Acetoacetate Production in Starvation Ketosis," *Nutr. Rev.,* **26**:147–49, 1968.
———: "Fat and Cholesterol in the Diet," *Nutr. Rev.,* **23**:3–6, 1965.
———: "Glyceride Structure and Fat Absorption," *Nutr. Rev.,* **27**:18–20, 1969.
———: "Safety of Used Frying Fats," *Nutr. Rev.,* **26**:210–12, 1968.
Scheig, R.: "What Is a Dietary Fat?" *Am. J. Clin. Nutr.,* **22**:651–53, 1969.

7 Energy Metabolism

The amount of available energy has become a crucial issue in our times, whether it be the oil, gas, coal, or electrical power to heat, air-condition, or light our homes, drive our automobiles, run our factories, and so on; or whether, in direct human terms, it be the amount of available food to yield the energy required to accomplish the involuntary and voluntary activities of the body. Sufficient food to meet the energy needs is the first nutritional priority. When the supply of calories is moderately reduced, the capacity to work is also reduced, and in children growth is retarded or ceases. As the energy available to the body continues to decrease, the body's own substance will be utilized until eventually no more of the body mass can be sacrificed and death ensues.

Energy transformation. Energy is the capacity to do work. The sun is the original source of all energy, arising from nuclear reactions. Through the action of chlorophyll with sunlight, by the process known as photosynthesis, plants synthesize carbohydrates from carbon dioxide and water. The carbohydrates stored by the plants are then available as energy to animals and to man. All of man's energy is derived from the plant and animal foods he eats. Carbohydrates, fats, and proteins are the energy-yielding substances. In a typical American diet carbohydrate furnishes 45 to 55 per cent of the calories, fats, 35 to 45 per cent, and proteins about 15 per cent.

Forms of energy. Potential (storage) energy is continuously available in the body from the small amounts of glycogen in muscle and liver, the sizable fat depots, and the cellular mass itself. The potential energy is transformed to other forms to accomplish the work of the body: for example, *mechanical* energy for muscle contraction; *osmotic* energy to maintain the transport of fluids and nutrients; *electrical* energy for the transmission of nerve impulses; *chemical* energy as in the synthesis of new compounds; and *thermal* energy for heat regulation.

Whenever one form of energy is produced, another form is reduced by exactly the same amount. This is known as the law of *conservation of energy,* which states that energy can be neither created nor destroyed. When foods supply more energy than is needed for the work of the body, the excess is stored as fat; it has resulted in weight gain. This store of energy is available at such a time as the food supply might furnish too few calories for the body's activities.

Transformation to ATP. If the potential energy of glucose, fatty acids, and amino acids were released in one step, much of it would be lost and wasted as heat. The cell utilizes energy efficiently by releasing small amounts of it at a time in a series of steps that occur in the mitochondria of the cell. The energy liberated in these steps is trapped in the form of adenosine triphosphate (ATP). This compound has two high-energy phosphate bonds, one of which is released in the innumerable transactions of the body that require energy (ATP→ADP). For example:

$$Glucose + ATP \rightarrow Glucose\text{-}6\text{-}phosphate + ADP$$

The reactions that occur in the catabolism of glucose, fatty acids, and amino acids liberate energy, and thereby ATP is again formed (ADP→ ATP). ATP is sometimes called the "legal tender" or "currency" for energy of the living organism, for, like the convenience of small coins of money, it is the convenient form for small bursts of energy.

The formation of ATP occurs in the metabolic

pathways described in the preceding chapters on carbohydrates, fats, and proteins. Initially these nutrients are oxidized independently to the "common denominators," namely pyruvic acid, acetyl coenzyme A, and alpha-ketoglutaric acid. In this first phase some of the reactions require ATP for their initiation; other reactions release small amounts of energy so that ATP is regenerated from ADP, but the net yield of energy is not great.

The common denominators enter the tricarboxylic acid (TCA) cycle, which is the common pathway for the oxidation of carbohydrates, fats, and proteins. About 90 per cent of the energy liberated from food occurs by this pathway.

Hydrogen transport. Each turn of the TCA cycle results in the removal of four pairs of hydrogen ions and the liberation of energy; the combination of hydrogen with oxygen to form water; the formation of carbon dioxide, which is removed by the respiration; and the production of another molecule of oxalacetate to initiate another turn of the cycle. The hydrogen ions are removed from the compounds in the cycle by the action of enzymes known as *dehydrogenases*. As the hydrogen ions are liberated they are passed, step by step, along a series of enzymes and coenzymes, some of which contain the B complex vitamins niacin and riboflavin. Finally, the pairs of hydrogen ions reach the stage where they combine with oxygen to form water. By this *electron transport system* small amounts of energy are liberated at each step; the energy is trapped in the form of a high-energy phosphate bond added to ADP to form ATP. Each turn of the TCA cycle yields 12 molecules of ATP.

Measurement. The potential energy value of foods and the energy exchanges of the body are expressed in terms of the calorie, which is a heat unit. By definition, the large Calorie, or kilocalorie (kcal), is the amount of heat required to raise the temperature of 1 kg water 1° C (from 15° to 16°). This unit is always used in nutrition and is 1000 times as large as the small calorie used in chemistry and physics. Some attempts have been made to use the term *kilocalorie* in writings on nutrition, but most of the nutrition literature continues to use the short-

ened form, *calorie;* this form will be used in this text.

The fuel value of foods is readily determined by means of an apparatus known as a bomb calorimeter. (See Figure 7–1.) A weighed sample of food is placed in a heavy steel container called a "bomb." After the bomb is charged with oxygen, the sample is ignited and the heat is dissipated into a known volume of water surrounding the bomb. By noting the change in the temperature of the water, one can calculate the energy value of the food by applying the definition for a calorie.

The joule. The joule, abbreviated J, is the unit of energy in the metric system. It is used internationally in the sciences, and it is logical that it also be used for expressing energy values in nutrition which is so closely related to chemistry and physics. The VIIIth International Congress of Nutrition in Prague in 1969 and the

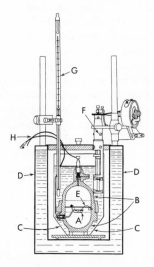

Figure 7–1. Diagram of bomb calorimeter with bomb in position. (Courtesy, the Emerson Apparatus Company, Boston, Mass.)

  (*A*) Platinum dish holding weighed food sample.
  (*B*) Bomb filled with pure oxygen enclosing food sample.
  (*C*) Can holding water of known weight in which the bomb is submerged.
  (*D*) Outer double-walled insulating jacket.
  (*E*) Fuse, which is ignited by an electric current.
  (*F*) Motor-driven water stirrer.
  (*G*) Thermometer calibrated to 1/1000° C.
  (*H*) Electric wires to send current through fuse.

Committee on Nomenclature of the American Institute of Nutrition in 1970 have recommended the adoption of the joule in place of the calorie.

The conversion of tables of food composition and dietary allowances from calories to joules will require a considerable period of time. For those who are accustomed to thinking in terms of calories some adjustment is also required. Although calories will continue as the unit of measurement for a number of years, it is essential that today's student of nutrition be aware of the forthcoming change and be prepared to make it. Young students in the nation's schools will be familiar with the joule but less so with the calorie.

One calorie is equivalent to 4.184 joules; a kilocalorie is equivalent to 4.184 kilojoules (kJ). Thus, a dietary allowance of 2000 kilocalories is 8368 kilojoules. It is anticipated that measurements in kilojoules will replace those in kilocalories when the metric system is fully adopted.

Physiologic fuel factors. The caloric values of foods burned in the bomb calorimeter are somewhat higher than those realized in the body. First, certain small losses occur in digestion for all three nutrients. For the typical mixed American diet, 98 per cent of the carbohydrate, 95 per cent of the fat, and 92 per cent of the protein are digested and absorbed. The carbohydrates and fats which are absorbed are entirely oxidized in the body as they are in the bomb calorimeter. In the case of proteins, however, the end products of metabolism are partly eliminated as urea and other organic nitrogen compounds which are combustible. In other words, the body loses part of the potential energy value of protein so that the net value is less than that measured by the calorimeter.

The "physiologic fuel factors" proposed by Atwater are based upon the corrections for losses of unabsorbed nutrients in the feces and for the caloric equivalent of the nitrogenous products in the urine. These factors are

1 gm of pure protein will yield 4 calories
1 gm of pure fat will yield 9 calories
1 gm of pure carbohydrate will yield 4 calories

Specific fuel factors. Each food has a specific coefficient of digestibility, and thus the fuel value likewise would be specific for each given food. For example, the coefficient of digestibility for the protein in milk, eggs, and meat is 97 per cent, but for the protein of whole ground corn meal it is only 60 per cent; the coefficient of digestibility for the carbohydrate of wheat is 98 per cent when white flour (70 to 74 per cent extraction) is used, but is 90 per cent when whole-wheat flour (97 to 100 per cent extraction) is used. The errors introduced by the variations in digestibility are small for the typical mixed American diet, and for any calculations the student is likely to make Atwater's physiologic fuel values are sufficiently reliable.

Whenever the diet differs markedly from the typical diet on which Atwater based his data, considerable error is introduced with the use of average fuel values. For example, the caloric value of a diet which is predominant in cereal foods would be overestimated. This can be a serious problem when it involves suitable allocation of food to populations where the food supply is short. The Nutrition Division of FAO[1] has made a study of specific factors applicable to foods and has published a table for estimating calories based on these specific factors rather than on the average values. The energy values listed in tables of food composition developed by the U.S. Department of Agriculture employ specific fuel factors for each food.

MEASUREMENT OF ENERGY
EXCHANGE OF THE BODY

Direct and indirect calorimetry. *Direct calorimetry* is the measurement of the amount of heat produced by the body. By this method the individual is placed in a specially constructed chamber called a respiration calorimeter. The chamber is so well insulated that no heat can enter into or escape through the walls. The heat given off by the individual is picked up by water flowing through coils in the chambers. Measurements are made of the temperature of the water at the beginning of the study, at intervals, and

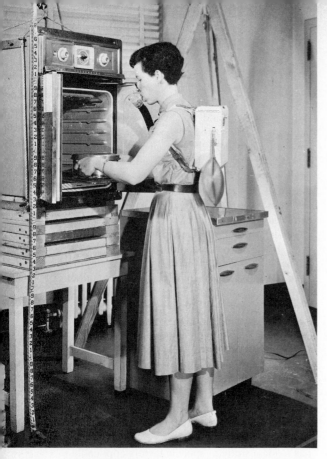

Figure 7–2. The energy expenditure for various kinds of activity may be measured by means of a portable respirometer. (Courtesy, U.S. Department of Agriculture.)

at the termination of the study. The volume of water flowing through the coils is also measured, and the calories expended can be calculated from these data.

The respiration calorimeter is so designed that the oxygen consumption and the carbon dioxide excretion can be measured at the same time the heat production is measured. From numerous studies the relationship of oxygen usage to heat production under varying conditions has been established. Therefore, it is possible to determine the level of energy metabolism by the less time-consuming and far less costly procedures of *indirect calorimetry*. Respiration calorimeters are used in only a few research centers.

Indirect calorimetry measures the amount of oxygen consumed in a given time period and, in other than basal conditions, the amount of car-

bon dioxide excreted. The amount of oxygen consumed is proportional to the amount of heat that is being produced. Numerous experiments on people of all ages have shown that 1 liter of oxygen is equal to 4.825 calories when the conditions for a basal metabolism test, described below, are met.

A portable apparatus is used for measuring the energy expenditure for various types of activity. This is a lightweight piece of equipment, weighing 8 lb or less, and consists of a meter for measuring the volume of expired air and a bag for collecting the sample of expired air. The air samples are analyzed for their amounts of oxygen and carbon dioxide, and from the data it is possible to determine the caloric equivalents. (See Figure 7–2.)

Basal metabolism test. The amount of energy required to carry on the involuntary work of the body is known as the *basal metabolic rate*. It includes the functional activities of the various organs such as the brain, heart, liver, kidneys, and lungs, the secretory activities of the glands, the peristaltic movements of the gastrointestinal tract, the oxidations occurring in resting tissues, and the maintenance of muscle tone. The basal metabolic rate is measured by indirect calorimetry under the following specific conditions.

1. Postabsorptive state: 12 to 16 hours after the last meal; usually performed in the morning.

2. Reclining, but awake: one-half to one hour of rest before the test is necessary if there has been any activity in the morning.

3. Relaxed and free from emotional upsets or fear of the test itself.

4. Normal body temperature.

5. Comfortable room temperature: about 70° to 75° F. Under these conditions, normal individuals fall within ± 15 per cent of standards established for their body size, sex, and age.

Suppose a young woman consumes 1200 cc oxygen in a six-minute test period; in a 24-hour period her basal heat expenditure is calculated as follows:

$$\frac{10 \times 1200 \times 24}{1000} = 288 \text{ liters oxygen in 24 hours}$$

$$288 \times 4.825 \text{ calories} = 1390 \text{ calories}$$

Factors influencing the basal metabolic rate. The adult basal metabolic rate is approximately 1 calorie per kilogram per hour for men and about 0.9 calorie per kilogram per hour for women. Thus, the range of basal metabolism for normal adults is about 1300 to 1700 calories. This accounts for the largest proportion of the total energy requirement for most people. The rate of basal metabolism is influenced by size, shape, and weight of the individual, sex, age, rate of growth, the activity of the endocrine glands, sleep, body temperature, and state of nutrition.

Surface area. Heat is continuously lost through the skin by radiation. Since the heat loss is proportional to the skin surface, the basal heat production is directly proportional to the surface area. A tall, thin person has a greater surface area than an individual of the same weight who is short and fat, and the former therefore will have a higher basal metabolism.

Sex. Women have a metabolic rate about 6 to 10 per cent lower than that of men. Formerly this was attributed to the fact that women had relatively higher proportions of adipose tissue, believed to be metabolically inert. However, this explanation is not fully satisfactory inasmuch as adipose tissue is now known to be metabolically active. The influence of the sex hormones may account for some of the difference.

Age. Per unit of surface area the basal metabolic rate is at its highest during the first two years of life. It declines gradually throughout childhood and accelerates slightly in adolescence. Thereafter the decline continues throughout life with somewhat more rapid decrease in the later years. The rapid growth rate explains the high metabolic rate in early childhood. In later years the lessened muscle tone and the reduction in muscle mass account for the lower rate.

Sleep. During the sleeping hours the basal metabolism is about 10 per cent lower than in the waking state. However, this is quite variable depending upon the amount of motion of the individual while asleep.

Body temperature. An elevation of the body temperature for each degree F increases the basal metabolism by 7 per cent.

Race. Some reports have indicated that the metabolic rates in Indians and other peoples of Asia are lower than those in Caucasians. Whether this is a racial effect or is caused by environmental factors is not certain.

Endocrine glands. The thyroid gland regulates the rate of energy metabolism, and any change in thyroid activity is reflected in the metabolic rate. If the thyroid is overactive (hyperthyroidism), the metabolism may be speeded up as much as 75 to 100 per cent; if the activity of the gland is decreased (hypothyroidism), the metabolism may be reduced by 30 to 40 per cent.

The measurement of *protein-bound iodine* has now largely replaced the basal metabolism test as a measure of thyroid activity. This test is based upon the fact that the level of protein-bound iodine circulating in the blood is proportional to the degree of thyroid activity. The basal metabolism test is still the method of choice for nutritional studies.

Other endocrine secretions may have a more transitory effect on the basal metabolism. An increased excretion of epinephrine during excitement or fear temporarily raises the metabolic rate. Disturbances of the pituitary gland may also modify the metabolic rate. Just prior to the onset of the menstrual period the metabolism is increased slightly, but it is a little lower than normal during the period. These slight changes are of no overall significance in determining the energy requirement.

State of nutrition. An individual who has been chronically undernourished is likely to have a lower basal metabolic rate. Analyses of metabolism in naturally occurring starvation and of experimental starvation "indicate that the oxidative rate of the active tissues deviates little, if at all, from the metabolic rate of the active mass under normal conditions. The observed decrease in basal metabolism is almost completely accounted for by the decrease in mass of active tissues."[*]

Depending upon the circumstances, undernourished children may have an increase or a

[*]Review: "The Metabolic Rate in Semistarvation," *Nutr. Rev.*, **6**:311, 1948.

decrease of the basal metabolic rate. Underweight school children sometimes show an increased rate because of the high percentage of active lean tissues. When undernutrition is severe, the destruction of body tissues is likely to lower the rate.

Pregnancy. During the last trimester of pregnancy the basal metabolism increases from 15 to 25 per cent. This increase can be accounted for almost entirely by the increase in weight of the woman and the high rate of metabolism of the fetus.

Factors influencing the total energy requirement. Superimposed upon the energy expenditure for maintaining the involuntary activities of the body are such factors as voluntary muscular activity, the effect of food, and the maintenance of the body temperature.

Muscular activity. Next to the basal metabolism, activity accounts for the largest energy expenditure; in fact, for some persons who are vigorously active, the energy needs for activity may exceed those for the basal metabolism. Sedentary work, which includes office work, bookkeeping, typing, teaching, and so forth, calls for less energy than more active and strenuous occupations such as nursing, homemaking, or gardening. A still greater amount of energy is required by those individuals who do hard manual labor such as ditch digging, shifting freight, and lumbering.

The energy expenditure for many activities has been measured in adults and children,[2,3] and the data serve as a guide in setting standards for various groups of people. A wide range of activities has been classified in five groups in Table 7–1. The calorie expenditures listed for each category include the basal metabolism and are representative for adults. The lower figure for each category would apply to women, and the higher figure to men. Of course it must be realized that these would vary from one indi-

Table 7–1. Calorie Expenditure for Various Kinds of Activity*

Type of Activity	Calories per Hour†
Sedentary	80 to 100
Reading; writing; eating; watching television or movies; listening to the radio; sewing; playing cards; typing; and miscellaneous office work and other activities done while sitting that require little or no arm movement	
Light	110 to 160
Preparing and cooking food; doing dishes; dusting; handwashing small articles of clothing; ironing; walking slowly; personal care; miscellaneous office work and other activities done while standing that require some arm movement; and rapid typing and other activities done while sitting that are more strenuous	
Moderate	170 to 240
Making beds; mopping and scrubbing; sweeping; light polishing and waxing; laundering by machine; light gardening and carpentry work; walking moderately fast; other activities done while standing that require moderate arm movement; and activities done while sitting that require more vigorous arm movement	
Vigorous	250 to 350
Heavy scrubbing and waxing; handwashing large articles of clothing; hanging out clothes; stripping beds; other heavy work; walking fast; bowling; golfing; and gardening	
Strenuous	350 and more
Swimming; playing tennis; running; bicycling; dancing; skiing; and playing football	

*Adapted from Page, L., and Fincher, L. J.: *Food and Your Weight.* Home and Garden Bulletin No. 74, U.S. Department of Agriculture, 1960, p. 4.

†Lower figures apply to women, higher figures to men. The figures include the metabolism at rest as well as for the activity.

vidual to another not only on the basis of body size but especially because of variations of intensity of effort expended.

If an exact record of activity for a given 24-hour period were kept, it would be possible with data such as those in Table 7–1 to estimate the daily caloric requirement of an adult. However, such calculations are time consuming and give, at best, only rough approximations since individuals vary widely in the efficiency of their work and in their muscle tone.

The figures in Table 7–1 illustrate the value of exercise in weight control, for it is quite evident that the student who sits quietly watching television, for example, is expending only half as many calories as one who is walking leisurely, and only one fourth as many calories as one who swims for an hour.

Not infrequently the question is raised as to the reason for the differing caloric needs of two people of the same build and body weight who are doing the same kind of work. The energy needs will be greater for the person who wastes many motions in the performance of a piece of work, who works under greater muscle tension, or who finds it difficult to relax completely even when at rest.

Mental effort. The nervous system is continuously active, and its energy requirement is a significant part of the basal rate. However, the energy expenditure beyond the basal rate for intense mental effort as in problem solving or writing examinations does not add appreciably to the caloric requirement. Some students become tense and restless in the solving of problems, but the increased expenditure of energy in such a situation is not primarily that of mental work.

Calorigenic effect of food. The ingestion of food results in increased heat production known as the *calorigenic effect* or *specific dynamic action* of food. The mechanisms that cause this increase are poorly understood. Protein when eaten alone has been shown to increase the metabolic rate by 30 per cent, whereas carbohydrates and fats will produce much smaller increases in metabolism. On the basis of the mixed diets usually eaten, the specific dynamic action is approximately 6 per cent of the energy requirement.[4]

Maintenance of body temperature. Under normal conditions the temperature of the body is controlled by the amount of blood brought to the skin. When the surrounding temperature is low, most of the heat is lost by radiation and conduction, but when the environmental temperature is high, the body heat is lost chiefly through evaporation. It is a well-known fact that more heat is lost by evaporation when the air is dry than when it is humid.

During cold weather, man avoids excessive heat losses from his body by the use of suitable clothing and the heating of his home or place of work. Moreover, body heat is conserved if there is a layer of adipose tissue under the skin. The subcutaneous fat serves to keep heat in the body rather than allowing it to be dissipated through the skin—an advantage in cold weather, but a disadvantage in warm weather.

When the body is subjected to extreme cold, the body temperature is maintained by an increase in involuntary and often voluntary activity. The blood vessels constrict so that there is less blood reaching the skin surface; the muscles become tense; and shivering follows. These involuntary activities result in a considerable increase in the metabolic rate. As anyone knows who has been exposed to a cold winter day, one is not likely to stand still. In addition, then, to the increased energy expenditure occasioned by the involuntary activities, the individual increases his voluntary activity.

Growth. The building of new tissue represents a storage of energy in one form or another; for example, every gram of protein in body tissue represents about 4 calories. When growth is rapid, as during the first year of life, the energy allowance must be high. In fact, the caloric need is greater per unit of body weight than at any other time in life. In pregnancy, likewise, the energy needs are increased to cover the building of new tissues. These needs are discussed in more detail in Chapters 21, 22, and 23.

CALORIC ALLOWANCES

Daily allowances. The Recommended Dietary Allowances[5] for calories take into account sex, body size, age, climate, and activity. They are based on the maintenance of desirable body weight or a suitable rate of growth and must be adjusted upward or downward to meet individual needs. The allowances are a rough guide in dietary planning for groups; they may vary widely for any given individual. The bases for these allowances are described in the following paragraphs.

Reference standard. The allowances for men and women are stated in terms of persons who are in good health, who live in an environment with a mean annual temperature of 20° C (68° F), and who weigh 70 kg (154 lb) and 58 kg (128 lb), respectively. Their physical activity is "light" and they are engaged in occupations that could be described neither as sedentary nor as heavy physical activity. The allowances for the American man and woman have been adjusted downward from the recommendations made by the Committee on Calorie Requirements of the Food and Agriculture Organization. For the man 23 to 50 years the calorie allowance is 2700, and for the woman the allowance is 2000 calories.

Adjustments for body size. Calorie allowances should be based upon the desirable weight for height and health. For example, for women 23 to 50 years who have similar activity but who vary in height and in desirable weight the following adjustments are typical:

kg	lb	kilocalories
50	110	1800
55	121	1950
58	128	2000
60	132	2050
65	143	2200
70	154	2300

Adjustments for age. The highest caloric requirement for males occurs between ages 15 and 22, and for females between ages 11 and 14. Beginning in early adulthood there is a gradual decline in basal metabolism and physical activity. Since the desirable weight at 25 years is a goal to maintain throughout life, the calorie intake needs to be correspondingly reduced. The Basic Diet pattern (Table 13–2) furnishes almost 1200 calories. Thus, it becomes

Table 7–2. Recommended Daily Dietary Allowances for Energy*

	Age years	Weight kg	Weight lb	Energy kcal		Age years	Weight kg	Weight lb	Energy kcal
Infants	0.0–0.5	6	14	kg x 117	Males (cont.)	23–50	70	154	2700
	0.5–1.0	9	20	kg x 108		51+	70	154	2400
Children	1–3	13	28	1300	Females	11–14	44	97	2400
	4–6	20	44	1800		15–18	54	119	2100
	7–10	30	66	2400		19–22	58	128	2100
Males	11–14	44	97	2800		23–50	58	128	2000
	15–18	61	134	3000		51+	58	128	1800
	19–22	67	147	3000	Pregnancy				+300
					Lactation				+500

Recommended Dietary Allowances, Food and Nutrition Board, National Academy of Sciences—National Research Council, Washington, D.C., 1973.

apparent that older persons, especially women, must restrict calorie-rich desserts and snacks if they are to avoid obesity.

Adjustment for climate. In summer and winter most Americans live in an environmental temperature of 20° to 25° C. In winter they wear warm clothing, live and work in well-heated buildings, and travel by heated means of transportation. Likewise, in summer many of them live and work in air-conditioned buildings. Therefore, adjustments for temperature are not usually necessary.

A small increase in calories (2 to 5 per cent) may be necessary in winter for the person carrying a weight of heavy clothing. When a person is inadequately clothed, the calorie expenditure may increase considerably.

When men are physically active at high environmental temperatures, an increase in the calorie allowance of 0.5 per cent for each degree above 30° C is indicated. This increase is necessary to cover the slight increase that occurs in the metabolic rate and in the extra energy expenditure to maintain normal body temperature. In warm climates, most individuals tend to reduce their activity and thus their caloric needs.

Adjustments for activity. Today the average work week is 35 to 40 hours; sleep may account for 50 to 60 hours; eating and travel to and from work may consume 20 hours, more or less; and leisure time may amount to 50 or 60 hours in a given week. The leisure activities may range from reading, watching television, movies, or stamp collecting, on the one hand, to such vigorous activities as tennis, gardening, golf, and swimming, on the other hand. Obviously, to set up a caloric allowance in terms of one's activity at work alone is to ignore a large part of one's day.

The recommended allowances are set up in terms of the general average of the population, but individuals will differ widely. Only rarely will these allowances need to be increased by more than 1500 calories for the healthy adult. For many Americans who are sedentary in their occupations and who are also inactive in their leisure, the allowances are too high.

The best guide to the adequacy of the caloric allowances lies in the maintenance of desirable weight. Individuals should be encouraged to weigh themselves at regular intervals. Thus, the insidious and undesirable increases in body weight over desirable levels may be checked by appropriate reduction in the intake of energy-rich foods. Likewise, suitable rates of growth may be maintained. The dangers of excessive weight gain, or of underweight, are discussed in Chapter 31.

Selecting foods for energy. The inclusion of minimum amounts of each of the Four Food Groups provides energy at approximately basal levels for the adult (see Figure 7–3). To com-

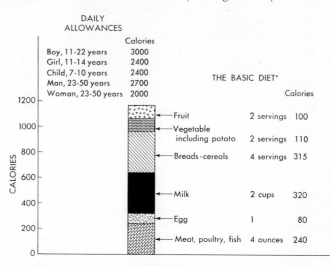

Figure 7–3. The Basic Diet provides just about half of the energy requirement of the teen-age girl and almost three fifths of that for the woman of 23 years. See Table 13–2 for complete calculations.

DAILY ALLOWANCES

Calories
Boy, 11-22 years   3000
Girl, 11-14 years   2400
Child, 7-10 years   2400
Man, 23-50 years   2700
Woman, 23-50 years   2000

THE BASIC DIET*

		Calories
Fruit	2 servings	100
Vegetable including potato	2 servings	110
Breads-cereals	4 servings	315
Milk	2 cups	320
Egg	1	80
Meat, poultry, fish	4 ounces	240

plete the caloric requirement, any foods desired may be selected. More foods from the bread-cereals group will not only increase the caloric intake at low cost, but will enhance the protein, iron, and B complex vitamin level of the diet. The selection of additional foods from the other three groups will increase the caloric level of the diet in varying degree and provide further nutritional benefits in protein, minerals, and vitamins.

Fats and sugars are concentrated sources of energy and may be used to rapidly increase the caloric level of the diet. They have a legitimate place in the diet, but it must be borne in mind that fats (except butter and fortified margarine) and sugars do not contain protein, minerals, and vitamins. When they constitute a large proportion of the total calories in the diet, there is danger that other nutrient needs will not be met. Too many Americans select diets in which fats and sugars provide one third or more of the calories. This is an important area for nutrition education.

Some Points for Emphasis in Nutrition Education

1. The calorie is a unit of heat. It measures the amount of energy available from foods and the energy exchange taking place in the body.

2. A calorie is the same whether it comes from carbohydrates, fats, or proteins. Carbohydrates and proteins furnish 4 large calories (kcal) per gram and fats 9 large calories per gram.

3. Weight for weight, foods that are dry or greasy are relatively high in calories: for example, cereals, cookies, cakes, pastries, sweets, butter, fatty meats. Foods that have a high concentration of water are much lower in calories: for example, fruits and vegetables.

4. The basal metabolism is the amount of energy the body uses at rest. It ranges from about 1300 to 1700 calories for adults and accounts for about half or more of the total calories needed by the average American.

5. The amount of activity is the important factor determining the number of calories needed above the basal metabolism. For the average young woman in America about 2000 calories are needed daily; the average young man needs about 2700 calories. Sedentary young adults require less than this, and older persons require considerably fewer calories.

6. In addition to furnishing the needed amounts of protein, minerals, and vitamins, the Four Food Groups in the recommended amounts provide almost 1200 calories. Thus, a young woman can use a reasonable amount of desserts, fats, and sugars without exceeding her energy requirement, but the older woman has very little leeway in using these foods if she is also going to meet her nutritional requirements.

7. The body is in energy balance when the calories supplied by food are exactly equal to the energy needed for all the involuntary and voluntary activities of the body. Weight is neither gained nor lost.

8. If the calorie intake is greater than the body needs, weight is gained, and if the calorie intake is less than the body needs, weight is lost.

Problems and Review

1. Define or explain what is meant by calorie; basal metabolism; bomb calorimeter; respiratory calorimeter; physiologic fuel factor; joule.
2. *Problem.* Using data from Table A-1, calculate the number of grams required of each of the following foods to furnish 100 calories: butter, milk, cheese, egg, potato, apple, banana, orange, sugar, bread, lean beef, cooked rice, chocolate cake.

3. Why are the physiologic fuel factors not suitable for calculating calorie values for the staple foods used in Asia and Africa?
4. What are the standard conditions for performing a basal metabolism test? What factors might make the basal metabolism of two adult individuals of the same age vary? How does age itself affect the basal metabolism?
5. Explain how the following factors affect the total energy requirement: muscular activity; food; climate; clothing; growth; muscle tension; endocrine secretions. Which of these has the greatest effect?
6. *Problem.* Calculate your own calorie intake for one day. What percentage of your calories was derived from each of the Four Food Groups? What percentage from sweets, fats, desserts, and snack foods?
7. Why would you expect the caloric requirement of many poor people to be higher during cold weather than that of people in better economic circumstances?
8. What is the best indication of adequate caloric intake?

Cited References

1. Committee on Calorie Conversion Factors and Food Consumption Tables: *Energy Yielding Components of Food and Computation of Calorie Values.* Food and Agriculture Organization, 1947.
2. Taylor, C. M., and MacLeod, G.: *Rose's Laboratory Handbook of Dietetics,* 5th ed. The Macmillan Company, New York, 1949, p. 73.
3. Passmore, R., and Durnin, J. V. G. A.: "Human Energy Expenditure," *Physiol. Rev.,* **34**:801–40, 1955.
4. Swift, R. W., *et al.:* "The Effect of High Versus Low Protein Equicaloric Diets on the Heat Production of Human Subjects," *J. Nutr.,* **65**:89–102, 1958.
5. Food and Nutrition Board: *Recommended Dietary Allowances,* 8th ed. National Academy of Sciences–National Research Council, Washington, D.C., 1973.

Additional References

Ames, S. R.: "The Joule—Unit of Energy," *J. Am. Diet. Assoc.,* **57**:415–16, 1970.
Buskirk, E. R., *et al.:* "Human Energy Expenditure Studies in the National Institute of Arthritis and Metabolic Diseases Metabolic Chamber. I. Interaction of Cold Environments and Specific Dynamic Action. II. Sleep," *Am. J. Clin. Nutr.,* **8**:602–13, 1960.
Buskirk, E. R., and Mendez, J.: "Nutrition, Environment and Work Performance with Special Reference to Altitude," *Fed. Proc.,* **26**:1760–67, 1967.
Calorie Requirements. FAO Nutritional Studies No. 15, Food and Agriculture Organization, Rome, 1957.
Consolazio, C. F., *et al.:* "Energy Requirements of Men in Extreme Heat," *J. Nutr.,* **73**:126–34, 1961.
Durnin, J. V. G. A.,: "The Use of Surface Area and of Body Weight as Standards of Reference to Studies on Human Energy Expenditure," *Br. J. Nutr.,* **13**:68–71, 1959.
Durnin, J. V. G. A., and Brockway, J. M.: "Determination of the Total Daily Energy Expenditure in Man by Indirect Calorimetry: Assessment of the Accuracy of a Modern Technique," *Br. J. Nutr.,* **13**:41–53, 1959.
Groen, J. J.: "An Indirect Method for Approximating Calorie Expenditure of Physical Activity. A Recommendation for Dietary Surveys," *J. Am. Diet. Assoc.,* **52**:313–17, 1968.
Harper, A. E.: "Remarks on the Joule," *J. Am. Diet. Assoc.,* **57**:416–18, 1970.
Konishi, F.: "Food Energy Equivalents of Various Activities," *J. Am. Diet. Assoc.,* **46**:186–88, 1965.

Lehninger, A. L.: "Energy Transformation in the Cell," *Sci. Am.,* **202**:102–14, 1960.

Nutrition and Working Efficiency. Base Study No. 5, Food and Agriculture Organization, Rome, 1962.

Richardson, M., and McCracken, E. C.: *Energy Expenditures of Women Performing Selected Activities.* Home Econ. Res. Rep. No. 11, U.S. Department of Agriculture, Washington, D.C., 1960.

Whedon, G. D.: "New Research in Human Energy Metabolism," *J. Am. Diet. Assoc.,* **35**:682–86, 1959.

Wilder, R. M.: "Calorimetry, The Basis of the Science of Nutrition," *Arch. Intern. Med.,* **103**:146–54, 1959.

8 Mineral Elements

The full story of each mineral element required by the human being is every bit as dramatic as that of proteins, or vitamins, or the energy-yielding components. New developments in laboratory technology now permit tracing minute amounts of mineral elements in living tissues, and many an element formerly considered to be a contaminant has joined the ranks of the essential nutrients. Fortunately, for those who must plan daily meals for individuals and families, present knowledge indicates that diets which include recommended amounts of foods from the Four Food Groups are likely to meet the needs for the many mineral elements—except for iron for adolescent girls and women.

This chapter is concerned with calcium, phosphorus, magnesium, sulfur, iron, and iodine and includes a brief discussion of other equally important but seldom deficient mineral elements. Sodium, potassium, and chlorine together with water balance and acid-base balance are discussed in Chapter 9.

Mineral composition of the body. About 4 per cent of the body weight is made up of the elements usually designated as minerals. These may be defined as those elements which remain largely as ash when plant or animal tissues are burned. Calcium and phosphorus account for three fourths of the mineral elements in the body, and five other elements account for most of the rest. Many of the elements are present in such minute amounts that they are generally referred to as *trace elements* or *micronutrients*. Some of the trace elements are essential to body functions; others may be present as contaminants. Table 8–1 summarizes the mineral composition of the body, including approximate concentrations of many of the minerals.

General functions. Mineral elements are present in organic compounds such as phosphoproteins, phospholipids, hemoglobin, and thyroxine; as inorganic compounds such as sodium chloride and calcium phosphate; and as free ions. They enter into the structure of every cell of the body. Hard skeletal structures contain the greater proportions of some elements such as calcium, phosphorus, and magnesium, and soft tissues contain relatively higher proportions of potassium.

Mineral elements are constituents of enzymes such as iron in the catalases and cytochromes; of hormones such as iodine in thyroxine; and of vitamins such as cobalt in vitamin B_{12}. Their presence in body fluids regulates the permeability of cell membranes; the osmotic pressure and water balance between intracellular and extracellular compartments; the response of nerves to stimuli; the contraction of muscles; and the maintenance of acid-base equilibrium.

The amount of an element present gives no clue to its importance in body functions. For example, a few milligrams of an element such as iodine can make a critical difference in the health of an individual.

Dynamic equilibrium. For the normal adult a balance usually exists between the intake of an element and its excretion. On the one hand, absorption and excretion are constantly adjusted to guard against an overload that might produce toxic effects. On the other hand, precise mechanisms carefully conserve needed amounts of mineral elements.

Homeostasis is maintained in spite of the fact that a continuous flow of nutrients into the cell and away from the cell is taking place. For example, bone, often thought of as being inert, is an exceedingly active tissue in its constant uptake and release of mineral constituents. Never-

Table 8–1. Mineral Composition of the Body

	Amount in the Body*		Micronutrients (no estimates of amounts)	
	Per Cent	Per 70 Kilograms Gm		
Major Elements			*Essential for Body Functions*	
Calcium	1.5–2.2	1050–1540	Cobalt	
Phosphorus	0.8–1.2	560–840	Selenium	
Potassium	0.35	245	Zinc	
Sulfur	0.25	175		
Sodium	0.15	105	*Probably Essential*	
Chlorine	0.15	105	Chromium	
Magnesium	0.05	35	Fluorine	
			Molybdenum	
Micronutrients			*No Known Function*	
Iron	0.004	2.8	Aluminum	Cadmium
Manganese	0.0003	0.21	Arsenic	Lead
Copper	0.00015	0.105	Barium	Nickel
Iodine	0.00004	0.024	Boron	Silicon
			Bromine	Strontium
				Vanadium

*Calculations are on the basis of elementary composition of the body as stated by H. C. Sherman in *Chemistry of Food and Nutrition*, 8th ed. The Macmillan Company, New York, 1952, p. 227.

theless, a state of balance or *dynamic equilibrium* is maintained, provided that the supply of nutrients is adequate. (See Figure 8–1.)

Foods as sources of mineral elements. Four factors need to be considered when selecting foods for their mineral content: (1) the concentration of the mineral in the food; (2) how much of a given food is ordinarily consumed; (3) whether the food has lost some of its minerals through refinement or in cooking processes; and (4) whether the food contains the mineral in available form.

Each of the Four Food Groups furnishes important amounts of several minerals. Fats and sugars are practically devoid of mineral elements, and highly refined cereals and flours are poor sources of most of them. Even a good selection of foods to meet nutritional requirements does not guarantee sufficient iodine in many parts of the world. Many women and adolescent girls are unable to obtain sufficient iron even from a good diet and still keep within their caloric requirement.

CALCIUM

Distribution and functions. Of the approximately 1200 gm of calcium in the adult body, 99 per cent is combined as the salts that give hardness to the bones and teeth. The bones not only provide the rigid framework for the body, but they also furnish the reserves of calcium to the circulation so that the concentration in the plasma can be kept constant at all times.

The remaining 1 per cent of calcium in the adult—about 10 to 12 gm—is widely distributed in body fluids where it fulfills many functions. Calcium is a catalyst for the conversion of prothrombin to thrombin, this being one of the several steps in the clotting of blood; it increases the permeability of cell membranes; it activates a number of enzymes including lipase, adenosine triphosphatase, and some proteolytic enzymes; it has a role in the transmission of nerve impulses; and it is directly related to muscle contraction. In the absence of calcium, muscles lose their ability to contract.

NUTRIENT INTAKE BELOW RECOMMENDED ALLOWANCE
Average Intake of Group Below Recommended Dietary Allowance, NAS-NCR, 1968

U.S. Diets of Men, Women, and Children, One Day in Spring 1965

Sex-Age Group	Protein	Calcium	Iron	Vitamin A value	Thiamine	Riboflavin	Ascorbic acid
Male and Female							
Under 1 year			● ● ● ●				Below by:
1-2 years			● ● ● ●				1-10% ●
3-5 years			● ●				11-20% ● ●
6-8 years							21-29% ● ● ●
							30% or more ● ● ● ●
Male:							
9-11 years		●					
12-14 years		● ●	● ● ●	●			
15-17 years		●	●				
18-19 years							
20-34 years							
35-54 years		●					
55-64 years		● ●					
65-74 years		● ●					
75 years and over		● ● ●		●		● ●	●
Female:							
9-11 years		● ● ●	● ● ● ●	●			
12-14 years		● ● ●	● ● ● ●	●	●		
15-17 years		● ● ● ●	● ● ● ●		● ●		
18-19 years		● ● ●	● ● ● ●	●	●		
20-34 years		● ● ●	● ● ● ●		●	●	
35-54 years		● ● ● ●	● ● ● ●		●	● ●	
55-64 years		● ● ● ●			●	●	
65-74 years		● ● ● ●	●	●	● ●	● ●	
75 years and over		● ● ● ●	●	● ●	● ●	● ● ●	

Figure 8–1. According to the 1965 dietary survey of the U.S. Department of Agriculture, calcium and iron were the nutrients that were most frequently below Recommended Dietary Allowances. Note that females were much more frequently below recommendations than were males. (Courtesy, U.S. Department of Agriculture.)

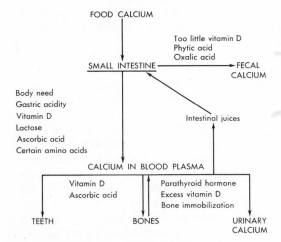

Figure 8–2. The utilization of calcium.

Absorption. Body need is the major factor governing the amount of calcium that will be absorbed. Healthy adults receiving a diet that meets recommended allowances absorb about 30 per cent of the calcium contained in their diets; the absorption from individual foods may vary from 10 to 40 per cent. At high intakes of calcium, the percentage that is absorbed is decreased. Growing children and pregnant and lactating women absorb 40 per cent or more of the calcium in their diets. (See Figure 8–2.)

People who customarily ingest low-calcium diets absorb high proportions of the total intake. The ability to efficiently utilize a limited intake of calcium, especially in favorable climates where the vitamin D supply is ample, explains why many people have satisfactory calcium nutrition despite the low intakes. On the other hand, individuals who have been accustomed to liberal intakes of calcium may show negative calcium balances for several weeks to several months before they become adjusted to lower levels.

Calcium salts are more soluble in acid solution, and hence most of the absorption occurs from the duodenum. Once bile and pancreatic juices have mixed with the chyme, the solubility of the calcium salts and hence the absorption are reduced. Because of the prevalence of achlorhydria, elderly persons may have a reduced absorption. An increase in the motility of the gastrointestinal tract also decreases the percentage of absorption.

Many dietary factors enhance or interfere with the absorption of calcium. Vitamin D facilitates the entrance of calcium into the mucosal cells and also improves the absorption from the duodenum. Calcium absorption is increased with high-protein diets, presumably because of the influence of specific amino acids, especially lysine, serine, and arginine. Lactose is also believed to improve the rate of absorption. Greenwald and his associates[1] found no beneficial effect by adding lactose to a high-calcium diet consumed by two osteoporotic women and one postsurgical hypoparathyroid man.

Oxalic acid, phytic acid, excess fat, and excess phosphate reduce the absorption of calcium because of the formation of insoluble complexes with calcium. Although these effects can be clearly demonstrated in experimental animals, the amounts of these factors in typical American diets are not believed to be sufficiently great to interfere seriously with the absorption of calcium. Oxalic acid is found in spinach, Swiss chard, beet tops, cocoa, and rhubarb. Spinach, for example, contains sufficient calcium to bind the oxalic acid, and none of the calcium in other foods eaten at the same meal would be adversely affected.[2] The amount of cocoa that could be ingested at a time is too small to reduce the absorption of calcium significantly; thus, there is no reason to avoid chocolate milk since the calcium will be as well utilized as that in plain milk.

Phytic acid is an organic phosphate compound found in the outer layers of cereal grains. It binds calcium into an insoluble complex, but the effect would be important only when whole-grain cereals comprised a major part of the diet and when the calcium intake was also low.

Contradictory reports have been given on the effect of fats. On the one hand, fats reduce intestinal motility so that there is longer contact with the absorbing surfaces. On the other hand, free fatty acids combine with calcium to form insoluble soaps that are excreted. Foods high in unsaturated fatty acids have little effect, whereas those high in saturated fatty acids are more likely to yield some soaps. In malabsorption syndromes such as sprue and celiac disease, the amount of unabsorbed fat is great and the calcium losses are then also serious.

Metabolism. The concentration of calcium in the plasma is kept within the narrow range of 9 to 11 mg per 100 ml, of which about 40 per cent is bound to plasma protein and 60 per cent is diffusible. Calcium is constantly being withdrawn from the circulation to effect mineralization of bone and for the many regulatory activities listed on page 104. When the plasma concentration of calcium falls, the parathyroid gland secrets parathormone, which brings about release of calcium from bone, thereby restoring the blood to its normal level. Parathormone also increases the reabsorption of calcium by the renal tubules and increases the excretion of phosphates in the urine, thereby maintaining normal calcium-to-phosphorus ratios in the blood.

The maintenance of the plasma calcium is not directly dependent upon the diet inasmuch as the bones are continuously releasing calcium. In the healthy adult bone mineralization and demineralization (resorption) are equal. During growth, the addition of mineral to bone exceeds the amounts that are removed. When the dietary intake is inadequate, the readily available stores at the ends of the bones, known as *trabeculae*, are first used up; then calcium from the shaft of the bone is withdrawn. Up to 40 per cent of the calcium may be withdrawn from bone over a long period of time before the rarefaction of bone can be detected by x-ray. By this time, bones are fragile and fracture easily.

Bone. Bone consists of organic and inorganic substances. The principal organic substance is the protein collagen, and the ground substance consists of small amounts of mucoproteins and mucopolysaccharides, especially chondroitin sulfate. The formation of bone is initiated early in fetal life with the development of the cartilagenous matrix. During the latter part of pregnancy some mineralization of the fetal skeleton takes place so that the infant at birth has a body calcium content of about 28 gm.

Bone hardness consists of a gradual mineralization of the cartilage. The process is referred to as calcification, mineralization, or ossification. Sufficient mineralization occurs during the first few months of life so that the skeleton can support the weight of the baby when he begins to walk. During childhood and adolescence the bones increase in length and in diameter, this increase in size depending upon the adequacy of the protein supply to form the matrix. The bones continue to increase in hardness for the first 20 years or so of life. Thus, at maturity the calcium content of the body is about 1000 to 1200 gm, depending upon body size; most of this is in the bone.

The complex mineral substance in bone consists of crystals that are ultramicroscopic in size, and that resemble apatite—$Ca_{10} (PO_4)_6 (OH)_2$. Small amounts of the calcium can be replaced by magnesium, sodium, potassium, lead, or strontium. Likewise the anions sulfate, fluoride, citrate, carbonate, and chloride may enter into the structure.

A number of factors influence the mineralization and resorption of bone. Vitamin D is essential for the deposit of minerals into the matrix. On the other hand, parathormone brings about resorption of bone. The emotions have an important bearing upon the calcium balance. Several studies have shown that persons who are under nervous strain or worry have negative calcium balances even though the dietary intake may be good.

Teeth. Like bones, teeth are complex structures consisting of a protein matrix and mineral salts, principally calcium and phosphorus as hydroxyapatite. In the fetus the development of teeth begins by the fourth month and calcification proceeds during the growth of the fetus. Prenatally and during infancy and childhood tooth development requires adequate supplies of many diet factors including not only calcium and phosphorus, but also vitamins A and D, and protein. The deciduous teeth of the infant are fully mineralized by the end of the first year of life, but the calcification of permanent teeth is completed at various times during childhood and adolescence; for some teeth the mineralization is not completed until early adult years.

The turnover of calcium in teeth is very slow, but, unlike calcium in bone, once the calcium in teeth is lost it cannot be replaced. Thus, any factor that increases the solubility of mineral salts at the tooth surfaces will lead to decay: for example, the activity of microorganisms when sugars stick to the teeth. On the other hand, the presence of fluoride in the salts of tooth enamel increases the hardness, thereby reducing their decay. (See page 118.) Because of the slow rate of turnover of calcium in teeth, the fetus does not take much calcium from the mother's teeth, and the popular notion of the loss of "a tooth for every child" is false.

Excretion. The daily losses of calcium in the urine average 175 mg in the adult, but individuals vary widely. In addition, about 20 mg calcium is excreted in the sweat, with considerably increased amounts during heavy perspiration. Fecal calcium includes (1) approximately 125 mg derived from the digestive juices and (2) unabsorbed dietary calcium. The total endogenous losses are about 320 mg daily.

Daily allowances. The Food and Nutrition Board[3] has set the calcium allowance for the adult at 800 mg. This assumes that 40 per cent of the dietary calcium will be absorbed, thus fully covering the 320 mg lost in urine, feces, and sweat each day.

The calcium allowance for infants one to six months is 360 mg, and for infants 6 to 12 months is 540 mg. The allowance for children from one to ten years is 800 mg. Boys and girls from 11 to 18 years should have 1200 mg. During pregnancy and lactation 1200 mg calcium is recommended.

The recommendations of the FAO/WHO Expert Committee[4] for calcium are somewhat lower than the levels cited above. This committee has recommended 400 to 500 mg calcium as a "practical allowance" for adults.

Food sources of calcium. The calcium content of some typical foods is shown in Table 8–2, and the calcium contribution of the basic diet pattern is charted in Figure 8–3. Milk is the outstanding source of calcium in the diet; without it, a satisfactory intake of calcium is extremely difficult. Whole or skimmed, homogenized or nonhomogenized, plain or chocolate-flavored, sweet or sour milks are equally good. For the adult 2 to 3 cups milk daily and for the child 3 to 4 cups daily will ensure adequate calcium intake. Cheddar cheese is an excellent source of calcium. Cottage cheese and ice cream are good sources but will not adequately substitute for milk. The dairy products, excluding butter, account for three fourths of the calcium in the American dietary.

All of the foods other than dairy products when considered together contribute not more than 200 to 300 mg calcium daily. Certain green leafy vegetables such as mustard greens, turnip greens, kale, and collards are important sources of calcium when they are eaten frequently. Canned salmon with the bones, clams, oysters, and shrimp are likewise good sources, but they are not eaten with frequency. Meats and cereal grains are poor sources. The use of nonfat dry milk in bread enhances the calcium value of the diet. Calcium is also an optional enrichment ingredient in flours and breads.

Various calcium salts such as calcium gluconate, lactate, carbonate, and sulfate are sometimes prescribed by a physician to supplement the dietary intake, especially when milk cannot be taken for one reason or another. Calcium in organic compounds and in inorganic salts is well utilized, but it must be remembered that the substitution of salts for milk as a source of calcium deprives the diet of important amounts of riboflavin, protein, and other milk nutrients.

Effect of calcium deficiency. Suboptimal in-

Table 8–2. Calcium Content of Some Typical Foods

	Household Measure	Calcium mg	Per Cent of Adult Daily Allowance*
Milk, fresh	1 cup	288	36
Milk, nonfat dry, low-density	1/3 cup	288	36
Cheese, American process	1 ounce	198	25
Salmon, pink, canned	3 ounces	167†	21
Collards, cooked	1/2 cup	145	18
Turnip greens, cooked	1/2 cup	126	16
Clams or oysters	1/2 cup	113	14
Mustard greens, cooked	1/2 cup	97	12
Shrimp	3 ounces	98	12
Ice cream	1/8 quart	87	11
Cottage cheese, uncreamed	3 ounces	77	10
Kale, cooked	1/2 cup	74	9
Broccoli, cooked	1/2 cup	66	8
Molasses, light	1 tablespoon	33	4
Egg, whole	1 medium	27	3
Cabbage, raw, shredded	1/2 cup	22	3
Carrots, cooked	1/2 cup	24	3
Bread, 4 per cent nonfat dry milk	1 slice	21	3

*Recommended Dietary Allowance of calcium for the adult is 800 mg.
†Includes bones packed with salmon.

takes of calcium may result in retarded calcification of bones and teeth in the young. Acute
deficiency of calcium is not usually seen unless
there is a concurrent lack of phosphorus and
vitamin D. Such deficiency leads to stunted
growth and rickets, as evidenced by bowing of
the legs, enlargement of the ankles and wrists,
and a hollow chest (see page 154).

It is a misconception that adults are not subject to calcium deficiency. The gradual drainage
from the bones to replace calcium ions that are
lost from the body daily leads to thin, fragile
bones which break easily and which heal with
difficulty. Osteomalacia is discussed in more
detail on page 155, and osteoporosis in Chapter 40.

Hypercalcemia. The milk-alkali syndrome is
characterized by an excess of calcium in the
blood and the soft tissues and by vomiting, gastrointestinal bleeding, and high blood pressure.
It occurs occasionally in patients who have peptic ulcer and who have used excessive alkali
therapy in conjunction with large amounts of
milk over a period of years. It does not occur in
the absence of alkali therapy even though large
amounts of milk are consumed, nor does it occur
when nonabsorbable antacids are used in ulcer
therapy.

Hypercalcemia also occurs in infants who are
given an excess of vitamin D. Gastrointestinal
upsets are noted, and growth is retarded. The
condition is corrected by the removal of vitamin D.

PHOSPHORUS

Distribution. Phosphorus accounts for about
1 per cent of body weight or one fourth of the
total mineral matter in the body. About 85 per
cent of the phosphorus is in inorganic combination with calcium as the insoluble apatite of
bones and teeth. In bones the proportion of
calcium to phosphorus is about 2 to 1. Soft tissues contain much higher amounts of phosphorus than of calcium. Most of this phosphorus
is in organic combinations.

Functions. Perhaps no mineral element has
as many widely differing functions as does
phosphorus. In fact, reference has been made to
phosphorus compounds at many points in preceding chapters of the text, and some of the
many roles are listed here for review purposes:

1. Phosphorus is a constituent of the sugar-
phosphate linkage in the structures of DNA and
RNA, the substances that control heredity (see
page 52).

2. Phospholipids are constituents of cell membranes, thus regulating the transport of solutes
into and out of the cell. The phosphorus-
containing lipoproteins facilitate the transport of
fats in the circulation.

3. Phosphorylation is a key reaction in many
metabolic processes: for example, the phosphorylation of glucose for absorption from the intestine, the uptake of glucose by the cell, and the
reabsorption of glucose by the renal tubules.

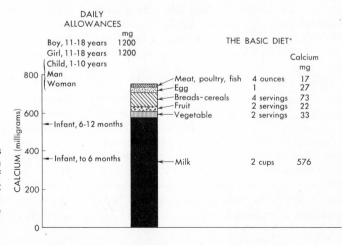

Figure 8–3. The milk group furnishes
almost three fourths of the calcium
allowance of the adult. The addition of
1 to 2 cups milk ensures sufficient
calcium during periods of growth, in
pregnancy, and in lactation. See Table
13–2 for complete calculation.

Likewise, monosaccharides are phosphorylated in the initial stages of metabolism to yield energy (see page 69).

4. Phosphorus compounds are essential for the storage and controlled release of energy—the ADP-ATP system (see page 69); in the niacin-containing coenzymes required for oxidation-reduction reactions—NADP-NADPH (see page 174); and for the active form of thiamine for decarboxylation reactions—TPP (see page 168).

5. Inorganic phosphates in the body fluids constitute an important buffer system in the regulation of body neutrality (see page 137).

Metabolism. Much of the phosphorus in foods is in organic combinations that are split by intestinal phosphatases to free the phosphate. The phosphorus is absorbed as inorganic salts. About 70 per cent of dietary phosphorus is normally absorbed. In general, the factors that govern calcium absorption also regulate phosphorus utilization.

The inorganic phosphorus content of blood serum ranges from 3 to 5 mg per cent and is slightly higher in children. The level is kept constant through regulation by the kidney. All of the plasma inorganic phosphate is filtered through the renal glomeruli but most of it is reabsorbed. Vitamin D increases the rate of reabsorption by the tubules, and parathormone decreases the reabsorption.

Daily allowances. The phosphorus allowances recommended by the Food and Nutrition Board[3] are the same as those for calcium, except for infants. With ordinary diets, the phosphorus intake exceeds the calcium intake, but within a relatively wide range of calcium-to-phosphorus ratios there are no adverse effects in children and adults.

During the first six months of life the phosphorus allowance is 240 mg and during the remainder of the first year the allowance is 400 mg or about 67 to 74 per cent of the calcium allowance. By keeping the phosphorus allowance below that of calcium during the first weeks of life, hypocalcemic tetany is avoided.

Food sources. Phosphorus is widely distributed in foods, the milk and meat groups being important contributors. Thus, a diet that fur-

nishes enough protein and calcium will also provide sufficient phosphorus. Whole-grain cereals and flours contain much more phosphorus than refined cereals and flours; however, much of this occurs in phytic acid, which combines with calcium to form an insoluble salt that is not absorbed. Vegetables and fruits contain only small amounts of phosphorus. (See Table A–2.)

MAGNESIUM

Distribution. The amount of magnesium in the body is much smaller than that of calcium and phosphorus. Of the 20 to 35 gm in the adult body, about 60 per cent is present as phosphates and carbonates chiefly at the surfaces of the bones. Most of the remaining magnesium is within the cells where the ratio of magnesium to calcium is about 3 to 1.

Extracellular fluids account for about 2 per cent of the body's magnesium. The normal concentration of magnesium in blood serum ranges from 1.7 to 3 mg per cent, about 80 per cent of this being ionized; the remainder is bound to protein.

Functions. Magnesium is essential for all living cells. It is a catalyst for numerous biologic reactions. For example, it is required as an activator for the enzymes involved in the oxidative phosphorylation of ADP to ATP (see page 69), and also for all enzymes that bring about the transfer of phosphate from ATP to a phosphate acceptor. These reactions are essential whenever energy is expended, as in active transport across cell membranes, the synthesis of innumerable substances, and the accomplishment of physical work.

Magnesium is one of four cations that must be in balance in extracellular fluids so that the transmission of nerve impulses and the consequent muscle contraction can be regulated.

Metabolism. The absorption of magnesium varies widely depending upon the conditions prevailing in the intestinal lumen. Many of the factors that enhance absorption of calcium (see page 106), such as acidity, or that interfere with absorption, such as oxalic and phytic acids, also affect the absorption of magnesium. However, neither vitamin D nor the parathyroid hormone is involved in the regulation of absorption, metabolism, or excretion of magnesium. The average absorption of dietary magnesium is about 40 per cent. Calcium and magnesium compete for the same carrier sites in the intestinal mucosa. Consequently, a high calcium intake increases the requirement for magnesium.

The body's level of magnesium is controlled largely by the kidneys. Magnesium is filtered from the blood by the glomeruli and is reabsorbed by the renal tubule. The daily urinary excretion of magnesium in adults usually ranges between 100 and 200 mg. Almost all of the magnesium in the feces represents unabsorbed dietary magnesium.

Daily allowances. The Food and Nutrition Board[3] has recommended a daily allowance of magnesium for men at 350 mg and for women at 300 mg. During pregnancy and lactation a daily allowance of 450 mg is recommended. The allowances range from 60 to 70 mg during the first year of life and thereafter gradually increase from 150 mg for the toddler to 250 mg for the child of 7–10 years.

Food sources. The average mixed American diet supplies about 120 mg magnesium per 1000 calories. Thus, it would appear that typical diets, especially those eaten by girls and women within their caloric allowances, would fall somewhat short of the recommended allowances. There is no evidence, however, that magnesium deficiency occurs except under conditions described below.

In the food supply available for consumption in the United States, dairy products excluding butter furnish about 22 per cent of the total magnesium, and flour and cereal products about 18 per cent (see Table 13–1). Dry beans and peas, soybeans, and nuts are excellent sources of magnesium as are also green leafy vegetables. (See Table A–2 for magnesium content of foods.)

Effects of imbalance. Under normal conditions of health and food intake magnesium deficiency is not likely to occur. Unlike calcium, magnesium is only slowly mobilized from bone. Therefore, a generally poor intake of magnesium if it is also accompanied by increased excretion

leads to rapid lowering of the plasma magnesium. The ionic imbalance thus produced in the extracellular fluid upsets the regulation of nervous irritability and muscle contraction. Characteristic symptoms of magnesium deficiency include muscle tremor, paresthesias, and sometimes convulsive seizures and delirium. Since these symptoms are similar to hypocalcemic tetany, a differentiation can usually be made by determining the blood levels of the two cations.

Among the circumstances under which magnesium deficiency is encountered are these: chronic alcoholism, cirrhosis of the liver, malabsorption syndromes such as sprue, kwashiorkor, severe vomiting, prolonged use of magnesium-free parenteral fluids, diabetic acidosis, and diuretic therapy. In most of these instances the deficiency has occurred because of curtailment of food intake or lowered absorption or both. The loss of magnesium from the body is increased during diuretic therapy, and also in diabetic acidosis.

High blood magnesium levels are sometimes encountered when there is an unusual increase in absorption or a marked reduction in urinary excretion. The symptoms of such excess include extreme thirst, a feeling of excessive warmth, marked drowsiness, a decrease in muscle and nerve irritability, and atrial fibrillation. The early stages of hypermagnesemia are readily corrected by giving calcium gluconate.

SULFUR

Distribution. Sulfur accounts for about 0.25 per cent of body weight, or 175 gm in the adult male. It is present in all body cells, chiefly as the sulfur-containing amino acids methionine, cystine, and cysteine. Sulfur is a constituent of thiamine and biotin, two vitamins that must be present in the diet. Connective tissue, skin, nails, and hair are especially rich in sulfur.

Functions and metabolism. Sulfur is an essential element for all animal species inasmuch as they all require the sulfur-containing amino acid methionine. Almost all of the sulfur absorbed from the intestinal tract is in organic form, principally as the sulfur amino acids. Inorganic sulfates, present in only small amounts in foods, are poorly absorbed.

Sulfur is a structurally important constituent of mucopolysaccharides such as chondroitin sulfate found in cartilage, tendons, bones, skin, and the heart valves. Sulfolipids are abundant in such tissues as liver, kidney, the salivary glands, and the white matter of the brain. Other important sulfur-containing compounds are insulin (page 69) and heparin, an anticoagulant.

Sulfur compounds are essential in many oxidation-reduction reactions. Included among these compounds are a number of coenzymes discussed elsewhere in this text: thiamine (page 168); biotin (page 179); coenzyme A (page 179); and lipoic acid (page 184). Glutathione, an important compound in oxidation-reduction reactions, is a tripeptide of glutamic acid, cysteine, and glycine. The concentration of glutathione is especially high in the red blood cells.

The metabolism of the sulfur amino acids within the cells yields sulfuric acid, which is immediately neutralized and excreted as the inorganic salts. One of the important reactions of sulfuric acid is the conjugation with phenols, cresols, and the steroid sex hormones, thereby detoxifying compounds that would otherwise be harmful.

Excretion. About 85 to 90 per cent of the sulfur excreted in the urine is in the inorganic form, being derived almost entirely from the metabolism of the sulfur amino acids. The ratio of nitrogen to sulfur excreted in the urine is about 13 to 1. The range of excretion by the adult is 1 to 2 gm. On a low-protein diet the excretion would be much less than on a high-protein diet.

From 5 to 10 per cent of the sulfur excreted is in the form of organic esters produced in the detoxification reactions. The fecal excretion of sulfur is about equal to the inorganic sulfur content of the diet.

Cystinuria is a relatively rare hereditary defect in which large amounts of cystine as well as lysine, arginine, and ornithine are excreted because of a failure of renal reabsorption. Being somewhat insoluble, the cystine forms renal calculi.

Requirements and sources. The daily requirement for sulfur has not been determined. A diet that is adequate in methionine and cystine is considered to meet the body's sulfur needs.

The sulfur content of foods depends upon the concentration of methionine and cystine. Food proteins vary from 0.4 to 1.6 per cent in their sulfur content, with an average of 1 per cent for a typical mixed diet. Thus, meat, milk, eggs, and legumes may be considered to be important sources.

TRACE ELEMENTS OR MICRONUTRIENTS

IRON

Distribution. The amount of iron in the body of the adult male is about 50 mg per kilogram, or a total of 3.5 gm; in the woman it is about 35 mg per kilogram, or a total of 2.3 gm. Approximately 70 to 80 per cent of the iron is functioning and the rest is held in storage as *ferritin* or *hemosiderin* by the liver, spleen, and bone marrow. In healthy men the iron reserve is about 1000 mg, but in menstruating women it is not more than 200 to 400 mg.

Of the functioning iron, 80 per cent is in the hemoglobin, and the remainder is in the myoglobin and iron-containing enzymes. All body cells contain some iron as constituents of the many enzymes. Iron circulates in the plasma bound to a β-globulin, *transferrin*—also known as *siderophilin*. Normally, the saturation of transferrin with iron ranges from 20 to 40 per cent. The concentration of plasma iron in men ranges from 50 to 180 mcg per 100 ml and in women from 40 to 135 mcg per 100 ml.[5]

Functions. Hemoglobin is the principal component of the red blood cells and accounts for most of the iron in the body. It acts as a carrier of oxygen from the lungs to the tissues and indirectly aids in the return of carbon dioxide to the lungs.

Myoglobin is an iron-protein complex in the muscle which stores some oxygen for immediate use by the cell. Enzymes such as the catalases, the cytochromes in hydrogen ion transport (see page 92), and xanthine oxidase contain iron as an integral part of the molecule. Iron is required as a cofactor for other enzymes.

Metabolism. The amount of iron that will be absorbed from the intestinal tract is governed by (1) the body's need for iron, (2) the conditions existing in the intestinal lumen, and (3) the food mixture that is fed (See Figure 8–4).

The absorption of iron is meticulously regulated by the intestinal mucosa according to body need. An increase in erythropoiesis leads to withdrawal of iron from the iron-transferrin complex in the circulation, and the lowering of transferrin saturation in turn brings about an increase in the amount of iron that is absorbed. Thus, growing children, pregnant women, and anemic individuals will have a higher rate of absorption than healthy males. The absorptive mechanism is also highly effective in preventing an overload of iron entering the body and causing toxic reactions. Although excess iron can be absorbed, extremely large intakes would be necessary for a long period of time before toxic reactions would result.

In the acid medium of the stomach and upper duodenum ferric iron is reduced to ferrous iron, a more soluble form that is readily absorbed. Achlorhydria, observed in many elderly persons and present in pernicious anemia, reduces the absorption of iron. Likewise, the surgical removal of the portion of the stomach that produces acid will also result in lower absorption of iron. The alkaline reaction of pancreatic juice reduces the solubility of iron so that little absorption takes place from the jejunum and ileum. Absorption of iron is also hindered in malabsorption syndromes.

The absorption of iron from foods varies widely, but in the healthy adult it averages about 5 to 10 per cent. From animal foods the absorption ranges from 10 to 30 per cent, whereas for vegetables it may be as little as 2 to

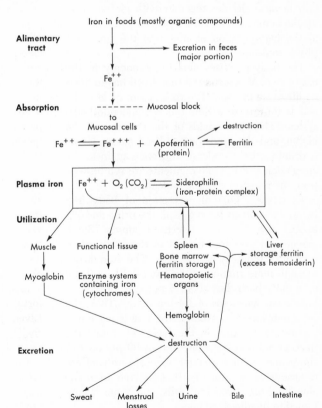

Figure 8–4. The utilization of iron.

10 per cent.[6] Absorption from plant sources improves when animal foods are simultaneously fed, probably because the amino acids released from the proteins enhance solubility. The presence of ascorbic-acid-rich foods also increases the absorption of iron in that ferric iron is reduced to ferrous iron.

Transport and utilization. Iron in the plasma is made available from three sources: (1) absorption from the intestinal tract, (2) release from body reserves, and (3) release from the breakdown of hemoglobin that takes place constantly. Within a 24-hour period the turnover of iron is about 27 to 28 mg.[7] Only 1 to 1.5 mg of this has been available from absorption.

Iron is withdrawn from the plasma into the bone marrow for the synthesis of hemoglobin, which is a complex substance composed of a basic protein, *globin,* linked to a prosthetic group, *heme.* The heme molecule consists of protoporphyrin with reduced iron at its center; four heme molecules together with globin make up the hemoglobin. Copper plays a catalytic role in the incorporation of iron into the protoporphyrin molecule.

The body exercises amazing economy in the use of iron. When the red blood cell has fulfilled its life cycle of about 120 days, more or less, the cell is destroyed within the reticuloendothelial system. The amino acids of the stroma and the globin, and the lipids, are utilized again. Heme is disintegrated to release iron once again to the circulation and the bile pigments are synthesized from the remainder of the molecule.

Excretion. The daily excretion of body iron by adults is about 0.1 mg from the urine and 0.3 to 0.5 mg into the intestinal lumen. Small amounts of iron are also lost in the perspiration and by exfoliation of the skin. The iron losses through menstruation range from 0.3 to 1.0 mg on a daily basis, but about 5 per cent of women have losses in excess of 1.4 mg daily.[3] Thus, the total iron losses by women are 1 to 2 mg daily.

Most of the iron in the feces represents the unabsorbed iron from the diet, or 90 per cent of the intake. A small amount of fecal iron is of endogenous origin, namely, that derived from the sloughing off of mucosal cells, and some is contained in the digestive juices.

Daily allowances. Dietary iron is required for (1) replacement of the daily losses of all individuals; (2) an expanding blood volume and increasing amounts of hemoglobin in growing children; (3) replacement of the varying losses through menstruation; (4) development of the fetus and to avoid anemia in pregnant and lactating women; and (5) a reserve of iron that is available when blood loss occurs from any cause whatsoever. The amounts of iron required for most of these needs have not been adequately studied for all age categories.

Table 8–3 lists the amounts of iron that must be absorbed to replace losses and to meet the synthetic requirements of various age groups. Assuming an average absorption of 10 per cent, the amounts of iron that must be provided in the diet are also listed. These values are compared with the recommended allowances of the Food and Nutrition Board.

Food sources. Of all nutrients, the iron allowance is the most difficult to provide in the diet. The iron content of typical diets adequate in other respects is estimated to be 6 mg per 1000 calories.[3] (See Figure 8–5.) Thus, men and boys with their caloric requirements can easily meet their iron needs, but girls and women with their lower caloric requirements cannot supply their needs even with a good selection of diet. Proposals are now being considered for increasing the levels of fortification of foods, especially cereals and breads.

Much more research is required to determine the availability of iron from various food sources and the conditions that enhance or detract from that availability. Lean meats, deep-green leafy vegetables, and whole-grain or enriched cereals and breads are the foods of the daily diet that must be depended upon for their iron. Milk, cheese, and ice cream are poor sources of iron— a fact that explains why infant diets must be fortified with iron-rich foods at an early age. Liver, other organ meats, dried fruits, legumes, shellfish, and molasses are iron-rich foods that deserve frequent use.

Cooking procedures may be an important determinant in the amount of iron that is actually ingested. On the one hand, some mineral salts are leached out when large amounts of water are

Table 8–3. Daily Iron Requirements*

	Absorbed Iron Requirement mg/day	Food Iron Requirement† mg/day	Recommended Dietary Allowance mg/day
Normal men and nonmenstruating women	0.5–1	5–10	10
Menstruating women	0.7–2	7–20	18
Pregnant women	2 –4.8	20–48‡	18+
Adolescents	1 –2	10–20	18
Children	0.4–1	4–10	10–15
Infants	0.5–1.5	1.5 mg/kg§	10–15 mg

*Adapted from: Committee on Iron Deficiency, Council on Foods and Nutrition: "Iron Deficiency in the United States," *J.A.M.A.*, **203**:407–14, Feb. 5, 1968; and Food and Nutrition Board: *Recommended Dietary Allowances*, 8th ed. National Academy of Sciences–National Research Council, Washington, D.C., 1973.

†Assuming an absorption of 10 per cent.

‡This amount of iron cannot be derived from diet and should be met by iron supplementation in the latter half of pregnancy.

§To a maximum of 15 mg.

used and subsequently discarded. Cast-iron cookware was widely used many years ago, and the uptake of iron from such cooking vessels added appreciably to the daily intake. Today, iron skillets are about the only such cookware used frequently. There are substantial differences between the iron content of foods cooked in cast-iron ware and the same foods cooked in glass or aluminum vessels.[8]

Effects of imbalance. Iron-deficiency anemia is characterized by reduced red cell and hemoglobin levels in the blood and by small, pale cells (microcytic, hypochromic). It is widely prevalent in the United States and throughout the world, but the exact incidence is not known. Infants, preschool children, adolescent girls, and pregnant women are especially susceptible. See Chapter 45 for discussion of anemias.

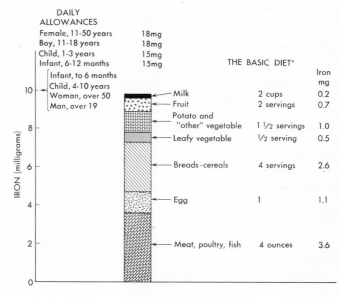

Figure 8–5. The Four Food Groups of the Basic Diet fulfill the iron allowance for the man. For teen-age girls and women it is difficult to meet the iron allowance without exceeding the calorie requirement. The allowances can be met with increased fortification of foods or by the use of iron supplements. See Table 13–2 for calculations.

Hemosiderosis is a disorder of iron metabolism in which large deposits of iron are made especially in the liver and in the reticuloendothelial system. The transferrin of the circulation becomes saturated and is unable to bind all of the iron that is absorbed. This disorder affects a high proportion of the adult Bantu population in South Africa and is believed to be caused by an overload of dietary iron.[9] Men commonly have an intake of 30 mg iron daily and frequently as much as 100 mg per day. The beer that they drink is fermented in iron pots, and likewise the acid-fermented cereal foods and sour porridge are cooked in these pots. The resulting foods have a high iron content.

Hemosiderosis also occurs when there is abnormal destruction of the red blood cells as in hemolytic anemia. It may also occur following prolonged iron therapy when it is not needed. The iron overload leads to deposits of iron in the liver cells, following which typical symptoms of cirrhosis develop. The excess iron may also be deposited in the lungs, pancreas, and heart.

IODINE

Endemic goiter, the iodine-deficiency disease, occurs in those areas where the iodine content of the soil is so low that insufficient iodine is obtained through food and water. Among the areas of iodine-poor soils are the Great Lakes, the Pacific Northwest, Switzerland, Central American countries, mountainous areas of South America, New Zealand, and the Himalayas. The World Health Organization has estimated that as many as 200 million people throughout the world may be affected. During World War I the prevalence of endemic goiter in young men drafted for service was high in the United States; with the use of iodized salt the incidence has decreased markedly.

Distribution and function. About one third of the iodine in the adult body, variously estimated from 25 to 50 mg, is found in the thyroid gland. The concentration in thyroid tissue is about 2500 times as great as that in any other tissue, all of which contain traces.

The only known function of iodine is as a constituent of thyroglobulin, a protein complex of several iodine-containing compounds. The thyroid hormone regulates the rate of oxidation within the cells and in so doing influences physical and mental growth, the functioning of the nervous and muscle tissues, circulatory activity, and the metabolism of all nutrients.

Metabolism. Iodine is ingested in foods as inorganic iodides and as organic compounds. In the digestive tract iodine is split from organic compounds and is absorbed as inorganic iodide. The degree of absorption is dependent upon the level of circulating thyroid hormone.

Iodine is transported by the circulation as free iodide and as protein-bound iodine. The protein-bound fraction (PBI) is sensitive to changes in the level of thyroid activity; it rises during pregnancy and with hypertrophy of the gland and falls with hypofunction of the gland. The measurement of PBI, therefore, is a specific diagnostic tool for thyroid activity and has largely replaced the basal metabolism test as a study of thyroid function.

Thyroid activity is controlled by the thyroid-stimulating hormone (TSH) secreted by the anterior lobe of the pituitary. When the blood level of the thyroglobulin is low, the activity of the thyroid is increased by TSH. By this action the thyroid gland withdraws iodide from the circulation, concentrates it, oxidizes it to iodine, and incorporates it into tyrosine to form diiodotyrosine, triiodothyronine, and thyroxine. These iodine-containing amino acids then become part of the thyroglobulin complex.

When thyroid hormone is utilized for cellular oxidation, iodine is released into the circulation. About one third of the released iodine is again incorporated into thyroid hormone and the remainder is excreted in the urine.

Daily allowances. The recommended allowance for iodine is 100 mcg for the reference woman and 130 mcg for the reference man. During pregnancy and lactation the allowances are 125 and 150 mcg, respectively. Infants should receive 35 to 45 mcg during the first year. The allowances gradually increase throughout childhood until the level reaches 150 mcg for the teen-age boy and 115 mcg for the teen-age girl.

Sources. Median values for the iodine content of foods used in a metabolic study were reported as follows:[10]

	Mcg per 100 gm Food
Seafood	54
Vegetables	28
Meat products	17.5
Eggs	14.5
Dairy products	13.9
Breads and cereals	10.5
Fruits	1.8

Although iodine is supplied by foods and water, the variations are wide depending upon the iodine content of the soils from which they come.

People living in coastal areas who eat salt-water fish and shellfish regularly as well as locally grown foods ingest enough iodine for their needs. However, the wide distribution of foods from one part of the country to another makes it difficult to rely upon food sources.

Iodized salt is the method of choice for supplying sufficient iodine intake because salt is an almost universally used dietary item, the addition of iodine does not affect flavor, and it is inexpensive. The concentration of iodine used in the United States is 0.5 to 1 part of sodium or potassium iodide per 10,000 parts (0.005 to 0.01 per cent) of salt. Since the usual daily intake of salt is 5 to 15 gm, the iodine intake would be 380 to 1140 mcg. Amounts in excess of 1000 mcg daily have not been shown to be harmful.[11]

Many nations of the world have adopted laws that require the iodization of all salt used. In the United States iodization is voluntary, but many people use salt without added iodine. The Food and Nutrition Board has recommended that federal legislation be enacted to make the iodization of salt mandatory.

Effects of deficiency. Iodine is the only nutrient for which a deficiency in the soil is known to have an adverse effect on human nutrition. The public health consequences of a lack of iodine in the food supply are endemic goiter, cretinism, and increased incidence of thyrotoxicosis and of thyroid cancer.[12] Simple, or endemic, goiter is an enlargement of the thyroid gland,

but with no other abnormal physical findings. The basal metabolism remains normal. The deficiency is more prevalent in females than in males and is more frequent during adolescence and in pregnancy.

The studies of Marine and Kimball[13] on schoolgirls in Akron, Ohio, showed the importance of sufficient iodine intake in a striking manner. Over a period of 2½ years they found 495 cases of goiter among 2305 girls who received no supplementary iodine, but only 5 cases among 2190 girls who received sodium iodide.

The most urgent reason for stressing iodine as a preventive measure is not the goiter itself but the cretinism which is its ultimate sequel in areas severely deficient in iodine. Cretinism occurs in the infant when the pregnant woman is so severely depleted that she cannot supply iodine for the development of the fetus. Cretinism is characterized by a low basal metabolism, muscular flabbiness and weakness, dryness of the skin, arrest of skeletal development and severe mental retardation. Desiccated thyroid given early enough to the infant results in marked improvement of physical development; mental retardation may be less severe, but any damage which has occurred to the central nervous system cannot be reversed. Endemic cretinism is rare or nonexistent in the United States today.[14]

Goitrogens. Certain substances in foods are known to interfere with the use of thyroxine and will produce goiters, at least in experimental animals, even though the iodine intake would normally be adequate. Such goitrogens are present in rutabagas,[15] peanuts—especially in the red skin,[16] and seeds of the *Brassica* family (cabbage, Brussels sprouts, cauliflower). The substances are inactivated by cooking, and there is currently no evidence that goiters in endemic regions are caused by them.

COPPER

Distribution. The presence of copper in blood was first recognized in 1875, but the nutritional significance was not established until Hart and Elvehjem at the University of Wisconsin found that traces of copper were essential for the formation of hemoglobin. The body of the human adult contains about 75 to 150 mg of copper. Traces of copper are found in all tissues, but by far the highest concentrations are found in the liver and brain. In the fetus and at birth the levels in these organs are several times as high, and they decrease during the first year.

Metabolism and function. Copper is absorbed from the stomach and from the upper gastrointestinal tract. About 95 per cent of the copper in blood plasma is firmly bound to a protein complex, *ceruloplasmin,* and 5 per cent is loosely bound to albumin. Molybdenum and zinc are antagonistic to copper; thus, an increased intake of these trace elements increases the requirement for copper. Almost all of the excretion of copper is in the feces, chiefly through the excretion of bile.

Copper is required for diverse functions, including melanin pigment formation, electron transport, integrity of the myelin sheath, phospholipid synthesis, bone development, and hemoglobin formation. Copper has been identified as a constituent of a number of enzymes: butyryl coenzyme A dehydrogenase required for the oxidation of fatty acids; tyrosinase required for melanin pigment formation; uricase in purine metabolism; and in the cytochrome oxidation system for energy production. Copper facilitates the formation of the hemoglobin molecule. The functions of several copper-containing proteins such as hepatocuprein and erythrocuprein are not known.

Daily allowances. A daily allowance of 2 mg copper is considered to be satisfactory for the adult. For infants an allowance of 0.08 mg per kilogram daily is sufficient.

Food sources. Typical diets furnish from 2 to 5 mg copper. Even a diet that is poor in other nutrients is likely to furnish enough copper. The copper content of foods is somewhat dependent upon the copper content of soil. Among rich sources are organ meats, shellfish, whole-grain cereals, legumes, and nuts. Milk is a poor source.

Effects of imbalance. Dietary deficiency of copper is not likely in humans. Low blood levels of copper have been observed in kwashiorkor, the nephrotic syndrome, and sprue, and occasionally in patients with iron-deficiency anemia.

In excessive amounts copper is toxic. A rare hereditary disorder known as Wilson's disease is characterized by a marked reduction of blood ceruloplasmin and greatly increased deposits of copper in the liver, brain, and other organs. The excess copper in these tissues leads to hepatitis, lenticular degeneration, renal malfunction, and neurologic disorders.

FLUORINE

Fluorine occurs normally in the body primarily as a calcium salt in the bones and teeth. It is not essential to life but small amounts of fluoride bring about striking reductions in tooth decay, probably because the tooth enamel is made more resistant to the action of acids produced in the mouth by bacteria.

Mottling of the teeth (chronic dental fluorosis) had long been observed in some Texas and Colorado communities and was associated with naturally occurring high concentrations of fluoride in the drinking water. If the drinking water contains fluoride in excess of 1.5 parts per million (1.5 ppm), the tooth enamel becomes dull and unglazed with some pitting. When the fluoride concentration of the water is greater than 2.5 ppm, the incidence increases, and the mottled areas of the teeth may become stained a dark brown.

Although esthetically undesirable, mottled teeth were found to be surprisingly free from decay. In a study reported from Galesburg, Illinois, there were only 236 decayed, missing, and filled teeth per 100 children, whereas in Michigan City, Indiana, there were 1037 decayed, missing, and filled teeth per 100 children.[17] The level of fluoride in the drinking water in Galesburg was approximately twice as high as that in Michigan City.

Over and over again, carefully controlled studies in a number of cities for more than 10 years have established that fluoridation of the water supplies at a level of 1 ppm may be expected to reduce the incidence of dental caries in children by approximately 50 to 60 per cent. Several thousand communities have now initiated water fluoridation as an effective public

health measure. Children who have been drinking fluoridated water since infancy show the
greatest benefits; those who begin the ingestion
of fluoridated water in later school years are
helped to a lesser extent.

Recent studies have shown that osteoporosis
occurs less frequently in elderly persons who
live in areas supplied with fluoridated water.[18]
Apparently the fluoride salts of calcium are less
readily lost from bone during immobilization or
following the menopause. Large excesses of
fluorine in the water (over 8 ppm) eventually
lead to bone fluorosis, with symptoms resembling
arthritis.

Foods as well as water contain varying
amounts of fluorine, with milk, eggs, and fish
being particularly important. The daily diet will
furnish about 0.3 to 0.5 mg, and six glasses of
water containing 1 ppm will provide an additional 1.2 mg. The amounts in water and from
the diet are not great enough to produce any
toxic manifestations. Up to 3 mg fluorine is excreted daily by the kidneys and sweat glands.

OTHER TRACE ELEMENTS

Manganese, zinc, molybdenum, selenium,
chromium, and cobalt are trace elements required for the functions of enzymes. In some
instances the element is an integral part of the
enzyme molecule (metalloenzymes) and the
removal of the mineral element would inactivate
the enzyme. In others the mineral element is independent of the enzyme molecule but forms a
loose combination (metalloenzyme complex),
thus exerting catalytic activity.

Except for zinc, no recommended allowances
have been set for these elements since only a
few studies have been conducted on the requirements. Data on the distribution of these elements
in foods are also limited. A diet that is reasonably adequate in other nutrients is considered to
satisfy the needs for these trace elements.
Dietary deficiency of these trace elements is
not likely in humans.

Experimental studies on animals have shown
that the mineral elements are closely interrelated. Thus, an excess of one element may in-

crease the need for another. Excessive amounts
of trace elements produce symptoms of toxicity
in animals.

Manganese. About 6 to 8 mg manganese are
supplied in the daily diet of the adult. Seeds of
plants—nuts, legumes, and whole-grain cereals
—are good sources, but animal foods are much
lower in their content. Manganese is rather
poorly absorbed from the small intestine by a
mechanism similar to that for the absorption of
iron. It is loosely bound to a protein and transported as *transmanganin*. Tissues that are rich in
mitochondria take up manganese readily from
the blood. A dynamic equilibrium exists between
intracellular and extracellular manganese. Most
of the metabolic manganese is excreted into the
intestine as a constituent of bile, but much of
this is again reabsorbed, indicating an effective
body conservation. Very little manganese is excreted in the urine.

Studies on experimental animals have shown
that manganese is required for normal bone
growth and development, normal lipid metabolism, reproduction, and regulation of nervous irritability. Manganese is an activator for a number of enzymes including arginase, which is
required for the formation of urea, and a number of peptidases that bring about the hydrolysis
of proteins in the intestine. Manganese can substitute for magnesium in a number of enzymes
required for oxidative phosphorylation.

Zinc. The recommended allowance for zinc
for adults is 15 mg, for pregnancy is 20 mg, and
for lactation is 25 mg. Diets that supply sufficient animal protein will also furnish enough
zinc, but vegetarian diets may be somewhat low.

Zinc is poorly absorbed from the intestine, and
most of that from the diet is excreted in the
feces. A high calcium and phytate intake interferes with zinc absorption, apparently because
calcium complexes with zinc and phytate to
form an insoluble compound. This effect is less
pronounced when the phytate content of the diet
is low.

The body's content of zinc is 2 to 3 gm, with
traces found in all body tissues. The highest
concentrations of zinc occur in organs such as
the liver, pancreas, kidney, and brain. The zinc
content of red blood cells is approximately 10

times that of blood serum. Most of the zinc derived from metabolic processes is excreted into the intestine, and only small amounts are excreted in the urine.

Zinc is a constituent of numerous enzymes, among them being carbonic anhydrase, which brings about the transfer of carbon dioxide; carboxypeptidase, which hydrolyzes proteins in the intestinal tract by removing the carboxyl group; and lactic dehydrogenase, which brings about the reduction of pyruvic acid to lactic acid in the anaerobic oxidation of glucose (see page 71). Zinc combines with insulin but it is not required for the activity of insulin.

Zinc deficiency has been rarely observed in humans, although it is readily produced in animals. (See Figure 8–6.) In human patients in Egypt and Iran zinc deficiency has been described in dwarfs who consumed a diet consisting primarily of bread and beans. Among the

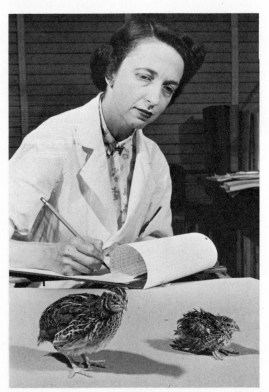

Figure 8–6. Nutritional studies with Japanese quail show the effects (*right*) of a diet without zinc. (Courtesy, Food and Drug Administration.)

findings were hepatomegaly and hypogonadism. Zinc metabolism is also altered in a number of disease states such as postalcoholic cirrhosis, chronic myeloid leukemia, and pernicious anemia.

Molybdenum. A precise balance of molybdenum is essential for plant and animal life. Nitrogen-fixing bacteria require this metal for their growth, and thus the synthesis of proteins and utimately animal life are affected. A deficiency of molybdenum will adversely affect the growth of legumes. Also, in molybdenum deficiency the growth of certain fungi that produce mycotoxins is favored. These mycotoxins have been shown to be carcinogenic in animals. (See also Chapter 19.)

Molybdenum is found especially in legumes, whole-grain cereals, and organ meats. It is absorbed as molybdate and is concentrated especially in the liver, adrenal, and kidney. It is a cofactor for a number of flavoprotein enzymes and is found in xanthine oxidase, an enzyme that brings about the oxidation of xanthine to uric acid.

Molybdenum competes with copper for the same metabolic sites, and an excess of molybdenum will result in symptoms of copper deficiency. Cattle grazing on lands that have a high molybdenum content develop a condition known as *teart* and characterized by diarrhea, brittle bones, loss of pigmentation, and weight loss. When the sulfate content of the diet is increased, the symptoms of toxicity are avoided inasmuch as the excretion of molybdenum is increased. This affords an interesting example of the interrelationship of sulfur, copper, and molybdenum.

Selenium. Foods may contain an excess or deficiency of selenium, thus leading to signs of toxicity or of deficiency disease. "Alkali disease" in cattle occurs when grains and forages containing high levels of selenium are ingested. It is characterized by anemia, emaciation, and stiffness and lameness. The area of selenium-rich soils in the United States are well known, and the hazards of toxicity are thus small. A level of selenium in excess of 5 ppm in foods is considered to be hazardous. Organic selenium compounds are quite unstable, and the cooking of foods results in losses of volatile selenium to the air.

The need for selenium in animals has been clearly established and is also probable for humans although the functions are not clearly understood. Selenium is readily absorbed and deposited in all tissues and is especially found in liver and kidney. It is related to the function of vitamin E and is able to cure some, but not all, of the deficiency symptoms produced in animals by lack of vitamin E. (See page 157.) Selenium, like vitamin E, is effective as an antioxidant. Selenium is related to sulfur metabolism in a number of ways and competes with sulfur for reactive sites in enzymes. A number of studies have indicated that a high intake of selenium may increase the incidence of dental caries.

Chromium. This element is present in the body at birth, a fact that suggests its essential nature. Typical diets supply about 80 to 100 mcg daily, of which only 2 to 5 mcg are absorbed. Chromium disappears rapidly from the blood and is stored in the tissues. It reenters the circulation following the ingestion of glucose.

Chromium appears to be required for maintaining a normal glucose tolerance. In patients with diabetes mellitus, the glucose tolerance has improved following treatment with chromium. The body content of chromium decreases with age, thus leading to speculation that lack of it may be related to the increased incidence of diabetes mellitus in later life.

Cobalt. This element is an essential constituent of vitamin B_{12} and must be ingested in the form of the vitamin molecule inasmuch as humans cannot synthesize the vitamin. No other function of cobalt has been established.

A summary of mineral elements and review questions appear at the end of Chapter 9.

Cited References

1. Greenwald, F., *et al.:* "Effect of Lactose on Calcium Metabolism in Man," *J. Nutr.,* 79:531–38, 1963.
2. Johnston, F. A.: "Calcium Retained by Young Women Before and After Adding Spinach to the Diet," *J. Am. Diet. Assoc.,* **28**:933–38, 1952.
3. Food and Nutrition Board: *Recommended Dietary Allowances,* 8th ed. National Academy of Sciences–National Research Council, Washington, D.C., 1973.
4. FAO/WHO Expert Committee: *Calcium Requirements.* WHO Tech. Rep. Series No. 230, 1962.
5. Wright, A. W., ed.: *Rypins' Medical Licensure Examination,* 11th ed. J. B. Lippincott Company, Philadelphia, 1970, p. 204.
6. Finch, C. A.: "Iron Metabolism," *Nutr. Today,* 4:2–7, Summer 1969.
7. Gubler, C. J.: "Absorption and Metabolism of Iron," *Science,* 123: 87–90, 1956.
8. White, H. S.: "Current Use and Changes in Use of Cast-Iron Cookware," *J. Home Econ.,* **60**:724–27, 1968.
9. deBruin, E. J. P., *et al.:* "Iron Absorption in the Bantu," *J. Am. Diet. Assoc.,* **57**:129–31, 1970.
10. Vought, R. L., and London, W. T.: "Dietary Sources of Iodine," *Am. J. Clin. Nutr.,* **14**: 186–92, 1964.
11. Astwood, E. B.: "Iodine in Nutrition," *Bordens Rev. Nutr. Res.,* **16**:53–68, 1955.
12. Scrimshaw, N. S.: "Endemic Goiter," *Nutr. Rev.,* **15**:161–64, 1957.
13. Marine, D., and Kimball, O. P.: "Prevention of Goiter in Man," *J.A.M.A.,* **77**:1068–70, 1921.
14. Nelson, W. E.: *Textbook of Pediatrics,* 8th ed. W. B. Saunders Company, Philadelphia, 1964, p. 1276.
15. Greer, M. A: "Goitrogenic Substances in Food," *Am. J. Clin. Nutr.,* **5**:440–44, 1957.
16. Srinivasin, V., *et al.:* "Studies on Goitrogenic Agents in Food. I. Goitrogenic Action of Groundnut," *J. Nutr.,* **61**:87–95, 1957.

17. Review: "Present Knowledge of Fluorine in Nutrition," *Nutr. Rev.,* **5:**322–26, 1947.
18. Rich, C., and Ensinck, J.: "Effect of Sodium Fluoride on Calcium Metabolism of Human Beings," *Nature* (Lond.), **191:**184–85, 1961.

ADDITIONAL REFERENCES

General

Cohn, N. L., and Briggs, G. M.: "Trace Minerals in Nutrition," *Am. J. Nurs.,* **68:**807–11, 1968.
Comar, C. L., and Bronner, F., eds.: *Mineral Metabolism,* 3rd ed. Vols. 1, 2. Academic Press, New York, 1964.
Consolazio, C. F., *et al.:* "Excretion of Sodium, Potassium, Magnesium, and Iron in Human Sweat and the Relation of Each to Balance Requirements," *J. Nutr.,* **79:**407–15, 1963.
Davis, T. R. A., *et al.:* "Review of Studies of Vitamin and Mineral Nutrition in the United States (1950–1968)," *J. Nutr. Educ.,* **1** (Suppl.): 41–57, Fall 1969.
Gormican, A.: "Inorganic Elements in Foods Used in Hospital Menus," *J. Am. Diet. Assoc.,* **56:**397–403, 1970.
Hegsted, D. M.: "Some Consequences of Overnutrition with Minerals," *Am. J. Clin. Nutr.,* **9:**548–52, 1961.
Present Knowledge in Nutrition, 3rd ed. The Nutrition Foundation, Inc., New York, 1967, Chaps. 28–33.
Underwood, E. J.: *Trace Elements in Human and Animal Nutrition,* 2nd ed. Academic Press, New York, 1962.
White, Hilda S.: "Inorganic Elements in Weighed Diets of Girls and Young Women," *J. Am. Diet. Assoc.,* **55:**38–43, 1969.

Calcium and Phosphorus

Bronner, F., and Harris, R. S.: "Absorption and Metabolism of Calcium in Human Beings Studied with Calcium[45]," *Ann. N.Y. Acad. Sci.,* **64:**314–25, 1956.
Council on Foods and Nutrition: "Symposium on Human Calcium Requirements," *J.A.M.A.,* **185:**588–93, 1963.
Garn, S., *et al.:* "Bone Loss as a General Phenomenon in Man," *Fed. Proc.,* **26:**1729–36, 1967.
Hankin, J. H., *et al.:* "Contribution of Hard Water to Calcium and Magnesium Intakes of Adults," *J. Am. Diet. Assoc.,* **56:**212–24, 1970.
Holemans, K. C., and Meyer, B. J.: "A Quantitative Relationship between the Absorption of Calcium and Phosphorus," *Am. J. Clin. Nutr.,* **12:**30–35, 1963.
Johnson, F. A., and Thorangkul, D.: "Effect of Low-Calcium Intake on Phosphorus Retention," *J. Am. Diet. Assoc.,* **35:**31–33, 1959.
Leitch, I., and Aitken, F. C.: "The Estimation of Calcium Requirement: Reexamination," *Nutr. Abstr. Rev.,* **29:**393–411, 1959.
Lotz, M., *et al.:* "Evidence for a Phosphorus-Depletion Syndrome in Man," *N. Engl. J. Med.,* **278:**409–15, 1968.
Mack, P. B., and LaChance, P. A.: "Effects of Recumbency and Space Flight on Bone Density," *Am. J. Clin. Nutr.,* **20:**1194–1205, 1967.
Spencer, H. J., *et al.:* "Effect of High Phosphorus Intake on Calcium and Phosphorus Metabolism in Man," *J. Nutr.,* **86:**125–32, 1965.

Magnesium

Flink, E. B.: "Magnesium Deficiency Syndrome in Man," *J.A.M.A.,* **160:**1406–1409, 1956.
Hathaway, M. L.: *Magnesium in Human Nutrition.* Home Econ. Res. Rep. 19. U.S. Department of Agriculture, Washington, D.C., 1962.
Hunt, E., *et al.:* "Magnesium Balance and Protein Intake Level in Adult Human Female," *Am. J. Clin. Nutr.,* **22:**367–73, 1969.

Jones, J. E., *et al.:* "Magnesium Requirements in Adults," *Am. J. Clin. Nutr.,* **20:**632–35, 1967.
Nelson, G. V., and Gram, M. R.: "Magnesium Content of Accessory Foods," *J. Am. Diet. Assoc.,* **38:**437–38, 1961.
Review: "Hypermagnesemia," *Nutr. Rev.,* **26:**12–15, 1968.
————: "Magnesium Toxicity in the Newborn," *Nutr. Rev.,* **26:**139–40, 1968.
Shils, M. E.: "Experimental Human Magnesium Depletion. I. Clinical Observations and Blood Chemistry Alterations," *Am. J. Clin. Nutr.,* **15:**133–43, 1964.
Sullivan, J. F., *et al.:* "Magnesium Metabolism in Alcoholism," *Am. J. Clin. Nutr.,* **13:**297–303, 1963.
Wacker, W. E. C.: "Magnesium Metabolism," *J. Am. Diet. Assoc.,* **44:**362–67, 1964.
Wacker, W. E. C., and Parisi, A. F.: "Magnesium Metabolism," *N. Engl. J. Med.,* **278:**658–63; 712–17; 772–76, 1968.

Iron
Beaton, G. H., *et al.:* "Iron Requirements of Menstruating Women," *Am. J. Clin. Nutr.,* **23:**275–83, 1970.
Burroughs, A. L., and Huenemann, R. L.: "Iron Deficiency in Rural Children," *J. Am. Diet. Assoc.,* **57:**122–28, 1970.
Conrad, M. E.: "Iron Balance and Iron Deficiency States," *Bordens Rev. Nutr. Res.,* **28:**49–68, 1967.
Elwood, P. C., and Waters, W. E.: "The Vital Distinction," *Nutr. Today,* **4:**14–19, Summer, 1969.
Hegsted, D. M.: "The Recommended Dietary Allowances for Iron," *Am. J. Public Health,* **60:**653–58, 1970.
Kuhn, I. N., *et al.:* "Observations on the Mechanism of Iron Absorption," *Am. J. Clin. Nutr.,* **21:**1184–88, 1968.
Layrisse, M., *et al.:* "Effects of Interaction of Various Foods on Iron Absorption," *Am. J. Clin. Nutr.,* **21:**1175–83, 1968.
Review: "Fortification of Bread with Iron," *Nutr. Rev.,* **27:**138–39, 1969.
————: "Iron and Erythropoiesis," *Nutr. Rev.,* **27:**227–31, 1969.
Schade, S. G., *et al.:* "Effect of Hydrochloric Acid on Iron Absorption," *N. Engl. J. Med.,* **279:**672–74, 1968.
Scott, D. E., and Pritchard, J. A.: "Iron Deficiency in Healthy Young College Women," *J.A.M.A.,* **199:**897–900, 1967.
White, H. S.: "Iron Deficiency in Young Women," *Am. J. Public Health,* **60:**659–65, 1970.

Other Trace Elements
Behar, M.: "Progress and Delays in Combating Goiter in Latin America," *Fed. Proc.,* **27:**939–44, 1968.
Blayney, J. R., and Hill, I. N.: "Fluorine and Dental Caries," *J. Am. Dent. Assoc.,* **74:**233–302, 1967.
DeGroot, L. J.: "Current Views on Formation of Thyroid Hormones," *N. Engl. J. Med.,* **272:**243–50; 297–303; 355–62, 1965.
Dowdy, R. P.: "Copper Metabolism," *Am. J. Clin. Nutr.,* **22:**887–92, 1969.
Frieden, E.: "Ceruloplasmin, a Link between Copper and Iron Metabolism," *Nutr. Rev.,* **28:**87–91, 1970.
Hadjimarkos, D. M.: "Effect of Selenium on Dental Caries," *Arch. Environ. Health,* **10:**893–99, 1965.
Hill, C. H.: "A Role of Copper in Elastin Formation," *Nutr. Rev.,* **27:**99–102, 1969.
Krehl, W. A.: "Selenium—the Maddening Mineral," *Nutr. Today,* **5:**26–32, Winter 1970.
Matovinovic, J.: "Endemic Goiter," *J. Am. Med. Wom. Assoc.,* **17:**427–30; 495–97; 571–76; 646–52, 1962.
Mills, C. F., *et al.:* "Metabolic Role of Zinc," *Am. J. Clin. Nutr.,* **22:**1240–49, 1969.
North, B. B., *et al.:* "Manganese Metabolism in College Women," *J. Nutr.,* **72:**217–23, 1960.

Prasad, A. D., *et al.*: "Zinc and Iron Deficiencies in Male Subjects with Dwarfism and Hypo-gonadism But Without Ancylostomiasis, Schistosomiasis, or Severe Anemia," *Am. J. Clin. Nutr.*, **12**:437–44, 1963.

Review: "Chromium and Glucose Tolerance," *Nutr. Rev.*, **26**:281–82, 1968.

———: "Copper and the Aorta," *Nutr. Rev.*, **27**:325–28, 1969.

———: "Copper and Taste Sensitivity," *Nutr. Rev.*, **26**:175–77, 1968.

———: "Dietary Iodine and Goiter in Ceylon," *Nutr. Rev.*, **27**:108–10, 1969.

———: "Physiological Distribution of Fluoride," *Nutr. Rev.*, **26**:103–104, 1968.

———: "Zinc in Hair as a Measure of the Zinc Nutriture of Human Beings," *Nutr. Rev.*, **28**:209–11, 1970.

Richards, L. F., *et al.*: "Determining Optimum Fluoride Levels for Community Water Supplies in Relation to Temperature," *J. Am. Dent. Assoc.*, **74**:389–97, 1967.

Sandstead, H. H., *et al.*: "Human Zinc Deficiency, Endocrine Manifestations, and Response to Treatment," *Am. J. Clin. Nutr.*, **20**:422–42, 1967.

Schroeder, H. A.: "The Role of Chromium in Mammalian Nutrition," *Am. J. Clin. Nutr.*, **21**:230–44, 1968.

Staff Report: "Iodized Salt," *Nutr. Today*, **4**:22–25, Spring 1969.

9 Fluid and Electrolyte Balance

The interchange that constantly takes place between the body and its external environment, and within the body between cells, tissues, and organs and their environment, is dependent upon the fluid medium that is precisely regulated in its volume, composition, and concentration. The electrolytes and nonelectrolytes held in solution in this aqueous medium maintain normal osmotic pressure relationships, control nervous irritability and muscle contraction, regulate acid-base balance, and facilitate movement of nutrients into cells and removal of wastes from cells.

This chapter includes a discussion of the role of water; the electrolyte composition of body fluids; three important electrolytes, namely, sodium, potassium, and chloride; the role of the kidney; mechanisms for fluid-electrolyte balance; and acid-base balance.

WATER

The body's need for water is second only to that for oxygen. One can live for weeks without food, but death is likely to follow a deprivation of water for more than a few days. A 10 per cent loss of body water is a serious hazard, and death usually follows a 20 per cent loss.

Distribution. The water content of an infant's body is as much as 70 per cent. About 65 per cent of body weight of lean adults is accounted for by water, and 55 per cent or less of weight in obese adults is water.

All body tissues contain water, but the variations in tissue contents are wide. For example, the approximate percentage of water in teeth is 5; fat and bone, 25; and striated muscle, 80.

Fluid compartments. Body fluids exist in two so-called compartments that are disseminated throughout the entire body. The *intracellular* fluid is that which exists within the cells. It accounts for about 45 per cent of body weight. The *extracellular* fluid is subdivided as follows: (1) the plasma fluid, accounting for 5 per cent of body weight, which contains protein as well as numerous substances that easily penetrate the capillary membrane; and (2) the interstitial fluid, representing about 15 per cent of body weight, which is similar to plasma fluid except in its much lower concentration of protein. Also included in the extracellular fluids are the lymph circulation and secretions such as those of the lacrimal glands, pancreas, liver, gastrointestinal mucosa, and others.

Functions. Most of the many functions of water are self-evident. Water is a structural component and a cushion of all cells. Each gram of protein holds about 4 gm water, and each gram of fat is associated with about 0.2 gm water. In some instances, as in bone, water is tightly bound, but in most tissues a constant interchange between intracellular and extracellular fluid is occurring in order to maintain osmotic pressure relationships.

Water is the medium of all body fluids including the digestive juices, the lymph, the blood, the urine, and the perspiration. All the physiochemical changes that occur in the cells of the body take place in the precisely regulated environment of the body fluids. Water enters into many essential reactions, such as hydrolysis that occurs in digestion. In oxidation-reduction reactions water is often the end product as in the oxidation of glucose.

Water is a solvent for the products of digestion, holding them in solution and permitting them to pass through the absorbing walls of the intestinal tract into the bloodstream. Because nutrients and cellular wastes are soluble in water, it is the means whereby nutrients are carried to the cells and wastes are removed to the lungs, kidney, gut, and skin. The metabolic wastes are diluted by water, thereby preventing cellular injury.

Water regulates body temperature by taking up the heat produced in cellular reactions and distributing it throughout the body. About 25 per cent of the heat lost from the body occurs by evaporation from the lungs and skin. Water is essential as a body lubricant: the saliva that makes possible the swallowing of food; the mucous secretions of the gastrointestinal, respiratory, and genitourinary tracts; the fluids that bathe the joints; and so on.

Sources of water to the body. Water to meet the body's needs is supplied by the ingestion of water and beverages, the preformed water in foods, and the water resulting from the oxidation of foodstuffs.

As may be seen below, water is the principal constituent by weight of almost all foods, pure sugars and fats being the important exceptions.

	Per Cent Water
Milk	87
Eggs	75
Meat, well done	40
Meat, rare	75
Fruits, vegetables	70–95
Cereals, ready to eat	1–5
Cereals, cooked	80–88
Breads	35

The oxidation of nutrients results in the release of water, as may be seen in the following example:

$$C_6H_{12}O_6 + 6\,O_2 \rightarrow 6\,H_2O + 6\,CO_2$$

The following amounts of water are produced in the oxidation of foodstuffs:[1]

	ml Water
100 gm fat	107.1
100 gm carbohydrate	55.5
100 gm protein	41.3

Using these equivalents, the water of oxidation for a 2100-calorie diet consisting of 80 gm pro-

tein, 90 gm fat, and 220 gm carbohydrate is approximately 250 ml.

Daily losses of water. The daily losses of water include:

	ml
Feces	100–200
Urine	1000–1500
Lungs	250–400
Insensible perspiration	400–600
Visible perspiration	None to 10,000

Some losses of water are *obligatory*, that is, they are essential for the maintenance of physicochemical equilibrium. The losses in the feces, through the lungs, and in the insensible perspiration occur regardless of intake. The amount of water loss from the kidney that is obligatory depends upon the amount of wastes that must be dissolved. Under normal circumstances it is about 600 ml. Urea and sodium chloride are the principal solids that are excreted, and thus any reduction in their production will correspondingly reduce the obligatory loss of water in the urine. A diet that is high in carbohydrate to minimize tissue catabolism and low in protein is one that reduces the formation of urea and thus will spare body water.

Insensible perspiration accounts for a relatively constant amount of water loss that is proportional to the surface area of the body. It is so called because the evaporation takes place from the skin immediately and the water loss is not noticeable. This evaporation is an important means by which body temperature is maintained. An infant weighing 10 pounds or so has a surface area that is about one third that of the adult, and thus the infant is much more vulnerable to water losses from the skin and rapid changes in body temperature.

The water losses by visible perspiration are highly variable, ranging from zero in cool weather to several liters during very warm weather under conditions of strenuous activity. Whenever a great deal of water is lost by perspiration, body water is conserved by the elimination of a much more concentrated urine.

Air expired from the lungs also contains water. Any condition that would increase the rate of respiration likewise increases the water loss by this route. The individual engaged in vigorous activity will lose more water by this route than the one who is sedentary.

Requirement. The 24-hour water requirement is that amount that replaces the losses by the kidneys, lungs, skin, and bowel. Ordinarily, thirst is an accurate guide to supplying the necessary amounts of water. Under ideal conditions including a low-solute diet, a minimum of physical activity, and absence of sweating, the water need for the adult is about 1.5 liters from beverages, food, and water of oxidation.[2] Although conditions are variable, the daily requirement is about 1 ml per calorie for adults and 1.5 ml per calorie for infants.

Table 9–1 illustrates a typical balance between water intake and water losses from the body. The mechanisms for the regulation of fluid balance and some of the problems of imbalance are discussed on pages 133 through 135.

Electrolytes

Definitions and measurement. An electrolyte is any substance that dissociates into its component ions when dissolved in water. It is so named because an electrical current can be transmitted by a solution containing any one of these substances. The dissociation for a given substance is constant, but the degree of dissociation varies widely from one substance to another. Strong electrolytes are those substances such as inorganic acids or bases that dissociate almost completely.

Cations carry positive electrical charges; they are electron donors. *Anions* carry negative electron charges; they are electron acceptors. In any solution the total cations are exactly equal to the total anions.

The concentrations of physiologic solutions are expressed, and most easily compared, in milliequivalents (mEq) rather than in weights per 100 ml or per liter. Snively and Brown[3] have used a dance analogy to describe this concept. For a dance one would invite equal numbers of boys and girls—not 1400 pounds of boys and 1400 pounds of girls. It is the number of boys to pair off with girls that is important, not their weight. With an equal number of boys and girls, any boy could dance with any girl.

Likewise, with cations and anions; any cation can pair off with any anion. For example, 1 milliequivalent of sodium combines with 1 milliequivalent of chloride. Expressed in weight, 23 mg sodium have combined with 35 mg chloride. But 1 milliequivalent of potassium can also combine with 1 milliequivalent of chloride; in this instance, 39 mg potassium have combined with 35 mg chloride. Another example: calcium, with two positive charges, can pair off with two chloride ions; it can, instead, pair off with one phosphate ion, since phosphate carries two negative charges. Thus, it is the *chemical combining power* rather than the weights of the substances that is most convenient in measuring electrolyte concentrations. The calculation of milliequivalents of an electrolyte, when the concentration in milligrams is known, may be expressed as follows:

$$mEq/liter = \frac{mg \text{ per liter}}{Equivalent \text{ weight}}$$

$$Equivalent \text{ weight} = \frac{Atomic \text{ weight}}{Valence \text{ of the element}}$$

Table 9–1. Normal Water Balance*

Available Water	gm	Excreted Water	gm
Water intake as such	1100	In urine	1000
Water in diet	900	In stool	200
Water of oxidation	200	In vapor (skin and lungs)	1000
Total	2200	Total	2200

*Newburgh, L. H., and MacKinnon, F.: *The Practice of Dietetics.* The Macmillan Company, New York, 1934.

Suppose the concentration of calcium in blood serum is 9.5 mg per 100 ml. Since the atomic weight of calcium is 40 and the valence is 2, the equivalent weight is $40 \div 2 = 20$.

$$\text{mEq/liter} = \frac{9.5 \times 10}{20} = 4.75$$

Electrolyte composition of body fluids. The electrolyte balance of the body is studied principally by determining the electrolyte concentrations in blood plasma. The electrolyte compositions of plasma and of cellular fluid are compared in Table 9–2. The electrolyte patterns for plasma and interstitial fluid are almost identical except for the much greater concentration of protein in the plasma. Note that within each fluid compartment the total milliequivalents' of cations exactly balance the total milliequivalents of anions. There are remarkable differences in the electrolyte composition of plasma and intracellular fluid, yet the concentrations are such that osmotic balance is maintained. Because of the higher protein within the cell, the total of all

electrolytes is higher than that in extracellular fluid. Each protein molecule carries eight negative charges thus combining with eight potassium ions; the protein molecule and the eight potassium ions would thus yield only nine osmotically active particles.

Sodium accounts for over 90 per cent of the cations in plasma; potassium, magnesium, and calcium are found in very small, though physiologically important, concentrations. The principal anion of plasma is chloride; there are smaller concentrations of bicarbonate and proteinate and very small amounts of phosphate, sulfate, and organic acids.

By contrast, potassium is the principal cation in intracellular fluid, with magnesium, sodium, and calcium accounting for the remainder. Phosphate as the organic phosphate in adenosine triphosphate, creatine phosphate, and sugar phosphate as well as inorganic phosphate is the principal balancing anion. Proteinate accounts for about one fourth of the anions in intracellular fluid, and the amounts of bicarbonate, chloride, and sulfate are small.

Table 9–2. Electrolyte Composition of Body Fluids*

	Blood Plasma		Cellular Fluid
	mg per 100 ml	mEq per liter	mEq per liter
Cations			
Sodium (Na$^+$)	327	142	10
Potassium (K$^+$)	19	5	148
Calcium (Ca^{++})	10	5	2
Magnesium (Mg^{++})	3.6	3	40
Total cations		155	200
Anions			
Chloride (Cl$^-$)	365	103	
Bicarbonate (HCO$_3$$^-$)	165	27	8
Phosphate (HPO$_4$$^{--}$)	9.6	2	
including other nonprotein ions			136
Sulfate (SO$_4$$^{--}$)	4.8	1	
Organic acids$^-$		6	
Proteinate$^-$		16	56
Total anions		155	200

*Adapted from Tables 17–3 and 17–4 in West, E. S., *et al.: Textbook of Biochemistry*, 4th ed. The Macmillan Company, New York, 1966, pp. 689, 690.

SODIUM

Throughout the history of man salt has occupied a unique position. Mosaic law prescribed the use of salt with offerings made to Jehovah, and there are frequent Biblical references to the purifying and flavoring effects of salt. Greek slaves were bought and sold with salt, and a good slave was said to be "worth his weight in salt." Because salt was scarce and greatly prized, the Via Salaria of Rome was a carefully guarded artery for the transport of salt. Salt served as a medium of exchange; thus the word *salary* from the Latin *salaria*. To own salt was a privilege, and royal banquet halls had imposing salt cellars. Important persons were invited to "sit above the salt" and those of lesser importance were seated "below the salt." Today salt is so commonplace that only those who are denied its free use give more than casual thought to it.

Distribution. About 50 per cent of the body's sodium is present in the extracellular fluid, 40 per cent in bone, and 10 per cent or less in intracellular fluid. Much of the sodium in bone is readily interchangeable with extracellular fluid, but some of it is located deeply in dense long bones. In terms of concentration, the sodium content of blood plasma is about 14 times that of intracellular fluid. (See Table 9–2.)

Functions. Sodium is the principal electrolyte in extracellular fluid for the maintenance of normal osmotic pressure and water balance. It is the largest component of the extracellular total base and supplies the alkalinity of the gastrointestinal secretions. It functions mutually with some and antagonistically with other ions in maintaining the normal irritability of nerve cells and the contraction of muscles, and in regulating the permeability of the cell membrane. The sodium "pump" maintains electrolyte differences between intracellular and extracellular fluid compartments. (See page 134.)

Metabolism. Most of the sodium in the diet is in the form of inorganic salts, principally sodium chloride. The absorption of sodium from the gastrointestinal tract is rapid and practically complete, there being only small amounts of sodium in the feces. The kidneys regulate the sodium level in the body. When the intake of sodium is high, the excretion is likewise high. But if the intake of sodium is low, the excretion of sodium is likewise decreased. An analysis of a 24-hour collection of urine is a good measure of the level of intake in the normal individual. When sodium is drastically restricted in the diet, the excretion of sodium by the normal kidney practically reaches the vanishing point, and sodium is almost completely conserved.

Sodium excretion is regulated primarily by the adrenocortical hormone aldosterone. An increase in aldosterone production increases the reabsorption of sodium, and a diminution of aldosterone secretion permits greater excretion of sodium. Indirectly the kidney influences the concentration of sodium through its regulation of water excretion under the influence of the antidiuretic hormone. The mechanisms for these controls will be discussed further on page 135.

The losses of sodium in perspiration depend upon the concentration and the total volume of sweat. In very warm weather the initial losses may be so high that the sodium depletion syndrome occurs unless compensation is made by increasing salt and fluid intake. With acclimatization there is a gradual reduction in the concentration of sodium in perspiration and hence the amount of sodium that will be lost through the skin. Concentrations of sodium in sweat ranging from 12 to 120 mEq per liter have been reported.[4]

Requirements. The average daily intake of salt is 6 to 15 gm, equivalent to 2500 to 6000 mg sodium. This is far in excess of physiologic requirements and reflects the desire for salt. Some people desire so much salt that they add salt to food without even tasting it, whereas others prefer only a light salting of food. The exact requirements for sodium are not known, but in the absence of visible perspiration the need is very low. Patients who are consuming diets restricted to 500 mg sodium daily, or even less, have been able to maintain sodium balance.

Food sources. The principal source of sodium in the diet is sodium chloride by virtue of its universal use in food preservation, in cookery, and at the table. Numerous sodium compounds are also used in food processing and preparation: baking soda and baking powder as leavening agents; sodium alginate, sodium propionate, sodium citrate, sodium sulfite, and numerous others to enhance some quality of a food product.

Sodium is a naturally occurring constituent of animal foods including milk, eggs, meat, poultry, and fish, and of certain salt-loving vegetables such as spinach, celery, chard, beet greens, and others. Most vegetables, fruits, cereals, and legumes are naturally low in sodium. (See also Table A–2.)

Sodium imbalance. Any disturbance in the concentration of sodium in extracellular fluids has a serious effect on osmotic pressure and on acid-base balance.

In cardiac or renal failure the excretion of sodium is reduced. Consequently, sodium and fluids are retained in tissues and the condition is known as edema. An excessive excretion of cortical hormones, as by adrenal tumors, leads to increased retention of sodium. Likewise adrenocorticotropic hormone used therapeutically in a variety of conditions also increases the retention of sodium.

Excessive sodium losses during hot weather have already been mentioned. A deficiency of adrenocortical hormone that is characteristic of Addison's disease is characterized by such large losses of sodium that the patient hungers for salt.

POTASSIUM

Distribution. About 97 per cent of the potassium in the body is within the tissue cells with the remainder being distributed in the extracellular fluid compartment. From Table 9–2 it may be seen that the concentration in cellular fluid is about 30 times that in the plasma.

Functions. Potassium is an obligatory component of all cells and increases in proportion to increase in the body's cell mass. Within the cell potassium is the principal cation for the maintenance of osmotic pressure and fluid bal-

ance just as sodium is the principal cation in extracellular fluid.

A portion of potassium is bound to protein. Thus, protein synthesis is accompanied by entrance of potassium into the cell, whereas tissue catabolism is accompanied by proportionate losses of nitrogen and of potassium.

Potassium is required for enzymatic reactions taking place within the cell. Some potassium is bound to phosphate and is required for the conversion of glucose to glycogen; this potassium is released during glycogenolysis.

The small concentration of potassium in extracellular fluid is essential, together with other ions, for the transmission of the nerve impulse and for contraction of muscle fibers.

Metabolism. Potassium is readily absorbed from the gastrointestinal tract. Although the digestive juices contain relatively large amounts of potassium, most of this is reabsorbed and the losses in the feces are small.

Under conditions of protein synthesis, glycogen formation, and cellular hydration, potassium is rapidly removed from the circulation. With the removal of sodium from the cell to the extracellular fluid by the sodium pump, potassium ions move in, thus balancing the cations between the fluid compartments. Potassium leaves the cell during protein catabolism, dehydration, or glycogenolysis.

Excess potassium is excreted by the kidney. Aldosterone secretion increases potassium excretion. Although the normal kidney readily excretes excess potassium, the ability to conserve potassium in the face of a deficit is much less rigid than that for sodium. Even in the absence of any potassium intake and with low tissue levels, the urinary losses may be 15 to 30 mEq per day.[5]

Requirements. The exact requirements for potassium are not known, but on the basis of obligatory losses it is estimated that 1 to 3 mEq per kilogram per day will suffice.[2] The daily intake on typical diets far exceeds this level.

Food sources. Because potassium is widely distributed in foods, the daily intake increases as the calorie intake increases. Meats, poultry, and fish are good sources. Fruits, vegetables, and whole-grain cereals are especially high in potassium. Bananas, potatoes, tomatoes, carrots, celery, orange juice, grapefruit juice, and broth are rich sources. (See Table A–2 for potassium values in foods.)

Effects of imbalance. Potassium deficiency is not primarily of dietary origin but there are numerous circumstances under which it can occur. One of these is defective food intake such as that in severe malnutrition, chronic alcoholism, anorexia nervosa, or some illness that seriously interferes with the appetite. Any condition that reduces the availability of nutrients for absorption can lead to potassium depletion: for example, prolonged vomiting, gastric drainage, and diarrhea. Potassium losses may exceed replacement in severe tissue injury, following surgery, in burns, and during prolonged fevers. Some therapeutic measures may also initiate potassium deficiency: for example, prolonged parenteral feeding without potassium in the parenteral fluids or excessive adrenocortical steroid therapy. Rapid infusions of glucose and insulin in diabetic acidosis bring about such rapid shifts of potassium into the cell that the plasma potassium levels may be reduced to levels that could bring about cardiac failure.

Potassium deficiency is characterized by low plasma levels of potassium (hypopotassemia or hypokalemia). The symptoms of deficiency include nausea, vomiting, listlessness, apprehension, muscle weakness, paralytic ileus, hypotension, tachycardia, arrhythmia, and an altered electrocardiogram. The heart may stop in diastole.

Potassium excess (hyperpotassemia or hyperkalemia) is a frequent complication in renal failure, in severe dehydration, following too rapid parenteral administration of potassium, and in adrenal insufficiency. Hyperkalemia is characterized by paresthesias of the scalp, face, tongue, and extremities; muscle weakness; poor respiration; cardiac arrhythmia; and changes in the electrocardiogram. Cardiac failure may follow with the heart stopping in systole. Hyperkalemia is corrected by using a low-potassium, low-protein, liberal-carbohydrate diet. Carbohydrate intake results in the formation of glycogen and the movement of potassium into the cells.

CHLORIDE

Distribution. Chlorine exists in the body almost entirely as the chloride ion. Most of the 100 gm or so of chloride in the body is present in the extracellular fluid but it also occurs to some extent in the red blood cells and to a lesser degree in other cells.

Functions. Chloride accounts for two thirds of the total anions of extracellular fluid. It is important in the regulation of osmotic pressure, water balance, and acid-base balance. It is the chief anion of gastric juice and is accompanied by the hydrogen ion rather than the sodium ion, thus providing the acid medium for the activation of the gastric enzymes and the digestion in the stomach. Chloride is one of several activators of salivary amylase.

Metabolism. For the secretion of gastric juice chloride is withdrawn from the blood circulation, and changes in dietary intake do not modify its production. The gastric juice mixes with foods and moves along the intestinal tract. The chloride from foods and that from the gastric juice is readily absorbed into the circulation.

The *chloride shift* between the red blood cells and the plasma is a mechanism whereby changes in pH are minimized. When the blood reaches the lungs, the blood CO_2 tension is decreased, the bicarbonate ions in the red blood cells decrease, bicarbonate ions move from the plasma into the cells, and chloride and OH ions move from the cells into the plasma. When the blood returns to the tissues, the partial pressure of CO_2 increases and these ionic shifts are reversed.

Chloride, like other ions, is filtered by the glomerulus and selectively reabsorbed from the renal tubules. Excess chloride is readily excreted. The chloride excretion usually parallels the excretion of sodium, but when it is essential to conserve sodium the kidney will substitute the ammonium ion. Sweat and feces contain variable amounts of chloride accompanied by sodium or potassium.

Dietary intake. The requirement for chloride has not been determined, but the liberal intake of sodium chloride assures more than adequate intake under normal circumstances. Most of the chloride ingested is from the salt used in food processing and preparation.

Chloride imbalance. Severe vomiting, drainage, or diarrhea leads to large losses of chloride and an alkalosis because of the replacement of chloride with bicarbonate.

ROLE OF THE KIDNEY

Structural unit. The nephron, of which there are approximately one million in each kidney, is the functioning unit of the kidney. (See Figure 9–1.) Each nephron consists of the *glomerulus,* which is a tuft of capillaries surrounded by a capsule (Bowman's capsule), and a *tubule,* including (1) the proximal convoluted tubule, (2) the loop of Henle, and (3) the distal convoluted tubule. The nephrons finally empty into collecting tubules.

Blood flows into the glomerulus through an *afferent arteriole* and leaves through an *efferent arteriole* and then flows through a system of *peritubular capillaries* that surround the tubules.

Functions of the kidney. The primary function of the kidneys is to maintain the constant composition and volume of the blood. This in-

cludes the regulation of the osmotic pressure, the electrolyte and water balance, and the acid-base balance. By regulation of the composition of the blood homeostasis in the interstitial and intracellular fluid compartments of the body is achieved. The production of urine permits the elimination of excess water and solutes such as sodium, chloride, and others, the by-products of metabolism such as urea, and ingested substances that may be toxic. A large intake of water is accompanied by increased excretion of urine, and a small intake of water results in the excretion of a much more concentrated urine. The kidney thus helps the individual to survive water or electrolyte depletion or to get rid of excess.

Glomerular filtration. Each minute about 1200 ml of blood flow through the kidneys, this being about one fifth to one fourth of the total cardiac output. The total amount of glomerular filtrate produced by the kidneys is about 125 ml per minute for a 24-hour total of 180 liters. The glomerular filtrate has essentially the same composition as the blood plasma except that it contains no protein or other large colloidal particles.

Functions of the tubules. The tubules control the concentration of blood constituents by selective reabsorption. As the glomerular filtrate moves through the proximal convoluted tubule all of the glucose, amino acids, ascorbic acid, acetoacetic acid, and a number of other substances are completely reabsorbed. About 80 to 85 per cent of the water and electrolytes (Na^+, K^+, Cl^-, HCO_3^-, HPO_4^{--}, and SO_4^{--}) are also reabsorbed into the circulation. The proximal tubules, however, are almost impermeable to the waste products of the body.

By the time the filtrate has reached Henle's loop, marked changes in composition have occurred. Most of the remaining sodium and some of the remaining water are reabsorbed into the circulation from Henle's loop.

About 3 per cent of the electrolytes and 13 per cent of the water still remains in the filtrate that reaches the distal convoluted tubule, which plays a major role in controlling the concentration of the solutes in the blood. When blood plasma sodium levels are low, sodium reabsorption is increased under the stimulus of aldo-

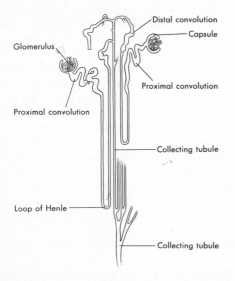

Glomerulus

Distal convolution

Capsule

Proximal convolution

Proximal convolution

Collecting tubule

Loop of Henle

Collecting tubule

Figure 9–1. Diagram of the course of two renal tubules. (Courtesy, Miller, M. A., and Leavell, L. C.: *Kimber-Gray-Stackpole's Anatomy and Physiology,* 16th ed. The Macmillan Company, New York, 1972.)

sterone. If the plasma concentration of sodium is high, very little sodium will be reabsorbed. Under the influence of the antidiuretic hormone, the permeability of the tubular cells is increased to permit more water to be reabsorbed.

By the time the filtrate has reached the collecting tubules only a small amount of the glomerular filtrate still remains. Water and electrolyte reabsorption continues at a variable rate depending upon the need.

Composition of urine. As the glomerular filtrate passes through the tubules, the metabolic wastes—unlike water and electrolytes—are poorly reabsorbed. Their concentration therefore increases as the filtrate moves along the tubules with the resultant formation of urine. Urine consists of about 95 per cent water and 5 per cent solids. The kidney can produce a urine varying in specific gravity from about 1.008 to 1.035 depending upon the proportions of water and solids to be excreted. The average daily excretion of solids is about 50 to 70 gm, with three fifths of this being nitrogenous and two fifths inorganic salts. Urea is the predominating nitrogenous substance in the urine, along with much smaller amounts of uric acid, ammonia, and creatinine. Sodium chloride is the principal inorganic salt excreted, this varying according to intake. In addition, chloride, phosphate, and sulfate salts of calcium, sodium, potassium, and magnesium are excreted. (See Table A–15.)

For an average load of solids, about 600 ml fluid must be excreted, this being referred to as the *obligatory* fluid excretion. With an increase in solid wastes, the fluid required for their excretion would also be increased. Among the situations in which increased solid wastes are produced are the following: (1) protein intake in excess of tissue needs so that large amounts of amino acids are deaminized and the urea production is increased; (2) increased tissue catabolism following any stress such as surgery, injury, burns, or fever; and (3) increased intake of salt. Whenever the kidney is unable to concentrate urine, the fluid requirement for excretion of wastes is greatly increased.

Metabolic activities. Only the liver exceeds the kidney in its metabolic activities. The energy production of the kidney is high. Water and urea pass through the membranes by *diffusion* and this passive reabsorption does not require energy. However, most substances are reabsorbed by *active transport*, thus entailing energy expenditure. Fatty acids are probably the principal source of energy in the aerobic oxidations occurring in the cortex, but glucose, fructose, and other substrates can also be oxidized. In the renal medulla oxidation is principally by anaerobic glycolytic pathway, glucose thus being the chief substrate.

The tubules have important secretory roles. Hydrogen ions are continually released from carbonic acid by the action of carbonic anhydrase into the tubules. The tubules synthesize ammonia (NH_3), which combines with the hydrogen ion to form the ammonium ion (NH_4^+), thus releasing bicarbonate ions to be reabsorbed into the blood and replacing the alkali reserve.

REGULATION OF FLUID AND ELECTROLYTE BALANCE

Fluid exchange. Although the sources of water to the body and the losses from the body are in balance, the fluid exchanges that take place in a 24-hour period are of tremendous magnitude and impressive in the precision of their regulation. For the digestive process alone the estimated daily volume of fluid that enters and leaves the gastrointestinal tract is estimated to be about 10 liters and is made up of the following:[6]

	ml
Water intake as beverage and in food	2,000
Saliva	1,500
Gastric juice	2,500
Bile	500
Intestinal juice	3,000
Pancreatic juice	700
	10,200

The fluid exchanges between the gastrointestinal tract and the blood circulation are variable from hour to hour; yet they are so balanced that normally the volume of the blood and the fluids within the tract are in equilibrium. Inasmuch as the daily losses from the bowel are no more than 100 to 200 ml, it is evident that the out-pouring of digestive juices into the intestinal tract is continuously balanced by the reabsorption of water from the gut. That the kidneys are highly efficient conservators of body water has been pointed out on page 132. The magnitude of water exchange that occurs between the blood circulation, the interstitial fluid, the lymph vessels, and the cells is no doubt very great.

Factors influencing fluid and electrolyte balance. The movements of water and solutes from one compartment to another are influenced by many factors: (1) the permeability of membranes to water and other substances; (2) the hydrostatic pressure within the capillaries; (3) the colloid osmotic pressure exerted by large molecules such as proteins; (4) the osmotic effect of electrolytes in the fluids of extracellular and intracellular fluids; (5) the lymph flow; (6) the mechanisms for active transport; (7) the competition of substances for carriers to transport materials across cell membranes; and (8) the hormonal and nervous controls influencing each of these factors.

Water and some particles of low molecular weight such as urea and chloride can move into and out of cells by diffusion. The transport of most solutes across cell membranes has been described on page 27. The filtration of water and solutes from the capillaries into the interstitial fluid is governed by the existing hydrostatic pressure, which is determined by the arterial blood pressure, the rate of blood flow through the capillary, and the venous pressure.

Proteins influence the equilibrium between plasma and interstitial fluids, and likewise between the cell and its surrounding fluid. Within the capillaries plasma albumin especially is the principal force that maintains fluid equilibrium between the interstitial fluid and the plasma. The plasma albumins exert a constant pull of fluid from the interstitial fluid to the plasma. Thus, the osmotic pressure opposes and balances the flow of materials out of the capillaries that is exerted by filtration pressure. When the concentration of plasma albumins is reduced, the osmotic pressure is reduced and the fluid remains in the tissue spaces; this is sometimes referred to as "nutritional edema."

Sodium has little effect on the osmotic pressure between the capillaries and the interstitial fluid because its concentration in the two fluids is about equal. However, sodium is the principal cation in interstitial fluid and potassium in the intracellular fluid so that these electrolytes effect important osmotic controls between these fluid compartments. A reduction of extracellular sodium, for example, results in the entrance of fluid into the cell, whereas an increase in extracellular sodium results in the withdrawal of fluid from the cell.

Mechanisms for the regulation of water balance. The sensation of thirst is one means whereby the body meets its water need. When the ionic concentration of the extracellular fluid is increased, the cells in the *drinking center* of the hypothalamus become dehydrated and the desire to drink water is initiated.

Water reabsorption from the renal tubule is modified according to the extracellular fluid concentration. This depends upon the *osmoreceptor system,* which is effective in two ways. One of these is the change in osmotic pressure that occurs in the interstitial fluid of the renal medulla. The loops of Henle of the renal tubules extend into the medulla. Because rapid, active absorption of sodium and chloride occurs, the interstitial fluid of the medulla has a high concentration of sodium and chloride and hence exerts increased osmotic pressure. As the tubular fluid passes into the collecting ducts located in the medulla, water is rapidly absorbed from the ducts.[7]

Water reabsorption by the tubules is also controlled by the secretion of antidiuretic hormone by the posterior pituitary gland. Osmoreceptors especially in the supraoptic nuclei of the hypothalamus are sensitive to increases in the osmolarity of the extracellular fluid. Under conditions of increased concentration, impulses are initiated that stimulate production of ADH. The hormone enters the circulation and passes to the kidney where it increases the permeability of the distal and collecting tubules so that the amount of water that is reabsorbed is greatly increased. If the concentration of electrolytes is low, no stimulation of the osmoreceptors occurs and hence the hormone is not produced. The cell permeability is then decreased so that more water will be excreted, thereby restoring normal electrolyte concentration.

Regulation of ionic balance. The regulation of sodium concentration in the extracellular fluid is better understood than that of other ions, but it is believed that the mechanisms that control the concentrations of other electrolytes are similar. These mechanisms are under nervous and hormonal control.

A low concentration of sodium in the extracellular fluid stimulates the secretion of aldosterone and, to a lesser extent, other mineralocorticoids by the adrenal cortex. The sequence for the stimulation of the adrenal is believed to be as follows: with a drop in blood pressure of the juxtaglomerular cells, the kidney is stimulated to produce *renin,* an enzyme, which in turn acts on a globulin substance in blood, *angiotensinogen,* to convert it to *angiotensin I,* an inactive substance. An enzyme in the plasma converts angiotensin I to angiotensin II; the latter substance in the blood circulation stimulates the production of aldosterone by the adrenal cortex. Upon reaching the renal circulation, aldosterone increases the permeability of the distal and collecting tubules so that more sodium is reabsorbed into the peritubular capillaries. When the extracellular sodium concentration is high, the adrenal cortex stops secreting aldosterone, and thus greater amounts of sodium will be excreted. When sodium is reabsorbed it carries positive electrical charges which draw negative ions, principally chloride, through the tubular membrane. Thus, the reabsorption of chloride closely parallels that of sodium.

Potassium ions are passively secreted into the distal and collecting tubules. This secretion is greater when the potassium content of the extracellular fluid is high. The retention of sodium under the influence of aldosterone is accompanied by an increased loss of potassium.

Fluid imbalance. A deficiency of fluid may occur because of inadequate intake, or abnormal loss, or a combination of the two. Abnormal loss of water occurs from prolonged vomiting, hemorrhage, diarrhea, protracted fevers, burns, excessive perspiration, drainage from wounds, and so on. It leads to decrease in peristaltic action,

reduced blood volume, poor absorption of nutrients, impairment of renal function, and circulatory failure. Loss of fluid is accompanied by electrolyte losses as well. Thus, the adjustment of fluid balance requires also the consideration of electrolyte concentration.

In some pathologic conditions the body is in *positive* water balance; that is, the intake of fluids is greater than the excretion, and the patient is said to have an *edema.* The effect of the lowered plasma albumin has been mentioned (see page 134). Congestive heart failure, cirrhosis of the liver, nephritis, and nephrosis are examples of cardiovascular and renal disturbances in which sodium excretion is reduced, thereby contributing to the retention of water.

ACID-BASE BALANCE

Acid-base balance refers to the regulation of the hydrogen ion concentration of body fluids. Normal metabolic processes result in the continuous production of acids that must be eliminated. On a given day, the equivalent of 20 to 40 liters of 1 N acid are eliminated by the lungs and 50 to 150 ml 1 N acid are excreted by the kidney.[8] The mechanisms for maintaining body neutrality are so efficient that the healthy individual does not need to give any thought whatsoever to the nature of his diet insofar as acid-producing or alkali-producing elements are concerned.

Many pathologic conditions, however, are characterized by serious disturbances in acid-base balance: for example, acidosis in uncontrolled diabetes mellitus, following severe dehydration, and in renal failure. Through the study of physiology and biochemistry the student has gained an understanding of electrolyte and fluid balance, the chemistry of respiration, and the regulation of acid-base balance. The scope of this text and the limitations of space permit only a brief summary of this important subject. Several references at the end of the chapter may be consulted by the student who desires a review or more extensive study.

Definitions and measurement. An *acid* is a substance that gives off or donates protons

(H^+ ions); a *base* is a substance that combines with or accepts protons. For example, HCl, a *strong* acid, dissociates almost completely in water to H^+ and Cl^-; the chloride ion is a very *weak* base because it has practically no capacity for combining with the hydrogen ions in the solution. Carbonic acid (H_2CO_3) is a *weak* acid; it dissociates only slightly in solution to H^+ and HCO_3^-. The bicarbonate ion is a relatively *strong* base because it combines readily with hydrogen ions to form a weak acid.

The acidity of a fluid is measured by its concentration of hydrogen ions; the greater the concentration of hydrogen ions, the greater the acidity. The weight of hydrogen ions in a liter of plasma is exceedingly small, and concentrations would be expressed as decimal fractions or as negative exponents, for example, $10^{-7.45}$ mole H^+ per liter. In order to avoid this cumbersome designation, the symbol pH is used. It is not important to understand all the mathematics involved in deriving pH but the student should be able to interpret changes in pH.

In an aqueous solution at room temperature where the concentration of hydrogen ions and hydroxyl ions is equal, the pH is designated as 7.0 and the solution is said to be "neutral." An alkaline reaction is expressed as a pH above 7.0—for example, 7.1. With increasing acidity, the pH value decreases; for example, a pH of 6.9 is slightly acid.

The pH of blood plasma is maintained within very narrow limits of 7.35 to 7.45—a slightly alkaline reaction. The extremes of pH compatible with life are 6.8 and 7.8; obviously, at these extremes individuals are very ill and prompt therapeutic measures must be instituted if the person is to survive.

Acids formed in metabolism. The principal end products of metabolic activities are acid, chiefly carbonic acid. The oxidation of carbohydrates, fatty acids, and amino acids in the Krebs cycle (see page 71) yields carbon dioxide and water; carbonic acid is the hydrated form of carbon dioxide. Intermediate products in metabolism are also acid such as lactic and pyruvic acid formed in carbohydrate metabolism, keto acids formed in fatty acid oxidation, and amino acids resulting from the hydrolysis of proteins. Urea synthesis is an acid-producing process, and nucleoproteins give rise to uric acid. Sulfuric acid is formed in the body from the sulfur-containing amino acids and phosphoric acid from the phospholipids and phosphoproteins.

The reaction of foods. If the cations (Na^+, K^+, Mg^{++}, and Ca^{++}) remaining in the body on the metabolism of a food exceed the anions (PO_4^{--}, SO_4^{--}, and Cl^-), the food is said to produce an "alkaline ash" and the excess cations will allow the body to retain more bicarbonate ions, thus producing an alkaline reaction. Vegetables, fruits, milk, and some nuts yield excess cations.

Meat, fish, poultry, eggs, cheese, cereals, and some nuts when metabolized yield an excess of anions that are not removed from the body immediately. These foods are said to produce an "acid ash." The excess anions carrying a negative charge must be balanced approximately with some cations. This yields an acid reaction because less bicarbonate, which also carries a negative charge, can exist in the body. The excess bicarbonate ions form carbonic acid, increasing the acidity.

Fats, sugar, and starches contain no mineral elements and are metabolized quickly to carbon dioxide and water which are rapidly removed from the body. These foods, therefore, do not form excess cations or anions which would disturb the neutrality regulation.

Although lemons, oranges, and certain other fruits contain some free organic acids that give them a taste of an acid (sour), they yield an alkaline ash because the body quickly oxidizes the anions of the acid to carbon dioxide and water and leave excess cations that are removed more slowly from the body. Plums, cranberries, and prunes contain aromatic organic acids that are not metabolized in the body, and therefore they increase the acidity of the body fluids.

The regulation of body neutrality. The reaction of the body fluids is kept within a narrow range by the following mechanisms:

1. Dilution is an important defense against the effects of the metabolic acids. The total volume of body fluid, representing about two thirds of body weight, is so great that the con-

siderable amounts of carbon dioxide produced result in only a slight increase in the bicarbonate concentration because of the distribution throughout the fluid system.

2. The presence of certain mixtures, called buffers, minimizes the change in pH when hydrogen ions are increased in the body fluids. They consist of weak acids in the presence of their sodium or potassium salts. The carbonic acid-bicarbonate (H_2CO_3-HCO_3^-) is one important buffer of the blood in maintaining the neutrality. The ease and speed with which the body can get rid of carbon dioxide obtained from this buffer mixture constitute one of the first lines of defense. The plasma bicarbonate is an indicator of the alkaline reserve of the body. Serious disturbances may occur if the alkaline reserve is depleted to a low level. Proteins, including hemoglobin in the blood, and phosphates also form important buffer mixtures.

3. Besides its buffer action hemoglobin aids in the transport of carbon dioxide in two ways which prevent great changes in reaction. The acid strength of hemoglobin is decreased when oxyhemoglobin loses oxygen whereby an extra amount of carbon dioxide can be transported without any change of reaction (isohydric transport). Hemoglobin can also transport a limited amount of carbon dioxide by forming a carbamate, which releases most of the carbon dioxide from the hemoglobin complex at the lung as the hemoglobin takes up oxygen.

4. In one minute the resting individual will have lost about 200 cc carbon dioxide and absorbed about 250 cc oxygen. Any increase in activity will raise the exchange of gases taking place by a very large amount. This is accomplished by increasing the respiratory rate. If the hydrogen ion concentration is increased, the respiratory center in the brain causes an increase in the rate of pulmonary ventilation. The increased ventilation increases the loss of carbon dioxide, and the hydrogen ion concentration of the body fluids returns to normal. If the hydrogen ion concentration is lowered, the respiratory center is inhibited and the rate of ventilation is reduced; thus, the carbonic acid concentration of the body fluids rises.

5. The kidney makes the final adjustment that keeps the body pH within normal limits. The glomerular filtrate has a pH of 7.4, but the kidney can excrete a urine that is as acid as pH 4.5 or as alkaline as pH 8; normally, the average urine pH is 6.0. Bicarbonate ions are filtered into the tubular fluid and their loss from plasma represents loss of alkali. Hydrogen ions are secreted into the tubules, and their loss from plasma represents a loss of acid. When the hydrogen ions of the plasma are increased, the secretion of the hydrogen ions into the tubular fluid also increases and exceeds the loss of bicarbonate, thus permitting the return of plasma to its normal pH. The urine excreted is then more acid. Conversely, in alkalosis the hydrogen ion secretion into the tubules is decreased, thus allowing greater loss of bicarbonate. The urine then becomes more alkaline.

The kidney cannot excrete strong acids such as HCl and H_2SO_4. The hydrogen ions secreted into the lumen of the tubule are excreted by combining with disodium phosphate to form monosodium acid phosphate. By excreting practically all of the phosphate as acid phosphate ($H_2PO_4^-$, instead of HPO_4^{--}) only one phosphate is lost instead of two, thus reducing by half the number of milliequivalents of fixed anions that are excreted; this permits the return of more fixed anions to the circulation.

The kidney is also able to synthesize ammonia from glutamine and other amino acids. The ammonia combines with hydrogen ions to form the ammonium ion (NH_4^+), which can then replace cations such as sodium or potassium. The latter are exchanged for the hydrogen ions so that they can be returned to the blood to carry more carbon dioxide as the bicarbonate ion.

Acidosis and alkalosis. The acid-base balance of the body can be upset by an increase in hydrogen ions, a loss of hydrogen ions, an increase in base, or a loss of base. In each instance the treatment can be instituted only after evaluation of symptoms that are present, the determination of the carbon dioxide content of the blood plasma and the pH, and the cause of the imbalance.

An *acidosis* is a condition in which the hydrogen ion concentration is increased or there is an excessive loss of base (mineral cations); the ratio of bicarbonate to carbonic acid is less than 20:1 and the pH is below 7.35. An *alkalosis* is a condition in which the hydrogen ion concentration is decreased or the base is increased; the ratio of bicarbonate to carbonic acid is greater than 20:1, and the pH is above 7.45.

With changes in concentrations of hydrogen ions and base, the lungs and kidneys attempt to compensate. Ventilation by the lungs is increased when there is an increase in hydrogen ions, and the kidney attempts to adjust by excreting a more acid urine and conserving base with the synthesis of more ammonia. When there is an increase in base, the respiration is depressed, and the hydrogen ions are retained and more base is excreted by the kidneys. If these adjustments succeed in keeping the bicarbonate-carbonic acid ration at 20:1, the pH remains at 7.35 to 7.45; the acidosis or alkalosis is said to be "compensated." When the pH is outside these limits, the acidosis or alkalosis is "uncompensated."

Respiratory acidosis or alkalosis results from an abnormality of the control of the normal CO_2 tension. Hypoventilation such as that seen in pneumonia, pulmonary edema, suppression of breathing as with morphine, and asphyxia lead to acidosis. The kidneys partially compensate by increasing the excretion of hydrogen ions and the synthesis of ammonia, thereby increasing the return of bicarbonate to the blood.

Respiratory alkalosis occurs when there is overventilation of the lungs so that excessive amounts of carbonic acid are lost. This may result from hysteria, from salicylate poisoning, in fevers and infections, and at high altitudes. By reducing the excretion of hydrogen ions and the synthesis of ammonia and by increasing the excretion of sodium, the kidneys compensate in part.

Metabolic acidosis or alkalosis refers to changes resulting from faulty intake or output of acids or bases other than carbonic acid. Metabolic acidosis occurs in a variety of circumstances: the rapid production of ketones in uncontrolled diabetes mellitus; the inability of the kidney to excrete acid phosphates in chronic renal failure; the ketosis of starvation; or the loss of bicarbonate and sodium that occurs with severe diarrhea. Ventilation of the lungs is greatly increased, and air hunger is characteristic of the patient in diabetic acidosis. The synthesis of ammonia by the kidney may increase tenfold in an effort to conserve base.

Metabolic alkalosis occurs when there is a severe loss of hydrochloric acid as a result of vomiting, or by the ingestion of soluble alkalinizing salts such as sodium bicarbonate.

SOME POINTS FOR EMPHASIS IN NUTRITION EDUCATION

1. Mineral elements perform varied and interrelated functions in the body. Among these functions are:

a. The hardness of bones and teeth especially by calcium and phosphorus.

b. The association with proteins in numerous ways: potassium with protein within cells; iron with hemoglobin; phosphorus with phosphoproteins; and so on.

c. The regulation of the transmission of the nerve impulse and the contraction of muscles; contraction of the heart muscle is one example.

d. The maintenance of the proper environment around and within all cells and tissues of the body—acid-base balance.

2. Mineral elements do not yield energy, as do carbohydrates, fats, and proteins; yet they are essential in the processes whereby the body derives its energy from foods.

3. Only calcium, iron, and iodine require particular attention in the planning of diets for normal individuals. Diets that are adequate in protein and calories and that include normal amounts of fruits and vegetables can be expected to supply all the other mineral elements in satisfactory amounts.

4. For most persons the calcium allowance can be met only when the diet includes 2 to 4 cups of milk, depending upon age. Cheese may be substituted for part of the milk allowance.

5. A deficiency of calcium may not become apparent for a long time because the bones supply the blood with its needs. Eventually, sufficient calcium is withdrawn from bones so that they become brittle and break easily, and osteoporosis may occur later in life.

6. Iron-deficiency anemia is widely prevalent, especially in infants, preschool children, teen-age girls, and pregnant women.

The only practical way by which these groups can obtain their iron needs is through the use of foods highly fortified with iron or by oral supplements of iron salts.

7. Iodine deficiency leads to endemic goiter. It can be prevented by the use of iodized salt.

8. Variations in the intake of acid-producing or alkali-producing foods do not result in acidosis or alkalosis in healthy individuals.

Problems and Review

1. Give several examples of the ways in which minerals function together in the body structure; in regulatory activities.
2. List four functions of calcium; of phosphorus.
3. What anions may combine with calcium in the intestinal tract and thus interfere with absorption? In which foods do these predominate? Of what practical significance is this in American diets?
4. Many adults believe that their needs for calcium are low because their bones are fully developed. Explain why this reasoning is wrong.
5. Iron is essentially a one-way substance. What does this mean? How does this affect the daily requirement?
6. *Problem.* Calculate your daily intake of calcium and iron for two days. Compare your intake with the recommended allowances. What were the important sources of calcium in your diet? Of iron?
7. *Problem.* Using the basic diet calculation on page 205, show how the iron level can be increased to 18 mg. Include your calculations for iron and for calories.
8. What is the principal function of iodine? What happens if the intake is inadequate?
9. To which groups of individuals is the prophylactic use of iodine especially important?
10. If you consume 10 gm of iodized salt in a day, how much iodine would you ingest if the level of iodization is 0.005 per cent?
11. What is the significance of fluorine in nutrition? What levels of fluorine are recommended in drinking water?
12. What is meant by dental fluorosis? At what levels of intake does it occur?
13. Name the principal mineral elements that contribute to an alkaline ash. Which foods are classed as alkali producing?
14. Name the principal mineral elements that contribute to an acid ash. Which foods are classed as acid producing?
15. What is the metabolic effect of an excess of acid-producing or of alkali-producing foods?
16. Describe the ways in which the lungs function to maintain the normal blood pH. Describe how the kidneys make the final adjustments to maintain acid-base balance.
17. Describe the water compartments of the body in terms of (a) relative size; (b) electrolyte composition.
18. What are the daily sources of water to the body? What are the routes of excretion by the healthy individual?
19. Describe the functioning parts of the kidney in terms of the results achieved by each of these parts.
20. What hormones control the excretion of water? Of sodium and potassium?
21. What is meant by obligatory water loss? If you found yourself in a situation where drinking water was extremely limited in supply, how could you reduce the loss of water from your body?

Table 9–3. Summary of the Minerals

Minerals	Functions in the Body	Metabolism	Food Sources	Daily Allowances
Calcium	Hardness of bones, teeth Transmission of nerve impulse Muscle contraction Normal heart rhythm Activate enzymes Increase cell permeability Catalyze thrombin formation	*Absorption*: about 5–10 per cent, according to body need; aided by gastric acidity, vitamin D, lactose; excess phosphate, fat, phytate, oxalic acid interfere *Storage*: trabeculae of bones; easily mobilized *Utilization*: needs parathyroid hormone, vitamin D *Excretion*: 60–90 per cent of diet intake in feces; small urinary excretion *Deficiency*: retarded bone mineralization; fragile bones; stunted growth; rickets; osteomalacia; osteoporosis	Milk, hard cheese Ice cream, cottage cheese Greens: turnip, collards, kale, mustard, broccoli Oysters, shrimp, salmon, clams	Children: 800 mg Teen-agers: 1200 mg Adults: 800 mg Pregnancy: 1200 mg Lactation: 1200 mg
Phosphorus	Structure of bones, teeth Cell permeability Metabolism of fats and carbohydrates: storage and release of ATP Sugar-phosphate linkage in DNA and RNA Phospholipids in transport of fats Buffer salts in acid-base balance	*Absorption*: about 70 per cent; aided by vitamin D *Utilization*: about 85 per cent in bones; controlled by vitamin D, parathormone *Excretion*: about one third of diet in feces; metabolic products chiefly in urine *Deficiency*: poor bone mineralization; poor growth; rickets	Milk, cheese Eggs, meat, fish, poultry Legumes, nuts Whole-grain cereals	Infants: 200 to 400 mg Children: 800 mg Adults: 800 mg Pregnancy: 1200 mg Lactation: 1200 mg
Magnesium	Constituents of bones, teeth Activates enzymes in carbohydrate metabolism Muscle and nerve irritability	*Absorption*: parallels that of calcium; competes with calcium for carriers *Utilization*: slowly mobilized from bone *Excretion*: chiefly by kidney *Deficiency*: seen in alcoholism, severe renal disease; hypo-magnesemia, tremor	Cereals, legumes Nuts Meat Milk	Infants: 60 to 70 mg Women: 300 mg Men: 350 mg Pregnancy and lactation: 450 mg

Element	Functions	Metabolism	Food Sources	Requirement
Sulfur	Constituent of proteins, especially cartilage, hair, nails Constituent of melanin, glutathione, thiamine, biotin, coenzyme A, insulin High-energy sulfur bonds Detoxication reactions	Absorbed chiefly as sulfur-containing amino acids Excreted as inorganic sulfate in urine in proportion to nitrogen loss	Protein foods rich in sulfur amino acids Eggs Meat Milk, cheese Nuts, legumes	Not established Diet adequate in protein meets need
Sodium	Principal cation of extra-cellular fluid Osmotic pressure; water balance Acid-base balance Regulate nerve irritability and muscle contraction "Pump" for glucose transport	*Absorption*: rapid and almost complete *Excretion*: chiefly in urine: some by skin and in feces; parallels intake; controlled by aldosterone *Deficiency*: rare; occurs with excessive perspiration and poor diet intake; nausea, diarrhea, abdominal cramps muscle cramps	Table salt Milk Meat, fish, poultry Egg white	Not established Probably about 500 mg except with excessive perspiration Diets supply substantial excess
Potassium	Principal cation of intracellular fluid Osmotic pressure; water balance; acid-base balance Nerve irritability and muscle contraction Regular heart rhythm Synthesis of protein Glycogenesis	*Absorption*: readily absorbed *Excretion*: chiefly in urine: increased with aldosterone secretion *Deficiency*: following starvation, correction of diabetic acidosis, adrenal tumors; muscle weakness, nausea, tachycardia, glycogen depletion, heart failure	Widely distributed in foods Meat, fish, fowl Cereals Fruits, vegetables	Not established Diet adequate in calories supplies ample amounts
Chlorine	Chief anion of extracellular fluid Constituent of gastric juice Acid-base balance; chloride-bicarbonate shift in red cells	*Absorption*: rapid and almost complete *Excretion*: chiefly in urine; parallels intake *Deficiency*: with prolonged vomiting, drainage from fistula, diarrhea	Table salt	Not established Daily diet contains 3 to 9 gm, far in excess of need

Table 9-3. Summary of the Minerals (Cont.)

Minerals	Functions in the Body	Metabolism	Food Sources	Daily Allowances
Iron	Constituent of hemoglobin, myoglobin, and oxidative enzymes: catalase, cytochrome, xanthine oxidase	*Absorption:* about 5 to 10 per cent; regulated according to body need; aided by gastric acidity, ascorbic acid *Transport:* bound to protein, transferrin *Storage:* as ferritin in liver, bone marrow, spleen *Utilization:* chiefly in hemoglobin; daily turnover about 27 to 28 mg; iron used over and over again *Excretion:* men, about 1 mg; women, 1 to 2 mg; in urine, perspiration, menstrual flow: fecal excretion is from unabsorbed diet *Deficiency:* anemia: frequent in infants, preschool children, teen-age girls, pregnant women	Liver, organ meats Meat, poultry Egg yolk Enriched and wholegrain breads, cereals Dark-green vegetables Legumes Molasses, dark Peaches, apricots, prunes, raisins Diets supply about 6 mg per 1000 calories	Infants: 10 to 15 mg Children: 10 to 15 mg Men: 10 mg Women: 18 mg Pregnancy and lactation: 18+ mg
Iodine	Constituent of diiodotyrosine, triiodothyronine, thyroxine; regulate rate of energy metabolism	*Absorption:* controlled by blood level of protein-bound iodine *Storage:* thyroid gland; activity regulated by thyroid-stimulating hormone *Excretion:* in urine *Deficiency:* simple goiter; if severe, cretinism—rarely seen in U.S.	Iodized salt is most reliable source Seafood Foods grown in non-goitrous coastal areas	Infants: 35–45 mcg Men: 130 mcg Women: 100 mcg Pregnancy: 125 mcg Lactation: 150 mcg
Manganese	Activation of many enzymes: oxidation of carbohydrates, urea formation, protein hydrolysis Bone formation	*Absorption:* limited *Excretion:* chiefly in feces *Deficiency:* not known	Legumes, nuts Whole-grain cereals	Not established

Mineral	Functions	Metabolism	Food Sources	Requirements
Copper	Aids absorption and use of iron in synthesis of hemoglobin Electron transport Melanin formation Myelin sheath of nerves Purine metabolism Metabolism of ascorbic acid	*Transport*: chiefly as protein, ceruloplasmin *Storage*: liver, central nervous system *Excretion*: bile into intestine *Deficiency*: rare; occurs in severe malnutrition Abnormal storage in Wilson's disease	Liver, shellfish Meats Nuts, legumes Whole-grain cereals Typical diet provides 2 to 5 mg	Infants: 0.08 mg per kg Adults: 2 mg
Zinc	Constituent of enzymes: carbonic anhydrase, carboxypeptidase, lactic dehydrogenase	*Absorption*: limited; competes with calcium for absorption sites *Storage*: liver, muscles, bones, organs *Excretion*: chiefly by intestine *Deficiency*: only in severe malnutrition	Seafoods Liver and other organ meats Meats, fish Wheat germ Yeast Plant foods are generally low Usual diet supplies 10 to 15 mg	Infants: 3–5 mg Children: 10 mg Adults: 15 mg Pregnancy: 20 mg Lactation: 25 mg
Fluorine	Increases resistance of teeth to decay; most effective in young children Moderate levels in bone may reduce osteoporosis	*Storage*: bones and teeth *Excretion*: urine Excess leads to mottling of teeth	Fluoridated water: 1 ppm	Not required for growth; not considered to be a dietary essential
Molybdenum	Cofactor for flavoprotein enzymes; present in xanthine oxidase	Absorbed as molybdate Stored in liver, adrenal, kidney Related to metabolism of copper and sulfur	Organ meats Legumes Whole-grain cereals	Not established
Selenium	Antioxidant Substitutes for some of functions of vitamin E	Stored especially in liver, kidney High intake may increase incidence of dental caries	Foods grown on selenium-rich soils may contain hazardous levels	Not established

CITED REFERENCES

1. Magnus-Levy, A., quoted in Rowntree, L. G.: "The Water Balance of the Body," *Physiol. Rev.*, **2**:116, 1922.
2. Food and Nutrition Board: *Recommended Dietary Allowances*, 7th ed. Pub. 1694. National Academy Sciences–National Research Council, Washington, D.C., 1968.
3. Statland, H., cited by Snively, W. D., Jr., and Brown, B. J.: "In the Balance," *Am. J. Nurs.*, **58**:55–57, 1958.
4. West E. S., *et al.*: *Textbook of Biochemistry*, 4th ed. The Macmillan Company, New York, 1966, p. 686.
5. Krehl, W. A.: "The Potassium Depletion Syndrome," *Nutr. Today*, **1**:20, June 1966.
6. Brook, C. E., and Anast, C. S.: "Oral Fluid and Electrolytes," *J.A.M.A.*, **179**:792–97, 1962.
7. Wright, A.: *Rypins' Medical Licensure Examination.* J. B. Lippincott Company, Philadelphia, 1970, p. 98.
8. Frisell, W. R.: *Acid-Base Chemistry in Medicine.* The Macmillan Company, New York, 1968, p. 51.

ADDITIONAL REFERENCES

Abbey, J. C.: "Nursing Observations of Fluid Imbalance," *Nurs. Clin. North Am.*, **3**:77–86, 1968.
Anthony, C. P.: "Fluid Imbalance—Formidable Foe to Survival," *Am. J. Nurs.*, **63**:75–77, 1963.
Baker, E. M., *et al.*: "Water Requirements of Men as Related to Salt Intake," *Am. J. Clin. Nutr.*, **12**:394–98, 1963.
Bugg, R.: "Your Body's Silent Partners," *Today's Health*, **7**:54, Jan. 1969.
Burgess, R. E.: "Fluids and Electrolytes," *Am. J. Nurs.*, **65**:90–95, 1965.
Camien, M. N., *et al.*: "A Critical Reappraisal of 'Acid-Base' Balance," *Am. J. Clin. Nutr.*, **22**: 786–93, 1969.
Earley, L. E., and Daugharty, T. M.: "Sodium Metabolism," *N. Engl. J. Med.*, **281**:72–86, 1969.
Fenton, M.: "What to Do About Thirst," *Am. J. Nurs.*, **69**:1014–17, 1969.
Frazier, H. S.: "Renal Regulation of Sodium Balance," *N. Engl. J. Med.*, **279**:868–75, 1968.
Kleeman, C. R., and Fichman, M. P.: "The Clinical Physiology of Water Metabolism," *N. Engl. J. Med.*, **277**:1300–1307, 1967.
Krehl, W. A.: "Sodium: A Most Extraordinary Dietary Essential," *Nutr. Today*, **1**:16, Dec. 1966.
"Potassium Balance," *Am. J. Nurs.*, **67**:343–66, 1967.
Review: "Sodium Intake and Blood Pressure," *Nutr. Rev.*, **27**:280–82, 1969.
Smith, J. R.: "Salt," *Nutr. Rev.*, **11**:33–36, 1953.
Strong, C. G.: "Hormonal Influence on Renal Function," *Med. Clin. North Am.*, **50**:985–95, 1966.
Wolf, A. V.: "The Castaway at Sea," *Nutr. Rev.*, **14**:161–64, 1956.

10 The Fat-Soluble Vitamins

INTRODUCTION TO THE STUDY OF THE VITAMINS

The story of the vitamins—their discovery, their positive functions in maintaining health, and their usefulness in healing deficiency diseases—is fascinating and deserving of considerable study. Popular interest was early aroused by the discovery of the role of vitamins in preventing such severe deficiency diseases as scurvy, pellagra, beriberi, and others. It is now known that vitamins function primarily in enzyme systems which facilitate the metabolism of amino acids, fats, and carbohydrates. Those who understand the functions of vitamins do not minimize their importance in relation to the utilization of food. However, it is important that no one be misled into believing that vitamins are "cure-alls" for disease. The properties of vitamins, their functions in metabolism, their distribution in foods, and the effects of deficiency will be discussed in the sections below.

Definition and nomenclature. The term *vitamine* was first coined by the Polish chemist, Funk, who believed that the water-soluble anti-beriberi substance he was describing was a "vital amine." The final "e" was soon dropped, but *vitamins* is the name given to a group of potent organic compounds other than protein, carbohydrate, and fat which occur in minute quantities in foods and which are essential for some specific body functions of maintenance and growth. Many of them cannot be synthesized, at least in adequate amounts, by the body and must be obtained from the diet.

Early classifications listed two groups of vitamins, namely, those that are water soluble and those that are fat soluble. This classification has been generally accepted, but it is arbitrary inasmuch as the vitamins within each group are not similar in their properties, functions, or distribution. Vitamins were first named for their curative properties or were given a convenient letter designation. Today, chemically descriptive names are now used for many of the vitamins; letter designations are still applied in some instances.

Measurement. Before the chemical nature of vitamins was discovered, their potency could be measured only by their ability to promote growth or to cure a deficiency when test doses were fed experimental animals such as rats, guinea pigs, pigeons, and chicks. Such measurement is known as "bioassay" and has been expressed in terms of units. Vitamins A and D are still measured in international units (I.U.). Other vitamins, formerly measured in units, are now measured by chemical assay in milligrams (mg) or micrograms (mcg or μg), 1 milligram being equal to 1000 micrograms. Still other vitamins are measured by their ability to promote growth of microorganisms; this is known as microbiologic assay.

Selection of foods for vitamin content. In selecting the foods to furnish vitamins in the diet it is well to keep in mind the following points: (1) under normal circumstances it is better to use common food sources than concentrates, because foods furnish other essential factors as well; (2) it is important to determine how often any given food will be used in the dietary; (3) the amount of food which would ordinarily be used must be ascertained; (4) the effects of processing and preparation of foods on the vitamin retention must be clearly understood; and (5) economic factors such as availability and cost must be considered. For example, 100 gm of parsley furnish about 8500 I.U. of vitamin A, whereas 100 gm of milk supply only 140 I.U. of vitamin A. Parsley, as a garnish, will have limited use, whereas 1 pint of milk a day, essential in an adequate diet, furnishes about 10 per cent of the day's needs for vitamin A.

Vitamin supplementation of the diet. Any diet selected on the basis of the Four Food Groups will provide the necessary amounts of vitamins. Vitamin supplements are not necessary for healthy persons. As a matter of fact, the water-soluble vitamins in excess of body need will be excreted in the urine. Vitamin A, being fat soluble, is stored in appreciable amounts in the liver; other fat-soluble vitamins are stored to a lesser degree. As a matter of fact, excessive intakes of vitamins A and D have been shown to be toxic.

Vitamin D supplementation for infants, growing children, and pregnant or lactating women is an important exception to the above statement since the diet does not supply sufficient amounts of the vitamin if fortified foods are not used.

Physicians may recommend supplementation of the diet when physical or emotional illness prevents the consumption of a fully adequate diet. Sometimes through ignorance or through poor eating habits a serious dietary deficiency of vitamins may pertain, in which instance a supplement is sometimes prescribed. However, such supplementation should never replace efforts toward the correction of the factors leading to the dietary inadequacy.

Undoubtedly, the sale of vitamin supplements far exceeds the need for them. The potency of preparations on the market varies widely, and the number of nutrients contained differs from one product to another. The consumer is unable, as a rule, to interpret the label information in terms of his own requirements. Under consideration by the Food and Drug Administration are regulations which would define the levels of nutrients to be used in such preparations and the appropriate labeling for these products. Such regulations are urgently needed.

VITAMIN A

Discovery. In 1913 McCollum and Davis of the University of Wisconsin and Osborne and Mendel of Yale University independently discovered that rats consuming purified diets with lard as the only source of fat failed to grow and developed soreness of the eyes. When butterfat or ether extract of egg yolk was added to the diet, growth resumed and the eye condition was corrected. The term *fat-soluble* A was applied by McCollum to the organic complex present in the ether extracts that was necessary for normal growth.

A few years later Steenbock at the University of Wisconsin demonstrated that the yellow pigments in plants, the carotenes, had vitamin A activity. The carotenes are now known as *provitamins* A or *precursors* of vitamin A.

Chemistry and characteristics. Vitamin A occurs in several forms: as *retinol* (an alcohol); as *retinal* (also known as retinene), an aldehyde; and as *retinoic acid*. It may be esterified and is known as *retinyl ester*. These several forms may be referred to as vitamin A. (See Figure 10–1.)

In its pure form vitamin A is a pale-yellow crystalline compound. It occurs naturally in the animal kingdom and has been synthesized so that it is available commercially. It is soluble in fat and fat solvents but insoluble in water, and it is relatively stable to heat and to acids and alkalies. It is easily oxidized and rapidly destroyed by ultraviolet irradiation.

The ultimate source of all vitamin A is in the carotenes which are synthesized by plants. Animals in turn, and man as well, convert a considerable proportion of the carotene of the foods they eat into vitamin A. The carotenes are dark-red crystalline compounds. Alpha-, beta-, and gamma-carotene and possibly cryptoxanthin are of nutritional significance. Upon hydrolysis each molecule of beta-carotene ($C_{40}H_{56}$) yields 2 molecules of vitamin A, while each molecule of the other three carotenes yields only 1 molecule of vitamin A.

Measurement. For many years vitamin A has been measured in international units. One unit of vitamin A is defined as the activity of 0.344 mcg crystalline retinyl acetate (0.300 mcg retinol). Retinol equivalents (R.E.) are proposed as a more precise designation, and it is expected that values in tables of dietary allowances and food composition will eventually be expressed as

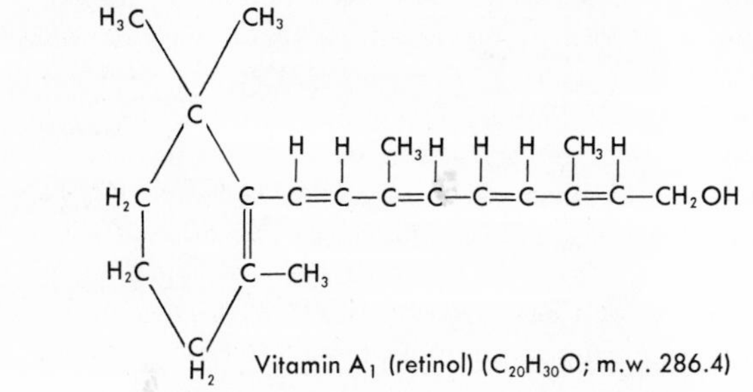

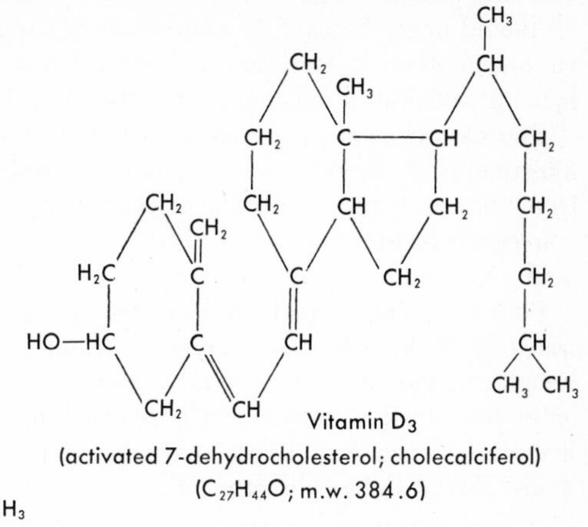

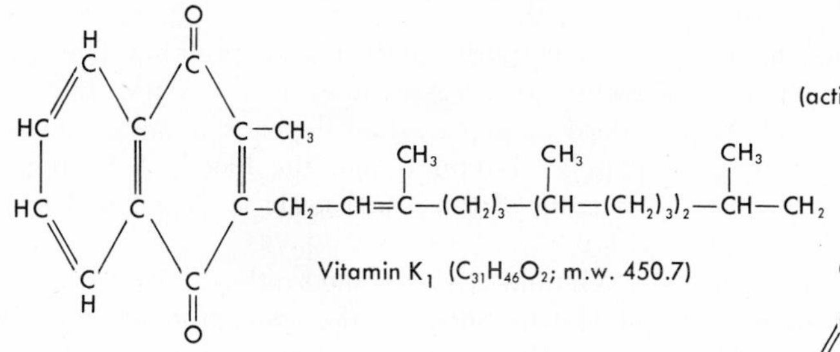

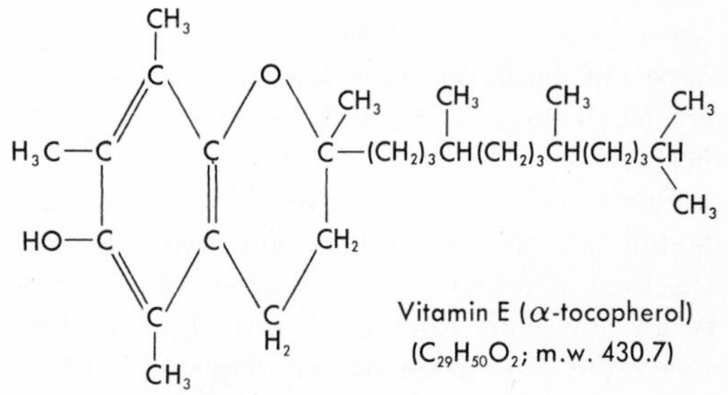

Figure 10–1. Each of the fat-soluble vitamins exists in several forms, only one of which is shown here. Note the similarity of structure of vitamin D to cholesterol.

R.E. rather than I.U.[3] Note these comparisons:

　1 R.E. = 1 mcg retinol, or 6 mcg beta-carotene, or 12 mcg other carotenes
　1 R.E. = 3.33 I.U. retinol or 10 I.U. beta-carotene

Absorption, storage, and transport. Foods supply vitamin A in the form of carotenes, as vitamin A esters, and as free vitamin A. The biologic availability of carotenes is much less than the theoretic yield and varies widely. Since carotenes are the principal source of vitamin A in the developing countries, it is important to have information on their availability. Studies on an Indian male population showed a range of absorption of carotenes from vegetables to be 33 to 58 per cent, with an average absorption of 50 per cent or more.[1] Another study on undernourished children showed that carotene absorption was not impaired when protein-calorie malnutrition was mild.[2] Not all of the carotene

absorbed will be converted to vitamin A. The FAO-WHO group has estimated that half of the absorbed carotene is converted to vitamin A, and that only one sixth of the carotene content of food is eventually utilized.

Vitamin A esters are hydrolyzed in the intestinal lumen before absorption takes place. The simultaneous presence of vitamin E in the intestinal tract prevents the excessive oxidation of vitamin A that would otherwise occur.

The absorption of vitamin A and the carotenes, like that of fat, is facilitated by bile. When a diet is very low in fat, or when there is an obstruction of the bile duct, the absorption of vitamin A and the carotenes is seriously impaired. The thyroid hormone facilitates vitamin A absorption.

The presence of mineral oil in the intestinal tract reduces the absorption of vitamin A. Since mineral oil is not absorbed and since it holds carotenes and vitamin A in solution, the vitamins are lost through excretion. Therefore, mineral oil should never be used as a substitute for regular fats in food preparation and should not be taken at mealtimes when it is used as a laxative.

The carotenes are converted to retinol in the intestinal mucosa. Within the mucosa the retinol from dietary sources or that derived from the conversion of carotene is esterified with palmitic acid.

Retinyl esters, retinal, and retinoic acid are transported in the chylomicrons through the lymph circulation to the thoracic duct and then enter the blood circulation to be carried to the liver for storage. Significant amounts of vitamin A are also absorbed directly into the portal circulation.[4] About 95 per cent of the body's vitamin A stores are held in the liver. The healthy adult has a store that is adequate for his needs for as long as a year. Infants and young children have not built up such reserves and therefore are much more susceptible to the effects of deficiency.

Retinol is carried in the blood circulation bound to a specific protein. The liver maintains the level of retinol in the blood so long as there is an adequate reserve of retinyl ester. Only when the liver reserves are depleted will the blood concentration be lowered.

Functions. Although vitamin A has been known for about 50 years, its functions have not been fully explained. Retinyl esters, retinol, and retinal are readily converted from one form to another, but retinoic acid cannot be converted to other forms. Retinoic acid fulfills some of the functions of vitamin A but does not function in the visual cycle.

The best understood function of vitamin A is related to the maintenance of normal vision in dim light. The retina of the eye contains two kinds of light receptors: the rods for vision in dim light and the cones for vision in bright light and color vision. The rods produce a photosensitive pigment, rhodopsin or visual purple, and the cones produce iodopsin or visual violet. In both these pigments vitamin A aldehyde is the prosthetic group, but the proteins to which the aldehyde is attached are different. When light strikes the pigments, they are split to the constituent parts, retinal and protein. The pigments are regenerated in the dark, but the speed of regeneration depends upon a constant supply of retinol from the blood. A simplified diagram of the visual cycle is shown in Figure 10–2.

Vitamin A effects the synthesis of constituents of mucus such as the mucoproteins and the mucopolysaccharides. The mucus secretions maintain the integrity of the epithelium, especially the membranes that line the eyes, the mouth, and the gastrointestinal, respiratory, and genitourinary tracts. These membranes maintained in their optimum condition offer resistance to bacterial invasion; to that extent vitamin A gives protection against infection, but the designation *anti-infective* is unfortunate. Large intakes of vitamin A do not confer additional protective benefits.

Vitamin A is essential for normal skeletal and tooth development. With a deficiency of vitamin A bones do not grow in length and the normal remodeling process does not take place. Studies on experimental animals have shown

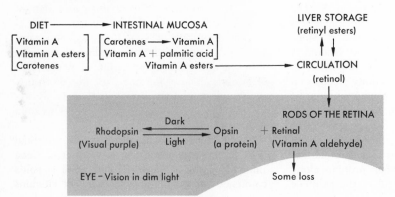

Figure 10–2. Metabolism of vitamin A for vision in dim light.

that vitamin A is essential for spermatogenesis in the male and normal estrus cycle in the female. If vitamin A is not available during fetal development many malformations result. The synthesis of hydrocortisone from cholesterol is facilitated in the adrenal cortex by vitamin A. The stability of biologic membranes appears to be maintained by an interaction of vitamins A and E.

Daily allowances. The recommended allowances for vitamin A are stated in retinol equivalents and international units.[3] When international units are calculated to retinol equivalents, it is assumed that one half of the vitamin A is retinol and one half is beta-carotene. Thus, 5000 I.U. = 1000 R.E.:

$$2500 \text{ I.U.} \div 3.33 = 750 \text{ R.E.}$$
$$2500 \text{ I.U.} \div 10 = 250 \text{ R.E.}$$
$$\overline{1000 \text{ R.E.}}$$

The vitamin A allowance for males over 11 years is 1000 R.E. or 5000 I.U. and for females over 11 years is 800 R.E. or 4000 I.U. The allowances for infants over 6 months and children up to 10 years are 400 to 700 R.E., for pregnancy 1000 R.E., and for lactation 1200 R.E.

Food sources. Only animal foods contain vitamin A as such, fish-liver oils being outstanding. These oils are generally not classed with common foods, but milk, butter, fortified margarines, whole-milk cheese, liver, and egg yolk contain vitamin A.

The principal source of vitamin A in the diet is likely to be from the carotenes which are widespread in those plant foods which have high green or yellow colorings. There is a direct correlation between the greenness of a leaf and its carotene content. Dark-green leaves are rich in carotene, but the pale leaves, in lettuce and cabbage for example, are insignificant sources. Abundant sources of carotene are found in foods such as:

Green leafy vegetables—spinach, turnip tops, chard, beet greens
Green stem vegetables—asparagus, broccoli
Yellow vegetables—carrots, sweet potatoes, winter squash, pumpkin
Yellow fruits—apricots, peaches, cantaloupe

The vitamin A contribution of the Four Food Groups is indicated in Figure 10–3. The meat group contributes only when liver or an organ meat is served once every week to 10 days. One egg provides about one tenth of the daily allowance.

Retention of food values. Since vitamin A is stable to the usual cooking temperatures, only slight losses are likely to occur in food preparation. The wilting of vegetables or dehydration of foods results in considerable losses. Canned and frozen foods retain maximal values for nine months or longer. Vitamin A activity is rapidly lost in rancid fats.

Effects of vitamin A deficiency. In the United States vitamin A deficiency should be practically nonexistent inasmuch as there are abundant

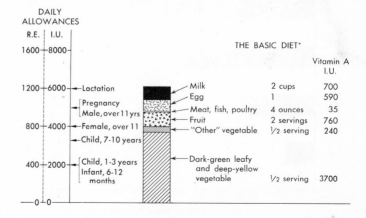

Figure 10–3. The Four Food Groups of the Basic Diet provide a liberal allowance of vitamin A for all age categories. Note the contribution made by dark-green, leafy, and deep-yellow vegetables. Breads, cereals, flours, and white potato do not provide vitamin A. See Table 13–2 for complete calculations.

dietary sources of vitamin A available. Nevertheless, the 1965 household survey of diets showed that one diet in every four failed to supply the recommended allowances and that one diet in every 10 supplied less than two thirds of the recommended allowances. (See Figure 1–4.) The National Nutrition Survey conducted on low-income groups disclosed that serum vitamin A levels were less than adequate in about 13 per cent of the population surveyed.[5] The predominance of low serum levels was in young children. About one fourth of the children six to nine years of age had low levels and one third of preschool children had unacceptable serum levels of vitamin A. (See Figure 10–4.)

Vitamin A deficiency and protein malnutrition are the principal nutritional problems throughout the world today. When the two conditions are present in the same child, the prognosis is very poor. In most countries of the world ample supplies of carotene are available, but people need to be educated to use the plant food sources containing it.

In addition to inadequate dietary intake, vitamin A deficiency may result from faulty absorption and metabolism such as chronic diarrhea in sprue and colitis, liver disease, abnormal fat metabolism as in pancreatic dysfunction, or incomplete absorption because of the use of mineral oil.

Night blindness. One of the earliest signs of vitamin A deficiency is night blindness, or nyctalopia (see Figure 10–5). This is a condition in which the individual is unable to see well in dim light, especially on coming into darkness from a bright light as in entering a darkened theater. Drivers who are easily blinded (glare blindness) by the headlights of other automobiles and who consequently see road markers, pedestrians, etc., with difficulty constitute a special traffic hazard. Nyctalopia occurs when there is insufficient vitamin A to bring about prompt and complete regeneration of visual purple. Dark-adaptation tests with a biophotometer, blood carotene and vitamin A levels, and a substantiating dietary history are useful in establishing a diagnosis of vitamin A deficiency. Other causes of night blindness must be ruled out. If a therapeutic dose of vitamin A does not bring about relief of night blindness after a few weeks' trial, it may be assumed that the condition is not a vitamin A deficiency.

Epithelial changes. An inadequate supply of vitamin A may lead to definite changes in the epithelial tissues throughout the body: *keratinization,* or a noticeable shrinking, hardening,

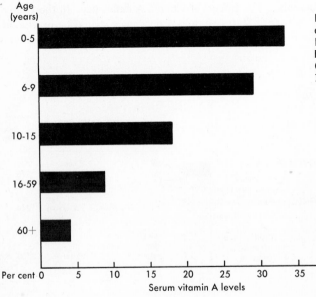

Figure 10–4. This chart shows the percentage of persons of low income in the National Nutrition Survey that had low serum vitamin A levels. (Courtesy, Drs. A. E. Schaefer and O. C. Johnson. Reprinted from *Nutrition Today,* **4**:6 [Spring], 1969 by permission.)

Figure 10–5. Night blindness. (*A*) Safe driving at night depends, in part, on the ability of one's eyes to adjust to the glare of lights. (*B*) Properly focused headlights of an approaching automobile do not impede a good view of the road when the eye has an adequate supply of vitamin A. (*C*) The edge of the road and distances far ahead cannot be seen immediately after meeting an automobile when there is insufficient vitamin A available to the eye. (Courtesy, The Upjohn Company, Kalamazoo, Mich.)

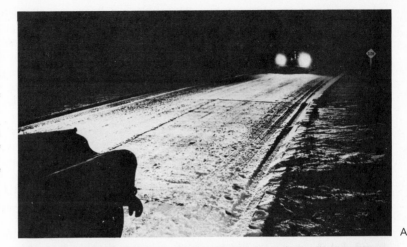

A

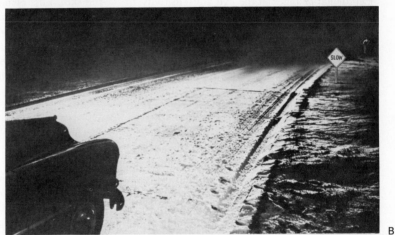

B

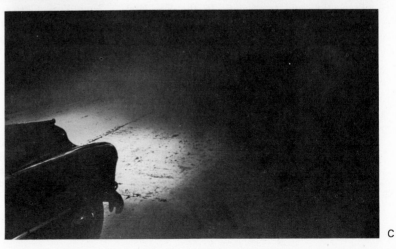

C

and progressive degeneration of the cells, occurs, which increases the susceptibility to severe infections of the eye, the nasal passages, the sinuses, middle ear, lungs, and genitourinary tract.

Skin changes in severe vitamin A deficiency known as *follicular hyperkeratosis* have been described. The skin becomes rough, dry, and scaly. The keratinized epithelium plugs the sebaceous glands so that goose-pimple-like follicles appear first along the upper forearms and thighs, and then spread along the shoulders, back, abdomen, and buttocks.

Epithelial changes in the eye. The epithelium of the eye may be so profoundly affected during vitamin A deficiency that the condition finally becomes irreversible. The first mild symptoms of epithelial changes in the eye are sensitivity to bright light (photophobia), itching, burning, and sometimes inflammation of the lids. The eyes and the eyelids become dry and inflamed owing to impairment of the lacrimal glands, whose function it is to secrete fluid to keep the surface moist and wash away bacteria and other foreign agents. *Xerophthalmia* is the most serious disturbance in the eye and occurs only after deficiency has been severe and prolonged. The cornea becomes dry and then inflamed and edematous. This is later followed by cloudiness and infection which leads to ulceration. The absence of the usual eye secretions provides a favorable medium for infection. The final stage of the disease, *keratomalacia,* is a softening of the cornea with permanent blindness resulting.

Prevention and treatment. In the Far East where xerophthalmia is a major cause of blindness, vitamin A deficiency is often attributed to ignorance since dietary sources of carotene are locally available. The very low fat intake by many of these people reduces the efficiency of absorption.

Vitamin A deficiency may become manifest in children who are fed skim milk for the treatment of kwashiorkor. As the child responds to the protein in the milk, the liver is rapidly depleted of its small store of vitamin A, thus precipitating the symptoms of deficiency. Therefore, it is important that the treatment for protein malnutrition include vitamin A supplements.

The recommended allowances for vitamin A

fully protect the normal individual against evidences of deficiency. Once deficiency has appeared, therapy consists of (1) correcting the diet so that vitamin A once again becomes adequate, (2) removing or curing any condition that interferes with absorption, and (3) prescribing therapeutic doses of vitamin concentrates.

Hypervitaminosis A. Therapeutic doses of vitamin A in excess of 50,000 I.U. daily over prolonged periods may be toxic to adults. Lesser doses will produce symptoms in children. Infants who received 18,500 to 60,000 I.U. daily showed signs of toxicity within 12 weeks.[6] The common symptoms of toxicity are anorexia, hyperirritability, and drying and desquamation of the skin. Loss of hair, bone and joint pain, bone fragility, headaches, and enlargement of the liver and speen are quite frequent. When vitamin A is discontinued, recovery takes place. Far too frequently excessive dosages are prescribed, and some individuals use supplements with uncalled-for zeal.

VITAMIN D

Cod-liver oil has been recommended as a remedy for rickets ever since the Middle Ages but does not appear to have been used with any consistency until the present century. During World War I, Hess and Unger noted the effect of cod-liver oil in protecting Negro children in New York City against rickets. Then in 1919 Mellanby found that the skeletal structure of puppies was influenced by some fat-soluble substance in food. McCollum, Steenbock, and Drummond simultaneously reported that cod-liver oil in which vitamin A had been destroyed still retained its antirachitic properties, and hence it was shown that vitamin A was not the antirachitic factor. Steenbock and Hess in 1924 independently found that foods that had been exposed to ultraviolet rays possessed antirachitic properties. Pure vitamin D was isolated in crystalline form in 1930 and was called calciferol.

Chemistry and characteristics. Vitamin D is a group of chemically distinct sterol compounds possessing antirachitic properties, but it is customary to speak of the group as though it were one vitamin. The vitamins are produced by irradiating a precursor or provitamin D with ultraviolet light; in other words, substances like ergosterol are exposed to ultraviolet light to form calciferol. Of the 10 or more forms of this vitamin which are known, only two are of nutritional interest: (1) vitamin D_2 (ergocalciferol)—ergosterol being the chief vitamin D precursor found in plants; and (2) vitamin D_3 (cholecalciferol)—the chief form occurring in animal cells and developed in the skin on exposure to ultraviolet light from sunshine or from a machine. (See Figure 10–1.) Pure vitamins D are white, odorless crystals which are soluble in fats and in fat solvents. They are insoluble in water, and they are stable to heat, alkalies, and oxidation.

Measurement. One international unit (I.U.) of vitamin D is the activity of 0.025 mcg of pure crystalline vitamin D. The I.U. and U.S.P. unit are identical.

Rachitic rats are the standard test animals for measuring the potency of vitamin D in materials. Young rats from mothers having a deficient supply of vitamin D are kept on a rachitogenic diet so that no calcification occurs in the ends of the long bones. When a test material is fed, its value as a source of vitamin D is measured by the amount which must be fed for 7 to 10 days to produce a good calcium line (line test) in the ends of the long bones. Standard cod-liver oil is fed to a similar group of animals and is used as a basis of comparison. No satisfactory chemical or microbiologic assay is yet available. (See Figure 10–6.)

Physiology. Vitamin D from the dietary or from concentrates is absorbed from the intestine together with the fats. Bile salts appear to be necessary for absorption. Man can synthesize provitamin D_3 in the body, and activation takes place in the skin on exposure to ultraviolet light. Vitamin D_3 from the skin or vitamin D_2 absorbed from the intestine is stored primarily in the liver, although some is also found in the skin, brain, lungs, spleen, and bones. The body conserves its stores of vitamin D carefully.

Function. Vitamin D regulates the absorption of calcium and phosphorus from the intestinal tract and also the calcification of bones and

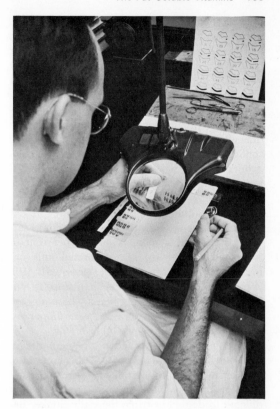

Figure 10–6. The line test is still used for determination of vitamin D. On charts in background, the darker the line, the better the healing. The amount of healing is related to the amount of vitamin D supplied to the test animal by the diet. (Courtesy, Food and Drug Administration.)

teeth but the mechanisms by which this is accomplished is not known. It is believed that vitamin D renders the intestinal mucosa more permeable to calcium and phosphorus and that in some way the active transport of calcium across cell barriers is facilitated.

Vitamin D improves the calcification of bone by regulating the amount of phosphorus that is available. The reabsorption of phosphate by the kidney tubules is increased by the influence of vitamin D. Also, the release of phosphate from organic compounds is dependent upon an enzyme, *alkaline phosphatase*, which may be regulated by vitamin D.

Daily allowances. At little as 100 I.U. vitamin D will promote bone development and prevent rickets. The recommended allowance of 400 I.U. is well documented for full-term and premature infants. Additional amounts do not confer greater benefits and are not required. Vitamin D should be supplied to bottle-fed and breast-fed infants.

The allowances for growing children, adolescents, and pregnant and lactating women are difficult to establish because of the exposure to sunlight, but 400 I.U. are recommended daily. Adults with normal exposure to sunlight do not require a dietary supplement.

Sources. Natural foods are poor sources of vitamin D, although small amounts are present in egg yolk, liver, and fish such as herring, sardines, tuna, and salmon. About 85 per cent of fresh milk and almost all evaporated milk are fortified with 400 I.U vitamin D per quart. Milk is especially suitable for fortification since it contains the calcium and phosphorus whose absorption it facilitates, and because it is an important food consumed by growing children.

Vitamin D has been added to a number of foods such as infant foods, cereals, margarines, and breads. If one consumes a quart of milk daily plus one or more of these foods it is not difficult to double or triple the daily intake. Because small excesses of the vitamin may be toxic to some, this is not desirable.

Fish-liver oils (cod, halibut, percomorph, and others) or water-miscible vitamin D preparations may be prescribed when fortified milk is not available. The concentration of these supplements is stated on the label for the product, and this should be carefully noted so that dosages are not excessive. The possibility that oils can be aspirated into the lungs thereby causing lipoid pneumonia is a deterrent to their use.

Sunlight cannot always be depended upon to supply the body with adequate ultraviolet rays to manufacture vitamin D, because these rays are so easily strained out by dust, smoke, fog, clothing, and ordinary window glass—all of which act as barriers to prevent the rays from reaching the skin.

Hypervitaminosis D. The tolerance for vitamin D varies widely. As little as 1800 I.U. over a long period of time may be mildly toxic to children,[7] whereas massive doses of 100,000 I.U.

may be necessary and tolerated by those rare individuals who have refractory rickets. Generally speaking, daily doses ranging from 1000 to 3000 I.U. per kilogram are toxic. The symptoms of toxicity include nausea, diarrhea, weight loss, polyuria, and nocturia. As the toxicity becomes more severe, renal damage, and calcification of the soft tissues such as the heart, blood vessels, bronchi, stomach, and tubules of the kidney occur.

Effects of vitamin D deficiency. A deficiency of vitamin D leads to inadequate absorption of calcium and phosphorus from the intestinal tract and to faulty mineralization of bone and tooth structures. The inability of the soft bones to withstand the stress of weight results in skeletal malformations.

Rickets. Infantile rickets is rarely seen in the United States because of the widespread use of fortified milk or of fish-liver oils in prophylaxis. When such preventive measures are not taken, rickets is more prevalent in northern regions than in warm, sunny climates. It is more likely to develop in dark, overcrowded sections of large cities where the ultraviolet rays of sunshine, especially in the winter months, cannot penetrate through the fog, smoke, and soot. Poverty and ignorance may account for failure to obtain enough vitamin D from concentrates, fortified milk, or skin exposure. Dark-skinned children are more susceptible to rickets than those of the white race.

Premature infants are more susceptible to rickets than full-term infants since the growth rate and the calcification of the skeleton impose additional demands for vitamin D.

Fully developed cases of rickets present the following characteristics (see Figure 10–7):

1. Delayed closure of the fontanelles, softening of the skull (craniotabes), and bulging or bossing of the forehead, giving the head a box-like appearance.

2. Soft, fragile bones leading to widening of the ends of the long bones; bowing of the legs; enlargement of the costochondral junction with rows of knobs or beads forming the *rachitic rosary;* projection of the sternum as in "pigeon breast"; narrowing of the pelvis; spinal curvature.

3. Enlargement of wrist, knee (knock-knees), and ankle joints.

4. Poorly developed muscles; lack of muscle tone—pot belly—being the result of weakness of abdominal muscles; weakness, with delayed walking.

5. Restlessness and nervous irritability.

6. High serum phosphatase; lowered inorganic blood phosphorus.

Rickets is treated by giving relatively large amounts of vitamin D concentrates, the dosage being prescribed by the physician.

Tetany. "Tetany is a syndrome manifested by a sharp flexion of the wrists and ankle joints, muscle twitchings, cramps, and convulsions. It is due to abnormal calcium phosphorus metabolism."* Tetany may result from insufficient dietary calcium or vitamin D, from failure of absorption of calcium or vitamin D, or from a disturbance of the parathyroid gland. The physician prescribes calcium salts to control the acute spasms, a diet liberal in calcium, and vitamin D concentrates.

Dental caries. A deficiency of vitamin D may lead to delayed dentition and to malformation of the teeth. There may be a predisposition to dental caries. It has been shown that children who have received an abundance of milk, eggs, meat, vegetables, and fruits and who have consistently had liberal intakes of vitamin D have fewer carious lesions than do children on suboptimal intakes.[8] Thus, protection against dental caries would seem to depend, at least in part, on adequate intakes and utilization of calcium, phosphorus, and vitamin D. The influence of fluoride has been discussed in Chapter 8 and that of carbohydrate in Chapter 5.

Osteomalacia. Frequently referred to as "adult rickets," osteomalacia represents a failure of the process of calcification to keep up with the rest of the metabolic processes. It is caused by simple vitamin D lack and calcium inadequacy. It occurs in the Orient especially in pregnant and lactating women who subsist on meager cereal diets and who are indoors most of the time.

*Sebrell, W. H.: "Preventive Medicine," in *Handbook of Nutrition.* American Medical Association, Chicago, 1943, p. 473.

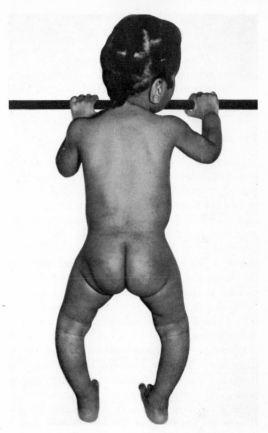

Figure 10–7. Early skeletal deformities of rickets often persist throughout life. Bowlegs that curve laterally, as shown here, indicate that the weakened bones have bent after the second year, as the result of standing. (Courtesy, Dr. Rosa Lee Nemir, Professor of Pediatrics, New York University–Bellevue Medical Center, and *The Vitamin Manual*, published by The Upjohn Company.)

Osteomalacia may occur when there is interference with fat absorption. A third type of this disease resembles resistant rickets in that the individual has an inherent resistance to vitamin D so that normal metabolism does not take place.[9]

The following changes take place in osteomalacia:

1. A softening of the bones, which may be so severe that the bones of the legs, spine, thorax, and pelvis bend into deformities.

2. Pain of the rheumatic type in bones of the legs and lower part of the back.

3. General weakness with difficulty in walking; there is especial difficulty in climbing stairs, and a waddling gait is frequent.

4. Spontaneous multiple fractures.

Since general malnutrition is no doubt present, osteomalacia is treated with a high-protein, high-calorie diet and therapeutic doses of vitamin D.

VITAMIN E

Discovery. Evans and Bishop established the fact that a fat-soluble factor was necessary for reproduction in rats. They showed that absence of vitamin E, or the antisterility factor, as it was designated, led to irreparable damage of the germinal epithelium in male rats, and female rats which had diets deficient in vitamin E were unable to carry their young to term. In severe deficiency the fetus dies and is resorbed completely. In the female the damage is not permanent; that is, normal reproduction could again take place if the diet were once more adequate in this factor.

Chemistry and characteristics. Vitamin E activity is exhibited by a number of compounds of related chemical structure including alpha-, beta-, and gamma-tocopherol. Alpha-tocopherol is the compound possessing the greatest vitamin E activity. (See Figure 10–1.) Vitamin E and the sex hormones are chemically related.

High temperatures and acids do not affect the stability of vitamin E, but oxidation takes place readily in the presence of rancid fats or lead and iron salts. Decomposition occurs in ultraviolet light. Vitamin E itself acts as an antioxidant.

Measurement. Vitamin E is expressed in international units or in milligrams of α-tocopherol. One international unit of vitamin E is equal to 1 mg synthetic *dl*-α-tocopherol acetate. The activity of the natural form, d-α-tocopherol acetate, is 1.36 I.U. per milligram; and that of the free alcohol, d-α-tocopherol, is 1.49 I.U. per milligram.[3] Ordinarily the dietary evaluation of tocopherols other than the alpha form is disregarded because of the lower potency of these factors.

Physiology. Vitamin E requires the presence of fat and of bile salts for absorption into the intestinal wall. It is absorbed into the lymph circulation and carried to the thoracic duct and the liver. Small amounts are present in all body tissues, with the highest concentrations in the pituitary, adrenal gland, and testes. The bulk of the body stores of vitamin E is in the muscle and adipose tissue. No toxicity to vitamin E, even in large amounts, has been shown.

There is little transfer of vitamin E across the placenta to the fetus. Hence, newborn infants have low tissue stores.

Functions. The principal role of vitamin E appears to be as an antioxidant. By accepting oxygen it helps to prevent the oxidation of vitamin A in the intestinal tract, thereby sparing vitamin A. In the tissues vitamin E reduces the oxidation of the polyunsaturated fatty acids, thereby helping to maintain the integrity of the cell membranes.

Vitamin E is probably involved in some synthetic processes. One of these is the incorporation of pyrimidines into nucleic acid, especially in the formation of the red blood cells in the bone marrow. Vitamin E is also required for the synthesis of coenzyme Q, a factor that is essential in the respiratory chain that releases energy from carbohydrates and fats.

Daily allowances. The Food and Nutrition Board recommends a daily intake of 4 to 5 I.U. during the first year of life, 12 I.U. for women, 15 I.U. during pregnancy and lactation, and 15 I.U. for men. These allowances are based upon metabolic body size.

The need for vitamin E is higher when the intake of polyunsaturated fatty acids is increased. Since the principal source of vitamin E is from vegetable oils and margarines, the increased intake of linoleic acid from these fats is accompanied by a satisfactory intake of vitamin E.

Sources. About 64 per cent of the tocopherol in American diets is supplied by salad oils, shortening, and margarine, 11 per cent by fruits and vegetables, and 7 per cent by grain foods. The vitamin E content of oils varies widely depending upon the source of the oil, whether or not it is hydrogenated, and the conditions of storage. Although many oils are good sources of the tocopherols they are also high in polyunsaturated fatty acids. Appreciable concentrations of vitamin E are present in dark-green leafy vegetables, nuts, and legumes. Foods of animal origin are low in vitamin E. Human milk provides adequate vitamin E for the infant, but cow's milk is low. (See Table A–2 for vitamin E content of foods.)

Effects of deficiency. Vitamin E deficiency has been observed in some infants with severe kwashiorkor. There was increased hemolysis of the red blood cells, macrocytic anemia, and creatinuria. These conditions were corrected by the administration of vitamin E.[10] Premature infants show an extremely low level of tocopherol in the serum and increased capillary fragility.

Long periods of time on experimental diets extremely low in tocopherols have produced increased hemolysis of red blood cells in men.[11] When polyunsaturated fat intake is increased the length of time required for the onset of hemolysis is much less. Vitamin E deficiency in human beings is not frequently reported.

In many species of animals vitamin E deficiency has resulted in reproductive failure, macrocytic anemia, shorter life-span of the red blood cells, creatinuria, liver necrosis, encephalomalacia, and muscular dystrophy. Based upon these findings numerous trials of vitamin E as a possible therapeutic agent have been made for menstrual disorders, the prevention of abortion, the improvement of lactation, the alleviation of muscular dystrophy, and cardiovascular disease. None of these has proved effective in the human being.

Vitamin K

The existence of vitamin K was first suggested by Dr. Dam of Copenhagen who in 1935 found that a "Koagulations Vitamin" was necessary to prevent fatal hemorrhages in chicks by promoting normal blood clotting.

Chemistry and characteristics. Vitamin K consists of a number of related compounds: the K_1 group first isolated from alfalfa, and the K_2 group from putrefied fish meal and produced in the intestine by bacterial synthesis. (See Figure 10–1.) The terminology adopted by an international committee is *phylloquinone* (K_1), *menaquinone* (MK_n), and *menadione*, a synthetic compound that is about three times as potent as vitamin K. Vitamin K is fat soluble, resistant to heat, but easily destroyed by irradiation, acids, and alkalies.

Measurement. The activity of test materials is measured in micrograms by its ability to prevent hemorrhage in young chicks. Menadione is used as the standard for measuring vitamin K potency.

Physiology. Vitamin K can be synthesized by bacteria of the lower intestinal tract. Being fat soluble, vitamin K requires the presence of bile for its absorption, most of which occurs in the upper part of the small intestine. Probably only a small amount of the intestinal synthesis is actually utilized. A large amount of vitamin K is excreted in the feces. Limited stores of vitamin K are maintained by the liver.

The newborn infant has a very limited supply of vitamin K, and synthesis by the relatively sterile intestinal tract does not take place for several days. Human milk supplies about one fourth as much vitamin K as does cow's milk. Thus, the first few days may be critical for the infant.

Function. Vitamin K is essential for the formation of prothrombin and other clotting proteins by the liver. A high prothrombin level of the blood indicates good ability to coagulate blood, whereas low blood levels of prothrombin are associated with a slow rate of coagulation. Vitamin K probably also participates in oxidative phosphorylation in the tissues.

Daily allowances. The variations in intestinal synthesis and in the diet have made it impossible to establish a daily allowance. Dietary deficiency is not believed to be a problem.

Sources. Green leaves of plants such as spinach and kale are excellent sources of vitamin K as are also cabbage, cauliflower, and pork liver. Cereals, fruits, and other vegetables are poor sources.

Effects of deficiency. A low blood level of prothrombin and other clotting factors leads to increased tendency to hemorrhage. Premature infants, anoxic infants, and those whose mothers have been taking anticoagulants are most susceptible to deficiency. The hemorrhagic disease of the newborn can be prevented by a single

Table 10–1. Summary of the Fat-Soluble Vitamins

Nomenclature	Important Sources	Physiology and Functions	Effect of Deficiency	Daily Allowances*
Vitamin A Retinol Retinal Retinyl ester Retinoic acid Provitamin A alpha-, beta-, gamma-carotene, cryptoxanthin	*Animal* Fish-liver oils Liver Butter, cream Whole milk Whole-milk cheeses Egg yolk *Plant* Dark-green leafy vegetables Yellow vegetables Yellow fruits Fortified margarines	Bile necessary for absorption Stored in liver Maintains integrity of mucosal epithelium, maintains visual acuity in dim light Large amounts are toxic	Faulty bone and tooth development Night blindness Keratinization of epithelium—mucous membranes and skin *Xerophthalmia*	Children: 400–700 R.E. (2000–3300 I.U.) Men: 1000 R.E. (5000 I.U.) Women: 800 R.E. (4000 I.U.) Pregnancy: 1000 R.E. (5000 I.U.) Lactation: 1200 R.E. (6000 I.U.)
Vitamin D Vitamin D₂ Ergocalciferol Vitamin D₃ Cholecalciferol Antirachitic factor	Fish-liver oils Fortified milk Activated sterols Exposure to sunlight Very small amounts in butter, liver, egg yolk, salmon, sardines	Synthesized in skin by activity of ultraviolet light Stored chiefly in liver Regulates absorption of calcium, phosphorus, and normal utilization in bones and teeth Large amounts are toxic	*Rickets* in children Soft, fragile bones Enlarged joints Bowed legs Chest, spinal, pelvic bone deformities Delayed dentition *Tetanic* convulsions in infants *Osteomalacia* in adults	Need is small for adults Children, pregnant or lactating women: 400 I.U.
Vitamin E Alpha-, beta-, gamma-tocopherol Antisterility vitamin	Plant tissues—vegetable oils; wheat germ, rice germ; green leafy vegetables; nuts; legumes Animal foods are poor sources	Not stored in body to any extent Related to action of selenium *Humans*: reduces oxidation of vitamin A, carotenes, and polyunsaturated fatty acids; hemopoiesis *Animals*: normal reproduction; utilization of sex hormones, cholesterol	*Humans*: hemolysis of red blood cells; mild anemia; deficiency is not likely *Animals*: sterility in male rats; resorption of fetus in female rats; muscular dystrophy; creatinuria; macrocytic anemia	Men: 15 I.U. Women: 12 I.U. Pregnancy: 15 I.U. Infants: 4–5 I.U.
Vitamin K Phylloquinone (K₁) Menaquinone (MKₙ) Menadione	Green leaves such as alfalfa, spinach, cabbage Liver Synthesis in intestine	Bile necessary for absorption Formation of prothrombin Sulfa drugs and antibiotics interfere with intestinal absorption Large amounts are toxic	Prolonged clotting time Hemorrhagic disease in newborn infants	Not known

*See Recommended Dietary Allowances for complete listing, Table 3–1.

dose of vitamin K_1 administered to the infant immediately after birth. The practice of giving vitamin K to the mother prior to delivery has been questioned since too much may lead to hemolytic anemia in the infant.

Deficiency may occur in adults because of a failure in absorption, or interference with the synthesis in the intestine, or inability to form prothrombin by the liver. Oral therapy with sulfa drugs and antibiotics interferes with the synthesis of the vitamin in the intestine. Obstruction of the biliary tract and severe diarrhea as in sprue, celiac disease, and colitis may seriously interfere with absorption. In severe disease of the liver the synthesis of the clotting factors is impaired even though the source of vitamin K is adequate.

If absorption is inadequate, vitamin K may be prescribed orally together with bile salts. Parenteral administration may be required when there is severe intestinal disease. Vitamin K_1 may be used for oral therapy, but menadione taken orally leads to vomiting.

Dicumarol is an anticoagulant often used to treat coronary thrombosis. It is antagonistic to the action of vitamin K and prevents the formation of prothrombin. Anticoagulant therapy carries the risk of hemorrhage. When an excessive amount of anticoagulant is given, vitamin K may be administered to counteract it.

PROBLEMS AND REVIEW

1. What is the relationship of carotene to vitamin A? What are the important sources of carotene?
2. Why are young children more susceptible than adults to deficiency of vitamin A or D? Describe the signs of deficiency that may be seen in children.
3. *Problem.* Calculate the vitamin A content of your own diet for two days. What percentage of your daily allowance is provided by sources rich in vitamin A? By sources rich in the provitamin?
4. Why is the fortification of milk with vitamin D generally recommended? Why is the fortification of other foods not desirable?
5. Which of the fat-soluble vitamins are toxic? What intakes are likely to lead to toxicity? What are the manifestations of the toxicity?
6. What interrelationship exists between these factors: vitamin A and E; vitamin D and phosphorus; vitamin D and calcium; vitamin E and selenium; vitamin E and polyunsaturated fatty acids?
7. What is the relation of vitamin K to blood clotting? Under what circumstances is a deficiency of vitamin K likely to occur?
8. What is the principal function of vitamin E? What conditions are necessary to produce a deficiency of vitamin E?

CITED REFERENCES

1. Rao, C. N., and Rao, B. S. N.: "Absorption of Dietary Carotenes in Human Subjects," *Am. J. Clin. Nutr.,* **23**:105–109, 1970.
2. Lala, V. R., and Reddy, V.: "Absorption of α-carotene from Green Leafy Vegetables in Undernourished Children," *Am. J. Clin. Nutr.,* **23**:110–13, 1970.
3. Food and Nutrition Board: *Recommended Dietary Allowances,* 8th ed. National Academy of Sciences–National Research Council, Washington, D.C., 1973.
4. Ganguly, A. J.: "Absorption of Vitamin A," *Am. J. Clin. Nutr.* **22**:923–33, 1969.
5. Schaefer, A. E., and Johnson, O. C.: "Are We Well Fed? The Search for the Answer," *Nutr. Today,* 4:2–11, Spring 1969.
6. Review: "Vitamin A Intoxication in Infancy," *Nutr. Rev.,* **23**:263–65, 1965.

7. Council on Foods and Nutrition: "Vitamin Preparations as Dietary Supplements and as Therapeutic Agents," *J.A.M.A.*, **169**:41–45, 1959.

8. Boyd, J. D.: "Nutrition as It Affects Tooth Decay," *J. Am. Diet. Assoc.*, **18**:211–15, 1942.

9. Review: "Osteomalacia Due to Increased Resistance to Vitamin D," *Nutr. Rev.*, **6**:79–80, 1948.

10. Roels, O. A.: "Present Knowledge of Vitamin E," *Nutr. Rev.*, **25**:33–37, 1967.

11. Horwitt, M. K., *et al.*: "Effects of Limited Tocopherol Intake in Man with Relationships to Erythrocyte Hemolysis and Lipid Oxidations," *Am. J. Clin. Nutr.*, **4**:408–18, 1956.

ADDITIONAL REFERENCES

Vitamin A

Arroyave, G.: "Interrelations between Protein and Vitamin A and Metabolism," *Am. J. Clin. Nutr.*, **22**:1119–28, 1969.

Bergen, S. S., Jr., and Roels, O. A.: "Hypervitaminosis A. Report of a Case," *Am. J. Clin. Nutr.*, **16**:265–69, 1965.

Breslau, R. C.: "Hypervitaminosis A. Acute Vitamin A Toxicity," *Arch. Pediatr.*, **74**:178–97, 1957.

High, E. G.: "Some Aspects of Nutritional Vitamin A Levels in Preschool Children in Beaufort County, South Carolina," *Am. J. Clin. Nutr.*, **22**:1129–32, 1969.

McCollum, E. V.: "Early Experiences with Vitamin A—A Retrospect," *Nutr. Rev.*, **10**:161–63, 1952.

McLaren, D. S.: "Xerophthalmia: A Neglected Problem," *Nutr. Rev.*, **22**:289–91, 1964.

McLaren, D. S., *et al.*: "Xerophthalmia in Jordan," *Am. J. Clin. Nutr.*, **17**:117–130, 1965.

Olson, J. A.: "The Alpha and the Omega of Vitamin A Metabolism," *Am. J. Clin. Nutr.*, **22**: 953–62, 1969.

Oomen, H. A. P. C.: "Clinical Epidemiology of Xerophthalmia in Man," *Am. J. Clin. Nutr.*, **22**: 1098–1105, 1969.

Pereira, S. M., *et al.*: "Vitamin A Therapy in Children with Kwashiorkor," *Am. J. Clin. Nutr.*, **20**:297–304, 1967.

Review: "Interrelationships of Vitamin A and E," *Nutr. Rev.*, **23**:82–84, 1965.

————: "Vitamin A Intoxication in Infancy," *Nutr. Rev.*, **23**:263–65, 1965.

Roels, O. A.: "Present Knowledge of Vitamin A," *Nutr. Rev.*, **24**:129–32, 1966.

Vitamin D

Avioli, L. B.: "Absorption and Metabolism of Vitamin D_2 in Man," *Am. J. Clin. Nutr.*, **22**:437– 46, 1969.

Committee on Nutrition, American Academy of Pediatrics: "The Prophylactic Requirement of Toxicity of Vitamin D," *Pediatrics*, **31**:512–25, 1963; **35**:1022–23, 1965.

————: "The Relation Between Infantile Hypercalcemia and Vitamin D: Public Health Implications in North America," *Pediatrics*, **40**:1050–61, 1967.

Dale, A. E., and Lowenberg, M. E.: "Consumption of Vitamin D in Fortified and Natural Foods and in Vitamin Preparations," *J. Pediatr.*, **70**:952–55, 1967.

Editorial: "Vitamin D, Another Frontier," *J.A.M.A.*, **210**:550, 1969.

Forbes, G. B.: "Present Knowledge of Vitamin D," *Nutr. Rev.*, **25**:225–28, 1967.

Review: "An Hypothesis for the Action of Vitamin D on Bone," *Nutr. Rev.*, **26**:183–85, 1968.

————: "Parathyroid Hormone and Hyperaminoaciduria of Human Vitamin D Deficiency," *Nutr. Rev.*, **26**:200–202, 1968.

————: "Rickets in Greece," *Nutr. Rev.*, **27**:51–52, 1969.

————: "Safe Levels of Vitamin D Intake for Infants," *Nutr. Rev.*, **24**:230–32, 1966.

Stearns, G.: "Early Studies of Vitamin D Requirement During Growth," *Am. J. Public Health*, **58**:2027–35, 1968.

Weick, Sr. M. T.: "A History of Rickets in the United States," *Am. J. Clin. Nutr.*, **20**:1234–41, 1967.

Vitamin E

Booth, V. H., and Bradford, M. P.: "Tocopherol Contents of Vegetables and Fruits," *Brit. J. Nutr.*, **17**:575–81, 1963.
Bunnell, R. H., *et al.:* "Alpha-Tocopherol Content of Foods," *Am. J. Clin. Nutr.*, **17**:1–10, 1965.
Dicks-Bushnell, M. W., and Davis, K. C.: "Vitamin E Content of Infant Formulas and Cereals," *Am. J. Clin. Nutr.*, **26**:262–69, 1967.
Dinning, J. S.: "Vitamin E Responsive Anemia in Monkeys and Man," *Nutr. Rev.*, **21**:289–91, 1963.
Green, J., and Bunyan, J.: "Vitamin E and the Biological Antioxidant Theory," *Nutr. Abstr. Rev.*, **39**:321–45, 1969.
Herting, D. C.: "Perspective on Vitamin E," *Am. J. Clin. Nutr.*, **19**:210–18, 1966.
Horwitt, M. K.: "Vitamin E in Human Nutrition—An Interpretative Review," *Bordens Rev. Nutr. Res.*, **22**:1–17, Jan. 1961.
Horwitt, M. K., *et al.:* "Polyunsaturated Lipids and Tocopherol Requirements," *J. Am. Diet. Assoc.*, **38**:231–35, 1961.
Oski, F. A., and Barnes, L. A.: "Vitamin E Deficiency: A Previously Unrecognized Cause of Hemolytic Anemia in Premature Infants," *J. Pediatr.*, **70**:211–20, 1967.
Review: "The Metabolic Role of Vitamin E," *Nutr. Rev.*, **23**:90–92, 1965.
———: "Vitamin E Status of Adults on a Vegetable Oil Diet," *Nutr. Rev.*, **24**:41–43, 1966.

Vitamin K

Johnson, B. C.: "Dietary Factors and Vitamin K," *Nutr. Rev.*, **22**:225–29, 1964.
Olson, R. E.: "The Mode of Action of Vitamin K," *Nutr. Rev.*, **28**:171–76, 1970.
Review: "Response of Human Beings to Vitamin K_1," *Nutr. Rev.*, **27**:287–89, 1969.
———: "Vitamin K Deficiency in Adults," *Nutr. Rev.*, **26**:165–67, 1968.
Vietti, T. J., *et al.:* "Observations on the Prophylactic Use of Vitamin K in the Newborn Infant," *J. Pediatr.*, **56**:343–46, 1960.
Wefring, K. W.: "Hemorrhage in the Newborn and Vitamin K Prophylaxis," *J. Pediatr.*, **63**:663–66, 1963.

11 The Water-Soluble Vitamins: Ascorbic Acid

Discovery. Scurvy has been known as a dread disease since ancient times. It particularly plagued the seagoing adventurers of the sixteenth and seventeenth centuries. Many factors were believed to be responsible for the disease such as too much salt meat, the influence of the sea air, an overflowing of black bile, and obstruction of the spleen. The remedies suggested were equally imaginative and bizarre, for example, vinegar or oil of vitriol. Even in these times there were those who advocated fresh herbs and fruits, but their advice was little heeded. Consequently, thousands of men lost their lives to the scourge.

Dr. James Lind, a British physician, in 1747 tested six remedies on 12 sailors who had scurvy. He found that oranges and lemons were curative. But it took another 50 years before the British Navy required rations of lemons or limes on the sailing vessels. From that day to the present the British sailor has been known as a "limey."

The scientific era of vitamin C began in 1907 when two Norwegian scientists, Holst and Frölich, produced scurvy in guinea pigs. The isolation and chemical nature of vitamin C, or ascorbic acid, was accomplished by Dr. Charles G. King and his coworkers at the University of Pittsburgh in 1932.

Chemistry and characteristics. Ascorbic acid is a white crystalline compound of relatively simple structure, and closely related to the monosaccharide sugars. It is synthesized from glucose and other simple sugars by plants and by most animal species. It can be prepared synthetically at low cost from glucose. Vitamin C activity is possessed by two forms: L-ascorbic acid (the reduced form) and L-dehydroascorbic acid (the oxidized form). (See Figure 11–1.) The latter is oxidized further with complete loss of activity.

Of all vitamins, ascorbic acid is the most easily destroyed. It is highly soluble in water. The oxidation of ascorbic acid is accelerated by heat, light, alkalies, oxidative enzymes, and traces of copper and iron. Oxidation is inhibited to a marked degree in an acid reaction, and when the temperature is reduced.

Measurement. The concentration of ascorbic acid is expressed in milligrams. In foods or body tissues it may be determined chemically, one method being based on the strong reducing action that will bring about a bleaching of a blue dye under specified conditions. The amount of decolorization that takes place is proportional to

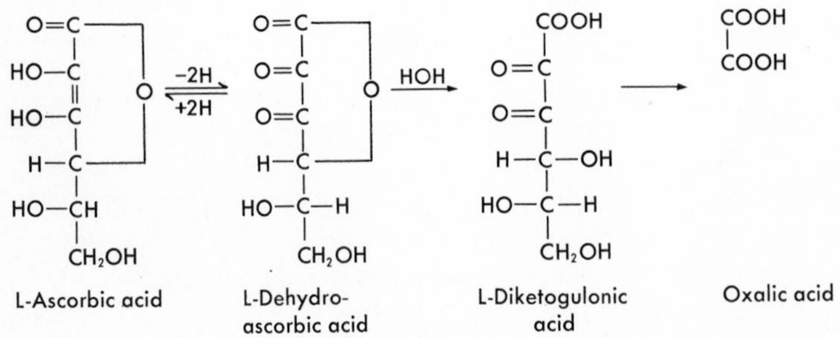

Figure 11–1. Ascorbic acid and dehydroascorbic acid are biologically active. These forms are easily converted to diketogulonic acid, which is inactive.

L-Ascorbic acid

L-Dehydro-ascorbic acid

L-Diketogulonic acid

Oxalic acid

Ascorbic acid, ($C_6H_8O_6$; m.w. 176.1)

the amount of vitamin present and may be determined quantitatively by means of a spectrophotometer or colorimeter.

Physiology. So far only five species are known to require a dietary source of ascorbic acid: man, monkeys, guinea pigs, Indian fruit bat, and the red-vented bulbul bird. Ascorbic acid is rapidly absorbed from the gastrointestinal tract and distributed to the various tissues of the body. The adrenal gland contains an especially high concentration of vitamin C, but other glandular tissues such as the pancreas, thymus, spleen, liver, pituitary, and kidney also contain appreciable amounts. The amount of ascorbic acid held by the tissue is limited. Once the tissues are saturated, any excess will be excreted in the urine. Thus, if one gives a large amount of vitamin C in one dose, most of it will be excreted if the diet has been good in the past, but a high proportion of the dose will be held in the tissues and a smaller amount excreted if the previous diet has been so poor that the tissues are impoverished.

A blood plasma concentration of 0.4 to 1.0 mg per 100 ml is satisfactory, but only the upper level indicates a state of tissue saturation. A reduction in the daily intake is quickly reflected in lower blood plasma levels, but the concentration of the vitamin in white blood cells is less subject to change.

Functions. The principal function of ascorbic acid is the formation of collagenous intercellular substances. Collagen is a protein widely distributed in fibrous tissue structures, cartilage, bone matrices, dentine, and the vascular endothelium. Ascorbic acid is essential for the hydroxylation of two amino acids, proline and lysine, to hydroxyproline and hydroxylysine, which are important constituents of collagen. The maintenance of this function helps to explain the importance of vitamin C in wound healing and in the ability to withstand the stresses of injury and infection.

Ascorbic acid is probably related to many functions involving cell respiration and to the functioning of enzymes, but the mechanisms for such action are not fully understood. Among these functions are (1) oxidation of phenylalanine to tyrosine; (2) reduction of ferric iron

to ferrous iron in the gastrointestinal tract so that iron is more readily absorbed; (3) release of iron from transferrin in the plasma for incorporation into tissue ferritin; and (4) conversion of folic acid into its active form, folinic acid.

As adrenocortical activity increases, the concentration of ascorbic acid and of cholesterol in the adrenal gland decreases. It thus appears that ascorbic acid may be involved in the synthesis of steroid hormones from cholesterol.

Daily allowances. The Food and Nutrition Board has recommended an allowance of ascorbic acid of 45 mg for males and females of all ages over 11 years, 35 mg for infants, 40 mg for children, and 60 mg for pregnancy and lactation.[1] The adult allowances are lower than the 1968 recommendations, and are in sharp contrast to the high levels advocated by some faddists.

The allowances for vitamin C vary widely in different countries. In Norway and Canada the allowance is 30 mg, and in East and West Germany it has been set at 70 to 75 mg. About 10 to 20 mg ascorbic acid will prevent scurvy, but the exact levels that promote optimum health are not known.

During infections such as tuberculosis, rheumatic fever, and pneumonia the requirements for ascorbic acid are increased.

Food sources. Almost all of the daily intake of ascorbic acid is obtained from the vegetable-fruit group. (See Figure 11–2.) Vitamin C has been called the "fresh-food vitamin," since it is found in highest concentrations just as the food is fresh from the plant. In general, the active parts of the plant contain appreciable amounts, and mature or resting seeds are devoid of the vitamin.

Raw, frozen, or canned citrus fruits such as oranges, grapefruit, and lemons are excellent sources of the vitamin. Orange sections including the thin white peel contain more vitamin C than an equal weight of strained juice.

Fresh strawberries, cantaloupe, pineapple, and guavas are also excellent sources. Other non-acid fresh fruits such as peaches, pears, apples, bananas, and blueberries contribute small amounts of the vitamin; when eaten in large amounts these fruits may be an important dietary

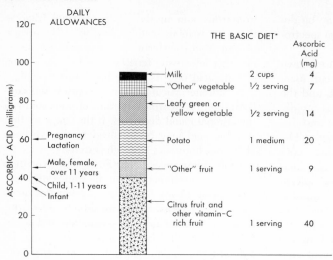

Figure 11–2. The vegetable-fruit group accounts for almost all of the ascorbic acid in the diet. See Table 13–2 for complete calculation of the Basic Diet.

source. The concentration of ascorbic acid in the nonacid canned fruits is considerably reduced.

Broccoli, Brussels sprouts, spinach, kale, green peppers, cabbage, and turnips are excellent-to-good sources even when cooked. The use of potatoes and sweet potatoes as staple food items enhances the vitamin C intake considerably provided that preparation methods have been good.

Milk, eggs, meat, fish, and poultry are practically devoid of vitamin C as they are consumed. If the mother's diet has been adequate, human milk contains four to six times as much ascorbic acid as cow's milk and is able to protect the infant from scurvy. Liver contains a small amount of vitamin C, but most of this is lost during cookery.

The simplest way to ensure adequate intake of ascorbic acid is to include a serving of orange or grapefruit or a double portion of tomato, preferably at breakfast. If other fruits or juices are used at breakfast, the day's allowance will be ample if two foods of fair concentration of ascorbic acid are included in the remaining meals.

Retention of food values. A warm environment, exposure to air, solubility in water, heat, alkali, and dehydration are detrimental to the retention of ascorbic acid in foods. The cutting of vegetables releases oxidative enzymes and increases the surfaces exposed to leaching by

water. Since the vitamin is so soluble, losses are considerable when large amounts of water are used. Vegetables should be added to a small quantity of boiling water, covered tightly, and cooked until just tender for high retention of ascorbic acid. Retention is also good when a pressure cooker is used, provided that the cookery time is carefully controlled. The practice of adding baking soda to retain green color of vegetables not only may reduce the vitamin C level but may also modify the flavor and texture of the vegetable. Leftover vegetables lose a large proportion of the ascorbic acid, although losses are reduced somewhat when the container is tightly covered in the refrigerator. On the other hand, citrus juices and tomatoes retain practically all the vitamin C value for several days.

Effects of deficiency. According to the 1965 dietary survey in the United States, 27 per cent of the diets provided less than the recommended dietary allowances for ascorbic acid; half of these diets furnished less than two thirds of the RDA. (See Figure 1–3.) The National Nutrition Survey showed that 12 to 16 per cent of people in all age categories had unacceptable serum levels of ascorbic acid.[2] Of all subjects surveyed in this study, 4 per cent had scorbutic gum lesions.

A deficiency of ascorbic acid results in the defective formation of the intercellular cement substance. Fleeting joint pains, irritability, re-

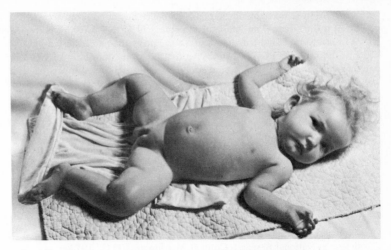

Figure 11–3. Child in scorbutic position. (Courtesy, Dr. Bernard S. Epstein, The Long Island Jewish Hospital, New Hyde Park, New York, and *The Vitamin Manual,* published by The Upjohn Company.)

tardation of growth in the infant or child, anemia, shortness of breath, poor wound healing, and increased susceptibility to infection are among the signs of deficiency, but none of these can establish a diagnosis. A dietary history, the concentration of ascorbic acid in the blood plasma and in the white blood cells, and a measure of the excretion of a test dose in the urine help to establish the diagnosis.

Scurvy. The classic picture of scurvy is rarely seen in adults in the United States. The incidence is also uncommon in infants, but a gross deficiency of ascorbic acid results in scurvy during the second six months of life. Infections, fevers, and hyperthyroidism may precipitate the symptoms when the intake has been inadequate. The symptoms are related to the weakening of the collagenous material.

Pain, tenderness, and swelling of the thighs and legs are frequent symptoms of infantile scurvy. The baby shows a disinclination to move and assumes a position with legs flexed for comfort (see Figure 11–3). He is pale and irritable and cries when handled. Loss of weight, fever, diarrhea, and vomiting are frequently present. If the teeth have erupted, the gums are likely to be swollen, tender, and hemorrhagic. Bone

calcification is faulty because of degeneration or lack of proper development of the bone matrix. The cartilage supporting the bones is weak, and bone displacement results. The ends of the long bones and of the ribs are enlarged somewhat as in rickets, but tenderness is a distinguishing characteristic in scurvy.

Scurvy in adults results after several months of a diet devoid of ascorbic acid. The symptoms include swelling, infection, and bleeding of the gums—gingivitis; tenderness of the legs; anemia; and petechial hemorrhages. The teeth may become loose and eventually may be lost. As the disease progresses, the slightest injury produces excessive bleeding, and large hemorrhages may be seen underneath the skin. There is degeneration of the muscle structure and of the cartilage generally.

Acute scurvy responds within a few days to the administration of 100 to 200 mg ascorbic acid given in the synthetic form or as orange juice. Chronic changes that have occurred, such as bone deformities and anemia, require much longer periods for their correction.

A summary of ascorbic acid is included with the B complex vitamins in Table 12–1.

PROBLEMS AND REVIEW

1. In what ways is ascorbic acid related to the functioning of each of these substances: iron, folic acid, cholesterol?

2. What are the clinical manifestations of a deficiency of ascorbic acid?
3. What is the effect of an intake of ascorbic acid in excess of the body's needs?
4. Why is a formula-fed baby more prone to scurvy than a breast-fed baby?
5. List the instructions you would give for the preparation and service of these foods in order that the maximum ascorbic acid would be retained: tossed green salad, buttered cabbage?
6. *Problem.* Calculate the ascorbic acid content of your own diet for two days. Compare your intake with the recommended allowances.
7. *Problem.* Calculate the amounts of each of the following foods necessary to furnish 25 mg of ascorbic acid: orange juice, tomato juice, sweet potato, cabbage, grapefruit, endive, strawberries, cantaloupe, apple, lettuce.
8. Mashed potatoes served in a restaurant probably should not be relied upon as a source of ascorbic acid. Give several reasons why this is true.

CITED REFERENCES

1. Food and Nutrition Board: *Recommended Dietary Allowances,* 8th ed. National Academy of Sciences–National Research Council, Washington, D.C., 1973.
2. Schaefer, A. E., and Johnson, O. C.: "Are We Well Fed? The Search for the Answer," *Nutr. Today,* 4:2–9, Spring 1969.

ADDITIONAL REFERENCES

Beeuwkes, A: "The Prevalence of Scurvy among Voyageurs to America 1493–1600," *J. Am. Diet. Assoc.,* 24:300–303, 1947.
Gordon, J., and Noble, I.: "Effect of Cooking Method on Vegetables," *J. Am. Diet. Assoc.,* 35:578–81, 1959.
Hodges, R. E., *et al.:* "Experimental Scurvy in Man," *Am. J. Clin. Nutr.,* 22:535–48, 1969.
Hood, J., and Hodges, R. E.: "Ocular Lesions in Scurvy," *Am. J. Clin. Nutr.,* 22:559–67, 1969.
King, C. G.: "Early Experiences with Ascorbic Acid—A Retrospect," *Nutr. Rev.,* 12:1–4, 1954.
————: "Present Knowledge of Ascorbic Acid (Vitamin C)," *Nutr. Rev.,* 26:33–36, 1968.
Lopez, A., *et al.:* "Influence of Time and Temperature on Ascorbic Acid Stability," *J. Am. Diet. Assoc.,* 50:308–10, 1967.
McDonald, B. S.: "Gingivitis—Ascorbic Acid Deficiency in the Navajo," *J. Am. Diet. Assoc.,* 43:331–35, 1963.
Noble, I.: "Ascorbic Acid and Color of Vegetables," *J. Am. Diet. Assoc.,* 50:304–307, 1967.
Pelletier, O.: "Smoking and Vitamin C Levels in Humans," *Am. J. Clin. Nutr.,* 21:1259–67, 1968.
Rivers, J. M.: "Ascorbic Acid in Metabolism of Connective Tissue," *N.Y. State J. Med.,* 65:1235–38, 1965.
Sherlock, P., and Rothschild, E. O.: "Scurvy Produced by a Zen Macrobiotic Diet," *J.A.M.A.,* 199:794–98, 1967.
Woodruff, C.: "Infantile Scurvy," *J.A.M.A.,* 161:448–56, 1956.

12 The Water-Soluble Vitamins: The Vitamin-B Complex

In areas of the world where polished rice is a staple food, beriberi, a serious disease affecting the nerves, has been known for generations. Takaki, a Japanese medical officer, studied the high incidence of the disease among men of the Japanese navy during the years 1878–1883. Among 276 men serving on one sailing vessel he found 169 cases of beriberi including 25 deaths at the end of nine months, but only 14 cases with no deaths occurred among a similar number of men on a second vessel who had received more meat, milk, and vegetables in their diet. Takaki believed this difference was related to the protein content of the diet.

About 15 years later (1897) Eijkman, a Dutch physician in the East Indies, noted that illness in fowls which ate scraps of hospital food was similar to beriberi seen in humans. He subsequently conducted a series of experiments which led to the first clear demonstration of a nutritional deficiency disease. He theorized that the starch of polished rice was toxic to the nerves, but that the outer layers of the rice kernel were protective. Another Dutch physician, Grijns, interpreted the findings as a deficiency of an essential substance in the diet.

A number of chemists demonstrated the effects of extracts from rice. Funk in 1911 coined the term *vitamine* for the substance which he found to be effective in preventing beriberi. Mc-Collum and Davis applied the term *water-soluble . B* to the concentrates which cured beriberi.

The water-soluble vitamin B described by Funk and others was soon discovered to be not a single substance but a group of compounds which we now designate as the vitamin-B complex. Many of these have now been synthesized, and their chemical and physical properties are fairly well understood. The role of these vitamins in metabolism is only partially known, but it is certain that they are essential for metabolic changes which take place in all cells. Principally these vitamins combine with specific proteins to function as parts of the various oxidative enzyme systems which are concerned with the breakdown of carbohydrate, protein, and fat in the body. Thus, they are interrelated and are intimately involved in the mechanisms which release energy, carbon dioxide, and water as the end products of metabolism.

THIAMINE

Discovery. Crystalline vitamin B_1 was isolated from rice bran by Jansen and Donath in Holland in 1926. The synthesis and structure were accomplished in 1936 by Dr. R. R. Williams, who had worked for a quarter of a century on studies of beriberi and on the factor in rice polishings which brought about cure of the disease. Because of the presence of sulfur in the molecule, the vitamin was named thiamine.

Chemistry and characteristics. Thiamine is available commercially as thiamine hydrochloride in a crystalline white powder. (See Figure 12–1.) It has a faint yeastlike odor and a salty nutlike taste, and is readily soluble in water. The vitamin is stable in its dry form, and heating in solutions at 120°C in an acid medium has little destructive effect. On the other hand, cooking foods in neutral or alkaline reaction is very destructive.

Measurement. Thiamine is now measured in milligrams or micrograms. It is determined by chemical or microbiologic methods, but in the past it was measured by using pigeons, rats, or chicks as assay animals.

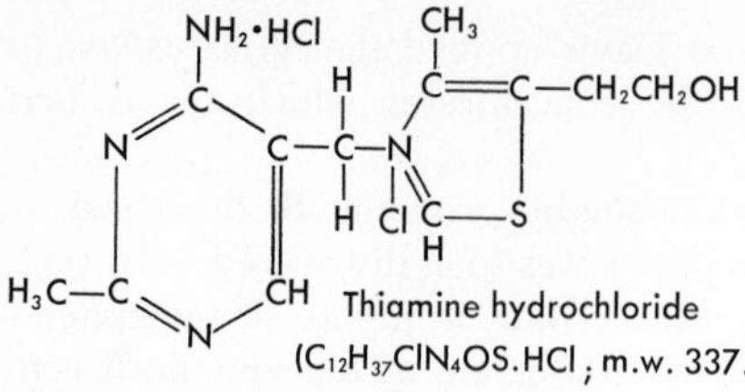

Thiamine hydrochloride
($C_{12}H_{37}ClN_4OS \cdot HCl$; m.w. 337.3)

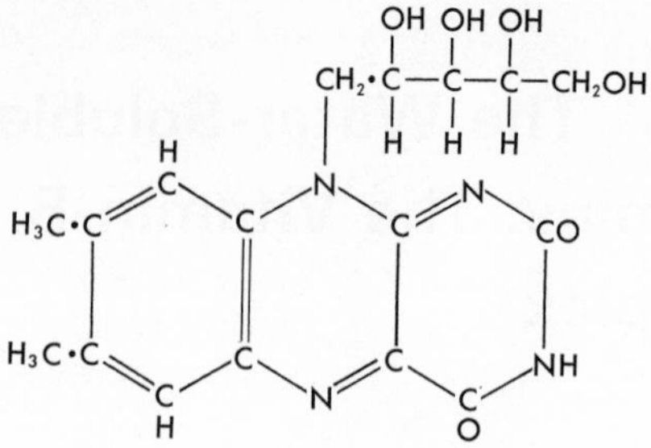

Riboflavin ($C_{17}H_{20}N_4O_6$; m.w. 376.4)

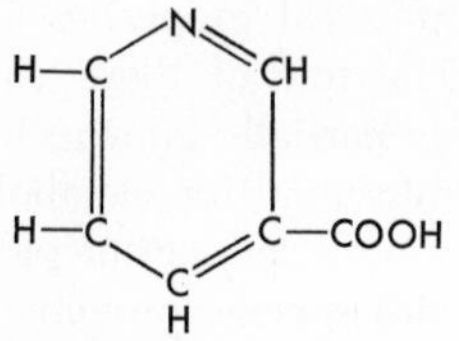

Niacin ($C_6H_5NO_2$; m.w. 123.1)

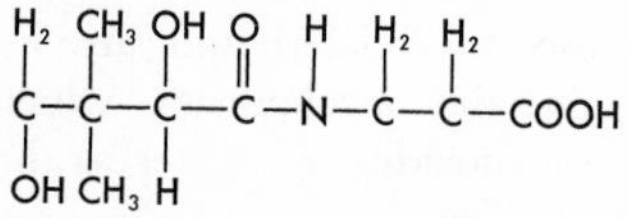

Pantothenic acid ($C_9H_{17}NO_5$; m.w. 219.2)

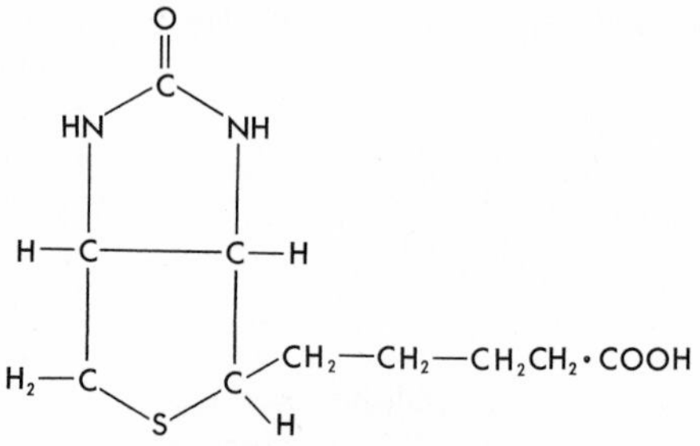

Biotin ($C_{10}H_{16}N_2O_3S$; m.w. 244.3)

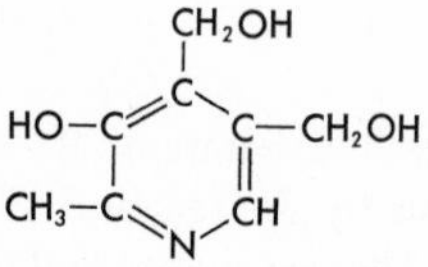

Pyridoxine ($C_8H_{11}NO_3$; m.w. 169) 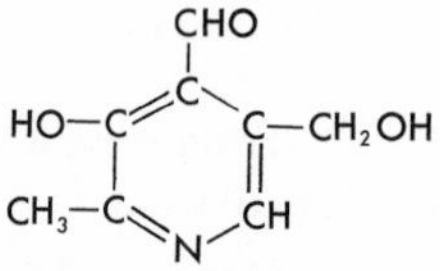   Pyridoxal 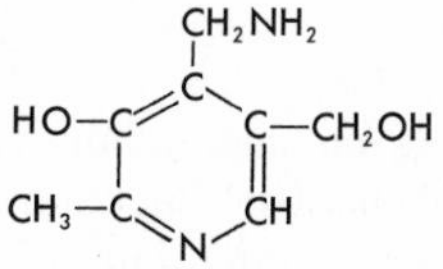   Pyridoxamine

Vitamin B6 (three forms shown)

Figure 12–1. These B-complex vitamins are essential for coenzymes in metabolic reactions involving carbohydrates, fats, and proteins. Note wide variations in structure.

Physiology. The thiamine ingested in food is available in the free form, or bound as in cocarboxylase, in a protein complex, or in a protein-phosphate complex. The bound forms are split in the digestive tract after which absorption takes place principally from the duodenum and jejunum. The amount of thiamine stored in the body is not great. The liver, kidney, heart, brain, and muscles have somewhat higher concentrations than the blood. The tissues are rapidly depleted during a deficiency.

The functioning form of thiamine is cocarboxylase, also known as thiamine pyrophosphate (TPP). The addition of two molecules of phosphate to thiamine is brought about by ATP.

Cocarboxylase in the presence of magnesium ions can combine with a specific protein to form carboxylase, the active enzyme. Cocarboxylase is the coenzyme for a number of enzyme systems.

If thiamine is ingested in excess of tissue needs, it is excreted in the urine. With a low dietary intake the urinary excretion promptly falls.

Functions. One of the critical points at which cocarboxylase functions in carbohydrate metabolism is in the oxidative decarboxylation of pyruvic acid and the subsequent formation of acetyl coenzyme A, which in turn enters the Krebs cycle. (See Figure 5–5.) This is one of the most complex reactions in carbohydrate metabolism and, in addition to TPP, also requires these co-factors: coenzyme A, which contains panto-thenic acid (see page 179); nicotinamide-adenine dinucleotide (NAD), which contains niacin (see page 174); magnesium ions; and lipoic acid (see page 184). Another point in carbohydrate metabolism that involves oxidative decarboxylation is in the Krebs cycle in the con-version of α-ketoglutaric acid to succinic acid. Because fats and amino acids as well as carbo-hydrate can contribute to α-ketoglutaric acid, thiamine and the other factors listed above are involved in the metabolism of the three energy-producing nutrients.

Thiamine pyrophosphate is also a cofactor for *transketolase,* an enzyme required to produce active glyceraldehyde through the pentose shunt. (See Figure 5–5.)

Daily allowances. The thiamine requirements for the various age categories are proportional to the calorie requirement. The minimum re-quirement is 0.33 mg of thiamine per 1000 calories, and the recommended allowance has been set at 0.5 mg per 1000 calories.[1] The margin of safety thus provided allows for indi-vidual variability and affords some protection during periods of stress such as infection.

The daily allowance for the reference man is 1.4 mg and for the reference woman is 1.0 mg. Elderly persons utilize thiamine somewhat less efficiently, and therefore an allowance of at least 1.0 mg is recommended even though the calorie requirement may be below 2000. The allowance for pregnant and lactating women is increased by 0.3 mg, beyond the normal require-ments for women. Infants should receive 0.3 to 0.5 mg, children up to 10 years 0.7 to 1.2 mg, teen-age boys 1.4 to 1.5 mg and girls 1.1 to 1.2 mg.

Sources. Grain products alone provide about one third of the thiamine of the daily diet in the United States and constitute the most im-portant single source in the diet. Because such a small portion of the grain foods is of the whole-grain variety, the cereal and flour enrich-ment program has been of special significance in improving the dietary level of thiamine dur-ing the last two decades. (See Table 20–1.)

Meats, poultry, fish, and eggs supply about one third of the daily intake of thiamine. Lean pork—fresh and cured—is especially high in its thiamine concentration; its frequent inclusion in the diet thus makes it a highly significant source. Liver, dry beans and peas, soybeans, and pea-nuts are also excellent sources. The thiamine in egg, a fair source, is concentrated in the yolk.

Although the concentration of thiamine in vegetables and fruits is low, the quantities of these foods eaten may be such that important contributions are made to the daily total. Milk is likewise a fair source because of the amounts taken in the daily diet and because milk is not subjected to treatment other than pasteurization, which does not materially reduce the thiamine level.

The thiamine contribution of the basic diet pattern is shown in Figure 12–2.

Retention of food values. Appreciable losses of thiamine occur in cookery as a result of (1) solubility of the vitamin in water, (2) the ready destruction in the presence of alkali, and (3) the prolonged exposure to heat.

Little loss occurs in the preparation of cooked breakfast cereals inasmuch as the water used in preparation is consumed. On the other hand, losses may be considerable when rice is washed before cooking and when it is cooked in a large volume of water that is later drained off. Pack-aged rice does not require preliminary washing, and losses are further minimized if rice is cooked in just enough water so that all of it is absorbed by the grains. "Converted" rice retains much more of the thiamine than does regular rice, because the parboiling of the rice in its process-ing distributes the water-soluble nutrients throughout the grain. In the baking of bread about 15 to 20 per cent of the thiamine content is lost.

When meats are broiled or roasted, the thia-mine losses may be 25 per cent or less. When meats are cooked in liquid, the losses may ap-proach 50 per cent if the liquid is discarded. If the liquids are used, the amount of thiamine remaining in the meat and liquid is about 75 per cent.

Thiamine losses in vegetable cookery are minimal if vegetables are cooked in a small amount of water for a short time without the

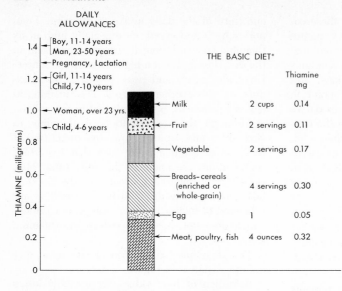

Figure 12–2. The Four Food Groups meet the recommended allowances for thiamine for women and children. The additional allowances for teen-agers and men are easily met by using increased amounts of these food groups. See Table 13–2 for complete calculation.

addition of alkali. When the principles for the retention of ascorbic acid are observed in food preparation, the maximum thiamine content will also be preserved.

Effects of deficiency. Thiamine deficiency is not rare in the United States but it is confined principally to the alcoholic population. The alcoholic ingests little thiamine in his limited food intake, but thiamine is required for the metabolism of alcohol as well as for carbohydrate.

Thiamine deficiency may also occur following gastrointestinal disturbances accompanied by persistent vomiting or diarrhea, or subsequent to febrile diseases or surgery when the dietary intake has been poor.

Beriberi still occurs in the Orient where high-carbohydrate diets are common and where enrichment of rice and wheat is not practiced. Williams demonstrated the effectiveness of rice enrichment in the Philippines, an area where the incidence of beriberi has been high.[2]

Diagnosis. The symptoms of mild deficiency are so vague that a diagnosis of thiamine lack is difficult. Some of the laboratory tests may be helpful but not necessarily conclusive. For example, an elevated level of pyruvic and lactic acids in the blood, especially after exercise and the administration of a standard amount of glucose, together with a low concentration of thiamine in the urine is suggestive of deficiency. If

such tests are further substantiated with a dietary history of thiamine lack plus the appearance of peripheral neuritis and disorders in the cardiovascular system, thiamine deficiency seems apparent.

The activity of an enzyme, erythrocyte transketolase, which is found in the red blood cells correlates closely with thiamine nutrition.[3] A measure of this activity is believed to be useful in detecting marginal deficiency before clinical symptoms have become apparent.

Mild thiamine deficiency. The individual who is deprived of small amounts of thiamine daily builds up an increasing deficiency state which may be characterized by fatigue, lack of interest in his affairs, emotional instability, irritability, depression, anger and fear, and loss of appetite, weight, and strength. As the deficiency becomes more marked, the patient may complain of indigestion, constipation, headaches, insomnia, and tachycardia after moderate exertion. There appears a feeling of heaviness and weakness in the legs which may be followed by cramping of the calf muscles and burning and numbness of the feet—an indication of the development of peripheral neuritis. The predominant symptoms thus concern the gastrointestinal, cardiovascular, and peripheral nervous systems.

Infantile beriberi. Infants in the Far East are especially susceptible to beriberi because the mother has a deficient intake of thiamine, and the milk she supplies to the infant consequently contains a very low level of thiamine. The onset is often sudden and is characterized by pallor, facial edema, irritability, vomiting, abdominal pain, loss of voice, and convulsions. The infant may die within a few hours. With thiamine therapy, recovery is equally dramatic.

Adult beriberi. When thiamine deficiency has been prolonged and severe, it progresses from the mild symptoms described above to the incapacitating and often fatal beriberi. In "wet" beriberi the chief manifestations are edema and cardiac failure; in "dry" beriberi cachexia and multiple neuritic symptoms are outstanding. Not infrequently the cardiac symptoms predominate and failure of the heart becomes imminent. Beriberi is characterized by the following symptoms:

1. Gastrointestinal disturbances resulting primarily from impairment of the motor processes throughout the gastrointestinal tract.

2. Muscular weakness or paralysis of the lower limbs caused by multiple neuritic conditions. The weakness affects first the foot, then the muscles of the calf, and then the thigh. The upper extremities are also affected in severe cases. The muscle degeneration may be so pronounced that coordination is impossible and a characteristic gait is present. The pain in the extremities at this stage is usually severe. The extent of muscular atrophy may be masked by edema in wet beriberi.

3. The heart becomes enlarged, and tachycardia, dyspnea, and palpitation occur on exertion. In the acute or pernicious type of beriberi, acute cardiac failure may be fatal before the seriousness of the disease has been fully appreciated.

4. Emaciation accompanies both dry and wet beriberi, but in the latter the edema may be so marked that the extent of malnourishment is not readily evident.

Treatment. Because beriberi is a complex vitamin-deficiency disease, patients make the greatest improvement when B complex vitamins rather than thiamine alone are prescribed. In addition to the B complex concentrates it is customary to prescribe a diet that is high in protein and calories.

RIBOFLAVIN

Discovery. As early as 1879 a pigment which possessed a yellow-green fluorescence had been discovered in milk. Other workers later obtained it from such widely varying sources as liver, yeast, heart, and egg white. The pigments which possess these fluorescent properties were designated as "flavins."

By 1928 the substance in yeast which prevented polyneuritis was shown to be more than one vitamin. The antineuritic fraction which was destroyed by heat was called vitamin B_1. Another fraction not destroyed by heat did not prevent or cure polyneuritis but it was needed for growth. It was designated as vitamin B_2 or vitamin G.

In 1932 a yellow enzyme necessary for cell respiration was isolated from yeast by Warburg and Christian, who also discovered that a protein and the pigment component were two factors in the enzyme. It then remained for Kuhn and his co-workers in 1935 to report on the synthesis of riboflavin and to note the relation of its activity to the green fluorescence, thereby establishing that lactoflavin and the vitamin are one and the same thing. Riboflavin is the preferred name for this vitamin, although the term vitamin B_2 is also used.

Chemistry and characteristics. Riboflavin was so named because of the similarity of part of its structure to that of the sugar ribose and because of its relation to the general group of flavins. (See Figure 12–1.) In its pure state, this vitamin is a bitter-tasting, orange-yellow, odorless compound in which the crystals are needle shaped. It dissolves sparingly in water to give a characteristic greenish-yellow fluorescence. It is quickly decomposed by ultraviolet rays and visible light. This vitamin is stable to heat, to oxidizing agents, and to acids, but it is sensitive to the effects of alkali, although to a lesser degree than is thiamine.

Measurement. Riboflavin is measured in terms of milligrams or micrograms. Chemical and microbiologic methods are both used extensively.

Physiology. Riboflavin is present in the free state in foods, or in combination with phosphate, or with protein and phosphate. Riboflavin is absorbed from the upper part of the small intestine and is phosphorylated in the intestinal wall. It is present in body tissues as the coenzyme or as flavoproteins.

The body guards carefully its stores of riboflavin so that even in severe deficiency as much as one third of the normal amount has been found to be present in the liver, kidney, and heart of experimental animals. Apparently the flavin content of the body tissues cannot be increased beyond a certain point since the urinary excretion increases markedly if a great elevation of intake occurs. On the other hand, a decided reduction in the supply leads to restriction or even curtailment of the urinary excretion.

Functions. Riboflavin is a constituent of two coenzymes: riboflavin phosphate or flavin mononucleotide (FMN) and flavin adenine dinucleotide (FAD). Both these coenzymes are prosthetic groups for aerobic dehydrogenases that act as hydrogen acceptors. The enzymes are required for the completion of several reactions in the energy cycle by which ATP is generated and in which hydrogen is transferred from one compound to another until eventually it reaches oxygen and forms water. Functionally, these enzymes are closely associated with the niacin-containing enzymes. (See Figure 5–5.)

Riboflavin is also a component of L- and D-amino acid oxidases that oxidize amino acids and hydroxy acids to α-keto acids, and of xanthine oxidase, an enzyme that catalyzes the oxidation of a number of purines.

Daily allowances. The allowances for riboflavin have been calculated at various times on the basis of the calorie intake, the protein allowance, and the metabolic body size. The resulting allowance is about the same regardless of the base used for the calculation. Based upon body size, infants and children require slightly higher allowances to promote growth.

The recommended allowance for the woman over 23 years is 1.2 mg and for the man is 1.6 mg. This corresponds to about 0.6 mg per 1000 kcal. The amount needed to prevent deficiency is about 0.3 mg per 1000 kcal. For pregnancy and lactation the allowances are, respectively,

1.5 and 1.7 mg. The infant's allowance is 0.4 to 0.6 mg, and for children to 10 years 0.8 to 1.2 mg are recommended.

Hyperthyroidism, fevers, the stress of injury or surgery, and malabsorption are among the factors that increase the requirement. Achlorhydria may precipitate deficiency because the vitamin is so quickly destroyed in an alkaline medium.

Food sources. In the American food supply, 42 per cent of the riboflavin is supplied by milk, 26 per cent by meat, poultry, and fish, and 14 per cent by cereal and flour products.

Liver, kidney, and heart contain considerable quantities of riboflavin, and other meats, eggs, and green leafy vegetables supply smaller, but nevertheless important, amounts. Cereals and flours are ordinarily low in riboflavin; their enrichment adds significantly to the riboflavin content of the diet.

Fruits, roots, and tubers are poor sources of riboflavin, and fats and oils are practically devoid of the vitamin. The contribution of the basic diet is shown in Figure 12–3.

Retention of food values. Pasteurization, irradiation for vitamin D, evaporation, or drying of milk accounts for loss of not more than 10 to 20 per cent of the initial riboflavin content of milk. On the other hand, milk that is bottled in clear glass loses a considerable proportion of its riboflavin if allowed to stand in direct sunlight—up to 75 per cent with 3½ hours exposure. The common practice of distributing milk in opaque containers prevents this loss.

Meats that have been stewed, roasted, or braised retain more than three fourths of the riboflavin; most of the remainder can be accounted for in the drippings. Because riboflavin is sparingly soluble, the usual cooking procedures for vegetables do not contribute to much loss, but the addition of sodium bicarbonate to preserve green color is destructive.

Effect of deficiency. Ariboflavinosis is believed to be one of the most common of deficiency diseases. It is rare that an individual seeks medical advice for it alone, but it may accompany other deficiencies especially of the B complex.

Symptoms. In 1939 Sebrell and Butler studied a group of women whom they placed upon a

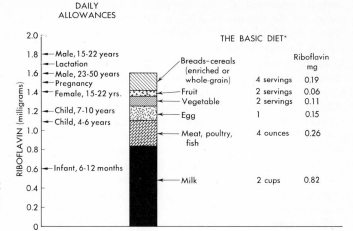

DAILY ALLOWANCES

THE BASIC DIET*

		Riboflavin mg
Breads-cereals (enriched or whole-grain)	4 servings	0.19
Fruit	2 servings	0.06
Vegetable	2 servings	0.11
Egg	1	0.15
Meat, poultry, fish	4 ounces	0.26
Milk	2 cups	0.82

RIBOFLAVIN (milligrams)

- Male, 15-22 years — 1.8
- Lactation
- Male, 23-50 years — 1.6
- Pregnancy
- Female, 15-22 yrs. — 1.4
- Child, 7-10 years — 1.2
- Child, 4-6 years
- Infant, 6-12 months — 0.6

Figure 12–3. Note the important contribution of milk to the riboflavin allowance. See Table 13–2 for calculation of the Basic Diet.

diet extremely low in riboflavin. This diet in the course of 94 to 130 days led to the development of definite symptoms such as "cracks in the skin at the corners of the mouth (cheilosis), a greasy eruption of the skin, changes in the tongue and keratitis caused by an invasion of the cornea by blood vessels."* (See Figure 12–4.) Glossitis caused by riboflavin deficiency may become apparent in pellagrins after therapy has corrected the acute manifestations of niacin deficiency. The lips and tongue assume a purplish-red and shiny appearance in contrast to the scarlet color seen in niacin deficiency. The mouth becomes increasingly sore.

Ocular manifestations are believed to be among the earliest signs of riboflavin deficiency. The eyes become sensitive to light and easily fatigued. There are also blurring of the vision, itching, watering, and soreness of the eyes. An increased number of capillaries develop in the cornea, and the eye becomes bloodshot in appearance. Not all corneal vascularization is caused by riboflavin deficiency, however.

NIACIN (NICOTINIC ACID AND NICOTINAMIDE)

Early studies. Pellagra, which means rough skin, is a disease which was described in Italy

*Sebrell, W. H., and Butler, R. E.: "Riboflavin Deficiency in Man," *Public Health Rep.*, **54**:2121, 1939.

in 1771. In the early part of this century it was one of the leading causes of mental illness and of death in this country. Its causes had been variously ascribed to toxic substances present in corn, infections from microorganisms, of toxicity produced by exposure to the sun.

Goldberger, of the United States Public Health Service, who was assigned to study the problem of pellagra in the South, early noted that the disease was almost always associated with poverty and ignorance, and that hospital at-

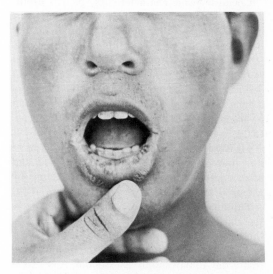

Figure 12–4. Cheilosis—lesions of the lips and fissures at the angles of the mouth. (Courtesy, Nutrition Section, National Institutes of Health.)

tendants who worked with the patients never contracted the disease. In 1915 he performed a classic experiment on 12 prisoners who were promised release in return for their cooperation in eating a diet representative of the poorer classes in the southern states. The diet consisted of sweet potatoes, corn bread, cabbage, rice, collards, fried mush, brown gravy, corn grits, syrup, sugar, biscuits, and black coffee. After a few weeks the prisoners developed headache, abdominal pain, and general weakness, and in about five months the typical dermatitis of pellagra appeared. Goldberger then suggested the existence of a pellagra-preventing (P-P) factor and related it to the B vitamins.

Identification of the vitamin. Goldberger in 1922 concluded that blacktongue in dogs was similar to pellagra in humans. Nicotinic acid had been known as a chemical substance since 1867, but it remained for Elvehjem and his coworkers in 1937 to discover its effectiveness as a curative agent for blacktongue in dogs. Following this discovery, Smith, Spies, and others were soon making reports of dramatic clinical improvement in pellagrous patients who had been given nicotinic acid. The term *niacin* was suggested by Cowgill to avoid association with the nicotine of tobacco.

Chemistry and characteristics. Niacin occurs in white, needlelike, bitter-tasting crystals. (See Figure 12–1.) It is moderately soluble in hot water but only slightly soluble in cold water. It is very stable to alkali, acid, heat, light, and oxidation; even boiling and autoclaving do not decrease its potency. Niacinamide occurs in animal tissues and is more soluble in water than is niacin. Both forms are of equal biologic activity.

Measurement. Niacin is measured in terms of milligrams. It may be determined in food and other materials by microbiologic assay or by chemical methods.

Physiology. Niacin is readily absorbed from the small intestine. Some reserves are found in the body, but, as with the other B complex vitamins, the amount appears to be rather limited so that a day-to-day supply is essential. Any excess of niacin which may be present is excreted in the urine in several forms so that it is somewhat difficult to account for all of it. In deficiency such as pellagra, the end products in the urine diminish markedly or are absent.

Tryptophan, one of the essential amino acids, is a precursor of niacin so that a diet which contains liberal amounts of tryptophan will provide enough niacin even though the diet itself may be low in preformed niacin. Vitamin B_6 is essential for this conversion. The experimental production of pellagra can be brought about only by diets low in both niacin and tryptophan.

Functions. Niacin, like other B complex vitamins, is a constituent of coenzymes involved in the metabolism of carbohydrates, fats, and proteins. Nicotinamide adenine dinucleotide (NAD, also known as coenzyme I) and nicotinamide adenine dinucleotide phosphate (NADP, or coenzyme II) are hydrogen acceptors involved in many reactions. For example, the complex reaction required for the decarboxylation of pyruvic acid and the formation of acetyl coenzyme A requires dehydrogenation by NAD (see also page 169); NAD and NADP are involved in dehydrogenation reactions in the Krebs cycle; hydrogen is transferred from NAD to FAD to cytochrome c in the respiratory chain in which ATP is liberated.

In the pentose shunt (see page 71) NADP is the hydrogen acceptor for two reactions, thereby forming NADPH. The latter is required for the synthesis of fatty acids and cholesterol, and for the conversion of phenylalanine to tyrosine.

Daily allowances. The symptoms of pellagra are prevented by a daily intake of 4.4 mg niacin per 1000 kcal. The recommended allowances provide about 50 per cent margin of safety, and are based upon 6.6 mg niacin per 1000 kcal. Although these levels are stated as niacin, it is recognized that 1 mg niacin is derived from each 60 mg dietary tryptophan as well as from preformed niacin in the diet.

For the reference man, 23–50 years, the allowance is 18 mg, and for the reference woman is 13 mg. The allowances for pregnancy and lactation are 15 and 17 mg, respectively. From 5 to 8 mg are recommended during the first year of life, and 9 to 16 mg for children to 10 years.

For boys and girls, 11 to 14 years, allowances are 18 and 16 mg, respectively.

As with the other B complex vitamins, the niacin requirements are increased whenever metabolism is accelerated as by fever and the stress of injury or surgery.

Sources. A diet that furnishes the recommended allowances for protein also provides enough niacin inasmuch as protein will supply tryptophan for conversion to niacin, and the protein-rich foods are generally, except for milk, rich sources of preformed niacin. Animal proteins contain about 1.4 per cent tryptophan, and plant proteins about 1 per cent tryptophan.[5] If one assumes that a mixed diet provides 1 per cent of the protein as tryptophan, then an intake of 65 gm protein is equivalent to 650 mg tryptophan, or 10.8 mg niacin.

Poultry, meats, and fish constitute the most important single food group insofar as preformed niacin is concerned. (See Figure 12–5.) Organ meats, peanuts, and peanut butter are rich sources, but are not ordinarily consumed in sufficient amounts to greatly affect the dietary level.

Whole grains are fair sources of niacin but most of this is in a bound form which may not be completely available.[5] The effect of cooking on the bound form is not known.

Potatoes, legumes, and some green leafy vegetables contain fair amounts of preformed niacin, but most fruits and vegetables are poor sources—as are also milk and cheese.

Enrichment of corn and rice, required in many states, has been a significant factor in reducing the incidence of pellagra.

Retention of food values. The cookery of foods does not result in serious losses of niacin, except insofar as part of the soluble vitamin may be discarded in cooking waters which are not used. The application of principles for the retention of ascorbic acid and thiamine which have been discussed earlier will result in maximum retention of niacin as well.

Effect of deficiency. Pellagra appears after months of dietary deprivation. The phenomenal decrease in the incidence of pellagra in the United States may be attributed to several factors including the enrichment program which is mandatory in some states, the concerted efforts in nutrition education, and the improvement in income. Pellagra is still a public health problem in some countries such as Spain, Yugoslavia, and certain areas of Africa.

Symptoms and clinical findings. Pellagra involves the gastrointestinal tract, the skin, and the nervous system. Although no two cases of pellagra are exactly alike, the following symptoms are characteristic.

1. Early signs include fatigue, listlessness,

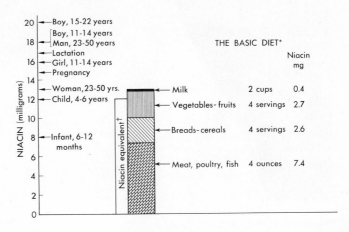

Figure 12–5. The meat group contributes most of the preformed niacin in the Basic Diet. Milk and eggs contain only small amounts of preformed niacin, but they are excellent sources of tryptophan. See Table 13–2 for complete calculation of Basic Diet.

headache, backache, loss of weight, loss of appetite, and general poor health.

2. Sore tongue, mouth, and throat, with glossitis extending throughout the gastrointestinal tract are present. The tongue and lips become abnormally red in color. The mouth becomes so sore that it is difficult to eat and swallow.

3. A deficiency of hydrochloric acid with a resultant anemia similar to pernicious anemia may be found.

4. Nausea and vomiting are followed by severe diarrhea.

5. A characteristic symmetric dermatitis especially on the exposed surfaces of the body—hands, forearms, elbows, feet, legs, knees, and neck—appears (see Figure 12–6). The dermatitis is sharply separated from the surrounding normal skin. At first the skin becomes red, somewhat swollen, and tender, resembling a mild sunburn; if the condition is untreated, the skin becomes rough, cracked, and scaly and may become ulcerated. Sunshine and exposure to heat aggravate the dermatitis.

6. Neurologic symptoms which include confusion, dizziness, poor memory, and irritability, and leading to hallucinations, delusions of persecution, and dementia are noted as severity increases.

The classic "D's" are the final stages of the disease—dermatitis, diarrhea, dementia, and death.

Treatment and prophylaxis. Niacinamide is given in therapeutic doses, many times in excess of the Recommended Dietary Allowances. With such therapy it is possible to progress rapidly from an all-fluid to a soft and then a high-protein regular diet. Obviously, prophylaxis must include careful and persistent education in dietary im-

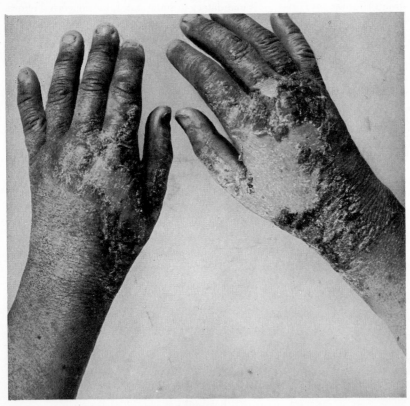

Figure 12–6. Dermatitis in pellagra.

provement, emphasis upon enrichment programs, and efforts to improve the economic status of affected populations.

Vitamin B₆

Discovery. Goldberger and Lillie in 1926 provided a description of dermatitis in rats that was recognized several years later to be characteristic of vitamin B_6 deficiency. In 1934 György reported that vitamin B_2 consisted of two factors—riboflavin, and another factor which he named vitamin B_6 that prevented rat acrodynia. In 1938 the isolation of a crystalline compound with vitamin B_6 activity was reported by several laboratories, followed by identification of the chemical structure by Harris and Folkers and its synthesis by Kuhn and Wendt in 1939.

Chemistry and characteristics. Vitamin B_6 consists of a group of related pyridines: pyridoxine, pyridoxal, and pyridoxamine. See Figure 12–1. These may appear in tissues and foodstuffs in the free form, or combined with phosphate, or with phosphate and protein. The preferred terminology is vitamin B_6; pyridoxine, being only one of the three active forms, is not entirely synonymous.

Vitamin B_6 is soluble in water and relatively stable to heat and to acids. Pyridoxal is destroyed in alkaline solutions. The vitamin is also sensitive to light. Of the three forms, pyridoxine is more resistant to food processing and storage conditions and probably represents the principal form in food products.

Measurement. Vitamin B_6 concentrations are expressed in milligrams or micrograms. The vitamin is determined in tissues and foods by chemical or fluorometric procedures. Because the vitamin occurs in various bound forms, some difficulties have been experienced in providing acceptable tabulations for food values.

Physiology. The active form of vitamin B_6 is the coenzyme pyridoxal phosphate, which can be formed from any of the three compounds. Since vitamin B_6 is water soluble, the body stores are small; about half of it is in the form of glycogen phosphorylase.

All forms of the vitamin may be excreted in the urine, but the principal metabolite is pyridoxic acid. In deficiency states pyridoxic acid disappears from the urine, and thus its presence or absence can be used to assess the state of vitamin B_6 nutrition.

Functions. Pyridoxal phosphate is the coenzyme for a large number of enzyme systems, most of which are involved in amino acid metabolism. A few examples are given below:

Decarboxylation. The removal of the carboxyl group from amino acids requires enzymes that contain pyridoxal phosphate. Each of the amino acids is decarboxylated by a specific enzyme. For example, the decarboxylation of tryptophan produces tryptamine and carbon dioxide. Serotonin is also produced by decarboxylation of tryptophan and is a potent vasoconstrictor as well as an agent in the regulation of brain and other tissues.

Transamination. Each of the many transaminases involves a distinct protein for which pyridoxal phosphate is the coenzyme. One example of transamination is shown on page 53. In the reaction, the amino group is removed from an amino acid and transferred to a keto acid, thus forming a new amino acid. This reaction is important in the formation of the nonessential amino acids.

Transulfuration. This involves the removal and transfer of sulfur groups from the sulfur-containing amino acids such as cysteine by transulfurases.

Tryptophan conversion to niacin. The importance of tryptophan as a source of niacin has been described on page 174. Several steps are required in this conversion, one of which is catalyzed by vitamin B_6.

Pyridoxal phosphate is also required for glycogen phosphorylase, an enzyme by which glycogen is broken down to glucose; for the formation of antibodies; for the synthesis of a precursor of the porphyrin ring which is part of the hemoglobin molecule; and possibly for the conversion of linoleic acid to arachidonic acid.

Daily allowances. The need for vitamin B_6 is proportional to the amount of protein metabolized. The recommended allowance for the reference man and woman is 2.0 mg daily.[1] This provides a reasonable margin of safety and permits a protein intake of 100 gm or more. Those who ingest a high-protein diet (125 to 150 gm) may need more, whereas those who have a low-protein diet (40 to 50 gm) may require only 1.2 to 1.5 mg.

The allowance for infants is 0.3 to 0.4 mg; for children from 1 to 10 years, it increases gradually from 0.6 to 1.2 mg; and for adolescents the range is 1.6 to 2.0 mg. During pregnancy and lactation 2.5 mg is recommended.

Food sources. The vitamin B_6 available in the American food supply per capita is 2.2 mg. The principal source is meat, poultry, and fish, with this group accounting for 47 per cent of the total amount available. Potatoes, sweet potatoes, and vegetables account for about 23 per cent of the total supply; dairy products, 9 per cent; and flour and cereals, 7 per cent. Whole grains are good sources of pyridoxine, but most of this is lost in the milling of the grains.

Effects of deficiency. Studies on a wide variety of animals have shown multiple effects of deficiency although the same symptoms do not appear in all species. Skin lesions, nervous symptoms, and blood disorders are characteristics of deficiency.

Vitamin B_6 deficiency was reported in the 1950's in infants who had received a commercial formula in which the pyridoxine had been inadvertently destroyed in the drying of the milk. The infants showed nervous irritability and convulsive seizures. Other related symptoms included weakness, ataxia, and abdominal pain. The convulsive seizures responded dramatically to the administration of pyridoxine.

Deficiency in adults. College students who ingested a vitamin-B_6-deficient diet for seven weeks showed rapid decreases in the blood levels of pyridoxine and increased excretion of xanthurenic acid with a tryptophan load test.[6] Xanthurenic acid is a metabolite resulting from the metabolism of tryptophan when there is insufficient vitamin B_6 to catalyze the reactions of the normal pathway. Thus, when vitamin B_6 is lacking, the excretion of xanthurenic acid will increase if a test dose of tryptophan is given.

Despite the decrease in blood pyridoxine and the increase in xanthurenic acid excretion, no clear-cut symptoms of deficiency have been observed in adults. When an antagonist to vitamin B_6 such as deoxypyridoxine is fed with a deficient diet, seborrheic dermatitis around the eyes, eyebrows, and angles of the mouth has been described.

Isonicotinic acid hydrazide (INH) is widely used in the treatment of tuberculosis. It is chemically related to pyridoxine and acts as an antagonist to vitamin B_6 activity. Patients who have been treated with this drug have experienced neuritic symptoms believed to be caused by imposed vitamin B_6 deficiency, and corrected when additional vitamin supplements were prescribed.

PANTOTHENIC ACID

Discovery. Pantothenic acid was isolated in 1938 by Dr. R. J. Williams and synthesized in 1940 by workers in the laboratories of Merck and Company. Although tests showed its vitamin nature by its ability to prevent certain deficiencies in animals, little interest was shown in this vitamin until about a decade later. In 1946 Lipmann and his associates showed that coenzyme A was essential for acetylation reactions in the body, and in 1950 reports from this same laboratory showed pantothenic acid to be a constituent of coenzyme A. The name for this vitamin is derived from the Greek word *panthos,* meaning "everywhere." The universal distribution of this vitamin in biologic materials suggests the key role that it plays in metabolism.

Characteristics. Pantothenic acid, as the free acid, is an unstable, viscous yellow oil, soluble in water. (See Figure 12–1.) Commercially, it is available as the sodium or calcium salt, which is slightly sweet, water soluble, and quite stable. There is little loss of the vitamin with ordinary cooking procedures, except in acid and alkaline solutions.

The pantothenic acid content of tissues and foods is determined by microbiologic methods, and values are expressed in milligrams or micrograms.

Functions. Coenzyme A is the form in which pantothenic acid functions in the body. Coenzyme A is a complex molecule consisting of a sulfur-containing compound, adenine, ribose, phosphoric acid, and pantothenic acid. The sulfur linkage is highly reactive. The formation of acetyl coenzyme A in the metabolism of carbohydrate has been referred to in Chapter 5 (see page 71). Acetyl coenzyme A, or active acetate as it is also known, combines with oxalacetate to form citrate, thus initiating the tricarboxylic acid cycle for the release of energy. Acetyl coenzyme A also is the unit from which fatty acids, cholesterol, steroids, the porphyrin part of the hemoglobin molecule, and acetylcholine are synthesized. The beta oxidation of fatty acids also requires coenzyme A.

Coenzyme A is synthesized in all cells and apparently does not cross cell membranes. Liver, kidney, brain, adrenal and heart tissues, being metabolically active, contain high concentrations, but there is none in the blood.

Requirement. The daily requirement for pantothenic acid is not known, but an allowance of 5 to 10 mg is believed to be satisfactory for adults and children.

Food sources. Most of the pantothenic acid in animal tissues is in the form of coenzyme A. As its name indicates, pantothenic acid is widely distributed not only in animal foods but also in whole grains and in legumes. Fruit, vegetables, and milk contain smaller amounts. The milling of flour results in loss of about 50 per cent, and dry processing of foods also leads to significant losses. Reports of dietary content indicate that the average American diet can be expected to provide 10 to 15 mg daily, with ranges from 6 to 20 mg.

Effects of deficiency. No clear-cut demonstration of pantothenic acid deficiency has been afforded by experimental diets low in pantothenic acid. When an antagonist, omega methyl pantothenic acid, was fed with deficient diets, the following symptoms were observed: loss of appetite, indigestion, abdominal pain; sullenness, mental depression; peripheral neuritis with cramping pains in the arms and legs; burning sensations in the feet; insomnia; and respiratory infections.[7] In these subjects there was an increased sensitivity to insulin, an increased sedimentation rate for erythrocytes, and marked decrease in antibody formation.

The neuropathy observed in alcoholics is possibly related to pantothenic acid deficiency. However, when diets are deficient in pantothenic acid, they are also deficient in many other factors, and therefore the separation of symptoms attributable to various nutrient lacks becomes exceedingly difficult.

BIOTIN

Discovery. In the 1920's a factor essential for the growth of yeast was described and named *bios*. In the 1930's Dr. Helen Parsons and her coworkers and others reported on the symptoms observed in rats that were fed a diet including raw egg white. The animals lost their fur, particularly around the eyes, giving a spectacle-like appearance; there was rapid loss of weight, paralysis of the hind legs, and eventual cyanosis and death. The symptoms did not occur when cooked egg white was used.

Small quantities of the active factor were isolated from egg yolk in 1936 by Kögl and were later established as being identical with the yeast growth factor and the anti-egg-white injury factor.

The substance in raw egg white has been found to be a glycoprotein that binds biotin and thereby prevents its absorption from the intestinal tract. It is called *avidin,* which means "hungry albumin." Heating of egg white inactivates the binding capacity of avidin.

Characteristics. Biotin is a relatively simple compound, a cyclic urea derivative and containing a sulfur grouping. (See Figure 12–1.) In its free form it is a crystalline substance, very stable to heat, light, and acids. It is somewhat labile to alkaline solutions and to oxidizing agents. In tissues and in foods it is usually combined with protein.

Functions and metabolism. Biotin is a coenzyme of a number of enzymes that participate in carboxylation, decarboxylation, and deamination reactions. For example, it is required in the synthesis of fatty acids. Another reaction catalyzed by biotin-containing enzymes is the fixation of CO_2 in the conversion of pyruvate to oxalacetate, an important reaction that generates the tricarboxylic acid cycle (see Figure 5–5). Within the TCA cycle, biotin is also required for the conversion of succinate to fumarate and oxalsuccinate to ketoglutarate.

Biotin is essential for the introduction of CO_2 in the formation of purines, these compounds being essential constituents of DNA and RNA. The deaminases for threonine, serine, and aspartic acid also require biotin as a coenzyme.

Biotin is stored in minute amounts principally in the metabolically active tissues such as the kidney, liver, brain, and adrenal. The biotin content of the feces and likewise of the urinary excretion is considerably greater than the dietary intake. This indicates the intestinal synthesis of biotin and the absorption of the vitamin from this source.

Dietary needs. The requirement for biotin has not been established, but it is believed to be about 150 mcg daily for adults. The average diet is estimated to contain 150 to 300 mcg daily.

Good dietary sources of biotin include organ meats, egg yolk, legumes, and nuts. Cereal grains, muscle meats, and milk contain only small amounts.

Effects of deficiency. Biotin deficiency has been described in human beings only when large amounts of raw egg whites were fed. Four volunteer subjects were fed an experimental diet containing approximately 3000 calories, low in biotin, and including 928 of the total calories from egg white (equivalent to about 60 egg whites!) for a period of 10 weeks. Beginning with the third to fourth weeks symptoms appeared approximately in this order: scaly desquamation, lassitude, muscle pains, hyperesthesia, pallor of skin and mucous membranes, anorexia, and nausea. The hemoglobin levels were lowered, the blood cholesterol levels were increased, and the urinary excretion of biotin dropped to about one tenth of the normal levels. All of these abnormalities were cured within five days when 150 mcg biotin was given daily.[8]

Recently biotin deficiency was reported in a 62-year-old woman with Laennec's cirrhosis who, on a physician's advice, had ingested six raw eggs daily for 18 months in an effort to regenerate liver tissue. Her symptoms included anorexia, nausea, vomiting, pallor, lassitude, scaly dermatitis, and desquamation of the lips. All these promptly disappeared or significantly improved within a few days following the daily parenteral administration of 200 mcg biotin.[9]

VITAMIN B_{12}

Discovery. Until the 1920's pernicious anemia was an invariably fatal disease. Then came the dramatic announcement by Minot and Murphy[10] that large amounts of liver—about a pound a day—would control the anemia and prevent the neurologic changes. To consume this amount of liver required heroic efforts on the part of the patient, and also challenged dietitians and nurses to find ways to help the patient to consume it.

Castle set forth the hypothesis that liver contained a substance which he termed the *extrinsic factor* and that its absorption required another principle in normal gastric secretion called the *intrinsic factor*. Patients with pernicious anemia were believed to be lacking in the intrinsic factor, but after consumption of very large amounts of liver some absorption of the extrinsic factor took place by simple diffusion.

The active principle in liver was extracted in the 1930's and provided the basis for the treatment of patients by injections. The factor was called erythrocyte maturation factor, anti-pernicious-anemia factor, animal protein factor, and extrinsic factor. Then in 1948 came the announcement by Rickes and his associates in the United States[11] and Smith and Parker in England[12] of the isolation of a few micrograms of a red crystalline substance that was shown to be dramatically effective in the remission of pernicious anemia. The structure of the compound was elucidated in 1955 and was established to be the same as that of the various factors listed above.

Characteristics. Vitamin B_{12} is the most complex of all vitamin molecules and contains a single atom of cobalt held in a structure similar to that which holds iron in hemoglobin and

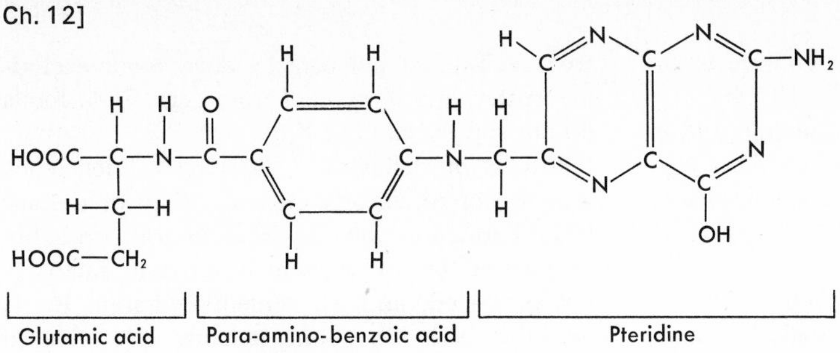

Glutamic acid | Para-amino-benzoic acid | Pteridine

Folic acid ($C_{19}H_{19}N_7O_6$; m.w. 441.4)

Figure 12–7. Folic acid and vitamin B_{12} are essential for the regeneration of red blood cells. Vitamin B_{12} has the most complex chemical structure of any of the vitamins; note the position of cobalt.

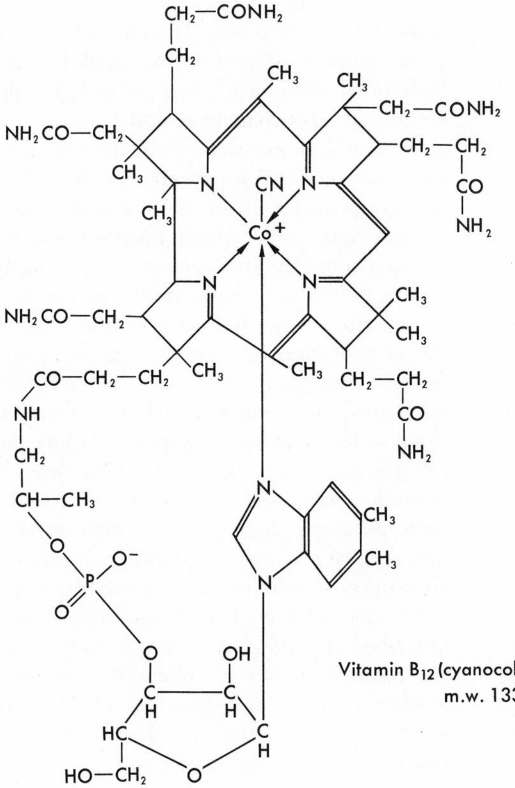

Vitamin B_{12} (cyanocobalamin shown; $C_{63}H_{88}CoN_{14}O_{14}P$; m.w. 1335.4)

magnesium in chlorophyll. (See Figure 12–7.) It occurs in several forms, designated as cobalamins; cyanocobalamin is one of the most active forms.

The deep-red needlelike crystals are slightly soluble in water, stable to heat, but inactivated by light and by strong acid or alkaline solutions. There is little loss of the vitamin by ordinary cooking procedures.

The synthetic vitamin is now produced inex-pensively as a by-product in the fermentation reactions required for the production of antibiotics such as penicillin and streptomycin. Vitamin B_{12} is assayed microbiologically and is measured in micrograms.

Function and metabolism. Intrinsic factor is produced by glands in the fundus and cardia of the stomach. Vitamin B_{12} is linked with intrinsic factor and carried through the small intestine to special sites in the ileum. There, in a manner not fully understood, the vitamin is attached to the special epithelial cells by the intrinsic factor in the presence of calcium and is transported across the cell into the blood circulation. The intrinsic factor remains in the intestine. In the blood circulation vitamin B_{12} is combined with serum proteins.

Intrinsic factor regulates the amount of absorption to about 2.5 to 3 mcg daily.[13] When the dietary intake is only 1 to 2 mcg daily, 60 to 80 per cent of the vitamin is absorbed, but with good diets the absorption for young men averages 10 per cent and for elderly men about 5 per cent. The absorption is greater if the vitamin B_{12} is present in three meals than if it is all provided in a single meal.

The liver is the principal site of storage for vitamin B_{12} and may contain from 2000 to 5000 mcg, a supply that is sufficient for three to five years.

Vitamin B_{12} is essential for the functioning of all cells but especially those of the gastrointestinal tract, the nervous system, and the bone marrow. Within the bone marrow a vitamin B_{12} coenzyme is essential for the synthesis of DNA. When DNA is not being synthesized the erythroblasts do not divide but increase in size, becoming megaloblasts which are released into the circulation. Whether the influence of vitamin B_{12} is a direct action or a facilitation of the use of folic acid is not understood.

Vitamin B_{12} is also required for enzymes that accomplish the synthesis and transfer of single-carbon units such as the methyl group, for example, the synthesis of methionine and choline, which are important lipotropic factors.

Dietary needs. A minimum intake of 0.6 to 1.2 mcg of vitamin B_{12} daily is sufficient for normal hematopoiesis and good health, but will not replenish liver stores. The recommended allowance for males and females over 11 years is 3 mcg daily, and for pregnancy and lactation is 4 mcg.[1] For infants, 0.3 mcg is recommended daily, and for children the allowance increases from 1.0 mcg at 1 to 3 years to 2.0 mcg at 7 to 10 years.

In 1970 the vitamin B_{12} available per capita in the American food supply was 9.6 mcg, of which 70 per cent was supplied by meats, poultry, and fish, 21 per cent by dairy foods excluding butter, and 9 per cent from eggs. Plant foods do not supply vitamin B_{12}.

Effects of deficiency. Vitamin B_{12} deficiency is a defect of absorption and rarely of dietary lack. Pernicious anemia is a disease, probably of genetic origin, in which intrinsic factor is not produced, and consequently vitamin B_{12} is not absorbed. The bone marrow is unable to produce mature red blood cells, but releases fewer number of large cells (macrocytes) into the circulation. Thus, the capacity to carry hemoglobin is reduced. The characteristic symptoms include lemon-yellow pallor, anorexia, abdominal discomfort, loss of weight, glossitis, neurologic disturbances including unsteady gait, and mental depression. Patients respond to as little as 1 mcg given parenterally; usually, initial therapy provides 15 to 30 mcg until the anemia is corrected, after which maintenance therapy is given monthly and averages 1 mcg daily.

Megaloblastic anemia from vitamin B_{12} deficiency also occurs following surgical removal of the part of the stomach that produces intrinsic factor, or the part of the ileum where the absorption sites are located. Such deficiency occurs three to five years following the surgery and can be prevented by injections of vitamin B_{12} at periodic intervals. Malabsorption syndromes such as sprue may also be characterized by megaloblastic anemias resulting from deficient absorption of vitamin B_{12} as well as folic acid.

Dietary deficiency of vitamin B_{12} has been described in vegetarians who consumed no animal foods whatsoever.[14] They showed low serum levels of vitamin B_{12}, glossitis, paresthesias, and some changes in the spinal cord, but did not have the characteristic anemia.

FOLIC ACID (FOLACIN; PTEROYLGLUTAMIC ACID)

Discovery. During the 1930's and 1940's many investigators had described water-soluble factors required by various animal species and microorganisms and given them names such as factor U (unknown factor required for chick growth); vitamin B_c (antianemia factor for chicks); Wills factor for treatment of tropical macrocytic anemia of pregnancy described by Dr. Lucy Wills; vitamin M, essential for monkeys; L-casei factor, citrovorum factor, and SLR factor for growth of various microorganisms. Folic acid was named in 1941 by Mitchell and his associates because of its prevalence in green leaves; *folium* is the Latin word for leaf. In 1945 the identification of the structure and the synthesis of folic acid by Angier and his coworkers at Lederle Laboratories established that these variously named factors were one and the same substance. That same year Dr. Tom Spies showed that folic acid was effective in the treatment of megaloblastic anemia of pregnancy and of tropical sprue.

Characteristics. Folic acid consists of three linked components: a pteridine grouping; para-aminobenzoic acid, sometimes classed as a B complex vitamin; and glutamic acid, an amino acid. (See Figure 12–7.) It may contain one, three, or seven glutamate groupings and is thus designated as mono-, tri-, or hepta-pteroylglutamate. Pure folic acid occurs as bright yellow crystals only slightly soluble in water. It is easily oxidized in an acid medium and is susceptible to sunlight. Appreciable losses of folic acid occur in foods stored at room temperature and in ordinary cooking procedures.

Folic acid is measured in micrograms and may be assayed by microbiologic, colorimetric, or fluorometric methods.

Physiology and functions. The several forms of folic acid are utilized in the body. The fecal and urinary excretions are usually greater than can be accounted for by the dietary intake. This indicates intestinal synthesis and also absorption of folic acid from dietary and intestinal sources. Most of the folic acid is stored in the liver. The conversion of folic acid to *folinic acid,* the biologically active form, is believed to occur in the liver. Ascorbic acid facilitates this conversion.

Folinic acid is the coenzyme for a number of enzyme systems. An important function is the biosynthesis and transfer of 1-carbon units such as methyl groups. This makes possible the synthesis of methionine, choline, and the introduction of the methyl group to the pyrimidine *thymine.* The latter is an essential component of DNA. The role of folinic acid in the synthesis

of the nucleoproteins is a key to the production of normal red blood cells in the bone marrow; its action is interrelated with that of vitamin B_{12}. Folic acid is also required for the oxidation of phenylalanine to tyrosine.

Dietary needs. The recommended allowance for adults is 400 mcg folic acid daily. For pregnancy the allowance is 800 mcg and for lactation it is 600 mcg; during the first year of life the needs are met with 50 mcg daily.

Folic acid is widely distributed in foods in both free and conjugate form. Liver, kidney, yeast, and deep-green leafy vegetables are excellent sources; lean beef, veal, eggs, and whole-grain cereals are good sources; and root vegetables, dairy foods, pork, and light-green vegetables are relatively low in the vitamin.

Effects of deficiency. Folic acid deficiency may result from inadequate dietary intake or secondary to disease. With a deficiency the serum folate level is reduced and changes take place in the production of red blood cells in the bone marrow. The anemia that results from folic acid deficiency is characterized by a reduction in the number of red blood cells, the release into the blood circulation of large nucleated cells (hence the designation macrocytic, or megaloblastic, anemia), low hemoglobin levels but a high color content of each cell, and lowered leukocyte and platelet levels.

The anemia has been observed in elderly patients who have had poor diets and who have various organic diseases, in pregnant women, and in infants whose formulas may be inadequate in folic acid or ascorbic acid. It frequently accompanies disease conditions in which the requirement for the vitamin is greatly increased, as in Hodgkin's disease and leukemia. Malabsorption syndromes, notably tropical sprue, are characterized by the presence of megaloblastic anemias.

The administration of folic acid to patients with megaloblastic anemia brings about dramatic reversal of the changes in the bone marrow. The red blood cells become normal in size, their number increases, the total hemoglobin increases, and the leukocyte levels return to normal. Many of the patients have a glossitis and diarrhea especially associated with malabsorption; these too are improved.

Folic acid will produce remission of the anemia in pernicious anemia, but it has no effect on the neurologic symptoms, which become progressively worse. Multiple-vitamin preparations, by regulation of the Food and Drug Administration, can provide no more than 0.1 mg folic acid daily. This is an amount that meets the daily need, but is insufficient to correct an anemia. Thus, these dosages would not mask a pernicious anemia and delay diagnosis until the serious problems of neurologic changes arise.

OTHER FACTORS

Choline. All living cells contain choline, $C_5H_{15}NO_2$, principally in phospholipids. Choline is known as a lipotropic factor in that it prevents the deposit of fat in the liver. It is an important constituent of acetylcholine and thus is essential for the transmission of nerve impulses. One of the important functions of choline is the donation of methyl groups that can be utilized in numerous reactions. Vitamin B_{12} and folic acid also aid in the biosynthesis and transfer of methyl groups.

Choline has been shown to be essential for various animal species, but the need for it by human beings has not been clearly established. Probably synthesis of choline within the body is sufficient.

Egg yolk is especially rich in choline, but legumes, organ meats, milk, muscle meats, and whole-grain cereals are also good sources. A typical diet furnishes from 200 to 600 mg daily. These relatively large amounts indicate that choline is probably not a true vitamin.

Inositol. Inositol, $C_6H_{12}O_6$, is a water-soluble, sweet-tasting substance distributed in fruits, vegetables, whole grains, meats, and milk. It possesses lipotropic activity but its significance in human nutrition has not been established.

Lipoic acid. Lipoic acid is a sulfur-containing, fat-soluble substance also known as *thioctic acid* and *protogen*. Strictly speaking, it is not a vitamin because it is not necessary in the diet of animals. It functions, however, in the same manner as many of the B-complex vitamins. It is a component of the complexes involved in the

decarboxylation of keto acids such as pyruvic acid and α-ketoglutaric acid. (See page 71.)

SOME POINTS FOR EMPHASIS IN NUTRITION EDUCATION (A GENERAL SUMMARY)

1. Vitamins are compounds of known chemical nature occurring in minute amounts in foods. They have exact functions in the body for the use of carbohydrates, fats, and proteins for energy and for the synthesis of tissues, enzymes, and other body regulators. Thus, vitamins help to maintain healthy tissues and normal functions of all organs.

2. Each vitamin has specific functions and cannot substitute for another. Many reactions in the body require several vitamins, and a lack of any one can interfere with the function of another.

3. Synthetic vitamins and the vitamins occurring naturally in foods have the same chemical formulas and, weight for weight, are of equal use in the body.

4. A diet that includes recommended amounts of the Four Food Groups will furnish sufficient amounts of all the vitamins (except vitamin D) required by healthy persons of all age categories.

5. Each food group makes a special vitamin contribution to the diet. All the vitamin needs are not easily met if one or more of these food groups are omitted. For example, fruits and vegetables are the principal sources of ascorbic acid; dark-green leafy vegetables and deep-yellow vegetables and fruits are a major source of carotene; milk is a principal source of riboflavin; meats, poultry, and fish are outstanding for niacin, vitamin B_6, vitamin B_{12}, and thiamine; and whole-grain and enriched breads and cereals are especially important for thiamine and niacin.

6. Vitamin D is present in natural foodstuffs in only small amounts. Infants, children, pregnant and lactating women, and people who have little exposure to sunlight should use vitamin D milk or a supplement.

7. All vitamins are susceptible to destruction under certain conditions. However, for practical purposes, if the homemaker observes rules for the preservation of ascorbic acid, thiamine, and riboflavin, all other vitamins are likely to be satisfactorily retained. For riboflavin, the principal destruction comes about when milk in clear-glass bottles is allowed to stand in direct sunlight. The retention of ascorbic acid, thiamine, and other vitamins is assured if (1) some raw foods such as salads are freshly prepared and used daily, (2) cutting and exposure of surfaces are reduced to the shortest possible period of time, (3) cookery takes place in a small volume of liquid, (4) the use of alkali to retain green color is avoided, (5) foods are cooked only to the point of tenderness, and (6) foods are served promptly after preparation.

8. Vitamins A and D are toxic, and high-potency supplements should be used only when prescribed by a physician for specific deficiencies.

9. If taken in greater amounts than the body needs, the water-soluble vitamins are excreted in the urine; hence, supplements in addition to a good diet are probably an economic waste.

10. Vitamin deficiencies can be diagnosed only by means of accurate dietary and medical history, physical examination, and laboratory studies. Self-diagnosis and therapy are wasteful and can be dangerous.

11. Vitamin deficiency diseases can occur (1) if the dietary intake is generally poor, (2) if a food group is consistently omitted without making appropriate compensation for such omission, and (3) when there is too little money to buy an adequate diet.

12. A large proportion of vitamin deficiencies in the United States are secondary to disease, including anorexia and vomiting and failure to eat, malabsorption as in diarrhea, sprue, and other conditions, and increased metabolic requirements because of fever and other stress factors.

13. Specific vitamin deficiencies require therapy with the vitamins that are lacking. Usually, synthetic vitamins are used to correct the deficiency inasmuch as large dosages can bring about rapid improvement.

PROBLEMS AND REVIEW

1. Explain how the following nutrients are interrelated:

riboflavin and niacin	pyridoxine and protein	cobalt and vitamin B_{12}
tryptophan and niacin	tryptophan and vitamin B_6	folic acid and ascorbic acid
glucose and thiamine	folic acid and folinic acid	choline and fat

2. What is the effect on carbohydrate metabolism of a deficiency of thiamine? What are clinical signs of such deficiency?

3. What is the role of niacin in metabolism? What clinical symptoms are observed in a niacin deficiency?

4. How can you explain the fact that milk is a pellagra-preventive food even though it contains very little niacin?

5. The dietary intake of vitamins may appear to be satisfactory when compared with recommended allowances, but a physician may prescribe a vitamin supplement. Under what circumstances would you expect such a supplement to be necessary?

6. What is the possible significance of each of the following in human nutrition: folic acid; choline; biotin; pantothenic acid; pyridoxine; inositol; vitamin B_{12}?

7. *Problem.* Examine the label information on three packages of dry cereals. Calculate the percentage of the recommended allowances provided by 1 ounce of each cereal, using your own allowances as the basis for calculation. How do these percentages compare with those indicated on the label? Explain any differences.

Table 12–1. Summary of Water-Soluble Vitamins
(*see also Points for Emphasis, page 184*)

Nomenclature	Important Sources	Physiology and Function	Effects of Deficiency	Recommended Allowances*
Ascorbic acid Vitamin C	Citrus fruits; tomatoes; melons; cabbage; broccoli; straw- berries; fresh potatoes; green leafy vegetables	Very little storage in body Formation of intercellular cement substance; synthesis of collagen Absorption and use of iron Conversion of folic acid to folinic acid	Weakened cartilages and capillary walls Cutaneous hemorrhage Sore, bleeding gums Anemia Poor wound healing Poor bone and tooth development **Scurvy**	Men: 45 mg Women: 45 mg Pregnancy: 60 mg Lactation: 60 mg Infants: 35 mg Children under 10: 40 mg Boys and girls: 45 mg
Thiamine Vitamin B$_1$	Whole-grain and enriched breads, cereals, flours; organ meats, pork; other meats, poultry, fish; legumes, nuts; milk; green vegetables	Limited body storage Thiamine pyrophosphate (TPP) is coenzyme for decarboxylation and transketolation; chiefly involved in carbohydrate metabolism	Poor appetite; atony of gastrointestinal tract, constipation Mental depression, apathy, polyneuritis Cachexia, edema Cardiac failure **Beriberi**	Men: 1.4 mg Women: 1.0 mg Pregnancy: 1.3 mg Lactation: 1.3 mg Infants: 0.3–0.5 mg Children under 10: 0.7–1.2 mg Boys and girls: 1.1–1.5 mg
Riboflavin Vitamin B$_2$	Milk; organ meats; eggs; green leafy vegetables	Limited body stores, but reserves retained carefully Coenzymes for removal and transfer of hydrogen; flavin mononucleotide (FMN) and flavin adenine dinucleotide (FAD)	Cheilosis (cracks at corners of lips) Scaly desquamation around nose, ears Sore tongue and mouth Burning and itching of eyes Photophobia	Men: 1.6 mg Women: 1.2 mg Pregnancy: 1.5 mg Lactation: 1.7 mg Infants: 0.4–0.6 mg Children under 10: 0.8–1.2 mg Boys and girls: 1.3–1.8 mg

Vitamin	Food Sources	Physiologic Functions	Deficiency Symptoms	Recommended Allowance
Niacin Nicotinic acid Nicotinamide	Meat, poultry, fish; whole-grain and enriched breads, flours, cereals; nuts, legumes Tryptophan as a precursor	Coenzyme for transfer of hydrogen in energy metabolism: nicotinamide adenine dinucleotide (NAD) and nicotinamide adenine dinucleotide phosphate (NADP)	Anorexia, glossitis, diarrhea Dermatitis Neurologic degeneration **Pellagra**	Men: 18 mg Women: 13 mg Pregnancy: 15 mg Lactation: 17 mg Infants: 5–8 mg Children under 10: 9–16 mg Boys and girls: 14–20 mg
Vitamin B$_6$ Three active forms: pyridoxine, pyridoxal, pyridoxamine	Meat, poultry, fish; potatoes, sweet potatoes, vegetables	Pyridoxal phosphate is coenzyme for transamination, decarboxylation, transulfuration Conversion of tryptophan to niacin Primarily concerned with protein metabolism	Nervous irritability, convulsions Weakness, ataxia, abdominal pain	Adults: 2.0 mg Pregnancy: 2.5 mg Lactation: 2.5 mg Infants: 0.3–0.4 mg Children under 10: 0.6–1.2 mg Boys and girls: 1.6–2.0 mg
Pantothenic acid	Meat, poultry, fish; whole-grain cereals; legumes Smaller amounts in fruits, vegetables, milk	Constituent of coenzyme A: thus, energy metabolism, fat and cholesterol synthesis	Deficiency seen only with severe multiple B complex deficits; then, gastrointestinal disturbances, neuritis, burning sensations of feet	Not known; probably about 5–10 mg
Biotin	Organ meats, egg yolk, nuts, legumes	*Avidin*, a protein in raw egg white blocks absorption; large amounts of raw eggs must be eaten Coenzyme for deamination, carboxylation, and decarboxylation	Deficiency only when many raw egg whites are consumed for long periods of time Dermatitis, anorexia, hyperesthesia, anemia	Not known; probably about 150 mcg

*See also Table 3–1 for complete listing of allowances.

Table 12-1. (Cont.)

Nomenclature	Important Sources	Physiology and Function	Effects of Deficiency	Recommended Allowances*
Vitamin B_{12} Cyanocobalamin Hydroxycobalamin	In animal foods only: organ meats, muscle meats, fish, poultry; eggs; milk	Requires intrinsic factor for absorption Biosynthesis of methyl groups Synthesis of DNA and RNA Formation of mature red blood cells	Lack of intrinsic factor leads to deficiency: pernicious anemia, following gastrectomy Macrocytic anemia Neurologic degeneration	Adults: 3 mcg Pregnancy: 4 mcg Lactation: 4 mcg Infants: 0.3 mcg Children: 1–2 mcg Boys and girls: 3 mcg
Folic acid Folacin Pteroylglutamic acid	Organ meats, deep-green leafy vegetables; muscle meats, poultry, fish, eggs; whole-grain cereals	Active form is folinic acid; requires ascorbic acid for conversion Coenzyme for transmethylation; synthesis of nucleoproteins; maturation of red blood cells Interrelated with vitamin B_{12}	Megaloblastic anemia of infancy, pregnancy, tropical sprue	Adults: 400 mcg Pregnancy: 800 mcg Lactation: 600 mcg Infants: 50 mcg Children under 10: 100–300 mcg Boys and girls: 400 mcg
Choline	Egg yolk, meat, poultry, fish, milk, whole grains	Probably not a true vitamin Donor of methyl groups: lipotropic action Component of acetylcholine	Has not been observed in humans	Not known; typical diet supplies 200–600 mg
Lipoic acid Thioctic acid Protogen		Probably not a true vitamin Coenzyme for decarboxylation of keto acids		Not known
Inositol	Widely distributed in all foods	Lipotropic agent Vitamin nature not established	Has not been observed in humans	Not known

8. *Problem.* Mrs. Smith has asked for your guidance in the selection, storage, and preparation of food so that maximum nutritive value will be retained. On the basis of your information concerning the stability of vitamins, indicate briefly a set of instructions for guiding Mr. Smith. Show how these rules apply to the preparation of a meal that includes roast beef, potatoes, green beans, cole slaw, milk, and fruit cup. Which vitamin or vitamins are especially concerned in each rule you have laid down?

9. *Problem.* Calculate the thiamine, riboflavin, and niacin content of your own diet for two days. Compare your intake with the recommended allowances. If there are any deficits, show how you could correct them.

10. *Problem.* A dietary calculation showed an intake of 80 gm protein and 12 mg niacin. Calculate the total niacin equivalent of this diet.

11. *Problem.* Calculate the percentage of your own daily requirement for thiamine and riboflavin which 3 cups of milk would supply. For each of these nutrients list two foods which would serve as effective supplements to the milk in supplying your daily needs.

CITED REFERENCES

1. Food and Nutrition Board: *Recommended Dietary Allowances,* 8th ed. National Academy of Sciences–National Research Council, Washington, D.C., 1973.
2. Williams, R. R.: "The World Beriberi Problem," *J. Clin. Nutr.,* 1:513–16, 1953.
3. Brin, M.: "Erythrocytes as Biopsy Tissue for Functional Evaluation of Thiamine Adequacy," *J.A.M.A.,* 187:762–66, 1964.
4. Horwitt, M. K.: "Niacin-Tryptophan Requirements of Man," *J. Am. Diet. Assoc.,* 34:914–19, 1958.
5. Mickelson, O.: "Present Knowledge of Niacin," in *Present Knowledge of Nutrition.* The Nutrition Foundation, Inc., New York, 1967, pp. 96–100.
6. Cheslock, K. E., and McCully, M. T.: "Response of Human Beings to a Low-Vitamin B_6 Diet," *J. Nutr.,* 70:507–13, 1960.
7. Glusman, N.: "The Syndrome of 'Burning Feet' (Nutritional Melalgia) as a Manifestation of Nutritional Deficiency," *Am. J. Med.,* 3:211–23, 1947.
8. Sydenstricker, V. P., *et al.:* "Preliminary Observations on 'Egg White Injury' in Man and Its Cure with a Biotin Concentrate," *Science,* 95:176–77, 1942.
9. Baugh, C. M., *et al.:* "Human Biotin Deficiency. A Case History of Biotin Deficiency Induced by Raw Egg Consumption in a Cirrhotic Patient," *Am. J. Clin. Nutr.,* 21:173–82, 1968.
10. Minot, G. R., and Murphy, W. P.: "Treatment of Pernicious Anemia by Special Diet," *J.A.M.A.,* 87:470–76, 1926.
11. Rickes, E. L., *et al.:* "Crystalline Vitamin B_{12}," *Science,* 107:396–97, 1948.
12. Smith, E. L., and Parker, L. F. J.: "Purification of Anti-pernicious Anemia Factors from Liver," *Biochem. J.,* 43:viii–ix, 1948.
13. Heyssel, R. M., *et al.:* "Vitamin B_{12} Turnover in Man," *Am. J. Clin. Nutr.,* 18:176–84, 1966.
14. Smith, A. D. M: "Veganism: A Clinical Survey with Observations on Vitamin B_{12} Metabolism," *Br. Med. J.,* 1:1655–58, 1962.

ADDITIONAL REFERENCES

Thiamine, Riboflavin, and Niacin

Ariaey-Nejad, M. R., *et al.:* "Thiamin Metabolism in Man," *Am. J. Clin. Nutr.,* 23:764–78, 1970.

Elvehjem, C. A.: "Early Experiences with Niacin—A Retrospect," *Nutr. Rev.,* 11:289–92, 1953.

FAO/WHO: *Requirements of Vitamin A, Thiamine, Riboflavin, and Niacin.* FAO Rep. Series No. 41, FAO, Rome, 1967.

Goldsmith, G. A.: "Experimental Niacin Deficiency," *J. Am. Diet. Assoc.,* 32:312–16, 1956.

György, P.: "Early Experiences with Riboflavin—A Retrospect," *Nutr. Rev.,* 12:97–100, 1954.

Henshaw, J. L., *et al.*: "Method for Evaluating Thiamine Adequacy in College Women," *J. Am. Diet. Assoc.,* 57:436–41, 1970.

Horwitt, M. K.: "Nutritional Requirements of Man, with Special Reference to Riboflavin," *Am. J. Clin. Nutr.,* 18:458–66, 1966.

Noble, I.: "Thiamine and Riboflavin Retention in Cooked Variety Meats," *J. Am. Diet. Assoc.,* 56:225–28, 1970.

Review: "Gastric and Pancreatic Function in Pellagra," *Nutr. Rev.,* 27:136–38, 1969.

———: "Nicotinamide Deficiency and Adrenocortical Steroids," *Nutr. Rev.,* 26:343–45, 1968.

———: "Riboflavin—Transport and Excretion," *Nutr. Rev.,* 27:285–87, 1969.

Sydenstricker, V. P.: "History of Pellagra. Its Recognition as a Disorder of Nutrition and Its Conquest," *Am. J. Clin. Nutr.,* 6:409–14, 1958.

Tanphaichitr, V., *et al.*: "Clinical and Biochemical Studies of Adult Beriberi," *Am. J. Clin. Nutr.,* 23:1017–26, 1970.

Williams, R. R.: *Toward the Conquest of Beriberi.* Harvard University Press, Cambridge, Mass., 1961.

———: "Recollections of the 'Beriberi-Preventing Substance,'" *Nutr. Rev.,* 11:257–59, 1953.

Vitamin B₆, Pantothenic Acid, and Biotin

Baker, E. M., *et al.*: "Vitamin B$_6$ Requirement for Adult Men," *Am. J. Clin. Nutr.,* 15:59–66, 1964.

Bridgers, W. F.: "Present Knowledge of Biotin," *Nutr. Rev.,* 25:65–68, 1967.

Chung, A. S. M., *et al.*: "Folic Acid, Vitamin B$_6$, Pantothenic Acid, and Vitamin B$_{12}$ in Human Dietaries," *Am. J. Clin. Nutr.,* 9:573–82, 1961.

Coursin, D. B.: "Present Status of Vitamin B$_6$ Metabolism," *Am. J. Clin. Nutr.,* 9:304–14, 1961.

Frimpter, G. W., *et al.*: "Vitamin B$_6$ Dependency Syndromes: New Horizons in Nutrition," *Am. J. Clin. Nutr.,* 22:794–805, 1969.

György, P.: "The History of Vitamin B$_6$," *Am. J. Clin. Nutr.,* 4:313–17, 1956.

Hines, J. D., and Harris, J. W.: "Pyridoxine-Responsive Anemia. Description of Three Patients with Megaloblastic Erythropoeisis," *Am. J. Clin. Nutr.,* 14:137–146, 1964.

Lepkovsky, S.: "Early Experiences with Pyridoxine—A Retrospect," *Nutr. Rev.,* 12:257–60, 1954.

Linkswiler, H.: "Biochemical and Physiological Changes in Vitamin B$_6$ Deficiency," *Am. J. Clin. Nutr.,* 20:547–57, 1967.

Review: "Vitamin B$_6$ Deficiency Following Isoniazid Therapy," *Nutr. Rev.,* 26:306–308, 1968.

Williams, R. J.: "Early Experiences with Pantothenic Acid—A Retrospect," *Nutr. Rev.,* 12:65–68, 1954.

Woodward, J. D.: "Biotin," *Sci. Am.,* 204:139–46, June 1961.

Vitamin B₁₂ and Folic Acid

Herbert, V.: "Biochemical and Hematologic Lesions in Folic Acid Deficiency," *Am. J. Clin. Nutr.,* 20:562–69, 1967.

———: "Nutritional Requirements for Vitamin B$_{12}$ and Folic Acid," *Am. J. Clin. Nutr.,* 21:743–52, 1968.

Kitay, D. Z.: "Folic Acid in Pregnancy," *J.A.M.A.,* 204:79, 1968.

Meindok, H., and Dvorsky, R.: "Serum Folate and Vitamin B$_{12}$ Levels in the Elderly," *J. Am. Geriatr. Soc.,* 18:317–26, 1970.

Review: "Anticonvulsant Therapy and Serum Folate," *Nutr. Rev.,* 27:78–79, 1969.

———: "Folic Acid and Pregnancy," *Nutr. Rev.,* 26:5–8, 1968.

Schweigert, B. S.: "The Role of Vitamin B_{12} in Nucleic Acid Synthesis," *Bordens Rev. Nutr. Res.,* **22**:19–28, April 1961.

Smith, E. L.: "Vitamin B_{12}. Part I," *Nutr. Abstr. Rev.,* **20**:795–809, 1951.

Ungley, C. C.: "Vitamin B_{12}. Part II. A Review of Clinical Aspects," *Nutr. Abstr. Rev.,* **21**:1–26, 1951.

West, R.: "Activity of Vitamin B_{12} in Addisonian Pernicious Anemia," *Science,* **107**:398, 1948.

Wilson, T. H.: "Intrinsic Factor and B_{12} Absorption—A Problem in Cell Physiology," *Nutr. Rev.,* **23**:33–35, 1965.

Unit III

Food Selection for Nutritional, Psychologic, and Cultural Values

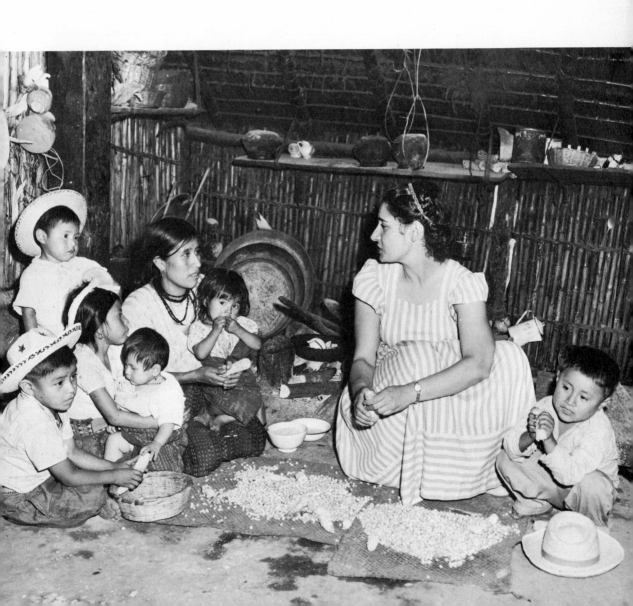

13 Nutritional Characteristics of the Food Groups and Their Contribution to a Basic Dietary Pattern

Food energy	3290 calories
Protein	100 gm
Fat	155 gm
Carbohydrate	381 gm
Calcium	0.93 gm
Phosphorus	1.52 gm
Iron	17.2 mg
Magnesium	344 mg
Vitamin A value	7800 I.U.
Thiamine	1.84 mg
Riboflavin	2.26 mg
Niacin	22.6 mg
Vitamin B_6	2.19 mg
Vitamin B_{12}	9.6 mcg
Ascorbic acid	108 mg

One instrument does not make up an orchestra; neither does one food, no matter how good it is, make up a well-balanced diet. The emphasis in the preceding unit was on the metabolic roles of specific nutrients and on food sources that would supply these nutrients. Foods, however, are complex substances that make a variety of nutritive contributions and therefore should be evaluated in terms of their total composition and not only for single nutrients for which they may be outstanding. The discussion in this chapter aims to show how each food group contributes to the total nutritional intake and to describe a dietary pattern for the adult that is based upon the Four Food Groups.

The national food supply. Are national food supplies adequate for the population needs? What is the relative contribution that may be expected of each of the major food groups to the nutrient supplies? Answers to these questions are provided annually by the Consumer and Economic Research Division of the Agricultural Research Service of the U.S. Department of Agriculture. The per capita nutritive value of the available food supply in 1970 was as follows:[1]

The percentage of total nutrients contributed by each of the major food groups is shown in Table 13–1. From this table it is easy to see the relative importance of each food group in supplying a given nutrient. This table also demonstrates how some food groups are important suppliers of several nutrients. The following statements represent a summary of the contribution made by each of the major food groups.

1. Milk and dairy products far exceed other food groups for calcium and riboflavin; they are second only to the meat group for the protein and phosphorus contribution.

2. The meat group, including eggs and dry beans, peas, and nuts as well as meat, poultry, and fish, ranks first as a source of protein, phosphorus, magnesium, iron, thiamine, niacin, vitamin B_6, and vitamin B_{12}. Because of the high level of consumption, this group ranks second for energy, vitamin A, and riboflavin.

3. Fruits and vegetables are the only important sources of ascorbic acid and contribute about half of the vitamin A; they supply roughly one fifth of the iron and about one fourth of the magnesium and vitamin B_6.

4. The flour-cereal group takes second place as a source of calories, iron, thiamine, and niacin. This group becomes increasingly important for these nutrients as the income is lowered and the consumption of them is increased.

5. Sugars and sweets and fats and oils each contribute about one sixth of the energy value of the diet but do not add appreciably to the protein, mineral, or vitamin levels.

194

Table 13–1. Contribution of Major Food Groups to Nutrient Supplies Available for Civilian Consumption, 1970*†

Food Group	Food Energy %	Protein %	Fat %	Carbo-hydrate %	Calcium %	Phos-phorus %	Iron %	Magne-sium %	Vita-min A Value %	Thia-mine %	Ribo-flavin %	Niacin %	Vita-min B6 %	Vita-min B12 %	Ascorbic Acid %
Dairy products, excluding butter	11.3	22.1	12.7	6.9	75.8	36.0	2.3	21.8	11.3	9.7	42.4	1.6	9.4	20.6	4.5
Meat (including pork-fat cuts), poultry, and fish	20.3	41.5	34.9	0.1	3.6	26.2	30.8	13.7	23.3	29.5	25.5	47.1	47.1	70.1	1.1
Eggs	2.2	5.8	3.3	0.1	2.6	6.0	6.0	1.4	6.8	2.5	5.9	0.1	2.2	9.3	0
Dry beans and peas, nuts, soya flour	2.9	5.0	3.5	2.1	2.7	5.7	6.4	10.9	‡	5.6	1.8	6.8	4.2	0	‡
Citrus fruits	0.8	0.4	0.1	1.7	0.8	0.6	0.8	1.9	1.3	2.5	0.5	0.8	1.1	0	24.5
Other fruits	2.4	0.6	0.3	5.1	1.3	1.2	3.7	4.0	6.6	2.0	1.6	1.9	5.8	0	12.0
Potatoes and sweet potatoes	2.8	2.4	0.1	5.5	1.0	4.0	4.6	7.3	5.7	6.6	1.8	7.4	12.0	0	20.3
Dark-green and deep-yellow vegetables	0.2	0.4	‡	0.5	1.5	0.6	1.6	2.0	20.8	0.9	1.0	0.6	1.7	0	8.4
Other vegetables, including tomatoes	2.4	3.2	0.4	4.5	4.8	4.8	9.2	10.2	15.3	7.0	4.5	5.9	9.2	0	29.2
Flour and cereal products	19.8	18.1	1.4	35.8	3.4	12.6	26.6	18.1	0.4	33.7	14.3	22.5	7.0	0	0
Sugars and other sweeteners	16.6	‡	0	37.1	1.1	0.2	5.6	0.4	0	‡	‡	‡	0.1	0	‡
Fats and oils, including butter	17.7	0.1	42.3	‡	0.4	0.2	0	0.4	8.4	0	0	0	0.1	0	0
Coffee and cocoa§	0.7	0.4	1.2	0.6	1.0	1.8	2.6	7.8	‡	0.1	0.7	5.2	0.1	0	0
Total ‖	100.0	100.0	100.0	100.0	100.0	100.0	100.0	100.0	100.0	100.0	100.0	100.0	100.0	100.0	100.0

*Adapted from Friend, B.: "Nutritional Review," *National Food Situation*, NFS–134. U.S. Department of Agriculture, Washington, D.C., Table 14, November 1970. Preliminary data for 1970.
†Percentages were derived from nutrient data which include quantities of iron, thiamine, and riboflavin added to flour and cereal products; quantities of vitamin A value added to margarine and milk of all types; quantities of ascorbic acid added to fruit juices and drinks.
‡Less than 0.05 per cent.
§Chocolate liquor equivalent to coca beans.
‖Components may not add to total owing to rounding.

MILK GROUP

Milk serves as the sole food for the young during the most critical period of life for some 8000 species. Although the milk of various mammals is used for food, cow's milk is by far the most common and will be discussed here. The milk group includes fresh and processed milks, cheese, and ice cream.

Importance of milk as a food. There is no adequate substitute for milk. No food has a wider acceptability or offers a greater variety of uses. Adults of all ages should include about 2 cups of fluid milk daily, or its equivalent as evaporated milk, dry milk, or hard cheese. This allowance should be raised to 3 cups or more for schoolchildren and pregnant women, and to 4 cups or more during the adolescent years and for the nursing mother.

Milk is a complex substance in which over 100 separate components have been identified.[2] It is fluid in spite of the fact that it contains more solids than many solid foods. Fresh cow's milk contains 87 per cent water and 13 per cent solids, whereas such foods as cabbage, strawberries, and summer squash, to name but a few examples, are lower in solids content and higher in water content.

The exact composition of milk varies with the breed of cattle, the feed used, and the period of lactation. Pooled market milk has a uniform composition which may be varied slightly by local or state regulations for butterfat and solids content.

Energy. Too many people become concerned about the caloric value of milk and will sometimes eliminate milk from their diets for this reason. From Figure 13–1 it may be seen that 2 cups of whole milk furnish about 15 per cent of the calories for the moderately active young woman, but the percentage contribution for most of the nutrients is considerably greater. By adjusting the fat level of milk, caloric modifications can be made for low-calorie and high-calorie diets.

1 cup skim milk = 90 calories
1 cup whole milk = 160 calories
½ cup whole milk + ½ cup light cream
= 330 calories

Protein. One cup of whole, skim, or diluted evaporated milk contains 9 gm protein. Thus, 2 cups daily furnish almost one third of the adult protein allowance.

The essential amino acids present in milk proteins are supplied in almost ideal proportions for maximum tissue synthesis. Casein accounts for four fifths of the protein in milk, and various whey proteins, including lactalbumins and lactoglobulins, constitute the remaining protein fractions. The latter proteins are especially rich in tryptophan.

Milk supplements cereal proteins in an excellent fashion, for it supplies the amino acids lysine and tryptophan, which are limited in the cereals. The biologic value of proteins in white wheat flour is only 50 per cent when used alone, but this is raised to 75 per cent when milk is used with the wheat flour.[3]

Fat. The fat of milk is highly emulsified and is easily digested. In the homogenization of milk the fat globules are still further reduced in size

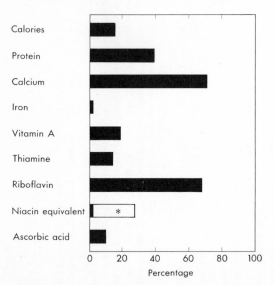

*Unshaded area represents niacin equivalent from tryptophan.

Figure 13–1. Percentage contributions of 2 cups of milk to the Recommended Dietary Allowances for the woman of 23 to 50 years.

to give a perfect emulsion. Milk fat contains a high proportion of short-chain fatty acids which are especially well tolerated. About 60 to 75 per cent of the fatty acids in milk are saturated, 24 to 40 per cent are monounsaturated, and 2 to 10 per cent are polyunsaturated. In modified-fat diets, when saturated fats must be kept to a minimum, skim milk may be substituted for whole milk.

Carbohydrate. Lactose is a carbohydrate occurring only in milk. This sugar is peculiarly adapted to making milk an ideal food for the young because it is much less sweet, less soluble, and more stable than sucrose and other sugars. It gives to milk a bland flavor. Lactose favors the growth of lactic-acid–producing bacteria which are believed to retard or prevent the growth of putrefying bacteria. Lactose probably favors the absorption of calcium and phosphorus and the synthesis of some B complex vitamins in the small intestine.

Minerals and vitamins. Milk supplies several mineral elements abundantly. Only the milk group provides a practical basis for meeting the recommended allowance for calcium. Phosphorus occurs in correct proportions with calcium to support optimum skeletal growth. Milk contains appreciable amounts of sodium, potassium, and magnesium, but it furnishes very little iron, so that the infant's diet must be supplemented at an early age to prevent anemia.

Milk is an outstanding dietary source of riboflavin and also supplies fair amounts of vitamin A, thiamine, vitamin B_6, and vitamin B_{12}. It is low in preformed niacin but is an excellent source of tryptophan, which functions as a precursor of niacin. About 85 per cent of market milk today is fortified with vitamin D to a level of 400 I.U. per quart, which is the recommended allowance for children. Milk furnishes only small amounts of ascorbic acid.

Cheese. The composition of cheese depends upon the kind of milk used—whole or skim—and the amount of water present. A pound of hard cheese contains the casein and fat of 1 gallon of milk. One ounce of Cheddar cheese is about equal to ¾ cup milk for its protein, calcium, and calories. The proteins (principally casein) in cheese contain all the essential amino acids and are therefore of high biologic value. Only a trace of the lactose present in milk remains in the cheese. Varying amounts of calcium, thiamine, and riboflavin are lost depending upon the method of preparation.

Soft cheeses vary widely in their composition. If made with skim milk, cottage cheese will contain as little as 1 per cent fat; the protein content is about 19 per cent. Creamed cottage cheese is made by mixing the curd with cream or a cream-milk mixture; the fat content of the final product is about 4 per cent. The caloric values of creamed and uncreamed cottage cheeses do not differ greatly, being 120 and 98 per ½-cup serving, respectively. Cottage cheese is considerably lower than Cheddar cheese in its calcium content since some of the calcium is lost in the whey with acid coagulation. Almost 11 oz of cottage cheese are needed to provide the calcium of 1 cup of milk.

Cream cheese, which is made from whole milk with cream added, contains approximately 9 per cent protein and 37 per cent fat. It is therefore high in calories but is not a good substitute for cottage or hard cheese in terms of protein. Its calcium content is low.

MEAT GROUP

The meat group includes the flesh of animals such as beef, veal, mutton, lamb, and pork. It also includes poultry, fish, eggs, legumes, and nuts. The daily recommendation from this group is two servings, the equivalents for one serving being:

2 or 3 oz edible portion lean cooked beef, veal, pork, lamb, poultry, or fish
2 eggs
1 cup cooked dry beans, peas, or lentils
4 tablespoons peanut butter

Place of meat in the diet. Since the days of the cave man and all through ancient and medieval history, meat has occupied a position of first importance in the diet. Today meat is the most expensive item of the daily menu and accounts for about one third of the food budget.

Even at lower income levels many families manage to have a fairly liberal allowance of meat.

Per capita consumption. On the basis of available food supplies, the per capita consumption each year of meat is about 182 pounds; of poultry, 47 pounds; and of fish, 11 pounds.[1] More than half of the meat consumed is beef, and pork accounts for almost two fifths. Thus, veal, lamb, and mutton together account for about 5 per cent of the meat consumed (see Figure 13–2).

The use of variety meats depends to no small extent on family traditions and beliefs. The tongue, liver, brain, and heart of beef, lamb, veal, or pork, the sweetbreads or thymus gland of calves, and tripe of beef are all useful and highly nutritious meats.

Fish and poultry in the diet. Fish and shellfish are gradually gaining in popularity. However, some reasons for the more limited use of fish may be the idea held by some people that fish is inferior food because it is used on fast days instead of meat; that it is a food selected by the poor; that it has not always been available far away from the seacoast, lake, or river regions; and that it is so often poorly cooked and unpalatable. As a food, fish is equal in nutritive value to meat except that the caloric value is usually lower by reason of the lower fat concentration. The small amount of connective tissue in fish makes it especially suitable for diets of the sick. Some people are allergic to shellfish in particular, and this fact must be kept in mind.

Chicken and turkey have become increasingly popular during recent years. Young chickens suitable for broiling or frying are available during the entire year, and turkeys of smaller size are being produced in greater numbers for year-round use by the average family.

Acceptability of meat and fish. Aside from its high nutritive value, meat is an important dietary item because the aromas and flavors given by meat extractives stimulate the appetite. Meat and fish have a high satiety value because the protein and fat content prolong the digestive period. The often heard comment "It doesn't seem like a meal without meat" attests to the importance of this food on a popular and psychologic basis.

Eggs. As breakfast, luncheon, or dinner main dishes, eggs may be used in numerous ways. They are essential ingredients in many desserts and in baked foods. In fact, the individual who is allergic to eggs soon discovers that a diet without eggs poses many problems in choice and in variety.

Legumes and nuts. Dried peas, beans, and soybeans are not widely used in this country. Peanuts, which are also leguminous seeds, are popular not only as a snack food but also as peanut butter. These foods can be important contributors to the protein, iron, and niacin levels of the diet as well as being inexpensive and interesting variations for menus.

Nutritive values of the meat group. Variations in the composition of meat, from one cut to another, and from one kind to another, are due largely to the proportion of lean and fat tissue. Considering the entire carcass, the proportion of fat is greater in older animals than in young animals; it is also higher in pork than in beef, and in lamb than in veal, and so on.

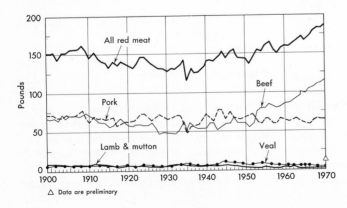

Figure 13–2. Per capita consumption of meat. (Courtesy, Consumer and Economic Research, U.S. Department of Agriculture.)

△ Data are preliminary

Moreover, one cut of meat may be extremely lean, that from another part of the animal may be well marbled with fat—that is, tiny fat streaks are intertwined with the muscle fibers and inseparable from them, and that from still another part may be high in adipose tissue and low in muscle fiber.

Such considerations as the above do not necessarily modify the nutritive value of meat as consumed since (1) fat may be trimmed off and discarded before meat is cooked, (2) fat loss in drippings may not be used, and (3) surrounding fat on meat may be left as plate waste. Obviously, it is important to know the values for cooked meat as it is actually consumed. Leverton and Odell[4] have conducted extensive analyses of cooked meat and have suggested the following values as a guide in dietary planning:

	Calories	Protein	Fat
	(per 100 gm cooked meat)		
		gm	gm
Extremely lean portion	200	32	8
Lean-plus-marble portions	255	28	16

The extremely lean portion would represent a selection of meat suitable for fat-restricted diets; it would contain no visible traces of fat. The lean-plus-marble portion represents meat as it is usually consumed.

Leverton and Odell[4] found that no one kind of cooked lean meat or of lean-plus-marble meat was significantly different from other kinds. Cooked pork was no higher in fat than similar portions of beef, veal, or lamb. For most dietary purposes, then, the four kinds of meat may be used interchangeably on a protein, fat, and caloric basis.

Protein. On a cooked basis, 1 oz lean meat, one egg, ½ cup dried beans or peas, and 2 tablespoons of peanut butter are about equal in quantity of protein furnished, that is, approximately 7 gm.

The proteins of eggs are so well proportioned in their amino acid composition that a nutrition committee of the Food and Agriculture Organization has recommended whole egg as a reference standard for comparing the quality of protein in other foods.

Regardless of the species, the amino acid composition of the proteins in flesh foods is relatively constant and of such balance and quality that meats, fish, and poultry rank only slightly below eggs and milk in their ability to effect tissue synthesis. The protein differences between so-called red and white meats are insignificant. The proteins in legumes and nuts are of somewhat lesser quality because the amounts of methionine and lysine are below optimum levels.

Fats. The fatty acids in beef, veal, and lamb are more saturated than those in pork, poultry, and fish. Depending upon the diet of the animal, pork and poultry may contain appreciable amounts of linoleic acid. Fatty acids in fish are more highly unsaturated, with a more generous proportion of polyunsaturated fatty acids.

Some legumes, such as peas and beans, are very low in fat, but soybeans and peanuts provide much more liberal amounts. An important proportion of the fatty acids is polyunsaturated.

The meat group is the principal source of cholesterol in the diet, but this lipid is not uniformly present in all flesh foods. Egg yolk, liver, brains, and shellfish are the outstanding sources.

Minerals. The mineral element of especial importance in the meat group is iron, all foods of this group being valuable. Light meats, including fish and light meat of poultry, are somewhat lower in iron content than the red muscle meats of beef. Meats are also rich in phosphorus, sulfur, and potassium, moderately high in sodium, and poor in their calcium content. Some shellfish and canned salmon with the bones contain appreciable amounts of calcium. Saltwater fish is a good source of iodine.

Vitamins. All foods of the meat group are good sources of the B complex vitamins. Pork, liver, and other organ meats and legumes are excellent for their thiamine content; poultry, veal, peas, and peanuts are rich in niacin. Vitamin B_{12} is supplied by organ meats, muscle meats, and eggs, but it is not found in the legumes.

Liver is an outstanding source of vitamin A; other organ meats and egg yolk are good sources of vitamin A. Otherwise, meats do not provide vitamin A, and they are not a source of ascorbic acid.

Extractives and purines. Various nonprotein nitrogenous substances, especially the purines, give meat its characteristic flavor. They are readily extracted from meat with water, as in the preparation of broth. They have very little nutritive value.

VEGETABLE-FRUIT GROUP

No group of foods lends greater variety to the diet in terms of color, flavor, and texture than does the vegetable-fruit group. This group is unique for its contribution to the ascorbic acid value of the diet; it is the major source of vitamin A value; it makes an excellent contribution to the iron level of the diet; and it is a fair source of other minerals and B complex vitamins.

The vegetable group includes practically every part of the plant—leaves, stems, roots, tubers, bulbs, flowers, and seeds. Mature seeds of the grasses are included in the cereal group, and those of leguminous plants such as peas and beans are included in the meat group.

In order to ensure optimum vitamin and mineral contributions the daily recommendation of four servings from the vegetable-fruit group should be governed as follows:

1 serving citrus fruit or other source of vitamin C
1 serving at least every other day of dark-green or deep-yellow vegetables for vitamin A
2 servings other vegetables and fruits, including potatoes

A serving is equivalent to ½ cup cooked vegetable or a whole piece of vegetable or fruit such as a banana, an apple, or medium-sized potato. Teen-agers should have larger servings of each, and young children may have smaller-size servings.

Nutritive characteristics. The composition of vegetables and fruits covers a wide range depending upon the part of the plant represented. Moreover, the handling of the food from farm to table may be so variable that the amounts of vitamins and minerals retained may be high or low. The vitamin concentration is affected by the

season, the degree of maturity, and the storage conditions.

Water. As the chief constituent of fruits and vegetables water constitutes 75 to 95 per cent of the weight. Foods relatively high in carbohydrate such as bananas and potatoes are lower in water content than those which are low in carbohydrate such as tomatoes, lettuce, melons.

Energy. As a group, these foods are not important contributors to the caloric value of the diet, although potatoes and sweet potatoes when eaten in quantity may make an appreciable contribution in low-cost diets. Many vegetables such as tomatoes, celery, asparagus, salad greens, and others furnish no more than 20 calories per serving. Potatoes, Lima beans, fresh corn, and bananas, for example, are slightly below 100 calories per serving unit. Other vegetables and fruits range from 40 to 80 calories per average serving.

Protein and fat. The protein concentration of most fresh vegetables ranges from 1 to 2 per cent and is even lower in fruits. Fresh peas and Lima beans are slightly above these levels. All foods of this group are extremely low in fat with the exception of avocados and olives.

Carbohydrate. The carbohydrate composition of this group ranges widely, being as low as 3 to 5 per cent for rhubarb, greens, summer squash, tomatoes, and others, to more than 30 per cent for a few foods such as sweet potatoes. Dried fruits contain about 65 per cent carbohydrate.

The exchange lists (Table A-4) provide a convenient classification for fruits and vegetables according to carbohydrate content. Fruits (list 3) are listed in the amounts required to furnish 10 gm carbohydrate. The group A vegetables in list 2 are those which, for practical purposes, are of negligible carbohydrate and calorie value; the group B vegetables are those which contain about 7 gm carbohydrate per ½-cup serving. A few vegetables (potatoes, sweet potatoes, corn, Lima beans) are included in the bread list since their carbohydrate value is more comparable to that of 1 slice of bread.

Starches, dextrins, sucrose, fructose, glucose, and cellulose occur in vegetables and fruits. The starch content of immature fruits is converted to sugars during ripening. The skins, seeds, and fibers of fruits and vegetables contribute variety to the textures of the diet and are also of value in the maintenance of normal gastrointestinal motility. Some fruits are also rich in pectin.

Minerals. Turnip greens, mustard greens, collards, kale, and broccoli are excellent sources of calcium. The calcium of spinach, poke, dock, beet greens, chard, and lamb's quarters is probably not nutritionally available because of the high oxalic acid content of those plants which results in insoluble calcium salts that are not absorbed. Some fruits contribute small amounts of calcium, but the daily contribution cannot be considered important.

The dark-green leafy vegetables are fair-to-good sources of iron. Likewise, fresh and dried apricots, raisins, prunes, dates, figs, peaches, and berries are good sources of iron.

Fruits and vegetables are rich sources of potassium, but the sodium content is negligible except for a few vegetables such as beets, carrots, spinach, celery, and chard.

Fruits and vegetables contribute to an alkaline ash. The acid or sour taste of some fruits, including citrus fruits, peaches, and others, is accounted for by several organic acids (citric, malic, tartaric) which are fully oxidized in the body. The mineral content of these fruits is such that they also yield an alkaline ash. Plums, prunes, rhubarb, and cranberries, on the other hand, contain benzoic acid, which cannot be utilized by the body; hence, they contribute to an acid reaction.

Vitamins. Among the best contributors to ascorbic acid are the citrus fruits, fresh strawberries, cantaloupe and honeydew melon, broccoli, and dark-green leafy vegetables. Potatoes and sweet potatoes contain lesser concentrations of this vitamin, but the amounts eaten daily by some people may appreciably add to the total intake.

Dark-green leafy vegetables and deep-yellow vegetables and fruits are outstanding for their carotene content. The concentration of the vitamin is directly proportional to the depth of the color. Lightly colored foods such as lettuce, cabbage, and white peaches are poor sources of the vitamin, although the outer green leaves of lettuce may contain 30 times as much vitamin A as the inner pale leaves.

Vegetables and fruits are fair sources of the B complex vitamins.

BREAD-CEREAL GROUP

Today in nearly every country of the world some cereal grain is regarded as "the staff of life." Man's discovery thousands of years ago that he could cultivate the land and grow grains meant that he no longer had to lead the nomadic life of the hunter. The word *cereal* is derived from Ceres, the ancient Roman goddess of agriculture and harvest. Numerous references in the Bible attest to the importance of cereals. For example, in Psalm 65:13 we read, "The pastures are clothed with flocks; the valleys also are covered with corn: they shout for joy; they also sing." In the Bible and other early literature *corn* referred to grains such as wheat, millet, and barley.

By reason of its availability, high yield per acre, low production cost, and excellent keeping qualities, grain is used more abundantly than any other food material. The bread-cereal group includes breads, breakfast cereals, flours and meals, rice, and pastas (macaroni, noodles, and spaghetti). Four servings or more of enriched or whole-grain cereal foods are recommended daily.

Rice is the chief dietary staple for half the world's population and constitutes as much as 80 per cent of the calories for most of Asia's peoples. Wheat ranks second to rice in worldwide use but is the principal cereal grain used in the United States and in some European countries. Corn is widely used in Central and South America. Millet, sorghum, rye, and barley are important in some parts of the world.

Nutritional value of cereal foods. The seed or kernel of the cereal grain (see Figure 13–3) is divided into three parts, the bran, germ, and endosperm. The aleurone layer just below the bran layer is sometimes identified as a fourth part. Although cereal grains vary somewhat in their composition, the average percentage composition of the whole grain is protein, 12; fat, 2;

carbohydrate, 75; water, 10; minerals, especially phosphorus and iron, and the B complex vitamins, especially thiamine, 1. The mineral

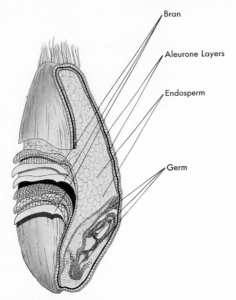

Figure 13–3. Whole wheat—cross section of grain. (Courtesy, the Ralston Purina Company, St. Louis, Mo.)

The Bran. The brown outer layers. This part contains:
1. Bulk-forming carbohydrates.
2. B vitamins.
3. Minerals, especially iron.

The Aleurone Layers. The layers located right under the bran. They are rich in:
1. Proteins.
2. Phosphorus, a mineral.

The Endosperm. The white center. This consists mainly of:
1. Carbohydrates (starches and sugars).
2. Protein.

This is the part used in highly refined white flours. Less refined flours and refined cereals are made from this part and varying amounts of the aleurone layer.

The Germ. The heart of wheat (embryo). It is this part that sprouts and makes a new plant when put into the the ground. It contains:
1. Thiamine (vitamin B1). Wheat germ is one of the best food sources of thiamine.
2. Protein. This protein is of value comparable to the proteins of meat, milk, and cheese.
3. Other B vitamins.
4. Fat and the fat-soluble vitamin E.
5. Minerals, especially iron.
6. Carbohydrates.

and vitamin compositions of market forms of cereal foods vary widely depending upon whether they are whole-grain, enriched, or unenriched. (See Chapter 17 for discussion of market forms.)

Energy. Cereal foods, it is well known, are the primary source of energy for most of the world's people. Many people infer from this fact that cereals per se are fattening, and so they omit this group of foods from their diets. By such omission they lose the many nutrient benefits provided by whole-grain and enriched products. Cereal grains contribute importantly to every nutrient need except calcium, ascorbic acid, and vitamin A. The average serving of a cereal food —1 slice bread, or ½ cup cooked cereal, or 1 cup ready-to-eat cereal—furnishes from 75 to 100 calories.

Protein. The quality of the protein of cereal grains is somewhat inferior to that of animal sources because some of the essential amino acids are present in less than needed amounts. Lysine is a limiting amino acid in wheat, rice, and corn, whereas tryptophan and threonine are also present in too small amounts in corn and rice, respectively. The aleurone layer of the grain contains protein which is superior to that found in the endosperm, whereas that found in the germ compares favorably in biologic value with animal protein. Unfortunately, these better-quality proteins are removed when cereals are refined. However, when even small amounts of milk, cheese, eggs, or meat are fed simultaneously with cereal foods, either whole-grain or refined, an economical protein intake of excellent biologic value results. Recent knowledge of the amino acid composition of foods is making it practicable to develop mixtures of cereals and other plant foods so that the protein approaches the quality of animal proteins.[5] Lysine is now being added to some cereals and breads, although the need for such supplementation of the American diet has not been demonstrated.

Minerals and vitamins. The greater part of the minerals, iron and phosphorus, and of the B complex vitamins occurs in the bran and germ of the grain. Consequently, most of these nutrients are lost when cereals are highly milled. Not only the American public, but people throughout the world, when given a choice, select white bread in preference to whole-grain breads. Whole-grain flours become rancid easily and are more subject to insect infestation if kept for any length of time so that a rapid turnover of this flour is essential. In view of these facts, it is of vast public health significance that refined cereals and breads be enriched with thiamine, riboflavin, niacin, and iron (see page 236).

Cereal grains are poor sources of calcium. Breakfast cereals are ordinarily consumed with milk, and commercial breads commonly include certain calcium salts, which are yeast foods or dough conditioners, and calcium propionate, which is a mold inhibitor. Many commercial breads also contain 4 per cent nonfat dry milk resulting in further improvement of the calcium level as well as of the quality of the protein.

Nutritive efficiency of bread. In one form or another bread has been used for thousands of years and is referred to both as unleavened and leavened loaves and cakes in the Old Testament. The grains from which bread is made are grown in almost every quarter of the globe and are therefore available as a foodstuff for practically all peoples. The nutritive contribution of bread is illustrated in Figure 13–4.

That bread is an important dietary constituent was convincingly demonstrated in a study reported by Widdowson and McCance.[6] These eminent British investigators observed the progress of 169 undernourished children, 4 to 15 years of age, for a year in a German orphanage at a time when food supplies were limited. The calories in the diets consumed by the children were distributed in these percentages: bread, 75; potatoes, 6; soups, vegetables, fruits, butter, margarine, 15; and milk, cheese, meat, fish, 4. Whole-wheat, enriched, and unenriched white breads were tested. The diets were not low in protein, but only 8 to 9 gm were derived from animal sources. Supplements of vitamins A, D, and C were included.

At the end of one year the children had made more rapid gains in height and weight than would be expected of normal children at the same age level; bone development was somewhat more rapid than normal; skin conditions had improved; and muscle tone had increased. The

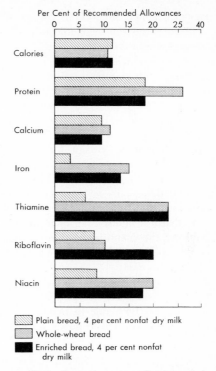

Per Cent of Recommended Allowances

Plain bread, 4 per cent nonfat dry milk

Whole-wheat bread

Enriched bread, 4 per cent nonfat dry milk

Figure 13–4. Percentage contribution of 4 slices (1/5 pound) of bread to Recommended Dietary Allowances for the woman of 23 to 50 years.

children were stated to be in excellent physical condition. No differences were observed in growth, development, or health with any of the breads tested, but the B-vitamin reserves were somewhat better in those children who had eaten bread enriched to the whole-wheat levels. These results clearly demonstrated the nutritive efficiency of unusually large amounts of bread.

OTHER FOOD GROUPS

Fats and oils. Butter, margarine, hydrogenated fats, lard and vegetable oils constitute the visible fats used in the diet. All the fats are concentrated sources of energy, but margarine and butter are the only fats that contain vitamin A. Margarine is fortified with 15,000 I.U. vitamin A per pound, thus equalling the year-round average for butter.

Butter, regular margarine, and hydrogenated

fats contain higher proportions of saturated fatty acids than do the vegetable oils. Cottonseed, corn, soybean, sesame, and safflower oils are rich in linoleic acid, but olive and coconut oils are poor in this polyunsaturated acid.

Sugars and sweets. Cane and beet sugars comprise the primary source of sweets in America; corn sugar (glucose), corn syrup, molasses, honey, and maple syrup are other sweetenings of varying importance. Except for honey and maple syrup they are an inexpensive source of energy, but since they are almost 100 per cent carbohydrate they make no appreciable contribution to any other nutrient. Molasses is an exception in that it contains a fair concentration of iron; however, the quantities used in the average diet are too small to make this a contribution of significance.

Sugars and sweets are valued for the way in which they enhance the acceptability of some cooked fruits and their role in making possible the many desserts and baked goods we enjoy so much.

A Basic Dietary Pattern

A dietary pattern based on the Four Food Groups of the Daily Food Guide (page 34) has been referred to time and again in the chapters pertaining to the nutrients. The nutritive values for foods in each of these groups are summarized in Table 13–2. The values assigned to each food group give consideration to the per capita consumption of foods in the United States. For example, the consumption of beef and pork is much higher than is that of lamb, veal, poultry, or fish; thus the values cited for meat, poultry, and fish are based on a greater weighting for beef and pork.

The basic dietary pattern provides the Recommended Dietary Allowances for the woman of 23–50 years for all nutrients except iron (see Figure 13–5). Sufficient calories to maintain optimum body weight are obtained by eating larger amounts of any of the foods in the basic diet, or by adding fats, sweets, desserts, and other foods. Usually the foods added for a satisfactory caloric level will also contain some protein, minerals, and vitamins, but it is necessary to emphasize that an excessive use of fats and sweets may jeopardize the satisfactory intake of essential nutrients.

Alternate basic pattern. Many basic plans could be constructed for individual needs. The plan in Table 13–2 permits considerable flexibility in day-to-day choice of foods and is applicable in any part of the United States. Never-

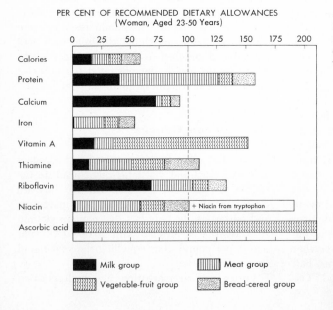

PER CENT OF RECOMMENDED DIETARY ALLOWANCES
(Woman, Aged 23-50 Years)

Calories
Protein
Calcium
Iron
Vitamin A
Thiamine
Riboflavin
Niacin   + Niacin from tryptophan
Ascorbic acid

■ Milk group   ▥ Meat group
▨ Vegetable-fruit group   ▦ Bread-cereal group

Figure 13–5. The Four Food Groups of the Basic Diet meet, or nearly meet, the recommended allowances in all respects except calories and iron for the woman of 23 to 50 years.

Table 13–2. Nutritive Value of a Basic Diet Pattern for the Adult in Health*

Food	Measure	Weight	Energy	Protein	Fat	Carbo-hydrate	Minerals		A	Vitamins			
							Ca	Fe		Thia-mine	Ribo-flavin	Niacin	Ascorbic Acid
		gm	calories	gm	gm	gm	mg	mg	I.U.	mg	mg	mg	mg
Milk	2 cups	488	320	18	18	24	576	0.2	700	0.14	0.82	0.4	4
Meat Group													
Egg	1	50	80	6	6	tr	27	1.1	590	0.05	0.15	tr	0
Meat, fish, poultry (lean cooked)†	4 ounces	120	240	33	10	0	17	3.6	35	0.32	0.26	7.4	0
Vegetable-Fruit Group													
Leafy green or deep yellow	1/4–1/3 cup‡	50	15	1	tr	3	14	0.5	3700	0.03	0.04	0.3	14
Other vegetable	1/4–1/3 cup§	50	15	1	tr	3	10	0.4	240	0.03	0.03	0.3	7
Potato	1 medium	122	80	2	tr	18	7	0.6	tr	0.11	0.04	1.4	20
Citrus fruit‖	1 serving	100	40	1	tr	10	10	0.2	160	0.07	0.02	0.3	40
Other fruit#	1 serving	100	60	1	tr	16	12	0.5	600	0.04	0.04	0.4	9
Bread-Cereal Group													
Cereal, enriched or whole grain**	3/4 cup	30 (dry)	105	3	tr	22	10	0.8	0	0.12	0.04	0.8	0
Bread, enriched or whole grain	3 slices	75	210	6	3	39	63	1.8	tr	0.18	0.15	1.8	tr
			1165	72	37	135	746	9.7	6025	1.09	1.59	13.1††	94
Recommended Dietary Allowances													
Woman (23–50 years)			2000	46			800	18	4000	1.0	1.2	13	45
Man (23–50 years)			2700	56			800	10	5000	1.4	1.6	18	45

*Values for foods in the meat, vegetable-fruit, and bread-cereal groups are weighted on the basis of the approximate consumption in the United States.

†Calculations based upon an average weekly intake for meat of 11 ounces beef, 7 1/2 ounces pork, 6 1/2 ounces poultry, 1 1/2 ounces lamb and veal, and 1 1/2 ounces fish.

‡Dark-green leafy and deep-yellow vegetables include carrots, green peppers, broccoli, spinach, endive, escarole, and kale. It is assumed that an average serving of 1/2 cup is eaten at least every other day.

§Other vegetables include tomatoes, lettuce, cabbage, snap beans, Lima beans, celery, peas, onions, corn, cucumbers, beets, and cauliflower. It is assumed that an average serving of 1/2 cup is eaten at least every other day.

‖Citrus fruit includes fresh, canned, and frozen oranges, orange juice, grapefruit, and grapefruit juice.

#Other fruit includes apples, peaches, pears, apricots, grapes, plums, prunes, berries, and bananas.

**Cereals include corn flakes, wheat flakes, macaroni, oatmeal, shredded wheat, and enriched rice.

††The protein in this diet contains about 720 mg trytophan, equivalent to 12 mg niacin; thus, the niacin equivalent of this diet is 25 mg.

205

Table 13–3. Alternate Low-Cost Basic Diet Pattern for the Adult in Health (Southern)*

Food	Measure	Weight	Energy	Protein	Fat	Carbo-hydrate	Minerals		A	Vitamins			
							Ca	Fe		Thia-mine	Ribo-flavin	Niacin	Ascorbic Acid
		gm	calories	gm	gm	gm	mg	mg	I.U.	mg	mg	mg	mg
Nonfat dry milk†	3/8 cup	30	110	11	tr	16	390	0.2	10	0.11	0.54	0.3	2
Meat Group													
Egg	1	50	80	6	6	tr	27	1.1	590	0.05	0.15	tr	0
Pork, lean and fat	2 ounces	60	215	13	17	0	6	1.7	0	0.30	0.14	2.7	—
Cowpeas, cooked, immature	1 cup	160	175	13	1	29	38	3.4	560	0.49	0.18	2.3	28
Vegetable-Fruit Group													
Greens‡	1/2 cup	75	20	2	tr	3	110	.8	4460	0.10	0.14	0.7	40
Sweet potato	1 medium	147	170	2	1	39	47	1.0	11,610	0.13	0.09	0.9	25
Fruit, noncitrus	1 serving	100	60	1	tr	16	12	0.5	600	0.04	0.04	0.4	9
Bread-Cereal Group													
Corn grits, degermed, enriched, cooked	1/2 cup	121	60	2	tr	14	1	0.3	75	0.05	0.04	0.5	0
Corn meal, degermed, enriched, dry	1/2 cup	72	260	6	1	57	5	2.1	320	0.32	0.19	2.6	0
Flour, enriched, self-rising	1/2 cup	55	190	5	1	41	146	1.6	0	0.25	0.15	2.0	0
			1340	61	27	215	782	12.7	18,225	1.84	1.66	12.4§	104
Recommended Dietary Allowances													
Woman (23–50 years)			2000	46			800	18	4000	1.0	1.2	13	45
Man (23–50 years)			2700	56			800	10	5000	1.4	1.6	18	45

*Nutritive values have been calculated using Table A–1 in the Appendix. Calories have been rounded off to the nearest 5; protein, fat, and carbohydrate to the nearest gram; and vitamin A to the nearest 10 units.
†Nonfat dry milk may be used in cooking or as a beverage. The liquid milk equivalent is 1 1/3 cups.
‡The average of collards, kale, mustard greens, and turnip greens has been used.
§The protein in this diet contributes about 610 mg tryptophan, equivalent to 10 mg niacin; thus the niacin equivalent of this diet is about 22 mg.

theless, it might be desirable to use a plan which includes greater or lesser amounts of meat, cereals and bread, milk, fruits, vegetables, and so on, and still achieve nutritive adequacy. An alternate low-cost basic diet is presented in Table 13–3. This includes a selection of foods typical of the low-income groups in the southeastern states.

There are several points of interest in the low-cost plan. It will be noted that there is less milk and meat and no citrus fruit. Larger amounts of plant foods, including corn grits, cornmeal, self-rising flour, cowpeas, and sweet potato, are included.

Nonfat dry milk has been used in this plan because of low cost and excellent keeping qualities in the dry state without refrigeration. This addition to the present dietary practices of low-income groups would greatly improve nutrition. Whenever whole milk or buttermilk is available, it may be substituted for the nonfat dry milk.

Egg is the only animal source of vitamin A. Although the carotene is less well utilized than true vitamin A, the levels in this diet provide a wide margin of safety for the person in health.

The allowances for the B complex vitamins are satisfactory because of the use of enriched cereal foods. If unenriched products are used, the diet would not fully meet the recommended allowances.

PROBLEMS AND REVIEW

1. *Problem.* Calculate the nutritive values for three foods that you eat regularly. Which of these foods provides the greatest nutritive value per 100 calories?
2. Why is milk not a perfect food?
3. *Problem.* Compare the nutritive value of 1 cup whole milk, 1 ounce Swiss cheese, 2 ounces cottage cheese, ⅛ quart ice cream, 1 ounce cream cheese. Use Table A-1.
4. *Problem.* Compare the nutritive values of 2 ounces lean roast beef, 2 ounces lean roast pork, 2 eggs, 4 tablespoons peanut butter, and ½ cup baked beans. Use Table A-1.
5. How does the protein quality of peanut butter and baked beans compare with that of meat?
6. *Problem.* List five fruits and five vegetables that are excellent sources of ascorbic acid. See Table A-1.
7. *Problem.* What nutrients are abundantly supplied by oatmeal, strawberries, prunes, broccoli, tomatoes, cowpeas, buttermilk, ham, eggs? See Table A-1.
8. Why is enrichment of breads and cereals of great importance? How can you be sure that the bread you buy is enriched?
9. Cereal proteins are of lower biologic value than milk proteins. Explain.

CITED REFERENCES

1. Friend, B.: "Nutritional Review," *National Food Situation.* Economic Research Service, U.S. Department of Agriculture, Washington, D.C., November 1970, p. 22.
2. Macy, I.G., *et al.: The Composition of Milks.* Pub. 254. National Academy of Sciences–National Research Council, Washington, D.C., 1953.
3. Brody, S., and Sadhu, D. P.: "The Nutritional Significance of Milk with Special Reference to Milk Sugar," *Sci. Month.,* **64**:5–13, 1947.
4. Leverton, R. M., and Odell, G. V.: *The Nutritive Value of Cooked Meat.* Misc. Pub. MP-49. Oklahoma Agricultural Experiment Station, Oklahoma State University, 1958.
5. Behar, M., *et al.:* "Principles of Treatment and Prevention of Severe Protein Malnutrition in Children (Kwashiorkor)," *Ann. N.Y. Acad. Sci.,* **69**:954–68, 1958.
6. Widdowson, E. M., and McCance, R. A.: "Studies on the Nutritive Value of Bread and on the Effect of Variations in the Extraction Rate of Flour on the Growth of Undernourished

Children." Her Majesty's Stationery Office, Privy Council, Medical Research Council Special
Report Series No. 287, London, 1954.

ADDITIONAL REFERENCES

Hughes, O.: *Introductory Foods,* 5th ed. The Macmillan Company, New York, 1970.
Newer Knowledge of Cheese, 2nd ed. National Dairy Council, Chicago, 1967.
Newer Knowledge of Milk, 3rd ed. National Dairy Council, Chicago, 1965.
Phipard, E. F., and Page, L.: "A Guide to Good Eating," *Food—The Yearbook of Agriculture
1959.* U.S. Department of Agriculture, Washington, D.C., pp. 266–70.
Rusoff, L. L.: "The Role of Milk in Modern Nutrition," *Bordens Rev. Nutr. Res.,* **25**:17–49,
April, 1964.
Siedler, A. J.: "Nutritional Contributions of the Meat Group to an Adequate Diet," *Bordens
Rev. Nutr. Res.,* 24:29–41, July 1963.
Stiebeling, H. K.: "Foods of the Vegetable-Fruit Group—Their Contribution to Nutritionally
Adequate Diets," *Bordens Rev. Nutr. Res.,* **25**:51–65, Oct. 1964.

PUBLICATIONS ESPECIALLY FOR THE HOMEMAKER

Consumer and Food Economics Research Division: *Nutrition—Food at Work for You.* U.S.
Department of Agriculture, Washington, D.C., 1968.
Eat to Live. Wheat Flour Institute, Chicago, 1968.
Facts about Nutrition. Pub. 917. U.S. Public Health Service, Department of Health, Education,
and Welfare, Washington, D.C., 1968.
McMillan, T. J.: "Your Basic Food Needs: Nutrients for Life, Growth." *Yearbook of
Agriculture 1969,* Washington, D.C., 1969, pp. 254–59.

14 Factors Influencing Food Habits and Their Modification

Just as "you can lead a horse to water, but you can't make him drink," so the presentation of well-prepared, highly nutritious food to people does not mean that they will eat it. Food is a common denominator to all people throughout the world. Not only is it essential for their physiologic needs but it also fulfills social, psychologic, and emotional needs. Although food meets common needs for all people, food habits are infinitely complex, being derived from man's earliest experiences and being influenced by his family, as well as by the social, economic, geographic, ethnic, and religious environment. Thus, if one studies food habits one also learns much about the culture of a people. One cannot study the culture of any group of people without some understanding of the food habits.

To understand fully the factors that determine food acceptance requires the multidisciplinary approach of the anthropologist, psychologist and psychiatrist, educator, social worker, and nutritionist. It is beyond the scope of a single chapter, such as this, to provide the depth of understanding of all factors influencing food acceptance. The objectives of the discussion that follows are (1) to create for the reader an awareness of the complexity of factors that determine food acceptance; (2) to provide some basis for understanding that the same food may have quite different meanings to different individuals; and (3)

to develop attitudes of respect and tolerance for individuals who may have food habits differing widely from those of others.

PHYSIOLOGIC BASES FOR FOOD ACCEPTANCE

Hunger. Probably several mechanisms serve to explain hunger. Physiologic studies have established that contractions of the empty stomach are governed by the hypothalamus, and that hunger sensations are associated with a drop in the blood sugar level. Food intake is regulated by two areas in the hypothalamus often referred to as the "feeding" and the "satiety" centers. In experimental animals the bilateral destruction of the ventromedial nucleus leads to obesity. On the other hand, if an area lateral to the ventromedial nucleus is destroyed, eating stops and the animal will starve. Mayer and his associates have shown that chemoreceptors in the ventromedial center of the hypothalamus have an affinity for glucose and are activated by it.[1] According to their *glucostatic theory*, when glucose utilization is high, these receptors respond by acting as a brake upon the lateral nucleus (the feeding center) and also exercising some control over the hunger contractions of the stomach. When glucose utilization is low, these receptors are not stimulated and the sensation of hunger causes the individual to eat.

Starving people will usually, but not always, accept anything edible that will fill the stomach. This might even be that which would normally be quite repellent. It is also true that people may refuse food for the relief of acute hunger when religious or cultural taboos are strongly entrenched.

Man does not choose by instinct that which is best for him. In different environments, he eats what is available and sometimes learns through experience that some foods may be better for him than others. This method of trial and error, at best, is time consuming and may, in the meantime, jeopardize one's state of health. It could also lead to gross misconceptions concerning foods. Quite obviously the scientific planning of diets, rather than guidance by hunger and instinct, is the only sound basis for being sure that physiologic needs are being met.

Sensations produced by food. The palatability of food is a composite of taste, smell, texture, and temperature. It is further conditioned by the surroundings in which food is consumed.

Sweet, sour, salty, and bitter are terms used to describe the sensations that result when foods placed in the mouth produce specific stimuli to the taste buds on the tongue. (See Figure 14–1.) The sense of taste is more highly developed in some individuals than in others; foods may be too salty for one individual and just right for another; or they may be too sweet for one, but not quite sweet enough for another. Some persons can detect slight differences in taste, others cannot. The number of taste buds varies not only from individual to individual, but also from age to age. Korslund and Eppright found that preschool children who had low taste sensitivities tended to accept more foods than did those with high taste sensitivities.[2] As the taste buds diminish in number later in life, foods that are more highly flavored tend to be preferred, whereas children voluntarily select bland or sweet foods. Taste sensitivity is decreased in those who smoke tobacco.

The taste and smell of foods are directly

linked. If one were to hold the nose while eating a piece of fruit, much of the enjoyment would be lost. As a matter of fact, odor is the most important component of flavor, and an individual would derive limited pleasure from food if the tongue were the sole source of the sensations. The stimulation of the olfactory organs is brought about by certain volatile oils. Foods may be accepted because of their aromas, or they may be rejected because of their repulsive odors. No doubt, the odors of certain cheeses, for example, are the determinants in their acceptance by some and their rejection by others.

The sense of touch is highly developed in the tongue. Temperature, pain, and variations in texture or "feel" are experienced. Steaming hot foods are necessary to enjoyment by some, but children usually prefer foods that are lukewarm. A choice of ice cream may be influenced as much by its texture—smooth, creamy, and velvety, or crystalline and grainy—as by its other flavor qualities. Children may reject foods that are slippery such as baked custard or a gelatin dessert only later to learn to enjoy this texture sensation. The stringiness of certain vegetables, the stickiness of some mashed potatoes, the greasiness of fried foods may be important factors in rejection.

Social and Emotional Factors Influence Food Acceptance

Role of culture. Montagu,[3] Lee,[4] and many other writers have pointed out that the circumstances under which one eats are largely determined by one's culture. Used in this sense, culture is "the sum total of ways of living built up by a group of human beings and transmitted from one generation to another."[*] Food habits may have existed among a given ethnic group for centuries, and such a heritage may account for great conservatism in accepting change. These patterns reflect the social organization of the people, including their economy, religion, beliefs about the health properties of food, and

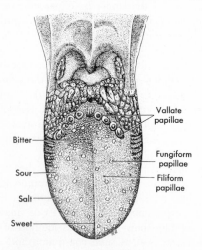

Figure 14–1. The upper surface of the tongue, showing kinds of papillae and areas of taste. (Courtesy, Miller, M. A., and Leavell, L. C.: *Kimber-Gray-Stackpole's Anatomy and Physiology*, 16th ed. The Macmillan Company, New York, 1972.)

Vallate papillae

Bitter

Fungiform papillae

Sour

Filiform papillae

Salt

Sweet

---

[*]*The Random House Dictionary of the English Language.*

attitudes toward the various members of the family. The emotional reactions to the consumption of certain foods may be so deeply rooted that effecting acceptance of them is almost impossible.

The family. No influence upon food habits is greater than that existing within the home. The mother especially sets the pattern for the food habits that will be developed by the children, for she is the one who plans the meals, purchases the food, prepares it, and serves it. Her values have been developed in the environment in which she grew up and they are based upon income, geographic region from which she came, level of education, superstitions, and taboos.

The mother who creates within the home an atmosphere of security and contentment reinforces the positive values of food.[5] On the other hand, in an environment of hostility, anger, and tension unpleasant images are created for food, often leading to their rejection. In this atmosphere, also, there may be excessive concern about "pure" foods, "pure" morals, and so on.[5]

Meal patterns. People in the United States are likely to think in terms of a three-meal pattern. Yet, there are many people both in the United States and in other countries who eat but two meals a day, whereas others have four or five meals daily. Certainly, in America the coffee break is prevalent in business and industry. Mid-afternoon and evening snacks are also commonplace in the home.

Rural Americans usually enjoy a hearty breakfast, but many Americans prefer a light breakfast; in European countries breakfast often consists of only a roll and beverage. The rural American usually prefers dinner at noon, but urban dwellers are more likely to eat dinner at night.

A good deal of ritual is part of the mealtime in some homes. Bread becomes the "staff of life" to some people; rice is the basic food for others, and corn to still others. (See Figure 14–2.) The meal would not be complete if these foods were not included. The art of food preparation is exercised, and food is highly valued for its many properties. Meals are to be enjoyed and relaxation is encouraged. A siesta following meals is customary in some countries. In other homes, mealtime is hurried. It may become the time when members of the family air their problems and when tensions are created.

Communications. The influence of the mass media on food habits can scarcely be overestimated. Those who enjoy an abundant variety of food can no longer be ignorant of the malnutrition and hunger that exist even in the United States as well as in the underdeveloped nations of the world. By these media the poor are also exposed to food products which they are unable to purchase. The affluent and the poor alike know that the distribution of food is decidedly

Figure 14–2. Indian homemaker preparing chappatties. In those parts of India where wheat is the staple grain, this unleavened bread forms an important part of the meal. The dough is baked in thin cakes. (Courtesy, The Rockefeller Foundation.)

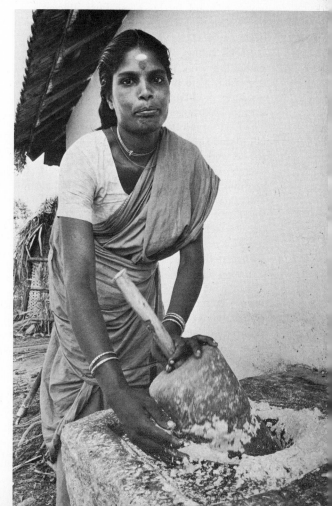

uneven, and that the capability exists to feed all people better.[6]

Manufacturers usually create desires for their products by appealing to the emotions. Foods are pictured in forms highly appealing to the eye and in situations that suggest fun, social status, and group acceptance. Foods will consequently be purchased to fulfill these emotional needs rather than their nutritional content.

Political-economic significance. The surplus foods available through agricultural policies have not always coincided with the nutritional needs or the tastes of the poor. Consequently, foods have often been wasted. During a war food supplies may be rationed and people are forced to substitute one food for another. The scarcity of a food sometimes creates a tremendous desire to possess that food. Throughout history people have gone on "hunger strikes" to achieve some political gain. Gandhi, the great Indian leader, comes to mind for his many fasts. Recently, in the United States, some people have fasted as a protest against the Vietnam war.

Social values of food. "To break bread" together has been from time immemorial an act of friendship. One provides food for friends during a visit in the home; one likewise extends friendship to the stranger by inviting him to share food. The food served to guests is the best that one can afford and the table appointments are as beautiful as one can make them. Important family events are joyously celebrated with meals: the wedding breakfast or reception; birthday parties; Christmas dinner; a Fourth of July picnic. To eat together, whatever the occasion, is to provide friendly relaxation and conversation. The loneliness of eating by oneself, day after day, is not appreciated by those who have never tried it.

Eating together also has connotations of status. Throughout history one's place at the table has been governed by his social standing. To be placed "above the salt" at a medieval banquet, to sit at the "head" table at a banquet today, and to be invited to eat at the captain's table while on board ship are marks of social distinction. In some societies women are considered to be inferior to men and must wait to eat until the men and boys have finished the meal. In other authoritarian situations, children may not be permitted to eat until the father has had his meal; in such a society, the father is always served the choicest foods. Many bonds of business or of politics are cemented at businessmen's luncheons or political dinners.

Prestige, it would appear, may be ensured when one serves foods that are costly, difficult to obtain, distinctive in flavor, or time consuming in preparation. Caviar, lobster, filet mignon, champagne, flaming crepes suzette are examples of such prestige foods. In the nineteenth century, the purchase of white sugar and white flour conveyed the idea that one could afford to buy that which was refined and therefore "better." Is the purchase today of the more costly breads prepared from hand-ground flours an expression of status with respect to one's supposed knowledge of nutrition, or to one's ability to buy or bake that bread which is distinctive from the more commonly available loaf?

Children too are highly influenced by the foods that are popular with their peer groups. Sometimes they come to scorn certain foods that they have liked because they are different from the prevailing pattern of other children. On the other hand, they are also susceptible to the suggestions of their teachers and classmates and learn to like foods with which they have not been familiar in their homes. (See Figure 14–3.)

Some foods are looked down upon by many people as lacking status; thus a delicious stew, or ground meat, or fish—no matter how good they may be—are considered by some to be food for the poor. However, these attitudes also are subject to change. Tourists to seacoast cities now seek out restaurants that specialize in seafoods and may be willing to spend considerable amounts of money for a specialty.

Some people delight in being epicures or gourmets. They derive a certain satisfaction from adventurous eating of food which is unusual, or which might be, in fact, unacceptable to most people—rattlesnake meat, for example. Others make a specialty of dining at unusual or expensive restaurants, or in becoming known for their abilities to prepare complex, unusual dishes.

Religious and moral values attributed to foods. Almost all religions place some regulations on the use of foods. The association of a

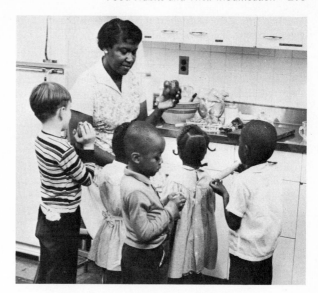

Figure 14–3. Preschool children learn about new foods by looking at them, touching them, and seeing them used in food preparation. (Courtesy, Project Head Start, Office of Child Development, U.S. Department of Health, Education, and Welfare.)

food with religion may give some clue to its importance in daily living. In the Middle East, bread becomes a symbol in the religious ceremonies of the people; to the Indians of Mexico, corn, the staple food, is invested with religious significance. Christians use bread and wine as symbols of Christ's body and blood in the Eucharist (Lord's Supper or Holy Communion). Religious significance is attached to a number of foods by the Jewish people. (See page 218.)

Certain foods are forbidden by religious regulation. Pork is forbidden to the Orthodox Jews and to the Islamites. Strict Hindus and Buddhists are vegetarians; they will eat no flesh of any animal, and many of them also abstain from eggs and milk. Seventh Day Adventists are lactovegetarians; that is, they will eat milk, cheese, eggs, nuts, and legumes but they eat no flesh foods.

Fasting is common to most, if not all, religions. On fast days one food may be substituted for another or foods may be abstained from altogether. A substitute food, such as fish for meat, is likely to be associated with denying oneself, and so when one wishes enjoyment, he doesn't choose to eat fish!

Moral attributes—"good" and "bad"—are often ascribed to foods. A child may be told to eat liver even if he doesn't like it because it is

"good" for him; he may also be told not to eat candy, which he does like, because it is "bad" for him. Or he might be told that he may have candy if he eats some liver!

Food is often used as a reward, punishment, or means of bribery. Thus, if a child has behaved well he is often rewarded with a prized food— candy, ice cream, cake; but if he has behaved badly he may be punished by being deprived of a food such as dessert. Adults, too, may reward themselves after a strenuous day or a trying experience by eating a special food or an expensive meal, often saying as they do so, "I certainly earned this today!" The family may feel a sense of reward, as well as the expression of a mother's love, when they sit down to a meal of their favorite foods; they may feel punished and unloved when the meal includes foods they dislike.

Age and sex influence food choices. Too often foods are categorized as being suitable for a given age group, or as more suitable for one sex than the other. Peanut butter, jelly, and milk are looked upon as foods for children, but olives and coffee are appropriate for adults! Teen-agers adopt current fashions in foods—hot dogs, hamburger, pizza, ice cream with many sauces and toppings. Women are said to prefer light foods such as soufflés, salads, fruits, and vegetables, whereas filling meals such as meat, potatoes, and pie represent the more usual choice of men.

Emotional outlets provided by food. Eating provides gratification for life stresses—the difficult examination in school; the homely adolescent who has no date to take her to the movies; the quarrel with a friend; the frustration and loneliness of having no friends; the profound grief at the death of a dear one; and countless others.

Food is a symbol of security to many. Milk, the first food of the infant, may be associated with the security of the infant held lovingly in his mother's arms. A person may be away from home, or may be ill, and look upon milk as expressing the comfort and security of the home; or, milk might be refused because the individual drinking it experiences a feeling of dependence which he does not want to admit, and so he says he doesn't "want to be treated like a baby."

Food may be used as a weapon. An insecure child may refuse to eat food so that his mother will be concerned about him. The ill and the lonely may impose dietary demands upon those caring for them in an effort to gain as much attention as possible.

Illness modifies food acceptance. Disease processes and drug therapy often modify the appetite. The anxiety of illness, the loneliness experienced if one eats from a tray alone, the lack of activity, and perhaps a modified diet are likely to interfere with food intake. (See also Chapter 27.)

REVIEW

1. How do you feel about food? List insofar as you are able the meanings which you clearly associate with foods. List the foods you especially like; those you especially dislike. Can you give any specific reason for placing the food in one category or another?
2. Note for one day the comments made by people around you about food. Do any of these fall within the physiologic or psychologic categories discussed in this chapter? Do they give you any clue concerning readiness to change food habits?
3. Suppose you were trying to introduce nonfat dry milk to a group of people who were entirely unfamiliar with it. How would you go about gaining their acceptance?
4. What is the difference between hunger and appetite?
5. Describe the physical factors in food acceptance.

CITED REFERENCES

1. Mayer, J.: "Why People Get Hungry," *Nutr. Today,* 1:2–8, June 1966.
2. Korslund, M., and Eppright, E. S.: "Taste Sensitivity and Eating Behavior of Preschool Children," *J. Home Econ.,* 59:168–70, 1967.
3. Montagu, M. F. A.: "Nature, Nurture, and Nutrition," *Am. J. Clin. Nutr.,* 5:237–44, 1957.
4. Lee, D.: "Cultural Factors in Dietary Choice," *Am. J. Clin. Nutr.,* 5:166–70, 1957.
5. Bruch, H.: "The Allure of Food Cults and Nutritional Quackery," *J. Am. Diet. Assoc.,* 57:316–20, 1970.
6. Mead, M.: "The Changing Significance of Food," *Am. Sci.,* 58:176–81, 1970.

ADDITIONAL REFERENCES

Babcock, C. G.: "Attitudes and the Use of Food," *J. Am. Diet. Assoc.,* 38:546–51, 1961.
Blackburn, M. L.: "Who Turns the Child 'Off' to Nutrition?" *J. Nutr. Educ.,* 2:45–47, Fall 1970.
Dickens, D.: "Factors Related to Food Preferences," *J. Home Econ.,* 57:427–30, 1965.

Fathauer, G. H.: "Food Habits—An Anthropologist's View," *J. Am. Diet. Assoc.*, **37**:335–38, 1960.

John, H. J.: "Hunger," *Am. J. Dig. Dis.*, **22**:197–200, 1965.

Labecki, G., and Merrow, S.: "How Wisely Do Students Select Their Diets?" *Nurs. Outlook*, **7**:471–73, 1959.

Lamb, M.: "Food Acceptance, a Challenge to Nutrition Education—A Review," *J. Nutr. Educ.*, **1**:20–22, Fall 1969.

Lowenberg, M. E., *et al.: Food and Man*. John Wiley & Sons, Inc., New York, 1968.

Pumpian-Mindlin, E.: "The Meanings of Food," *J. Am. Diet. Assoc.*, **30**:576–80, 1954.

Pyke, M.: "Food Technology and Society," *Nutr. Rev.*, **28**:31–34, 1970.

Simoons, F. J.: "The Geographic Approach to Food Prejudices," *Food Technol.*, **20**:274–76, March, 1966.

15 Cultural Food Patterns in the United States

Dietary planning for various ethnic groups. Nurses, dietitians, and teachers come in contact with people from many ethnic origins. Today, in America, most of the population are those whose forebears have been here for many generations. They have come not only to accept but also to enjoy the abundance and endless variety of foods available. The pressures of advertising, the nutrition education in the classroom and through the school lunch program, and the frequency with which people today eat in restaurants have done much to unify the food patterns. (See Figure 15–1.) Many people, however, continue to relish favorite dishes associated with holidays and religious customs even though their food habits as a whole can no longer be described in the light of those prevailing in the country of their origin. It is quite important to make allowance for the inclusion of such dishes in menu plans in order to gain the fullest acceptance of the meals.

The physical development of any people depends upon the available supply of energy foods, protein, minerals, and vitamins. Food the world over supplies these nutrients, although the agriculture and technologic development of a country may be such that the supply is inadequate to meet fully the needs of the population. It is important for the health worker to recognize that widely varying patterns may provide the essentials of good nutrition and that she should learn to build upon the desirable characteristics of any given diet. She needs to remember that people who have had little education, who are economically underprivileged, or who are ill are less readily motivated to effect change in their existing food habits.

In describing the food patterns of a given ethnic group it is sometimes assumed that all people adhere to that pattern. This is by no means true. The American Indian of North Dakota is likely to follow a somewhat different pattern than the Indian of the Southwest because of differences in food availability. Black people who have migrated from the South to the northern cities continue to enjoy at least some of the foods to which they have been accustomed, such as blackeyed peas, greens with pot liquor, chitterlings, biscuits, and many others. On the other hand, black people who have lived in the North for several generations may prefer other northern dishes. Within a given ethnic group one will also find individuals who differ widely in their food habits.

Food habits change rapidly. With the mobility of people, the rapid communication with all parts of the world, the changes in agriculture and food technology, and advances in education it is not surprising that food habits often change rapidly—that is within a generation or less. One of the dramatic examples of changing food habits is that of the Japanese in Hawaii as described by Wenkam and Wolff.[1] The Japanese who came to Hawaii at the end of the nineteenth century were mostly agricultural workers who were employed on the plantations. For them, the family was the important social unit. They achieved status through it and were guided by respect for the family, ancestral worship, and so on. Individual desires were subordinated.

The early Japanese immigrants retained the vegetarian food habits of Japan, a diet in which rice, barley, and soybeans were the staple foods. They also used peas and mung beans, cabbage, marine algae, vegetables, roots, and tubers. Those who lived near the seacoast consumed fairly large amounts of fish, but it was not available inland. Scarcely any meat was eaten.

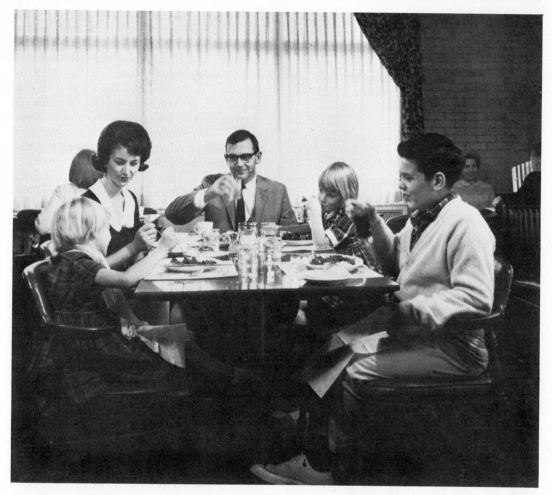

Figure 15–1. More frequent meals away from home help to introduce new foods to the family, thereby effecting some changes in food habits. (Courtesy, U.S. Department of Agriculture.)

As the immigrants associated with Caucasians and other Orientals they began to include new foods such as Chinese pork, Hawaiian poi, and Portuguese sweet bread. The changing diet was accelerated during World War II when Nisei soldiers were in contact with soldiers of other ethnic groups.

The largest group of Japanese living in Hawaii today have drastically changed their diets. This cosmopolitan group have replaced rice with white flour, bread, and crackers. The consumption of animal foods has increased conspicuously. They have substituted the American breakfast for the traditional rice, soup, and pickled vegetables.

A second smaller group, mostly older Japanese, are those who have retained the traditions of the Japanese diet, although they eat some American foods. A third group, also small, has become so completely "Americanized" that some of them have even changed their names. To them, the Japanese traditions hold no meaning.

The single most important influence on the food habits has been the American system of education with its emphasis on democracy and the individual.[1] The family controls have also been weakened, and hence the restrictions placed on the use of food, for example, animal foods, are no longer honored. A desire for higher status has been important, and so rice was given up because it no longer was a prestige food. The early immigrants to Hawaii expected to return to Japan as soon as they had earned enough money, and so they retained their Japanese food habits. However, for the present generation of Japanese, Hawaii is the permanent home. Finally, the inter-mingling of ethnic groups and the availability of foods have contributed to the evolution of the food habits.

REGIONAL FOOD PATTERNS OF THE UNITED STATES

Perhaps nowhere in the world can one find so great a variety of foods and methods of prep-aration as in the United States. The dietary patterns are an amalgamation of the foods native to the region and the habits and customs handed down by generations of foreign born. The foods vary from the wheat of the North Central plains to the rice of Louisiana, the potatoes of Maine to the citrus fruits of Florida, the dairy products of Minnesota and Wisconsin to the beef of the western ranges, the fish of the seacoast to the fruits of the Far West. One might associate baked beans with New England, chile con carne with the Southwest, and fried chicken with the South, but today these dishes are served every-where in the United States.

In addition to the baked beans and brown bread on a Saturday night, in New England one is likely to encounter such favorite dishes as codfish cakes, lobster, clam chowder, and other seafood specialties. Pumpkin pie, squash, Indian pudding, and turkey originated with the Pilgrim fathers, who made adaptations of foods used by the American Indian.

The Pennsylvania Dutch are known for many rich foods including potato pancakes, many kinds of sausage, Philadelphia scrapple, sticky cinna-mon buns, pickles and relishes ("seven sweets and seven sours"), and shoofly pie.

Fried chicken, country ham, and hot biscuits

are specialties of the South. Green vegetables such as turnip tops, collards, kale, and mustard greens are well liked; they are likely to be cooked for a relatively long time with fat pork as a flavoring agent. The water in which the vegetables are boiled (pot liquor) is often con-sumed, thus retaining some of the minerals and vitamins that would otherwise be lost. Sweet potatoes are preferred to white potatoes, and corn is the cereal of choice, although rice and wheat are also widely used. Corn appears in such forms as corn pone, corn bread, hominy grits, spoon bread, and hush puppies—in Florida and Texas, especially.

Dairy products, meat, and eggs abound in the Middle West. Here one finds dietary patterns similar to those of Scandinavia, Germany, Po-land, England, and other northern European countries.

New Orleans is noted for its fine restaurants, which show the influence of French and Creole cookery. Soups and fish dishes are often highly seasoned, and sauces are used for many meats and vegetables.

The Mexican and Spanish influences are felt in the Southwest where pinto beans, tortillas made from flour or lime-treated corn, and chili, a hot pepper, are important constituents of the diet. Usually these staple food items are served with highly seasoned sauces (see Mexican die-tary patterns, page 221).

The abundance of luscious fruits and vege-tables in the Far West leads to a much greater consumption of salads as main dishes as well as accompaniments of the meal. The Oriental in-fluence is especially noted in the delicious vege-tables of Japanese and Chinese cookery. Sea-foods abound in great variety on the West Coast, as in the East, but the salmon of the Pacific Northwest is especially prized.

ORTHODOX JEWISH FOOD HABITS

Outstanding characteristics. The description of the dietary pattern of the Jewish people pre-sented here is based, in large part, on a recent article by Kaufman.[2] Orthodox Jews observe

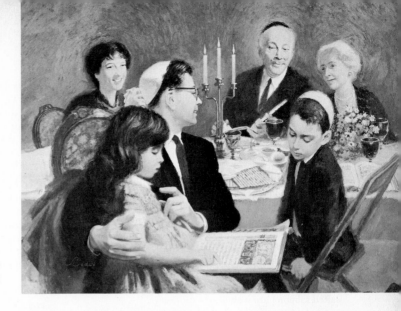

Figure 15–2. Jewish family at a Seder table. (Courtesy, The B. Manischewitz Company, Newark.)

dietary laws based on Biblical and rabbinical regulations (the rules of Kashruth). These laws pertain to the selection, preparation, and service of food. Conservative Jews nominally observe the laws but make distinctions within and without the home, while Reform Jews minimize the significance of dietary laws. Food habits of the Jewish people may also be influenced by the country of origin—for example, Russia, Poland, or Germany.

Milk and its products are never eaten in the same meal as meat. Usually two meals contain dairy products and one meal contains meat and its products.

Religious festivals include certain food restrictions. No food is cooked or heated on the Sabbath. Yom Kippur (Day of Atonement) is a 24-hour period of fasting from food and drink. The Passover, sometimes also referred to as "The Feast of Unleavened Bread," lasts for eight days and commemorates the release of the Israelites from the slavery of Egypt. During this period only unleavened bread is used (Exod. 12:15–20; 13:3–10; 23:15). Only utensils and dishes that have made no contact with leavened foods may be used during this time. Thus, the Orthodox Jewish home would have four sets of dishes: one for meat and one for dairy meals during the Passover, and one for meat and one for dairy meals during the rest of the year when leavened breads and cakes may be used.

The Passover begins with the Seder when everyone sits down to a beautifully set table. On a platter are foods that commemorate the Exodus from Egypt: matzoth, the unleavened bread the Jews ate when they left Egypt; a bone as a reminder of the sacrifice of the lamb by the Jews; bitter herbs for the bitterness of slavery; and *harosseth,* a mixture of apples, nuts, cinnamon, and wine to look like the clay of which the Jews made bricks in Egypt. (See Figure 15–2.)

The diet is generally rich in pastries, cake, many preserves, and relishes. Breads, cereals, legumes, fish, and dairy products are used abundantly. Encouragement should be given to the inclusion of more fruits and vegetables.

TYPICAL FOODS AND THEIR USES

Milk Group

Milk, cottage and cream cheese, sour cream used abundantly. Milk and its products may not be used at same meal as meat (Exod. 23:19; 34:26; Deut. 14:21). Milk may not be taken until six hours after eating meat. Separate dishes and utensils must be used for milk and meat dishes.

Meat Group

ALLOWED FOODS

All quadruped animals that chew the cud and divide the hoof (Lev. 11:1–3; Deut. 14:3–8): cattle, deer, goats, sheep. Organs of these animals may be used.

Animals must be killed in prescribed manner for minimum pain to animal, and for maximum blood drainage. Blood is associated with life and may not be eaten (Gen. 9:4; Lev. 3:17; 17:10–14; Deut.

12:23–27). Meat is made *kosher* (clean) by soaking it in cold water, thoroughly salting it, allowing it to drain for an hour, and then washing it in three waters.

Hindquarters of meat may be used only if the part of the thigh with the sinew of Jacob is removed (Gen. 32:33).

Poultry: chicken, duck, goose, pheasant, turkey. Chicken is common for Sabbath eve meal.

Fish with fins and scales (Lev. 11:9; Deut. 14:9–10): cod, haddock, halibut, salmon, trout, tuna, whitefish, etc.

Eggs. Fish and eggs may be eaten at both meat and milk meals.

Dried beans, peas, lentils, in many soups.

Corned beef, smoked meats, herring, *lox* (smoked, salted salmon) are well liked.

Cholent: casserole of beef, potatoes, and dried beans. Served on the Sabbath.

Gefillte fish: chopped, highly seasoned fish; a first course for the Sabbath meal.

Kishke: beef casings stuffed with rich filling and roasted.

Knishes: pastry filled with ground meat.

Kreplach: noodle dough filled with ground meat or cheese filling.

PROHIBITED FOODS

Animals which do not chew the cud or divide the hoof (Lev. 11:4–8): pork.

Diseased animals or animals dying a natural death (Deut. 14:21).

Birds of prey (Lev. 11:13–19; Deut. 14:11–18).

Fish without fins or scales (Lev. 11:10–12): eels, shellfish such as oysters, crab, lobster.

Egg with blood spot.

Vegetable-Fruit Group

All kinds used without restriction.

Cucumber, lettuce, tomato very frequently used.

Cabbage, potatoes, and root vegetables are often cooked with the meat.

Borsch: soup with meat stock and egg, or without meat stock and with sour cream; includes beets, spinach, cabbage.

Dried fruits are used in many pastries.

Bread-Cereals Group

All kinds used without restriction. Rye bread (pumpernickel), white seed rolls; noodles and other egg and flour mixtures.

Bagel: doughnut-shaped hard yeast roll.

Blintzes: thin rolled pancakes filled with cottage cheese, ground beef, or fruit mixture; served with sour cream.

Bulke: light yeast roll.

Challah: braided loaf or light white bread.

Farfel: noodle dough grated for soup.

Kasha: buckwheat groats served as cooked cereal or as potato substitute.

Kloese: dumplings, usually in chicken soup.

Latkes: pancakes.

Matzoth: flat, unleavened bread.

Other Foods

Unsalted butter preferred.

Chicken fat or vegetable oils for cooking.

Rich pastries are common.

Cheese cake.

Kuchen: coffee cake of many varieties.

Leckach: honey cake for Rosh Hashana (New Year).

Strudel: thin pastry with fruit, nut filling.

Teiglach: small pieces of dough cooked in honey, with nuts.

Sponge cake and macaroons at Passover.

Many preserves, pickled cucumbers, pickled green tomatoes, relishes.

Many foods are highly salted.

PUERTO RICAN FOOD HABITS

Outstanding characteristics. Most of the Puerto Ricans now living in the mainland of the United States were born here, but many of them retain the food habits of their parents who came from the island. Because of unfamiliarity with the English language, expensive imported foods are often bought in stores managed by other Puerto Ricans. Some familiarity with the American supermarket would help these people to obtain similar, if not identical, foods more in keeping with their limited income. The typical dietary pattern of the Puerto Rican has been described by Torres.[3]

Rice, legumes, and *viandas* (starchy vegetables) are basic to all diets. Dried codfish (*bacalao*) and milk are used as the income permits. Meat is well liked, but it is too expensive except for the well-to-do. Fruits on the island are abundant and provide ample ascorbic acid; green vegetables are also abundant. Neither fruits nor vegetables are eaten as much as they should be. The diet is high in carbohydrate and fat. Increased amounts of protein, vitamin A, and ascorbic acid should be provided.

A typical breakfast for the very poor consists of *café con leche* with or without bread; oatmeal and egg are included when income permits. Lunch in the rural areas is a plateful of viandas with codfish and oil; rice and stewed beans might be used in the city. Dinner in urban and rural areas consists of rice and beans, and viandas or bread. Between-meal eating is frequent.

Families with a more liberal income add meat to the daily meals. Chicken, pork, and beef are well liked. Desserts are not always used, but fruits cooked in syrup are especially well liked.

TYPICAL FOODS AND THEIR USES

Milk Group

Milk is well liked but very little is used. Nonfat milk solids well accepted; people must be shown how to use it.

Most of the milk is used in strong coffee, (*café con leche*); 2–5 ounces milk per cup. Many drink this several times a day.

Cocoa and chocolate used widely.

Meat Group

Chicken, pork especially well liked. Seldom used by low-income groups, but liberally by the prosperous.

Chicken often cooked with rice (*arroz con pollo*). Codfish used frequently; served with viandas.

Legumes (*granos*): chick peas, kidney beans, navy beans, dried peas, pigeon peas, and other varieties. Stewed and dressed with sauce (*sofrito*). About 3–4 ounces legumes eaten daily.

Vegetable-Fruit Group

Viandas (starchy vegetables): green bananas and green plantain most common; *batata amarillo* (yellow sweet potato); *batata blanca* (white sweet potato); ripe plantain; white *ñame;* white *tanier; panapen* (breadfruit) in some parts of the island; yautia; *yuca* (cassava), occasionally. Viandas are boiled and served hot with oil, vinegar, and some codfish—often as a one-dish meal in rural areas.

Beets and eggplant most commonly used vegetables.

Carrots, green beans, okra, and tomatoes in small amounts.

Some spinach and chard but insufficient succulent vegetables eaten.

Yellow squash (*calabaza*) used in soups or fritters.

Fruits usually eaten between meals rather than at meals. Include: acerola (richest known source of vitamin C), cashew nut fruit, grapefruit, guava, mango, orange, papaya, pineapple.

Preference often shown for imported canned peaches, pears, apples, fruit cocktail.

In the United States, potatoes and sweet potatoes may be used instead of tropical viandas. Citrus fruits should be stressed.

Bread-Cereals Group

Rice (*arroz*) used once or twice daily by all (7 ounces per capita daily). Enriched by Puerto Rican law. May be boiled and dressed with lard or combined with legumes, chopped pork sausages, dry codfish, or chicken.

Cornmeal mush made with water or milk is popular.

Oatmeal may be cooked in thin gruel for breakfast. Cornmeal may substitute for rice, and may be eaten with beans and codfish.

Wheat bread, noodles, spaghetti are widely used. Cream of Wheat and other cereals imported by the well-to-do.

In the United States suggest whole-grain and enriched cereals and potatoes for some of the rice.

Other Foods and Seasonings

Sofrito: sauce made of tomatoes, onion, garlic, thyme, and other herbs, salt pork, green pepper, and fat. This is basis for much of cooking.

Annato: yellow coloring used with rice.

Lard, oil, salt pork, or ham butts used in cooking. Lard is used on bread.

Sugar in large amounts in coffee, cocoa, chocolate; molasses.

Coffee (Mocha, never a blend) is very strong; consider American coffee to be very weak and dislike it. Coffee usually served with hot milk.

Carbonated beverages are being used more frequently.

MEXICAN-AMERICAN FOOD HABITS

Outstanding characteristics. The chief foods of the Mexican-Americans are dried beans, chili peppers, and corn, but wheat is gradually replacing corn. Many families eat one good meal daily at noon, such as lentil-noodle vegetable soup, and breakfast and supper consist of a sweet coffee or sometimes milk and tortillas. Those of low income use very little meat, usually for flavoring beans, soups, and vegetable stews.

The National Nutrition Survey in the Southwest showed that a high proportion of Mexican-Americans had low blood levels of vitamin A,

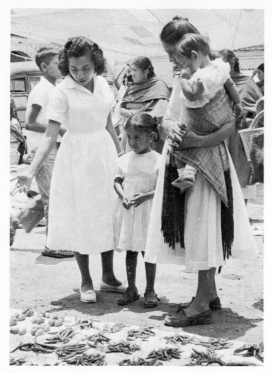

Figure 15–3. Clinic nurse in Mexico has opportunity on market day to point out the importance of fruits and vegetables to supplement the diet of tortillas and black beans. (Courtesy, UNICEF.)

riboflavin, and hemoglobin.[4] Deficiencies of thiamine, ascorbic acid, and protein were less frequent but of sufficient magnitude to constitute a problem. (See Figure 15–3.)

The diets of these people would be improved with greater emphasis on inexpensive variety meats, tomatoes, chili peppers, cheese, and evaporated milk.[4] Beans are an important source of protein but the people need to learn to supplement the beans with milk. Enriched flours and breads, citrus fruits, and cooking in iron pots are also recommended.

TYPICAL FOODS AND THEIR USES[4, 5]

Milk Group

Very little milk is used; some evaporated milk for infant feeding.

Meat Group

Beef and chicken well liked; meat used only two or three times weekly.

Eggs: two or three times a week.

Fish: infrequently.

Pinto or calico beans: refried (*frijoles refritos*); used daily by some; two or three times weekly by others.

Chile con carne: beef with garlic seasoning, beans, chili peppers.

Enchiladas: tortilla filled with cheese, onion, shredded lettuce, and rolled.

Taco: tortilla filled with seasoned ground meat, lettuce, and served with chili sauce.

Tamales: seasoned ground meat placed on masa, wrapped in corn husks, steamed, and served with chili sauce.

Topopo: corn tortilla filled with refried beans, shredded lettuce, green or ripe olives.

Vegetable-Fruit Group

Corn: fresh or canned; *chicos,* corn steamed while green and dried on the cob; *posole,* similar to hominy.

Chili peppers: fresh, canned, or frozen are good source of ascorbic acid.

Beets, cabbage, many tropical greens, peas, potatoes, pumpkin, squash, string beans, sweet potatoes, turnips.

Bananas used frequently. *Chayotes* (cactuslike fruit), oranges.

Nopalitos: leaf or stem of prickly pear cactus; diced as vegetable.

Bread-Cereals Group

Corn is staple cereal with wheat gradually replacing it. Rice, macaroni, spaghetti. Some yeast bread; sweet rolls very popular. Increasing use of ready-to-eat cereals.

Atole: cornmeal gruel.

Masa: dried corn which has been heated and soaked in lime water, washed, and ground while wet into puttylike dough; contains appreciable amounts of calcium.

Sopaipillas: puffs of deep-fried dough. Use as bread or dessert, usually with honey.

Tortilla: thin, unleavened cakes baked on hot griddle, using masa; wheat now replacing lime-treated corn.

Other Foods and Seasoning

Ground red chili powder is essential to most dishes; garlic and onion very common; salt in abundance.

Cinnamon, coriander, lemon juice, mint, nutmeg, oregano, parsley, saffron.

Butter rarely used.

Coffee with much sugar used in large amounts.

Sugar and sweets in large amounts.

Italian Food Habits

Outstanding characteristics. The favorite foods for the Italian diet are readily available, and the nurse or dietitian should experience no difficulty in adapting the diet of a given locality to the Italian pattern. Cantoni[6] has recently summarized the prevailing pattern for Italian people in the United States.

Pastas, available in a great variety of shapes, are an important staple of the Italian diet. They are prepared from durum wheat of high-gluten content. Crusty white bread is widely used. The Italians use fruits, vegetables, and cheese liberally and should be encouraged in continuing to do so. Milk is not as widely used as it should be, although cheese will substitute in part. Dietary instruction should include emphasis on the use of enriched flour for bread and pastas.

The typical breakfast consists of fruit, Italian bread with butter, and coffee with hot milk and sugar. The main meal of the day comes at noon if all members of the family are at home but will come in the evening when some members are away from home all day. The main meal may consist of broth with noodles, meat or chicken or pasta with sauce, vegetables, green salad, bread without butter, fruit, and coffee with milk. The evening meal (or lunch) includes a substantial soup as a main dish, Italian bread, coffee with milk and sugar, sometimes cold cuts or cheese or salad, and sometimes wine.

Typical Foods and Their Uses

Milk Group
Goat milk is preferred. Most adults drink little milk; usually with coffee or chocolate; dislike plain milk.

American cheese disliked. Prefer expensive Italian cheeses: *Mozzarella* and *Ricotta* for cooking and with bread; *Parmesan* and *Romano* for grating; *Gorgonzola.*

Meat Group
Chicken: roast; baked with oil, garlic, salt, pepper; *cacciatora,* browned in oil, simmered in wine, tomato sauce.

Lamb.

Pork: roasted or fried sausages; baked or fried chops.

Veal: cutlets, *scallopine* or with tomato sauce.

Cold cuts: *coppa* (highly peppered), *mortadella* (bologna), *prosciutto* (cured ham), salami.

Meats often browned in salt pork or oil and simmered in a sauce with combinations of celery, garlic, onion, parsley, green pepper, tomato purée, wine; meat balls; meat loaf. Smaller quantities of meat eaten than by some other groups.

Fish: fresh preferred; canned: anchovies, sardines, tuna. Fish sauces (anchovy, clam, tuna) for spaghetti on fast days.

Chick peas, kidney beans, lentils, split peas in soups. *Pastafasiole:* bean soup. *Minestrone:* substantial soup of vegetables, chick peas, pasta.

Frittata: omelet with eggs, cheese, bread crumbs, seasonings.

Vegetable-Fruit Group
Favorite vegetables: artichoke, asparagus, broccoli, eggplant, escarole, peppers, squash (zucchini and others), string beans, tomatoes in sauce. Vegetables are cooked in water, drained, dressed with olive oil or oil and vinegar or lemon juice.

Insalata: salad of greens; may be mixed with celery, onions, green peppers, tomatoes. Dressed with olive oil, vinegar (often wine vinegar), garlic, pepper, salt.

Fruits are well liked and eaten abundantly when available: apricots, cherries, dates, figs, grapes, melons, peaches, plums, quinces.

Bread-Cereals Group
White crusty bread forms substantial part of meal. Made of high-protein flour, water, yeast, salt, and little if any fat. Flour not likely to be enriched except where state law requires it.

Pasta: includes macaroni, spaghetti, noodles in many forms and shapes. Used two to three times a week. Spaghetti is usual pasta of southern Italy, but rice, cornmeal, and noodles are more common in northern Italy.

Pastasciutta: pasta with gravy or sauce.

Noodle doughs filled with meat, vegetable, or cheese mixtures: *cannelloni, lasagne, manicotti, ravioli, tortellini.*

Polenta: thick cornmeal mush served plain, or in casserole with sausages, tomato sauce, grated cheese.

Risotto alla Milanese: rice cooked in broth, flavored with Parmesan cheese, onion, mushroom, saffron, wine.

Other Foods and Seasonings
Butter, olive oil, salt pork. Oil in cooking; preference for olive oil.

Pies and pastry used more in America than in Italy.

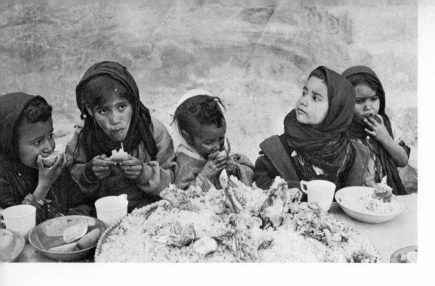

Figure 15–4. Traditional meal of Jordanian children is supplemented with milk. (Courtesy, George Holton and UNICEF.)

Cannoli: filled pastries.
Farfalleti dolci: dough mixture fried in fat.
Torta: cake.
Zabaglione: soft custard with egg yolks, white wine, sugar.
Tutti-frutti ice creams.
Seasonings: basil, celery, garlic, nutmeg, onion, oregano, parsley, pepper, green pepper, hot peppers, rosemary, saffron, tomato purée, wine.

DIETARY PATTERNS OF THE NEAR EAST—ARMENIA, GREECE, SYRIA, TURKEY

TYPICAL FOODS AND THEIR USES[7]

Milk Group

Cow's, goat's, or sheep's milk; fermented preferred to sweet (yogurt); little used by adults. Often served hot and sweetened to children.
Soft and hard cheeses.

Meat Group

Lamb is preferred; also pork, poultry, mutton, goat, beef.
Fish: fresh, salted, or smoked; octopus, squid, shellfish, roe.
Eggs often used as main dish but not at breakfast.
Beans, peas, and lentils.
Nuts may be used with wheat and rice in place of meat; pignolias, pistachios.
Ground or cut meat often cooked with wheat or rice, or in stews with cereal grains and vegetables. For example:
Breast of lamb stuffed with rice, currants.
Squash stuffed with chopped meat, onions, rice, parsley.
Cabbage rolls with ground meat, rice, and baked in meat stock; served with lemon juice.
Barbecued meats on special occasions: skewered meats are broiled.
Shashlik: mutton or lamb marinated in garlic, oil, vinegar; roasted on skewers with tomato and onion slices.

Vegetable-Fruit Group

Eggplant, greens, onions, peppers, tomatoes; also cabbage, cauliflower, cucumbers, okra, potatoes, zucchini.
Vegetables cooked with olive oil and served hot or cold; cooked in meat or fish stews; stuffed with wheat, meat, nuts, beans; salads with olive oil, vinegar.
Grapes, lemons, oranges; also apricots, cherries, dates, figs, melons, peaches, pears, plums, quinces, raisins. Fresh fruits widely used in season; fruit compotes.

Bread-Cereals Group

Bread is staff of life; used at every meal. Baked on griddles in round, flat loaves.
Cracked whole wheat (*bourglour*) and rice used as starchy food, or with vegetables, or with meat (*pilavi*). (See Figure 15–4.)
Corn in *polenta.*

Other Foods and Seasonings

Olive oil and seed oils used in cooking. Butter is not much used.
Nuts (hazel, pignolia, pistachio) used for snacks, in desserts, pastries.
Paklava: pastry with nuts and honey.
Black olives.
Herbs, honey, sugar, lemon juice, seeds of caraway, pumpkin, and sesame.
Apricot candy, Turkish paste.
Wine, coffee.

Dietary Patterns of the Chinese

Typical Foods and Their Uses

Milk Group
Milk and cheese are well liked but need to be emphasized.

Meat Group
Pork, lamb, chicken, duck, fish and shellfish, eggs, and soybeans. Organ meats including brain and spinal cord, blood, and bone are used.

Egg rolls: shrimp or meat and vegetable filling rolled in thin dough, and fried in deep fat.

Egg foo yung: combination of eggs, chopped chicken, mushrooms, scallions, celery, bean sprouts cooked similar to an omelet.

Sweet and pungent pork: pork cubes coated with batter and fried in oil; then simmered in a sauce of green pepper, cubed pineapple, molasses, brown sugar, vinegar, and seasonings.

Chow mein: veal, chicken, shrimp, with celery, mushrooms, water chestnuts, bamboo shoots, in sauce; served with soy sauce. A popular dish made for American tastes.

Vegetable-Fruit Group
Cabbage, cucumbers, many greens, mushrooms, bamboo shoots, soybean sprouts, sweet potatoes.

Vegetables are thinly sliced or chopped; cooked in a little oil for a short time before water is added to seal in flavor, preserve crispness, and fresh green color. Any juice remaining is served with the vegetable.

Bread-Cereals Group
Rice is staple food served with every meal.

Wheat and millet are widely used.

Other Foods and Seasonings
Lard, soy, sesame, and peanut oils used in cooking.

Soy sauce present in almost every meal contributes to high salt intake.

Almonds, ginger, sesame seeds for flavoring.

Tea is beverage of choice.

Problem and Review

1. What factors must be kept in mind in teaching normal nutrition to people whose food habits differ widely from our own?
2. What technologic advances of the twentieth century have tended to eliminate regional differences in food patterns of the United States?
3. *Problem.* Select any one ethnic group and plan menus for one day including recipes for special dishes.
4. Make a survey of the ethnic groups represented in the class. List favorite dishes for each of these ethnic groups. Discuss the nutritive values of these dishes. What foods require emphasis in the patterns of these ethnic groups?
5. What problems in dietary adjustment would you expect to encounter for a Puerto Rican child; a student from India who is a strict vegetarian?
6. Compare the principal cereal foods and meats used by the Chinese, the Mexicans, and the Greeks.

Cited References

1. Wenkam, N. S., and Wolff, R. J.: "A Half Century of Changing Food Habits Among Japanese in Hawaii," *J. Am. Diet. Assoc.*, **57**:29–32, 1970.
2. Kaufman, M.: "Adapting Therapeutic Diets to Jewish Food Customs," *Am. J. Clin. Nutr.*, **5**:676–81, 1957.
3. Torres, R. M.: "Dietary Patterns of Puerto Rican People," Am. J. Clin. Nutr., **7**:349–55, 1959.
4. Bailey, M. A.: "Nutrition Education and the Spanish-speaking American," *J. Nutr. Educ.*, **2**:50–54, 1970.
5. Hacker, D. B., and Miller, E. D.: "Food Patterns of the Southwest," *Am. J. Clin. Nutr.*, **7**:224–29, 1959.

6. Cantoni, M.: "Adapting Therapeutic Diets to the Eating Patterns of Italian-Americans," *Am. J. Clin. Nutr.,* 6:548–55, 1958.
7. Valassi, K. V.: "Food Habits of Greek Americans," *Am. J. Clin. Nutr.,* 11:240–48, 1962.

ADDITIONAL REFERENCES

Berkowitz, P., and Berkowitz, N. S.: "The Jewish Patient in the Hospital," *Am. J. Nurs.,* 67:2335–37, 1967.
Food Customs of New Canadians. Toronto Nutrition Committee, Toronto, Ontario, 1967.
Forbes, J. D.: *Mexican-Americans. A Handbook for Educators.* Far Western Laboratory for Educational Research and Development, Berkeley. Superintendent of Documents, Washington, D.C., 1969.
Hiemstra, S. J.: "Telescoping 20 Years of Change in the Food We Eat," in *Food for Us All— Yearbook of Agriculture 1969.* Superintendent of Documents, Washington, D.C.
Ho, G. P., *et al.:* "Adaptation to American Dietary Patterns by Students from Oriental Countries," *J. Home Econ.,* 58:277–80, 1966.
Kight, M. A., *et al.:* "Nutritional Influences of Mexican-American Foods in Arizona," *J. Am. Diet. Assoc.,* 55:557–61, 1969.
King, A.: *Extension Guide to Good Eating. Acceptable Foods of Some Racial and Ethnic Groups in the United States.* Dairy Council of California, San Francisco, 1969.
Korff, S. I.: "The Jewish Dietary Code," *Food Technol.,* 20:926–28, 1966.
Kraus, B.: *The Cookbook of the United Nations,* Revised. Simon and Schuster, New York, 1970.
Longman, D. P.: "Working with Pueblo Indians in New Mexico," *J. Am. Diet. Assoc.,* 47: 470–73, 1965.
Pangborn, R. M., and Bruhn, C. M.: "Concepts of Food Habits of 'Other' Ethnic Groups," *J. Nutr. Educ.,* 2:106–10, Winter 1971.
Understanding Food Patterns in the United States of America. The American Dietetic Association, Chicago, 1969.
Vayda, A. P., *et al.: Environment and Cultural Behavior.* Natural History Press, Garden City, N.Y., 1969.
Wuerffel, S.: "Nutrition Work among the Sioux," *J. Am. Diet. Assoc.,* 53:113, 1968.

Unit IV

Meal Planning, Food Selection, and Food Preparation

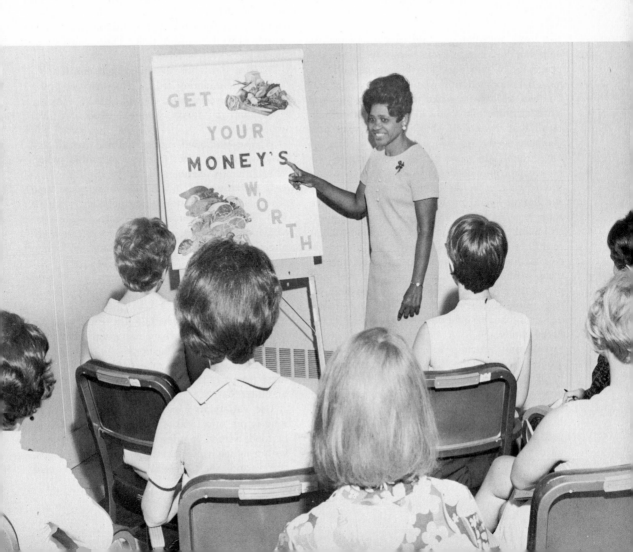

16 Meal Planning for the Family

Nurses, nutritionists, and home economists help families in numerous ways to apply the principles of nutrition. The lessons of nutrition have been learned only when the individual and families are able to make the best use of their material, time, and financial resources to obtain meals that meet their physical, social, and psychologic needs. No two individuals or families have exactly the same needs. For example, one homemaker may need suggestions on how to get the most value for the limited amount of money she has to spend on food; another would like some ideas on how to use donated food supplies; still another needs some help in planning meals that fit in with a busy work schedule. An elderly woman living alone might need some help in meal planning with limited facilities for food preparation. Or the professional person may be responsible for the supervision of a homemaker or a home health aide during a period of illness in the family.

This unit provides a brief but basic background for individuals who are concerned with helping families to better food habits through good meal planning, food selection, and food preparation. Additional resource materials are listed at the end of each chapter.

Meal patterns must fit the family. Planning meals for the family group entails consideration of the needs of each individual. Specific require-

ments for various periods of the life cycle are detailed in Chapters 21 through 24. One can readily adapt the family menu to meet these needs if care is exercised in planning meals. For example, if steak appears on the menu for the adult members of the family, a meat patty would be suitable for the young child and might be preferred by some elderly persons. A baked apple is readily prepared for the child at the same time an apple pie is being baked. The same salad can usually be used for both the overweight and underweight members of the family if the dressing is omitted for the former.

Save time in food preparation. Time, like money, needs to be budgeted for its best use. Time management in the preparation of food is essential for the homemaker who is also employed outside the home. It also means additional hours for care of the children and home duties as well as leisure time. These suggestions may help:

1. Plan meals for several days at one time.

2. Write a market order and restrict shopping to once or twice a week.

3. Shop at hours when markets are less crowded.

4. Use simplified menus suitable for all age groups. Do not cater to every individual whim of each family member.

5. Make use of convenience foods when time saved is more important than the slightly higher cost of the item, but compare costs. Some convenience foods are no more expensive; most are slightly more expensive; and some are quite costly.

6. Arrange the kitchen in terms of efficient work units, keeping utensils and food supplies at the point of first use.

7. Plan a work schedule for each day. In time this will show where important savings in minutes and hours can be made.

8. Include other members of the family in meal preparation tasks according to their skills and interests.

Use variety in meals. Variety in meal planning is the sum total of many kinds and classes of foods served in pleasing color combinations, with a judicious mixture of soft and crisp foods, bland and sharp flavors, and hot and cold dishes—all prepared in the best tradition of American cookery. It ensures better nutrition and enhances the interest in the meal.

Four Food Groups. A very common error in meal planning is emphasizing one type of food to the exclusion of others. A meal consisting of roast beef, macaroni and cheese, and custard predominates in protein, whereas spaghetti, potatoes, and cake in another meal would be equally poor because of the preponderance of carbohydrate. First, then, variety means selecting foods each day from each of the basic food groups. Thus, a breakfast of orange juice, egg, toast, butter, and milk includes foods from the Four Food Groups. The orange juice contributes ascorbic acid not found in any of the other foods, egg and milk are the chief sources of protein, egg and bread provide most of the iron, milk is the outstanding contributor of calcium and riboflavin, and so on. Used together these foods comprise a good breakfast, but used singly some nutrients would be provided in less than desirable amounts.

Color. The first appeal to the appetite is through the eye. Attractive color combinations are important, for food must look good enough to eat. Chicken à la king, mashed potato, and cauliflower are monotonous in appearance, whereas changing the cauliflower to green peas or beans would add color appeal. Sometimes color appeal consists merely in using a garnish such as chopped parsley and paprika on fish, radish roses, green pepper rings, or some red jelly in a tiny lettuce cup. One need not restrict garnishes to the much overworked cherry or to the wilted sprig of parsley!

Texture. Texture variation is equally important. For example, a meal made up of meat loaf, mashed potatoes, stewed squash, white bread, and baked custard would be greatly improved by changing the vegetable to one requiring some mastication and by adding a green salad and crusty rolls. Children will not eat well if all the foods in a given meal require a lot of chewing, whereas most adults rebel against all soft foods. (See Figures 16–1 and 16–2.)

Flavor. Taste appeal depends on the blending of bland and sharp flavors. Creamed onions, spicy cole slaw, pickles, and sharp cheese rep-

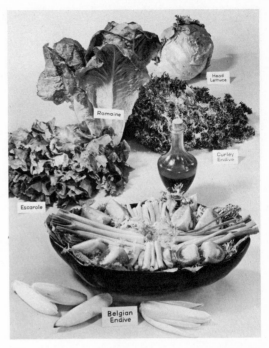

Figure 16–1. A variety of salad greens adds crisp texture and mild to tangy flavors to a meal. (Courtesy, United Fresh Fruit and Vegetable Association.)

resent too many strongly flavored foods in a single meal; on the other hand, boiled potatoes, mashed squash, and vanilla pudding are all bland and lack interest unless contrasted with some sharper flavor. Spicy foods and marked flavors should not dominate the meal, but should provide the accent. Flavor variety precludes using the same food in two forms at one meal; for example, tomato juice and tomato salad would not be a good choice.

Climate. Even the season of the year requires some consideration, for on a cold winter day hearty soups and stews may seem especially desirable. Summer meals also require that the same nutrients be provided, but one is likely to prefer less of heavy and rich foods. One should not make the mistake, however, of serving cold foods only, or of planning salad meals that do not include protein.

Preparation. Variety can be introduced by using many methods of preparation. For example, eggs may be soft cooked, poached, in

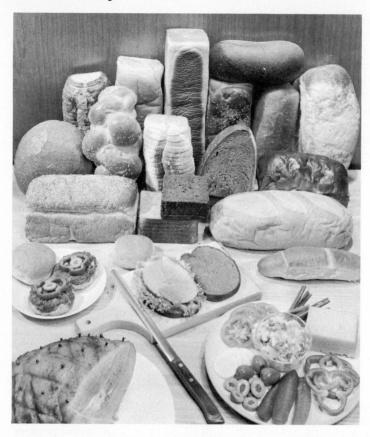

Figure 16–2. Breads of many shapes, textures, and flavors add interest to any meal. (Courtesy, General Mills, Inc., Minneapolis.)

omelets of various kinds, creamed, or deviled, to mention but a few methods of preparation; likewise, tomatoes may be fresh in salads, broiled, stewed, escalloped, fried green or ripe, in cream soups, in tomato juice, and so on.

Provide satiety value. A satisfying meal is one that will allay the sense of hunger until almost time for the next meal. A breakfast of orange juice and toast is digested in such a short time that a sense of hunger and fatigue quickly appears. The addition of cereal and milk or eggs will, however, postpone these sensations.

Protein foods are high in satiety value as are foods cooked with fat. Carbohydrate foods, fruits, vegetables, and liquids are somewhat low in their staying power. The choice of foods will depend upon the interval between meals, long intervals demanding those of higher satiety value.

Begin with a good breakfast. Over a period of six years, a series of experiments was conducted by the Departments of Physiology and Nutrition at the State University of Iowa to determine the effectiveness of various breakfast plans on physical and mental efficiency.[1] In brief, the results of these studies showed that (1) efficiency in physiologic performance, as measured by bicycle ergometer, treadmill, and maximum grip strength, decreased in late morning hours when breakfast was omitted; (2) attitude toward school work and scholastic achievement was poorer when breakfast was omitted; (3) the content of the breakfast did not determine its efficiency so long as it was nutritionally adequate; (4) a basic breakfast providing one fourth of the daily caloric requirement and one fourth of the daily protein allowance was superior to smaller or larger breakfasts for maintaining efficiency in the late morning hours; (5) a protein intake of 20 to 25 gm was most suitable for the maintenance of the blood glucose level during the late morning hours; and (6) the omission of breakfast was of no value in weight reduction. In fact, those who omit breakfast while on a weight reduction regimen experience greater hunger in addition to being physiologically inefficient.

A change to better breakfast habits means (1) planning simple, easy-to-prepare, but varied meals; (2) arising sufficiently early so that there is time for eating breakfast; (3) eating breakfast with the family group so that it, like other meals, has pleasant social associations.

Breakfast should provide at least one fourth of the daily nutritive needs. It may include some protein food such as egg or milk, cereal or breadstuff, or both, and a beverage. Children and teen-agers should include milk for breakfast. If citrus fruit or another good source of ascorbic acid is included at breakfast, the day's allowance is assured. Cereal may be hot or cold; breads may vary from plain white enriched or whole grain to muffins, griddle cakes, waffles, or sweet rolls, as the occasion warrants. A break-

fast may be light or heavy depending upon the individual's activity and preferences. (See Figure 16–3.)

LIGHT BREAKFAST
Orange juice
Oatmeal with sugar and milk
Coffee with cream and sugar
Milk for children

MEDIUM BREAKFAST
Stewed prunes
Poached eggs (2) on buttered toast
Coffee with cream and sugar
Milk for children

HEAVY BREAKFAST
Cantaloupe
Griddle cakes with syrup
Sausages
Coffee with cream and sugar
Milk for children

Lunch is often neglected. Thousands of workers eat lunches in facilities that have a selection limited to sandwiches, pastries, and beverages. All too common a pattern is a sandwich, perhaps a piece of pie, and a glass of carbonated beverage or a cup of coffee. This pattern can often be improved by including a salad and a

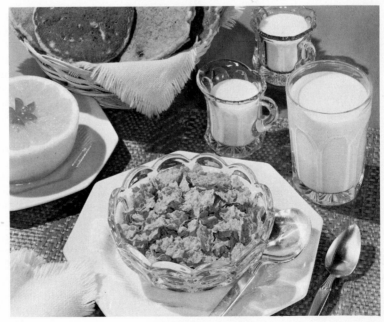

Figure 16–3. A good breakfast supplies one fourth to one third of the day's nutrient needs. (Courtesy, Cereal Institute, Inc., Chicago.)

glass of milk. Sometimes the food choice is so limited that the only way to improve the luncheon pattern would be to carry a packed lunch. This option is not available to the man or woman who lives in a room and who has no opportunity for food preparation. When the choice of food is restricted at lunch, the basic foods must be included in the morning and evening meals.

Through school food services lunches are made available to children and teen-agers in a large proportion of the nation's schools. These lunches are appetizing, nutritious, low in cost, and designed to improve the food habits. (See Chapter 23.)

The homemaker and preschool children often have less satisfactory luncheon patterns than workers or schoolchildren. Often the lunch is a means to use leftovers or a day-to-day monotony of sandwiches or canned foods because the

Figure 16–4. A satisfying lunch for the figure-conscious young woman can be packed at home for school or work. (Courtesy, Sunkist Growers.)

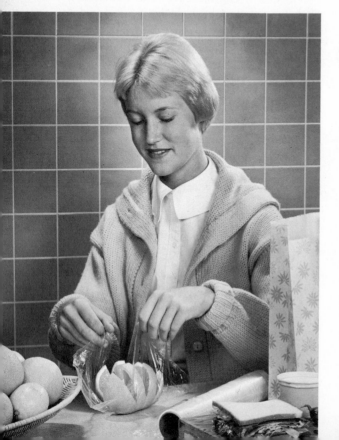

homemaker does not take time for planning or adequate preparation. Luncheons at home can be inexpensive, easy to prepare, tasty, and nutritionally adequate with a little foresight and planning. (See Figure 16–4.) The following menus illustrate good luncheons or suppers that require a minimum of preparation time.

Spanish omelet
Buttered green cabbage
Fresh fruit cup
Cookie
Milk

Sandwich:
    Chopped egg, celery, mayonnaise on
        Whole-wheat bread
Carrot and cucumber sticks
Potato chips
Fresh plums
Spice cupcake
Milk

Salad bowl with mixed greens, diced ham, cheese,
    tomato wedges
French dressing
Whole-wheat muffin with butter and jelly
Pumpkin pie
Milk

Dinner patterns are many. The chief meal of the day may be served at noon or at night, depending upon family custom. In terms of minerals and vitamins it must make up any lack that may have occurred in the other meals. The American custom of making the dinner meal much larger than the other two however, is not a good practice. When one meal provides a large share of the day's carbohydrate and calories, the normal metabolic mechanisms are overloaded. As a result, alternate metabolic pathways may be used. These alternate paths favor the synthesis of adipose tissue and of cholesterol, both of which are likely to be undesirable.

Meat, fish, fowl, or occasionally a cheese, egg, or legume dish comprises the main dish at dinner. Potatoes or a starchy food and a green or yellow vegetable are generally served with the meat. If no salad has been included in the luncheon, it should be given here. The dessert may consist of puddings, cake, ice cream, pastries, or fruit. Milk should again be given to the

Figure 16–5. This colorful meal is rich in all nutrients and balances the day's meals. Dessert might be cake or pastry, but for those who need to watch their weight, fruit or gelatin dessert would be a better choice. (Courtesy, U.S. Department of Agriculture.)

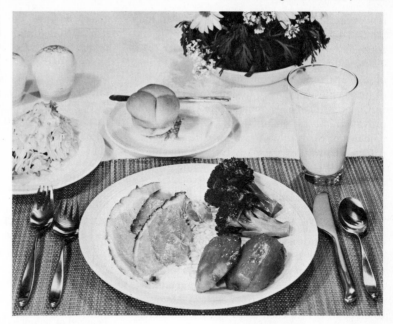

children. For more elaborate meals one may also include an appetizer such as a clear soup or fruit cup. (See Figure 16–5.)

Meal Pattern for Dinner	Sample Menu
Meat, fish, or poultry	Broiled salmon
Potato or substitute	Creamed whole potatoes
Vegetable, green or yellow	Fresh peas
Salad, if none at lunch	Lettuce, grapefruit, and celery salad
Bread, whole-grain or enriched	French dressing
	Parker House rolls
Butter or fortified margarine	Vanilla ice cream
Dessert	Coffee
Beverage	Milk for children

Dinner is often a good time to balance the calories for the day. The active person may eat heartily of potatoes, rolls, desserts as well as of meat, vegetables, and milk, whereas the individual who needs to watch calories can eat meat, vegetables, and milk and more sparingly of the calorie-rich foods. The calorie intake each day should be such that it balances with a normal weight for one's height and body build.

Snacks are often useful. There can be no rigid rule concerning between-meal eating. Active children often benefit by having a midmorning or midafternoon snack, provided that it is of such a nature that the appetite at mealtime is not lessened. Workers in industry, nurses, students, and others experience a "lift" with a snack. This does not imply a continuous pattern of nibbling and raiding the refrigerator at any and all times.

It is the quality of the snack that is important. Concentrated sweets and carbonated beverages may contain little other than carbohydrate and may destroy mealtime appetite; but fruits, fruit juices, milk, or a sandwich, depending upon the individual's activity and the interval between meals, carry many valuable nutrients. Between-meal snacks, properly chosen, may actually aid some persons to maintain weight by reducing the tendency to overeat at mealtime.

MASTER FOOD PLANS

Need for quantitative plans. The Daily Food Guide is a convenient basis for planning nutritionally adequate menus but it does not provide the quantitative information necessary for a number of situations. For example, nutritionists, nurses, and social workers must be able to help families set up food plans that will provide nutritionally adequate meals within their incomes. To establish the cost of adequate diets in terms of the available food supply at varying levels of income, it is necessary to have information on the amounts of specific food groups that must be provided. Such quantitative information on amounts of foods to purchase for various age-sex categories provides the basis for the amount of money to be included for food in the welfare allowances to the poor.

The Consumer and Economic Research Division of the U.S. Department of Agriculture has set up master food plans at five cost levels: low cost; moderate cost; liberal cost; low cost especially adapted to the southeastern states; and economy plan for temporary use when funds are limited. These plans include recommendations for the amounts of food from each of 11 groups to be provided for each of 20 age-sex categories. The amounts of food listed for each category will provide the Recommended Dietary Allowances.

The low-cost and moderate-cost plans are presented in Tables 16–1 and 16–2. The low-cost plan has more flour, cereals, baked foods, potatoes, dry beans, and peas. The moderate-cost and liberal-cost plans allow more meat, eggs, fruit, and vegetables other than potatoes. All plans include generous amounts of milk. Within each plan more or less expensive selections can be made. The moderate-cost plan will cost roughly 25 to 35 per cent more than the low-cost plan, whereas the liberal-cost plan will cost an additional 10 to 20 per cent or even more.

How to use the food plans. To use these plans, follow these steps:

1. List the quantities of food required for one week from each food group for each member of the family. Total the amounts for the family. These totals serve as a guide for the family from week to week.

2. Plan menus for the week, keeping the amounts of the 11 food groups in mind.

3. Prepare the market order, listing the kinds and amounts of foods required for each of the 11 food groups.

4. Compare the amounts of foods in the market order with the totals required for the family from each group (see step 1). If the amounts required for the menus are substantially different from the totals needed by the family revise the menus as needed.

With a little practice the food plans are very easy to use. One example of a week's menus for a family using the low cost plan is given below[*]

SUNDAY
Grapefruit juice
Wheat griddlecakes with syrup
Milk for children

Roast shoulder of pork with stuffing
Sweet potatoes (roasted in pan with meat)
Green beans
Coleslaw
Bread
Apple gingerbread
Milk

Poached or scrambled eggs
Cottage-fried potatoes
Apple-and-celery salad
Toast
Ice cream

MONDAY
Orange juice
Hot wheat cereal with milk
Toast
Milk for children

Egg salad sandwich
Peanut butter and shredded-lettuce sandwich
Gingerbread
Milk

Pork pie with potatoes (pork left from Sunday roast)
Sour beets and beet greens
Bread
Raisin-rice pudding
Milk for children

TUESDAY
Stewed prunes
Ready-to-eat cereal with milk
Toast
Milk for children

Meat turnover (ground beef)
Potato salad

[*]*Food for Families with School Children.* Home and Garden Bulletin No. 13, U.S. Department of Agriculture, Washington, D.C., 1963.

Table 16–1. Low-Cost Family Food Plan*

Weekly Quantities of Food‡ for Each Member of Family

Sex-Age Group†	Milk, Cheese, Ice Cream§ Qt	Meat, Poultry, Fish‖ Lb	Oz	Eggs No.	Dry Beans, Peas, Nuts Lb	Oz	Flour, Cereals, Baked Goods# Lb	Oz	Citrus Fruit, Tomatoes Lb	Oz	Dark-Green and Deep-Yellow Vegetables Lb	Oz	Potatoes Lb	Oz	Other Vegetables and Fruits Lb	Oz	Fats, Oils Lb	Oz	Sugars, Sweets Lb	Oz
Children																				
7 months to 1 year	4	1	4	5	0	0	1	0	1	8	0	4	0	8	1	0	0	1	0	2
1 to 3 years	4	1	12	5	0	1	1	8	1	8	0	4	0	12	2	4	0	4	0	4
3 to 6 years	4	2	0	5	0	2	2	0	1	12	0	4	1	4	3	4	0	6	0	6
6 to 9 years	4	2	4	6	0	4	2	12	2	0	0	8	2	4	4	4	0	8	0	10
Girls																				
9 to 12 years	5 1/2	2	8	7	0	6	2	8	2	4	0	12	2	4	5	0	0	8	0	10
12 to 15 years	7	2	8	7	0	6	2	12	2	4	1	0	2	8	5	0	0	8	0	12
15 to 20 years	7	2	12	7	0	6	2	8	2	4	1	4	2	4	4	12	0	6	0	10
Boys																				
9 to 12 years	5 1/2	2	8	6	0	6	3	0	2	0	0	12	2	8	5	0	0	8	0	12
12 to 15 years	7	2	8	6	0	6	4	4	2	0	0	12	3	4	5	4	0	12	0	12
15 to 20 years	7	3	8	6	0	6	4	12	2	0	0	12	4	4	5	8	0	14	0	14
Women																				
20 to 35 years	3 1/2	3	4	7	0	6	2	8	1	12	1	8	2	0	5	0	0	6	0	10
35 to 55 years	3 1/2	3	4	7	0	6	2	4	1	12	1	8	1	8	4	8	0	4	0	10
55 to 75 years	3 1/2	2	8	5	0	4	2	0	2	0	1	0	1	4	3	12	0	4	0	6
75 years and over	3 1/2	2	4	5	0	4	1	8	2	0	1	0	1	4	3	0	0	4	0	4
Pregnant**	5 1/2	3	12	7	0	6	2	12	3	4	2	0	1	8	5	8	0	6	0	6
Lactating**	8	3	12	7	0	6	3	12	3	4	1	8	3	4	5	8	0	10	0	10
Men																				
20 to 35 years	3 1/2	3	8	6	0	6	4	4	1	12	0	12	3	4	5	8	0	12	1	0
35 to 55 years	3 1/2	3	4	6	0	6	3	12	1	12	0	12	3	0	5	0	0	10	0	12
55 to 75 years	3 1/2	3	0	6	0	4	2	12	1	12	0	12	2	4	4	8	0	10	0	10
75 years and over	3 1/2	2	12	6	0	4	2	8	1	8	0	12	2	0	4	4	0	8	0	8

*Family Food Plans 1964. Consumer and Food Economics Research Division, U.S. Department of Agriculture, Hyattsville, Maryland, 1964.
†Age groups include the persons of the first age listed up to but not including those of the second age listed.
‡Food as purchased or brought into the kitchen from garden or farm.
§Fluid whole milk, or its calcium equivalent in cheese, evaporated milk, dry milk, or ice cream.
‖Bacon and salt pork should not exceed 1/3 pound for each 5 pounds of meat group.
#Weight in terms of flour and cereal. Count 1 1/2 pounds bread as 1 pound flour.
**Three additional quarts of milk are suggested for pregnant and lactating teen-agers.

Table 16–2. Moderate-Cost Family Food Plan*

Weekly Quantities of Food‡ for Each Member of Family

Sex-Age Group†	Milk, Cheese, Ice Cream§ (Qt)	Meat, Poultry, Fish‖ (Lb)	(Oz)	Eggs (No.)	Dry Beans, Peas, Nuts (Lb)	(Oz)	Flour, Cereals, Baked Goods# (Lb)	(Oz)	Citrus Fruit, Tomatoes (Lb)	(Oz)	Dark-Green and Deep-Yellow Vegetables (Lb)	(Oz)	Potatoes (Lb)	(Oz)	Other Vegetables and Fruits (Lb)	(Oz)	Fats, Oils (Lb)	(Oz)	Sugars, Sweets (Lb)	(Oz)
Children																				
7 months to 1 year	5	1	8	6	0	0	0	14	1	8	0	4	0	0	1	8	0	1	0	2
1 to 3 years	5	2	4	6	0	1	1	4	1	8	0	4	0	0	2	12	0	4	0	4
3 to 6 years	5	2	12	6	0	1	1	12	2	0	0	4	1	0	4	0	0	6	0	8
6 to 9 years	5	3	4	7	0	2	2	8	2	4	0	8	1	12	4	12	0	10	0	14
Girls																				
9 to 12 years	5 1/2	4	4	7	0	4	2	8	2	8	0	12	2	0	5	8	0	8	0	12
12 to 15 years	7	4	8	7	0	4	2	8	2	8	1	0	2	4	5	12	0	12	0	14
15 to 20 years	7	4	8	7	0	4	2	4	2	8	1	4	2	0	5	8	0	8	0	12
Boys																				
9 to 12 years	5 1/2	4	4	7	0	4	2	12	2	4	0	12	2	4	5	8	0	10	0	14
12 to 15 years	7	4	12	7	0	4	4	0	2	4	0	12	3	0	6	0	0	14	1	0
15 to 20 years	7	5	4	7	0	6	4	8	2	8	0	12	4	0	6	8	1	2	1	2
Women																				
20 to 35 years	3 1/2	4	12	8	0	4	2	4	2	4	1	8	1	8	5	12	0	8	0	14
35 to 55 years	3 1/2	4	12	8	0	4	2	4	2	4	1	8	1	4	5	0	0	6	0	8
55 to 75 years	3 1/2	4	4	6	0	2	1	8	2	4	0	12	1	4	4	4	0	6	0	8
75 years and over	3 1/2	3	8	6	0	2	1	4	2	4	0	12	1	0	3	12	0	4	0	8
Pregnant**	5 1/2	5	8	8	0	4	2	12	3	4	2	0	1	8	5	12	0	6	0	8
Lactating**	8	5	8	8	0	4	3	12	3	8	1	8	2	12	6	4	0	12	0	12
Men																				
20 to 35 years	3 1/2	5	0	7	0	4	4	0	2	4	0	12	3	0	6	8	1	0	0	4
35 to 55 years	3 1/2	4	12	7	0	4	3	8	2	4	0	12	2	8	5	12	1	14	1	0
55 to 75 years	3 1/2	4	8	7	0	2	2	8	2	4	0	12	2	4	5	8	0	12	0	14
75 years and over	3 1/2	4	8	7	0	2	2	4	2	4	0	12	2	0	5	4	0	8	0	12

*Family Food Plans 1964. Consumer and Food Economics Research Division, U.S. Department of Agriculture, Hyattsville, Maryland, 1964.

†Age groups include the persons of the first age listed up to but not including those of the second age listed.

‡Food as purchased or brought into the kitchen from garden or farm.

§Fluid whole milk, or its calcium equivalent in cheese, evaporated milk, dry milk, or ice cream.

‖Bacon and salt pork should not exceed 1/3 pound for each 5 pounds of meat group.

#Weight in terms of flour and cereal. Count 1 1/2 pounds bread as 1 pound flour.

**Three additional quarts of milk are suggested for pregnant and lactating teen-agers.

236

Vegetable slaw: Cabbage, minced onion, radish
  slices, and dressing
Peanut butter cookies
Milk

Lima bean–tomato casserole
Spinach
Cornmeal muffins
Sweet-potato custard
Milk for children

WEDNESDAY
Grapefruit juice
French toast   Syrup
Milk for children

Cheese and lettuce sandwiches
Beet and green bean salad
Graham crackers
Milk

Spaghetti with meat balls
Salad bowl: Lettuce, celery, carrot, cabbage
French bread
Baked apple with milk

THURSDAY
Tomato juice
Hot wheat cereal with milk
Toasted rolls
Milk for children

Lima bean soup
Cottage cheese and lettuce sandwich on raisin bread
Oatmeal cookies
Milk

Oven-fried chicken
Scalloped potatoes
Carrots
Orange, chopped prune, and cabbage salad
Bread
Butterscotch pudding

FRIDAY
Stewed prunes
Oatmeal and milk
Toast
Milk for children

Corn and onion soup
Deviled-egg sandwich, or deviled egg salad for those
  at home
Celery
Bread
Orange
Milk

Baked perch fillets
Mashed potatoes
Green peas and onions
Biscuits
Hot apple pie
Milk for children

SATURDAY
Orange juice
Fried cornmeal mush with syrup
Milk for children

Cold chicken
Potato cakes
Shredded carrot salad
Pickles
Bread
Oatmeal cookies
Milk

Braised liver
Riced potatoes
5-minute cabbage
Jellied tomato and cottage cheese salad
Bread
Sliced peaches
Cookies
Milk for children

PROBLEMS

Problems 1 to 4. Use the following family group for the problems listed, or substitute
another family grouping:
  Father: 36 years old; 25 pounds underweight; works in a factory; carries lunch to work.
  Mother: 32 years old; pregnant (seventh month); does all her own housework.
  Boy: 10 years; in school; very active; comes home at noon for lunch.
  Girl: three years.
1. *Problem.* Tabulate the daily nutritional requirements for each member of the family by
   referring to the table of allowances on page 31.
2. *Problem.* Using the moderate-cost food plan on page 236, tabluate the amounts of foods
   needed for one week from each of the food groups for the entire family.

3. *Problem*. Plan menus for a week on the basis of the amounts of foods tabulated in problem 2.
4. *Problem*. Prepare a market list for the menus, being sure that the amounts in the market order and the food allowances from each group correspond.
5. *Problem*. Select a series of menus from any popular magazine. Check them against the Four Food Groups for dietary adequacy. Point out good examples of menu planning.
6. *Problem*. Plan breakfast and supper menus for three days for a woman who lives alone and who works in a department store. She is of normal weight and 47 years old. She eats a lunch consisting of soup, crackers, ice cream or pie, and coffee. She has a refrigerator at home, but only a two-burner hot plate on which to cook.

CITED REFERENCE

1. *Breakfast Source Book.* Cereal Institute, Chicago, 1959.

ADDITIONAL REFERENCES

Asprey, G. M., *et al.:* "Effect of Eating at Various Times on Free-Style Swimming Performance," *J. Am. Diet. Assoc.,* **47**:198–200, 1965.
Henthorn, F. Y.: "Better Breakfasts," *Am. J. Nurs.,* **63**:98–100, Aug. 1966.
Ohlson, M. A., and Hart, B. P.: "Influence of Breakfast on Total Day's Food Intake," *J. Am. Diet. Assoc.,* **47**:282–86, 1965.
Thornton, R., and Horvath, S. M.: "Blood Sugar Levels After Eating and After Omitting Breakfast," *J. Am. Diet. Assoc.,* **47**:474–77, 1965.

MEAL PLANNING AIDS FOR FAMILIES

Publications by U.S. Department of Agriculture, Washington, D.C.
Eat a Good Breakfast, Leaflet 268.
Family Fare: Food Management and Recipes, G 1.
Food for Families with School Children, G 13.
Food for Families with Young Children, G 5.
Food Guide for Older Folks, G 17.
Food for the Young Couple, G 85.
"A Food Guide for the Ages, from Baby to Gramps," in *Food for Us All—Yearbook of Agriculture 1969,* pp. 294–303.
"Food Planning for Families at 3 Different Cost Levels," *ibid.,* pp. 279–85.

17 Quality and Economy Factors in Food Selection

Today's homemaker has more money to spend, spends less time in food preparation, and serves better meals than at any time in history. She married at a younger age, has a better education, and enjoys more leisure than did her mother. She lives longer and returns to the work force when her children are in school, if not sooner. All these factors influence the numerous judgments she must make as a shopper, concerning quality, brand, nutritive value, price, convenience, variety, and glamor. During a given year she will purchase about one ton of food for each teen-ager and adult in her family. On this food she will spend, on a national average, about 17 per cent of the family income. (See Figure 17–1.)

Today's foods are more wholesome, are more nutritious, and lend more variety to the diet than foods at any previous time have. Although food costs are higher than 10 years ago, incomes have risen rapidly; hence one hour of a man's labor today will buy more food than it would have 10 years ago. Food is the largest single item in the budget of most families. Obviously the proportion spent for food varies widely in different circumstances. One can be adequately nourished at many cost levels, but to be so when

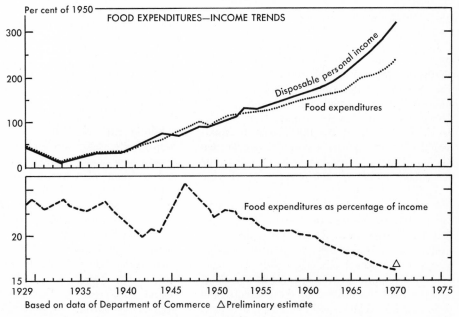

Figure 17–1. The amount of money spent for food has risen steadily, but the percentage of total income spent for food has declined to 17 per cent. At low-income levels, however, much higher proportions of total income must be spent for food. (Courtesy, U.S. Department of Agriculture.)

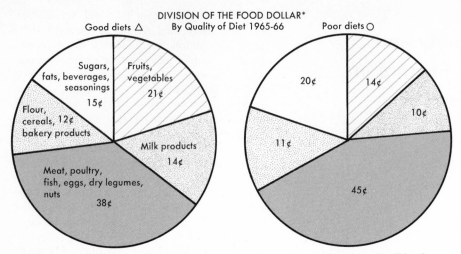

DIVISION OF THE FOOD DOLLAR*
By Quality of Diet 1965-66

Good diets △   Poor diets ○

* By families using $9-$12 worth of food per person a week; just above U.S. average for all families.
△ Had recommended dietary allowances (1963) for 7 nutrients.   U.S. households, data for one year.
○ Had less than 2/3 RDA for 1 to 7 nutrients; is not synonymous with hunger and malnutrition

Figure 17–2. The quality of the diet is influenced by the allotment of the food dollar to various food groups. In good diets a larger share of the food dollar is spent for milk and fruits and vegetables; a smaller share of the dollar is spent for the meat group and for sugars, fats, and beverages. (Courtesy, U.S. Department of Agriculture.)

the income is low requires careful planning, considerable ingenuity, and time to make the less varied diet interesting.

The amount of money required for food for any given family depends on the size of the family, the number of children and their ages, the activities of the various members, special needs for pregnancy and lactation, and possible therapeutic requirements. The cost of food is decidedly influenced by the choice of foods within each group, the amount of preparation the food has undergone before its sale, the type of market, packaging, and so on. (See Figure 17–2.)

Convenience foods. Homemakers today take for granted the built-in services in many foods that have been cleaned, trimmed, and made ready for cooking, such as poultry, washed greens, and frozen foods. They purchase many items that require only the opening of a package or a can and the heating of the contents, and others, such as cake or pudding mixes, that need one or two simple steps in mixing before cooking. Among the great variety of convenience foods in today's markets are

Canned foods: fruits, vegetables, seafood, meats, stews, spaghetti, gravy, soups
Dehydrated foods: instantized milk, instant potatoes, instant coffee, soups
Frozen foods: fruits, vegetables, breads, pastries, cakes, ready-to-eat or ready-to-bake poultry, meat, and fish dishes, complete dinners, pizza, Chinese egg rolls, appetizers, and so on.

Studies on costs[1,2] have shown that canned soups, fruits, vegetables, and citrus juices, frozen orange juice and vegetables, and muffin, cake, and pudding mixes compare favorably in cost with home-prepared fresh products. Items that are appreciably more expensive are usually those that involve much preparation or that have a short shelf life, for example, ready-to-eat salads, packaged salad greens, ready-to-bake rolls, pastries, frozen entrees, and frozen vegetables in sauces. For some homemakers the somewhat higher costs may be less important than the appreciable savings in time that convenience foods afford.

Ten recommendations for effecting economy. The quality characteristics for specific food groups must be understood if wise selections are to be made. In general, appreciable savings can be made if the following suggestions are observed in the purchase and use of food.

1. Plan meals for several days at one time. Use the Four Food Groups as the basis for menu planning to assure good nutrition.

2. Read newspapers for reports of the U.S. Department of Agriculture on foods in plentiful supply. When planning menus, take advantage of advertised specials. (See Figure 17–3.)

3. Use a market list. Be prepared to make substitutions when other foods of equal nutritive value are cheaper. Resist the temptation to purchase many luxury foods now available in markets. Avoid impulse buying.

4. Purchase foods the family will eat. Uneaten foods are no bargain. The wise homemaker, however, introduces new foods from time to time so that her family may learn to enjoy a wide variety.

5. Read labels on packages and cans. Know what the specifications mean. Compare weights and costs of various brands. The private label of a market is often less expensive than nationally advertised brands.

6. Purchase grades according to intended use in the menu.

7. Buy large-size packages only if the price per unit is less, if there is space to properly store the food, and if the food can be used before it spoils.

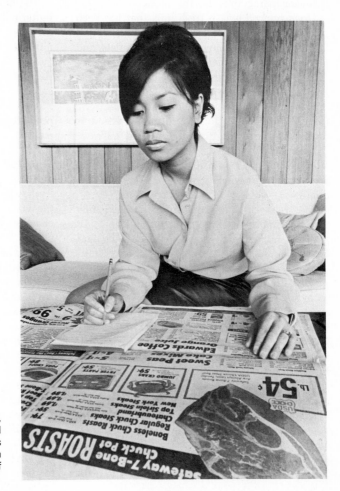

Figure 17–3. Before going to the market, this homemaker checks the advertised food prices in her newspaper. She adjusts her menu plans accordingly and prepares a market list. (Courtesy, U.S. Department of Agriculture.)

8. Provide storage conditions that maintain the wholesomeness and nutritive value of the food.

9. Use foods when they are in optimum condition. If there are leftovers, plan for their prompt use, usually within 24 hours.

10. Eat meals at home or carry lunch whenever practical. Meals in restaurants or at lunch counters generally cost more than twice as much as similar food prepared at home.

MILK GROUP

Types of milk. Among the kinds of milk available in the market, those described in the following paragraphs are the most common.

Homogenized milk is fresh milk that has been pasteurized and subjected to a process that breaks up the fat into very fine droplets and mixes them so completely as to make it impossible for the fat to rise as cream. It now accounts for most of the fluid milk sold. This milk has a "richer" taste, but it is not different in food value from plain milk. It gives a softer curd and is more easily digested than a firm curd milk.

Skim milk is fresh pasteurized milk from which the fat has been removed. It contains all the nutrients of whole milk except fat and vitamin A.

Two per cent milk is fresh pasteurized milk which contains only 2 per cent fat and up to 10 per cent milk solids to give a richer body and flavor than skim milk.

Fortified milks are those to which one or more nutrients have been added. Vitamin D is added to most evaporated and fresh whole milks to a level of 400 I.U. per quart. Vitamin A is sometimes added to skim milk. Multiple fortified milk incorporates multivitamin preparations including vitamins A, D, and the B complex; it must conform to local or state regulations.

Chocolate milk is whole milk to which chocolate syrup has been added and chocolate-flavored milk drink is skim or partially skimmed milk to which the chocolate syrup has been added. The nutrients of milk are diluted in proportion to the amount of chocolate syrup used. The syrup adds caloric value without a corresponding addition of protective nutrients. These flavored milks are nutritious and wholesome, but they should not become the sole way in which milk is taken. Some children refuse to take white milk when they become accustomed to the sweetness of these forms of milk.

Cultured milks are prepared from pasteurized milk to which certain desirable microorganisms have been added. They have a nutritive value equal to that of the milk from which they are made. The fermentation of the milk results in a formation of lactic acid from the lactose and some coagulation of casein. Lactic acid, in turn, is believed to encourage a favorable intestinal flora. The consistency of the milk is less fluid, and the flavor is much desired by some people.

The most widely used of the cultured milks is buttermilk, produced by culturing skim milk, partly skimmed milk, or reconstituted nonfat dry milk with *Streptococcus lactis* and incubating it. Salt is usually added to bring out the flavor. *Acidophilus milk,* of very limited distribution, is cultured with *Lactobacillus acidophilus* under standard conditions. *Yogurt* is a pasteurized milk product of custardlike consistency which is fermented by using a mixed culture of organisms. It may be prepared from whole milk, skim milk, or partially skimmed milk.

Evaporated milk is the product obtained from fresh whole milk after a little more than half the water has been removed. The protein is so changed that a softer, finer curd results. The milk is homogenized, usually fortified with vitamin D, and sterilized. When diluted with water to its original volume, it has a composition like that of whole sweet milk. Evaporated milk is easily digested, free from bacteria until the can is opened, and lends itself particularly well to the preparation of infant formulas.

Condensed milk is prepared by adding sugar to milk and reducing its water content by evaporation. It owes its keeping qualities to its high sugar content (42 per cent) rather than to the application of heat. It has found wide use in the preparation of desserts.

Dried milk results from the removal of 95 to 98 per cent of the water from fresh milk. *Nonfat dry milk* is made from skim milk and accounts for most of the dry milk on the market. Dried milks are made by spraying partially evaporated milk into warm dry air (spray process). The *instantizing* process produces a fine powder that dissolves instantly. One pound of nonfat dry milk is equivalent to about 5 quarts of fresh skim milk and is therefore a concentrated source of protein, calcium, riboflavin, and other nutrients. Dried milks are easily stored and transported for they require no refrigeration. Nonfat dry milk has excellent keeping qualities, but whole dried milk is subject to oxidation and consequent rancidity.

Filled milk is any milk or cream in which the butterfat has been removed and replaced with a vegetable fat (usually coconut oil). The nutritive value is similar to that of whole milk.

Imitation milk is a product resembling milk but it contains no milk products such as skim milk or nonfat dry milk. Typical constituents of an imitation milk are a protein source such as sodium caseinate or soy protein, corn syrup solids, sugar, and a vegetable fat (usually coconut oil). Additives for color, flavor, and stability are normally added. The nutritive values vary from brand to brand, but they are generally lower in protein, calcium, and vitamins and are not a replacement for whole milk.

Cream is the fat of milk which has been separated by centrifugation or by gravity. It is sold as light or "coffee" cream, which has a fat content of 18 to 20 per cent, and as heavy or "whipping" cream, which has a fat content of 35 to 40 per cent. *Half-and-half*, often used in high-calorie diets, consists of half milk and half light cream with a final fat content of about 11.5 per cent. *Sour cream* is light cream which has been cultured under controlled conditions.

Cheese. Cheese is a milk product representing the solids or curd of milk. The curd may be produced by the action of rennet or of lactic acid. As the milk casein coagulates and becomes semisolid, the whey separates out. The difference in varieties of cheese is due to the kind of milk used—cow (most common), goat, or sheep; the method used for curding the milk—rennet or lactic acid; the temperature and humidity for ripening; the amount of salt and seasonings used; the amount of moisture retained; and the type of bacteria or mold used for ripening.

More than 400 varieties of hard, semihard, and soft cheeses are marketed, but American, Cheddar, cottage, cream, and process cheeses account for the bulk of the consumption in this country. Cheeses with little curing are mild in flavor and less expensive; those cured for six months or longer are mellow to sharp in flavor. Good-quality cheese has a smooth, waxy texture, uniform color, and a nutty, slightly acid flavor. Cheeses that have been aged for six months or longer have better cooking qualities.

Process cheese consists of a blending of mild American cheese with other cheeses, followed by pasteurization. An emulsifying agent, such as disodium phosphate or sodium citrate, gives a smooth texture and keeps the fat from separating out. The process cheeses have a consistently uniform flavor and texture, and they keep well; they do not have the fine flavor of an aged Cheddar.

Purchase of milk and cheese. Whole milk purchased in half-gallon or gallon containers in supermarkets is less expensive than milk delivered to the door. Nonfat dry milk costs about one third as much as fresh milk, and its use for cooking can result in worthwhile savings. Many people find that mixing one part reconstituted nonfat milk with one part whole milk gives a highly acceptable beverage. Evaporated milk is also less expensive than fresh milk and lends itself well to cooking. American, Cheddar, process, and cottage cheese are economical buys. Among the expensive items in the dairy group are cream, ice cream, aged cheese, and imported cheeses.

MEAT GROUP

Quality of meat. The standards for various grades of beef, veal, and lamb established by the U.S. Department of Agriculture are based upon the amount of surface fat and marbling (fat interspersed among the muscle fibers), color, firmness of flesh, texture, and maturity. (See Table 17–1.) No comparable grading standards have been set up for pork.

Prime beef, which is very tender and has a considerable amount of surface fat and generous

Table 17–1. Government Grades for Meat

Beef	Veal	Lamb
Prime	Prime	Prime
Choice	Choice	Choice
Good	Good	Good
Standard	Standard	—
Commercial	—	—
Utility	Utility	Utility
Cutter	Cull	Cull
Canner	—	—

U.S. CHOICE

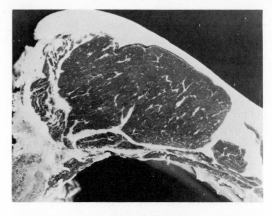

U.S. GOOD

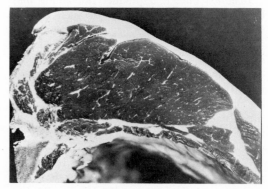

Figure 17–4. Two grades of meat. Note the greater amount of separable fat and the generous marbling of the choice cut. (Courtesy, U.S. Department of Agriculture.)

marbling, is sold chiefly to hotels and restaurants. Many retail markets sell only one grade of meat —either choice or good, depending upon location. These grades are less generously marbled with fat than prime meat, but they are juicy and flavorful. Standard beef has very little fat, is less tender and juicy, but is quite rich in flavor. (See Figure 17–4.)

Beef is the flesh of cattle over one year old. Good-quality beef has a bright, cherry-red color; a fine-grain texture marbled with fat; solid creamy-white layers of fat surrounding the muscle bundles; and porous red bones.

Choice veal is the flesh of a calf six weeks to three months old. It has a fine-grain texture; grayish-pink color; clear, hard fat sparsely distributed; and porous red bones.

Lamb is the flesh of sheep two to three months old, but a well-fed animal may still be classed as lamb, rather than mutton, at one year. The flesh is firm and fine grained and pink in color; and the fat is firm, white, and flaky.

Pork includes the flesh of a suckling pig to a mature medium-size pig. Its flesh is fine and firm with a minute layer of fat coating the fibers; the color is grayish pink; the fat is smooth and white; and the bones are soft and tinged with red.

Poultry of best quality has these characteristics: flexible breastbone and well-fleshed breasts; short, fleshy legs; flexible wings which spring back into place when pulled out; fat well distributed but not abundant; dry, firm skin without cuts, tears, or bruises. The class of the bird may be designated as "broiler," "roaster," or "stewing hen."

Selection of meat for economy. Although meat is relatively more costly than some of the other foods, the homemaker can keep costs down by intelligent selection. Prime and choice grades are more expensive per pound than good and standard cuts; they also yield less lean edible portion per pound. When there is a choice of grades available, good or standard grades for many purposes will yield delicious dishes at considerable less cost than prime or choice grades. When comparing costs per pound, one must consider the number of lean, edible portions. For example, 1 pound of spare ribs will serve only two persons, whereas 1 pound of lean round steak will serve three to four. (See Figure 17–5.)

COST OF 1/3 OF A DAY'S PROTEIN*
Meats and Meat Alternates, June 1970

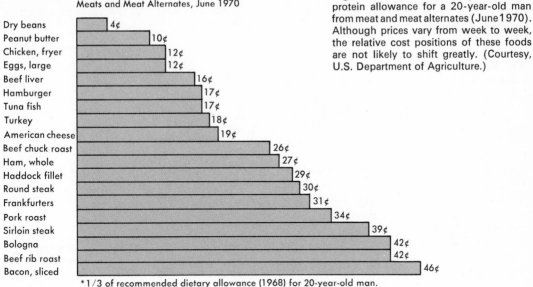

Dry beans — 4¢
Peanut butter — 10¢
Chicken, fryer — 12¢
Eggs, large — 12¢
Beef liver — 16¢
Hamburger — 17¢
Tuna fish — 17¢
Turkey — 18¢
American cheese — 19¢
Beef chuck roast — 26¢
Ham, whole — 27¢
Haddock fillet — 29¢
Round steak — 30¢
Frankfurters — 31¢
Pork roast — 34¢
Sirloin steak — 39¢
Bologna — 42¢
Beef rib roast — 42¢
Bacon, sliced — 46¢

*1/3 of recommended dietary allowance (1968) for 20-year-old man.
BLS prices, average for U.S. cities

Figure 17–5. The cost of 1/3 of a day's protein allowance for a 20-year-old man from meat and meat alternates (June 1970). Although prices vary from week to week, the relative cost positions of these foods are not likely to shift greatly. (Courtesy, U.S. Department of Agriculture.)

The homemaker should learn to recognize the various cuts of meat and be able to select them according to their use in the menu. (See Figure 17–6.) The less tender cuts that require moist heat in preparation are less expensive than those cooked by dry heat, such as oven roasts, steaks, and chops. By using flavoring aids, including vegetables, spices, and herbs, many delicious dishes may be prepared.

Expenditure for meat can be reduced if the selection is made according to market supply. Pork may be less costly at one time and beef at another. Poultry and fish have been good buys in recent years, although shellfish is a luxury item. If a freezer is available, it may be a good idea to purchase additional cuts when they are on sale.

The supply of meat may be stretched by using it in casseroles, stews, hearty soups, meat loaf, or creamed dishes. Main dishes using eggs,

Figure 17–6. Seven basic cuts of meat. This diagram may be used for beef, lamb, veal, or pork. (Courtesy, National Live Stock and Meat Board, Chicago.)

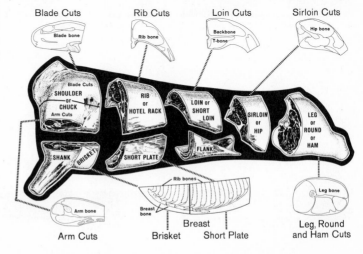

cheese, dry peas and beans, or peanut butter may be substituted occasionally for meat.

Quality of eggs. A strictly fresh egg has a thick, gelatinous white, a round, firm, upstanding yolk, and gives a delicate flavor. As the egg ages, the yolk and white become more watery so that the egg flattens out over a large surface when broken. Eggs may be graded as AA, the finest quality, new laid, especially good for poached or fried eggs where delicacy of flavor is desirable; A, of excellent quality for all table use and cooking; B, useful for all cooking and some table purposes; C, with thin whites and weakened yolks which break easily, but quite suitable for baking and cooking. (See Figure 17–7.) Cracked eggs are likely to be contaminated by *Salmonella* and should be used only in foods that are to be thoroughly heated. They are not suitable for table use or for foods such as custards cooked at low heat.

Selection of eggs for economy. The price of eggs is related to the grade, size, and color. For each size the following minimum weights have been set up:

Size	Minimum Weight Per Dozen
	ounces
Jumbo	30
Extra large	27
Large	24
Medium	21
Small	18
Peewee or pullet	15

Small eggs are often a better buy in the fall, whereas large eggs may cost only a few cents more during winter and spring months. To determine whether one size egg is a better buy than another, the prices may be compared on the basis of the above weights. A practical guide is this:[3] if the difference in cost is less than seven cents between one size and the next smaller size, the larger egg is a better buy.

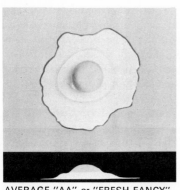

AVERAGE "AA" or "FRESH FANCY"

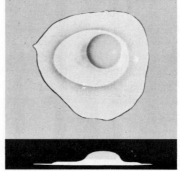

AVERAGE "A"

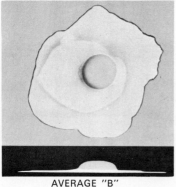

AVERAGE "B"

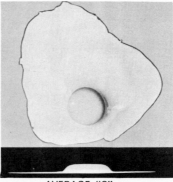

AVERAGE "C"

Figure 17–7. Interior quality of eggs. Note round yolk and thick white of grade AA and A eggs, flat yolk and thin white which spread out on the plate of grade B and C eggs. (Courtesy, U.S. Department of Agriculture.)

People in some communities prefer brown eggs (Boston, for example), whereas others prefer white eggs (New York and Philadelphia). The color of the shell has nothing to do with the nutritive values; so there is no merit in paying an additional amount for eggs of one color or another.

VEGETABLE-FRUIT GROUP

Quality of vegetables and fruits. Fresh, canned, frozen and dehydrated vegetables and fruits provide a broad selection on a year-round basis.

Crisp, ripe, but not overmature vegetables that are firm in texture and free from blemishes should be selected. As vegetables become too mature, the lignocellulose which is formed gives the characteristic stringy or woody texture which cannot be overcome by cookery. Wilted vegetables are lower in carotene and ascorbic acid content than the crisp vegetables. Vegetables deteriorate rapidly in palatability and nutritive value unless proper storage facilities are provided.

Fruits improve in flavor and aroma with ripening. As the fruit ripens, there is an increase in the sugar content and the volatile flavoring compounds and a decrease in the starch and organic acid. Unripe fruits lack flavor, and the sugar content will not have been fully developed. Some fruits such as peaches and pears bruise so easily that they are customarily picked before fully ripe. They should be allowed to ripen fully at room temperature before refrigeration.

Bananas are high in starch content when green. During the ripening at room temperature, this starch is changed to more digestible sugars. Bananas have the best flavor when the skin shows speckles of brown (not bruised or decayed spots). A tinge of green at the stem end of a banana is an indication that the fruit is not sufficiently ripe for use in its raw form.

Canned fruits and vegetables are usually sold by grade, using the grading of the U.S. Department of Agriculture or, more frequently, similar grade standards maintained by the manufacturer. Grade A products are of excellent quality,

uniform in color and size of pieces, practically free of blemishes, and of the proper degree of maturity. When serving fruits or vegetables in a way where size and and color are important, this grade is the preferable choice. Grade B fruits and vegetables are of less uniform color and size of pieces, slightly less tender, and less free of defects. They are just as nutritious as grade A vegetables.

Commercially canned fruits and vegetables closely approximate cooked fresh products in their nutritive values since vacuum closure of the cans reduces the rate of oxidation. There is some unavoidable loss of ascorbic acid and thiamine.

The water-soluble nutrients distribute themselves in canned foods so that the concentration is about equal in the liquid and solid phases. Thus, if the contents are in the proportion of two-thirds solid and one-third liquid, two thirds of the vitamin C, for example, would be in the solids and one third in the liquid. If the liquid is not used, one third of the original vitamin C value would be lost. When vegetables are used, the liquid should be drained off first into a saucepan and reduced in volume by heating before the solids are added.

The nutritive values of the frozen products are equal to the fresh foods; in fact, frozen fruits and vegetables that have been packed immediately after harvesting may be superior to fresh foods that have been improperly handled from farm to market to consumer. Frozen foods require storage at O° F, and thus a freezer or a separate freezing compartment in the refrigerator is essential if the foods are to be kept for more than a few days. When frozen foods are to be used within a week, it is satisfactory to keep them in the ice-cube section of the refrigerator. The consumer should select frozen foods only in markets which appear to use care in the display of these foods. If foods are stored above the freezing line indicated in the cabinet, or if frozen foods have thawed, they will lose some of the qualities of texture and may even spoil because of the growth of organisms.

Purchase of vegetables and fruits. Fresh fruits and vegetables locally grown and in season are usually less expensive. Apples, cabbage, and root vegetables in fall, citrus fruits in winter, and peaches, tomatoes, and melons in mid-summer to fall represent examples of good buys. The cost of canned and frozen products should be compared with the fresh food in terms of edible portions per purchase unit. Fresh peas, for example, will yield about two servings per pound, and even in season are likely to be more expensive than frozen or canned peas.

Canned foods should be selected according to use. For service as dessert, peach halves may be preferred, but pieces will serve as well at less cost in a fruit cup or salad.

Fruits and vegetables are highly perishable, so that they should be used before deterioration takes place. The liberal use of these foods in their raw state ensures maximum nutritive values.

BREAD-CEREAL GROUP

Flour. Wheat is superior to other flours in giving a light, porous quality to leavened products and is consequently the grain of first importance in the United States. Two proteins in wheat provide for the development of a high gluten content when moisture is added. The elasticity of the gluten permits the ready expansion by gas and consequent lightness of the finished product. The development of gluten depends upon the extent of mixing and the amount and type of liquid used. Long mixing tends to toughen gluten and makes the leavening process more difficult. Gluten develops more quickly in a batter than in a dough. All-purpose flours find widest usefulness for the multiple purposes for which flour is used in the home.

The wheat flour used in the United States is usually a 70 per cent extraction; this means that 70 per cent of the grain, namely the endosperm, is used, and the bran and germ layers are discarded for animal feeds. Practically all of the flour sold in retail markets is now enriched.

The ancient civilizations of the Incas in Peru, the Mayas in Mexico, and the Indians of North America used corn or maize—a food unknown to the Spanish adventurers and the English colonists. Even today cornmeal is widely used in the southern states where it is prominent in

corn bread as well as in spoon bread and mush, and in the Southwest corn is used for the preparation of tortillas.

Rye and barley flours are used much more extensively in Europe than in America. These flours produce a heavier loaf of bread than that of wheat.

The flours of potato, soybean, oats, rice, banana, and taro find some usefulness in specialty products; they are a great help to the individual who is allergic to wheat.

Kinds of bread. The Food and Drug Administration has established standards of identity for five kinds of bread: white, enriched, milk, raisin, and whole wheat. Under these regulations specified levels of certain ingredients must be included for bread offered for interstate sale.[4] For numerous other breads on the market no standards of identity have been developed. However, interstate trade requires that the ingredients of such breads be listed on the label in the order of the amounts used in the formula.

About 85 per cent of all white bread and rolls sold to the American public are enriched. The B vitamins and iron are included at levels to equal whole-wheat bread (see Figure 13–4).

Whole-wheat flour is the only flour that may be used in bread labeled as "whole-wheat," "graham," or "entire-wheat" bread. This bread accounts for only a small proportion of bread sold in America today. Nutritively speaking, whole-wheat and enriched breads are so similar that one can be guided by taste preferences and cost of the loaf in making one's selection. On the other hand, many people buy breads labeled as "cracked wheat," "wheaten," "wheat," and "rye" in the mistaken belief that they are made with the whole grain. These breads, in fact, are made with white flour and varying proportions of cracked wheat, whole-wheat, or rye flours, as the case may be.

Numerous specialty breads are available in bakeries and supermarkets. Often these are labeled as being low in calories or possessing other special nutritional qualities. On a weight-for-weight basis, however, the caloric value of white, rye, whole-wheat, protein, and many specialty breads is so similar that there is no need to consider them separately.[5] Although soy flour, wheat germ, molasses, and other ingredients increase the nutritive value of bread, these additions are important only in relation to the amounts used in the formula and to the amounts of nutrients contributed to the daily intake.

Breakfast cereals. Hot or cold, enriched or whole grain, from wheat, corn, rice, or oats, cereals are a mainstay of the breakfast. Cereals also find usefulness as ingredients in many desserts, as extenders for main dishes such as meat loaf, as crumb toppings for casserole dishes, and in place of part of the flour in quick breads and yeast breads.

Cereals vary widely in their protein, mineral, and vitamin content. Some cereals are fortified to supply substantial proportions of the daily allowance for vitamins and iron; others are improved in the quantity and quality of protein that they contain. A wide variety of sugar-coated cereals—some fortified, some not—is intended to appeal particularly to children's tastes.

Breakfast cereals vary widely in cost per serving, and the cost is not, of itself, always related to the nutritive value. Labels need to be read and interpreted with care in order to determine which products are the best buy in nutritional value. Generally, cereals that require cooking are more economical than ready-to-serve cereals. Almost all cereals are now of the quick-cooking variety and require only a few minutes of cooking. Individual packets of precooked cereals to which hot water is added are convenient but the per-serving cost is somewhat greater than that of cereals that are cooked in the home. Likewise, individual-serving-size packages of cereal are more expensive than family-size packages.

Bulgur. This has been a popular staple among people of the Near East for centuries. Large quantities of bulgur have been donated by the government in the Food for Peace Program, and lesser amounts have been included in the foods distributed to the poor in the United States. Bulgur is a wheat product of whole or cracked grains with a nutlike flavor and a slightly chewy texture. The wheat is parboiled and dried, and some of the bran is removed. Present methods of processing retain 75 per cent or more of the minerals and vitamins in the wheat.

Pastas. A special kind of hard wheat flour—durum—is used in the manufacture of some 150 different shapes of pastas, including macaroni, spaghetti, vermicelli, and noodles. The pastas are used in many side dishes for the main meal or as a main dish in combination with cheese, meat, fish, or poultry.

Rice. About 95 per cent of the world's rice is grown in the Orient. Rice was first introduced into South Carolina in 1685 and has been an important crop in Louisiana, Texas, Arkansas, and California.

Brown rice is the whole-grain rice with the hull and a little of the bran removed. White rice is milled to remove the hull, bran, and germ. In the milling some of the minerals and vitamins are removed. Since white (polished) rice is a staple for so many of the world's people, enrichment is of major importance. Rice may be enriched by coating the kernels with a premix of vitamins. It should not be washed prior to cooking. The amount of cooking water should be no more than can be absorbed by the rice kernels.

Parboiled rice is steamed by a special process so that the thiamine and other vitamins and minerals are distributed throughout the kernel with only a slight loss taking place in washing and cooking. *Converted rice* is parboiled by a patented process. *Precooked rice* requires the addition of hot water and a short period of standing before it is ready to be served; it is more costly than uncooked rice.

OTHER FOODS

About 15 to 20 per cent of the food expenditure is for fats, sweets, beverages, and foods other than those included in the Four Food Groups. (See Figure 17–2.) In the selection of fats, margarines are much less costly than butter. Hydrogenated fats, lard, and oils are suitable for cooking and frying. Corn, cottonseed, soybean, and safflower oils possess the advantage of being high in linoleic acid and are also inexpensive. Olive oil, prized by some for its flavor, is not a good source of linoleic acid and its cost is greater than that of other oils.

Cane and beet sugars, corn syrup, and corn sugar are inexpensive sources of calories. Confectioners' and brown sugars are slightly more expensive than granulated sugar. Colored sugars for cookie decoration and cinnamon sugar usually sold in shakers are a convenience item, but they are easily prepared in the home at a fraction of the cost. Honey, maple syrup, maple sugar, candies, and cake icings are among the more costly items in the sweets category.

Coffee, tea, cocoa, and carbonated beverages are included in the budget allotment for beverages. It goes without saying that a high consumption of carbonated beverages adds greatly to the grocery bill while yielding no nutritional values other than calories.

Spices, herbs, pickles, and relishes add interest and variety to meals. Spices and herbs lose much of their flavor if kept too long; therefore, one should purchase the size container that will be used up within about a six-month period. Preserves, pickles, and relishes may be expensive, and their use will be sharply restricted when the food budget is limited. Fancy cookies, cakes, pretzels, and many tempting snack items can substantially increase the amount of the grocery bill without adding significantly to the intake of essential nutrients.

PROBLEMS AND REVIEW

1. Prepare a chart that shows the kinds of milk available in a supermarket near your home. Include the following information: size of container; price; principal characteristics of each kind. Write a summary of your study.
2. *Problem.* Assuming that a given family requires 3 quarts of milk per day, calculate the cost of milk for one month, using current prices and purchasing the milk in these ways: (1) as fresh, grade A homogenized milk; (2) as fresh milk for half of the supply and nonfat dry milk equivalent to half of the supply.
3. Determine the kinds of cheeses available in your market. Have you tasted all of these at one time or another? What are their characteristics?
4. What factors determine the grading of eggs? What changes occur in eggs with age?
5. Obtain the prices of various grades and sizes of eggs in local markets and discuss the relative economy of each.
6. List the factors that determine the quality of meat.
7. Why are not all so-called cheap cuts of meat economical?
8. *Problem.* Complete the following table:

	Cost per pound	Protein per Pound as Purchased, Grams	Cost per 100 Grams Protein
Lamb chop		83	
Lamb neck		66	
Pork shoulder		59	
Pork loin chop		70	
Beef rib roast		69	
Beef round		88	
Frankfurter		65	
Frying chicken		69	

9. *Problem.* Calculate the cost of 25 mg ascorbic acid from each of five fresh fruits available in your market.

10. *Problem.* Compare the cost of three brands of canned peaches, canned peas, canned to-matoes. Note labeling information concerning grade. How do you account for the differ-ences?

11. *Problem.* Obtain the prices and weights of family-size packages of ready-to-eat cereals, including the following: cornflakes; puffed wheat; rice flakes; two brands of sugar-coated cereals; two brands of cereals that are fortified with vitamins and minerals. Calculate the cost per ounce. Tabulate the nutritive values stated for one ounce on the label. What conclu-sions can you draw from this study?

12. *Problem.* Compare the label information and cost per pound for five kinds of bread avail-able in your local market.

Cited References

1. Economic Research Service: *Comparative Costs to Consumers of Convenience Foods and Home-Prepared Foods.* Marketing Research Report No. 609, U.S. Department of Agriculture, Washington, D.C. 1963.
2. Martin, K. M., and Robinson, C. H.: *Comparison of Preparation Time and Costs for Con-venience and Home Prepared Foods.* Drexel University, Philadelphia, 1963.
3. *Eggs in Family Meals.* G 103. U.S. Department of Agriculture, Washington, D.C., 1969.
4. *Bread—Facts for Consumer Education.* U.S. Department of Agriculture, Washington, D.C., 1955.
5. Bradley, W. B.: "Breads for Special Dietary Purposes." American Institute of Baking, Chi-cago, 1953.

Additional References

Captain, O. B., and McIntire, M. S.: "Cost and Quality of Food in Poverty and Nonpoverty Urban Areas," *J. Am. Diet. Assoc.,* **55**:569–71, 1969.
Economic Research Service: *What Makes Food Prices.* ERS 308. U.S. Department of Agricul-ture, Washington, D.C., 1969.
Gunderson, F. L., *et al.: Food Standards and Definitions in the United States.* Academic Press, New York, 1963.
Lessons on Meat. National Live Stock and Meat Board, Chicago, 1964.
Moore, M. L.: "When Families Must Eat More for Less," *Nurs. Outlook,* **14**:66–69, April 1966.
Myers, T.: "Food Goes to Market," *J. Home Econ.,* **58**:377–41, 1966.

Budgeting and Buying Aids for Families

Publications by Consumer and Marketing Service, U.S. Department of Agriculture, Washing-ton, D.C.:
Family Food Budgeting for Good Meals, G 94.
How to Buy Beef Roasts, G 146.
How to Buy Beef Steaks, G 145.
How to Buy Eggs, G 144.
How to Buy Fresh Fruits, G 141.
How to Buy Poultry, G 157.
How to Buy Fresh Vegetables, G 143.
How to Use U.S.D.A. Grades in Buying Foods, PA 708.
More Food, Better Diets for Low-Income Families, PA 930.
Hayes, J., ed.: *Food for Us All—Yearbook of Agriculture 1969.* U.S. Department of Agriculture, Washington, D.C., 1969, pp. 45–50; 55–61; 94–252.

18 Basic Principles and Practices in Food Preparation

Importance of quality standards in food preparation. The nutrition of the individual is profoundly influenced by the quality of the food preparation. Highly nutritious foods can be seriously reduced in nutritive values, most especially in the levels of soluble vitamins, when improper methods of preparation are used. When the food resources of a family or of a community are limited, such losses can be of major consequence. Good cookery encourages high acceptance of food, whereas poor cookery leads to excessive plate waste. Many a vegetable, rich in minerals and vitamins, has been left on the plate because it was neglected or abused in its preparation. Generally speaking, food preparation that leads to the highest level of acceptability is also characterized by the highest level of nutrient retention.

The principles of food preparation are based upon the physical and chemical characteristics of the various food groups, which range from those foods high in sugars, starches, and cellulose to those high in proteins and fats. Environmental factors such as heat, light, air, water, and the particular combinations of ingredients must be considered.

Food preparation is much more than a science. It is an art, for it is linked with the total cultural pattern of people. Food preparation requires a sense of discrimination in the blending of flavors, as well as of textures, colors, and shapes. Food preparation, like any skill, requires a considerable amount of practice in order to achieve a high quality of product with efficient use of time, money, and materials.

Methods of cookery. Foods may be cooked by moist heat, by dry heat, or by frying.

Moist heat. Cookery by moist heat includes boiling, stewing, braising, and steaming.

BOILING is cooking in water at 212° F, or 100° C. The bubbles break rapidly on the surface of the water.

SIMMERING is cooking at a temperature below the boiling point—approximately 200° F, or 93° C. The bubbles of steam rise slowly to the surface of the vessel.

STEWING is cooking for a long time at about 200° F. It is used for less tender cuts of meat. The liquid is sometimes thickened.

BRAISING is cooking over direct heat or in an oven in a small amount of liquid at a low temperature with the pan tightly covered.

STEAMING is cooking by the heat of direct steam or in a steam-jacketed vessel such as a double boiler or bain-marie. The pressure cooker employs increased pressure of steam, thus raising the temperature and shortening the cooking time.

Dry heat. Cooking by dry heat includes broiling, baking, and roasting.

BROILING is cooking by direct heat from a gas flame, electric wires, or live coals. It is usually used for tender cuts of meat, and the temperature is high enough quickly to sear the surface.

PAN BROILING is cooking in a hot metal pan on top of the stove with just enough fat to keep the food from sticking; fat is poured off as it accumulates.

BAKING is cooking in an oven using an open or covered pan. The oven *roasting* of meats is really a baking process.

Frying. DEEP FRYING is cooking by immersion in hot fat at 350° to 400° F.

SAUTÉING is cooking in a small amount of fat in a frying pan, the food being turned frequently.

FRICASSEEING is cooking in a small amount of fat and then serving with a sauce.

Microwave cookery. Microwave cookery is gradually gaining in popularity, particularly in institutions, but the equipment is still too expensive for most home use. The food to be cooked is placed in an electronic oven where it is exposed to the penetration of microwaves produced by a magnetron tube. The absorbed microwaves cause agitation of molecules within the food so that heat is generated. Cooking time is one half to one tenth that needed by conventional methods.

Foods are cooked in china, pyrex, ceramic, or paper dishes since these materials permit the microwaves to pass through to be absorbed by the food. Metal utensils are not used since they reflect the microwaves and cause damage to the magnetron.

Only small quantities of food may be cooked at one time. One important disadvantage of microwave cookery is that foods do not brown. Meats, especially, are an unattractive gray color unless subsequently browned. Cakes must be carefully watched since there is a tendency to overbake them, thus resulting in a dry product. The flavor, color, and nutritive values of vegetables compare favorably with other methods of cooking.

EFFECTS OF COOKERY UPON FOOD QUALITIES

Some raw foods, especially fruits and vegetables, are delightful and necessary constituents of the daily diet. Nevertheless, most foods must be cooked to make them acceptable to human beings.

Digestibility. One of the most important reasons for cooking food is to enhance the digestibility. Cooking softens the connective tissue of meat and the coarse fibers of fruits and vegetables so that irritation of the gastrointestinal tract is minimized. Cooking also bursts the starch granule of vegetables and cereals so that hydrolysis of starch is more rapid and complete.

Microbiologic changes. The cooking of food destroys microorganisms and parasites that may be present, but the limitations of cookery in making food safe to eat must also be recognized. Pork, often infested with *Trichinella*, is safe only when the meat is cooked until no tinge of

pink remains in the meat. Some foods are not cooked at sufficiently high temperatures to destroy all microorganisms, or the toxins produced by them, and illness could result. Thus, cooking of food should never be used as an excuse for poor practices in food handling prior to cookery. (See also Chapter 19.)

Enzymatic effects. All plant and animal cells contain enzymes that are released when the cell walls are ruptured as in peeling, cutting, chopping, or grinding food. Subsequently, rapid changes take place in the physical and chemical qualities of the food. For example, because of enzyme action, fresh peaches darken rapidly when they are sliced and exposed to the air. However, if the peaches are cooked, no such darkening takes place because the enzymes, being protein in nature, are inactivated by heat. Also, if some ascorbic acid or lemon juice is sprinkled over the raw peach slices darkening can be delayed because acid retards the enzyme action.

Color changes. Foods undergo many color changes during cookery, some of which enhance the desirability of the product whereas others do not. The color of vegetables and fruits especially is influenced by the pH of the cooking medium. The green pigments in plants change to an olive green and finally brown if subjected to long cooking, especially in an acid medium. If the water is slightly alkaline, the green color is maintained, hence the practice by some of adding a pinch of baking soda to the cooking water for green vegetables. Unfortunately, such addition of alkali is destructive of vitamin C and thiamine, and also results in a product that tends to be mushy.

Some authorities advocate that green vegetables be cooked in an uncovered saucepan for better color, whereas others leave the pan uncovered only for the first few minutes of cooking. White vegetables such as cauliflower, onions, and potatoes become yellow if cooked in water that is alkaline but remain white if a small amount of an acid (cream of tartar) is added.

Red pigments as in fruits—strawberries, plums, raspberries—bleach out into the cooking fluid, and the food itself sometimes appears pale. The color remains red in a slightly acid medium but turns blue in an alkaline medium. The vinegar in pickled beets or with red cabbage helps to retain the attractive red color.

The red color of meat changes to pink, gray, or brown upon exposure to heat. Beef is the only meat served with tinges of red, varying from the bright red of rare beef to the faint pink of fairly well-done meat. Veal, pork, and chicken are cooked until well done with the color being gray to white.

The attractive brown crusts of breads and cakes result from the linkage of certain amino acids in the flour with a sugar when subjected to high heat. This is referred to as the browning reaction. The brown color is also achieved in part by the dextrinization of starch on the surface of the food.

Texture changes. The texture of foods is importantly modified in food preparation. If meat needs to be chewed a great deal before it is swallowed, it is said to be tough. Since proteins become tough when cooked too long or at too high temperatures, it is apparent that the texture would be adversely affected. Meats that contain much connective tissue are tough when cooked by dry heat, but they will be tender if cooked with moist heat. The marination of meat with vinegar, wine, tomato juice, or French dressing prior to cooking has a tenderizing effect upon the meat and connective-tissue fibers and is often recommended for less tender cuts of meat.

The texture of cereals, fruits, and vegetables is related to the structural fibers. The cellulose is quickly softened by cooking, and some cellulose, in fact, may disintegrate. However, in the case of vegetables no amount of cooking will result in a tender product if the vegetable was overmature when prepared for cooking.

Protein denaturation. Perhaps you have seen a notation on the menu card in some restaurants which states that the tenderness of a steak cannot be guaranteed if it is cooked to the "well-done" stage. Such a statement illustrates the principle of protein cookery. Proteins coagulate at relatively low cooking temperatures and are toughened when the temperature is too high or the time is prolonged. Thus, directions for the preparation of protein dishes usually specify

"moderately low oven temperature," "cook in a double boiler," "cook at simmering, not boiling temperature," as the case may be. Coagulation of proteins occurs at a lower temperature when salt or acid is added to the food. The temperature at which coagulation occurs is increased in the presence of sugar.

Starch gelatinization. This is the important action in cereal cookery. When starch is heated in water, there is rapid penetration of the starch granule with water. Since large quantities of water are enmeshed, the effect is thickening. Maximum gelatinization occurs only at boiling temperatures. Slow stirring as gelatinization is taking place helps to prevent lumping. However, excessive mechanical agitation can cause rupture of the starch granules so that the mixture becomes sticky.

The ability of starch to absorb water is seen in the large increase in volume of oatmeal, rice, macaroni, noodles, and spaghetti when they are cooked. Likewise, a small amount of cornstarch or somewhat larger amounts of flour have great thickening power for the preparation of puddings.

Vitamin retention. Carotenes in vegetables and vitamin A in eggs, milk, and organ meats are not adversely affected by the cookery of foods. Ascorbic acid and thiamine are the vitamins most readily destroyed by cooking procedures. Therefore, if attention is given to the preservation of these nutritive values, there is assurance that other vitamins are also retained.

Meat. Braising and stewing result in greater losses of all the B vitamins than do broiling, roasting, and pan frying. This is explained in part by the solubility of these vitamins in water and emphasizes the necessity for using liquids and drippings from meat cookery in either gravies, sauces, or soups. Losses are much higher for thiamine than for riboflavin and niacin. In the latter vitamins the losses can be explained almost entirely on the basis of extraction into drippings.

When meats are roasted or broiled, they retain 65 and 70 per cent of the thiamine, respectively; pan-fried meats still contain 90 per cent of the initial thiamine. On the other hand, stewed meats retain only 25 per cent of the thiamine, and an additional 25 per cent is present in the liquid. (See Figure 18–1.)

Vegetables. As much as 90 per cent of the ascorbic acid is retained if a vegetable such as cabbage is cooked in a small amount of water for the proper length of time. If a vegetable is cooked in a large amount of water, as little as 50 per cent of the vitamin may be retained.

Potatoes baked in the skin retain practically all of the ascorbic acid and lose only small amounts when boiled in their skins. When they are mashed, about 50 per cent of the vitamin has been lost. Dehydrated potatoes contain practically no ascorbic acid.

COOKERY OF PROTEIN FOODS

Milk. When milk is heated, some of the lactalbumin sticks to the bottom and sides of the pan so that scorching occurs readily. A scum

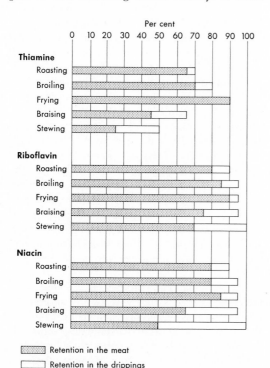

Figure 18–1. Vitamin retention after cooking meat by various methods. (Courtesy, National Live Stock and Meat Board, Chicago.)

forms on the surface of the milk as it is being heated; this makes it difficult for steam to escape and causes milk to boil over easily. These problems can be reduced by stirring while it is heating slowly over a direct flame or by using a double boiler.

Cheese. Cheese softens and melts at low temperatures but rapidly becomes rubbery and stringy when it is cooked too long or at too high a temperature. The fat tends to separate out from the other constituents. When cheese is mixed with other ingredients as in sauces, there is less separation of fat. Processed cheeses blend well with other ingredients and retain a soft, smooth texture.

Eggs. Eggs are easily overcooked resulting in toughened products or unappetizing curdled mixtures. Egg white is largely composed of albumen, which begins to coagulate at 140° F (changes from the raw state to a tender, jellylike substance) and solidifies at a temperature of 147° to 149° F. The yolk of egg coagulates at a little higher temperature than the white. When the temperature of cooking is increased, the egg proteins are toughened.

Salt and dilute acid such as vinegar hasten coagulation, and one or the other is sometimes added to water in which eggs are poached. The presence of sugar, as in custards, elevates the coagulation temperature somewhat and thus helps to avoid curdling. (See Figure 18–2.)

Soft-cooked, hard-cooked, and poached eggs should be simmered, not boiled. Custards and soufflés are usually placed in a pan of hot water and baked until just set. Soft custards and puddings with egg are cooked in a double boiler. When egg is to be added to a hot mixture, a small amount of the hot mixture is gradually mixed with the beaten egg until the egg is fairly well diluted. The diluted egg is then combined with the remaining mixture in the double boiler and cooking is continued with constant stirring just long enough for thickening to occur.

Meat. The proteins of muscle fibers are coagulated by heat at temperatures much below the boiling point of water; boiling toughens albumin and hardens the globulin.

The tenderness of meat cuts and hence the method of cookery depend upon the amounts

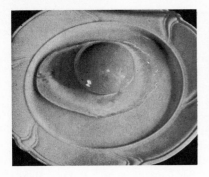

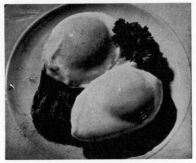

Figure 18–2. (*A*) Egg of best quality. Note round upstanding yolk, thick white and small area covered. (*B*) Eggs of best quality poach well. (Courtesy, the Poultry and Egg National Board, Chicago.)

A   B

and kinds of connective tissue that are present. The proteins of connective tissue are insoluble and are of two kinds, collagen and elastin. Collagen is the chief constituent of white connective tissue which binds the muscle fibers to each other and to the bones. It is changed to gelatin when subjected to moist heat for a prolonged cooking time but is hardened by dry heat. The change from collagen to gelatin may be hastened by the use of acid; thus, tomato juice, as in the preparation of Swiss steak, or vinegar, sometimes used in the marination of meat, helps to give a more tender product in a shorter cooking time.

Elastin, the main component of yellow connective tissue found in the ligaments, walls of the blood vessels, and between the muscle fibers, is not affected by moist heat but is hardened by dry heat.

Tender cuts of meat require only a short cooking time, but less tender cuts with much connective tissue require longer cookery. Fish contains such a small amount of connective tissue that the cooking time is very short.

Cooking tender cuts of meat. Roasting, broiling, pan broiling, or frying is used for tender cuts of meat. (See Table 18–1.) A low temperature used throughout the cooking period results in less shrinkage, more juiciness, more attractive appearance, and greater tenderness. Searing is not only unnecessary, but it is undesirable.

Roasting. Large tender cuts of beef, veal, pork, or lamb are roasted in an uncovered pan with a rack to permit circulation of heat around the meat. The fat side is placed up so that the

meat bastes itself. No water is used. The meat may be seasoned with salt and pepper at the beginning of the roasting or later, since salt penetrates only to a depth of about ½ inch. An oven temperature of 300° F is used for all meats except pork, which requires a temperature of 350° F. Pork must be cooked so thoroughly that no tinge of pink remains in the meat itself or along the bone. A meat thermometer inserted into the center of the thickest muscle of the roast is the only reliable guide.

Broiling. Broiling is used for tender chops, steaks, meat patties, ham slices, fish, or poultry. The meat is placed 2 or 3 inches away from the heat and is broiled until the top surface is browned. Thick pieces of meat and poultry are placed further from the heat so that the surface will not become dried out before the center is cooked. Salt and pepper are added to the browned surface of the meat just before turning; to add salt at the beginning would extract considerable amounts of juices and thus retard browning and detract from flavor. If fish, liver, and veal are broiled, they should be brushed with butter, margarine, or oil to prevent dryness.

Pan broiling. Pan broiling is cooking in a heavy uncovered skillet without the addition of fat. The meat is turned occasionally as it browns. Fat is poured off as it accumulates; otherwise the meat would be fried rather than broiled.

Cooking less tender cuts of meat. Braising, simmering, or stewing is used for less tender cuts of meat. (See Table 18–1.) Braising is also recommended for liver and steaks and chops of pork and veal. The meat may be dredged with flour or coated with egg and crumbs, if desired. It is browned in fat, after which liquid is added with salt, pepper, herbs, spices, and vegetables, depending upon the dish which is being prepared. The meat may be cut in small pieces to increase the surface area and to give a highly flavored broth. The flavor is further developed by long, slow cooking over a flame or in an oven. (See Figure 18–3.)

Table 18–1. Methods of Cookery for Various Cuts of Meat

	Dry Heat		Moist Heat	
Type	Broiling	Roasting	Braising	In Liquid
Beef	Steaks	Loaf	Brisket	(Large cuts and stews)
	Club	Rib	Plate	Brisket
	Hamburg	Rolled	Pot roast	Corned beef
	Loin tip	Standing	Shank	Flank
	Porterhouse	Rump	Short ribs	Heel of round
	Rib		Steaks	Neck
	Sirloin		Arm	Plate
	T bone		Blade	Shank
	Tenderloin		Flank	Short ribs
	Top round		Round	Stew meat
Veal	Too lean for broiling	Leg	Breast	Breast
		Loaf	Chops	Flank
		Loin	Rib	Heel of round
		Rack	Loin	Neck
		Shoulder, bone in or rolled	Cubes	Riblets
			Steaks	Shank
				Shoulder
				Stew meat
Lamb	Chops	Leg	Breast	Breast
	Loin	Loaf	Chops, shoulder	Flank
	Rib	Shoulder, bone in or rolled	Neck slices	Neck
	Shoulder		Shank	Riblets
	Sirloin			Shank
	Patties			Stew meat
	Steaks			
Pork	Bacon	Boston butt	Chops	Smoked
	Canadian bacon	Loin	Hocks	Ham
	Ham slice	Sirloin	Shoulder steaks	Picnic ham
	Smoked shoulder slice	Spareribs	Spareribs	Shank
	Thin pork chops	Ham, fresh or smoked	Tenderloin	Shoulder butt
		Picnic ham, fresh or smoked		
		Ham loaf		
Variety	Brains		Brains	Brains
	Kidney		Heart	Heart
	Liver, lamb, or veal		Kidney	Kidney
	Sweetbreads		Liver	Sweetbreads
			Sweetbreads	Tongue

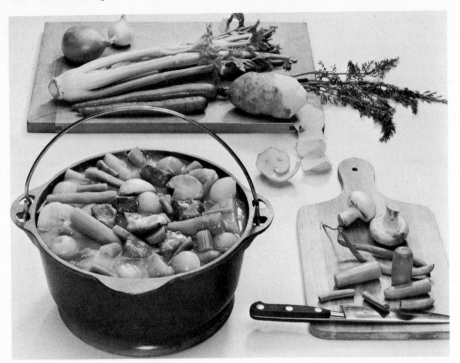

Figure 18–3. Moist heat, as in the preparation of a stew, is used for less tender cuts of meat. With fresh vegetables, such a dinner meal is delicious. (Courtesy, United Fresh Fruit and Vegetable Association.)

PREPARATION AND COOKERY OF VEGETABLES

Principles of cookery. Properly cooked vegetables should be tender yet firm and crisp, rather than hard and tough or soft and soggy. Some color change in green vegetables is unavoidable because heat decomposes the chlorophyll, but this can be kept to a minimum if overcooking is avoided.

Appreciable amounts of vitamins and minerals are lost when peelings and skins are discarded, since vitamins and minerals occur in greatest concentration near the skin. Moreover, the exposure to air hastens oxidation, with the result that dicing in small pieces, chopping, grinding, and stirring during cookery greatly hasten destruction.

Vitamin and mineral losses through solubility can be materially lessened by (1) keeping pieces

as large as practical in order to avoid excessive surface exposure, (2) cooking with skins on whenever possible, (3) avoiding long soaking in water that is later discarded, (4) using a minimum quantity of water in cookery, and (5) saving water in which vegetables were cooked or canned for use in soups, sauces, or gravies whenever practical.

Some destruction of vitamins during cookery is unavoidable, but this can be kept to a minimum. The water in which vegetables are cooked should be rapidly boiling before vegetables are added and should be quickly brought to the boiling point again. This facilitates prompt destruction of enzymes which may oxidize the vitamins. Continuous boiling rather than simmering is most effective in giving a tender product in the shortest length of time. This does not mean that excessively high heat, with consequent rapid escape of steam and danger of scorching, is necessary. For most vegetables a tightly covered pot, using a minimum quantity of water, is desirable. Even such strongly flavored vegetables as cabbage may be cooked in this way.

Methods used for cooking vegetables. Boiling, steaming, and baking are the most commonly used methods of cooking vegetables.

1. Boiling. Many vegetables such as string beans, turnip and mustard greens, spinach, carrots, and green peas may be cooked in a covered vessel with a small amount of water to preserve the flavor, reduce nutrient losses, and keep oxidation at a minimum. Washed greens require no additional water.

2. Steaming. Spinach, chard, broccoli, and asparagus are especially adapted to this method. A basket to hold the vegetables is placed over a pan of rapidly boiling water. The vessel is tightly closed, thus permitting steam to circulate around the vegetables. Although vegetables retain their shape and nutritive values very well, the cooking time is much longer than by boiling.

3. Pressure cooker. For preservation of flavor, color, and nutritive value the use of a pressure cooker is good. However, the cooking time must be carefully controlled, and the instructions of the manufacturer should be followed carefully since the cooking time is materially shortened and overcooking can readily occur.

4. Baking, with or without removing the skin. This method retains the nutrients which lie close to the skin, if the vegetables are not pared. Potatoes, eggplant, and squash are well suited to baking.

5. Sautéing. Eggplant, green or ripe tomatoes, and cucumbers are cooked to advantage with this method. The slices of vegetable are rolled in crumbs and browned in small amounts of fat. They should be drained to remove excess grease.

6. Broiling. Vegetables may be cooked under an open flame for a short time at high temperature. Tomatoes lend themselves well to broiling.

7. Panning consists in cooking vegetables in a heavy covered frying pan with a small amount of fat. Finely shredded cabbage, kale, collards, and sliced summer squashes are especially delicious when cooked by this method.

COOKERY OF CEREALS AND PASTES

Cereals. Breakfast cereals are cooked with just enough water to give a smooth, thick consistency. Disodium phosphate added to quick-cooking cereals during manufacture enhances the ability of the granule to take up water and hence the cooking time is reduced. Fine-grain cereals require less cooking time than those of coarser texture.

The dry cereal should be added slowly to rapidly boiling salted water so that boiling does not stop. If very fine cereals are to be cooked, lumping can be avoided by mixing the cereal with a small amount of cold water before adding it to the boiling liquid. It is necessary to stir constantly while cooking over direct heat; however, quick-cooking cereals require cooking for only a few minutes. Well-cooked breakfast cereal is free from lumps, neither too thick nor too thin, and full-flavored.

Rice is preferably cooked with just enough water so that all the water will be absorbed—usually 2 to 2½ times the volume of rice. A minimum of stirring yields fluffy whole grains which remain separated rather than becoming stuck together.

Various paste products—macaroni, spaghetti, noodles—are cooked in a large volume of water until just tender. They need not be fully cooked when they are to be used in dishes requiring further heating. Excessive cooking results in a pasty, gummy, sticky product.

PROBLEMS AND REVIEW

1. *Problem.* List three ways in which each of the following foods may be used in meals: eggs, milk, American cheese, potatoes, apples, carrots, cabbage, beef. Consult any cookbook or popular magazine for interesting ideas.

2. What is the effect of each of the following practices in food preparation? Which practice is good? Which is poor?
   a. Marinating meat in wine, oil, and herbs for 24 hours.
   b. Adding a little vinegar to the water in which beets are cooked.
   c. Adding a tiny pinch of baking soda to the water in which green beans are cooked.
   d. Adding salt to water before poaching eggs.
   e. Boiling eggs.
   f. Searing a roast at 500° F and then turning heat down to 350° F to complete the roasting.
3. *Problem.* Outline the steps in the preparation of the following meal so that maximum nutritive values will be retained: pot roast with carrots, potatoes, onions; tossed green salad; baked custard with fresh peach slices. List the principles of cookery involved in this meal preparation.
4. Why is home-prepared coleslaw likely to be a good source of ascorbic acid whereas commercially prepared slaw is unreliable for this vitamin?
5. What is meant by denaturation, coagulation, sautéing, simmering?

References

"Buying and Cooking Food," in *Food for Us All—Yearbook of Agriculture 1969.* U.S. Department of Agriculture, 1969, Washington, D.C., pp. 94–252.

Dawson, E. H.: "When You Cook," in *Food—Yearbook of Agriculture 1959.* U.S. Department of Agriculture, Washington, D.C., pp. 495–509.

Eheart, M. S., and Gott, C.: "Conventional and Microwave Cooking of Vegetables," *J. Am. Diet. Assoc.,* **44:**116–19, 1964.

Gordon, J., and Noble, I.: "Effect of Cooking Method on Vegetables. Ascorbic Acid Retention and Color Difference," *J. Am. Diet. Assoc.,* **35:**578–81, 1959.

————: "Waterless vs. Boiling Water Cooking of Vegetables," *J. Am. Diet. Assoc.,* **44:**378–82, 1964.

Lee, D. C., and Spader, M.: "Chinese Cooking of Vegetables Preserves Color, Texture, Flavor," *J. Home. Econ.,* **51:**43–44, 1959.

Lushbough, C. H., *et al.:* "Thiamine Retention in Meats After Various Heat Treatments," *J. Am. Diet. Assoc.,* **40:**35–38, 1962.

Noble, I.: "Thiamine and Riboflavin Retention in Braised Meat," *J. Am. Diet. Assoc.,* **47:**205–208, 1965.

Schlosser, G. C., and Gilpin, G. L.: "What and How to Cook," in *Food—The Yearbook of Agriculture 1959.* U.S. Department of Agriculture, Washington, D.C., pp. 519–54.

Consumer Information on Foods and Recipes

Publications by the U.S. Department of Agriculture, Washington, D.C.
Beef and Veal in Family Meals, G 118.
Cereals and Pastas in Family Meals, G 150.
Cheese in Family Meals, G 112.
Eggs in Family Meals, G 103.
Family Fare: Food Management and Recipes, G 1.
Food for Us All—Yearbook of Agriculture, 1969.
Fruits in Family Meals, G 125.
Milk in Family Meals, G 127.
Pork in Family Meals, G 160.
Poultry in Family Meals, G 110.
Vegetables in Family Meals, G 105.

Unit V
Safeguarding the Food Supply

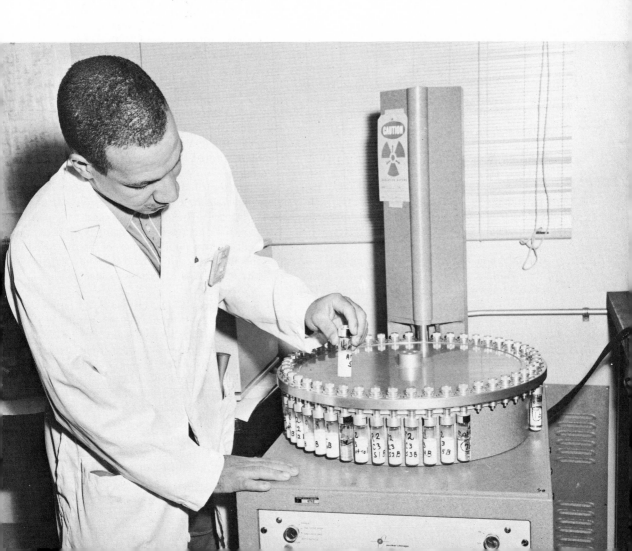

19 Preservation and Sanitary Handling of the Food Supply

ILLNESS CAUSED BY FOOD

Following the exodus of the Jews from Egypt, the people had a great craving for meat. When quails were brought in large numbers by winds from the sea, the people gathered them and ate them. This is what happened:*

While the meat was yet between their teeth, before it was consumed, the anger of the Lord was kindled against the people, and the Lord smote the people with a very great plague. Therefore the name of that place was called Kibrothhattaavah,†, because there they buried the people who had the craving.

Recently among some people living on the island of Lesbos (Greece) a syndrome has been observed following the eating of quail.[1] The symptoms include muscular pain, paralysis of used muscles, excretion of myoglobin in the urine, and oliguria. Apparently this illness occurs only in persons who have some enzymatic abnormality and who have become physically fatigued before eating the quail. It is theorized that the eating of quail elicits the abnormality in these persons, thus producing the symptoms. The author of this report believes that this twen-

*The Holy Bible, Numbers 11:33–34.
†Graves of craving.

tieth-century syndrome is the same as that which afflicted the Jews during the exodus.

The ancient Egyptians realized that the meat of animals that had died a natural death was unfit for human food. Greek records of many centuries ago note that the wife, daughter, and two sons of the Greek poet Euripides died after having eaten poisonous fungi. For centuries kings were protected against poisoning by employing official food tasters. Thus, history records on numerous occasions the role of food in producing illness.

Illness resulting from the eating of food may be caused by contamination of the food by bacteria, molds, and fungi, by the presence of some natural toxicant in the food, by the contamination of food by a toxic chemical, or by sensitivity of a given individual to one or more foods. Bacterial, parasitic, and chemical contaminations are considered in this chapter.

Food-borne diseases as a public health problem. When one considers the total population of the United States and the amount and variety of foods consumed each day, it becomes evident that the reported incidence of outbreaks of illness from the food supply is indeed very low. In 1966 the National Communicable Disease Center instituted a program for the control of food-borne diseases. During the first two years the "big three" reported as causes of illness were *Salmonella, Clostridium perfringens,* and *Staphylococci.*[2] The number of cases reported is believed to represent not more than 1 to 2 per cent of the total number of persons who became ill as a result of food poisoning.[3] Thus, millions of persons experience some food-borne illness each year.

For most people in good health an outbreak of food poisoning from the organisms listed above results in an illness of short duration leading to discomfort and absence from work or school. But for the very young, the elderly, and those who are debilitated from other illness, these seemingly mild infections can lead to serious complications or even death. The outbreak of an infection in a child-caring institution or in a nursing home is especially life threatening. Therefore, to protect the vulnerable, every precaution must be taken to minimize the occurrence of infection among the more vigorous who in turn become the agents for transmission of organisms.

Other diseases transmitted by foods are typhoid fever, bacillary dysentery, tuberculosis, scarlet fever, streptococcic sore throat, botulism, undulant fever, amebic dysentery, and trichinosis.

Food-borne diseases result from eating food (1) from an animal or plant that has been infected, (2) that has been contaminated by organisms transmitted by insects, flies, roaches, or rodents, (3) that has had contact with sewage polluted water (shellfish, for example), or (4) that has been contaminated by a food handler who has not observed good personal hygiene or acceptable food-handling practices.

Some illnesses are enteric in that the symptoms are confined to the gastrointestinal tract with mild to severe nausea, vomiting, abdominal pain, and diarrhea. Other food-borne diseases are systemic; that is, the organisms invade the circulation and produce symptoms in organs and tissues.

Bacterial food infections. A bacterial *infection* results from the ingestion of food that has been contaminated with large numbers of bacteria. The bacteria continue to grow in the favorable intestinal environment and produce irritation of the mucosa with symptoms occurring in 12 to 36 hours after ingestion of the food.

Salmonellosis. About 1300 serotypes of the *Salmonella* genus have been identified, each of which is capable of causing infection in man.[4] The symptoms may last for two or three days, but the organisms may be eliminated for two or three weeks thereby providing a continuing source of contamination for others.

Typhoid fever, fortunately rare in the United States, is the most serious of the *Salmonella* infections. The symptoms of the gastrointestinal tract may be severe with ulcerations of the mucosa occurring. Unlike most infections by *Salmonella,* typhoid fever is systemic. The organisms particularly affect the liver and gallbladder, but they may also localize in the bone marrow, kidney, spleen, and the lungs where bronchitis and pneumonia may result.

Meat, poultry, fish, eggs, and dairy products that are eaten raw or that have been inadequately heated are most frequently implicated in salmonellosis. Contaminated cake mixes, bakery foods, coloring agents, powdered yeast, and chocolate candy have also caused outbreaks of the infection.

Animals including cattle, swine, poultry, fish, dogs, and birds harbor the organisms. They are usually infected by contact of one animal with another or by animal feeds. A single egg that is infected can contaminate a whole batch of eggs being frozen or dried. A butcher block or kitchen counter with which infected meat has been in contact is a source of contamination for any food placed upon it. Flies and rodents coming in contact with feces of animals or man are responsible for contamination of food. Food handlers who do not observe good personal hygiene or who do not follow essential directions in the preparation of food are a major source of contamination of the food supplies.

Shigellosis (bacillary dysentery). The *Shigella* genus includes pathogenic organisms widely distributed and capable of producing severe illness. Bacillary dysentery is characterized by fever, abdominal pain, vomiting, and diarrhea. The intestinal mucosa may become ulcerated, and stools often contain blood and mucus. Fatalities from the infections are ordinarily low, but in tropical countries where sanitation is poor and malnutrition is prevalent the disease may be fatal to as many as 20 per cent of persons affected.

Infected human feces are the source of the infection, which is transmitted by the direct fecal-oral route or through contamination of food or water.

Clostridium perfringens, the gas gangrene organism, ordinarily inhabits the intestinal tract and in usual numbers does not produce illness. However, when a food is consumed which has been contaminated with large numbers of bacteria, illness results. In 1968 this food-borne illness accounted for 28 per cent of all outbreaks reported to the National Communicable Disease Center.[5]

Clostridium perfringens appears normally in the soil, in the intestinal tract of man and animals, and in sewage. The bacteria are destroyed by heat, but the spores they produce will survive boiling for as long as five hours. If foods are allowed to remain at temperatures between 50° and 140° F for several hours, the spores germinate and prodigious numbers of bacteria are then present in the food. Refrigeration of food immediately after heating will prevent rapid germination of the spores. However, a large mass of food may cool so slowly even at refrigerator temperatures that considerable bacterial growth occurs.

Bacterial food intoxication. Food poisoning frequently results from the ingestion of a food in which a bacterial toxin has been produced. The preformed toxin is responsible for the symptoms, which may be mild to severe. Usually the symptoms are apparent from one to six hours following a meal.

Staphylococcal poisoning occurs abruptly after the ingestion of food containing the enterotoxin. The gastrointestinal symptoms are often severe but usually the illness lasts for only one to three days.

Staphylococci are found in the air and occur especially in infected cuts and abrasions of the skin, boils, and pimples. They may be present in the nose and throat of food handlers. Rapid growth of the bacteria occurs in contaminated food if it is held at temperatures ranging between 50° and 140° F for three to four hours. Semisolid foods such as custards, cream fillings in pastries, cream puffs, cream sauces, mayonnaise, chicken and turkey salads, croquettes, potato salad, ice cream, poultry dressing, ham, ground meat, stews, and fish provide the ideal culture media for bacterial growth.

Staphylococci are killed at high temperatures, but the toxin is not inactivated with temperatures ordinarily used in food preparation. The contaminated food usually does not smell, taste, or appear to be spoiled. The best safeguard against staphylococcal poisoning is prompt refrigeration of food.

Botulism is an extremely rare type of food poisoning but of such serious consequences that its occurrence is quite newsworthy. About 65 per cent of all instances of ingestion are fatal. The symptoms usually, but not always, begin with the gastrointestinal tract. Dizziness, head-

ache, double vision, and paralysis of the muscles occur. Death usually is the result of respiratory paralysis and cardiac failure.

Clostridium botulinum is found in soils all over the world and consequently infects the vegetables grown thereon. The spores produced by the bacteria are quite heat resistant, and they will germinate rapidly under anaerobic (without oxygen) conditions such as found in canned foods. As the spores germinate the deadly toxin is produced by the bacteria.

Most instances of botulism are traced to the ingestion of home-canned nonacid vegetables and meats. A few outbreaks in recent years have been reported from commercially processed tuna fish, whitefish, and soup.

Canned foods which contain little or no acid such as meat, beans, asparagus, corn, and peas are very good media for the growth of the bacillus botulinus, whereas acid-containing foods such as tomatoes and certain fruits are not favorable for growth. The processing of canned vegetables in boiling water is not adequate for destruction of spores, and therefore the use of sterilization with steam under pressure should be urged for the home as well as for commercial establishments.

Botulinus-infected foods do not necessarily taste or smell spoiled, so that home-canned vegetables should always be brought to a vigorous boil before being used since the toxin is inactivated in 10 minutes by heat at 80° C. It goes without saying that any food that shows gas production or change in color or consistency should be destroyed without even tasting it. The contents of any can that has bulging ends should likewise be discarded. It is important that such foods be burned since animals eating them will otherwise be poisoned.

Parasitic infestations of food. Many protozoa and helminths (worms) gain admission to the body by means of food and parasitize the bowel, thereby causing injury to the intestinal lining. Some of them also invade other tissues of the body.

Among the parasitic protozoa are *Endamoeba histolytica,* which causes amebic dysentery. The source of infection is human feces, and infection may be transmitted by a food handler who is a carrier or by contaminated water supplies. The symptoms may be acute, chronic, or intermittent. Erosion of the intestinal mucosa sometimes occurs with profuse bloody diarrhea. The individual with a chronic infection may experience only mild discomfort of diarrhea or constipation. The liver, lung, brain, and other tissues may be infected and abscesses may form. Preventive measures include maintenance of sanitary controls of the water supply and sewage disposal, as well as supervision of public eating places by health agencies.

The helminths that frequently invade the intestinal tract include *nematodes* (roundworms), *cestodes* (tapeworms), and *trematodes* (liver, intestinal and lung flukes). Trichinosis, one of the more serious infestations, results from the ingestion of raw or partially cooked pork infected with *Trichinella spiralis,* a very minute roundworm barely visible to the naked eye. In the intestinal tract the larvae are set free from their cysts during digestion of the meat and develop into adults within a few days. The females deposit larvae in the mucosa and invade the lymph and blood circulation. The muscles of the diaphragm, the thorax, the abdominal wall, the biceps, and the tongue are frequently involved, there being muscular pain, chills, and weakness.

Trichinella is destroyed by cooking pork until no trace of pink remains. The recommended internal temperature for cooked pork is 170° F, which allows a margin of about 30° F above the lethal point of the organisms. Trichinella is also destroyed by freezing at 0° F or below for at least 72 hours. Government inspection does not include examination for *Trichinella* at the present time. The cooking of all garbage fed to hogs will go a long way toward reducing *Trichinella* infestation.

Hookworm infestation is a serious problem in children in tropical countries of the world, and in some parts of the United States. The larvae penetrate the exposed skin and reach the lymphatics and blood circulation. They are carried to the lungs and migrate into the alveoli, trachea, epiglottis, and pharynx and are swallowed. They may also be carried from soil to hands to mouth.

It has been estimated that a single hookworm may remove almost 1 ml blood per day as it carries on its blood-sucking activity in the intestine. The loss of blood produces an anemia with symptoms of weakness, fatigue, and growth retardation. Usually the infestation is present in children who also are malnourished. A good nutritious diet is always important for these children, but the eradication of hookworm infestation depends upon sanitary measures for disposal of feces so that the cycle of parasite growth in the soil is broken.

Naturally occurring toxicants in foods. Numerous naturally occurring chemical substances in foods produce some toxic manifestations in animals and in man. One class of compounds long known to be poisonous is the alkaloids such as strychnine, atropine, scopalamine, solanine, and others. The green part of sprouting potatoes contains sufficient solanine to produce pain, vomiting, jaundice, diarrhea, and prostration. Ordinarily, these green parts are removed with the peel of the potato. Varieties of hemlock have been mistaken for parsley, horseradish, or wild parsnip and eaten in salads and soup only to produce immediate, often fatal, illness. Monkshood, foxglove, and deadly nightshade have from time to time been mistaken for edible plants and have caused violent illness.

Legumes and seeds. Because legumes are important sources of protein and energy in some parts of the world, the presence of toxic factors in them is of nutritional and economic importance. Soybeans are a most valuable source of protein when they are heated. Raw soybeans contain a trypsin inhibitor and probably some other factors that interfere with metabolism and with growth in animals. In addition, the phytic acid content of soybeans binds zinc so that animals fed a diet in which soybeans are the source of protein develop a severe zinc deficiency. This can be corrected by supplementing the diet with zinc. Soybeans also contain a goitrogen, but this is not believed to be a factor in endemic goiter.

Lathyrism has been known since the time of Hippocrates. It is a neurologic disease characterized by weakness of the leg muscles, dragging of the feet, loss of sensation to heat and pain, and spinal cord lesions. It is observed in India and in Mediterranean countries following the ingestion of large amounts of the lathyrus plants for periods of six months or more. These legumes grow under adverse conditions of drought and hence they may be ingested extensively during a famine.

Favism is an inherited sensitivity to fava or broad beans and is fairly common in the Mediterranean area, and in Asia and Formosa. Sensitive individuals have a deficiency of glucose-6-phosphate dehydrogenase and reduced glutathione content of the red blood cells. An unidentified substance in the fava beans leads to hemolysis of the red blood cells and thus hemolytic anemia in the sensitive individuals.

Gossypol is a toxicant in cottonseed that must be removed before the meal can be used in protein mixtures (see page 374). Some strains of cottonseed are now being developed that are free of this toxic substance.

Mushroom poisoning. A few species of mushrooms are so toxic that eating them may be fatal, others are mildly toxic, and many species are harmless and greatly enjoyed. The *Amanita* is the most poisonous of the mushrooms and produces severe abdominal pain, prostration, jaundice, and death in more than half the people who ingest it. This source of poisoning can be eliminated if people will use only the commercially grown mushrooms.

Mycotoxins. Many molds growing on grains and nuts can produce illness in animals and probably in man. A class of substances of extreme toxicity to cattle, swine, poultry, and laboratory animals is the aflatoxins produced by the mold *Aspergillus flavus.*[6] Much attention has been focused on peanuts and Brazil nuts[7] since they are subject to the mold growth. Practically all of the growth is associated with peanuts that have been allowed to remain in contact with damp ground. If broken shells and discolored, shriveled, and rancid kernels are removed, the remaining nuts are practically free of aflatoxins. There has been no evidence of contamination of domestically produced peanut butter and peanut products. However, the importance of peanuts as a source of protein in some African countries emphasizes the need to improve methods of

harvesting and to remove nuts that may have been contaminated.

Interference with nutritive properties. The adverse effect of some chemical substances is an interference with the utilization of a nutrient and thus the imposition of a deficiency. One of the best known examples of this is the oxalic acid content of certain green leafy vegetables such as spinach, beet tops, and chard that interferes with the absorption of calcium. If these vegetables are eaten frequently by those whose calcium intake is otherwise marginal, a problem of calcium inadequacy could arise. Rhubarb leaves are so high in oxalic acid content that their ingestion leads to gastrointestinal upsets, and in severe intoxications to hematemesis, hematuria, noncoagulability of the blood, and convulsions.

Goitrogens are substances that interfere with the utilization of iodine. They are found in cabbage, Brussels sprouts, cauliflower, kohlrabi, rutabagas, and soybeans. There is little evidence that the ingestion of these foods has produced any increase in endemic goiter.

Thiaminase, an enzyme antagonistic to thiamine, is present in bracken fern, raw fish, and a variety of fruits and vegetables. In an ordinary mixed diet this is of no concern. The enzyme is destroyed by heat.

Excess of nutrients. The toxic effects of vitamins A and D are well known. The ingestion of seal or polar bear liver leads to symptoms of acute vitamin A toxicity, inasmuch as 1 pound of the liver contains about 10 million I.U. of vitamin A. On a practical basis in the United States the hazards of vitamin A toxicity relate to the indiscriminate use of vitamin supplements and not to excesses in the diet itself. If several foods that are fortified with vitamin D are consumed each day, the intake could be in excess of requirements, and hypercalcemia is a possible outcome. (See Chapter 10.)

Selenium, a nutritional essential in trace amounts, is toxic to animals that graze in pastures with selenium-rich soils. People living in seleniferous areas also appear to have a higher incidence of dental caries.[8]

Tyramine toxicity. Cheddar cheese and Chianti wine contain appreciable amounts of tyramine, which is produced by the decarboxylation of tyrosine. Tyramine is a potent vasopressor substance but it is normally metabolized in the body by the action of monoamine oxidase. Patients with depressive states are frequently treated with monoamine oxidase inhibitor because of its ability to produce euphoria. Since the inhibitor interferes with the metabolism of tyramine, the ingestion of tyramine-containing foods leads to nausea, vomiting, headache, and severe hypertension, and sometimes death. A glass of Chianti wine or as little as 1 ounce of Cheddar cheese contains enough tyramine to produce some toxic effects, and large amounts may be dangerous for some.

Chemical poisoning. Lead is a particularly dangerous metal since it accumulates in the body and results in chronic illness characterized by severe anemia and changes in the kidneys and arteries, death occurring in some cases. A minute quantity of lead occurs naturally in food and is ingested daily, but whenever the daily intake is 1 mg or more, the eventual accumulations may become toxic. Food may become contaminated with lead if it is exposed to dust containing lead, or if it is kept in containers in which solders, alloys, or enamel containing lead have been used. Canned foods were formerly subject to lead contamination, but the canning industry has long since devised containers that are entirely safe for food.

Cadmium, zinc, and antimony are readily soluble and will quickly produce illness if ingested. They are not used in the manufacture of utensils or cans.

Accidental poisonings have occurred when chemicals have been mistaken for powdered milk, flour, or baking powder. Some years ago in a state institution 47 deaths resulted when roach powder containing sodium fluoride was mistaken for dry milk powder and used as such.[9] In another instance boric acid was used in place of lactic acid for the preparation of infant formulas. Even common table salt became a deadly poison a few years ago when it was mistaken for sugar in the preparation of infant formulas.

The coloring of pesticides green or some other color unusual to foods could prevent accidental poisonings. It goes without saying that insecti-

cides, lye, moth balls, and numerous other poisons should be placed where small children cannot reach them.

The metals used in cooking utensils and in food containers have been a source of much controversy. Many studies have shown that glass, stainless steel, aluminum, agate, and tin are suitable containers for food since these materials are practically insoluble or, when dissolved to a slight degree, are not harmful to health. Acid foods may dissolve some of the tin from cans so that a change of flavor results from the iron underneath the tin coating, but the ingestion of these foods is not harmful. It is recommended that acid foods be transferred from the can to a covered glass container if the food is to be refrigerated after opening. The intentional use of chemicals in foods is discussed on pages 272–73.

Radioactive fallout. Man has always been exposed to the radiation of naturally occurring radioisotopes in the environment. With the advent of the nuclear bomb the amount of such exposure has increased, although to date the annual exposure of the population from this source is very small when compared to that which occurs naturally. No change in food habits is currently indicated by the amounts of radioactive contamination.

Following a nuclear detonation there are several pathways by which the radionuclides eventually are ingested by man. (See Figure 19–1.) For example, contaminated plants may be eaten by cows; much of the element is excreted in the urine of the cow, but some will be secreted in the milk which, in turn, is consumed

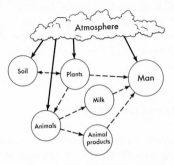

Figure 19–1. Pathways of radioactive fallout. (Courtesy, National Dairy Council Chicago.)

by man. Some of the consumed element will be excreted in the feces of man, but some will be absorbed and will enter the metabolism in a manner similar to that of the element with which it is related. Strontium-90 is related to calcium and is deposited chiefly in the bones; cesium-137, like potassium, is distributed throughout the body in the soft tissues; and within 48 hours of ingestion iodine-131 is accounted for in the thyroid gland and in the urine. Excessive deposits of radioactive elements carry the threat of cancer—of the thyroid with iodine-131, and of the bone with strontium-90.

Each radioisotope has a specific *physical half-life*. This is the amount of time that elapses before half of the element is decayed. The element thus emits radiations to the external environment with consequent exposure of man, animals, and plants over this period of time. The *biologic half-life* refers to the length of time before half of the element is excreted from the body. Thus, some elements may be rapidly excreted causing little harm, whereas others are retained. Strontium-90 and cesium-137 have a physical half-life of 28 years. Strontium-90 is of much more serious biologic consequence since its rate of turnover is slow in the body, whereas cesium-137 has a biologic half-life of about 140 days.

The Federal Radiation Council has established guidelines which define the potential hazards of radiation.[10] The U.S. Public Health Service, Atomic Energy Commission, and U.S. Department of Agriculture are among the groups that periodically analyze foods from all over the country to determine levels of radioactivity. About one third to one half of the dietary strontium-90 is present in milk; however, the high calcium intake helps to ensure a preferential use of calcium rather than strontium by the body. The current levels in foods present no risks whatsoever.

PRESERVATION OF FOODS

Factors contributing to food spoilage. Foods are made unsafe to eat or become esthetically undesirable or both by the actions of bacteria, yeasts, and molds; by enzymatic action; by chemical or physical changes; and by contact with insects and rodents. In food spoilage these factors often coexist. Unsafe foods do not necessarily show any changes in appearance and palatability, and hence the danger from them is great. Foods that are rancid, moldy, or rotting are less likely to be consumed and therefore may not be a direct threat to health, but the economic waste is considerable.

Temperature and growth of organisms. Bacteria, yeasts, and molds grow rapidly at temperatures of 50° to 140° F; within this range the rate of growth increases tenfold for each 10° C (18° F) increase in temperature. Thus, the bacteria produced in a food left at room temperature for three or four hours can reach astronomical numbers.

Growth of microorganisms is retarded at refrigerator temperatures and is stopped at freezing temperatures. Many molds and some bacteria known as *psychrophils* grow even at refrigerator temperatures, leading to spoilage of food. Pathogenic bacteria do not grow at these temperatures. Many bacteria are not killed by freezing—an important fact to remember when frozen foods are thawed and allowed to stand at room temperatures. (See Figure 19–2.)

Some bacteria known as *thermophils* thrive at relatively high temperatures. They are responsible for the "flat sour" which occurs in some home-canned foods.

Many bacteria produce spores that are very resistant to heat. In fact, several hours of boiling

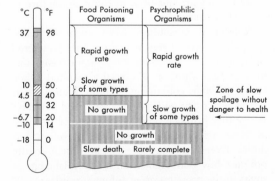

Figure 19–2. Low-temperature limits on growth of food poisoning and psychrophilic organisms. (Courtesy, Dr. Horace K. Burr and the *Journal of the American Medical Association*, **174**: 1178–80, 1960.)

may not destroy them. Under favorable conditions such spores will germinate rapidly.

Physical and chemical changes. Appearance, texture, flavor, and the chemical constituents of foods are modified by the influence of air, heat, light, moisture, and time. These changes are accelerated by enzyme action and by the presence of minute traces of mineral catalysts such as copper and iron. All plant and animal tissues contain enzymes that are highly active at room temperatures and above.

The rate of chemical change doubles for each 10° C (18° F) rise in temperature. Rancidity of fats is one example of undesirable oxidation and contributes to the deterioration of flavor even in foods that contain only small amounts of fat. Oxidation also leads to loss of ascorbic acid.

Plant and animal tissue fibers are softened, and the surface of cut nonacid fruits are oxidized and become darkened as a result of enzyme action, thereby changing the texture, color, and nutritive value. Some nutrients may be lost by discarding fluids in which they have been dissolved. The exposure of milk to sunlight leads to a tallowy flavor and loss of riboflavin and vitamin B_6. With storage, changes in texture also occur: sugar may crystallize out of jellies; ice cream becomes gummy and granular; and frozen meats and poultry become dry.

Food preservation. The criteria for successful food preservation, whether it be for a day or two or for months, are these: (1) safety from contamination by pathogenic organisms or toxicity through chemicals; and (2) maintenance of optimum qualities of color, flavor, texture, and nutritive value.

Methods of food preservation that destroy bacteria are *bactericidal;* these include the application of heat by cooking, canning, preserving, and irradiation sterilization. Other methods such as dehydration, freezing, treatment with antibiotics, salting, and pickling retard the growth of bacteria, molds, and yeasts; they are *bacteriostatic.*

Pasteurization. Of all foods, milk is perhaps most susceptible to contamination. Yet, milkborne diseases are now rare because pasteurization is employed for more than 90 per cent of all milk consumed in the United States. The milk used for the preparation of cheese, butter, and ice cream is also pasteurized. The inspection of cows, barns, milk handlers, and dairy-processing plants is also essential to the production of milk of high quality.

Milk is pasteurized by (1) the *holding* process in which milk is heated to at least 143° F and kept at that temperature for at least 30 minutes, or by (2) the *high-temperature short-time* method in which milk is heated to 160° F and kept at that temperature for at least 15 seconds.

Milk may be sterilized by boiling it for a specified time as in the preparation of infant formulas or by heat as in the processing of evaporated milk. Pasteurization does not appreciably change the color or flavor of milk, but sterilization deepens the color and gives to milk a slightly carmelized flavor.

Cooking and baking. Boiling temperature (212° F), if maintained sufficiently long for heat to completely penetrate the food, will kill bacteria. When low-heat cookery is used as in the preparation of custards or when heat penetrates food masses very slowly as in casseroles or stuffed poultry, bacteria may not be killed. Such foods may cause food poisoning if they have been carelessly handled prior to cookery.

The spores of *Clostriduim perfringens* and *Clostridium botulinum* are highly resistant to heat, and temperatures above boiling, as with a pressure cooker, are necessary to destroy them. The enterotoxin produced by staphylococci is not inactivated by boiling; on the other hand, botulin is inactivated by boiling for at least 10 minutes. Cooked foods that are improperly handled are rapidly subject to spoilage.

Canning. Commercial firms now employ standard methods for canning each food. Sterilization is brought about by means of steam under pressure. By means of agitation of the cans during processing, heat penetration of the can contents is accelerated and the heating time is shortened with a great improvement in flavor and in color.

Aseptic canning is an application of the high-temperature short-time processing. The product is first sterilized at 275° to 350° F in a matter of seconds, cooled, and filled aseptically into presterilized containers in a sterile atmosphere.

The method has been used for fluid products such as soups, sauces, fruit juices, milk, and baby foods and appears to be applicable to other foods in small pieces. The resultant product is of better color and flavor and retains more of the heat-labile vitamins.

Some nutritive losses, especially of heat-labile vitamins, occur during canning, but the newer techniques have reduced these losses considerably. The manner of storage is probably the major factor in nutrient retention or loss. As much as 25 per cent of ascorbic acid and thiamine may be lost from fruits and vegetables stored for a year at 80° F, but with storage at 65° F these losses may be reduced to 10 per cent. Meats, likewise, lose 20 to 30 per cent of their thiamine content after six months' storage at 70° F, but the riboflavin content is not adversely affected. Carotene losses in fruits and vegetables are small even after months of storage. Water-soluble nutrients distribute themselves evenly throughout the solids and liquids; thus, if the solids constitute two thirds of the total, one third of these water-soluble nutrients will be lost if the liquid is not used.

Home canning. When foods are canned in the home, a pressure canner should always be used for low-acid foods, including most vegetables, poultry, and meat, in order that bacteria and their heat-resistant spores may be destroyed. Fruits and tomatoes, being acid foods, may be safely canned at boiling temperatures.

Cool storage and refrigeration. Modern refrigeration has been largely responsible for the tremendous variety of foods available all over the country, in season and out. By means of it foods can be kept for long periods of time in commercial cold-storage rooms at the proper humidity, or may be transported from coast to coast without danger of loss from spoilage or freezing, or may be kept in the home refrigerator to reduce the number of trips the homemaker makes to the market.

Fruits except bananas and vegetables are kept just above the point at which they will freeze. Butter and meats may be kept at much lower temperatures.

Cool storage is being gradually extended to canned and dehydrated foods to retain optimum color, flavor, and nutritive values. (See page 268.)

Freezing. In the quick freezing of foods, first developed as a practical method of processing some 40 years ago, bacteria are unable to grow and enzymes are inactivated. Today an almost endless variety of frozen foods is available—fruits, vegetables, juices, meats, poultry, fish, pies, cakes, cookies, rolls, stews, casseroles, and complete meals.

Foods to be frozen must be carefully selected for quality and maturity. No frozen product is ever any better than the raw materials from which it was frozen. Because ready-to-eat foods involve mixtures and are subject to more handling prior to freezing, special care must be taken to enforce the most rigid sanitary practices. Some foods such as raw salad vegetables and tomatoes cannot be frozen satisfactorily because of texture changes. Fruits are softened by the freezing process.

Before freezing, vegetables are blanched to inactivate the oxidative enzymes. The darkening of fruits is prevented by immersion in a sugar syrup or by using ascorbic acid. Foods are packed in consumer-size moisture-vapor-proof containers and placed between metal plates at −40° F where freezing begins almost immediately and is complete within an hour. Pieces of foods such as shrimp, green beans, peas, and carrots may also be spread on a wire mesh belt that is moved slowly through a freezing tunnel at −40° F and subsequently packaged. In a modification of this method, known as "fluidized freezing," a current of air is passed through the belt thus lifting the food up into the air and quickly freezing it on all sides.

Cryogenic freezing utilizes liquid nitrogen (−320° F), liquid or solid carbon dioxide (−109° F), or some other refrigerant. With this method some foods can be frozen that were not satisfactory with sharp freezing, for example, tomatoes, watermelon, onion rings, and green pepper. Liquid nitrogen systems are in extensive use for the transportation of frozen foods.

Frozen foods should be stored at temperatures below 0° F. Ascorbic acid losses are greater than those for other nutrients. Orange juice held at

32° F for a year loses no more than 5 per cent of its ascorbic acid content, but nonacid foods lose appreciable amounts at 0° F and much lesser amounts at −10° to −20° F. Frozen foods should be kept for only a few days in the freezing compartment of a refrigerator.

If frozen foods are allowed to stand for some time at room temperature subsequent to their thawing, microorganisms multiply rapidly. Fully thawed foods should not be frozen again because further deterioration will take place. Fruits retain the best color if they are thawed in the container before it is opened. Most vegetables are cooked by dropping the frozen vegetable directly into a small quantity of boiling water and rapidly returning it to the boiling point. Corn on the cob should be thawed before it is cooked. Meats may be cooked while still frozen or may be thawed prior to cooking; the former procedure requires a considerable increase in the cooking time.

Dehydrofreezing, a relatively new process, consists in evaporating about half the water from fruits and vegetables and then freezing the product. The costs of packaging, shipping, and storage are thus reduced. Water is added to reconstitute the food when it is cooked.

Freeze-drying consists in placing the frozen food under a vacuum to remove the water and packaging in the presence of an inert gas such as nitrogen. The product retains its original volume and shape and rehydrates readily. Freeze-dried coffee is probably the most widely used product prepared by this technique. Seafoods, beef, pork, chicken, soups, and several food mixtures have been found acceptable in taste tests conducted by the U.S. Department of Agriculture.[11] They rated somewhat lower than frozen or canned foods but possessed the advantages of long shelf life, storage, and refrigeration, and light weight. The process is currently quite costly and only limited supplies are available in the general market.

Dehydration. Drying of foods is an effective means of avoiding spoilage since microorganisms cannot grow in the absence of water. Dried foods possess the special advantages of light weight and small volume and are easily transported and stored. The dehydration of certain fruits such as prunes, peaches, apricots, apples, figs, dates, and raisins, as well as meat, fish, and legumes, has been practiced for centuries. Every market today features numerous dried foods: nonfat dry milk; quick bread, yeast bread, cake, cookie, and pudding mixes; dehydrated soups; instant coffee; instant mashed potatoes; citrus juice powders; precooked rice and beans; cereals; and many others. Dried whole eggs and egg whites are used extensively in the baking industry.

Chemical preservation. Sugar is employed in high concentrations for the preparation of jams, jellies, and preserves. The water is made unavailable to the microorganisms, and hence spoilage will not occur. However, molds will grow on the surface of these foods if sterility is not maintained. Sodium chloride and vinegar are also good preservative agents as employed in brining and pickling.

The number of chemicals that may be used for preservation is now strictly limited by government regulations. Sodium benzoate may be used in some foods up to a concentration of 0.1 per cent if labels specifically indicate its use. Sulfur dioxide may be used in the drying of apples to lessen darkening. Meats may be cured with smoke that contains phenols. Older methods of curing meat employed considerable amounts of salt so that preservation was possible at ordinary room temperature. Recent processes employ less salt and more uniform though shorter curing periods, but it is important to emphasize that hams so cured are perishable and require refrigeration. Failure to refrigerate hams has caused a number of outbreaks of food poisoning in recent years. Spices such as cloves and cinnamon have been much overrated for their preservative properties, since concentrations sufficient to inhibit bacterial growth would render food inedible. See also food additives on page 272.

Antibiotics in food preservation. The uncontrolled use of antibiotics in foods or as drugs is a potential hazard to approximately 10 per cent of the population who react unfavorably to contact with them with symptoms ranging from a mild skin rash to fatal anaphylactic shock.[12] The repeated ingestion of antibiotics may produce an immunity in other individuals so that they do not respond to therapeutic doses required in the treatment of disease conditions. It is, therefore, a prime requirement that the food supply that may have had any contact with antibiotics contain no residues when eaten.

Antibiotics are used in food production. The farmer adds antibiotics to feeds to stimulate the growth of swine and poultry, or he may employ antibiotics to prevent and treat illness in animals. Crops are sometimes sprayed with antibiotics. Since no residues of the antibiotics are present in the foods as eaten, these practices constitute no health hazard. One possible source of antibiotic residues has been milk from cows which have been treated for mastitis. Regulations of the Food and Drug Administration now specify that milk obtained for three days following treatment for mastitis with antibiotic drugs must not be used for human consumption.

The shelf life of poultry and fish treated with an antibiotic is increased two to three times because of the reduced growth of microorganisms. Chlortetracycline (Aureomycin) and oxytetracycline (Terramycin) have been used in the cooling water for dressed poultry, allowing a maximum residue of 7 ppm in the uncooked poultry. Likewise, these antibiotics may be used in the ice slush for packing raw fish and shellfish, the maximum of residue allowed in the uncooked fish being 5 ppm. The cooking of poultry and fish destroys the antibiotic residues at these levels of use. With improved methods of food handling the Food and Drug Administration has recommended that the use of antibiotics to prolong shelf life be prohibited.

Preservation of foods by irradiation. One of the potential peacetime uses of atomic energy is in the radiation preservation of foods. Microorganisms can be destroyed by using gamma rays or high-speed electrons, both types of radiation being referred to as ionizing radiations. The unit of absorbed dose is the *rad,* which is the energy absorption of 100 ergs per gram. One million rad will increase the temperature of a food by only about 2° C; therefore, the term *cold sterilization* is applied to radiation processing.

Low-level irradiation. Ionizing radiation at dosages between 5,000 and 20,000 rad is sufficient to depress the sprouting of potatoes, onions, and similar foods. With 25,000 to 50,000 rad insects that infest grains are destroyed. Presently, other methods are used to control these problems because of their lower cost and their known reliability. A dosage of 750,000 rad will eliminate *Trichinella* in pork, but 20,000 rad suffice to prevent maturation of the worm larvae.

At somewhat higher levels of irradiation, that is, 100,000 to 1,000,000 rad, most microorganisms are destroyed but the product is not sterile. Fruits and vegetables may be kept for a longer time; and meats, poultry, and fish may be kept under refrigeration for appreciable lengths of time without deterioration. Radiopasteurization with doses of less than 500,000 rad holds promise of market application in the not-too-distant future.

To effect sterilization, that is, complete destruction of bacteria, 4.8 to 6.0 million rad are required, the spores of *Clostridium botulinum* being especially resistant. The inactivation of enzymes requires such high levels that it appears some heat treatment, such as blanching prior to radiation, is the only practical solution. At high dosages of radiation such as are required for sterilization, adverse changes occur in color, flavor, and texture so that many products are no longer acceptable. Moreover, modifications of nutritive value also occur. Vitamins A and E, ascorbic acid, and thiamine are especially sensitive.

Irradiation does not make the food radioactive. Irradiated foods are not presently available in the market, nor are they approved for sale by the Food and Drug Administration. Many technologic problems must be overcome before irradiation becomes practical for commercial use. Long-term studies are being conducted by the Armed Forces Food and Container Institute at Natick, Massachusetts.

FOOD ADDITIVES

Intentional additives. An *intentional* additive is a substance of known composition that has been added to a food to improve the quality in some way. Without these substances it would not be possible to produce the high quality of food that the consumer has come to expect and to maintain this quality over normal periods of transit and storage from farm, to factory, to market, to consumer. More than 1000 such substances are currently in use. Among the many functions they perform are these: enhance the flavor; improve the color; stabilize and improve texture by emulsifying, retaining moisture, thickening, binding, leavening, preventing caking, or hardening, or sticking; enrich or fortify with minerals and vitamins; mature and bleach flour; prevent oxidation and spoilage; act as propellant for food in pressurized cans. Some additives perform a single function whereas others may serve several purposes. For example, salt is both a preservative and a flavoring agent. Ascorbic acid prevents discoloration of cut fruit and also adds to the nutritive value. Table 19–1 lists some examples of additives and the functions they perform.

Incidental additives. A food may contain minute traces of a chemical as a result of contact with a substance used in its production, processing, or packaging. Since its presence serves no useful purpose in the final food product, such a chemical is considered to be an *incidental* additive. For example, food may have picked up a substance from a wrapper or a container, either by dissolving it out or by abrasion from the container into the food. Or food may

Table 19–1. Typical Uses of Some Intentional Additives

Function	Chemical Compounds	Examples of Food
Acids, alkalies, buffers		
Enhance flavor	Acetic acid	Cheese, catsup, corn syrup
	Sodium hydroxide	Pretzel glaze
Leavening	Baking powder, baking soda	Cakes, cookies, quick breads, muffins
Antioxidants		
Preventing darkening	Ascorbic acid	Fruit to be frozen
	Sulfur dioxide	Apples, apricots, peaches to be dried
Prevent rancidity	Butylated hydroxyanisole (BHA); butylated hydroxytoluene (BHT)	Lard, potato chips, meat pies, cereals, crackers
	Lecithin	Margarine, candy
	Tocopherol	Candy, oils
Coloring	Annatto; carotene	Butter, margarine
	Certified food colors	Baked goods, soft drinks
Flavoring (over 300 compounds in use)	Aromatic chemicals, essential oils, spices	
Nutritional fortification	Mineral salts, vitamins	Iodized salt; enriched breads and cereals; fortified milk and margarine; see p. 286
Preservatives	Sodium chloride	Dried pickles, salted meats
	Sodium benzoate	Dried codfish; maraschino cherries
	Chlortetracycline	Antibiotic dip for fish and dressed poultry
Inhibit mold	Calcium propionate	Bread, rolls
	Sorbic acid	Cheese wrappers
Sweeteners, nonnutritive	Saccharin	Dietetic foods and beverages
Texture	Alum	Firm pickles
Anticaking agents, retain moisture, emulsifiers, give body, jelling, thickening, binding	Disodium orthophosphate	Evaporated milk, cheese
	Mono- and diglycerides	Margarine, chocolate
	Sodium alginate	Cream cheese, ice cream
	Pectin	Jelly, French dressing
Whipping agents	Carbon dioxide	Whipped cream in pressurized can
Yeast foods and dough conditioners	Calcium phosphate; calcium lactate	Bread

contain residues of detergents remaining on dishes or residues of pesticides used in crop control.

Of genuine concern in recent years has been the widespread use of pesticides not only by farmers but also by home gardeners and by communities. Without the use of some pesticides the farmer would not be able to realize the necessary yields of crops to feed the population. The pesticides in use are numerous and fulfill such functions as killing weeds, destroying insects and rodents, and controlling plant diseases.

By their very nature the chemicals used are toxic to some forms of life or they would not be effective in controlling the pests that peril crops. It is essential that the pesticide residues remaining on foods be at levels that do not constitute any danger to health of the consumer either immediately or through gradual buildup in the body over a long period of time. It is equally important that there be no appreciable increase from year to year in the concentration of pesticides in the environment to endanger animal, fish, or bird life or to increase the levels in soils and water so that future food supplies contain levels that are toxic. Some pesticides meet these criteria but others do not. The kinds and amounts of pesticides that may be used and the residues that may remain in foods are established by regulations formulated by the Food and Drug Administration, the U.S. Department of Agriculture, and the U.S. Department of Interior. (See page 282.)

SAFE FOOD PRACTICES

The slogan of the National Sanitation Foundation is "Sanitation is a way of life." It is not difficult to formulate standards to be observed in the preparation and serving of foods in the home and in the public eating place, but it is quite another matter to educate the food handler to apply the given rules with intelligence. The best guarantee for safe food practices is effective education of homemakers and food handlers in institutional kitchens.

Safe food practices pertain to the personal hygiene of the individual, the selection, care, and preparation of food, and the selection and care of equipment. Many booklets, posters, and films are available for education on these aspects of providing a wholesome supply of food. The following rules illustrate the application of the principles of safe food practices.

Personal hygiene. 1. Individuals who have colds, sore throat, flu, or pimples, boils, or carbuncles on face or hands should not handle food until recovered.

2. Work with clean hands and fingernails, clean hair, and clean clothing.

3. Always wash hands after using the toilet, scratching the head or other part of the body, or blowing the nose. Use soap and warm water.

4. Wash hands after handling raw meat, fish, poultry, or garbage.

5. Use tongs to lift food and spoons to mix food. Avoid handling food with hands as much as possible.

6. Avoid sneezing or coughing near foods. Cover the mouth and nose while coughing or sneezing.

7. Do not return tasting spoon to food without washing it.

Food selection and storage. 1. Select foods from markets that maintain high standards of sanitation.

2. Protect foods at home or in the market from flies, insects, rodents, or contamination by unnecessary handling, sneezing, or coughing.

3. Keep cereals, flours, packaged mixes, nonfat dry milk, sugars, and other dry foods in closed containers at room temperature.

4. Store root vegetables and tubers in a dark room at cool temperature. If such facilities are not available make purchases for only a week at a time.

5. Keep refrigerator temperature at 40° to 45° F.

6. Permit adequate circulation of air around foods in the refrigerator.

7. Keep the most perishable foods in the coldest part of the refrigerator. Use perishable foods within the prescribed time limits. (See Table 19–2.)

8. Refrigerate cooked foods promptly. If a fairly large amount is to be chilled, put it into shallow pans so that cooling is rapid.

Table 19–2. Guide to Refrigerator Storage*

Foods and Storage Space	Storage Time
Coldest Part of Refrigerator	
Loosely wrapped	
Roasts, steaks, chops	3 to 5 days
Ground meats, variety meats, poultry, fish	1 to 2 days
Tightly covered	
Milk, cream, cottage cheese, cream cheese	3 to 5 days
Hard cheese	Several weeks
Other Parts of Refrigerator	
Tightly covered	
Butter, margarine	2 weeks
Opened canned foods, fresh or reconstituted juice	1 to 2 days
Nuts	
Mayonnaise and other salad dressings (after opening jar)	
Peanut butter (after opening jar)	
Covered: eggs	1 week
Uncovered	
Ripe fruits: apples	1 week
Berries, cherries	1 to 2 days
Apricots, grapes, pears, peaches, plums, rhubarb	3 to 5 days
Some fresh vegetables	
Ripe tomatoes, corn in husk, Lima beans and peas in pods	
Crisper and/or Plastic Bag	
Most fresh vegetables	
Leafy green vegetables, asparagus, Brussels sprouts, cauliflower, summer squash, beets, broccoli, cabbage, carrots, celery, cucumbers, green onions, peppers, radishes, snap beans	

Consumers All. Yearbook of Agriculture, 1965. U.S. Department of Agriculture.

9. Keep cream-filled bakery products, sandwich spreads, and salads under constant refrigeration.

10. Use canned foods within six months. Store at temperatures below 70° F if possible.

11. Use a pressure cooker for canning nonacid vegetables, meats, and poultry. Boil home-canned vegetables and meat for 10 minutes before use.

12. Discard without tasting all foods from tin cans which bulge or from glass jars which spurt when opened.

13. Use frozen foods stored in the freezing compartment of a refrigerator within a week.

14. Keep frozen foods in the freezer at 0° F or lower. Use them within the time limits set for various categories. (See Table 19–3.)

15. Use frozen foods promptly after thawing.

16. Follow directions for heating frozen prepared foods to be sure that they are heated sufficiently to destroy organisms.

17. Label all insect powders, detergents, and other chemicals. Do not keep them near foods. Keep them out of reach of children.

Care of equipment. 1. Clean all kitchen equipment after each use. Inspect meat choppers, slicers, and mechanical mixers to be sure that they are thoroughly cleaned.

2. Scrub all surfaces with which raw meat, poultry, and fish have come in contact before placing any other food on them.

3. Keep dirty dishes away from clean dishes.

4. When using hand washing for dishes, use hot water and detergent, changing the water frequently. Place washed dishes in rinse water at 170° F for at least 30 seconds. Allow dishes to drain without drying with a towel.

5. Dishes are better sanitized when washed

Table 19–3. Maximum Storage Time for Some Frozen Foods (at 0° F)

	Months		Months
Beef or lamb roasts, steaks, chops	12	Cooked fish and shellfish	3
Pork or veal roast	8	Oysters	1
Poultry, cut up	6	Fruits	12
Chicken, whole	3	Fruit juices	12
Ground meat	3	Vegetables	8–10
Cooked meat, frozen dinners	3	Pie, unbaked	8
Sausage, ham	2	Cakes	2–3
Fish, shrimp, clams, raw	2–4	Bread, rolls, pastry	2–3
		Frozen desserts	1

in a dishwasher. In institutions public health regulations specify that dishes be washed at least 20 seconds at 140° F and then rinsed at 170° F for at least 10 seconds.

EMERGENCY FEEDING

Following a natural or man-made disaster, the goals of emergency feeding are "to keep people alive, to restore and maintain morale, and to provide adequate and familiar food that will keep people at work or enable them to return to work."* The American Red Cross assumes responsibility for emergency feeding in a natural disaster such as a flood, and the civil defense and welfare services carry out feeding during disaster from war.

Problems associated with emergency feeding. Disruption of one or more utilities may make it impossible to cook foods or to use water. Stockpiles must be so planned that some foods not requiring heating are available. The lack of water limits the kinds of foods which can be cooked and seriously interferes with cleaning and waste disposal.

The dietary needs of special groups require preplanning. Infants and young children are especially vulnerable to the lack of food, and parents are likely to become panic stricken if their children are not cared for. Dry and evaporated milk supplies are vital for infants and children. When no water is available for formula preparation, Bovee has suggested that canned fruit

*Bovee, D. L.: "Emergency Feeding in Disaster," *Am. J. Clin. Nutr.*, 6:77, 1958.

juices and even carbonated beverages might be used. The ill and the aged should also be considered. Most patients on modified diets can survive a short period when some foods needed by them are not available. For example, patients with peptic ulcer may get along quite satisfactorily if it is at all possible to eat a food such as bread at more frequent intervals. Every diabetic should be fully instructed on what to do when he is unable to get his food or his insulin.

The worker in a disaster—fire fighter, rescue worker, or the person restoring facilities—must receive sufficient food allowances so that he can keep his work at a maximum output; this may require 3000 to 3500 calories daily.

A disaster is no time to give unfamiliar foods, since the stress of the emergency will usually lead to refusal. Therefore, local foods which are familar and well liked should be used.

During the first few days following a disaster, food to allay hunger and to sustain morale takes precedence over meeting nutritional needs. A cup of hot coffee to the adult and milk to the child given as soon as possible are tangible evidence that someone is caring for them and that some community facilities are functioning. When an emergency is of more than a few days' duration, nutrient needs must be considered. The recommended allowances, however, are likely to provide unrealistic goals when there are food shortages; rationing priorities must be defined.

Safety of food supplies. Following a nuclear attack, the hazards of radioactive contamination of food and water must be appreciated. Foods which are in sealed, unbroken packages or in cans are safe for use, as are those in a refrigerator or freezer which has remained closed. However, the outside of the food container or utensil for cooking and eating must first be washed in detergent solution to remove the radioactive substances. Wash water and cloths used for cleaning must be buried.

If no refrigeration facilities are available, food spoilage occurs rapidly and food poisoning may affect large numbers of people. Infant formulas may be prepared from dry milk just before use if they cannot be refrigerated.

Guide for an Emergency Shelf for the Family*

General Considerations

1. Allow about 2 quarts liquid per person per day—fruit and vegetable juices, bottled water, soft drinks. Allow 2 additional quarts water for personal care.

2. Plan menus in advance using foods the family likes, and keeping these situations in mind: (1) no fuel available and water is limited; (2) no fuel available but there is sufficient water; (3) cooking facilities but little water; (4) cooking facilities and ample water.

3. Stock foods on the basis of menus planned. Avoid those foods which increase thirst. A two-week supply of foods is recommended.

4. Rotate food supplies at least every six months so that stock is always fresh.

5. Use only airtight containers—metal, plastic, or heavily waxed cardboard. Glass is not satisfactory since it may shatter.

6. Consider emergency cooking facilities.

Suitable Foods from Which to Select (all in airtight containers)

Liquids: fruit juices including citrus juices; vegetable juices; carbonated beverages; water

Milk: nonfat dry and evaporated

Canned foods: fruits; vegetables; soups; stews; baked beans; spaghetti and other pastes with sauces; chicken, meatballs, sea food, pressed pork; peanut butter; cheese; oils; shortening; jelly, jam, preserves

Dried foods: dried fruits; legumes

Cereals and breads: dry cereals; ready-to-eat cereals; spaghetti, macaroni, rice, noodles; flour; canned or frozen breads; cookies

Infant foods: dry milk, cereals, fruits, vegetables, strained meats

Miscellaneous foods: instant coffee, tea, salt, pepper, sugar, candy, pickles

Supplies: cooking and eating utensils, paper dishes, matches, candles, bottle and can openers, covered cans for waste disposal, water containers, paper towels and napkins, detergent powder

*Adapted from "Confidentially Speaking—A Report on Emergency Feeding," Nutrition Section, Louisiana Department of Health, August 1957.

Review

1. List several ways in which bacterial diseases may be transmitted by foods.
2. Give two examples of bacterial infections transmitted by foods; two examples of bacterial poisoning.
3. What organisms are responsible for most cases of summer food poisoning?
4. Explain what is meant by botulism. Which types of food are most likely to contain botulinus toxin? What measures are necessary to eliminate the possibility of botulinus poisoning?
5. Describe the effects of *Trichinella* infestation. How can it be avoided?
6. Lead and arsenic are especially poisonous to man. In what ways do they sometimes contaminate food supplies?
7. Name several plants that are poisonous to man. What types of chemical compounds produce this poisoning?
8. What are the causes of food spoilage?
9. Why are commercially canned foods likely to be superior in their vitamin content to home-canned foods?
10. Which method of canning is preferable for home use? Why?
11. What losses of nutritive value occur in dehydration?
12. Name five chemical agents frequently used for preservation.
13. What are the time and temperature requirements for the pasteurization of milk?

14. What is the nature of each of these in food preservation: irradiation, aseptic canning, dehydrofreezing, antibiotics? What advantages and disadvantages may be claimed for each?
15. Read the labels of a variety of packaged foods and list the additives. Try to determine the reason for each additive. What objections can you see to the use of additives? Would it be advisable to avoid the use of all additives? Explain your answer fully.
16. What is strontium-90? Cesium-137? Iodine-131? Of what significance are they to the health of man?
17. Why is a liberal intake of milk likely to be protective against the effects of strontium-90?
18. Each of the rules stated on page 274 for the selection, care, and preparation of food is based upon an important principle discussed in this chapter. Select any six of these rules and for each write a statement of the principle involved.
19. Prepare a menu for three days that could be used following a disaster when cooking facilities are available but the water supply is lacking. List the foods that would be necessary in the family stockpile for these menus.

Cited References

1. Ouzounellis, T.: "Some Notes on Quail Poisoning," *J.A.M.A.*, **211**:1186–87, 1970.
2. Woodward, W. E., *et al.*: "Foodborne Disease Surveillance in the United States, 1966 and 1967," *Am. J. Public Health*, **60**:130–37, 1970.
3. Foster E. M.: "Microbial Problems in Today's Foods," *J. Am. Diet Assoc.*, **52**:485–89, 1968.
4. Foltz, V. D.: "Salmonella Ecology," *J. Am. Oil Chem. Soc.*, **46**:222–24, 1969.
5. "Clostridium Perfringens," *FDA Papers*, **4**:19–22, Feb. 1970.
6. Milstead, K. L.: "Science Works Through Law to Protect Consumers," *J. Am. Diet. Assoc.*, **48**:187–91, 1966.
7. Campbell, A. D.: "Natural Food Poisons," *FDA Papers*, **1**:23–27, Sept. 1967.
8. Hadjimarkos, D. M.: "Geographic Variations of Dental Caries in Oregon," *J. Pediatr.*, **48**:195–201, 1956.
9. Lidbeck, W. L., *et al.*: "Acute Sodium Fluoride Poisoning," *J.A.M.A.*, **121**:826–27, 1943.
10. Dunning, G. M.: "Radioactivity in the Diet," *J. Am. Diet. Assoc.*, **42**:17–28, 1963.
11. Bird, K.: *Freeze-Dried Foods*. Marketing Research Report No. 617, U.S. Department of Agriculture, 1963.
12. Welch, H.: "Problems of Antibiotics in Foods," *J.A.M.A.*, **170**:2093–96, 1959.

Additional References

Anderson, E. C., and Nelson, D. J., Jr.: "Surveillance for Radiological Contamination," *Am. J. Public Health*, **52**:1391–1400, 1962.
Armstrong, R. W.: "Type E Botulism from Home-canned Gefilte Fish," *J.A.M.A.*, **210**:303–305, 1969.
Borgstrom, G.: *Principles of Food Science*. The Macmillan Company, New York, 1968, Vol. I, Chaps. 2, 3; Vol II, Chaps. 5, 6, 7, 12.
Brooke, M. M.: "Epidemiology of Amebiasis in the U.S." *J.A.M.A.*, **188**:519–21, 1964.
Browe, J. H.: "Principles of Emergency Feeding," in Wohl, M. G. and Goodhart, R. S.: *Modern Nutrition in Health and Disease*, 4th ed. Lea & Febiger, 1968, pp. 1183–95.
Coerver, R. M.: "One Man's Meat," *Am. J. Nurs.*, **58**:690–92, 1958.
Dack, G. M.: *Food Poisoning*. University of Chicago Press, Chicago, 1956.
Dolman, C. E.: "Botulism," *Am. J. Nurs.*, **64**:119–24, 1964.
Hodges, R. E.: "The Toxicity of Pesticides and Their Residues in Food," *Nutr. Rev.*, **23**:225–30, 1965.

Huppler, P. P., *et al.:* "Bacterial Implications of Holding Casseroles in Automatic Ovens," *J. Home Econ.,* **56:**748–51, 1964.

Longrée, K.: "Sanitation in Food Vending," *J. Am. Diet. Assoc.,* **54:**215–20, 1969.

Mickelsen, O.: "Present Knowledge of Naturally Occurring Toxicants in Foods," *Nutr. Rev.,* **26:**129–33, 1968.

Moses, W. R., and Pippin, H. N.: "Chemical Preservatives," *FDA Papers,* **4:**25–28, Feb. 1970.

Schroeder, S. A., *et al.:* "Epidemic Salmonellosis in Hospitals and Institutions" *N. Engl. J. Med.,* **279:**674–78, 1968.

Smillie, W. G., and Kilbourne, E. D.: *Preventive Medicine and Public Health,* 3rd ed. The Macmillan Company, New York, 1963.

Thatcher, F. S.: "Food-Borne Bacterial Toxins," *Can. Med. Assoc. J.,* **94:**582–90, 1966.

Werrin, M., and Kronick, D.: "Salmonella Control in Hospitals," *Am. J. Nurs.,* **66:**528–31, 1966.

Wogan, G. N.: "Current Research on Toxic Food Contaminants," *J. Am. Diet. Assoc.,* **49:**95–98, 1966.

20 Controls for the Safety and Nutritive Value of the Food Supply

You shall not eat anything that dies of itself.
DEUT. 14:21

You shall not have in your bag two kinds of weights, a large and a small. You shall not have in your house two kinds of measures, a large and a small. A full and just weight you shall have, a full and just measure you shall have.
DEUT. 25:13–15

These Biblical quotations are but two of the many laws concerning the use of food set down by Moses and others. Although examples may be found throughout history of efforts to exercise some controls over the food supply, the major advances have come in the present century.

FEDERAL LEGISLATION

Need for food laws. The growth of an urban society and the revolutionary developments in science and technology have necessitated numerous controls to protect the consumer. In the early days of this nation the consumer, for the most part, was also the producer. He grew the crops, raised the cattle, preserved the food by methods then available, and cooked the food in his own home. By and large, those not engaged in agriculture purchased food from sellers who were known on a personal basis. Even in colonial history, however, one can find examples of laws designed to protect the consumer against fraud.

With the industrial development and movement to cities people became dependent upon growers, manufacturers, and distributors for the food supply. Not all practices were honest. In fact, the conditions for sanitation in food processing and marketing by the end of the nineteenth century were often described as appalling. Far too common were fraudulent practices whereby the products were diluted with some cheap and unsafe ingredient so that a greater profit could be realized. Over these unsavory practices the consumer had little control.

Advances in science and technology. The twentieth-century developments in microbiology have provided the rationale for good practices in handling food and have served as the basis for setting up controls which might be exercised for a safe food supply. The chemist's laboratory has opened hitherto undreamed-of possibilities for variety in the food supply, preservation, and improvement of nutritional quality, but it has also created vast problems in controls from farm, to factory, to warehouse, and to market. Today's farmer fertilizes his soil with products purchased from a chemical plant; he dusts and sprays his crops; he uses hormones to accelerate the growth of animals. The manufacturer chooses from hundreds of chemical products to improve the color, flavor, texture, nutritional quality, and keeping properties of his product. Chemicals of some sort enter into the numerous steps in food production —from the sanitation of the plant machinery to the package in which the food is sold. Without these aids from the chemical industry, this country could not produce its abundant supply of high-quality food.

Role of the food industry. Much credit for the remarkable improvements in the food supply must be given to responsible growers, manufacturers, and distributors. A visit to a modern food plant can be an exciting experience. One is impressed with the systems developed for the quality grading of food as it is received, the complex machinery for handling food from raw product to package, the continuous emphasis upon sanitation, and the attractiveness of the finished product. The laboratories in such a plant are at the very center of the successful operation. On the one hand, they are concerned with quality control; on the other, they are developing products for tomorrow's market basket. Many specialists are employed in the maintenance of controls and development of new products—agricultural specialists, food scientists, chefs, microbiologists, chemists, biochemists, nutritionists, and home economists, to name but a few.

Good laws aid industry as well as the consumer, for they provide guidelines for good manufacturing practice and protect against unfair competition through dishonest labeling and adulteration. Federal agencies of the Department of Agriculture and of Health, Education, and Welfare work closely with manufacturers on problems which arise in food production.

Federal laws. One of the principal crusaders in the movement to secure legislation for a wholesome food supply was Dr. Harvey W. Wiley, who was a chief chemist for the U.S. Department of Agriculture. Through his writings and his public appearances he sought the cooperation of women's groups and was instrumental in the enactment in 1906 of the first "pure food" law, the Food and Drug Act. The law, signed by President Theodore Roosevelt, has been represented by some as the most significant peacetime legislation in the history of the country.[1]

Food, drug, and cosmetic act. With rapid advances in food technology and industry, the manufacture and distribution of food became increasingly complex and broader in scale so that the original law became inadequate. Many consumer pressures in the 1930's led to the enactment of the Food, Drug, and Cosmetic Act of 1938. The objectives of the law have been summarized as "safe, effective drugs, and cosmetics; pure, wholesome foods; honest labeling and packaging."[2] The Food and Drug Administration (FDA) is an agency of the Department of Health, Education and Welfare charged with the responsibility for the enforcement of this act and its amendments.

Amendments. The Food, Drug, and Cosmetic Act has been amended a number of times to meet new problems of control as they have arisen. Although additives are essential for high-

quality food in sufficient supply for a rapidly expanding population, the introduction of thousands of such products on the market necessitates legal controls for safety and usefulness. For such protection, these amendments to the 1938 law have been enacted:

1954: Pesticides Amendment.
1958: Food Additives Amendment, including intentional and incidental additives.
1960: Color Additive Amendments.

Before an additive may be marketed approval must be secured from the Food and Drug Administration, which has spelled out in some detail the requirements that must be met. Essentially, these amendments place the burden of proof for usefulness and safety of a food additive upon the manufacturer, who is required to submit full data which includes name, chemical properties, methods for manufacture, quantities to be used, the conditions for use, the effect of additions on the food, methods for detecting residues in foods, safety, and recommended tolerances. Data pertaining to safety must include toxicity tests on two or more species of animals, usually for a two-year period; estimates of the maximum amounts which might be consumed in a day; and the cumulative effects upon the body.

The Food and Drug Administration may conduct further tests after examination of the manufacturer's data. Approval will include specific limits for amounts and conditions of use. If a request is denied, the manufacturer may appeal the decision, submit additional data, and request a hearing.

Fair Packaging and Labeling Act. In 1966 the Congress authorized the FDA to set up requirements for complete information in labeling and for packaging that is not deceptive in terms of the contents. This act supplements the 1938 law. Included are these label regulations:[3]

1. A statement of identity of a food, under its usual or common name such as *peaches* or *beets*, must appear in bold type on the principal display panel. If a standard of identity (see page 285) has been established for the product, the name shall appear as it is stated in the standard. When a food is packed in various forms such as whole, sliced, or

chopped, the form shall be prominently shown with the name of the product except when a see-through container is used.

2. The name and full business address of the manufacturer, packer, or distributor shall be conspicuously shown, indicating "packed for" or "distributed by" if the name is not that of the manufacturer.

3. A statement of the net contents separated from other label information shall appear in legible boldface type within the bottom 30 per cent of the principal display panel. For packages containing more than 1 pound but less than 4 pounds the net contents shall be stated in ounces, followed in parentheses by the weight in pounds and ounces or in pounds and common or decimal fractions, for example, 35 ounces (2 pounds 3 ounces). For liquid measure of at least 1 quart but less than 1 gallon the volume shall be stated in fluid ounces, followed in parentheses by the measure in quarts or pints and fluid ounces or by common or decimal fractions of quarts or pints.

4. When a label includes a statement of the number of servings, the usual size of that serving shall be stated, for example, in cups or tablespoons.

5. When ingredient listing is required, the information shall appear in a single panel listing by common name in decreasing order of predominance. A listing is not required for products for which a standard of identity has been established.

Regulation of pesticides. That each citizen has a responsibility to be informed concerning matters of health and that he can be effective in bringing about change is well illustrated by the developments during the last decade on pesticide control. The public was little aware of the use of pesticides until the book *Silent Spring* by Rachel Carson was published in 1962. The wide concern created by the book led to the appointment by President Kennedy in 1963 of a Science Advisory Committee which later issued a report recognizing the advantages that pesticides had played in food production and disease control, but also calling for "orderly reduction in the use of persistent pesticides."* Intensive study of the effects of pesticides has been conducted by toxicologists and public health officials. Special interest groups such as the National Audubon Society, the Sierra Club, and the Environmental Defense Fund have pub-

*Ramsey, L. L.: "A Twilight for Persistent Pesticides," *FDA Papers*, 4:14–18, Feb. 1970.

licized the problems created by pesticides such as DDT. In March 1969 the Food and Drug Administration found that shipments of coho salmon from Lake Michigan contained DDT far in excess of safe tolerances. This was a threat to public health and also to the fishing industry, and a commission was appointed to study the problem. In November 1969 the Commission on Pesticides set forth these principles:

1. Chemicals, including pesticides used to increase food production, are of such importance in modern life that we must learn to live with them;

2. In looking at their relative merits and hazards we must make individual judgments upon the value of each chemical, including the alternatives presented by the nonuse of these chemicals. We must continue to accumulate scientific data about the effects of these chemicals on the total ecology; and

3. The final decision regarding the usage of these chemicals must be made by those governmental agencies with the statutory responsibilities for the public health, and for pesticides regulations.*

The Commission made 14 recommendations to the Secretary of Health, Education, and Welfare.[4] Some of these have been implemented and others require legislative action. Among the recommendations are these:

Close cooperation between the Departments of Agriculture, Health, Education, and Welfare, and Interior.

Elimination of the use of DDT and DDD within two years except where essential for human health and welfare.

Restriction on the use of other persistent pesticides.

Development of standards for pesticide content of foods, water, and air so that the public is protected from hazards, but also recognizing the need for an optimum food supply.

Reviewing adequacy of legislation pertaining to the labeling and instructions for use of pesticides, the packaging and transportation to avoid spillage and contamination of other materials, and control of effluents from plants manufacturing pesticides; and others.

Meat and poultry inspection. The "pure food" law of 1906 did not include meat and meat prod-

* *Ibid.*, pp. 16–17.

ucts. The Meat Inspection Act, passed in 1906, is enforced by the Meat Inspection Division of the Agricultural Research Service in the U.S. Department of Agriculture. The Poultry Inspection Act passed in 1957, with regulations similar to the Meat Inspection Act, requires the inspection of poultry and poultry products that enter interstate commerce. These laws provide for (1) the inspection of animals intended for slaughter; (2) the inspection of carcasses and all meat products; (3) enforcement of sanitary regulations; (4) guarding against the use of harmful preservatives. (See Figure 20–1.) Federal inspection stamps (see Figure 20–2) are placed upon the surface of the carcass if the meat is wholesome. The flesh of an animal that is diseased is stamped "inspected and condemned" and the carcass must be destroyed or may be used for nonfood purposes if warranted.

Two new laws have been recently enacted: the 1967 Federal Wholesome Meat Act and the 1968 Federal Wholesome Poultry Products Act.[5] These laws give authority to the U.S. Department of Agriculture to seize meat and poultry products moving illegally or that have become adulterated or misbranded after leaving official premises. An important part of these laws sets up a cooperative arrangement between state-federal inspection programs. This provides better protection for the consumer of meat and poultry products within a given state. Preventive sanitation is an important part of the inspection program.

ENFORCEMENT OF THE LAWS

Food and Drug Administration. In order to enforce the law the Food and Drug Administration must also be a scientific organization. Pharmacologists, bacteriologists, chemists, biochemists, entomologists, physicians, and veterinarians are among the specialists who work in Washington and in the 18 district offices to determine the physical and chemical characteristics of products and to develop improved methods to detect deviations from the standards which have been set up.

The Food and Drug Administration also con-

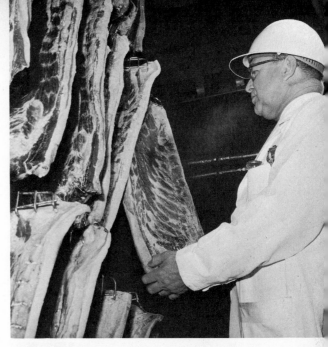

Figure 20–1. U.S. Department of Agriculture meat inspectors check for the wholesomeness of all meat products and meat produced in plants dealing in interstate or foreign commerce. An inspector examines bacon during processing at a smokehouse to make sure the processing is done according to approved formulas and procedures. (Courtesy, U.S. Department of Agriculture.)

ducts an educational program pertaining to voluntary compliance activities directed to the manufacturer. Most recently highly qualified nutritionists and dietitians have been appointed in many cities to serve as consumer consultants to the public.

Enforcement of legislation. The federal laws cover about 60,000 establishments that process foods which enter interstate commerce and foods

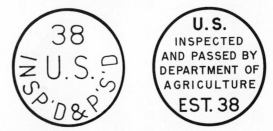

Figure 20–2. (*A*) Seal appearing as purple stamp on cuts of meat passed by U.S. Department of Agriculture inspector. (*B*) Seal appearing on labels of prepared meat products. (Courtesy, U.S. Department of Agriculture.)

which are imported. Inspectors visit factories, warehouses, and stores to see that the laws are being complied with. They are concerned with the raw materials used, the processes of manufacturing, the packaging and storage practices, and plant sanitation. (See Figure 20–3.)

If inspectors find violations of the law they may remove the food from the market or require that the labeling be revised. Depending on the circumstances, the food may be destroyed, or it may be reclaimed and relabeled under the supervision of the inspectors.

Court proceedings become necessary for those who flagrantly violate the laws. Fines or imprisonment, or both, may be imposed for each violation. Injunctions may be issued by the court to prevent repetition of a violation.

Adulteration and misbranding. Under the law, definitions of adulteration and misbranding have been developed. (See Figure 20–4.)

Adulteration of food has occurred if it contains any substance injurious to health; it contains any filthy, putrid, or decomposed substance; it is prepared, handled, or stored under unsanitary conditions; diseased animals have been used in preparation; the container is made of a poisonous substance which will render the contents harmful; valuable constituents have been omitted; substitutes have been used to conceal inferiority; it contains coal-tar colors other than those permitted by law; it contains pesticide residues or additives not recognized as safe.

Misbranding has occurred if the label is false

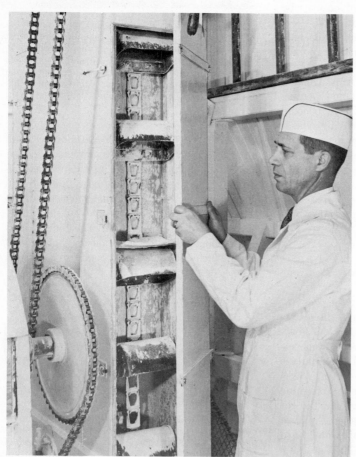

Figure 20–3. The FDA inspector knows that the interior of the elevator is a common place for insect development if flour is allowed to remain. (Courtesy, Food and Drug Administration.)

or misleading; the food is sold under another name; imitations are not clearly indicated; the size of the container is misleading; statement of weight, measure, or count is not given or is wrong; manufacturer, packer, or distributor is not listed on the package forms; it is below standard without indication of substandard quality on the label; it fails to list nutrient information when it is supposed to be for special dietary purposes; it fails to list artificial colorings, flavorings, and preservatives.

Standards. A *standard of identity* establishes what a product really is. A product which has been so defined must include specified ingredients, often with amounts restricted to designated minimum-maximum ranges. For example, the standard of identity for Cheddar cheese specifies a minimum of 50 per cent milk fat (on a moisture-free basis) and not more than 25 per cent moisture. Fruit jelly and preserves must contain not less than 45 parts by weight of fruit or fruit juice to 55 parts total sweetener. Optional ingredients listed in the standard may be used, but any ingredients that are not mentioned in the standard are forbidden.

The standards are set up after consultation with numerous sources for the customary practices in manufacture and preparation. Proposals for new standards are published in the Federal Register. Opportunity is then given for interested parties, including manufacturers and consumers, to study the proposed regulations and to recommend changes. If there is any controversy, public hearings may be held.

The label for a food for which a standard of identity has been set does not need to include a listing of required ingredients since these are defined within the standard. However, if optional ingredients are included they must be named.

Among the products for which standards of identity have been established are: chocolate and cocoa products; cereal flours and related products; macaroni and noodle products; bakery products; milk and cream; cheese and cheese products; frozen desserts; dressings for foods—mayonnaise, French dressing, salad dressing; canned fruit and canned fruit juices; fruit but-

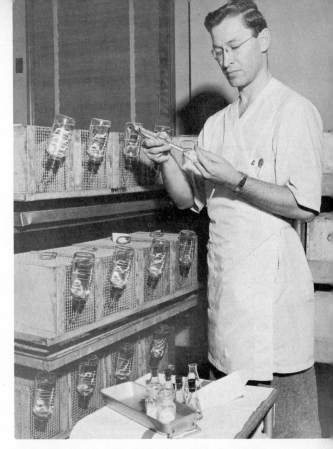

Figure 20–4. An FDA biochemist checks the vitamin D content of milk by feeding the test dose to a laboratory animal. After a given period of time, the bone calcification will be measured by the line test shown in Figure 10–6. (Courtesy, Food and Drug Administration.)

ters—jellies, preserves; shellfish; canned tuna; eggs and egg products; oleomargarine—margarine; vegetables and vegetable products.

Standards of quality indicate the minimum quality below which foods must not fall. Foods that do not meet the quality specifications must be labeled "Below Standard in Quality" followed by a statement such as "Good Food—Not High Grade" or "Excessively Broken," etc. Canned foods that do not meet standards of quality are seldom seen on the market.

Standards for fill aim to protect the customer against deception through the use of containers that appear to contain more food than they actually do. Specifications are set up for foods that tend to shake down in the package, or for number of pieces of food within a container.

REGULATIONS PERTAINING TO NUTRITIONAL VALUE

Enrichment of foods. Few nutritional programs have been of greater significance than the enrichment and fortification of foodstuffs. This venture in public health illustrates the effectiveness of the combined efforts of public and private agencies at state and national levels and of the food industry.

Policies for enrichment. In 1961 the Food and Nutrition Board of the National Research Council and the Council on Foods and Nutrition of the American Medical Association adopted jointly a statement of general policy regarding addition of specific nutrients to foods. They endorsed:

... the enrichment of flour, bread, degerminated cornmeal, corn grits, whole grain cornmeal, and white rice; the retention or restoration of thiamine, riboflavin, niacin, and iron in processed food cereals; the addition of vitamin D to milk, fluid skim milk, and nonfat dry milk; the addition of vitamin A to margarine, fluid skim milk, and nonfat dry milk; and the addition of iodine to table salt. The protective action of fluoride against dental caries is recognized and the standardized addition of fluoride to water is endorsed in areas in which the water supply has a low fluoride content.*

In 1968 the two groups reaffirmed the endorsement of enrichment and revised the policy statement. The addition of nutrients to foods is endorsed when all the following criteria are met:

1. The intake of the nutrient(s) is below the desirable level in the diets of a significant number of people.

2. The food(s) used to supply the nutrient(s) is likely to be consumed in quantities that will make a significant contribution to the diet of the population in need.

3. The addition of the nutrient(s) is not likely to create an imbalance of the essential nutrients.

4. The nutrient(s) added is stable under proper conditions of storage and use.

5. The nutrient(s) is physiologically available from the food.

6. There is reasonable assurance against excessive intake to a level of toxicity.*

In addition, the policy statement provides guidelines for the composition of imitation or fabricated foods. Essentially a new food should contain the same amounts and variety of nutrients on a comparable caloric basis as the food it replaces.

Enrichment standards. The enrichment of foods is not presently required by federal law, and many states do not require it. Although manufacturers have voluntarily enriched flours and breads and other foods, the products are not always available to people who are on marginal diets and who would benefit the most. A national program of enrichment is clearly desirable.

When nutrients are added voluntarily to flours and breads, the amounts used must come within minimum-maximum ranges set up by the Food and Drug Administration. (See Table 20–1.) The label must include a statement that spells out each vitamin and/or mineral that has been added.

Other standards for the voluntary additions of nutrients to food include:

1. Vitamin A fortification of margarine: 15,-000 U.S.P. units per pound to compare with the year-round average for butter.

2. Vitamin D fortification of milk: 400 U.S.P. units per quart or tall can of evaporated milk. Most of the evaporated milk and fluid milk is now fortified.

In 1966 the FDA set up regulations for foods for special dietary uses.[5] Some of these regulations are as follows:†

1. The Recommended Dietary Allowances for minerals and vitamins for four age groups and for pregnant and lactating women shall replace the Min-

---

*Council on Foods and Nutrition, American Medical Association and Food and Nutrition Board, National Research Council: "Statement of General Policy in Regard to Addition of Specific Nutrients to Foods," May 1961.

*Council on Foods and Nutrition: "Improvement of Nutritive Quality of Foods," *J.A.M.A.*, **205**:160–61, Sept. 16, 1968.

†Hearings on these regulations have not yet been completed and hence they are not yet in effect.

Table 20–1. Federal Standards of Identity for Enriched Foods

(*Minimum and Maximum Levels in Milligrams per Pound*)

Foods	Thiamine	Riboflavin	Niacin	Iron
Bread, rolls, and other baked foods	1.1–1.8	0.7–1.6	10.0–15.0	8.0–12.5
Flour*	2.0–2.5	1.2–1.5	16.0–20.0	13.0–16.5
Farina	2.0–2.5	1.2–1.5	16.0–20.0	13.0–—†
Macaroni, noodle, paste products‡	4.0–5.0	1.7–2.2	27.0–34.0	13.0–16.5
Cornmeal and grits	2.0–3.0	1.2–1.8	16.0–24.0	13.0–26.0
Rice§	2.0–4.0	1.2–2.4	16.0–32.0	13.0–26.0

*Calcium enrichment is also required for self-rising flour.

†A maximum level of iron enrichment for farina has not been established.

‡Levels of enrichment allow for 30 to 50 per cent losses in preparation.

§ Because of technical difficulties in the application of riboflavin, the enrichment levels for this vitamin in rice are optional pending further study and hearings.

imum Daily Requirements, inasmuch as the latter have often been misunderstood.

2. Definitions and standards of identity have been set for vitamin and mineral supplements, with the amounts permitted falling within a specified range.

3. Foods intended for modified diets must meet certain standards in their formulation and in labeling. For example, if a food is represented as "lower in calories," it must have at least 50 per cent fewer calories than the food with which it is compared. When artificial sweeteners are used, the label must indicate its presence and that it is nonnutritive. Foods for diabetic diets must be labeled "for the diets of diabetics" and must list the protein, fat, and carbohydrate value in grams and the calories in 100 grams of foods and in an average serving.

4. The levels of minerals and vitamins used to fortify nine classes of foods are defined:

. . . processed cereals; fruit or vegetable juices, drinks, nectars, etc.; infant and junior fruit products; fluid and powdered whole milk (or milk products) for drinking; fluid skimmed milk (or milk product) and fluid or powdered low-fat milk (or milk product) for drinking; salt; frozen dessert products; milk fortifiers; and meat substitutes.

OTHER AGENCIES

Role of the Food Protection Committee. To study the legitimate uses of chemical additives, the Food Protection Committee was established in 1950 as a permanent committee of the Food and Nutrition Board. The membership of the committee includes specialists who are qualified to establish criteria for the evaluation of additives on the basis of their chemical and physical properties, their toxicologic aspects when tested in several species, and their metabolic and nutritional aspects.

The Food Protection Committee acts as a clearing house for information on pesticides and intentional chemicals; it reviews the information and makes it available; it assists in the integration and promotion of research in foods; it aids regulatory agencies in the formulation of principles and standardized procedure; it aids in the dissemination of accurate information to the public. The committee cooperates closely with the Food and Drug Administration so that suitable legal controls may be enacted.

Federal agencies. *The U.S. Public Health Service.* The Public Health Service is also under the Department of Health, Education, and Welfare. It carries out research to establish effective procedures in ensuring a safe food supply. It recommends sanitary codes and ordinances. During outbreaks of food poisoning it conducts tests to determine the source and nature of the poisoning. One of its concerns is the effect of diet on nutritional status and health.

The Public Health Service has defined standards for milk production and quality that provide the basis for the codes used in most states and communities. It also certifies interstate milk shippers.

Federal Trade Commission. Consumers may be misled by advertising just as they are misled by the label or the appearance of a product. The FTC aims to prevent unfair methods of competition in commerce. An order may be issued to a company to "cease and desist" if its advertising is false, misleading, or exaggerated in its claims.

The Post Office Department. This Department enforces laws relating to false advertising and the use of the mails to defraud.

State and local regulations. Food that is produced and sold within state boundaries does not come under federal control. Therefore, states and communities must establish their own regulations for the safety and quality of foods. The identity of foods, the labeling, the inspection of plants, markets, and public eating places are subject to control set up by state departments of agriculture and of health. Some cities and states require periodic medical examination of food handlers. Most of the regulations are patterned after those of federal laws, but considerable variations exist from state to state.

PROBLEMS AND REVIEW

1. What reasons can you give for the need for federal legislation concerning the food supply?
2. What is the aim of the Food, Drug, and Cosmetic Act? Under its provisions what is meant by misbranding? By adulteration?
3. What provisions are included in the Meat Inspection Act?
4. In purchasing two foods manufactured in another state you find that all the ingredients are listed on the label of one product, but there is no such listing on the other label. How can you explain the difference?
5. *Problem.* Determine the governmental agency in your community that is responsible for controlling the sale of milk; the sale of meat sold within the state; the inspection of public eating places.
6. Examine the labels of several packages or cans of dietetic foods. What information is given? Does it agree with the requirements set up for dietetic foods?
7. Under recently enacted federal legislation, where does primary responsibility for providing the safety of an additive rest? What information is essential for establishing this safety?
8. *Problem.* Prepare a short paper (about 300 words) that describes the activities of any one of the following organizations in promoting a safe food supply: Food Protection Committee; U.S. Public Health Service; your state department of health; your state department of agriculture.

CITED REFERENCES

1. Hill, M. M.: "Labels on Food Products," *Nutrition Program News,* U.S. Department of Agriculture, Washington, D.C., March–June 1964.
2. Larrick, G. P.: "The Role of the Food and Drug Administration in Nutrition," *Am. J. Clin. Nutr.,* 8:377–82, 1960.
3. Friedelson, I.: "Fair Packaging," *FDA Papers,* 1:21–24, Oct. 1967.
4. Ramsey, L. L.: "A Twilight for Persistent Pesticides," *FDA Papers,* 4:14–18, Feb. 1970.
5. "New Meat Inspection Laws for Consumer Protection," *Public Health Rep.,* 84:214, 1969.
6. "Regulations for Foods for Special Dietary Uses," *FDA Fact Sheet,* U.S. Department of Health, Education, and Welfare, Washington, D.C., 1968.

ADDITIONAL REFERENCES

Anderson, O. E.: *The Health of a Nation: Harvey W. Wiley and the Fight for Pure Food.* University of Chicago Press, Chicago, 1958.

Chadwick, D. R.: "The Public Health Role in Controlling Radiation," *Am. J. Public Health,* **55**:731–37, 1965.

Council on Foods and Nutrition: "Improvement of Nutritive Quality of Foods," *J.A.M.A.,* **205**:868–69, 1969.

Darby, W. J.: "Man—His Environment and Health. Part II. Pesticides: A Contribution to Agriculture and Nutrition," *Am. J. Public Health,* **54** (Supplement): 18–23, Jan. 1964.

Duggan, R. E.: "Foods and Pesticides," *FDA Papers,* **2**:14, Sept. 1968.

Food Protection Committee, Food and Nutrition Board, Selected Publications:
Chemicals Used in Food Processing, Pub. 1274, 1965.
An Evaluation of Public Health Hazards from the Microbiological Contamination of Foods, Pub. 1195, 1964.
Radionuclides in Foods, Pub. 988, 1962.

Lennington, K. R.: "Status and Review of the Salmonella Program," *FDA Papers,* **2**:9, Feb. 1968.

Leverton, R. M.: "Fortification Broadened to More Foods Distributed by USDA," *J. Am. Diet. Assoc.,* **54**:317, 1969.

Moses, W. R., and Pippin, H. N.: "Chemical Preservatives," *FDA Papers,* **4**:25–28, Feb. 1970.

Patterson, M. I., and Marble B.: "Dietetic Foods" *Am. J. Clin. Nutr.,* **16**:440–44, 1965.

Ramstad, P. E.: "The Food Processor's Stake in Public Health—An Industry Viewpoint," *Am. J. Public Health,* **54**:2037–39, 1964.

Vinz, G. L.: "The Compleat Inspector," *FDA Papers,* **2**:4, Sept. 1968.

ESPECIALLY FOR THE LAYMAN

Bauer, W. W.: "Why Today's Bread Is Better," *Today's Health,* **44**:60–64, Dec. 1966.

Earl, H. G.: "Food Poisoning: The Sneaky Attacker," *Today's Health,* **43**:64, Oct. 1965.

Food and Drug Administration, U.S. Department of Health, Education, and Welfare:
Additives in Our Food, Pub. 43.
FDA—What It Is and Does, Pub. 1.
How Safe Is Our Food? Pub. 41.
Read the Label, Pub. 3.
48 Ways to Foil Food Infections. Channing L. Bete Co., Inc., Greenfield, Mass., 1967.

Martin, R.: "What You Don't See Can Hurt You," *Today's Health,* **43**:42, Nov. 1965.

Oser, B. L.: "How Safe Are the Chemicals in Our Food?" *Today's Health,* **44**:61–64, Mar. 1966.

U.S. Department of Agriculture:
Family Food Stockpile for Survival, G 77.
Keeping Food Safe to Eat. G 162.

Unit VI
Special Nutritional Needs Throughout the Life Cycle

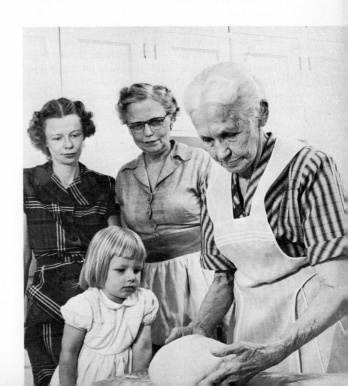

21 Nutrition During Pregnancy and Lactation

The concept of maternal care is described as follows by the World Health Organization:[*]

The object of maternity care is to ensure that every expectant and nursing mother maintains good health, learns the art of child care, has a normal delivery, and bears healthy children. Maternity care in the narrower sense consists in the care of the pregnant woman, her safe delivery, her postnatal care and examination, the care of her newly born infant, and the maintenance of lactation. In the wider sense, it begins much earlier in measures aimed to promote the health and well-being of the young people who are potential parents, and to help them to develop the right approach to family life and to the place of the family in the community. It should also include guidance in parentcraft and in problems associated with infertility and family planning.

The Committee on Maternal Nutrition of the Food and Nutrition Board has recently issued a comprehensive report on the role of nutrition in human reproduction.[1] Two summaries of this report may be read with profit by the student who does not have time to study the detailed report.[2,3]

Some vital statistics. Maternal deaths in the United States decreased from 367 per 100,000 live births in 1940 to 28 in 1967.[1] The toxemias of pregnancy caused 52.2 maternal deaths per 100,000 in 1940 and 6.2 in 1965. These remarkable improvements in the maternal mortality rate are not evenly distributed throughout the population. The mortality rate is about three times as high in nonwhite women and appears to be associated with low income; when white and nonwhite mothers of similar income were compared there was little difference. Maternal deaths were the highest in the teen-age group. The improvement in the rate of maternal deaths is attributed to the use of antibiotics and better overall treatment, and more attention to nutrition could further improve the record.[3]

Of 40 countries that were ranked for infant mortality, the United States fell thirteenth and Canada fourteenth. In the United States for 1967 there were 22.4 infant deaths for each 1000 live births. The mortality rate is much higher for infants born to mothers of low income and to teen-age mothers. The infant with a birth weight less than 2500 gm has less chance for survival than does the larger infant; presently, 1 in 12 infants has a birth weight below this level. In addition to infant mortality, one must also consider the number of infants who fail to grow satisfactorily and those who have some defects.

The Committee on Maternal Nutrition has listed the following factors of importance in the incidence of low-birth-weight infants and the related neonatal mortality: "socioeconomic status of the mother, . . . biological immaturity (under 17 years of age), high parity, short stature, low prepregnancy weight for height, low gain in weight during pregnancy, poor nutritional status, smoking, certain infectious agents, chronic disease, complications of pregnancy, and a history of unsuccessful pregnancies."[*] Many of these factors will be considered in more detail in the discussion that follows.

[*]World Health Organization: *The Organization and Administration of Maternal and Child Health Services.* Fifth Report of the World Health Organization Expert Committee on Maternal and Child Care, WHO Tech. Rep. Ser. No. 428, Geneva, 1969.

[*]Committee on Maternal Nutrition: *Maternal Nutrition and the Course of Pregnancy: Summary Report.* Food and Nutrition Board, National Academy of Sciences —National Research Council, Washington, D.C., 1970, p. 4.

Nutritional Studies

Folklore and diet in pregnancy. Since earliest times the diets of pregnant women have been considered to be of importance. The foods eaten by the pregnant woman were believed to convey to the unborn child not only certain physical characteristics but also desirable or undesirable attributes of behavior. Consequently, various societies set up rigid rules for the pregnant woman, including the foods she could eat, the foods she must not eat, and even the foods she must not touch lest she contaminate them for the rest of the community. Even today superstitions about foods and their desirability for the pregnant woman prevail among some people.

Some of the theories relating to nutrition that have been practiced by physicians are now known to be incorrect: the semistarvation of the mother with the view of a smaller baby and easier delivery; the restriction of salt and fluids to reduce the incidence of toxemia; and the theory the maternal organism will produce a healthy baby regardless of the mother's own state of nutrition.[3]

Prematernal nutrition. The *perinatal concept*[4] assumes that the mother is in a good nutritional state prior to conception, and that this status will be maintained throughout pregnancy, labor, and the period after birth. Fewer complications in pregnancy, fewer premature births, and healthier babies result when the mother is well nourished prior to conception.

The influence of the quality of prematernal nutrition was strikingly demonstrated in World War II.[5] In Holland food rations were severely restricted from October 1944 to May 1945 so that pregnant women early in 1945 had less than 1000 calories and 30 to 40 gm protein available. Prior to this period women had ingested diets that were reasonably adequate. The babies conceived before the hunger period and born during the hunger period were shorter and had lower birth weights than those born before this time, this being a direct result of the mother's diet during the latter half of pregnancy. However, there was no increase in the rate of still births, prematurity, and malformations but the rate of conception fell off markedly during the hunger period.

During the siege of Leningrad acute food shortages occurred between August 1941 and February 1942. Prior to this time the food supplies had been inadequate so that women were chronically undernourished. During 1942 the birth rate fell off markedly, the stillbirth rate was twice as high, and prematurity had increased 41 per cent. The infants had low vitality, had poor resistance to infection, and did not suckle well. The better outcome in Holland was directly related to the better diets of women prior to conception.

Tompkins' studies in Philadelphia showed that women who are underweight at the time of conception have the greatest probability of premature labor and toxemia. He found a strikingly high incidence of prematurity in infants born of mothers who were both underweight and anemic.[6]

Difficult deliveries are more frequent in short than in tall women, according to studies reported from Scotland.[7] The more frequent occurrence of "flat pelvis" in short women was believed to be related to inadequate diet in childhood. Thus, a short stature may mean that a woman has not achieved the full genetic possibilities of body structure because of dietary inadequacies.

Prenatal nutrition. Burke and her coworkers[8] studied 216 pregnant women over an extended period during which the women were examined and their diets analyzed. The diets were rated as excellent if they contained 100 per cent of the optimal standards for each of the nutrients. Ratings of good, fair, poor, and very poor were given to diets containing 80, 60, 50, and less than 50 per cent respectively of the optimal levels for the food constituents.

These studies of Burke and her associates indicate that a woman who has a poor or a very poor diet during pregnancy will in all probability have a poor infant; that is prematurity, congenital defects, and stillborn infants occurred almost entirely in this group. On the other hand, the women who had good-to-excellent diets almost invariably bore infants in good physical condition. Inadequate nutrition during pregnancy resulted in relatively greater harm to the fetus than to the mother. It is of further interest that no cases of eclampsia were noted in those women receiving excellent or good diets, whereas 50 per cent of those receiving poor or very poor diets developed toxemia of varying degrees of severity.

The Vanderbilt cooperative study of 2338 pregnant white women of low income showed the effects of weight status and hemoglobin levels of the mother on the infant.[9] Underweight women (less than 85 per cent of standard) produced smaller babies, prematurity occurred more frequently, and artificial feeding was more common. The overweight group (120 per cent of standard) had more stillborn children and a threefold increase in pre-eclampsia. Women who gained too much, especially during the second trimester, had more toxemia.

Low intakes of iron and ascorbic acid were correlated with lower hemoglobin levels and blood levels of vitamin C. However, during the first year of life the infants of these mothers maintained hemoglobin levels equal to those whose mothers had higher hemoglobin levels, showing that appropriate infant feeding practices can make up for the deficient infant stores of iron.

The Vanderbilt study did not fully establish nutritional deficiency as a primary causative factor in metabolic diseases of pregnancy. The investigators point out that the patient cannot be assured of freedom from complications simply through a satisfactory intake of nutrients. They did observe that diets which contained less than 50 gm protein and less than 1500 calories resulted in a greater frequency of complications of pregnancy and of the newborn, but they felt that the low levels of intake were a result of the complications rather than the cause.

Teen-age pregnancies. Each year in the United States there are about 200,000 live births to girls under 17 years of age. In every category the risks are greater for these young mothers and their babies. Toxemia occurs three to four times more frequently in teen-age pregnancies and is higher in younger girls than in older girls.[10] Fetal losses, low birth weights, neonatal deaths, and deaths of mothers are substantially higher in girls under 16 years than in older

girls and women. The risk is greater for nonwhite girls than for white girls. Those from low-income families have less successful pregnancies than those from higher-income families.

Many factors enter into the high risk in teen-age pregnancies. The nutritional needs of the girl during the period of maturation are considerable, but often are not met because many adolescents regardless of socioeconomic status are known to have unsatisfactory, often bizarre diets. When the nutritional demands of pregnancy are superimposed upon the immature girl who is inadequately nourished, the outcome for mother and infant may well be poor. Young girls who become pregnant may also be under severe emotional stress, especially if the pregnancy is out of wedlock. Society often takes a punitive attitude toward the girl. For example, she may be required to discontinue her education, or she may be kept in seclusion, perhaps with a relative in another community, in order to minimize the supposed hurt to the girl herself or the family. Under severe emotional stress brought about by such a situation, nutrient balances are often negative even when an adequate diet is consumed. Many teen-age pregnancies occur in low-income families where there is the least understanding of the nutritional needs during pregnancy, the least money to purchase the foods for an adequate diet, and the least prenatal care.

PHYSIOLOGIC AND BIOCHEMICAL CHANGES IN PREGNANCY

Three stages of pregnancy. Pregnancy may be considered in three stages:[4]

1. The preimplantation period, about two weeks following conception. The fertilized ovum becomes implanted in the wall of the uterus and the placenta begins to develop.

2. The period of organ formation, about two to eight weeks. All the major organs—heart, kidneys, lungs, liver, and skeleton—are formed during this period. Studies on experimental animals have shown that congenital malformations occur when the pregnant animal has had a diet grossly deficient in vitamins, for example vitamin A or riboflavin.[11] However, it is difficult

to correlate poor nutrition with malformations sometimes seen in humans.

3. The period of rapid growth of the fetus and the establishment of the maternal reserves in preparation for labor, the puerperium, and the production of milk from the eighth week to term.

The placenta. This is the organ to which the fetus is attached by means of the umbilical cord and by which the nutrition of the fetus is maintained. The placenta achieves its maximum size early in gestation. It is richly supplied with protein, fat, carbohydrates, minerals, vitamins, enzymes, and hormones, and by its large surface area, estimated to be between 10 and 13 sq m, it maintains contact between the maternal and fetal circulations. The composition of the placenta changes, and the transfer of nutrients is regulated selectively to correspond to the changing needs of the developing fetus.

Hormones. Progesterone, the estrogens, and the gonadotropins are the hormones primarily involved in reproduction. Progesterone is secreted by the corpus luteum and brings about increased secretion by the endometrium, as well as developing glycogen and lipid stores. It also inhibits contraction of the uterine smooth-muscle layers thereby preventing expulsion of the embryo. In these ways progesterone has prepared for the implantation of the fertilized ovum and its early growth. Between the second and third months of gestation the formation of progesterone is taken over by the placenta.

Gonadotropins are especially concerned with organ formation up to about the fourth month of pregnancy and with fetal growth. Chorionic gonadotropin is produced by the *trophoblastic* cells (outer layer of cells of the dividing ovum) and has the same effects on the corpus luteum as the luteinizing hormone and the luteotropic hormone from the pituitary gland. It keeps the corpus luteum from degenerating and keeps it secreting large quantities of estrogen and progesterone. The endometrium remains in the uterus and is gradually phagocytized by the growing fetal tissues, thereby furnishing a major portion of the nutrition to the fetus during the first weeks of pregnancy.

Estrogen production increases appreciably after about the one-hundredth day of gestation.

Estrogen and progesterone stimulate the growth of the mammary glands and also inhibit the lactogenic function of the pituitary gland until birth of the infant.

Steroid hormones are produced in greater amounts with the result that water and sodium are more readily retained in the body. The thyroid gland is less active during the first four months of pregnancy, and thereafter is somewhat more active than normal.

Blood circulation. A gradual increase in blood volume up to about 25 per cent by the end of pregnancy occurs. This increase is required in order to carry the essential nutrients to the placenta and also to remove the increased level of metabolic wastes. With the increase in blood volume there is a corresponding dilution of the blood constituents. For example, the hemoglobin concentration of healthy young women averages 13.7 gm per 100 ml blood with a range from 12.0 to 15.3 gm.[3] During pregnancy, women who have received supplemental iron have an average hemoglobin of 12.0 gm per 100 ml. This change is sometimes referred to as the "physiologic anemia of pregnancy." A level of 11.0 gm hemoglobin per 100 ml blood is considered to be the border below which a true anemia exists. The plasma albumin is also lowered during pregnancy. On the other hand, the serum alkaline phosphatase is increased considerably.

Gastrointestinal changes. Most women have an increase in appetite and thirst during the first trimester, although morning nausea may temporarily interfere with eating. Some women have cravings for certain foods and aversions to others. *Pica*, an appetite for such things as starch, clay, and chalk, is present in a surprising number of women and these abnormal items are sometimes consumed in large amounts.

Less acid and pepsin are produced by the stomach, and regurgitation of stomach contents into the esophagus (heartburn) sometimes occurs. The reduced motility of the intestinal muscles may contribute to constipation. However, there is no apparent impairment of absorption.

Weight gain. The gain in weight for the healthy woman who enters pregnancy at her desirable weight level should be about 20 to 25 pounds. However, the gains in weight vary widely, being greater in young women than in those who are somewhat older and greater in those who are having their first babies. (See Figure 21–1.)

The weight gain is accounted for by the weight of the full-term baby of about 7½ pounds; increase in size of the uterus, 2 pounds; placenta and membranes, 1¼ pounds; amniotic fluid, 2 pounds; increase in breast tissue, 1½ pounds. To this must be added the weight of the increased blood circulation and the reserves of nitrogen, calcium, phosphorus, and lipids that are built up in preparation for parturition and lactation.

Tompkins has emphasized that failure to gain at a normal rate during the first two trimesters as well as initial underweight status increases the probability of premature labor.[6] On the other hand, he stated that an excessive rate of gain during the second and third trimesters results in greater likelihood of preeclampsia and eclampsia.

The Committee on Maternal Nutrition[1] has indicated that weight gain during the first trimester should be 1.5 to 3.0 pounds and thereafter should be 0.8 pound weekly until the end of pregnancy.

Basal metabolism. The basal metabolism is slightly reduced during the early part of pregnancy, but thereafter it increases until it is as much as 25 per cent over the normal rate by the end of the term. This increase is accounted for in part by the gain in weight and also by the

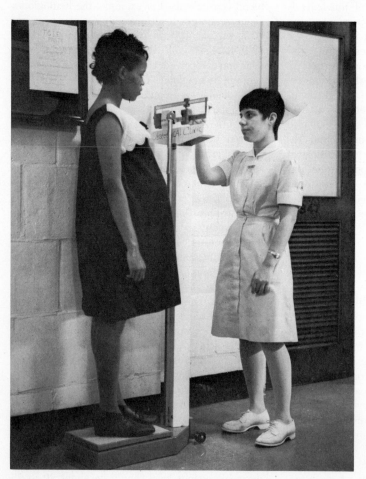

Figure 21–1. Weight is checked at each clinic visit. After the first trimester the weekly gain should be about 0.8 pound. (Courtesy, School of Nursing, Thomas Jefferson University.)

high metabolic activity of the placenta and the fetus.

NUTRITIONAL CONSIDERATIONS

Recommended allowances. There has been surprisingly little research in recent years on the nutritional requirements during pregnancy, and consequently for some nutrients the recommendations of the Food and Nutrition Board must be based upon scanty data.[12] Table 21–1 compares the nutritional allowances for the normal, pregnant, and lactating woman. The higher allowances of some nutrients for the teen-age pregnant girl should be noted.

Energy. The total caloric cost of producing the fetus, the placenta, and other maternal tissues and of establishing the reserves is about 80,000 calories. Part of this is made up by the fact that activity usually decreases during pregnancy. It is estimated that 300 calories daily in

excess of the normal requirement usually suffices for a normal weight gain of 20 to 25 pounds.

Although obesity is a hazard to pregnancy, weight reduction during pregnancy is not considered desirable.[1] Low-calorie diets, therefore, should be restricted to women prior to their pregnancy or following it. The indicator of correct caloric intake is the rate of gain each week, and this should be watched closely.

Protein. During the last six months of pregnancy about 950 gm of protein are deposited. An allowance of 30 gm protein added to the normal allowance for the nonpregnant woman is satisfactory.

Minerals. The efficiency of absorption of minerals such as calcium and iron improves during pregnancy, but the demands of the fetus and other developing tissues necessitate increases in the diet during the second and third trimesters. The full-term fetus contains about 28 gm calcium.[7] Some calcium and phosphorus deposition takes place early in pregnancy, but most of the

Table 21–1. Recommended Dietary Allowances During Pregnancy and Lactation

Nutrient	Normal Woman*	Pregnant Woman*	Pregnant Teen-age Girl 15–18 years†	Lactating Woman*
Energy, kcal	2000	2300–2400	2400	2500–2600
Protein, gm	46	76	78	66
Vitamin A, R.E.	800	1000	1000	1200
I.U.	4000	5000	5000	6000
Vitamin D, I.U.	—	400	400	400
Vitamin E, I.U.	12	15	15	15
Ascorbic acid, mg	45	60	60	60
Folacin, mcg	400	800	800	800
Niacin, mg	13	15–16	16	17–18
Riboflavin, mg	1.2	1.5–1.7	1.7	1.7–1.9
Thiamine, mg	1.0	1.3–1.4	1.4	1.3–1.4
Vitamin B$_6$, mg	2.0	2.5	2.5	2.5
Vitamin B$_{12}$, mcg	3.0	4.0	4.0	4.0
Calcium, mg	800	1200	1600	1200‡
Phosphorus, mg	800	1200	1600	1200‡
Iodine, mcg	100	125	140	150
Iron, mg	18	18+	18+	18
Magnesium, mg	300	450	450	450
Zinc, mg	15	20	20	25

*Reference woman: 65 inches tall, 128 pounds. Where a range is shown the higher values are for the woman 19 to 22 years.

†Girl, 65 inches, 119 pounds.

‡These levels would be further increased for the teen-age girl who nurses her baby.

calcification of bones occurs during the last two months of pregnancy. The first set of teeth begins to form about the eighth week of pre-natal life, and they are well formed by the end of the prenatal period. The six-year molars, which are the first permanent teeth to erupt, begin to calcify just before birth.

If the mobile reserve of calcium is lacking in the mother, the demands of the fetus can be met, perhaps inadequately, only at severe ex-pense to the mother. For many women it is ad-visable to increase the calcium intake early in pregnancy even though fetal calcification does not occur until later. The phosphorus allowance should be about equal to that for calcium and will be readily supplied through the calcium-rich and protein-rich foods.

From 700 to 1000 mg iron must be absorbed and utilized by the mother throughout preg-nancy.[9] Of this total, about 240 mg are spared by the cessation of the menstrual flow. The remainder must be made available from the diet. The recommended allowances indicate a daily intake of 18 mg iron, a level that is difficult to achieve even with well-selected diets. The Com-mittee on Maternal Nutrition recommends that an iron supplement of 30 to 60 mg daily be given during the second and third trimesters because of the widespread incidence of nutri-tional anemia.

The iodine allowance is 125 mcg daily and may be satisfied by using iodized salt. If sodium restriction is required, the physician may pre-scribe iodine supplementation since most foods cannot be relied upon for their iodine content.

Sodium restriction should be used rarely. Studies by Pike[13] have shown that such restric-tion had adverse effects on experimental animals. There is little evidence that sodium restriction modifies the course of toxemia.

Vitamins. For many of the vitamins the re-quirements during pregnancy have not been thoroughly studied. The allowances therefore are stated at levels considered to be safe for the pregnant woman. An increased conversion of tryptophan to niacin occurs in pregnancy. The niacin, thiamine, and riboflavin allowances have been increased in proportion to the caloric increase.

The placenta actively transports vitamin B_6 so that the concentration in the fetal circulation is five times that of the maternal circulation; thus the allowance in pregnancy has been con-siderably increased. Vitamin B_{12} levels often fall in the maternal circulation and may be twice as high in the infant circulation as in the mother; correspondingly, the allowance during pregnancy has been substantially raised.

Pregnancy apparently imposes an additional demand for folacin. Megaloblastic anemia occurs in a small number of women especially during the last trimester. This may be caused by a die-tary deficiency or may result from vomiting or a metabolic defect. If folacin deficiency is sus-pected, a supplement of 0.2 to 0.4 mg folate may be prescribed.

The pregnant woman should be assured of 400 I.U. vitamin D daily, an amount that is supplied by using fortified milk.

DIETARY COUNSELING

The basic diet. The Basic Diet plan, Table 13–2, provides ample allowances for protein, vitamin A, and ascorbic acid. The caloric level is just over half that needed by the preg-nant woman. (See Figure 21–2.) When 1½ to 2 cups milk are added the calcium, thia-mine, and riboflavin needs are fully met. Vitamin D will be provided as fortified milk or may be prescribed as a supplement. Except for iron and iodine, other minerals and vita-mins will be provided in sufficient amounts by the recommended amounts of foods. Since foods are a variable source of iodine, iodized salt should be used. A supplement of iron in the form of ferrous sulfate, fumarate, or glu-conate is recommended. (See Table 21–2.)

For the pregnant teen-ager the food al-lowances are the same as for the pregnant woman except that the intake of milk should be 5 to 6 cups daily.

Dietary management. Nutrition education may be especially effective during pregnancy, for the mother-to-be is usually anxious that her baby have the best opportunity for a

Figure 21–2. The Basic Diet provides ample vitamin A and niacin (not shown in chart) as well as protein, riboflavin, and ascorbic acid to meet the needs of the pregnant woman. The addition of 1 to 2 cups of milk supplies the needed calcium. The iron intake can be increased by including liver weekly and by eating more meat, eggs, dark-green leafy vegetables, and enriched bread. An iron supplement prescribed by the physician will be less costly than these additional amounts of food, and will not increase the calorie intake.

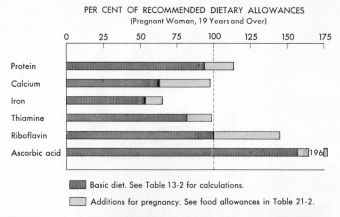

PER CENT OF RECOMMENDED DIETARY ALLOWANCES
(Pregnant Woman, 19 Years and Over)

Basic diet. See Table 13-2 for calculations.

Additions for pregnancy. See food allowances in Table 21-2.

healthy life. The father is also concerned about the well-being of his wife, and in encouraging her proper diet he may also improve his own food habits.

The pregnant teen-ager who is a happy homemaker is quite receptive to nutrition counseling, but when a pregnancy is unwanted, especially out of wedlock, the teen-ager may resist many efforts to help. She may use food as an outlet for her emotions, but in so doing she often selects those foods rich in calories but having little else to recommend them nutritionally. The motivation for better nutrition for this girl may be in terms of her own well-being.

As in all dietary counseling the dietary pattern must be based upon the woman's present food habits and her cultural and socioeconomic circumstances. (See Figure 21–3.) Women who are pregnant for the first time will require more counseling than those who have had successful pregnancies.

Table 21–2. Food Allowances for Pregnancy and Lactation

	Pregnant Woman	Pregnant Teen-Age Girl	Lactating Woman
Milk	3–4 cups, whole	5–6 cups, whole	6 cups, whole
Meat, fish, poultry (liver once a week)			
cooked weight	4 ounces	4 ounces	4 ounces
Eggs	1	1	1
Vegetables, including:			
Dark green leafy or deep yellow	1/2 cup	1/2 cup	1/2 cup
Potato	1 medium	1 medium	1 medium
Other vegetables	1/2–1 cup	1/2–1 cup	1/2–1 cup
One vegetable to be raw each day			
Fruits, including:			
Citrus	1 serving	1 serving	1 serving
Other fruit	1 serving	1 serving	1 serving
Cereal, enriched or whole grain	1 serving	1 serving	1 serving
Bread, enriched or whole grain	5 slices	5 slices	5 slices
Butter or fortified margarine	To meet caloric	To meet caloric	To meet caloric
Desserts, cooking fats, sugars, sweets	needs	needs	needs
Vitamin D supplement (or use fortified milk)	400 I.U.	400 I.U.	400 I.U.
Iodized salt	Daily	Daily	Daily

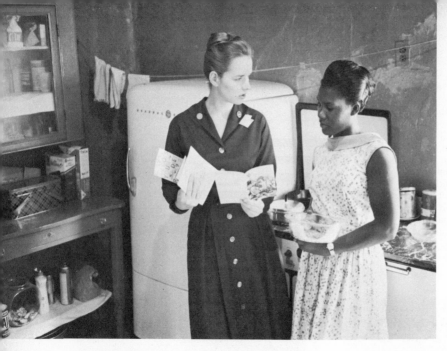

Figure 21–3. Within the home a public health nurse can provide practical suggestions for a satisfactory diet for the mother-to-be. Should any problems of planning arise, the nurse may consult a nutritionist. (Courtesy, United Fund and Community Nursing Services, Philadelphia.)

Those whose incomes are low may need help in budgeting their food expenditures. This means help for the entire family, for a mother is not likely to improve her own diet at the expense of that of other children in the family.

Some women dislike milk and find it difficult to consume the 3 cups or more that are required. The inclusion of milk in soups, puddings, and sauces may be suggested. Part of the milk may be used as nonfat dry milk in cooked foods or as a reinforcement of the fresh whole milk that is taken. Milk may be flavored with fruit or chocolate, vanilla, or molasses. Cheddar cheese may be substituted for part of the milk, using 1 ounce as an equivalent for 1 cup of milk.

As sources of protein, poultry, fish, legumes, and peanut butter are less expensive than meat. When legumes or peanut butter is used, the meal should include part of the day's allowance of milk so that all the essential amino acids will be available.

Canned or frozen citrus juices are less expensive ways to include ascorbic acid for the day. Fresh fruits in season—for example, cantaloupe—may be inexpensive sources of ascorbic acid.

Many women are especially concerned about maintaining their slender figures and may be reluctant to include such foods as milk, bread, and potatoes because of the belief that these foods are fattening. Some instruction concerning the caloric value of foods may be useful.

COMPLICATIONS OF PREGNANCY

Mild nausea and vomiting. During the first trimester, the physiologic and biochemical balances are often disturbed, possibly because of excessive hormone production. Gastrointestinal upsets, including loss of appetite, nausea, and vomiting, are relatively frequent; loss of weight occasionally takes place because of inability to eat sufficient food.

Mild early morning nausea may usually be overcome by the use of high-carbohydrate foods such as crackers, jelly, hard candies, and dry toast before arising. Frequent small meals rather than three large ones may be preferable. Fluids should be taken between meals rather than at mealtime. Fatty, rich foods such as pastries, desserts, fried foods, excessive seasoning, coffee in large amounts, and strongly flavored vegetables may be restricted or eliminated if the nausea persists or if the patient complains of heartburn or gastric distress.

Pernicious vomiting. Severe and persistent vomiting requires close supervision by the physician, and hospitalization may become necessary. Intravenous or tube feedings to provide some fluid, electrolytes, and calories are occasionally indicated. When oral feedings are resumed, it is of the utmost importance to proceed gradually with the kinds and amounts of foods which are offered.

High-carbohydrate, low-fat foods are best tolerated and include dry toast with jelly, crackers with jelly, baked potato, plain gelatin, cereal with milk and sugar, tomato juice, hard candy, and broth. Fasting aggravates the condition, and therefore feedings of 3 to 6 ounces should be offered every two hours. Dry foods are more likely to be retained than liquid foods. However, dehydration must be guarded against.

The psychologic factor is of some importance and little is gained by urging the woman to eat foods that do not appeal to her. She should be consulted about her likes and dislikes; a food that appeals to her is more likely to be retained.

When the high-carbohydrate foods are satisfactorily taken, the diet is gradually liberalized to include the foods customarily allowed on first a soft and then a normal diet. Generally speaking, foods high in fat, pastries, rich desserts, fried foods, and cream are poorly tolerated. Highly seasoned foods and strongly flavored vegetables may also cause some distress. It is usually desirable to give only dry foods at meals and to allow liquids one to two hours after meals.

Constipation. The occurrence of constipation especially during the latter half of pregnancy is common. The amount of pressure exerted by the developing fetus on the digestive tract, the limitation of exercise, and insufficient bulk may be contributing factors in its causation. The normal diet outlined on page 299 provides a liberal allowance of fruits, whole-grain cereals, and vegetables, and consequently of fiber. It is also necessary to stress the importance of adequate fluid intake and of regular habits of exercise, elimination, sleep, and recreation.

Overweight. Although obesity represents an added risk during pregnancy, it is now questioned whether the added stress of weight loss should be superimposed upon the stress of pregnancy.[1] Diets that provide 1500 calories or less may be planned to supply the essential protein allowance, but negative nitrogen balances occur because of increased tissue catabolism. It is now recommended that the emphasis be placed upon a consistent rate of weight gain during pregnancy and that weight loss be postponed until after the pregnancy has come to term.

Anemia. Iron-deficiency anemia is relatively common and it is corrected by prescribing oral iron supplements. The diet should be liberal in its protein content to furnish the essential amino acids for globin formation.

Megaloblastic anemia is not common in pregnant women in the United States. It is corrected by prescribing a supplement of folacin.

Toxemia. By toxemia is meant that combination of symptoms including hypertension, edema, and albuminuria. Preeclampsia is the appearance of hypertension, edema of the face and hands, and/or albuminuria about the twentieth week of pregnancy. It should be suspected when there is a sudden gain in weight, indicating fluid retention rather than tissue building. Eclampsia is the end result of preeclampsia; it includes the earlier symptoms but may culminate in convulsions.

The treatment of toxemias is highly controversial. In fact, toxemia has been called the "disease of theories."[1] As pointed out earlier in this chapter, Burke[8] and Tompkins and Wiehl[6] showed a relationship between nutrition and the incidence of toxemia, but these findings are disputed by others, especially the Vanderbilt group.[9] Protein and calorie restriction are no longer recommended, and sodium restriction should be used with caution.

LACTATION

Nutritive requirements. McGanity and his associates[9] found that women who had high intakes of calcium, phosphorus, and riboflavin from their diets nursed their babies more frequently than did women who drank less than 3 glasses of milk daily and who had calcium supplements. When one considers the nutritive value of human milk, and that the nursing mother will produce 20 to 30 ounces each day, it becomes apparent that the requirements for protein, minerals, vitamins, and calories are equal to or greater than they were in pregnancy. The recommended allowances for the various nutrients have been listed in Table 21–1.

The need for protein is greatest when lactation has reached its maximum, but it is a need which should be anticipated and planned for during pregnancy. The mechanics of converting food into milk protein are only about 50 per cent efficient, and thus about 2 gm of food protein are required to produce 1 gm of milk protein. This conversion takes place when there is a suitable mixture of all of the essential amino acids, and therefore the proteins of milk, eggs, meat, poultry, and fish should have priority.

Approximately 120 calories are required for each 100 ml of milk, and thus the daily production of 850 ml of milk (30 ounces) would necessitate an additional 1000 calories in the diet.

Even liberal intakes of calcium may not be successful in completely counteracting a negative calcium balance. Consequently, a high level of calcium intake and the building of considerable reserves throughout pregnancy cannot be overemphasized. The baby is born with a relatively larger reserve of iron since milk is not a good source of iron. A good allowance of iron in the mothers' diet during lactation does not convey additional iron to the infant. Nevertheless iron-rich foods are essential for the mother's own health, and supplements are included early in the infant's diet.

Selecting the daily diet. The pattern of diet used during pregnancy (page 298) may be used during lactation, provided the following additions are made: (1) 1 pint of milk; (2) foods as desired to provide the additional calories. Weight gain, beyond that desirable for body build, should be avoided. When the baby is weaned, the mother must reduce her food intake in order that obesity may be avoided.

The choice of foods during lactation may be wide. There are no foods that require restriction, except where distress may occur in individual cases following the taking of a particular food such as strongly flavored vegetables or highly seasoned or spicy foods. Successful lactation is dependent not only upon an adequate diet, but also upon sufficient rest for the mother, freedom from anxiety, and a desire to nurse the baby.

PROBLEMS AND REVIEW

1. What evidence exists that diet is of importance in the development of the fetus and the health of the mother?
2. What physiologic changes occur during the course of pregnancy?
3. Name the hormones which are especially important in controlling the changes occurring during pregnancy? What is the effect of an excess production?
4. In what way do the nutritional practices of teen-age girls affect the outcome of pregnancy?
5. What weight increases are recommended for each trimester? What are the dangers of underweight or insufficient weight gain?
6. What foods are especially important for their protein content in the diet during pregnancy and lactation?
7. What mineral elements require especial attention during pregnancy? What changes occur in the rate of absorption of calcium and iron?
8. Discuss the need for an increased vitamin intake. What foods would you recommend for this?
9. Mrs. A. does not like milk and is taking calcium gluconate to correct calcium deficiency. Why is this less desirable than taking milk? List ways by which she could incorporate milk into her diet.

10. What recommendations can you make to a woman with complaints of nausea, vomiting, and gastric distress?
11. What instructions are in order for the woman who complains of constipation?
12. What is meant by the "physiologic anemia of pregnancy"? What are the hazards of iron-deficiency anemia? What measures are essential for its prevention and treatment?
13. A woman secretes 800 ml milk daily. What amount of protein is here represented? What allowances must be made in the diet for protein?
14. *Problem.* Plan a low-cost diet for a woman of moderate activity during the second half of pregnancy. Calculate the nutrients in this diet and compare them with the recommended allowances.
15. *Problem.* Modify the diet in problem 14 for a woman who is lactating.

CITED REFERENCES

1. Committee on Maternal Nutrition, Food and Nutrition Board: *Maternal Nutrition and the Course of Pregnancy.* National Academy of Sciences–National Research Council, Washington, D.C., 1970.
2. ————: *Maternal Nutrition and the Course of Pregnancy: Summary Report.* National Academy of Sciences–National Research Council, Washington, D.C., 1970.
3. Shank, R. E.: "A Chink in Our Armor," *Nutr. Today,* **5**:3–11, Summer 1970.
4. Macy, I. G.: "Metabolic and Biochemical Changes in Normal Pregnancy," *J.A.M.A.,* **168**:2265–71, 1958.
5. Stearns, G.: "Nutritional State of the Mother Prior to Conception," *J.A.M.A.,* **168**:1655–59, 1958.
6. Tompkins, W. T., and Wiehl, D. G.: "Nutritional Deficiencies as a Causal Factor in Toxemia and Premature Labor," *Am. J. Obstet. Gynecol.* **62**:898–919, 1951.
7. Thomson, A. M., and Hytten, F. E.: "Nutrition in Pregnancy and Lactation," in Beaton, G. H., and McHenry, E. W., eds.: *Nutrition: A Comprehensive Treatise.* Vol. III. Academic Press, New York, 1966, pp. 103–45.
8. Burke, B. S., *et al.:* "Nutrition Studies During Pregnancy," *Am. J. Obstet. Gynecol.,* **46**: 38–52, 1943.
9. McGanity, W. J., *et al.:* "Vanderbilt Cooperative Study of Maternal and Infant Nutrition. XII. Effect of Reproductive Cycle on Nutritional Status and Requirements," *J.A.M.A.,* **168**:2138–45, 1958.
10. Gold, E. M.: "Interconceptional Nutrition," *J. Am. Diet. Assoc.,* **55**:27–30, 1969.
11. Warkany, J.: "Production of Congenital Malformations by Dietary Measures (Experiments in Mammals)," *J.A.M.A.,* **168**:2020–23, 1958.
12. Food and Nutrition Board: *Recommended Dietary Allowances,* 8th ed. National Academy of Sciences–National Research Council, Washington, D.C., 1973.
13. Pike, R. L.: "Sodium Intake During Pregnancy," *J. Am Diet. Assoc.,* **44**:176–81, 1964.

ADDITIONAL REFERENCES

Anderson, E. H., and Lesser, A. J.: "Maternity Care in the United States. Gains and Gaps," *Am. J. Nurs.,* **66**:1539–44, 1966.
Apte, S. V., and Iyengar, L.: "Absorption of Dietary Iron in Pregnancy," *Am. J. Clin. Nutr.,* **23**:73–77, 1970.
Chopra, J. G., *et al.:* "Anemia in Pregnancy," *Am. J. Public Health,* **57**:857–68, 1967.
Cooper, B. A., *et al.:* "The Case for Folic Acid Supplements During Pregnancy," *Am. J. Clin. Nutr.,* **23**:848–54, 1970.
Garnet, J. D.: "Pregnancy in Women with Diabetes," *Am. J. Nurs.,* **69**:1900–1902, 1969.

Hughes, E. C.: "Diabetes and Pregnancy," *Postgrad. Med.,* **42:**487–92, Dec. 1967.

Kitay, D. Z., and Marshall, J. S.: "Remission of Folic Acid Deficiency in Pregnancy," *Am. J. Obstet. Gynecol.,* **102:**297–303, 1968.

Pike, R. L., and Gursky, D. S.: "Further Evidence of Deleterious Effects Produced by Sodium Restriction During Pregnancy," *Am. J. Clin. Nutr.,* **23:**883–88, 1970.

Schram, M., and Raji, M.: "The Problem of Underweight Pregnant Patients," *Am. J. Obstet. Gynecol.,* **94:**595–96, 1966.

Shenolikar, I. S.: "Absorption of Dietary Calcium in Pregnancy," *Am. J. Clin. Nutr.,* **23:**63–67, 1970.

Streiff, R. R., and Little, A. B.: "Folic Acid Deficiency in Pregnancy," *N. Engl. J. Med.,* **276:**776–79, 1967.

Wallace, H. M.: "Teen-age Pregnancy," *Am. J. Obstet. Gynecol.,* **92:**1125–31, 1965.

Zackler, J., *et al.:* "The Young Adolescent as an Obstetric Risk," *Am. J. Obstet. Gynecol.,* **103:**305–12, 1969.

22 Nutrition During Infancy

Growth and development of the infant. Each infant's physical growth and development are determined by the characteristics acquired from his ancestors, the quality of the nutrition of his mother during pregnancy, and the adequacy of the breast feeding or formula and supplements offered throughout infancy. The development of personality patterns begins at birth and is closely related to feeding habits. The importance of satisfying feeding relationships between the mother and infant from the earliest days after birth can scarcely be overemphasized.

Each infant is individual and he best serves as his own control in the measurement of his progress. Although it is often useful to make comparisons with stated norms, such as height and weight, it is also dangerous to expect every infant to conform exactly to such norms. No single criterion of physical status is indicative of the quality of nutrition, but a series of measurements over a period of time are likely to be reliable indicators.

Several criteria may be applied to determine whether an infant is well nourished, namely: steady gain in height and weight, but some weekly fluctuations are to be expected; sleeps well, is vigorous, and happy; firm muscles and a moderate amount of subcutaneous fat are developed; teeth begin to erupt within five to six months, and from 6 to 12 teeth have come through by the end of the year; and elimination is normal for the type of feeding. The breast-fed baby usually has two to three soft, yellow stools each day and the formula-fed infant has one to two yellow, somewhat firmer stools.

During the first year the infant will grow and develop more rapidly than at any other time of life. At a weekly gain ranging from 5 to 8 ounces he will double his birth weight in the first five months. The weekly gain slows down to 4 to 5 ounces for the remainder of the year, and he will have tripled his birth weight by the time he is 10 to 12 months old.

The baby will increase his birth length of 20 to 22 inches by another 9 to 10 inches during the first year. At birth he has a large head in proportion to the rest of his body, but his short arms and legs will grow especially rapidly in the next 12 months.

The infant's body contains a much higher proportion of water than that of older children and adults; the muscles are poorly developed and the amount of subcutaneous fat is limited. Since the skin surface area is high in proportion to the total body weight, the loss of body water and of body heat is also relatively high. The skeleton contains a high percentage of water and cartilage and will be only gradually mineralized throughout childhood and adolescence. At birth the calcium content of the body is about 25 to 28 gm, and by the end of the first year this has tripled.

The gastrointestinal system of the full-term infant is able to digest protein, emulsified fats, and simple carbohydrates, but starches and most fats are poorly tolerated until some months later when the digestive enzyme production is more fully developed.

The kidneys reach their full functional capacity by the end of the first year. During the first few months the glomerular filtration rate is somewhat lower, and therefore the excretion of a high concentration of solutes is more difficult. Young infants also excrete greater amounts of some amino acids, apparently because of lower ability to reabsorb them from the tubules.[1] The reabsorption of other amino acids, such as phenylalanine, is high; thus, 97 to 98 per cent of phenylalanine may be reabsorbed even though blood levels may be high, as in phenylketonuria, one of many genetic diseases.

The hemoglobin level of the full-term infant at birth is about 17 to 20 gm per 100 ml. This level is gradually lowered as the infant grows and his blood circulation expands, but the levels remain satisfactory until about the third month when iron-rich foods should be introduced.

The brain develops rapidly in fetal life and during infancy and early childhood. By the age of four years the brain has reached 80 to 90 per cent of its adult size. The increase in the number of brain cells is most rapid during fetal life and in the first five to six months after birth, and thereafter the rate slows down markedly. If malnutrition is unusually severe during pregnancy and during the first few months of life, as in the marasmic infant, the number of the brain cells may be greatly reduced. It has not been established, however, that brain develop-

ment is in any way impaired when the level of undernutrition is less severe. (See also Chapter 25.)

NUTRITIONAL REQUIREMENTS

The Food and Nutrition Board has recognized that human milk is the best food for infants and will meet the nutritive requirements early in life when it is supplied in sufficient quantity. In order to plan formulas using cow's milk or other substitutes, the nutrient allowances are stated in Table 22–1.

Energy. The caloric requirement of the infant is high in terms of his body weight. The allowance of 120 calories per kilogram for the young infant is accounted for approximately as follows: basal metabolism, 60; specific dynamic action, 5; growth, 15; activity, 35; and fecal loss, 5. Since

Table 22–1. Recommended Allowances for Normal Infants*

Nutrient	0–6 Months	6–12 Months
Weight, kg	6	9
lb	14	20
Height, cm	60	71
in	24	28
Energy, kcal	kg × 117	kg × 108
Protein, gm	kg × 2.2	kg × 2.0
Vitamin A, R.E.†	420	400
I.U.	1400	2000
Vitamin D, I.U.	400	400
Vitamin E, I.U.	4	5
Ascorbic acid, mg	35	35
Folacin, mcg	50	50
Niacin, mg	5	8
Riboflavin, mg	0.4	0.6
Thiamine, mg	0.3	0.5
Vitamin B_6, mg	0.3	0.4
Vitamin B_{12}, mcg	0.3	0.3
Calcium, mg	360	540
Phosphorus, mg	240	400
Iodine, mcg	35	45
Iron, mg	10	15
Magnesium, mg	60	70
Zinc, mg	3	5

*Food and Nutrition Board: *Recommended Dietary Allowances*, 8th ed. National Academy of Sciences—National Research Council, Washington, D.C., 1973.

†Assumed to be all as retinol in milk during the first six months of life. All subsequent intakes are assumed to be one-half retinol and one-half as β-carotene when calculated from international units. As retinol equivalents, three-fourths are as retinol and one-fourth as β-carotene.

Figure 22–1. Spread of daily calorie requirements during the first year. Note that the largest babies would require a supplement to the formula by the end of the first month to meet their caloric requirements. For smaller babies a formula of 24 to 32 ounces per day would suffice for the caloric need for several months. (Courtesy, Gerber Products Company.)

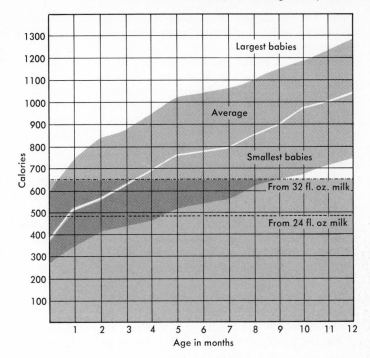

the activity of infants varies widely, an allowance that is correct for one infant may be too high or too low for others who are more or less active. During rapid growth the caloric storage is greater than during slow growth.

The wide spread of caloric requirements for large and small babies at a given age is shown in Figure 22–1. If the total formula is restricted to 32 ounces or less, large babies will require supplementary foods at an earlier age than will small babies in order to meet their caloric needs.

Protein. The recommended allowances for protein are based on the intakes and composition of human milk from which the protein is assumed to be 100 per cent utilized. Gradually foods are introduced in which the protein quality is less than that of human milk. Thus, when a regular mixed diet is fed, the allowance should be increased by applying the correction factor 100/70; for example, $100/70 \times 2.0 = 2.9$ gm per kilogram at six months to one year.

Fat. The intake of fat is important to maintain caloric adequacy. About 3 per cent of the total caloric intake should be supplied as linoleic acid in order to maintain the integrity of the skin and normal growth. Human milk supplies about 6 to 9 per cent of its calories as linoleate. Many pediatricians now recommend formulas in which vegetable fat has been substituted for butterfat. This increases the intake of linoleic acid and is also a prophylactic measure against elevated levels of blood cholesterol, which later in life are believed to increase the incidence of coronary disease. (See Chapters 6 and 42.)

Water. The normal daily turnover of water by the infant is about 15 per cent of his body weight. The water loss from the skin is large because of the greater surface area in relation to body weight. The ability of the kidneys of the young infant to concentrate urine is much less than that of older children or adults. Hence, to excrete a given amount of solute, chiefly urea and sodium chloride, a larger volume of fluid is required. The osmolar load of breast milk is well within the excretion capacity of the kidney, but more concentrated formulas could present an excessive osmolar load.

Infants require about 150 ml water per 100 calories. This requirement is met by breast milk, and by formulas containing 5 to 10 per cent sugar and enough water to give a concentration of 20 calories per ounce.

Minerals. A recent study has shown that infants receiving human milk absorbed 50 to 60 per cent of the total calcium, whereas those receiving a commercial formula absorbed about 25 to 30 per cent of the total calcium.[3] Inasmuch as the formula contained about twice as much calcium as human milk, the total amount of calcium absorbed was about equal.

The circulating hemoglobin of the well-nourished infant is ample during the first three months, after which foods providing iron must be added in order to meet the needs of the expanding blood volume. Those infants born of anemic women, as well as premature infants, will require iron supplementation at an earlier age in order to forestall anemia.

The sodium requirement is about 1 mEq per kilogram body weight, but by the end of the first year infants are ingesting as much as 6.3 mEq per kilogram.[4] This large increase in sodium intake results from the use of foods to which salt has been added in processing or in preparation within the home. Since there appears to be some correlation between high salt intakes and hypertension later in life, Mayer recommends that infants be given foods that contain lower amounts of salt.

Many trace mineral elements are required, but practical experience has shown that the diet will be adequate in these if the major nutrients are furnished in sufficient amounts. The use of fluoridated water for the dilution of infant formulas is recommended.

Vitamins. The dangers of toxicity of vitamins A and D must be kept in mind. The adverse effects of vitamin A are noted when very large amounts are ingested over a long period of time (see page 152), but the safe margin of intake for vitamin D is much narrower. The vitamin D content of the formula and of any foods should be taken into account before prescribing a supplement. Commercial formulas, evaporated milk, and most fresh milk contain sufficient vitamin D and a supplement is not required. It is customary to prescribe a supplement of 400 I.U. vitamin D for the breast-fed baby.

Human milk from the well-nourished mother supplies sufficient ascorbic acid for the infant's needs. Infants who are fed high-protein formulas early in life require as much as 50 mg ascorbic acid in order to avoid tyrosinemia and tyrosinuria.

The infant is born with a store of vitamin B_6 that protects him during the neonatal period inasmuch as human milk is very low in this vitamin. When the protein intake increases, the vitamin B_6 intake must also increase. An intake of 0.015 mg vitamin B_6 per gram of protein is adequate. Cow's milk contains proportionately higher concentrations of vitamin B_6 and formulas are ordinarily adequate in this vitamin. Symptoms of vitamin B_6 deficiency have been observed in infants breast fed by undernourished mothers, and in infants who received formulas in which vitamin B_6 had been destroyed in processing. (See page 178.)

The allowances for thiamine, riboflavin, and niacin have been set up proportionate to the caloric intake. These allowances are easily met by the human milk or the formula with the gradual additions of supplementary foods.

BREAST FEEDING

Approximately 87 per cent of all mothers can supply their infants with enough milk to justify the continuation of nursing if there is proper management.[5] In the United States, however, less than 20 per cent of all mothers breast-feed their babies. No doubt there are many reasons for this, including in some instances the mother's early return to work. If breast feeding is to be successful, the advantages must be sold to the mother early in pregnancy. An adequate diet, exercise, rest, and freedom from anxiety are important during the prenatal period as well as during lactation. The additional foods required by the mother to meet the demands of lactation will cost from $2.50 to $3.00 per week.[6] This is slightly more than the cost of evaporated-milk formulas prepared in the home.

Advantages of breast feeding. Human milk is the natural food for the infant. Breast feeding gives a safe and protected feeling to the infant and a sense of satisfaction to the mother. In lower economic groups breast-fed infants have a consistently lower mortality rate, probably because there is no problem of sanitation. As a rule, there are fewer and less serious illnesses and feeding problems among breast-fed infants; constipation also occurs less frequently. On a practical basis breast feeding eliminates preparation of a feeding; the milk is available at proper temperature; and errors in calculation and in formula preparation are avoided.

Contraindications to breast feeding. If the mother can supply less than half of the infant's needs, breast feeding is usually not practical. It must be discontinued when (1) chronic illnesses are present in the mother, such as cardiac disease, tuberculosis, severe anemia, nephritis, epilepsy, insanity, and chronic fevers; (2) another pregnancy ensues; (3) it is necessary for the mother to return to employment outside the home; or (4) the infant is weak or unable to nurse because of cleft palate or harelip. Temporary cessation is also indicated when the mother acquires an acute infection which the infant has not yet acquired; in such a situation the mother's breasts should be completely pumped at regular intervals so that the milk supply will not dwindle.

Colostrum. The clear, yellowish secretion from the breast during the first few days after delivery is not mature milk, but a substance richer in protein and in vitamin A than the milk secreted later. The levels of carbohydrate, fat, niacin, pantothenic acid, biotin, and riboflavin are low initially and reach mature milk levels by the tenth day. Both colostrum and mature milk contain the same levels of ascorbic acid.

The infant receives only 10 to 40 ml of colostrum during the first two to three days, but by the end of the first week the supply of milk will usually satisfy the full nutrient needs. While the nutritive contribution of colostrum seems to be small, the secretion apparently confers an immunity to certain infections during the first few months and aids in the development of the digestive enzymes.

Technique of feeding. Whether the baby is breast fed or bottle fed, the feeding satisfies at the same time the baby's needs for food, a feeling of safety and warmth, and love. The mother, likewise, gains a sense of satisfaction and a feeling of closeness to the baby. If these important needs are to be met, the mother must be comfortable and relaxed; she not only feeds the baby but talks and smiles. Anxiety or tension, on the other hand, are also communicated to the baby.

Breast feeding should be initiated within 24 to 48 hours after birth since the sucking of the hungry infant stimulates the flow of milk. At first the mother will probably hold the baby against the breast while reclining and supported by pillows. Later she should sit in a comfortable chair with armrests—perhaps a rocker. A footstool to support the feet is also helpful.

A publication by the Children's Bureau, *Infant Care*, gives practical advice to the new parents in an interesting, easy-to-understand manner. For example, to initiate breast feeding:

> To get the baby started, press a little milk onto the baby's lips. If he's frantically nuzzling about, stroke the cheek nearest the nipple and he will turn toward it. If you touch the opposite cheek he will turn away automatically.[*]

The baby may get enough food by emptying one breast but if he is still hungry he should be offered the other breast. At the next feeding the breast not emptied should be offered first.

When the baby stops sucking he should be held over the shoulder and patted on the back to release any air which may have been swallowed. Some babies "burp" best if they are laid across the knee, abdomen down, and patted. Some babies require two or three "burpings" for each feeding.

Intervals of feeding. Healthy infants will establish, after a few weeks, schedules of their own which are reasonably regular from day to day if they are fed when they indicate that they are hungry. This is sometimes referred to as *self-demand feeding.*

The success of self-demand feeding depends upon the mother's ability to determine when the

---

[*]*Infant Care*, Children's Bureau Pub. No. 8, U.S. Department of Health, Education, and Welfare, Washington D.C., 1963, p. 14.

child is hungry. The infant who cries at intervals much shorter than three hours may be underfed, may have swallowed too much air at the previous feeding, or may be crying because of other discomforts.

The very young infant may require as many as 10 or 12 feedings at first, but he soon establishes a rhythm of feeding which falls into approximately three- to four-hour intervals. After the second month, the night feeding usually may be discontinued. By the end of the fourth or fifth month, the infant sleeps through the night and will no longer require a feeding around 10 P.M.

Adequacy of feeding. About 2.5 ounces of human milk per pound of body weight result in satisfactory weight gain. The baby is getting enough milk if he is satisfied at the end of a 15- to 20-minute feeding, if he falls asleep promptly and sleeps quietly for several hours thereafter, and if he makes satisfactory gains from week to week. The infant should be weighed once a week in the same amount of clothing each time.

Insufficient milk intake is indicated when the infant is not satisfied at the completion of the feeding, when he is restless and fails to fall asleep quickly after nursing, when he awakens frequently if he does go to sleep, and when his gains are not satisfactory. In such cases, the physician may advise adding a supplementary food, or replacing one or more of the breast feedings with bottle feedings.

Even human milk is low in some nutrients required by the growing baby so that it is necessary to supplement the diet of the breast-fed infant according to the routine suggested in Table 22–4.

Weaning the baby. As a rule, weaning is started during the fifth to the ninth month by substituting a cup feeding for the breast at any convenient interval. When the baby has become accustomed to this—after about four to five days—the second cup feeding is offered and so continued in this way until the baby is entirely weaned. Weaning usually requires a period of two to three weeks. The transfer from breast to cup should be gradual.

If breast feeding must be terminated at an earlier age, it is usually necessary to substitute bottle feeding and subsequently to proceed with weaning to the cup. Breast feeding after nine months has no special advantages for the infant and may lead to serious depletion of the mother.

BOTTLE FEEDING

Although breast feeding is highly desirable and should be encouraged, the fact remains that most babies are now bottle fed. Who is to say that one method is greatly superior to another? The circumstances for each family must be considered in making the choice, and no mother should ever be made to feel guilty if she chooses bottle feeding instead of breast feeding.

Comparison of human and cow's milk. The most widely used substitute for human milk is cow's milk. Goat's milk is used in some countries, and occasionally in the United States when the infant is allergic to cow's milk. Milk of other mammals such as the water buffalo, llama, camel, and sheep is used in countries where such milk is available. Table 22–2 gives a comparison of the nutritive values of human, cow's, and goat's milk.

Cow's milk contains about three times as much protein as human milk. About 60 per cent of the protein in human milk is lactalbumin and the remainder is casein. In cow's milk only 15 per cent of the protein is lactalbumin, with the remainder being casein. The efficiency of the proteins in the two milks is about equal. Human milk forms fine flocculent curds and the emptying time of the stomach is more rapid than for cow's milk. The curd from cow's milk is larger, tougher, and more slowly digested; it may be modified by heating the milk, by homogenization, or by acidification.

The full-term infant utilizes well the fat of both human and cow's milk. Cow's milk, however, contains a larger proportion of volatile, short-chain fatty acids (such as butyric acid), which are somewhat more irritating than the long-chain fatty acids (such as oleic acid) found in human milk. Human milk contains almost twice as much lactose as cow's milk. Both kinds of milk provide about 20 calories per ounce.

Table 22–2. Composition of Human, Cow's, and Goat's Milk* (per 100 gm milk)

	Human†	Cow's	Goat's		Human	Cow's	Goat's
Water, gm	85.2	87.4	87.5	Sodium, mg	16	50	34
Energy, calories	77	65	67	Potassium, mg	51	144	180
Protein, gm	1.1	3.5	3.2	Vitamin A, I.U.	240	140	160
Fat, gm	4.0	3.5	4.0	Thiamine, mg	0.01	0.03	0.04
Carbohydrate, gm	9.5	4.9	4.6	Riboflavin, mg	0.04	0.17	0.11
Total ash, gm	0.2	0.7	0.7	Niacin, mg	0.2	0.1	0.3
Calcium, mg	33	118	129	Ascorbic acid, mg	5	1	1
Phosphorus, mg	14	93	106				
Iron, mg	0.1	tr	0.1				

*Watt, B. K., and Merrill, A. L.: *Composition of Foods—Raw, Processed, Prepared*. Handbook No. 8, U.S. Department of Agriculture, 1964, p. 39.
†U.S. samples.

The total ash content is more than three times as high in cow's milk, almost all of this being accounted for by the higher contents of calcium, phosphorus, sodium, and potassium. Some healthy full-term infants fed cow's milk have a syndrome of convulsions known as *neonatal tetany* about the sixth day of life.[7] This is believed to be due to the high blood phosphorus and low blood calcium levels observed in these infants and attributed to the high phosphorus level of cow's milk. Some dilution of the milk is desirable to reduce the phosphorus content.

Because of the lesser capacity of the infant's kidneys to excrete wastes, the high ash content of cow's milk may present too high a solute load. By dilution of the milk, this problem is corrected.

The vitamin contents of human and cow's milk vary considerably. Human milk from a well-nourished mother can meet the infant's ascorbic acid requirements, but cow's milk will need to be supplemented. Neither milk contains sufficient vitamin D or iron to meet the infant's needs for the first year.

Commercial formulas. Probably the majority of infants in the United States are now being fed commercially prepared formulas. Most of the widely used brands require only dilution with water. Their cost is moderate, and safety and convenience are important factors to consider. Some formulas are packaged ready to use in 4-ounce and 8-ounce disposable bottles; their cost is considerably greater.

Most premodified formulas use cow's milk as a base. For specific purposes such as allergy to milk or inborn errors of metabolism special formulas have been developed. The formulas for healthy babies are modified to simulate human milk and one or more of these modifications are usually included:

Protein content is usually lowered; the protein is treated to produce a fine, flocculent, easily digested curd.

Butterfat is removed, and vegetable oils, such as corn oil, are substituted to increase the linoleic acid content.

Lactose or other carbohydrate is added.

Calcium level is reduced by dilution.

Sodium level is reduced by dialyzing milk with a resin.

Vitamins A, D, and ascorbic acid are usually added.

Iron may be added.

Cost. One of the important considerations in the selection of a formula is its cost. A recent study in four Pennsylvania counties showed that commercially prepared formulas were most frequently used, with whole-cow's-milk formulas ranking second.[8] Many of the families in this study were in the low-income group. It may well be asked whether, by education, many families can be helped to get more for their money.

Studies of costs[6, 8] have shown that a formula

prepared from evaporated vitamin D milk, cane sugar, and ascorbic acid tablets is least expensive. Use of fresh whole milk, special sugars such as Dextri-maltose, and fresh orange juice increases the formula costs. In the studies cited, premodified formulas cost slightly more than fresh-milk formulas and about half again as much as the evaporated-milk formulas.

Planning the formula. Evaporated, fresh whole, and dried cow's milks are used frequently. The milk is modified by dilution, homogenization, heating, or acidulation to produce a finer, smoother curd which is more readily digested.

Evaporated milk is inexpensive, readily available, and stored without refrigeration until the can is opened. It contains fat in a finely divided form, produces a fine, soft curd, and is fortified with 400 I.U. vitamin D per tall can.

Plain or homogenized fresh milk may be used. The latter has a more finely divided fat and forms softer curds than plain milk.

Dried milk may be obtained as whole, skim, or protein milk. It does not require refrigeration, but once the can has been opened the milk powder should be kept in a cool place in a container with a tight lid. By correct dilution the milk may approximate fresh liquid milk, or it may be prepared in a more concentrated form.

Acid-milk formulas prepared from fresh or evaporated milk are occasionally prescribed. Certain advantages are claimed for these formulas: (1) the curd formed is fine and smooth; (2) less dilution is required so that infants with a small capacity may be more readily nourished; (3) the tendency to vomit is reduced; (4) the acid counteracts the neutralizing effect of cow's milk, and calcium and iron may be more completely absorbed.

Amount of milk. About 1.5 to 2 ounces of fresh whole milk ($\frac{3}{4}$ to 1 ounce evaporated milk) per pound of body weight is suitable for the healthy infant.

Sugar. Most of the day's caloric needs are met by milk. Since cow's milk is diluted, sugar is added to complete the caloric requirement. Sucrose and corn syrup are inexpensive, easily digested, and lend themselves readily to formula preparation, although they possess the slight disadvantage of sweetness. Lactose, the sugar of

milk, is expensive and is seldom used. Dextrinized products such as Dextri-maltose are less sweet and are sometimes prescribed.

During the first two weeks the amount of sugar added may be $\frac{1}{2}$ ounce; thereafter, 1 ounce is sufficient until other foods are added to the diet when the sugar in the formula may be discontinued.

Liquid. A baby will usually take 2 or 3 ounces more of fluid in a single feeding than his age in months. More than 7 ounces at one feeding is usually undesirable before the infant is seven months old. Feedings larger than 8 ounces are not needed after six months since the infant will be taking other foods as well. The total fluid requirement of the infant is met by offering water between feedings, and by fruit juices.

Intervals of feeding. As with breast feeding, the number of feedings and the amount taken at each feeding should be flexible. Formula-fed infants should not, as a rule, be fed at less than three-hour intervals since cow's milk remains for a longer time in the stomach than breast milk.

Calculation of the formula. An example of the calculation of a formula is given below.

Infant, 5 months old, weighs 14 pounds
Number of feedings: 5 (assuming approximately 4-hour intervals)
Size of feedings: age in months plus 2
   $5 + 2 = 7$ ounces
Daily total: 5×7 ounces $= 35$ ounces
Whole milk: 14×1.75 ounces $= 24.5$ ounces
Water: $35 - 24.5 = 10.5$ ounces
Sugar: 1 ounce

This formula provides 490 calories from milk and 120 calories from sugar, or a daily intake of about 44 calories per pound of body weight. Food supplements given at this age will further increase the caloric intake. The formula contains 24.5 gm protein, or about 1.7 gm protein per pound of body weight.

Technique of feeding. The feeding is usually given at body temperature, but no adverse effects have been noted when it is given at room temperature. To warm the formula the bottle should be placed in a deep saucepan full of warm water. Heat the water rapidly, and shake the bottle several times to assure that the mixture is uniformly heated. Test the temperature by letting a few drops of formula fall on the inner surface of the forearm; the formula is the correct temperature when the heat is barely felt.

As in breast feeding the baby should be held in a semireclining position. The baby should never be propped up and allowed to feed himself. (See Figure 22–2.)

An overly large hole in the nipple leads to rapid taking of the formula and excessive swallowing of air, discomfort, and perhaps regurgitation. On the other hand, a very small hole in the nipple will necessitate too long a period of feeding. During the feeding the nipple should be filled with fluid, and not air, so that less air is swallowed. Even so, the infant will need to be "burped" one or more times as experience shows to be necessary.

The baby should not be expected to finish the entire amount of formula in the bottle at each feeding. The mother soon learns how much the baby will usually take at each feeding and can adjust the amounts of formula in the bottle. Any formula remaining at the end of each feeding must be discarded.

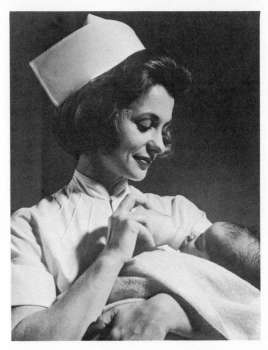

Figure 22–2. The young infant experiences security and comfort as he is held while being fed. (Courtesy, Ross Laboratories.)

FORMULAS FOR THE PREMATURE INFANT

Nutritive requirements. The premature infant is born with poorly developed muscle tissues, very little body fat, low stores of iron, and an inadequately mineralized skeleton. Regulation of the body temperature is difficult because of the very high surface area and the incomplete development of the sweat glands. The digestive ability is limited since the stomach can hold little food at the time, and the digestive enzymes are not sufficiently developed for satisfactory digestion and absorption of fat.

Very small infants are unable to suck, whereas somewhat larger infants may be overfatigued if sucking is prolonged. Feeding by medicine dropper or by gavage may be necessary.

The first need is for fluid, and in most instances, with a graduated program, the baby will be receiving his full nutritive requirements by the end of the first week to 10 days. The following allowances have been recommended for some of the nutrients:

Calories: 40 to 50 per pound by end of first week; then 50 to 60 per pound
Protein: 2.0 to 2.7 gm per pound
Vitamin D: 400 I.U. begun during the second or third week
Ascorbic acid: 50 mg begun during the second or third week

Intervals of feeding. Since very small babies can take only limited amounts of fluid, they are preferably fed at two-hour intervals for the first few days; thereafter, three-hour intervals may be used.

Choice of formula. Human milk, evaporated milk, or partially skimmed milk formulas are used. Human milk, however, contains insufficient protein, calcium, and phosphorus for the rate of growth required of the premature infant; it may be fortified by using skimmed cow's milk, Under careful supervision, better gains are obtained with mixtures of partially skimmed cow's milk or evaporated milk because of the somewhat greater protein and mineral content. Feeding mixtures which may be employed are illustrated in Table 22–3.

Suggested daily program. For infants weighing 1000 to 1200 gm (2 to 2½ pounds) the following schedule is typical:[9]

First 36 hours. Nothing by mouth.
Next 24 hours. Start with 4 ml 10 per cent sterile glucose solution; at two- to three-hour intervals increase this by 4 ml until 16 ml is taken. At the next feeding reduce the glucose solution to 12 ml and introduce 4 ml of breast milk or formula. Continue to increase the milk feeding by 4 ml at each feeding, correspondingly decreasing the glucose until only milk is being taken.

For infants weighing 1800 to 2000 gm (4 to 4½ pounds) the following schedule may be used:

First 24 hours. Nothing by mouth.
Next 24 hours. Start with 8 ml 10 per cent sterile glucose solution. At four-hour intervals increase the glucose feeding by 8 ml until 32 ml are being taken. At the next feeding, introduce 8 ml breast milk or formula and reduce the glucose feeding to 24 ml. Continue to increase the milk feeding at each interval by 8 ml and correspondingly reduce the glucose given. At the beginning of the next 24-hour period milk feedings only will be given.

PREPARATION OF THE FORMULA

Equipment needed. The usual equipment includes:

Bottles, 8 oz graduated, of heat-resistant glass or plastic which can be boiled; wide-mouthed bottles are easier to clean; provide one for each feeding plus two or three extra for water and orange juice
Nipples, one for each feeding, plus extra for orange juice and water
Bottle caps, glass, metal, plastic, or paper
Bottle sterilizer or large kettle with wire rack to hold bottles
Saucepan or pitcher with pouring lip, 2- or 3-quart size, for mixing formula
Standard measuring cup with pouring lip, graduated in ounces
Standard measuring spoons
Long-handled spoon
Funnel
Bottle brush with stiff bristles and long handle
Tongs are convenient
Jar for used nipples
Fine strainer
Can opener if evaporated milk is used

Care of equipment. Before starting to make the formula the hands should be scrubbed thoroughly and the work area should be scrupulously clean. Persons with a skin disease should not be permitted to prepare feedings.

Table 22–3. Feeding Mixtures Designed to Give 120 Calories per Kilogram
(55 Calories per Pound) *

	Per Kilogram	Per Pound	Grams/Kilogram			Percentage of Total Calories		
			Protein	Fat	Carbohydrate	Protein	Fat	Carbohydrate
Human milk	180 ml	2 1/2 oz	2.2	6.7	12.9	7	50	43
Evaporated milk	70 ml	1 oz	4.8	5.5	12.9	16	41	43
Carbohydrate	6 gm	3 gm						
Water to make	150 ml	2 1/4 oz						
Half skim milk powder	18 gm	1 tbsp	6.0	2.2	19.4	20	16	64
Carbohydrate	11 gm	5 gm						
Water to make	150 ml	2 1/4 oz						

*Gordon, H. H., *et al.*: "Feeding of Premature Infants. A Comparison of Human and Cow's Milk," *Am. J. Dis. Child.*, **73**: 442, 1947.

Immediately after each feeding rinse the bottle and nipple with cold water. Fill the bottle with cold water and allow to stand. Scrub all bottles at one time with detergent and water, using a long-handled brush which will reach into the corners of the bottles. Rinse bottles thoroughly in warm water. Scrub nipples inside and out with water and rinse. Test each nipple to be sure that the hole has not become plugged.

Mixing and sterilization. Measure the required amount of sugar, leveling off the spoon with a knife, and put into a large pitcher or saucepan. Add measured amounts of milk and water and mix well. Pour formula into bottles according to the amount required for each feeding. Put nipples on bottles and test the flow of milk. Cover loosely with nipple covers.

Place bottles on rack in sterilizer. Include one or two extra bottles of drinking water. Pour water into the sterilizer until water comes halfway up on the bottles.

Cover the sterilizer. Bring water to a boil and continue boiling gently for 25 minutes. Remove sterilizer from heat and let stand until bottles are cool enough to handle. Press nipple covers down firmly. Cool bottles to room temperature and then place in the refrigerator. (See Figure 22–3.)

SUPPLEMENTARY FOODS DURING THE FIRST YEAR

Supplements of vitamin D and of ascorbic acid are provided after the second or third week of life. Practices vary widely concerning the time when solid foods are introduced. Many infants are now given some solid food as early as six weeks, whereas others are fed the first solid foods at about three months or so. No clear advantage can be ascribed to one or the other, since babies thrive on either.

Introduction of new foods. A number of practical suggestions are offered for the introduction of new foods.

1. Introduce only one new food at a time. Allow the infant to become familiar with that food before trying to give another.

2. Give very small amounts of any new food —teaspoonfuls or even less—at the beginning.

3. Use a very thin consistency when starting solid foods. Gradually the consistency is made more solid as the infant learns how to use his tongue in propelling the food back. A small spoon is put into the baby's mouth so that the food is placed on the middle of the tongue and swallowing is more readily accomplished. The fact that a baby spits out his first feedings of solid food may indicate that he hasn't yet learned the tongue movements rather than that he doesn't like the food.

4. Never force an infant to eat more of a food than he takes willingly.

5. If, after several trials, it is apparent that a baby has an acute dislike for a food, omit that item for a week or two and then try it again. If the dislike persists it is better to forget about that food for a while and substitute another.

6. Food should be slightly seasoned with salt. Other seasonings are avoided.

7. Use foods of smooth consistency at first— strained fruits, vegetables, and meats.

8. When the baby is able to chew, gradually substitute finely chopped fruits and vegetables for puréed foods—usually at eight to nine months.

9. Infants may object to taking some foods by themselves but will take them willingly if they are mixed with another food. For example, egg may be mixed with formula, cereal, or vegetable; again, vegetables may sometimes be made into a soup with a little milk until the baby becomes accustomed to the new flavor.

10. Variety in choice of foods is important. The baby, like older persons, may tire of the repetition of certain foods, especially cereals and vegetables.

11. The mother or anyone feeding the infant must be careful to avoid showing in any way a dislike for a food which is being given. (See Figure 22–4.)

Sequence of additions. No uniformity of opinion exists concerning the time and sequence at which supplements are added. Some pediatricians introduce cereals, egg yolk, strained meats, fruits, and vegetables very early. In many infants the swallowing reflex is not fully established until the third or fourth month, and too early

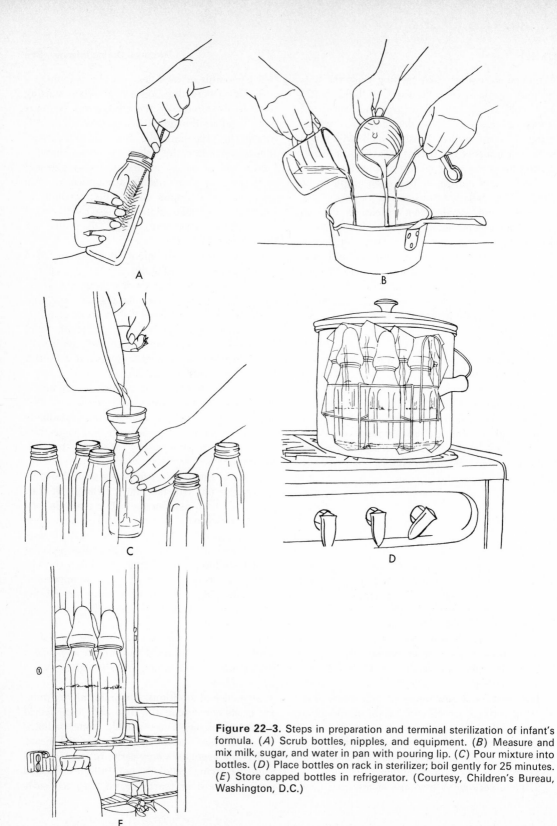

Figure 22–3. Steps in preparation and terminal sterilization of infant's formula. (*A*) Scrub bottles, nipples, and equipment. (*B*) Measure and mix milk, sugar, and water in pan with pouring lip. (*C*) Pour mixture into bottles. (*D*) Place bottles on rack in sterilizer; boil gently for 25 minutes. (*E*) Store capped bottles in refrigerator. (Courtesy, Children's Bureau, Washington, D.C.)

Figure 22–4. Feeding is also a means whereby happy relationships are established with others. (Courtesy, The Equitable Life Assurance Society of the United States.)

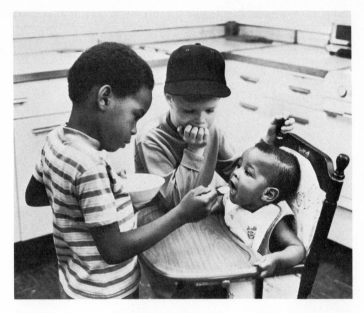

feeding, especially if forced, could lead to resistance and rebellion later on. The outline in Table 22–4 for feeding during the first year is typical of many.

Vitamins. Premodified formulas usually supply vitamins A and D and ascorbic acid without requiring further supplementation. When fortified evaporated or fresh milk is used for the preparation of the formula in the home, no further vitamin A or D is ordinarily required.

If, for any reason, vitamins A and D are prescribed as a supplement, the water-miscible preparation is preferable because of the lessened danger of aspiration. Since both vitamins are toxic when taken in excessive amounts, great care must be taken to see that the exact prescribed dosages are used.

Synthetic ascorbic acid is usually preferred initially because some babies may show an intolerance to orange juice. The ascorbic acid may be added to the formula just before it is given to the baby, or it may be given separately in a bottle of water. After several weeks orange juice is gradually introduced. One teaspoonful of strained orange juice (frozen, canned, or fresh) is diluted with an equal amount of boiled water. Gradually the amount is increased until the baby is taking 3 ounces of undiluted juice daily, at

about three months of age. Grapefruit juice or tomato juice may be used, but the latter must be given in twice as great amounts to provide the equivalent amount of vitamin C. The mother must be cautioned not to boil the juices.

Cereal foods. Cereals are often the first semi-solid foods given to the baby, at approximately two to four months. Specially formulated dry infant cereal foods possess the distinct advantage of enrichment with iron, thus bolstering the iron intake when body reserves have reached a low point. These cereal foods are mixed with a portion of the warm formula to the desired consistency.

Cooked cereals given to the rest of the family may also be used for the baby if they have been thoroughly cooked, are well strained, and are diluted with part of the formula. Cooking directions appear on the containers in which the cereal is purchased.

Crisp toast, zwieback, and graham crackers may be given when the teeth begin to appear, about five to eight months.

Egg yolk. The rich supplies of iron and of B complex vitamins, as well as vitamin A, are reasons favoring the introduction of egg yolk at the third to the fifth month. Hard-cooked egg yolk may be mashed with a fork and mixed with

Table 22–4. Typical Feeding Schedules for Normal Babies During the First Year*

Hour	Food	1 Month	3 Months	6 Months	10–12 Months
6 A.M.	Formula†	3–4 oz	5–6 oz	7–8 oz	6 A.M.
8 A.M.	Orange juice Vitamin D‡	1 oz 400 I.U.	3 oz 400 I.U.	3 oz 400 I.U.	Orange juice, 3 oz Zwieback, 1/2 piece
10 A.M.	Formula Cereal	3–4 oz	5–6 oz 1/4–2 tbsp	7–8 oz 2–4 tbsp	Breakfast, 7:30 A.M. Cereal, 2–5 tbsp Milk, 8 oz
2 P.M.	Formula Egg yolk Vegetable	3–4 oz	5–6 oz	7–8 oz 1 yolk 2–3 tbsp	Chopped fruit, 1–2 tbsp Vitamin D, 400 I.U.
6 P.M.	Formula Cereal Fruit	3–4 oz	5–6 oz	7–8 oz 2–4 tbsp 1/4–2 tbsp	Dinner, 11:30–12 Meat, 1/2–1 oz, or Egg, 1 whole Potato, 2–4 tbsp Chopped vegetable, 2–4 tbsp
10 P.M.	Formula	3–4 oz	5–6 oz	Discontinued	Milk, 8 oz
2 A.M.	Formula	3–4 oz	Discontinued		Supper, 5:30 P.M. Cereal or potato, 2–5 tbsp Milk, 8 oz Chopped fruit, 1–2 tbsp Toast or zwieback

*Feeding intervals, amounts of food, and age at which supplements are given are subject to individual variation.

†Formula or breast milk; plain milk after seven to nine months.

‡The appropriate concentrate for vitamin D is prescribed by the physician. Note exact measurements carefully.

part of the formula, cereal, or vegetable. Only ¼-teaspoon amounts should be given initially since some infants may be allergic to the egg protein. Soft custard is also a suitable way in which to introduce the egg yolk. Egg white, which leads to allergic manifestations more frequently, is not given until the infant is at least 8 to 10 months old and it then is introduced with extreme caution.

Fruits. Ripe banana and strained orange or grapefruit juice are the only raw fruits permitted during the first year. Cooked or canned prunes, pears, applesauce, peaches, and apricots are the fruits with which an infant first becomes acquainted, usually by the third to fourth month. These fruits are strained for the first few months they are offered, but they may be chopped by the end of the first year. Most babies accept fruits very well.

Vegetables. Strained carrots, green beans, spinach, squash, peas, asparagus, and tomatoes are all suitable for the infant from the fourth month or earlier. They are conveniently purchased in small cans, or the vegetables may be cooked at home until very soft, lightly seasoned with salt, and pressed through a sieve. The first feeding of less than 1 teaspoon is gradually increased to 3 or 4 tablespoons daily by the end of the year. Chopped vegetables are substituted for strained vegetables at 10 to 12 months. Baked or mashed potato may be included occasionally by the seventh month.

Meats. Canned strained baby meats may be used as early as the second month, although they are more usually introduced at the fifth to the seventh month. When the baby is accustomed to strained meats and meat soups, he may be given ground meat including beef, lamb, lean pork, thoroughly boned fish, chicken, and liver. The baby who is teething often enjoys a piece of crisp bacon.

Other foods. In some areas such as the Southwest, a variety of beans are widely used. They are a good source of protein, iron, and B complex vitamins and may be cooked and sieved for the infant. The infant may be given simple puddings toward the end of the first year. It is desirable that the amounts of sugar used in the preparation of fruits and puddings be kept small so that the infant does not develop a special craving for sweets.

PROBLEMS AND REVIEW

1. Select an article from the list of references pertaining to breast feeding and on the basis of your reading prepare a 200-word summary of viewpoints on breast feeding.
2. What vitamins are customarily prescribed for breast-fed infants?
3. Describe the procedures to follow to ensure satisfactory weaning.
4. What advantages can be claimed for the use of commercially prepared formulas?
5. Compare the composition of human and cow's milk. What adjustments can be made so that cow's milk simulates human milk?
6. *Problem.* Calculate a formula using evaporated milk for an infant who weighs 12 pounds and is four months old.
7. *Problem.* Examine the labeling of four popular brands of premodified formulas. How much of each would be required daily for the four-month infant weighing 12 pounds? Are any supplements required? Calculate the cost for the formula for one day, and compare with the cost of the formula calculated in problem 6.
8. What explanations might there be for the failure of an infant to gain weight at a satisfactory rate?
9. List the supplementary foods that are customarily introduced during the first year. What are the important nutritive contributions of each food added? At what approximate age is each usually introduced?
10. What functions, other than nutrition, are provided by the inclusion of supplementary foods during the first year? What are some guidelines you could give to the young mother for the satisfactory introduction of new foods?
11. Why is egg white customarily omitted from the infant's diet?
12. *Problem.* Outline a day's diet for an infant of seven months.
13. How do the nutritive requirements of premature infants differ from those of full-term infants? What feeding progression is recommended for these infants?
14. What recommendations could you offer for the preparation of a formula where no refrigeration is available.

CITED REFERENCES

1. Brodehl, J., and Gellissen, K.: "Endogenous renal transport of free amino acids in infancy and children," *Pediatrics*, **42**:395–404, 1968.
2. Food and Nutrition Board: *Recommended Dietary Allowances*, 8th ed. National Academy of Sciences–National Research Council, Washington, D.C., 1973.
3. Hanna, F. M., *et al.*: "Calcium-Fatty Acid Absorption in Term Infants Fed Human Milk and Prepared Formulas Simulating Human Milk," *Pediatrics*, **45**:216–24, 1970.
4. Mayer, J.: "Hypertension, Salt Intake, and the Infant," *Postgrad. Med.*, **45**:229–30, Jan. 1969.
5. Review: "The Vitamin Composition of Human Milk," *Nutr. Rev.*, **4**:134, 1946.

6. Heseltine, M. M., and Pitts, J. L., Chm.: "Economy in Nutrition and Feeding of Infants," *Am. J. Public Health,* **56**:1756–84, 1966.
7. Oppé, T. E., and Redstone, D.: "Calcium and Phosphorus Levels in Healthy Newborn Infants Given Various Types of Milk," *Lancet,* **1**:1045–48, 1968.
8. "Infant Formula Feeding," *Nutr. News,* Division of Nutrition, Pennsylvania Department of Health, Fourth Issue, 1969.
9. Nelson, W. E.: *Textbook of Pediatrics,* 9th ed. W. B. Saunders Company, Philadelphia, 1970.

ADDITIONAL REFERENCES

Adams, S. F.: "Use of Vegetables in Infant Feeding Through the Ages," *J. Am. Diet. Assoc.,* **35**:692–703, 1959.
Aldrich, R. A.: "Nutrition and Human Development," *J. Am. Diet. Assoc.,* **46**:453–56, 1965.
Beal, V. A.: "Breast- and Formula-Feeding of Infants," *J. Am. Diet. Assoc.,* **55**:31–37, 1969.
———: "Calcium and Phosphorus in Infancy," *J. Am. Diet. Assoc.,* **53**:450–59, 1968.
Berenberg, W., *et al.*: "Hazards of Skimmed Milk, Unboiled and Boiled," *Pediatrics,* **44**:734–37, 1969.
Children's Bureau: *Infant Care.* Pub. 400 Rev. U.S. Department of Health, Education, and Welfare, Washington, D.C., 1963.
Committee on Nutrition, American Academy of Pediatrics: "Appraisal of Nutritional Adequacy of Infant Formulas Used as Cow's Milk Substitutes," *Pediatrics,* **31**:329–38, 1963.
Dyal, L., and Kahrl, J.: "When Mothers Breast Feed," *Am. J. Nurs.,* **67**:2555, 1967.
Filer, L. J.: "Salt in Infant Foods," *Nutr. Rev.,* **29**:27–30, 1971.
Fomon, S. J.: *Infant Nutrition.* W. B. Saunders Company, Philadelphia, 1967.
Hytten, F. E.: "Is Breast Feeding Best?" *Am. J. Clin. Nutr.,* **7**:259–63, 1959.
O'Grady, R. S.: "Feeding Behavior in Infants," *Am. J. Nurs.,* **71**:736–39, 1971.
Owen, G. M.: "Modification of Cow's Milk for Infant Formulas: Current Practices," *Am. J. Clin. Nutr.,* **22**:1150–55, 1969.
Review: "Calcium, Phosphorus, and Strontium Metabolism in Infants," *Nutr. Rev.,* **27**:254–56, 1969.
———: "Excessive Weight Gain in Infancy," *Nutr. Rev.,* **28**:184–85, 1970.
Rose, H. E., and Mayer, J.: "Activity, Calorie Intake, Fat Storage, and the Energy Balance of Infants," *Pediatrics,* **41**:18–29 1968.
Schmitt M. H.: "Superiority of Breast Feeding. Fact or Fancy?" *Am. J. Nurs.,* **70**:1488–93, 1970.
Spock, B.: *Baby and Child Care.* Pocket Books, New York, 1955.
Whitten, C. F.: "Evidence That Growth Failure from Maternal Deprivation Is Secondary to Undereating," *J.A.M.A.,* **209**:1675–82, 1969.

23 Nutrition for Children and Teen-agers

Growth and development. The term *growth* refers to an increase in size because of cell multiplication; the term *development* denotes an increase in the complexity of function. The latter, for example, not only refers to the increasing ability to metabolize nutrients and to coordinate motor skills, but it also refers to the complex mental and behavioral changes that occur. The outstanding fact to remember is that each person is unique in every way. Although many factors influence his life, he is physically, biochemically, mentally, and emotionally like no other person.

Neither growth nor development occurs at a uniform rate. The rapid growth in overall size that occurred in fetal life and during infancy is followed by a long period of very gradual growth that accelerates again in the adolescent years. In organ development cellular growth occurs in three phases: (1) rapid cell division occurs (hyperplasia); (2) cell division slows down but protein synthesis continues so that the cells increase in size (hypertrophy); and (3) cell division ceases but protein synthesis continues for a time with further increase in size.[1] Eventually growth ceases. These phases follow a chronologic schedule for each . organ, but the timing of development differs for the organs and tissues of the body. The nervous system shows rapid growth early in life, with the size of the brain having achieved 80 to 90 per cent of its maximum size by the age of four years. However, the complexity of function continues to develop. On the other hand, the growth and development of the reproductive organs are negligible until the beginning of the adolescent years. Since each organ has a critical time for its development, it should be evident that interference with the supply of nutrients at any given period can be serious for the development of specific organs and systems as well as the organism as a whole.

Food habits and development. Foods to supply good nutrition are obviously fundamental to the physical growth and development of the child. But food means much more to the individual than nutrition alone. The infant's earliest relationships are associated with food, and throughout the growing years food continues to be a major factor in the development of the whole person. For each person food becomes a language of communication; it has cultural and social meanings; it is intimately associated with the emotions; and its acceptance or rejection becomes highly personal.

Food influences each stage of physical, mental, and emotional growth and development. But the food habits that result are also the consequence of the interrelated personal and environmental factors that surround the individual: the stages of physical and behavioral changes that occur and the rates of change; the widening circle of human relationships; and the economic, social, and cultural factors.

Good food habits have several characteristics. First, the pattern of diet permits the individual to achieve the maximum genetic potential for his physical and mental development. Second, the food habits are conducive to delaying or preventing the onset of degenerative diseases that are so prevalent in American society today. Third, the food habits are part of satisfying human relationships and contribute to social and personal enjoyment. The development of food habits is a continuous process in which each year builds upon what has gone before. The responsibility of parents and all who work with children goes far beyond assuring the ingestion of specified levels of nutrients. It requires the application of knowledge from the fields of human behavior and development, psychology, sociology, and anthropology.

NUTRITIONAL STATUS OF CHILDREN

Assessment of nutritional status. The determination of nutritional status can be made only by specialists qualified to give comprehensive physical and dental examinations, to make biochemical studies of the blood and urine, and to evaluate patterns of growth and measurements of body size. A single measurement at a given point in time may be of limited value, but a series of measurements at that time on a given individual are useful in measuring health status. When such measurements are repeated at regularly spaced intervals, the progress of the individual can be noted; thus, each person serves as his own control.

Height-weight charts indicate whether a given child falls within the range of heights and weights for other children of the same chronologic age, but they do not indicate anything about nutritional status. After all, one does not need a height-weight chart to determine gross obesity or severe underweight. Moreover, the chart could be misused by interpreting deviations of weight to be obesity or underweight, when, in fact, for that individual the level of weight might be entirely appropriate in terms of functioning tissue. Longitudinal-type grids (Wetzel grid) or percentile curves (Stuart-Meredith curves) are replacing height-weight tables for assessment of growth.

Stature is considered to be an important index of nutritional status because it is an indication of how well the individual has been able to achieve his genetic potential. The individual who is short may never have received the essential nutrients in sufficient quantity for the best development of his body, whereas the tall individual gives indication of full development. Mitchell[2] has reported on the changes in stature which occurred in boys and girls in Japan over a 10-year period following the war as compared with a similar group prior to the war. As a direct outcome of an improved diet the stature of the boys and girls following the war was significantly greater; the protein content of the diet was believed to be especially important in bringing about this increase.

Certain physical and behavioral characteristics may be noted by the mother, teacher, or nurse which would indicate that some children should be studied more carefully with respect to the adequacy of their nutrition. The well-nourished child may be expected to exhibit these characteristics:

Sense of well-being: alert; interested in activities usual for the age; vigorous; happy.

Vitality: endurance during activity, quick recovery from fatigue; looks rested; does not fall asleep in school; sleeps well at night.

Weight: normal for height, age, and body build.

Posture: erect; arms and legs straight; abdomen pulled in; chest out.

Teeth: straight, without crowding in well-shaped jaw.

Gums: firm, pink; no signs of bleeding.

Skin: smooth, slightly moist; healthy glow; reddish-pink mucous membranes.

Eyes: clear, bright; no circles of fatigue around them.

Hair: lustrous; healthy scalp.

Muscles: well developed; firm.

Nervous control: good attention span for his age; gets along well with others; does not cry easily; not irritable and restless.

Gastrointestinal factors: good appetite; normal, regular elimination.

Nutritional status of children. Numerous studies have shown that the nutritional status of most children in the United States is good. Because some of these studies have been limited to children from middle-income groups, the problems of undernutrition or malnutrition often seemed less serious than they, in fact, are. Longitudinal studies have been conducted by Beal and her associates at the Child Research Center in Denver[3] and by Burke and her coworkers at the Center for Research in Child Health and Development in Boston.[4] These studies have shown that children of a given age set up their individual patterns of growth, which may vary widely, just as their intakes of nutrients vary.

An extensive series of studies on approximately

4000 children 5 to 12 years of age and an equal number of adolescents 13 to 20 years was reported by more than 200 investigators between the years 1947 to 1958.[5] Among the important findings were these: at all ages the nutrient intakes by boys were better than those by girls; elementary-school children more nearly met their recommended allowances than did teen-agers; and the adolescent girl had the poorest record of nutrient intake. Below the age of 12 years, the mean nutrient intake exceeded the recommended allowances except for slightly low calcium intakes by girls. For boys from 13 to 20 years only vitamin C was below recommended standards, but for girls the intakes of calcium, ascorbic acid, and thiamine were seriously inadequate and the intake of protein was moderately low. Many of these studies did not include evaluation of nutritional status, and the intakes could not be equated with changes in health. In some of the studies a correlation was found between the dietary intake and the blood levels of ascorbic acid and vitamin A, and between the dietary protein and iron and the blood hemoglobin levels. Also found were some skin and eye changes, such as inflammation of the eyes and reddened gums, associated with low vitamin A and C levels of the blood.

The National Nutrition Survey in its first phase was directed to areas of low income in 10 states.[6] It uncovered an alarming amount of malnutrition that included every type of deficiency seen in underdeveloped countries. Although the number of cases of severe deficiency was few, one might well ask why kwashiorkor, rickets, goiter, and other preventable deficiencies should occur. The incidence of failure to gain at a satisfactory rate was high among preschool children. Anemia was highly prevalent in preschool children and in teen-agers, and dental decay was found to be practically universal. In many of the children unacceptable blood levels of ascorbic acid, vitamin A, riboflavin, protein, and thiamine were found. (See also Chapter 1.)

Failure to maintain normal weight is a frequently recurring problem. The cooperative studies indicated that overweight and underweight occurred with equal frequency in boys and girls prior to adolescence. During adolescence, girls were more often overweight and boys were more frequently underweight, the degree of overweight or thinness increasing with age. Studies on overweight girls have shown that the caloric intake, surprisingly, is not as great as that of girls of normal weight; however, the activity of the overweight girls has been less.[7,8]

Stresses of various kinds may have an adverse effect on nutrition. The incidence of tuberculosis is higher than it should be in the adolescent years and in early adulthood and is believed to occur more frequently in those who have had inadequate diets, especially with respect to protein and calcium. A large proportion of infants are born to young women who have not yet completed their own body growth and maturation. The stress of pregnancy can have serious effects on the girl who has had a poor intake of protein, calcium, and iron during the preceding years. Johnston[9] has called attention to the frequency with which slipping of the upper femoral epiphysis takes place in rapidly growing adolescent girls.

Common dietary errors. Studies of food habits of children have shown repreatedly that the foods requiring particular emphasis for the improvement of diets are milk, dark-green leafy and deep-yellow vegetables, and ascorbic-acid-rich fruits. Among the food habits that contribute to these deficiencies are these:

Poor breakfast or none at all: lack of appetite; getting up too late; no one to prepare breakfast; monotony of breakfast foods; no protein at breakfast, meaning that the distribution of good quality protein is poor even though the day's total may be satisfactory; too little fruit, meaning that ascorbic acid often is not obtained.

Poor lunches: failure to participate in school lunch program; poor box lunches; spending lunch money for snacks or other items; unsatisfactory management of school lunch program with resultant poor menus, poor food preparation, excessive plate waste.

Snacks: account for as much as ¼ of calories without providing significant amounts of protein, minerals, and vitamins; often eaten too near to mealtime thus spoiling the appetite.

Overuse of milk, especially by younger children: other foods are not eaten so that the intake of iron and certain vitamins may be low.

Self-imposed dieting, especially by teen-age girls:

caloric restriction but no consideration given to protein, minerals, and vitamins.

Irregular eating habits: few meals with the family group; no adult supervision in eating; children often prepare own meals without guidance.

NUTRITIONAL REQUIREMENTS

Changes in growth and development. Height and weight changes follow a general pattern throughout childhood, but the chronologic age at which these changes occur may vary considerably; hence, a child cannot be compared with others of the same age. By the end of the first year the rate of growth has slowed considerably. The toddler gains 8 to 10 pounds during the second year, thus quadrupling his birth weight. Thereafter, the yearly gains are approximately 4 to 7 pounds up to the preadolescent period.

For a year or two before adolescence and during adolescence the growth rate accelerates. The most rapid changes occur in girls between 11 and 14 years and in boys between 13 and 16 years. The rapid spurt in growth usually covers a period of two to three years. There are tremendous variations in the age at which maturation occurs so that the nutritional requirements for an 11-year-old girl who is maturing early, for example, will be quite different from those of the 11-year-old girl who has not yet begun to show these rapid changes.

The number, size, and composition of the bones change from birth to maturity. The skeleton has reached its full size in girls by the age of 17 years, and in boys at 20 years. The water content of the bones gradually diminishes as the mineralization increases. Provided that the diet remains good, bone mineralization continues for several years after the attainment of full size.

Dietary allowances. Because the anabolic activities are considerable during the entire period of childhood, the nutritional requirements in proportion to body size are much higher than they will be in the adult years. Moreover, childhood and adolescence are times of considerable physical activity and hence the energy requirement is greater. The Recommended Dietary Allowances are those levels of nutrients that are believed to support optimum growth and development (see Table 3–1). When using these allowances it is important to interpret them in terms of the child's size as well as with reference to age category.

Energy. The very young child has a high basal metabolic rate incident to intensive cellular activity and to a proportionately high surface area. Year by year the rate of metabolism decreases, then accelerates somewhat during adolescence, after which it again declines to the adult level. The basal metabolism of boys is higher than that of girls owing to the greater muscle mass.

The one- to three-year-old needs about 1300 calories daily; the seven- to ten-year-old should have 2400 calories, which is more than his mother is likely to need; and the 15- to 18-year-old boy requires 3000 calories. Boys engaged in competitive athletics or heavy labor must have considerably more calories if they are to grow satisfactorily. Macy and Hunscher[10] have shown that a deficit of as little as 10 calories per kilogram body weight resulted in failure to grow and depression of nitrogen retention even though the protein intake had been satisfactory.

Protein. The protein allowance for children at one to three years is 23 gm and increases to 36 gm for the 7- to 10-year-old. The allowance for teen-agers is approximately that of adult males and females. Based on body weight, the allowance decelerates from 1.8 gm per kilogram for the one- to three-year-old to 0.9 gm per kilogram for the teen-ager. About 12 to 15 per cent of the total calories should normally be obtained from protein.

Since the requirement for the essential amino acids is proportionately higher for children than for adults (see Table 4–2), one half to two thirds of the protein should be selected from complete protein foods.

Minerals. The recommended calcium and phosphorus allowances are 800 mg for children from one to ten years. During the teen years the allowance for boys and girls is 1200 mg. The greatest retention of calcium and phosphorus precedes the period of rapid growth by two years or more, and liberal intakes of these minerals before the age of 10 are a distinct advantage.[11] Children whose diets have been poor require a good diet for as long as six months before they can equal the calcium and phosphorus retention of children on a good diet.[12] Such a lag in retention can be a special hazard for the poorly nourished teen-age girl who becomes pregnant.

Adequacy of calcium intake is directly correlated with the intake of milk or milk foods. All nonmilk foods can be expected to yield only 0.2 gm calcium in the diet of young children, and 0.3 gm calcium in the diet of older children.

The data on magnesium requirements are limited, and hence the daily allowances are estimates based upon amounts of magnesium contained in milk.[13] For children the allowances range from 150 mg at one to three years to 250 mg at 7 to 10 years. Boys from 11 to 18 years should receive daily allowances of 350 to 400 mg and girls should receive 300 mg. One quart of milk furnishes about 120 mg magnesium, and dark-green leafy vegetables are also good sources. Many diets that are reasonably adequate in other nutrients may be somewhat lower than these allowances in magnesium; however, symptoms of magnesium deficiency have not been demonstrated on such intakes.

The recommended allowances of iron—from 10 to 18 mg, depending upon age—can be satisfied only when consistent emphasis is placed upon the inclusion of enriched or whole-grain cereals and breads, eggs, meats of all kinds, legumes, fruits, and green leafy vegetables. Far too often children of all ages consume minimum amounts of fruits and vegetables, thus leading to suboptimal iron intakes. Milk, which is low in iron, may be consumed in excessive amounts by some children, thus crowding out other essential foods.

Throughout childhood, but especially during adolescence, the use of iodized salt should be encouraged because the high-energy metabolism increases the activity of the thyroid gland and the corresponding likelihood of simple goiter.

Vitamins. The vitamin requirements of children have not been extensively studied. Throughout childhood and adolescence 400 I.U. vitamin D should be provided—an allowance easily met by using fortified milk. The vitamin A needs are related to body weight, and the allowance increases from 2000 I.U. at one to three years to 5000 I.U. for boys and 4000 I.U. for girls. Milk, butter and margarine, egg yolk, dark-green leafy, and deep-yellow vegetables and fruits are good sources.

The allowances for ascorbic acid range from 40 mg for the one- to three-year-old to 45 mg for the 11- to 18-year-old boy and girl. Thiamine and niacin allowances are 0.5 mg and 6.6 mg, respectively, per 1000 calories. Allowances for riboflavin range from 0.8 to 1.2 mg for children from 1 to 10 years; teen-age boys need up to 1.8 mg and girls 1.4 mg. The allowance for vitamin B_6 ranges from 0.6 mg for the toddler to 1.2 mg by 10 years of age. Teen-age boys and girls need 1.6 to 2.0 mg vitamin B_6.

Although allowances have been established for vitamin E, the data pertaining to requirements for children are limited. An increased intake of polyunsaturated fats increases the need for vitamin E. When diets are adequate in protein, minerals, ascorbic acid, and thiamine, the dietary allowances for folacin, vitamin B_{12}, and vitamin B_6 are likely to be met.

DIET FOR THE PRESCHOOL CHILD

Food selection correlated with behavioral changes. The nutritional requirements of the child cannot be satisfied apart from an understanding of behavioral changes which occur. During the second year the appetite tapers off corresponding to the slower rate of growth. Beal[14] found that healthy, well-nourished girls reduced their milk intake as early as six months and returned to higher intakes at two to three years of age. Boys also reduced their milk intake at about nine months, but started to increase their consumption between one and two years. An intake of 2 cups or less is not uncommon for a period of time. Some children's appetites improve by five years or earlier, but other children have poor appetites well into the school years.

Many mothers must be reassured that the child will remain well nourished provided that foods abundant in protein, minerals, and vitamins are offered, and that feeding does not become an issue between mother and child. Some compensation for the reduced consumption of milk may be made by incorporating milk into foods such as simple puddings. The occasional use of flavorings such as molasses, cocoa, or the use of vegetable colors may introduce additional interest. Children may sometimes be encouraged to drink milk if they are permitted to pour the milk into a small glass or cup from a small pitcher. Cottage cheese and mild American cheese are often well liked and help to increase the calcium and protein intake.

Preschool children prefer mildly flavored foods to those of strong flavor, or those which are spicy. Vegetables as a class of foods are frequently disliked. Most young children enjoy raw vegetables but they are unlikely to consume sufficient amounts because they become fatigued with chewing. Plain foods are generally well liked, but mixtures such as casserole dishes, creamed foods, and stews are not popular.

Fruits are well liked and may be given raw or cooked, although melons and berries should be used with discretion if at all. Simple desserts such as milk puddings, sherbets, ice cream, plain cakes, and cookies may be included.

The ability of the child to chew should determine the texture of foods he may be given. The toddler may be given chopped vegetables and ground meat, whereas the three- to five-year-old can manage diced vegetables and minced or bite-size pieces of tender meat. Children enjoy chewing some foods such as zwieback, crackers, and strips or wedges of vegetables. Foods that are stringy such as celery, sticky such as some mashed potatoes, or slippery such as custard are often disliked because the child is not familiar with the texture.[15] (See Figure 23-1.)

The gastrointestinal tract of the preschool child is easily irritated by very sweet or rich foods, fried foods, excessive amounts of cellulose, or foods inadequately chewed such as nuts. Foods of this nature may also displace dietary essentials and it is advisable to omit them in the diet of one- to three-year-olds, and to use them seldom for older preschool children.

Food jags are not uncommon, especially between the ages of two and four years. The child may shun all but a few foods, such as milk or peanut butter and jelly sandwiches. Such occurrences do not last too long, if the parent does not show concern, and if the foods which constitute the child's preference at the moment are nutritious in general.

The preschool child is almost constantly active. His interest is readily diverted from food. If he becomes overtired or excessively hungry, his appetite may lag a great deal.

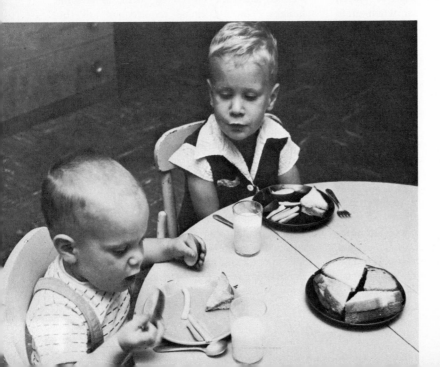

Figure 23–1. Children learn about foods by feeling them. Toddlers and preschool children enjoy foods that they can pick up with their fingers. Note also the small sandwiches and partly filled glasses of milk. (Courtesy, U.S. Department of Agriculture.)

Meal patterns. The Four Food Groups constitute a sound basis for planning the daily meals. Children of this age should consume each day:

2 cups milk
1 egg
1–3 ounces chopped meat, fish, or poultry
4 ounces orange juice or other source of ascorbic acid
2–4 tablespoons other fruit such as banana, peaches, pears, apple, apricot, prunes
2–4 tablespoons vegetables, including deep yellow and dark green leafy
1 potato
1 raw vegetable such as carrot sticks, cabbage slices, lettuce, tomato
⅓ to ⅔ cup enriched dry or cooked cereal
1–3 slices enriched or whole-grain bread
400 I.U. vitamin D, either as fortified milk or as a concentrate

The following meal patterns for a child from one to six* show that little adjustment needs to be made from the adult menu.

Breakfast

Fruit or juice
Cereal with milk
Toast
Butter or margarine
Milk

Lunch or Supper

Main dish—mainly meat, eggs, fish, poultry, dried beans or peas, cheese, peanut butter
Vegetable or salad
Bread
Butter or margarine
Dessert or fruit
Milk

Dinner

Meat, poultry, or fish
Vegetable
Relish or salad
Bread
Butter or margarine
Fruit or pudding
Milk

*Your Child from 1 to 6. Children's Bureau Pub. 30, Welfare Administration, U.S. Department of Health, Education, and Welfare, Washington, D.C., 1963.

Snacks. Most young children with a limited capacity for food are more likely to obtain all the dietary essentials if they are fed something in the middle of the morning and the afternoon. Moreover, very active children become excessively fatigued and hungry if they are not fed between meals. Snacks should make a liberal contribution to one or more of the nutrient needs. (See Figure 23-2.) Some which are suitable for preschool children are:

Fruit juices with little or no sugar
Milk and milk beverages
Fruit of any kind; raw vegetables
Small sandwiches; crackers with peanut butter
Molasses, oatmeal, or peanut butter cookies
Dry cereal from the box or with milk
Cheese wedge
Fruit sherbet or ice cream

Establishing good food habits. Suggestions have been made in the preceding chapter for the establishment of good food habits in the infant. In addition, the following considerations are conducive to the development of good food habits in the preschool child.

Meals should be served at regular hours in a pleasant environment. The child should be comfortably seated at a table. Deep dishes permit the child to get his food onto the fork or spoon with greater ease. A fork, such as a salad fork with blunt tines, and a small spoon can be handled comfortably. A small cup or glass should be only partially filled with liquid to minimize spilling; however, the coordination of eye, hand, and mouth is difficult and some spilling is to be expected.

Children enjoy colorful meals just as adults do. Their appetites also vary from day to day, and like adults they react strongly to portions that are too large. It is much better to serve less than the child is likely to eat and to let him ask for more.

Even favorite foods should not be served too often. Breakfasts do not need to be stereotyped. A hamburger or sandwich with an orange cut in sections to be picked up with the fingers is just as satisfactory as a juice, cereal, and egg breakfast.

Fewer difficulties are likely to be encountered if new foods are given at the beginning of the

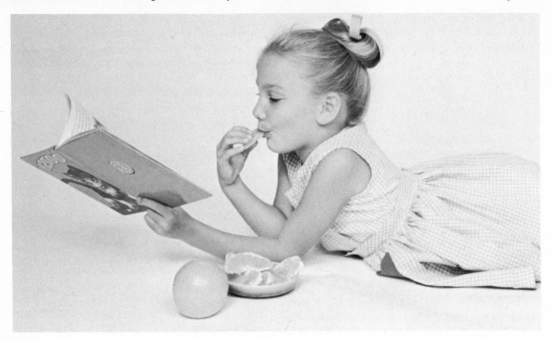

Figure 23–2. Snacks can provide valuable nutrients such as ascorbic acid. (Courtesy, Sunkist Growers.)

meal when the child is hungry. A food is more likely to be accepted if it is given in a form which can be easily handled, which can be chewed, and if some favorite food is also included in the same meal. The parent should assume that the child will also take some responsibility in accepting the offered food.

Whether or not the preschool child should eat with other members of the family or alone is a matter that each mother must determine for the child's greatest good and the family's convenience. If the father returns from work at such an hour that the evening meal must be late, if the child becomes overexcited about the family doings, or if the child is expected to live up to a code of behavior beyond his young years, it is better that he be allowed to eat before the rest of the family in a pleasant, quiet atmosphere with his mother nearby. Even so, an occasional meal with the family may be a treat for the child and parent if tension can be avoided. Since children are great imitators, they enjoy doing just as Daddy or Mother or the other children are doing.

The child may well learn early in life that he is expected to eat foods prepared for him, but this does not mean that nagging or bribery will accomplish anything. Children, like adults, enjoy attention, and they are quick to realize that food can be a powerful weapon for gaining such attention. It is therefore important to recognize that a display of concern or the use of force in getting a child to drink milk or to take any other food can have nothing but unfavorable effects. When a child refuses to take a food, the unwanted item should be calmly removed without comment after a reasonable period of time. If the child is refusing to eat because he thereby attracts attention, the mother should make certain that the child receives his full share of affection and companionship at other than mealtimes. By so doing the child will lose interest in using food as a weapon.

Diet for the Schoolchild

Characteristics of food acceptance. Elementary-school children are usually better fed than preschool children or adolescents. Group acceptance is extremely important at this time, and the child needs to be able to keep up with his classmates and to have a sense of accomplishment. When the child goes to school for the first time he makes acquaintance with food patterns that may be different from those he knows at home. He learns that certain foods may be acceptable to the peer group, whereas other foods from a different cultural pattern may be looked upon with disdain; as a result he may be unwilling to accept these foods at home—good though they may be. On the other hand, within a group he is willing to try foods with which he is unacquainted and which he would not try alone.

Schoolchildren have relatively few dislikes for food except possibly for vegetables, which are usually not eaten in satisfactory amounts. By the time children reach 8 to 10 years of age the ap-

petite is usually very good. Feeding problems are more likely to result because parents are unduly concerned with behavior at mealtime which does not come up to adult standards. Most children of this age are in a hurry, and don't like to take time for meals. Breakfast, especially, is likely to be skipped.

Schoolchildren may be subject to many stresses which affect the appetite. Communicable diseases occur often in this age group. They reduce the appetite on the one hand, but they increase body needs on the other. Schoolwork, class competition, and emotional stresses in getting along with many children may have adverse effects on appetite, as may also an unbalanced program of activity and rest.

Choice of foods. Table 23–1 lists the kinds and amounts of foods which may be taken in a day by healthy schoolchildren. A number of

Table 23–1. Foods to Meet Nutritional Needs of Elementary-School Children and Teen-agers

Food	6 to 10 Years	10 to 12 Years	12 to 16 Years
Milk	2–3 cups	3–4 cups	4 cups or more
Eggs	1	1	1 or more
Meat, poultry, fish	2–3 ounces (small serving)	3–4 ounces (average serving)	4 ounces or more (large serving)
Dried beans, peas, or peanut butter	2 servings each week. If used as an alternate for meat, allow 1/2 cup cooked beans or peas or 2 tablespoons peanut butter for 1 ounce meat		
Potatoes, white or sweet (occasionally spaghetti, macaroni, rice, noodles, etc.)	1 small or 1/3 cup	1 medium or 1/2 cup	1 large or 3/4 cup
Other cooked vegetable (green leafy or deep yellow 3 to 4 times a week)	1/4 cup	1/3 cup	1/2 cup or more
Raw vegetable (salad greens, cabbage, celery, carrots, etc.)	1/4 cup	1/3 cup	1/2 cup
Vitamin C food (citrus fruit, tomato, cantaloupe, etc.)	1 medium orange or equivalent	1 medium orange or equivalent	1 large orange or equivalent
Other fruit	1 portion or more, as: 1 apple, 1 banana, 1 peach, 1 pear, 1/2 cup cooked fruit		
Bread, enriched or whole grain	3 slices or more	3 slices or more	4–6 slices or more
Cereal, enriched or whole grain	1/2 cup	3/4 cup	1 cup or more
Butter or fortified margarine	1 tablespoon or more	1 tablespoon or more	1 tablespoon or more
Vitamin D	400 I.U. at all ages, using: fortified milk, fish-liver oil, or vitamin D concentrate		
Additional foods	Sweets, desserts, etc., to satisfy energy needs		

other equally satisfactory patterns could be devised for different cultural groups. A diet for adults which places emphasis first on the inclusion of protein, minerals, and vitamins is also a good one for schoolchildren. The amount of milk given to children should be greater than that for the adult. Although no foods need to be forbidden to this age group, it is extremely important that high-carbohydrate and high-fat foods not be allowed to replace essential items of the diet.

Food habits. The suggestions concerning good food habits for preschool children also apply to schoolchildren. A good school lunch program (see page 332) may introduce new foods in a setting where the child is anxious to conform to the group. The elementary teacher may integrate nutrition education with the total classroom experience so that good food habits are strengthened.

Since children are likely to be in a hurry, it is often wise to require that a certain time be spent at the table—say 15 or 20 minutes—so that the child will take time to eat. Children learn good manners by imitation of adults, and not by continuous correction at the table. During the elementary-school years, little can be gained by overemphasis on manners. In fact, the food

intake may be adversely affected. (See Figure 23–3.)

DIET FOR THE TEEN-AGER

Characteristics of food intake. Even boys and girls who have had an excellent dietary pattern are likely to succumb to bizarre, unbalanced diets during the adolescent years. Teen-agers have many concerns about their development such as the size and shape of the body, their attractiveness, skin conditions, their vitality, sexual development, and social approval by their peers. They feel independent and seek freedom to make their own decisions. It is a period in which family conflict is likely to increase.

Most teen-agers are concerned about their body weight.[16,17] Most girls want to weigh less and equate overweight with fatness which is undesirable. Generally, they want smaller hips, smaller thighs, and smaller waists but larger busts. Most boys want to weigh more and they equate overweight with muscle development which is desirable. They want a larger upper torso and arms, an indication of strength.

Teen-agers are often fatigued, anxious, and under emotional stress. These factors may have

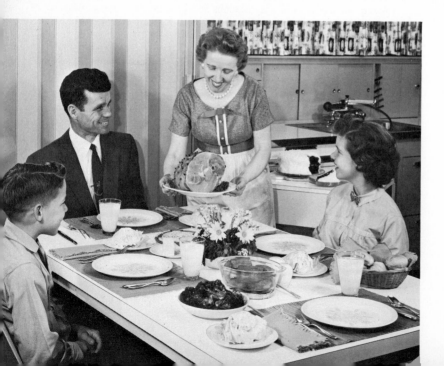

Figure 23–3. Mealtime should be a happy time for the family to share. In such an environment, the patterns established for good food habits in early childhood are reinforced throughout the school years. (Courtesy, U.S. Department of Agriculture.)

an adverse effect on the retention of nutrients. Students who were taking examinations and young women who were upset about a pregnancy were found to have negative nitrogen and mineral balances.[12,18] Emotional difficulties may stem from the feeling of social inadequacy or the pressures of schoolwork. When there is conflict within the home because of the teen-ager's food choices, failure to accept responsibilities, the use of money, dating hours, and so on, the emotions not only determine food intake for some adolescents but also modify the nutrient utilization.

Selection of foods. Milk, green leafy and deep-yellow vegetables, and citrus fruits are the foods which especially require emphasis. Moderate amounts of sweets, soft drinks, coffee, and tea cannot be considered harmful for this age group, provided that they do not replace essential foods in the diet. The list in Table 23–1 should serve as the starting point for the planning of meals at home and in the school lunch.

Snacks may be counted upon as supplying one fourth, or more, of the caloric requirement. They should also furnish an equivalent amount of the day's allowances for protein, minerals, and vitamins. Thus, sandwiches, hamburgers, fruit, and milk should be encouraged. Candy, rich pastries, cookies, and pretzels may be satisfying to the palate, but will not support their caloric content with important nutrients.

A study has shown that snack patterns may, in fact, be preferable to three meals a day, provided that the choice of snacks is good. In three boarding schools 226 boys and girls aged 6 to 16 years were fed for one year on one of three plans of meal frequency: in school A, three meals daily; in school B, seven meals daily; and in school C, five meals daily.[19] The average calorie intakes and food allowances did not differ significantly, but individual records were not kept. The older children, 11 to 16 years, who received only three meals per day showed increased tendency to deposit fat as demonstrated by the increase in the weight-to-height proportion and by caliper measurements of skinfold thickness. The differences were more marked in the girls than in the boys. These differences were not observed in the younger children.

Food habits. Good health in general is too abstract an approach to interest the teen-ager. Most of them have never known anything but good health. Girls can be appealed to on the basis of a better figure, an improved complexion, and glossy hair. Boys are especially interested in physical fitness and the greater ability to compete in athletic contests. They, too, are concerned about complexion problems. Adolescents are more anxious to improve their eating habits when they are reminded that their acceptance of foods makes them a more appreciated dinner guest.

Boys and girls give a surprisingly good performance when given responsibilities concerning meals at home. When they share in the planning of menus, in the purchase of foods, and in the preparation of meals, they take pride in showing their skills in shopping, or in trying a new recipe. Of course, it is good psychology to share these responsibilities as a privilege of growing up and not as a burden imposed by the parent. In their fulfillment, with subtle guidance and praise where merited, food habits are often improved.

CHILD NUTRITION PROGRAMS

In 1853 the Children's Aid Society of New York opened a vocational school for the poor and served meals to those who attended. School feeding was initiated in some elementary schools in Philadelphia in 1894. After the turn of the century many schools throughout the country provided meals or hot-dish supplements to carried meals.

The school lunch program has experienced rapid growth since the 1930's when surplus commodities were first distributed following the passage of a law in 1935. Although more than a third of all elementary- and secondary-school pupils receive plate lunches on any given school day, many of the most needy children do not have the program available to them. The existence of malnutrition in the United States was highlighted in the late 1960's, and as a result a considerable expansion of child nutrition pro-

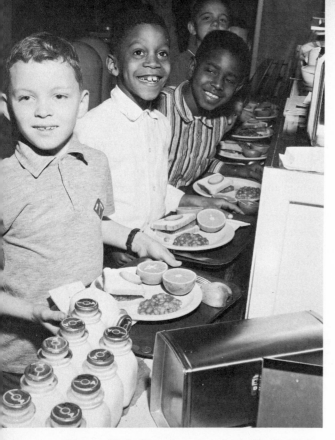

Figure 23–4. These boys in a Louisville, Kentucky, school are obviously ready to enjoy their type A lunch. (Courtesy, U.S. Department of Agriculture.)

grams supported by the U.S. Department of Agriculture has taken place.[20] (See Figure 23–4.)

National School Lunch Program. In 1946 the National School Lunch Act was passed to provide participating schools with (1) cash assistance; (2) donation of surplus food commodities; and (3) technical assistance in the purchase and use of foods and in the management and equipment of the school lunchroom. More recently, legislation has authorized higher-than-average rates of reimbursement for schools that have a large attendance from low-income areas. Financial assistance is also provided to help schools in these areas to purchase equipment needed for the lunch programs.

To participate in the program, a school must agree to: operate the program on a nonprofit basis; provide free or reduced-price lunches for needy children; serve all children regardless of race, color, or national origin; serve nutritious

lunches that meet the requirement for type A lunches as established by the Secretary of Agriculture; provide kitchen and dining facilities. No discrimination must be shown in any way to children who are eligible for free or reduced-price meals; that is, they must not be identified by placing them in separate lines, requiring them to sit in places set apart, or requiring them to provide service as a reimbursement for the meal.

Type A lunch. Five components are included in the Type A lunch:

1. Fluid whole milk, ½ pint, served as a beverage.

2. Protein-rich food such as: 2 ounces cooked or canned lean meat, fish, poultry; 2 ounces cheese; 1 egg; ½ cup cooked dry beans or peas; 4 tablespoons peanut butter; or an equivalent of any combination of these in a main dish.

3. Vegetables and fruits, at least ¾ cup, consisting of two or more servings. One serving of full strength juice may be counted as not more than ¼ cup of the requirement.

4. Whole-grain or enriched bread, 1 slice; or muffins, cornbread, biscuits, rolls made of enriched or whole-grain flour.

5. Butter or fortified margarine, 2 teaspoons, as a spread, as a seasoning, or in food preparation.

Nutritive value of type A lunch. When foods are served in the amounts specified, and additions are made to satisfy the appetite, the type A lunch provides, on the average, one third of the recommended allowances for the 10- to 12-year-old child. Larger portions must be provided for older children. Since the child eats but five meals in the school each week, the contribution represents about one fourth of his total nutritive needs.

Some care must be taken in the selection of fruits and vegetables. A vitamin-C-rich food should be served daily, and a vitamin-A-rich food at least twice a week. Well-managed school lunch programs seldom permit sales of soft drinks, candy, pretzels, and similar carbohydrate-rich foods because they contribute little except calories to the child's nutritional needs, and because the child's money may be used for these empty calories rather than the more nutritious foods. The American Medical Association, the American Dietetic Association, and the National Congress of Parents and Teachers have opposed the sale of candy and soft drinks within the schools.[21,22]

School breakfast program. Presently, the breakfast program is limited to schools that have a large number of needy children. Under the U.S. Department of Agriculture Program funds are provided to help schools pay for the foods purchased for the preparation of the breakfast, food commodities are donated, and financial assistance is provided in the purchase of kitchen equipment. The standard setup for the breakfast is:

1. One-half pint whole milk.

2. One-half cup fruit, or fruit or vegetable juice.

3. One serving bread or cereal; may be 1 slice whole-grain or enriched bread, or an equivalent amount of cornbread, biscuits, or muffins; or ¾ cup of whole-grain or enriched or fortified cereal.

4. As often as practicable, a serving of protein-rich food such as 1 egg, or 1 ounce meat, fish, or poultry, or 1 ounce cheese, or 2 tablespoons peanut butter.

Additional foods to round out the breakfast and to satisfy the appetite would include foods

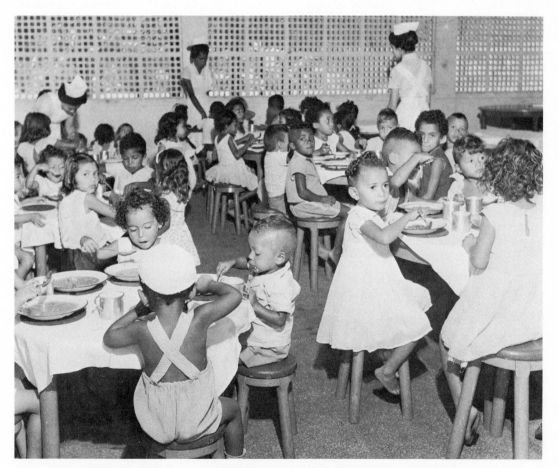

Figure 23–5. Child-care centers throughout the world are an effective means whereby the nutrition of preschool children can be improved. In such centers children also learn about new foods. This group of children in Brazil is provided with a thick soup and milk. (Courtesy, Jean Speiser and UNICEF.)

of popular appeal such as doughnuts, potatoes, or bacon; sweeteners; butter or margarine.

The standards for participation in the Program are similar to those of the National School Lunch Program.

Special food service program. This program provides assistance to day-care centers, recreation centers, settlement houses, and summer day camps. (See Figure 23–5.) It helps to improve the nutrition of preschool as well as school-age children. This program provides cash assistance up to a maximum of 15 cents for breakfast, 30 cents for each lunch or supper, and 10 cents for each supplemental feeding between meals; finances up to 80 per cent of operating costs in cases of severe need; supplies donated foods; furnishes financial assistance for purchase or rent

of necessary equipment; and provides technical assistance in setting up the program. The requirements for participation include meals served according to U.S. Department of Agriculture standards, operation of the program on a nonprofit basis for all children without discrimination, and free or reduced-price meals to needy children.

Special milk program. This provides reimbursement to schools, child-care centers, and camps for part of the cost of the milk served. Because the milk can be sold at low cost to the child, milk drinking is encouraged. In schools where there are many needy children the full cost of the milk served to these children is reimbursed.

PROBLEMS AND REVIEW

1. What criteria, other than height and weight, may be used to determine nutritional status?
2. What average yearly gains may be expected from the end of the first year until maturity is reached? How do these vary for boys and girls?
3. Compare the protein and caloric needs of the one- to three-year-old; seven- to ten-year-old; 11- to 14-year-old; and 15 to 18-year-old boy with those of the adult.
4. Why would you expect the calcium, phosphorus, and iron needs to be especially high during childhood?
5. How long should vitamin D supplementation be provided? Why?
6. In terms of food habits, what can be expected at each of these ages: 18 months to 2 years; 5 years; 7 years; 10 years; 15 years?
7. Discuss the role of cultural pressures on food habits and attitudes to food.
8. In what way may disturbances in the mother-child relationship be reflected in feeding difficulties?
9. What is meant by the type A lunch?
10. Why is skipping breakfast a serious problem? What factors may interfere with the child's appetite for breakfast?
11. What objections may there be to the use of fried foods in the diet of preschool children? To the sale of soft drinks and candy on school premises?
12. *Problem.* Record the food intake of a child for one day, and calculate the nutritive values. Are all the nutrients provided at recommended levels? What suggestions can you make for the improvement of the diet?
13. Plan three menus for packed lunches for an eight-year-old boy. Do these lunches provide ⅓ of the day's recommended allowances?
14. A mother asks you about the advisability of allowing her children to eat between meals. What suggestions can you make to her?
15. *Problem.* Plan a menu for one day for a family consisting of father, mother, 16-year-old boy, 13-year-old girl who tends to be overweight, eight-year-old girl, and three-year-old boy. Indicate in table form the approximate amounts of food for each, and include any modifications in preparation which may be required.
16. *Problem.* List several ways in which you, as a school nurse, could assist in bringing about the improvement of food habits of schoolchildren.

CITED REFERENCES

1. Winick, M.: "Nutrition and the Ultimate Makeup of Various Tissues," *Food and Nutrition News,* National Livestock and Meat Board, Chicago, April 1969.
2. Mitchell, H. S.: "Protein Limitation and Human Growth," *J. Am. Diet. Assoc.,* **44**:165–72, 1964.
3. Beal, V. A.: "Dietary Intake of Individuals followed Through Infancy and Childhood," *Am. J. Public Health,* **51**:1107–17, 1961.
4. Burke, B. S., *et al.:* "Longitudinal Studies of Child Health and Development, Harvard School of Public Health, Series II, No. 4. Calorie and Protein Intakes of Children between One and Eighteen Years of Age," *Pediatrics,* **24**:922–74, 1959.
5. Morgan, A. F., ed.: *Nutritional Status, U.S.A.* Bull. 769, California Agricultural Experiment Station, Berkeley, 1959.
6. Schaefer, A. E., and Johnson, O. S.: "Are We Well Fed? The Search for the Answer," *Nutr. Today,* **4** (No. 1): 2–11, 1969.
7. Eppright, E. S., *et al.:* "Very Heavy and Obese School Children in Iowa," *J. Home Econ.,* **48**:168–72, 1956.
8. Johnson, M. L., *et al.:* "Relative Importance of Inactivity and Overeating in the Energy Balance of Obese High School Girls," *Am. J. Clin. Nutr.,* **4**:37–44, 1956.
9. Johnston, J. A.: "Nutritional Problems of Adolescence," *J.A.M.A.,* **137**:1587–89, 1948.
10. Macy, I. G., and Hunscher, H. A.: "Calories—A Limiting Factor in the Growth of Children," *J. Nutr.,* **45**:189–99, 1951.
11. Stearns, G.: "Human Requirements of Calcium, Phosphorus and Magnesium," in *Handbook of Nutrition.* The Blakiston Company, Philadelphia, 1951, Chap. 4.
12. Ohlson, M. A., and Stearns, G.: "Calcium Intake of Children and Adults," *Fed. Proc.,* **18**:1076–85, 1959.
13. Food and Nutrition Board: *Recommended Dietary Allowances,* 8th ed. National Academy of Sciences–National Research Council, Washington, D.C., 1973.
14. Beal, V. A.: "Nutritional Intake of Children. II. Calcium, Phosphorus and Iron," *J. Nutr.,* **53**:499–510, 1954.
15. Lowenberg, M. E.: "Food Preferences of Young Children," *J. Am. Diet. Assoc.,* **24**:430–34, 1948.
16. Huenemann, R. L., *et al.:* "A Longitudinal Study of Gross Body Composition and Body Conformation and Their Association with Food and Activity in a Teen-Age Population. View of Teen-Age Subjects on Body Conformation, Food and Activity," *Am. J. Clin. Nutr.,* **18**:325–38, 1966.
17. Dwyer, J. T., *et al.:* "Adolescent Attitudes Toward Weight and Appearance," *J. Nutr. Educ.,* **1**(No. 2): 14–19, Fall 1969.
18. Stearns, G.: "Nutritional State of the Mother Prior to Conception," *J.A.M.A.,* **168**:1655–59, 1958.
19. Fabry, P., *et al.:* "Effect of Meal Frequency in School Children," *Am. J. Clin. Nutr.,* **18**: 358–61, 1966.
20. *Child Nutrition Programs. Handbook for Volunteers.* FNS 10. U.S. Department of Agriculture, Washington, D.C., 1970.
21. Council on Foods and Nutrition: "Confections and Carbonated Beverages," *J.A.M.A.,* **180**:1118, 1962.
22. Martin, E. A.: *Roberts' Nutrition Work with Children.* University of Chicago Press, Chicago, 1954.

ADDITIONAL REFERENCES

Balsley, M., *et al.:* "Nutritional Component in Some Problems of Adolescence," *J. Home Econ.,* **60**:648–52, 1968.

Begum, A., and Pereira, S. M.: "Calcium Balance Studies on Children Accustomed to Low Calcium Intakes," *Br. J. Nutr.*, **23**:905–11, 1969.

Cahn, A.: "Growth and Caloric Intake of Heavy and Tall Children," *J. Am. Diet. Assoc.*, **53**:476–80, 1968.

Christakis, G., *et al.:* "A Nutritional Epidemiologic Investigation of 642 New York City Children," *Am. J. Clin. Nutr.*, **21**:107–26, 1968.

Coussons, H.: "Magnesium Metabolism in Infants and Children," *Postgrad. Med.*, **46**:135–39, Dec. 1969.

Dayton, D. H.: "Early Malnutrition and Human Development," *Children* **16**:210–217, 1969.

Edwards, C. H., *et al.:* "Nutrition Survey of 6200 Teen-Age Youths," *J. Am. Diet. Assoc.*, **45**:543–46, 1964.

Eppright, E. S., *et al.:* "Eating Behavior of Preschool Children," *J. Nutr. Educ.*, **1**:16–19, Summer 1969.

Falkner, F.: "The Physical Development of Children. A Guide to Interpretation on Growth Charts and Development Assessments; and a Comment on Contemporary and Future Problems," *Pediatrics*, **29**:448–66, 1962.

———: "Some Physical Growth Standards for White North American Children," *Pediatrics*, **29**:467–74, 1962.

Huenemann, R. L., *et al.:* "Food and Eating Practices of Teen-Agers," *J. Am. Diet. Assoc.*, **53**:17–24, 1968.

Leverton, R. M.: "The Paradox of Teen-Age Nutrition," *J. Am. Diet. Assoc.*, **53**:13–16, 1968.

Myers, M. L., *et al.:* "A Nutrition Study of School Children in a Depressed Urban District," *J. Am. Diet. Assoc.*, **53**:226–33; 234–42, 1968.

Owen, G. K., and Kram, K. M.: "Nutritional Status of Preschool Children in Mississippi," *J. Am. Diet. Assoc.*, **24**:490–94, 1969.

Review: "Environment and Growth," *Nutr. Rev.*, **27**:282–83, 1969.

Roth, A.: "The Teen-age Clinic," *J. Am. Diet. Assoc.*, **36**:27–30, 1960.

Publications for Parents

American Heart Association: *Healthy Eating for Teenagers,* 1969.

Children's Bureau, U.S. Department of Health, Education and Welfare, Washington, D.C.:
The Adolescent in Your Family.
Your Child from 1 to 3.
Your Child from 3 to 4.
Your Child from 1 to 6.

Nutrition Foundation: *Food Choices: The Teen-age Girl.*

U.S. Department of Agriculture, Washington, D.C.:
Food for the Family with Young Children, HG 5.
Food for the Families with School Children, HG 13.

24 Nutrition in Later Maturity

Some characteristics of aging. One person in ten today in the United States is 65 years or older, thus accounting for some 20 million individuals. The average life-span for a girl born today is 75 years, and for a boy it is 68 years. Most of the increase in life-span since the first years of this century has resulted from the greatly reduced infant mortality and not from the lengthening of the life-span during the later years. Having reached the age of 65 years, an individual has a life expectancy of another 14 years; at age 70, the expectancy is another 10 years.

Aging is a continuous process that begins with conception and ends with death. The Greek word for *old man* is *geron* and that for *treatise* is *logos;* therefore, the term *gerontology* means the study of the aging process. The suffix *-iatrics* means *the treatment of;* thus, *geriatrics* is the specialty in medicine concerned with the prevention and treatment of disease in older persons.

Persons in later maturity fall into three sub-groupings: those in middle age are likely to be at the peak of their careers and the fulfillment of their hopes, but are beginning to think about retirement; those for whom retirement has become a fact rightfully should be able to live up to high expectations; those in old age experience a decline with increasing dependency based upon state of health, economics, and social change.[1] Vast differences may become apparent from one decade to another, but it is dangerous to generalize. It is just as wrong to place all persons over 65 years into one category as it is to consider all individuals under 21 years in the single category of children. One individual in his 80's may well fit into a group characteristic of the 60's, whereas another in his 60's can be "older than his years."

An individual may enter upon the later years of his life with sufficient income for the necessities and some of the amenities of life; good physical and mental health; the love and support of a wife or husband and children; a role in the community; satisfying hobbies and interests to keep him busy; outlets for recreation; a sense of security and a feeling of being needed; and strong personal goals and spiritual values. He who has these blessings is indeed fortunate. But, for the majority of persons in the later years one or more of these characteristics is missing. The older person often comes to resent the designation "golden age" or "senior citizen," for reality is far removed from these connotations.

Socioeconomic factors. In the dietary survey of 1965 half the families in which the head of the household was 65 years or over had incomes below $3645, a level that is not adequate to provide the necessities for life. Retirement from one's occupation brings reduced income, with the majority of persons dependent upon small pensions (or none at all) and upon Social Security. Relatively small numbers of older persons have savings to provide income or to meet emergencies. In the recent inflationary years, the older person with a fixed income has had an increasingly difficult time providing for his needs. Technologic changes have also led to earlier retirement for many people; the man who is retired at 60 years, or even 55 years, has had less time to accumulate savings and finds it difficult to find other employment in our youth-oriented culture.

Loneliness is the complaint of millions of older persons. The active, productive individual upon retirement often finds that he has been "put on the shelf"; he is no longer consulted for advice; he seldom sees his former coworkers, and when

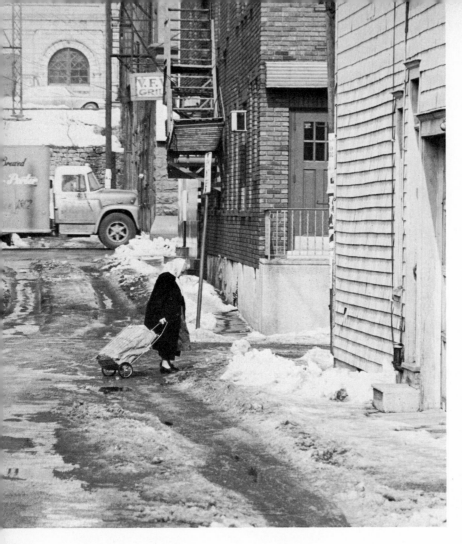

Figure 24–1. Reduced income often prevents older people from receiving an adequate diet. This older woman is returning home with a supply of food donated by the U.S. Department of Agriculture. (Courtesy, Kevin Shields and U.S. Department of Agriculture.)

he does he experiences a feeling of condescension—real or imagined. Loneliness also results from a change in the family situation. Children are often located in distant cities, and there is less communication with them. Most devastating of all is the loss of one's husband or wife. One of the major aspects of aging is that a larger and larger proportion of the older population consists of women who are widowed and living alone. By 1975 it is estimated that there will be about 3.3 million more older women than older men. (See Figure 24–1.)

Housing is a major problem for many older persons. Some older people remain in the large home that was desirable while the family was being raised, but they no longer have the physical stamina to take care of it and often lack the financial resources to maintain repairs and so on.

Those who live in apartments often find that they cannot afford the increasing rents so they are forced to move to less desirable places. Living in a single room with no facilities for food preparation is the lot of a very large proportion of the elderly.

PHYSIOLOGIC AND BIOCHEMICAL CHANGES

Cellular changes. For each species there appears to be a built-in limitation of the life-span. The forces that bring this about are by no means clear, but investigations of the aging process at the molecular level are beginning to shed some light on the process.

At least in part the changes in function that

occur with aging are believed to be caused by a loss in the number of functioning cells.[2] The cells of the liver, gastrointestinal mucosa, skin, and hair continue to divide and reproduce throughout life. On the other hand, muscle and nerve cells do not have this capacity, thereby leading to gradual decrease in function. The changes that occur in the glomerular filtration rate and renal blood flow are caused, at least in part, by a reduction in the number of functioning nephrons.

The study of changes in connective tissue, which is so abundant in the human body, is of especial note.[3] Collagen is one of the fibrous materials found in tendons, ligaments, skin, and blood vessels. With aging the amount of collagen increases and becomes more rigid; the skin loses its flexibility, the joints creak, and the back becomes bent.

Some investigators postulate that aging is due, at least in part, to free radical reactions occurring within the cell.[4,5] The free radicals are highly reactive and give rise to a variety of products, the reactions being irreversible. Within the cell, polyunsaturated fats are especially susceptible to peroxidation, and this may be the "mainspring of the aging process."[4] Lipid peroxidation is believed to bring about disintegration of the cell mitochondria, which are the energy powerhouse; thus, the ability to bring about electron transport and phosphorylation is lost. In addition, the lysosome membranes are broken, and the enzymes contained in these "suicide bags" bring about the hydrolysis of the cell.

If peroxidation of lipids is responsible for aging, then some inhibitor of the free radical reactions is required. There are, in fact, a number of effective antioxidants, the most important of which is probably vitamin E. Other antioxidants are glutathione, cysteine, and sulfhydryl proteins, as well as ascorbic acid. Possibly, then, the function of vitamin E is the delay in aging by reason of reduction of lipid peroxidation. This explains the necessity for increasing the intake of vitamin E when the intake of polyunsaturated fats is increased—a recommendation widely approved for the delay or prevention of atherosclerosis. See Chapter 6.

Energy metabolism. From 30 to 90 years the basal metabolism decreases about 20 per cent.[2]

There is an increasing proportion of body fat to protoplasmic tissue, lesser muscle tension, and sometimes a diminution of thyroid activity. The rate of basal metabolism was found to be higher in a group of vigorous, healthy women of middle age than it was for less active women of the same age.[6]

In the population as a whole the weight increases steadily throughout the years of maturity until it plateaus at the decade of 65 to 74 years.[7] Thereafter, a gradual decline takes place. In general the incidence of overweight and underweight after 65 years follows the pattern of the population as a whole. Undoubtedly, obesity increases the susceptibility to the degenerative diseases of middle age, becomes an extra burden on weight-bearing joints, and increases the likelihood of accidents.

Carbohydrate metabolism. Usually the fasting blood sugar is normal. Likewise, the absorption of carbohydrate is not impaired. However, when a carbohydrate load is presented, as in the glucose tolerance test, the blood sugar remains elevated for a longer period of time than it does in younger persons. Following exercise, the levels of blood lactic acid and pyruvic acid are often above normal limits.

Fat metabolism. With increasing age the blood cholesterol and blood triglyceride levels gradually increase. The kind and amount of fat and carbohydrate in the diet, the degree of overweight, the stresses of life, and many other factors are believed to be responsible for these changes. In turn, about 90 per cent of the deaths from heart disease, vascular accidents of the central nervous system, and malignancies occur in people over 45 years of age.

Function of the gastrointestinal tract. The senses of taste and smell are less acute in later life, thus interfering with the appetite for many foods. The loss of natural teeth and a seeming inability on the part of the individual to become accustomed to dentures make it difficult to chew food properly or to eat with comfort. Consequently, more and more carbohydrate-rich foods which require a minimum of chewing may be selected, leading to seriously deficient intakes of protein, minerals, and vitamins.

Digestion in later years is affected in a number of ways. A reduction of the tonus of the musculature of the stomach, small intestine, and colon leads to less motility so that the likelihood of abdominal distention from certain foods is greater, as is also the prevalence of constipation. The volume, acidity, and pepsin content of the gastric juice are often reduced, achlorhydria being observed in 35 per cent of those 65 years and older.[8] A reduction in acidity is known to have an adverse effect on the absorption of calcium and iron, and may also explain the lower vitamin B_{12} levels of blood observed in many older persons.

Fats are often poorly tolerated because they further retard gastric evacuation, because the pancreatic production of lipase is inadequate for satisfactory hydrolysis, and because chronic biliary impairment may interfere with the flow of bile to the small intestine.

Other changes. Many older persons, especially men, have an elevated blood urea nitrogen and blood uric acid, indicating some deterioration of kidney function. Nocturia is a common complaint, leading often to a reduction of the intake of fluid, and thus increasing the difficulty of satisfactory waste elimination.

Reduced blood levels of vitamin C and hemoglobin may reflect low intakes of ascorbic acid and iron. Some clinicians believe that the reduced levels of blood iron are the result of blood loss rather than inadequate iron intake.[9]

Hormonal imbalances occur rather frequently. In women, especially, these imbalances lead to disturbances in calcium and nitrogen metabolism and the resultant condition known as osteoporosis. Bone loss occurs with greater frequency in women who have been poor milk drinkers throughout their lives.[10] (See also Chapter 40.)

NUTRITIONAL REQUIREMENTS

Dietary deficiencies. Man's nutrition at age 60, 70, or 80 is the product of the influences of heredity, environment, and nutrition in the entire preceding years. Consequently, the variations in nutritional status are likely to be even more diverse than they are in the younger age groups which have been subject to the influences for a shorter period of time.

The individual who has had a lifetime of poor nutritional habits is not likely to be in as good health as the one who has enjoyed the benefits of a good diet. Good diet in later years cannot completely make up for the years of inadequacy or correct irreversible tissue changes. Furthermore, an older individual cannot completely change his whole pattern of eating. Nevertheless, even the individual with poor food habits who is in a poor state of nutrition can benefit greatly through the application of the principles of good nutrition.

A study in Syracuse, New York, of 283 households in which one member was at least 65 years old and receiving Social Security benefits reflects dietary inadequacies that are representative of many older persons.[11] Only half the households had food that provided the recommended allowances for all nutrients. Calcium and ascorbic acid were the nutrients most frequently in short supply, with 3 of every 10 persons failing to receive the recommended allowances. A third of those whose diets were poor lacked adequate levels of five or more nutrients. More than one third of the householders used some vitamin supplements, but only a small number effectively supplemented their diets with the missing nutrients. Hence, the choice of supplement was poor.

In the Syracuse study, householders in their 60's had more adequate diets than those in their 80's. The quality of diet was correlated with the level of income, with more fair and poor diets being found in the lowest income group. More persons in the good diet group were overweight than in the fair- to poor-diet group. As a rule, men had better diets than women.

Recommended allowances. Although some clinicians prescribe increased levels of some nutrients for the older person, there is no convincing evidence that the requirements for protein, minerals, and vitamins are increased.[2]

Energy. For each decade after 25 years the caloric allowance is reduced. After 50 years, the allowance for a man is 2400 calories and for a woman it is 1800 calories. Inasmuch as the allowances for other nutrients are not reduced, women especially must choose their diets with care lest they exceed their caloric requirements.

The Basic Diet (see Table 13–2) furnishes about three fourths of the woman's caloric need, so that in a given day approximately 500 calories can be obtained from foods that are often favorite dishes of older people.

Protein. A daily intake of 0.8 gm protein per kilogram body weight is satisfactory.

Minerals. The allowance for calcium is the same as that for younger adults, whereas the iron allowance for men and women is 10 mg. Because anemia is a common occurrence in many men and women, iron supplements are sometimes prescribed. A diet liberal in calcium may promote bone mineralization in those with osteoporosis.

Vitamins. The allowances for vitamin A and ascorbic acid are the same as those for younger adults. The B complex vitamins are needed in proportion to the caloric requirement, which means that the total daily needs for thiamine, riboflavin, and niacin are somewhat lower. (See Table 3–1.)

Water and fiber. About 6 to 8 glasses fluid is as essential for the older person as it is for the younger individual. The kidneys can function more adequately when there is sufficient fluid with which to eliminate the waste solids. Water stimulates peristalsis and thus aids in combating constipation. When nocturia is a problem, the individual should be encouraged to take as much water as possible early in the day.

Many older persons select diets that are smooth in character. This choice, together with an inadequate fluid intake, can lead to persistent constipation and often to the use of harmful laxatives and mineral oil. Although rough fiber is not advised for older persons, the fiber of tender vegetables, fruits, and whole-grain cereals will encourage normal peristalsis.

DIETARY MANAGEMENT

Food habits. The older person tends to follow dietary patterns of his earlier years. He has been influenced by the many factors which determine food acceptance from infancy throughout life (see Chapter 14). By the time he reaches middle age and later maturity, his pattern has become fixed and it is indeed difficult to introduce new foods or markedly to change the patterns of eating.

With increasing years the individual sees and hears less well, moves more slowly, and may be troubled by chronic illness. The frustrations and isolation from the people and work one loves and the feelings of being rejected and unwanted may be expressed by complaints against food and refusal to eat, or, on the other hand, by self-indulgence in favorite foods such as sweets.

Good food served in pleasant circumstances by people who care may indicate to the older person that someone cares for him and that he is important. Attention to holiday customs, for example, bolsters the morale and the food intake. On the contrary, food poorly prepared or carelessly served may be associated with lack of love and thus will be refused. (See Figure 24–2.)

Older persons who live alone often have no incentive to cook. They may eat carbohydrate foods to excess because they are easy to chew, require no preparation, and are inexpensive. Milk is taken poorly by many because of erroneous ideas concerning its value for adults, its supposed constipating or gas-producing effects, and its cost. Vegetables may be considered as too difficult to chew and too expensive. Fruits are often thought to be too "acid." Many older persons labor under the mistaken notion that their food needs are small because they no longer have growth needs, and because they are inactive.

Older persons are particularly susceptible to the claims of the food faddists. Having lost some sense of well-being they are likely to be misled by claims of unscrupulous persons concerning "miracle" diets and drugs. Although the foods recommended by these faddists may not in themselves be harmful, the undue emphasis placed upon them may mean that the necessary foods for nutritional adequacy are neglected and that the individual delays too long in seeking medical advice for his ills.

Daily meal plans. The Basic Diet outlined for the younger adult (Table 13–2) serves also as the foundation for the diet after 50 years. For the woman with her lower caloric requirements the remaining foods must be chosen with care

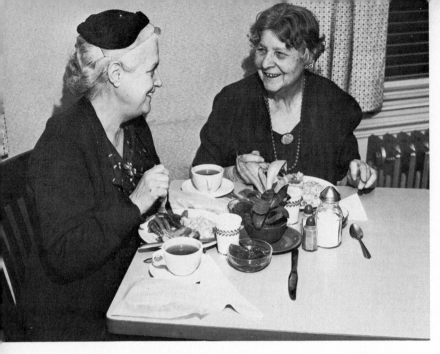

Figure 24–2. Pooling resources for food and companionship is one way for older people to solve the problems of lonely mealtimes when the temptation is to rely on snacks. Members of the Philadelphia Center for Older People demonstrate the principle. (Courtesy, The United Fund, Philadelphia.)

lest the caloric intake be excessive. Three menus for a low-cost diet suitable for an older couple are shown below.* In addition to the foods listed, a glass of milk should be included daily. Coffee or tea are used as desired.

SUNDAY

Orange juice
Scrambled egg
Toast

Swiss steak
Mashed potatoes
Broccoli
Bread
Chocolate pudding

Welsh rarebit
Crisp bacon strip
Apple-raisin salad
Ice cream
Cookies

MONDAY

Orange juice
Oatmeal
Milk
Toast

Frankfurters stuffed with mashed potatoes and cheese
Scalloped tomatoes

*From "Sample Menus for a Week" in *Food Guide for Older Folks*, HG 17, U.S. Department of Agriculture, Washington, D.C., 1963.

Hot rolls
Apple brown betty

Lamb stew with potatoes
Snap beans
Bread
Chocolate pudding

TUESDAY

Prunes
French toast
Syrup

Lamb stew
Beets
Tossed green salad
Bread
Rice-and-raisin pudding

Spaghetti, tomato, chopped meat casserole
Broccoli
Bread
Grapefruit segments

DIETARY COUNSELING

Most persons beyond 65 years live in their own homes and are able to take care of themselves. Any plans for the diet must give consideration to the individual's income, the facilities for food preparation, the physical ability to shop for food and prepare it, the social and cultural background, and the individual attitudes toward food together with the motivations for obtaining an adequate diet. With increasing age, the problems of meal management are greater.

Many people will improve their diets if they are given assistance in planning simple meals that meet their nutritional requirements; advice concerning best food buys for the money; recipes suitable for one or two people; and suggestions for simple food preparation. Because many older people fall prey to "health food" hucksters, nutrition education is essential pertaining to the nutritional values of foods available in food markets in relation to their specific needs. Many older people do not need mineral or vitamin supplements. Those who do are identified only by medical examination, following which a prescription for the specific supplements should be given. The following suggestions may enhance the enjoyment of meals:

1. Serve colorful foods attractively on a tray if eating alone.

2. Eat leisurely in pleasant surroundings.

3. Eat four or five light meals instead of three heavier meals.

4. Include essential foods first. Sweets may be taken in moderate amounts but excess may cause discomfort and lead to overweight.

5. Eat a good breakfast to start the day right.

6. Fats may retard digestion. If there is discomfort, avoid fatty meats and fish; fried foods; gravies, sauces, and salad dressings; rich cakes, doughnuts, pastries, and puddings.

7. Certain foods may cause distress for some people. These are most likely to be dried cooked beans, Brussels sprouts, cabbage, cantaloupe, cauliflower, cucumber, onions, radishes, turnips, watermelon. Do not arbitrarily omit these foods if the individual enjoys and tolerates them.

8. Eat the heaviest meal at noon rather than at night if sleeping is difficult.

9. Avoid tea and coffee late in the day if insomnia is a problem.

10. Drink hot milk just before going to bed.

Many older people are unable to chew their food well. Nevertheless, ground meats and puréed foods are quite unpopular. Older people in nursing homes were found to prefer roasts and chops even though they could not chew well, but they disliked steaks because they were difficult to cut and to chew; they also disliked ground meats.[12] With a sharp scissors or knife it is possible to finely mince meats and other foods for ease in swallowing and rapid digestive action. The following suggestions may help the person who has chewing difficulty to obtain a more adequate diet.

Milk as a beverage
Cottage or cream cheese; American cheese in sauces or casserole dishes
Eggs, soft-cooked, scrambled, poached
Tender meat, or poultry, finely minced or ground; flaked fish; finely diced meat in sauces often taken more readily
Soft raw fruits as banana, berries; canned or cooked fruits; fruit juices
Soft-cooked vegetables, diced, chopped, or mashed. Raw vegetables such as tomatoes can often be eaten if finely chopped—skin and seeds removed
Cooked and dry cereals with milk
Bread, crackers, and toast with hot or cold milk
Desserts: diced cake with fruit sauce; fruit whips; gelatin; ice cream and ices; puddings; pie, if crust is tender and cut up

Community services. Many older persons who are slightly handicapped can remain in their own homes provided that some services are available from the community. (See Figure 24–3.) One of the most difficult problems is that of shopping —the inability to get to a market or the inability to carry the supplies home. Many community charitable organizations might well investigate the need for providing such services to its older citizens. The Meals-on-Wheels program provides a hot meal and a packed lunch or supper daily to older people who can qualify, but the program reaches only a small segment of the population that could use the service. Geriatric cen-

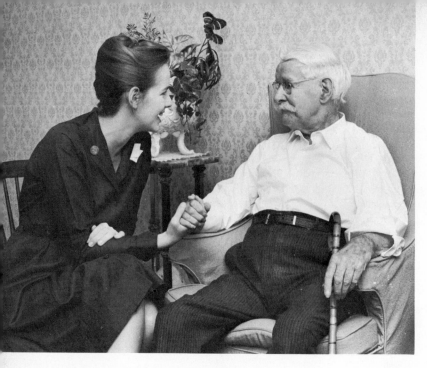

Figure 24–3. This public health nurse's warmth and genuine interest are important qualities for making diet instruction more likely to be followed. (Courtesy, The United Fund and Community Nursing Service, Philadelphia.)

ters in some cities serve meals to older people who are able to come to these centers; such meals also afford the much needed companionship. Through Medicare and Medicaid nutritional services are available for those who are ill. (See also Chapter 28.)

PROBLEMS AND REVIEW

1. What changes occur with aging which may modify the digestion of foods?
2. Compare the nutritional needs of the adult of 25 years with one of 65 years.
3. What reasons can you give for the difficulty many older women experience in the healing of a bone?
4. What are the dangers of overweight in the middle aged?
5. A widow has no cooking facilities in her room and eats dinner in a restaurant. Her income is limited. What are some foods she could eat at home which require no cooking, but which would be nutritionally valuable?
6. *Problem.* Plan menus for two days which could be prepared with only a single gas burner available for cooking.
7. *Problem.* Using the low-cost plan on page 235 plan a week's menus for a man and woman 65 years old.
8. Consult the suggestions for effecting economy in food purchasing in Chapter 18. Which of these might not be practical for a single person or an older couple? Why?

CITED REFERENCES

1. Tibbitts, C.: "Economic and Social Adequacy of Older People," *J. Home Econ.*, **54**:695–99, 1962.
2. Shock, N. W.: "Physiologic Aspects of Aging," *J. Am. Diet. Assoc.*, **56**:491–96, 1970.
3. "The Enigma of Human Aging," *Chem. Eng. News*, Pt. I, Feb. 12, 1962, pp. 138–146; Pt. II, Feb. 19, 1962, pp. 104–112.
4. Tappel A. L.: "Where Old Age Begins," *Nutr. Today*, **2** (4): 2–7, Dec. 1967.

5. Harman, D.: "Increasing the Useful Life Span," *Food & Nutr. News.* National Livestock and Meat Board, Chicago, March 1970.
6. Roberts, P. H., *et al.:* "Nutritional Status of Older Women—Nitrogen, Calcium, Phosphorus Retentions of Nine Women," *J. Am. Diet. Assoc.,* **24**:292–99, 1948.
7. Hollifield, G., and Parsons, W.: "Overweight in the Aged," *Am. J. Clin. Nutr.,* **7**:127–31, 1959.
8. Tuohy, E. L.: "Feeding the Aged," *J.A.M.A.,* **121**:42–48, 1943.
9. Ho, R.: "Disorders of Iron Metabolism in Geriatrics," *Geriatrics,* **23**:79–86, July 1968.
10. Whedon, D. G.: "Effects of High Calcium Intakes on Bones, Blood and Soft Tissue; Relationship of Calcium Intake to Balance in Osteoporosis," *Fed. Proc.,* **18**:1112–18, 1959.
11. Le Bovit, C.: "The Food of Older Persons Living at Home," *J. Am. Diet. Assoc.,* **46**:285–89, 1965.
12. Lane, M. M.: "Stereotyped Ideas about Food," *Nurs. Homes,* **16**:27, Dec. 1967.

ADDITIONAL REFERENCES

Breen, L. Z.: "Aging and Its Social Aspects," *J. Home Econ.,* **54**:685–91, 1962.
Brink, M. F., *et al.:* "Current Concepts in Geriatric Nutrition," *Geriatrics,* **23**:113–20, March 1968.
Butler, R. N.: "Why Are Older Consumers So Susceptible?" *Geriatrics,* **23**:83–88, Dec. 1968.
Davidson, C. S., *et al.:* "The Nutrition of a Group of Apparently Healthy Aging Persons," *Am. J. Clin. Nutr.,* **10**:181–99, 1962.
Esposito, S. J., *et al.:* "Nutrition in the Aged; Review of the Literature," *J. Am. Geriatr. Soc.,* **17**:790–806, 1969.
Frenay, Sr. A. C.: "Helping Students Work with the Aging," *Nurs. Outlook,* **16**:44–46, July 1968.
Guggenheim, K., and Margulec, I.: "Factors in the Nutrition of Elderly People Living Alone or as Couples and Receiving Community Assistance," *J. Am. Geriatr. Soc.,* **13**:561–68, 1965.
Lee, D.: "Attitudes and Values: Family, and Community, Individual," *J. Home Econ.,* **54**:691–94, 1962.
Nicholson, E.: "Physical and Psychological Adequacy," *J. Home Econ.,* **54**:700, 1962.
Pelcovits, J.: "Nutrition for Older Americans," *J. Am. Diet. Assoc.,* **58**:17–21, 1971.
Sebrell, W. H., Jr.: "It's Not Age That Interferes with Nutrition of the Elderly," *Nutr. Today,* **1**:15–18, June 1966.
Walker, D. M.: "New Findings in Nutrition of Older People," *Am. J. Public Health,* **55**:548–53, 1965.
Wolff, K.: "A New Conceptualization of the Geriatric Patient," *Geriatrics,* **23**:157–62, 1968.

POPULAR GUIDES FOR THE LAYMAN

Food Guide for Older Folks. HG 17, U.S. Department of Agriculture, Washington, D.C., 1963.
Irwin, T.: *Better Health in Later Years.* Pamphlet 446, Public Affairs Committee, Inc., New York, 1970.
May, E. E., *et al.: Homemaking for the Handicapped.* Dodd, Mead, and Company, New York, 1966.

Unit VII
Nutrition and Public Health

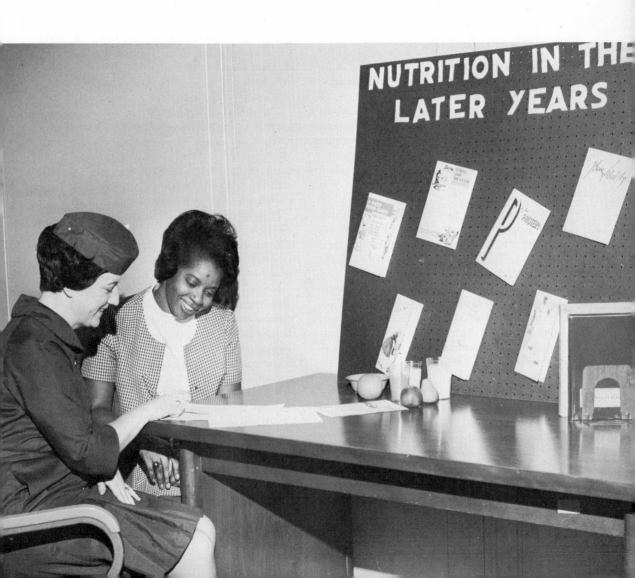

25 National and International Problems in Nutrition

Focus on community nutrition. The term *public health nutrition* is generally understood to be concerned with those problems of nutrition that affect large numbers and that can be solved most effectively through group action. The term *community* may be used to refer to any group of people—small or large; it might be, for example, a closely knit group such as the student community, or it might be certain areas of a city, state, or nation.

Physicians, nurses, dietitians, and nutritionists in their respective roles must be informed citizens regarding the nutritional concerns of the local community, the state, the nation, and even the world. Some of them will pursue careers in governmental or private agencies whose primary function is better health through better nutrition. All professional workers in health have a responsibility to assume leadership in finding solutions to nutritional problems of the community whether it be support of community organizations that are providing services, expansion of educational programs in nutrition, committee activities to develop new programs, or taking a position on proposed legislation that affects the nutritional well-being of the population.

The purposes of this unit are to give the reader an appreciation of the scope of nutrition problems in the nation and throughout the world; to create an awareness of the many resources that exist in official and voluntary organizations for working with these problems; to provide a few examples of nutrition programs in action; and to develop a sense of individual responsibility toward the improvement of nutrition and health.

Scope of Malnutrition

The nature of malnutrition. Malnutrition is an inclusive term that involves the lack, imbalance, or excess of one or more of some 40 or so nutrients that are required by the body. In the initial stages of development a deficiency is so mild that physical signs are absent and biochemical methods generally cannot detect the slight changes. As tissue depletion continues the biochemical changes can be measured in body fluids and tissues. With further depletion the physical signs become apparent until finally the full-blown signs of the predominating classic deficiency can be recognized.

Nutritional deficiencies rarely occur singly inasmuch as an inadequacy of food almost always reduces the intake of more than one nutrient. Moreover, the metabolic interdependence of nutrients means that a lack of one will interfere with the proper utilization of another, many examples of which have been cited in Unit II.

Primary nutritional deficiencies are those that are caused by inadequate or imbalanced intake of food. These conditions are the result of many environmental factors, some of which are discussed more fully on page 351.

Secondary deficiences are those that result from some fault in digestion, absorption, and metabolism so that tissue needs are not met even though the ingested diet would be adequate in normal circumstances. Thus, the restoration and maintenance of good nutrition are important concerns in clinical nutrition.

An overview of the principal nutritional problems in the United States and throughout the world was presented in Chapter 1. The nutritional deficiencies arising from lack of specific nutrients, the nutritional problems encountered at various stages of the life cycle, and the effects of disease upon nutrition are discussed in detail in appropriate chapters of this text. Table 25-1

Table 25–1. Summary of Diseases of Malnutrition

Principal Disease Conditions	Nutrient Imbalances
Obesity	Calorie excess (Chapter 31)
Underweight	Calorie deficit (Chapter 31)
Protein-calorie malnutrition	
Kwashiorkor	Principally protein lack (page 357)
Marasmus	Calorie-protein lack (page 357)
Dental caries	Calcium, phosphorus, fluorine, vitamins A and D, sugar in the diet (Chapters 5, 8, 10)
Anemia, microcytic, hypochromic	Iron (Chapters 8 and 45)
Macrocytic in infancy, pregnancy, malabsorption	Folacin (Chapters 12 and 45)
Pernicious (absorptive defect)	Vitamin B_{12} (Chapters 12 and 45)
Goiter, endemic	Iodine (Chapter 8)
Osteoporosis	Possibly calcium, vitamin D; endocrine factors (Chapter 40)
Osteomalacia	Vitamin D, calcium, phosphorus (Chapter 10)
Scurvy; hemorrhagic tendency; inflamed gums; loose teeth	Ascorbic acid (Chapter 11)
Beriberi; polyneuritis; circulatory failure; emaciation; edema	Thiamine (Chapter 12)
Pellagra; glossitis; dermatitis; diarrhea; nervous degeneration; dementia	Niacin (Chapter 12)
Cheilosis; scaling of skin; cracking of lips; light sensitivity; increased vascularization of eyes	Riboflavin (Chapter 12)
Growth failure, anemia, convulsions in infants	Vitamin B_6 (Chapter 12)
Night blindness; keratomalacia; xerophthalmia; blindness	Vitamin A (Chapter 10)
Rickets; bone deformities	Vitamin D (Chapter 10)
Hemorrhagic tendency in infants	Vitamin K (Chapter 10)

summarizes the principal nutritional deficiencies on the world scene today and includes a cross-reference to the chapters within this text where a fuller description is available.

Some signs of nutritional deficiencies. Classic deficiency diseases are diagnosed relatively easily because the physical and biochemical findings are prominent and specific. Nevertheless, the diagnosis of even these may be missed when the disease is seldom seen by clinicians, as is the case in the United States.

Many of the physical signs that suggest nutritional lack are also the result of other factors. For example, a student who obtains only five or six hours of sleep may complain that he is unable to concentrate well, is irritable, and always feels tired. These symptoms are also characteristic of a continuing dietary lack of B complex vitamins. A differential diagnosis and correct treatment can be arrived at only when there is a correlation of a complete medical and dietary history, a thorough physical examination, and laboratory studies. The latter include the blood concentration of many substances such as hemoglobin, plasma proteins, minerals, and vitamins, the urinary excretion of metabolic end products, and bone x-rays.

By being observant a teacher, nurse, or nutritionist can detect many signs in schoolchildren and in adults that suggest the possibility of nutritional deficiency and can hasten referral to a physician for diagnosis. These signs, of themselves, do not warrant a diagnosis of general or specific deficiency, and much harm can result when treatment is recommended by those not fully qualified to do so. Among the signs and complaints to which teachers and nurses may be alert are these:

Attendance: frequent absences from school or work.

Growth: deviation from standards by more than 10 per cent; appearance of excessive obesity or thinness; failure to grow in stature or gain in weight.

Behavior: easily fatigued; listless; apathetic; depressed; nervous; irritable; inability to concentrate; complaints of insomnia; lowered work capacity.

Skin: pallor; dermatitis; scaling around the nose and ear; wounds that fail to heal; bed sores.

Hair: dull, lifeless, thin; easily pulled out.

Eyes: swollen, congested eyelids; itching, burning; increased vascularization; poor vision in dim light.

Mouth: swollen, red lips; fissuring at the corners of the lips; sore, inflamed tongue; pale mucous membranes.

Teeth: dental caries; poor chewing; sore, bleeding gums.

Skeletal deformities: poor posture; deformities of the long bones, bones of the chest, spine, and pelvis.

Neuromuscular: poor coordination; flabby muscles; sore, painful muscles; muscle weakness.

Thyroid: enlarged.

Infections: frequent colds and other infections.

Gastrointestinal: poor appetite; diarrhea; fear of eating many foods.

Economic cost of malnutrition. The maintenance of health and the treatment of disease are important not only for humanitarian reasons but also in economic terms. What is good nutrition really worth? Can a preventive program in nutrition be economically justified? The answers are not easy to obtain. Preventive programs in nutrition entail costs of food assistance to the poor, the services of public health and welfare organizations, the education of professional personnel, and a vast educational program in nutrition for the public. Malnutrition and the resulting illness lead to even greater costs for medical services including hospital care, extended-care services, physician's fees, laboratory studies, drugs, and other expenses. Illness also means loss of income through absence from work and loss of time in school. In the marginally ill and the physically and mentally handicapped it means reduced efficiency at work, reduced ability to learn, and the ability to perform only a limited range of tasks.

Child wastage because of malnutrition has been singled out by Cook[1] as being especially restrictive in an economic sense. Children comprise up to half of the population in many developing countries, but most of them will never reach maturity. The costs involved in their short lives include extra food consumed by the mother during pregnancy, the costs of childbirth, the food, clothing, and shelter consumed by the child while living, and even the costs of burial. These malnourished children are consumers without ever reaching the status of producers and their own brief existence has usually been miserable.

When malnourished children survive to adulthood their stunted growth, retarded mental development, lessened ability to learn, reduced work efficiency, and physical defects including blindness are among the handicaps that beset them.

FACTORS CONTRIBUTING TO MALNUTRITION

The causes of malnutrition are complex. They include conditions that preexist within the individual—the *host*, the quality of the *environment*, and the specific *agents* that provoke the problem. Each element of this triad interacts with others. For example, many people in the United States suffer from some degree of malnutrition but the food supply, water, and waste disposal meet high standards of sanitation and safety so that health remains relatively good. On the other hand, people in some developing countries may suffer the same degree of malnutrition but may be exposed to grossly contaminated food and water so that life-threatening illness results.

Susceptibility of the individual. Within a given environment some individuals are more susceptible than others to malnutrition. Normal adults can usually survive moderate nutritional deficits rather well. Among the vulnerable groups are these:

1. Infants and preschool children: their nutritional requirements are high during rapid growth. When nutrients are not available for a given stage of development, the physical or mental retardation may be irreversible.

2. Pregnant women: inadequate diets compromise the development of the fetus and also the mother's own nutritional status and her freedom from the complications of pregnancy.

3. The elderly: malnutrition results from chronic ill health and long-standing nutritional deficiency; endocrine imbalances; inability to chew; physical handicaps that prevent adequate shopping or food preparation; loneliness and lack of interest in eating; and misconceptions concerning diet.

4. The sick: poor appetites; psychiatric disorders that prevent eating; infections; fevers and metabolic disorders that increase nutritional requirements; allergy; blood losses; injuries; gastrointestinal disorders that lead to fear of eating; diarrhea; malabsorption; and so on. (See Chapter 32.)

The vulnerability of these groups to malnutrition is considered when priorities are assigned to food assistance and to educational programs.

Environmental factors that favor malnutrition. In the United States and throughout the world poverty and ignorance are leading causes of malnutrition. Lack of available food is a principal cause of malnutrition in the underdeveloped and the developing countries of the world, but not in North America, Europe, and Oceania.

Poverty. On a worldwide basis a per capita annual income of $300 or less constitutes poverty, according to Simpson[2]; in the United States where the expectations of people are somewhat higher, the poverty level is about $750 per person annually. About 2.1 billion people—64 per cent of the world's population—have annual incomes below the poverty level; two thirds of these people live in India, Indonesia, Pakistan, and China. The per capita income in most African and Latin American countries ranges from moderate to extreme poverty.

Even in the United States approximately 30 million people are living at the poverty level. They are to be found in the slums of the cities and in rural areas as well. The American Indian living on reservations, Negroes, Puerto Ricans, Spanish Americans, and many people living in Appalachian regions constitute important segments of the poor population. Probably the plight of no group in the United States is less favorable

than that of migrant farm workers because they have few if any roots in a community and they do not have the continuing services of agencies that can provide assistance. (See Figure 25–1.)

Poverty means too few dollars to spend for food; competition between food and other necessities of life as well as things that give personal satisfaction for the available dollars; lack of food storage and preparation facilities; inability to purchase foods under the most favorable price conditions; and crowded, often unsanitary housing. Poverty results in a vicious cycle—poverty —inadequate diet—malnutrition—illness—inability to work—poverty.

In the 1965 household survey of food consumption by families in the United States four times as many diets were rated poor when family income was $3000 or less as they were when the income was $10,000. (See Figure 25-2.) With each increase in income there was a decrease in the number of diets that rated poor.

Lack of education. People of all income classes and at all educational levels lack knowledge regarding the essentials of an adequate diet. In the 1965 U.S. Department of Agriculture survey 9 per cent of affluent families (annual income over $10,000) had diets that were rated poor. (See Figure 25-2.) Those who are ignorant concerning nutrition are particularly susceptible to food faddism, superstition, and nutritional quackery. (See page 353.)

A limited education exacts a particularly severe toll from those who are also poor. It is, for many of them, the cause of their poverty inasmuch as people with minimal education and technical skills are unable to secure employment to earn a satisfactory living wage. Somehow, the poor must use each dollar more carefully but they have too little consumer information to help them. Moreover, inasmuch as the amount and quality of food available to them are limited, they need to employ the best techniques in food preparation to preserve nutritive values—but they lack the facilities and skills to do so.

Cultural factors. Malnutrition may result because people refuse to eat foods prohibited by religious beliefs or taboos and superstitions, those that lack prestige value, and those that are unfamiliar.

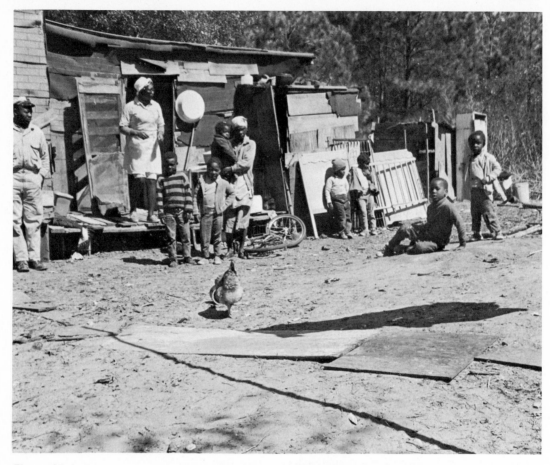

Figure 25–1. Poverty in a rural area, as shown here, or in a city ghetto is an important cause of malnutrition. (Courtesy, Larry Rana and U.S. Department of Agriculture.)

The taking of life is prohibited by some religions and no flesh foods may be eaten. This restriction excludes even eggs and milk for some. The prohibition against the taking of life may also mean that pesticides will not be used against rodents, thus resulting in high food losses in some countries. In India the sacred cows still compete seriously for the food supply of humans.[3]

Social customs, taboos, and superstitions may interfere with adequate food intake, especially by vulnerable groups. In some of the developing countries the father and other men in the family eat first and are given the choicest share of food. When food is scarce, women and children may get less than they need. Many primitive people believe that foods are endowed with specific qualities that can influence the personality of the unborn child or that can mark him physically. Thus, animal foods in particular may be taboo for pregnant and lactating women.

To be accepted food must be familiar. People to whom rice is the staple do not quickly change to a diet consisting principally of wheat. Even a change in a familiar food will reduce its acceptability. The new high-yielding varieties of rice and corn are less well liked by the people who use them because they are slightly different in color and texture and have somewhat different cooking qualities.[4]

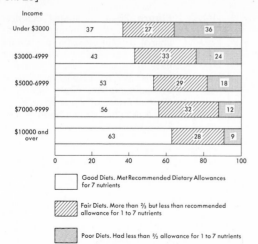

Income

Under $3000	37	27	36
$3000-4999	43	33	24
$5000-6999	53	29	18
$7000-9999	56	32	12
$10000 and over	63	28	9

0   20   40   60   80   100

☐ Good Diets. Met Recommended Dietary Allowances for 7 nutrients

▨ Fair Diets. More than ⅔ but less than recommended allowance for 1 to 7 nutrients

▨ Poor Diets. Had less than ⅔ allowance for 1 to 7 nutrients

Figure 25–2. With each increase in income, the percentage of good diets also increases. Even at liberal income levels, however, 1 diet in 10 is poor, and 3 in 10 are fair. (Courtesy, U.S. Department of Agriculture.)

In any society some foods have status and others do not. Some are for the rich and others for the poor. Plentiful foods may be ignored because they lack status value even though they are of excellent nutritive quality, whereas other foods of more marginal value may be selected because of their prestige value. Poor people often resent gifts of food that are classed as surplus. In the developing countries spices, fats, oils, sweets, tea, coffee, and cola beverages are often purchased because they are equated with a higher standard of living.[3]

Urbanization. Jelliffe[5] has described the flood of rural dwellers to the cities that is now occurring throughout the entire world as "disurbanization" because the influx is too rapid to accommodate people in terms of employment, housing, food, and services. The shanty towns and ghettos provide surroundings that are often worse than the rural areas left behind. Because they need cash to purchase food, people find themselves with diets that are more meager than their rural fare.

Infants and children suffer most from this trend. Infants are often weaned early, partly because the mother seeks employment and partly because she is trying to emulate the women of the Western world who do not breast-feed their babies. Unfortunately, the substitute feedings for the baby are insufficient in quantity, often poor in quality, and likely to be grossly contaminated with bacteria. Jelliffe deplores the use of highly advertised expensive proprietary infant formulas because few people in the developing countries can afford them and mothers use too little of the formula to meet the baby's needs.

Inadequate supply of food. The food-to-population ratio is critical in determining the quality of nutrition. On a worldwide basis the amount of food available today is just about sufficient to meet the energy needs of man, but the distribution is decidedly uneven. Moreover, where calorie deficits exist, the amount and quality of protein available are also in short supply. Although the total food supply has increased in recent years, the per capita supply is actually less in many countries because the population has increased even more rapidly. Many predict that the present rate of population increase can only mean widespread famine by the end of the century. (See Figure 25-3.)

In the developing countries the farmer lacks modern agricultural skills and has no money to purchase fertilizers or equipment to practice modern agriculture. (See Figure 25-4.) Food spoilage is excessively high because of a lack of processing, storage, and distribution facilities. Where agriculture is most primitive the diets are almost always at the subsistence level. Thus, there is no food left over for an emergency, and a drought can mean months of hunger until the next harvest. Governments in many developing countries are usually unable to finance the irrigation programs needed for crops, the industrial plants for food processing and storage, and the roads for food distribution.

Food Faddism and Nutritional Quackery

Food faddism and nutritional quackery may lead the unsuspecting and poorly informed individual to malnutrition and ill health. *A fad* is a fashion of the moment—here today and gone tomorrow. Thus it is with many food fads. A teen-age girl often follows a fad diet to lose

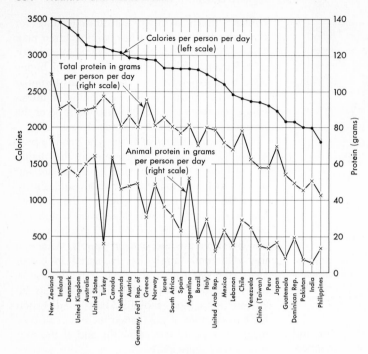

Figure 25–3. Estimated calories, grams of total protein, and grams of animal protein available per capita in 32 countries. The countries that have the lowest level of available calories also have the lowest level of available protein. (Data from *The State of Food and Agriculture*, Food and Agriculture Organization, Rome, 1965.)

weight whereas the boy relies upon fad diets to give him athletic prowess. The elderly individual looks to a food or fad diet as a panacea for poor health. Food fads stem from ignorance about food properties and the essentials of nutritionally adequate diets. They are subscribed to by the rich and poor, and the young and old.

Nutritional quackery refers to the misrepresentation and fraud practiced for financial gain by those who pose as authorities in nutrition but who have little or no preparation for their practice.

Types of food fads. Among the numerous fallacies foisted upon the unwary public are these.

1. *Fallacy.* Certain foods have specific properties in promoting health or in curing disease. For example, honey and vinegar is held to be useful in treating arthritis, and garlic is believed to reduce hypertension.

Facts. No single food has a unique health-giving property. Good nutritional status requires that the proper balance and quantities of essential nutrients be obtained from a mixed diet of many possible food combinations.

Diseases have numerous causes, among which poor diet may be contributory, as in the nutritional deficiencies. No food is known to cause

arthritis, nor is any specific food helpful in its treatment. Arthritis patients, like others, require a nutritionally adequate diet and should avoid becoming overweight. Chronic degenerative diseases such as cancer, diabetes, and others are not cured by specific foods. In some endocrine diseases such as diabetes mellitus a controlled diet planned to meet individual needs is essential therapy, but these pathologic conditions require medical advice and meticulous counseling by professionally qualified personnel.

2. *Fallacy.* Only foods grown on soils that have been organically fertilized are of high nutritive value.

Facts. Foods of high nutritive value are produced on soils fertilized chemically or organically. The amount of organic fertilizer available is totally inadequate to meet the farmer's needs. With chemical fertilizers the farmers of many nations are now beginning to produce increased yields of crops of high nutritional quality, thereby helping to improve the lot of people who too often get less food than they need.

3. *Fallacy.* Pesticides should never be used because the crops sprayed with them are poisonous.

Facts. Without some control of insects and

plant diseases, the food supply in many parts of the world would be so seriously threatened that the effects of food shortages and famine would surely outweigh the possible hazards of pesticides. Some pesticides, to be sure, have been shown to constitute a health hazard, and their use is being prohibited. The Food Protection Committee of the Food and Nutrition Board, the Food and Drug Administration, and the U.S. Department of Agriculture are concerned with setting standards for pesticides, testing new products, and developing safe controls for their use.

4. *Fallacy.* Processed foods are devoid of nutritive value. White bread, white sugar, canned foods, and pasteurized milk are held to be nutritionally impoverished.

Facts. Most white bread is now enriched with iron, thiamine, riboflavin, and niacin and is approximately equal to whole-grain bread in nutritive value. (See Figure 13-4.) Legislation is now being considered to require enrichment of all white breads and flours.

White sugar is an inexpensive source of carbohydrate and calories. Although it provides no protein, minerals, or vitamins, its moderate use in the diet can be justified. (See page 74.) Brown sugar, raw sugar, and honey are also good sources of carbohydrate and calories, but they are much more expensive than white sugar. They contain only insignificant traces of some minerals and vitamins.

All food processing has some effect on nutritive values, but modern techniques in the food industry maintain high nutritive values. In fact, vegetables and fruits frozen or canned at the peak of their quality may be superior to the fresh product that has been poorly handled from farm to market.

5. Reducing fads are so numerous that one may wonder whether some popular publications could survive without them! Their proponents often reap generous incomes from them before the unsuspecting public realizes that weight loss is simply a matter of adjusting calories below the energy requirement on an otherwise adequate diet. See Chapter 31.

Identifying the quack. The food faddist or charlatan is not always identified with ease, but he may have some of these characteristics and may employ some of these techniques.

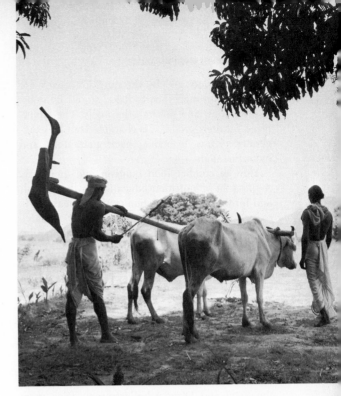

Figure 25–4. Primitive methods of agriculture restrict the amount of land that can be tilled and the yield per acre. (Courtesy, Jack Ling and UNICEF.)

He sells something—special foods, a dietary plan, cooking utensils, cookbooks, magazines, and books describing dietary regimens, or a series of lectures.

He appeals to the emotions rather than to the intellect. He plays upon the fears and hopes of people. Either he scares people about the dire consequences of failing to consume certain foods or to use certain products, or he makes fantastic claims for cure of disease, or for beauty, vitality, and long life.

He claims that he is persecuted by medical and nutritional groups. He generally attacks the medical profession, regulatory federal agencies, agricultural practices, and the food industry.

He glibly uses scientific terminology to confuse his audience and to impress upon them that he is learned in the science of nutrition. He often quotes reputable nutrition authorities, lifting their writings out of context.

He usually has no academic preparation in college or in a professional school that qualifies him to be an expert in nutrition, but he makes claim to diplomas, degrees, titles, and experience.

The products sold by the nutrition quack are dispensed through "health food" stores, by door-to-door sales, and through the mails. The advertising for their products is characterized by exaggerated claims, by money-back guarantees, and by testimonials.

How to combat food faddism and quackery. A program of nutrition education in the schools and for the adult population could immeasurably reduce the dangers of faddism but it is naïve to believe that faddism could be altogether avoided. There are always people who like to think that some special food or product can effect some miracle in their lives.

Several federal agencies are empowered to combat food faddism, but these powers are restricted to materials that cross state lines. Many states have also set up regulations comparable to those of federal groups. Among the legal channels to reduce food faddism are the regulations against adulteration and misbranding set up by the Food and Drug Administration. (See page 284.) Consumers should demand that such regulations be further strengthened and that the machinery for ensuring adherence to these regulations be sufficiently expanded to be more fully effective than it is at the present time.

The U.S. Post Office can prosecute individuals who solicit money through the mails by fraudulent advertising. The Federal Trade Commission is empowered to issue orders of cease and desist, and to prosecute those who engage in deceptive advertising through public communications media.

A few of the many publications available for combatting food faddism are listed at the end of this chapter. Many organizations involved in one or more aspects of community nutrition are also useful resources for information. (See Chapter 26.)

PROTEIN-CALORIE MALNUTRITION—A WORLD CONCERN

Protein-calorie malnutrition (P-CM), the world's most serious nutritional problem, to some degree affects up to 70 per cent of infants and preschool children in the developing countries of Central and South America, Africa, the Middle East, and southeastern Asia.[6] Millions die annually and millions more will go through life stunted in their physical growth and unable to achieve their potential mental development.

Etiology. P-CM is an inclusive term that embraces mild deficiency, kwashiorkor, and marasmus. Kwashiorkor was first described in the 1930's by Dr. Cicely Williams, a pediatrician, who observed the syndrome in infants and preschool children in Ghana. It is "the disease the child gets when the next baby is born."[7] The principal dietary deficiency is protein, with the calorie intake being satisfactory or almost so. In the developing countries babies are usually breast fed for 18 to 24 months, and sometimes longer. Upon the birth of another child, the older child is deposed from the breast and subsists largely on a high-carbohydrate low-protein diet provided by the staple foods of the country. The symptoms become apparent about three to four months after the child has been weaned and have their highest incidence between two and five years of age.

In Africa the staples to which the child is weaned are manioc, cassava, plantain, and millet; in Central America and South America they are corn and beans; and in Asia, rice and some legumes. These foods do not provide sufficient amino acids for the rapid growth needs of the infant. The ignorance of the mother concerning food needs of the baby may further reduce the intake of protein. In Iran, for example, many babies are given tea sweetened with as much as 40 gm sugar daily.[8] Condensed milk has been substituted for evaporated milk in some instances, thereby providing a high-carbohydrate low-protein formula. When diarrhea is present, the concerned mother often resorts to feeding of dilute gruels for extended periods of time.

Marasmus results from a deficiency of calories as well as protein. It occurs at an earlier age than does kwashiorkor and is usually evident by the second half of the first year. The incidence of marasmus is increasing with urbanization in the developing countries because infants are being weaned at a very early age. The low-protein formulas and other staple foods, poverty, poor sanitation, and cultural patterns all contribute to the high incidence.

Synergism between malnutrition and infection. When a diet is nutritionally inadequate but the sanitation is good and infections are minimal, the onset of deficiency symptoms is gradual. Likewise, when a well-nourished child succumbs to an infection, the period of illness is usually short, the residual effects are few, and the mortality rate is low. Conversely, the coexistence of malnutrition and infection vastly increases the severity of both; that is, a synergism exists between the two. (See Figure 25-5.) The child with prekwashiorkor rapidly advances to kwashiorkor if he also has gastroenteritis, measles, or some other infection. Infections that are ordinarily mild become so severe in the malnourished that the resulting death rate is high. In some countries the mortality from measles is 400 times greater than in the United States—not because of increase in virulence but because of coexisting malnutrition.[9]

Kwashiorkor. Moderate to severe growth failure is present in kwashiorkor. For the first few months of life the breast-fed infant in the developing countries grows at a rate that is comparable to that of well-fed infants in the Western world. Thereafter, the increase in stature and in tissue development is increasingly retarded. The muscles are poorly developed and lack tone. Edema is usually severe resulting in a large pot

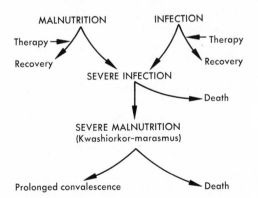

Figure 25–5. The prognosis in malnutrition or infection occurring independently is good if appropriate therapy is instituted. When malnutrition and infection interact, the severity of both is greatly increased and the prognosis is guarded.

belly and swollen legs and face and masking the muscle wasting that has occurred. (See Figure 4-9.) Anorexia and diarrhea are common. In fact, poor sanitation is likely to be the cause of the diarrhea, which, in turn, rapidly advances the child from moderate malnutrition to severe kwashiorkor.

One of the more striking features of the deficiency is the profound apathy and general misery of the child. He whimpers but does not cry or scream. He is not interested in or curious about his surroundings, but remains seated wherever he is put down. When he again begins to smile he is said to be on the road to recovery.

Pathologic and biochemical changes. Fatty infiltration of the liver is usually so extensive that the liver cells are all but obliterated. The serum levels of triglycerides, phospholipids, and cholesterol are reduced indicating an inability of the liver to manufacture and release these substances to the circulation. Atrophy of the pancreas results in a lessened production of amylase, lipase, and trypsin.

The total serum protein and albumin fractions are markedly reduced thus accounting for the severe edema that is present. Hemoglobin levels are low, especially if parasitism is also present. The serum vitamin A levels are usually reduced; profound vitamin A deficiency is a serious complication leading to blindness and death in some children.

Marasmus. Severe growth failure and emaciation are the most striking characteristics of the marasmic infant. The wasting of the muscles and the lack of subcutaneous fat are extreme. As in kwashiorkor, the incidence of diarrhea is high. (See Figure 25-6.)

Marasmus differs from kwashiorkor in several important respects: the onset is earlier, usually, within the first year of life; growth failure is more pronounced; there is no edema and the blood protein concentration is reduced less markedly; skin changes are seen less frequently; the liver is not infiltrated with fat; and the period of recovery is much longer.

Mental development. Possibly the most serious problem of P-CM may be in the mental retardation that occurs. It must be emphasized that the effects of malnutrition on mental develop-

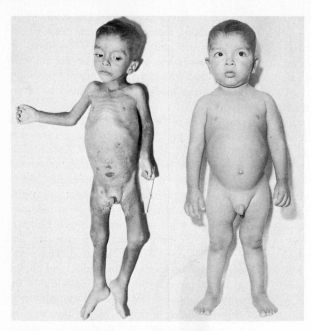

Figure 25–6. Severe protein-calorie malnutrition. Two-year-old child two weeks after admission and 10 weeks after treatment with INCAPARINA. (Courtesy, Institute of Central America and Panama and the *Journal of the American Dietetic Association.*)

ment and learning are exceedingly difficult to measure. As a rule, the malnourished child is also exposed to environmental influences that interfere with rapid learning. Moreover, the methods for testing children in one cultural environment are not applicable in an entirely different cultural setting. These problems are being actively studied by teams including pediatricians, social anthropologists, geneticists, psychologists, and others. If brain development is irreversibly retarded, this could mean that nations with large numbers of malnourished children might be unable to achieve their economic and social equality with the rest of the world.

Malnutrition can have two effects on the child's potential mental development. First, if the nutrients required for multiplication and growth of the brain cells are lacking during the period of most rapid development, it appears highly unlikely that the deficiency can be corrected by improved nutrition once the time cycle for brain development has gone by. (See Chapter 22.) In other words, the degree of mental retardation that has occurred will depend on the time when development was interrupted and how long the deficit has lasted. It would be expected that the effects would be most profound

in severe malnutrition during the first year of life. If nutrition is satisfactory during infancy and subsequently deteriorates, the effects are less devastating.

The second effect of malnutrition in the preschool years may be on the interference of learning that normally occurs in healthy preschool children at a truly fantastic rate. The apathy, lack of curiosity, and reduced activity of the malnourished child over a protracted period of time will greatly reduce the amount of learning. Thus, the development of behavioral characteristics expected of the normal child at any given age may be delayed for months or years and may sometimes never be fully corrected.

Prevention and treatment of P-CM. The prevention of P-CM by providing milk to the world's children is not feasible inasmuch as the milk supplies are totally inadequate. Over the course of time the most practical approach is to improve the food supply of the entire family because this is the best way to ensure that the preschool child will receive his needed share. Another approach is to develop food mixtures that contain sufficient quantities of essential amino acids to meet the needs of the growing child. These measures will be discussed further in Chapter 26. An indirect approach of considerable importance is the improvement of sanitation and programs of immunization so that the incidence of infections is greatly reduced, thereby avoiding the synergistic effects of malnutrition and infection.

Insofar as malnutrition itself is concerned a milk formula, when properly planned, is curative; but, as indicated above, some of the adverse effects of development may not be reversed. Successful therapy becomes apparent by weight gain, a return of appetite, and increased interest in the surroundings. The liver and pancreas rapidly return to normal and the blood proteins are replaced.

The prognosis for children with alterations in fluid and electrolyte balance is not good. A deficit of potassium is usually present in severe malnutrition and this may lead to cardiac failure if food therapy is too vigorous at the beginning. In children of Uganda cardiac failure was found to be a severe problem, usually developing after several days of apparently successful treatment.[10] It appeared that the cardiac failure was associated with a diet providing a liberal intake of sodium and was preventable by giving a formula low in sodium until diuresis had occurred.

When electrolyte imbalance is present, the initial therapy is directed to restoration of electrolyte and fluid balance. Thereafter, a half-strength formula of skim milk is fed, with gradual increases to normal concentration. Anemia and vitamin A deficiency may become more apparent as growth resumes and as the blood volume increases. These complications can be prevented by using formulas that are fortified with vitamins A and D, and with iron and folacin.

REVIEW

1. What problems of malnutrition are you aware of in your community? What factors may be contributing to these problems?
2. If the nutritional needs of the community are not known, how could you go about finding out?
3. On the basis of their records of food intake for three days, a teacher tells her pupils that many of them have nutritional deficiencies, especially of vitamin C. In what ways is this conclusion misleading?
4. What are some characteristics that a teacher might observe in the children in her class that would indicate the need for referral to a physician?
5. List some superstitions regarding food with which you are familiar. What facts can you cite to refute these ideas?
6. Examine some popular publications to see if you can find examples of food misinformation. Or visit a "health food" store or the "health food" department of a department store to determine what claims are being made for the products being sold.
7. Describe the differences between marasmus and kwashiorkor.
8. For what reasons is a dilute formula used in the early treatment of protein-calorie malnutrition?
9. The rapid urbanization of the world's population can be especially devastating to infants and preschool children. Explain why this is so.
10. What is meant by the synergism between malnutrition and infection?

CITED REFERENCES

1. Cook, R.: "The Financial Cost of Malnutrition in the Commonwealth Caribbean," *J. Trop. Pediatr.*, **14**:60–65, June 1968.
2. Simpson, D.: "The Dimensions of World Poverty," *Sci. Am.*, **219**:27–35, Nov. 1968.
3. Devadas, R. P.: "Social and Cultural Factors Influencing Malnutrition," *J. Home Econ.*, **62**:164–71, 1970.

4. Altschul, A. M.: "Food: Proteins for Humans," *Chem. Eng. News,* **47**:69–81, Nov. 24, 1969.

5. Jelliffe, D. B., and Jelliffe, E. F. P.: "The Urban Avalanche and Child Nutrition," *J. Am. Diet. Assoc.,* **57**:111–18, 1970.

6. Coursin, D. B.: "Nutrition and Brain Function," in Wohl, M. G., and Goodhart, R. S.: *Modern Nutrition in Health and Disease,* 4th ed. Lea & Febiger, Philadelphia, 1968, p. 1076.

7. "The Word 'kwashiorkor,'" *Am. J. Clin. Nutr.,* **3**:338, 1955.

8. Review: "Childhood Malnutrition in Iran," *Nutr. Rev.,* **27**:69–71, 1969.

9. Gordon, J. E.: "Nutritional Science and Society," *Nutr. Rev.,* **27**:331–38, 1969.

10. Wharton, B. A., *et al.:* "Cardiac Failure in Kwashiorkor," *Lancet,* **2**:384–87, Aug. 19, 1967.

ADDITIONAL REFERENCES

Ashworth, A., *et al.:* "Calorie Requirements of Children Recovering from Protein-Calorie Malnutrition," *Lancet,* **2**:600–603, Sept. 14, 1968.

Beeuwkes, A. M.: "Characteristics of the Self-styled Scientist," *J. Am. Diet. Assoc.,* **32**:627–30, 1956.

Bernard, V. W.: "Why People Become the Victims of Medical Quackery," *Am. J. Public Health,* **55**:1142–47, 1965,

Cravioto, J., *et al.:* "Nutrition, Growth, and Neurointegrative Development. An Experimental and Ecologic Study," *Pediatrics,* **38**:319–72, 1966.

Expert Committee on Medical Assessment of Nutritional Status. Tech. Rep. Series No. 258, World Health Organization, Geneva, 1963.

György, P.: "Protein-Calorie and Vitamin A Malnutrition in Southeast Asia," *Fed. Proc.,* **27**:949–53, 1968.

Huth, M. J.: "Malnutrition in Developing Countries: Some Causes and Solutions," *J. Home Econ.,* **61**:269–75, 1969.

Jalso, S. B., *et al.:* "Nutritional Beliefs and Practices," *J. Am. Diet. Assoc.,* **47**:263–68, 1965.

May, J. M., and Lemons, H.: "The Ecology of Malnutrition," *J.A.M.A.,* **207**:2401–2405, 1969.

Meyers, T.: "The Extra Cost of Being Poor," *J. Home Econ.,* **62**:379–82, 1970.

Mitchell, H. S.: "Don't Be Fooled by Fads," in *Food, the Yearbook of Agriculture 1959.* U.S. Department of Agriculture, Washington, D. C., p. 660.

Mönckeberg, F. B.: "Malnutrition and Mental Behavior," *Nutr. Rev.,* **27**:191–93, 1969.

New, P. K.-M., and Priest, R. P.: "Food and Thought: A Sociologic Study of Food Cultists," *J. Am. Diet. Assoc.,* **51**:13–18, 1967.

Pre-School Child Malnutrition. Primary Deterrent to Human Progress. Pub. 1282, National Academy of Sciences–National Research Council, Washington, D.C., 1966.

Review: "The Economics of Malnutrition," *Nutr. Rev.,* **27**:39–41, 1969.

———: "Malnutrition and Physical and Mental Development," *Nutr. Rev.,* **28**:176–77, 1970.

———: "Seasonal Hunger in Underdeveloped Countries," *Nutr. Rev.,* **26**:142–45, 1968.

———: "Sociological Techniques in Nutrition Studies," *Nutr. Rev.,* **26**:297–99, 1968.

Sandstead, H. H., *et al.:* "How to Diagnose Nutritional Disorders in Daily Practice," *Nutr. Today,* **4**:20–26, Summer 1969.

Scrimshaw, N. S.: "Ecological Factors in Nutritional Disease," *Am. J. Clin. Nutr.,* **14**:112–22, 1964.

Scrimshaw, N. S., and Behar, M.: "Malnutrition in Underdeveloped Countries," *N. Engl. J. Med.,* **272**:137–44; 193–98, 1965.

Sherlock, P., and Rothschild, E. O.: "Scurvy Produced by a Zen Macrobiotic Diet," *J.A.M.A.,* **199**:794–98, 1967.

Stare, F. J.: "Good Nutrition from Food, Not Pills," *Am. J. Nurs.,* **65**:86–89, Feb. 1965.

"The Syndrome of Poverty," *Am. J. Nurs.,* **66**:1749–61, 1966.

Winick, M.: "Nutrition and Cell Growth," *Nutr. Rev.,* **26**:195–97, 1968.

26 Nutrition Education and Services Through Community Action

The White House Conference on Food, Nutrition, and Health held in December 1969 recognized that the nutritional status of people of all ages at all levels of income and living in all parts of the United States was not as good as it should be.[1] The plight of the poor was especially emphasized because of the greater prevalence of malnutrition among them. Two major solutions proposed at this conference entailed numerous supporting recommendations: (1) the level of the income and the assistance available to poor people must be increased so that adequate diets for them are possible; and (2) a coordinated, comprehensive program of nutrition education must be initiated that will reach all segments of the population throughout their lives. Other important recommendations made at the conference included expansion of nutrition services through feeding in the schools, day-care centers, institutions, and so on; fortification of foods; surveillance of the food supply; informative labeling and advertising.

For people in the developing countries of the world, an adequate supply of food of high nutritive value is the first priority. Then, the improvement of nutrition must be supported by solving the problems of poverty and ignorance.

Public health nutritionists, dietitians, and nurses have direct roles to fulfill in implementing many of the community programs required for the improvement of nutrition. In addition they must be informed about programs involving research, legislation, food technology, and so on and lend their support to them. A few of the numerous activities designed to help people toward better nutrition will be described in this chapter.

MANY DOORS OPEN TO BETTER NUTRITION

Nature of services. In the hospital or clinic the nurse and dietitian give direct service to the individual. Nutrition services of the community are also provided on an individual basis, especially at the city-county level. For example, such direct services are given by a public health nurse, or a homemaker from a welfare agency, or a volunteer who delivers a hot meal to an aged person. Direct service may also be provided by a physician, nurse, or other member of a public health team which is setting up a study or a demonstration project in a given locality.

Community programs in nutrition seek to improve nutrition through research, education, improvement of the food supply, and feeding. The individual reaps the rewards of activities such as these: legislation which protects the food supply; research concerning the preventive and therapeutic aspects of diet with respect to disease; methods for preserving the food supply; the development of new and better foods through food technology; a more abundant food supply because of research on plant varieties, soil conservation, pest control; education for an adequate diet—and so on.

Facilities of the community. The problems of food production and of nutrition are being met by a large number of groups that work either cooperatively or independently. The partial listings in Tables 26–1 and 26–2 give the student some idea of the scope of efforts being made by many groups at local, state, and national levels. A number of categories are included: official agencies constitute those which have been authorized by the government and which are tax supported; voluntary agencies are supported by private funds, such as the United Fund, foundations, and

Table 26–1. A Partial List of Organizations at Local and State Levels Concerned Directly or Indirectly with Nutrition Problems

Official	*Voluntary (cont.)*
Department of agriculture (state)	Social agencies: church and community support
Department of health	Children's aid
Food sanitation	Community nursing
Nutrition	Family service
Regional medical programs	Salvation Army
Department of welfare	Settlement houses
Board of education	Welfare
Health education and services	Institutions:
Home economics	Children's camps, day nurseries, orphanages
School food services	Hospitals, nursing and convalescent homes
Extension services	Homes for the aged
Public libraries	Correctional institutions
State universities	Professional organizations: see Table 26–2
	Civic groups:
Voluntary	Chambers of commerce
Educational groups	Service organizations
Private elementary and secondary schools	Women's clubs
Private colleges and universities; home economics,	Industry-sponsored groups
medicine, nursing	Health centers and hospitals
Parent-teachers associations	Plant cafeterias and restaurants
Libraries	Demonstration programs of stores and utility companies

other means; professional organizations; and industrial groups, especially from the food industry.

Nutrition Education

Scope of educational programs. Education means change of behavior. It moves the individual from lack of interest and ignorance to increasing appreciation and knowledge and finally to action. Nutrition education offers a great opportunity to individuals to learn about the essentials of nutrition for health and to take steps to improve the quality of their diets and thus their well-being.

Nutrition education must become an essential component of the curriculum in elementary and secondary schools. The classroom instruction finds application in the meals provided through school food services. The implementation of nutrition education necessitates the development of coordinated, sequential curricula from kinder-garten through high school. Also essential is the initiation of college and in-service courses in nutrition for the nation's teachers.

Nutrition education must continue throughout the individual's life in order to accommodate for developments in nutrition science and for changing economic circumstances, health requirements, and the new food products being developed for the nation's markets. To reach the millions of citizens requires a greatly expanded use of the mass media, and the involvement of governmental and private agencies, universities, and food industries. Educational activities at the community level in health centers, maternal and child-care centers, day-care centers, Head Start programs, youth organizations, and women's clubs are also needed to reach the citizenry.

What knowledge is essential? The Interagency Committee on Nutrition Education developed basic concepts on the nutrition information needed to make wise choices of food for individuals and families. The concepts are not facts to be memorized as such, but they serve as

Table 26–2   A Partial List of Organizations at the National Level Concerned Directly or Indirectly with Nutrition Problems

Official	*Voluntary*
Department of Agriculture	American Red Cross
Agricultural Research Service	National Academy of Sciences–National Research
Consumer and Marketing Service	Council
Cooperative State Research Service	Food and Nutrition Board; committees on food
Economic Research Service	protection, dietary allowances, amino acids,
Federal Extension Service	food standards and fortification, iron nutri-
Foreign Agricultural Service	tional deficiency, marine protein resources
International Agricultural Development Service	development, international nutrition, and others
Department of Health, Education, and Welfare	Professional societies and voluntary health associa-
Children's Bureau	tions
Food and Drug Administration	American Academy of Pediatrics
Office of Education	American Dental Association
Public Health Service	American Diabetes Association
National Institutes of Health: allergy and infec-	American Dietetic Association
tion, arthritis and metabolic, cancer, heart,	American Heart Association
mental	American Home Economics Association
National Nutrition Program	American Institute of Nutrition
Department of the Interior	American Medical Association Council on Foods
Bureau of Commercial Fisheries	and Nutrition
Bureau of Indian Affairs	American Nurses' Association
Department of State	American Public Health Association
Agency for International Development	American School Food Service Association
	Institute of Food Technologists
	National League for Nursing
	Foundations
	Ford Foundation
	Kellogg Foundation
	National Vitamin Foundation
	Nutrition Foundation
	Rockefeller Foundation
	Williams-Waterman Fund of the Research
	Corporation
	Industry-sponsored groups
	American Institute of Baking
	Cereal Institute
	National Dairy Council
	National Livestock and Meat Board

guidelines for the selection of content, learning experiences, and teaching materials in a program of education.

BASIC CONCEPTS IN NUTRITION*

1. Nutrition is the food you eat and the how the body uses it.

*Hill, M. M.: "I.C.N.E. Formulates Some Basic Concepts in Nutrition," *Nutrition Program News*, Sept.– Oct. 1964, U.S. Department of Agriculture, Washington, D.C.

We eat food to live, to grow, to keep healthy and well, and to get energy for work and play.

2. Food is made up of different nutrients needed for health and growth.

All nutrients needed by the body are available through food. Many kinds and combinations of food can lead to a well-balanced diet. No food, by itself, has all the nutrients needed for full growth and health. Each nutrient has specific uses in the body. Most of the nutrients do their best work in the body when teamed with other nutrients.

3. All persons, throughout life, have need for the same nutrients, but in varying amounts.

The amounts of nutrients needed are influenced by age, sex, size, activity, and state of health. Suggestions for the kinds and amounts of food needed are made by trained scientists.

4. The way food is handled influences the amount of nutrients in food, its safety, appearance, and taste.

Handling means everything that happens to food while it is being grown, processed, stored, and prepared for eating.

Family counseling. Dietitians, nutritionists, and nurses devote a great deal of time to counseling individuals and families. (See Figure 26–1.) Certain important principles must guide the counselor throughout the process.[2,3] They apply to education for normal nutrition under varying cultural and economic situations, and also to the guidance essential for a modified diet. (See also Chapter 28.)

Become acquainted. The nurse or nutritionist must establish an environment of warmth, kindness, and genuine interest. The person needs to know that you are there to help him, that you think he can learn, and that he is worth something. What does the individual say first? How intense are his feelings? Ample time must be allowed to let him voice his problems without the frustration of interruptions.

Before you can help people with their food problems you must know something about their present food practices—what foods they use, how these foods are prepared, the facilities for food preparation, the meanings of food in terms of social, ethnic, and religious factors, the adequacy of income for the purchase of food, their concept of the importance of food to their total life style. The list of items for the dietary history on page 392 can be adapted to the interview for family counseling.

Build upon that which is good. Every diet has some good features about it, and the counselor should capitalize upon these. A negative, critical attitude toward current practices is rarely helpful.

Focus on a specific problem. People often feel overwhelmed by many problems and are unable to progress toward solving any of them. A small problem that seems urgent to the individual and toward which some success can be anticipated should be singled out for attention. Then, with time, other problems are attacked.

Establish realistic goals. Although the counselor suggests possible goals, the decision for action must be made by the individual. Some-

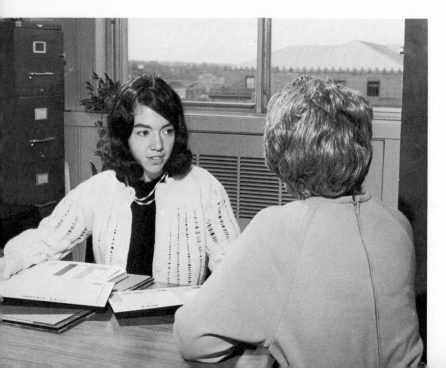

Figure 26–1. A public health nutritionist provides nutrition and diet counseling to a patient referred by a physician. (Courtesy, Division of Nutrition, Pennsylvania Department of Health.)

times the goals may seem to be quite limited and of no great importance; for example, learning how to cook a one-dish meal may be a genuine accomplishment to an unskilled homemaker. Each person being helped needs to feel that something is expected of him and that he can achieve the goals he has chosen. He needs to have a clear understanding of what he is to do before the next interview.

Learn to communicate effectively. Professional people must modify the scientific terminology they use so easily to the level of education of the individual. Counseling means talking together with the individual being helped—not lecturing; it means listening and answering questions as well as asking them; it means showing and doing as well. Learning has been described this way:

> Each remembers *best* what he does,
> Next best, what he *sees*,
> Least well what he hears.*

There is almost a surfeit of leaflets, bulletins, posters, slides and film strips, and movies available for family and group counseling. Most of these materials have been developed for middle-class families and are not useful to poor people who have little education. Films that portray affluence and lavish displays of food may create resentment rather than conveying information.

Printed materials are a supplement to counseling, never a substitute for it. Usually it is better to introduce only one leaflet or bulletin at a time, and to supplement this at latter interviews if needed.

Maintain continuity. Whenever possible the same person should follow through with an individual or family. This helps the person to know that someone is really concerned and looking after his welfare, and it helps to avoid misunderstandings.

Evaluate the results. An evaluation indicates to the counselor whether her techniques are satisfactory, or whether some changes will increase

her effectiveness. Sometimes the evaluation may show that an individual cannot be helped or does not want to be helped; this, too, should be recognized. From time to time the person being helped should evaluate his own progress, for by so doing he can reassess his goals and, if need be, change his direction.

HELPING PEOPLE WITH LOW INCOMES

Characteristics of the poor. The poor are often thought of as a single group that can be described in terms of a "culture of poverty." Although certain characteristics of behavior are enforced upon them by reason of poverty, it is a serious error to regard the poor as a homogeneous group.[2]

Variations in environment and culture. Poor people living in Appalachia, the Mexican-Americans of the Southwest, the Puerto Ricans, the American Indians, the black people in city ghettos, and many people in cities and in rural areas have one thing in common—lack of sufficient income to meet their basic needs. Their cultures, however, have little in common. Moreover, within each of these groups, individuals and families differ from one another in their values, aspirations, and style of living just as people of the more affluent society differ from one another. Some poor people come from families that have been poor for generations and have never known any other way of life; other people are poor because of changed circumstances brought about by unemployment, inflation, and health costs. Some of the poor have a fair level of education, whereas others are illiterate. Some homemakers are good managers and do a remarkable job in keeping the family together, whereas others lack even the simplest skills in homemaking and in child care. Some constantly strive for a better way of life, whereas others regard their present status as permanent and about which they can do little.

The limitations of poverty. A limited income restricts people to living in declining neighborhoods with deteriorating houses, inadequate sanitation, crowding, and lack of privacy. There is a

*Project Head Start: *Nutrition Instructors Guide*, 3 B. Office of Child Development, U.S. Department of Health, Education, and Welfare, Washington, D.C., 1967, p. 8.

constant fear of eviction because of loss of income and failure to pay the rent.

The poor are isolated from society. They move about from place to place—usually not by choice but by necessity—and therefore establish no roots in the community. Their participation in community activities is minimal and their contact with the outside world through newspapers and magazines is small. This isolation encourages suspicion of the motives of those who may try to help them; it also means that they are poorly equipped to cope with emergencies because they do not know what resources are available to them.

The poor must live from day to day and are unable to plan ahead. The future is uncertain, they are fatalistic about what is to come, and setting goals for the future seems pointless.

Lacking education, the poor may not be able to make the best use of the little money they have. They are often at the mercy of credit schemes that, over a period of time, exact large interest payments.

Poor people have known little success. They feel that people look down upon them and have little concern for them. They will often place more confidence in the advice of a neighbor, a faith healer, or a practitioner of folk medicine— all of whom are attuned to their way of living.

Social problems are not unique to the poor but they are likely to be more frequent. Many of the families have only one parent, usually the mother. Men in many households are unable to fulfill their roles as providers, and they leave their homes so that their families can qualify for public assistance.

Poverty and diet. The income is often inadequate to cover the period for which it is intended. At the beginning of the pay period the family may eat fairly well, even enjoying an occasional luxury. But as days go on the diet becomes more monotonous and inadequate, including inexpensive foods that may be good sources of calories but that are poor sources of protein, minerals, and vitamins.

The homemaker may lack transportation to a supermarket if one is not nearby and therefore food is purchased from a neighborhood grocer at prices that are almost certainly higher. Often the local grocer belongs to the same ethnic group, is someone to whom they can turn for advice, and is willing to extend credit.

Homemakers are unable to take advantage of bulk purchases or to stock their cupboards when food specials are advertised. It is sometimes said that the poor cannot afford to be thrifty.

Food preparation facilities are often limited. To tell people how to prepare foods that require an oven is not useful if there is only a hot plate. Sometimes the homemaker is unable to read a recipe and lacks even the simplest skills in food preparation. Donated foods such as nonfat dry milk, flour, beans, and fats have often been wasted because the homemaker did not know what to do with them.

Many homemakers are employed outside the home and children are left to fend for themselves. Sometimes the food supply is limited, but even with an adequate amount of food available children are not likely to select the foods that they need.

Better nutrition for the poor. Adequate income is basic to an adequate diet. Before you can tell people what foods they require and how to prepare them, there must be food in the home to prepare or money with which to purchase it. A recent study has shown that the welfare allowances in many states do not provide a sufficient allowance for food to provide the amounts of foods recommended for the low-cost plan (see page 235).[4] With the rising expectations of poor people these inequities will undoubtedly be corrected by legislation but that may well be several years away. Therefore, supplementary food programs supported by the U.S. Department of Agriculture will continue to be important.

Supplementary food programs. The Food Stamp Program is available in numerous communities and is gradually replacing the Commodity Distribution Program in other locations. Under the Food Stamp Program families whose incomes are below a certain level may trade the money they would ordinarily spend for food for food stamps that are worth a great deal more. The difference between the money spent for the stamps and their value in purchasing food is made up by the U.S. Department of Agriculture.

Purchases can be made with food stamps in any retail market that has been approved to accept stamps. Welfare workers, public health nurses, and nutritionists must be prepared to help families interpret the regulations for the use of the stamps and learn how to make the most effective use of them. Many people who are not receiving public assistance but who are living at subsistence levels do not realize that they can also purchase the stamps.

The Commodity Distribution Program makes surplus foods available to the needy at designated distribution centers. Food is also distributed to needy pregnant women and preschool children through maternal and child health centers. Surplus foods are also distributed to school lunch and breakfast programs, day-care centers, Head Start Programs, and institutions. The selection of foods from time to time has included such items as flour, rice, rolled wheat, rolled oats, cornmeal, bulgur, nonfat dry milk, canned chopped meat, peanut butter, dry beans, shortening, margarine, and raisins. Many homemakers in needy families do not know how to use some of the foods that are issued, and others who are employed outside the home do not have the time for food preparation.

Nutrition education for the poor. An adequate income alone does not guarantee improvement in nutrition. When incomes are supplemented, only a small fraction of the increase in money is usually spent for food; even that small amount may be spent for a luxury item rather than one that improves the diet. (See also Figure 25–2 and pages 361 to 363.)

The guidelines for family counseling described on pages 364 to 365 are applicable to working with the poor. In an effort to reach low-income families The Cooperative Extension Service of the U.S. Department of Agriculture developed an *Expanded Nutrition Education Program.*[5,6] This program uses program aides who are mature nonprofessional women selected from the community in which the people who are to be helped live. The program aide is given a period of intensive training by home economists and nutritionists from county extension services and is supervised on the job by staff aides and professionals. (See Figure 26–2.)

Program aides work with homemakers on an individual basis in their homes and give assistance on the problems associated with foods, child care, housekeeping and management, clothing repair, and so on. The assistance for better nutrition is on such practical points as how to use a commodity food, what to look for on a label, how to use the Daily Food Guide, and easily prepared breakfasts. The teaching includes the use of very simple booklets and demonstrations.

Because she comes from the community the program aide is aware of the problems of the family. She is able to make better contacts with people because she knows from experience what it means to have little money to spend for food. Her assistance is less likely to be viewed with suspicion than is that of a helper who comes from a middle-class environment with different standards and values.

SOME COMMUNITY PROGRAMS FOR NUTRITION EDUCATION AND SERVICES

State nutrition programs. A nutrition program in a state department of health is tailored to the needs of the population of that state and is dynamic. Nutritionists in state programs work closely with physicians, nurses, dentists, dental hygienists, social workers, administrators of institutions, food service managers, dietitians, and others. The activities below are representative of those included in state nutrition programs.

1. Define the place of nutrition in program areas.
   a. Conduct surveys of community needs.
2. Provide materials on nutrition information.
   a. Analyze and interpret findings of science.
   b. Prepare leaflets on topics such as: weight control; meal planning; infant feeding; food misinformation; recipes for use of special foods such as nonfat dry milk or for therapeutic diets; diet patterns for various cultural groups; teen-agers; senior citizens. (See Figure 26–3.)
   c. Prepare diet manuals, food value charts, exhibits, newspaper, magazine, radio, and television releases.
3. Consultant service to institutions: child care, nursing homes, small hospitals, mental hospitals, homes for the aged.
   a. Planning food service facilities.

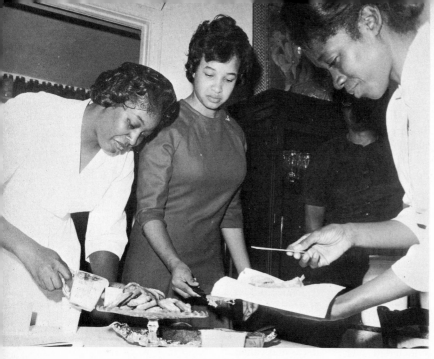

Figure 26–2. Nutrition aides prepare foods donated by the U.S. Department of Agriculture before holding a demonstration in a home. (Courtesy, Kevin Shields and U.S. Department of Agriculture.)

b. Personnel training; budgeting; menu planning; purchasing; sanitation; preparation and service of food; therapeutic diets.

4. Work with schools: elementary, secondary, college, medical, nursing.
   a. Plan and conduct dietary surveys as part of research program.
   b. Assist in developing programs in nutrition education.
   c. Conduct workshops for school faculty.
   d. Assist in training programs for school food service personnel; help to interpret educational value of school meals.

5. Cooperate with other health groups in rehabilitation and in chronic disease programs: cardiovascular disease, diabetes, tuberculosis, arthritis, cerebral palsy, orthopedic disabilities, mental retardation, etc.
   a. Preparation of materials for professional and lay instruction.
   b. Conduct of institutes for staff education of nurses, nutritionists, physicians.

6. Work with patients (usually on a demonstration basis with nurses).
   a. Clinics: child health, crippled children, cardiovascular, diabetes, prenatal, tuberculosis.
   b. Food budgets.
   c. Home visits.

7. Work with other groups:
   a. Social and welfare agencies on dietary standards and budgets.
   b. Public instruction.

8. Assist in programs of research with schools of home economics, medical schools, departments of health, federal and private agencies.

Project Head Start. Preschool children are especially vulnerable in meeting their physical and social needs, but until recently most of them have not been reached very effectively. They are too old for maternal-infant services and too young for school services.

Project Head Start initiated in the summer of 1965 by the Office of Economic Opportunity is of particular significance in that it aims to give underprivileged preschool children an opportunity to fulfill their potential in growth and physical and mental development. Head Start Child Development Centers are established through community action and involve educators, health workers, and parents who share the responsibility of getting children ready for school.

Nutrition is an essential element of each program. Children who attend a half-day session receive a snack and lunch, using the food plan in Table 26–3 as a guide. Breakfast is also provided in some programs and would include these food groups:

Fruit or fruit juice
Milk
Cereal, bread, or roll, plus one or more of these:
  Piece of cheese
  Egg, hard cooked or scrambled
  Peanut butter

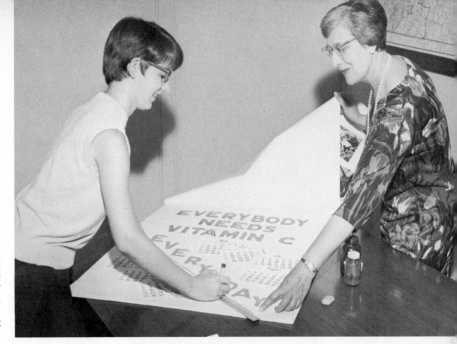

Figure 26–3. A public health nutritionist confers with the artist preparing visual aids for nutrition education programs. (Courtesy, Division of Nutrition, Pennsylvania Department of Health.)

When children are at the center for only two hours, a more substantial snack consisting of milk, a sandwich, and fruit should be provided.

An important aspect of this program is the parent participation and education. Guides have been developed for those who will teach nutrition, including such topics as the daily food guide, planning meals for preschool children, food habits of young children, how to buy food, sanitary practices in storage and handling of food. (See Figure 26–4.)

Dial-a-Dietitian. Sponsored by the American Dietetic Association and supported by state and district dietetic associations and community agencies in many cities, Dial-a-Dietitian is a telephone service to people who have questions regarding nutrition.[7] In each city the program has been publicized through newspapers and spot announcements on radio and television, giving a telephone number where people can call for information. A telephone answering service records the question, name, address, and telephone number of the person calling. Within 24 to 48 hours a dietitian returns the call and provides the information requested. (See Figure 26–5.)

Through the service dietitians clarify technical

Table 26–3. Food Plan for One Meal and One Snack—Project Head Start*

	Amount	Sample Menu
Morning Snack		
Fruit or fruit juice	1/3–2/3 cup	Orange juice
Bread and butter	1/2–1 slice	Whole-wheat bread and butter or margarine
Noon Meal		
Meat, poultry, or fish	1/2–1 ounce	Ground beef pattie
Vegetables	1–2 tablespoons cooked	Spinach
	2–4 strips raw	Carrot strips
Bread	1/2–1 slice	Whole-wheat bread and butter
Butter or margarine	1/2–1 teaspoon	
Fruit or pudding	1/4–1/2 cup	Vanilla pudding
Milk	1/2–1 cup	Milk

**Nutrition Guidelines for the Project Head Start Centers Feeding Program.* Office of Economic Opportunity, Washington, D.C., May 1965, p. 3.

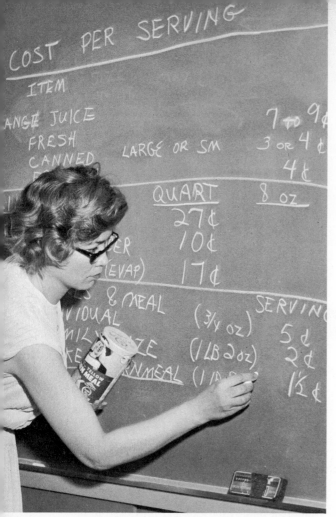

INTERNATIONAL AGENCIES FOR NUTRITION

Food and Agriculture Organization. Of all international agencies, the Food and Agriculture Organization of the United Nations (FAO) is most directly concerned with food. It was founded in Quebec, Canada, in October 1945, the aims being:

To help the nations raise the standard of living;

To improve the nutrition of the people of all countries;

To increase the efficiency of farming, forestry, and fisheries;

To better the condition of rural people;

And, through these means, to widen the opportunity of all people for productive work.*

The headquarters office of FAO is in Rome where the work of the organization is supervised by a director-general. FAO provides assistance to about 120 member states by maintaining an intelligence service which gathers, analyzes, and distributes information on which action can be based, and by acting in an advisory capacity to help governments decide what action to take. It has been engaged in a giant survey ("Indicative World Plan for Agricultural Development") to ascertain the needs and priorities for the next two decades on a country-by-country and region-by-region basis.

Technical assistance is provided in agriculture, economics, fisheries, forestry, and nutrition to member countries that request assistance. The participating countries supply technical experts so that a team going to a given locality truly has an international approach. The diversified projects in which local governments have shared costs have included: development of food storage, processing, and marketing facilities; land reclamation through irrigation and drainage; control of animal diseases; control of locusts; development of grains of higher nutritive quality, greater yield, and increased resistance to disease; inland fish culture in ponds and rice fields; estab-

Figure 26–4. A leader in a Head Start program shows mothers how to compare costs of foods per serving by using label and price information. (Courtesy, Project Head Start, Office of Child Development, U.S. Department of Health, Education, and Welfare.)

terminology, give specific information pertaining to normal diets, reinforce the teaching that a patient has received from a dietitian or physician, evaluate a product, disprove a fallacy, and urge medical advice if the individual gives indication that he has health problems not being treated. The questions asked fall into these categories: composition of foods especially calories, food sanitation, food preparation, food additives, food buying, and resource materials. Modified diets are not prescribed nor is a detailed instruction for them provided by telephone or mail; the person is advised to seek the help of a physician or dietitian.

*Food and Agriculture Organization—What It Is— What It Does—How It Works. Leaflet, Food and Agriculture Organization, Rome, 1956.

lishment of home economics programs in colleges; school feeding; and many others.

World Health Organization. The World Health Organization (WHO) was created in 1948 and is administered by a director-general with headquarters in Geneva, Switzerland, and with six regional offices, one of which is in Washington, D.C.

WHO is "the directing and coordinating authority for international health work." It is governed by two principles defined in its constitution:

Universality: The health of all peoples is fundamental to the achievement of peace and security. The enjoyment of the highest attainable standard of health is one of the fundamental rights of every human being without distinction of race, religion, political belief, economic or social condition.

Concept of health: Health is a state of complete physical, mental and social well-being and not merely the absence of disease or infirmity.*

The assistance which WHO renders to governments includes:

. . . strengthening national health services; establishing and maintaining epidemiological and statistical services; controlling epidemic and endemic diseases; maternal and child health; promotion of mental health to foster harmonious human relations; improvement of sanitation and of preventive and curative medical services.*

Major efforts of WHO have been directed to the eradication of malaria, tuberculosis, venereal diseases, and yaws. These crippling diseases yearly reduce by thousands the number of workers available to produce food; the return of these people to productivity has incalculable effects on improving the food supply. The improvement of the sanitary standards—pure water supplies, pure milk and other food, insect control, housing, waste disposal—is likewise concerned with the improvement of nutrition.

United Nations Children's Fund. To children in different countries UNICEF means different things. It may mean an injection to cure them of

World Health Organization—What It is—What It Does—How It Works. Leaflet, World Health Organization, Geneva, 1956.

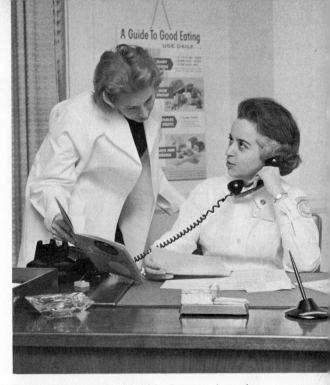

Figure 26-5. Dial-a-Dietitian Program in action. (Courtesy, The Nutrition Foundation.)

yaws, a crippling disease, or vaccination to protect against tuberculosis; but to all children in these countries UNICEF has come to mean milk (see Figure 26–6).

Organized in 1947, UNICEF continued the emergency feeding in war-devastated countries of Europe, with emphasis on protein-rich foods, especially milk. Now, all over the world, children are benefited by milk distribution through emergency relief, school feeding, and maternal and child health centers. Nonfat dry milk has been donated from the surplus in the United States, and UNICEF has provided for its transportation and distribution.

Although UNICEF continues to provide emergency relief, most of its funds are now diverted to long-range programs, for it is realized that countries must be able to solve their own nutritional problems. With UNICEF funds demonstration programs, such as acceptance tests of fish protein concentrate, have been initiated with the cooperation of FAO and WHO.

Food for Freedom Program. Public Law 480, first called the Food for Peace Program and now known as the Food for Freedom Program, was

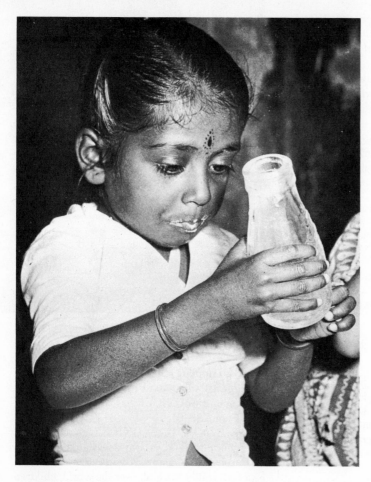

Figure 26–6. Undernourished children receive a daily ration of milk supplied by UNICEF. (Courtesy, UNICEF.)

adopted by the Congress in 1954 as a means of using agricultural surpluses for feeding the world's needy people. The program has been administered by the Agency for International Development (AID) in the Department of State.

Throughout the years the program has provided food through UNICEF, CARE, and other relief agencies working in maternal and child health centers. (See Figure 26–6.) Food has been available for refugees and to feed people in disasters such as floods, hurricanes, and crop failures. Surplus foods have also been used as part payment for laborers working on development programs: irrigation projects, dams, roads, drainage, and so on. Assistance has been given to business investors by providing guarantees

against losses of investments in developing countries through war, revolution, and expropriation. Loans have been made to the development of food industry in various countries including dairy plants, bakeries, fertilizer plants, and tractor manufacture.

INCREASING THE WORLD FOOD SUPPLY

Priorities. The rapid increase in the world's population without a comparable increase in wealth and in the production of food has been described by Altschul[8] as a "derangement of our ecosystem." At least 20 per cent of the people in less developed countries receive far too few calories and 60 per cent receive diets of poor quality.

Altschul lists three priorities for people who are poor and for whom the food supply is scarce. In descending order of need they are: (1) sufficient calories to sustain life; (2) protein of adequate quality and amount; and (3) esthetic qualities to satisfy social as well as nutritional needs of even the poorest people.

Important enterprises of AID and foundations such as the Ford and Rockefeller Foundations have included the development of better agricultural practices, improved strains of plants, and protein mixtures of high nutritive value. In turn the skills of the agriculturist, food technologist, nutrition scientist, marketing expert, anthropologist, and many others have been involved in the governmental research programs, in universities, and in the food industries.

Potential sources of food. Cereal grains today comprise the principal source of food for the world's people and will, undoubtedly, continue to rank first throughout the world. (See Figure 26–7.) In recent years the so-called "green revolution" has been taking place.[9] In many less developed countries high yields of cereals are being achieved by using improved strains of rice, wheat, and corn, and by emphasizing modern agricultural practices including fertilizers and equipment. Some nations such as India have increased their yields beyond any earlier record and others have produced enough grain to meet their own needs and to export some.

Improved cereal quality. Cereal grains are deficient in one or more of the essential amino acids and thus do not meet the needs for rapid synthesis of proteins required during growth. (See page 50.) An outstanding example of an improved cereal grain is opaque-2 corn, a hybrid variety that has been developed in which the lysine and tryptophan content of the endosperm is 50 per cent higher than in the regular varieties[8, 10] Also, the leucine content is lower so that the balance with isoleucine is improved. This development is of considerable significance to Central and Latin American countries where corn is a staple food. The new variety requires special handling in milling and baking. Tortillas made with it are softer and have a slightly

sweeter taste than those made with regular corn.[10]

Nitrogen balance studies on adults have shown that 300 gm of opaque-2 corn fed daily would be adequate for most men weighing 70 kg or less and for all women.[10] By contrast, 600 gm of regular African maize was required to maintain nitrogen equilibrium. In studies on healthy preschool children Bressani found that masa prepared from opaque-2 corn produced weight gains and nitrogen retention equal to those achieved with skim milk when fed at a level of 1.8 gm protein and 100 calories per kilogram.[11] When the level of intake was reduced to 1.5 gm per kilogram, milk was slightly superior.

Amino acid supplementation. To improve the protein quality of wheat requires additional

Figure 26–7. Rice is the principal food for more than half of the world's population. Methods of agriculture and harvesting are still primitive in many areas. With modern agricultural methods and seed that produces higher yields, some countries are now meeting their needs for this staple. (Courtesy, Food and Agriculture Organization.)

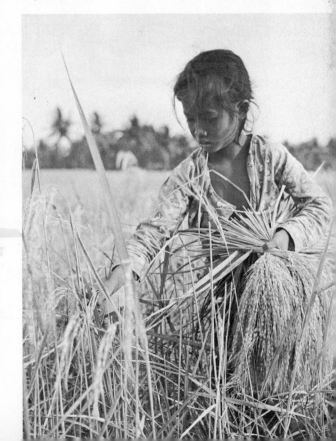

lysine; rice needs lysine and threonine; corn needs lysine and tryptophan; and legumes require methionine. The addition of lysine and methionine to low-cost foods is now economically feasible and in the not too distant future it is expected that the cost of tryptophan will also be sufficiently lowered to make its use practical.

Nutrition scientists have been cautious about amino acid supplementation because an excess of one amino acid can create an increased need for the next most limiting amino acid. Amino acid imbalances in low-protein diets can result in growth failure and other metabolic problems. *Modern Bread* is a lysine-enriched bread, also fortified with minerals and vitamins, that is pro-

duced in government-owned bakeries in India. The lysine enrichment increases the available protein by 33 per cent.[8] Lysine enrichment is now used in Japan and is underway in other countries of the Far East.

Other plant sources. Legumes, including chick peas, peanuts, and many varieties of beans, are important sources of protein and calories in Central America, Africa, and India. Soybeans contain protein of superior quality and probably have not been utilized as much as they might be. Cottonseed is a useful source of protein when the toxic pigment, gossypol, is removed.

Leaves of plants such as alfalfa and single-celled plants, including yeasts, fungi, and algae,

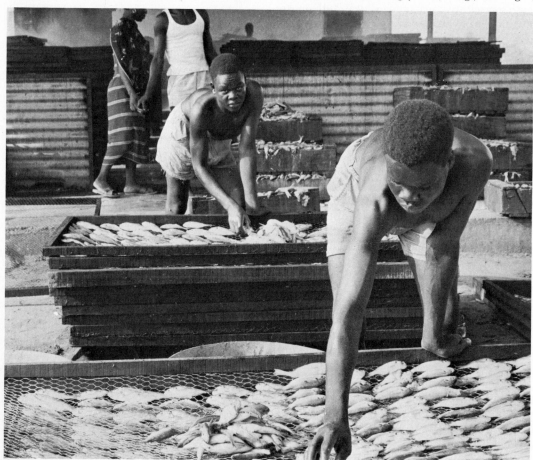

Figure 26–8. Fish is an excellent source of protein that can be used to supplement protein sources in many developing countries. In this illustration fresh fish is placed on trays to be smoked. (Courtesy, Priya Ramrakha and UNICEF.)

may become important sources of food at some time in the more distant future. The techniques for producing them at low cost are not yet known, and major problems remain in developing products that are esthetically acceptable. The high nucleic acid content leads to increased uric acid production and subsequent problems of excretion.

Protein isolates. Proteins can be isolated from foods such as wheat, soybeans, cottonseeds, and fish to give an almost pure protein in powder or fiber form. Soy protein isolates have been used to formulate foods that simulate chicken, bacon, ham, beef, and seafoods. The calorie and amino acid contents of these simulated foods are comparable to those of meat. Presently these foods are too expensive for the developing countries, but their future use appears to be good.

Fish. Undoubtedly the sea can supply a substantial part of the world's protein needs. Except for people living near the sea, the per capita consumption of fish is low. Fish farming in freshwater ponds is used to some extent in some Oriental countries. (See Figure 26–8.)

Fish protein concentrate is a low-fat, bland, practically odorless powder produced from whole fish. It contains in excess of 80 per cent protein and has been incorporated successfully into biscuits and other food combinations.

Food mixtures. Many food mixtures that apply the principle of the supplementary value of the proteins of various foods have been developed, particularly for the relief of protein-calorie malnutrition in children. These mixtures do not yet account for a sizable proportion of the world's protein needs. Among the mixtures that have been shown to be nutritionally satisfactory, economically feasible, and acceptable to the consumers are these:[8,12]

Incaparina: the first mixture to be developed; cottonseed and corn flours, vitamins, minerals, and torula yeast; protein efficiency equal to milk; 26 per cent protein; Central America.

Bal Ahar: a farina-like blend of bulgur wheat, peanut flour, nonfat dry milk, vitamins, minerals; 22 per cent protein; India.

Golden Elbow Macaroni (*General Foods*): corn, soy, and wheat flours; calcium carbonate, calcium phosphate, iron, B vitamins; 20 per cent protein; Brazil.

Leche Alim: a cereal food of toasted wheat flour, fish protein concentrate, sunflower meal, skim milk powder; 27 per cent protein; Chile.

Puma (Monsanto); *Saci* (Coca-Cola); and *Vitasoy* (Lo): beverages containing vegetable protein, sugar, vitamins; compete with soft drinks in price and are well accepted; 2.5 to 3 per cent protein; Brazil, Guiana, Hong Kong.

PROBLEMS AND REVIEW

1. List the public and private agencies in your own community that work for better nutrition in one way or another. If possible, arrange for an interview to learn more about the activities of one of these.

2. *Problem.* Plan a 20-minute discussion-demonstration for a group of parents of underprivileged preschool children on one of these topics: menus for preschool children; taking care of the food in the home; developing good food habits in children.

3. List a number of learning experiences that could be used for children in a Head Start program.

4. *Problem.* Plan a lesson on one of these topics to help a homemaker who has a low income:
   a. How to obtain and use food stamps.
   b. How to use nonfat dry milk in some cooked foods.
   c. What to look for on labels of packages.
   d. Buying some economical cuts of meat.

5. *Problem.* Determine the current regulations for assistance through food stamps in your community.

6. *Problem.* Determine the current public assistance allowance for food in your community for:
   a. A man and his wife who are over 65 years.

b. A mother with four children: girls, 6 and 10 years; and boys, 4 and 14 years. According to the current cost of food under the low-cost plan for this family, are these allowances adequate?

7. Write a 1000-word paper on any one of these topics, using at least four references in addition to the text:

Nutritional status in the United States.

Protein-calorie malnutrition.

Economic factors in malnutrition.

Cultural factors in malnutrition.

Food mixtures for better protein.

Program aides in nutrition education.

CITED REFERENCES

1. *Proceedings for the White House Conference on Food, Nutrition and Health,* 1969. Superintendent of Documents, Washington, D.C., 1970.
2. Shoemaker, L.: *Parent and Family Life Education for Low-Income Families.* Children's Bureau Pub. 434–1965. U.S. Department of Health, Education, and Welfare, Washington, D.C., 1965.
3. Matthews, L. I.: "Principles of Interviewing and Patient Counseling," *J. Am. Diet. Assoc.,* **50**:469–74, 1967.
4. Calloway, D. H.: "Malnutrition: Poverty or Education," *J. Nutr. Educ.,* 1(4):9–12, Spring 1970.
5. Spindler, E. P., *et al.:* " 'Program Aides' for Work with Low-Income Families," *J. Am. Diet. Assoc.,* **50**:478–86, 1967.
6. Cook, F.: "Nutrition Education via People to People," *J. Nutr. Educ.,* 1(2):9–11, Fall 1969.
7. Wagner, M. G., *et al.:* "Evaluation of the Dial-a-Dietitian Program. I. Program Organization. II. Impact of the Program on the Community," *J. Am. Diet. Assoc.,* **47**:381–84; 385–90, 1965.
8. Altschul, A. M.: "Food: Proteins for Humans," *Chem. Eng. News,* **47**:68–81, Nov. 24, 1969.
9. Brown, L. R.: *Seeds of Change: The Green Revolution and Development in the 1970's.* Praeger Publishers, Inc., New York, 1970.
10. Clark, H. E.: "Meeting Protein Requirements of Man," *J. Am. Diet Assoc.,* **52**:475–79, 1968.
11. Bressani, R.: "Protein Quality of Opaque-2 Maize in Children," Proc. High Lysine Corn Conference, Washington, D.C. Corn Industries Research Foundation, 1966, p. 34.
12. "Fortified Foods: The Next Revolution," *Chem. Eng. News,* **48**:36–43, Aug. 10, 1970.

ADDITIONAL REFERENCES

Community Programs

Barney, H. S.: "The Use of Nutrition and Home Economics Aides," *J. Home Econ.,* **62**:114–19, 1970.

Egan, M. C.: "Combating Malnutrition through Maternal and Child Health Programs," *Children,* **16**:67–71, March–April 1969.

Eisler, M., *et al.:* "The Nutrition Rehabilitation Center," *J. Am. Diet. Assoc.,* **55**:246–51, 1969.

Finch, R. H.: "Toward a Comprehensive Food and Nutrition Program," *Public Health Rep.,* **84**:667–72, 1969.

Juhas, L.: "Day-Care for Children: Recent Developments and Their Implications for Dietitians," *J. Am. Diet. Assoc.*, **57**:139–43, 1970.

Wagner, M.: "The Irony of Affluence," *J. Am. Diet. Assoc.*, **57**:311–15, 1970.

Walsh, H. E.: "The Changing Nature of Public Health," *J. Am. Diet. Assoc.*, **46**:93–95, 1965.

Low-Income Families

Coltrin, D. M., and Bradfield, R. B.: "Food Buying Practices of Urban Low-Income Consumers—A Review," *J. Nutr. Educ.*, **1**(3):16–17, 1970.

Herzog, E.: *About the Poor. Some Facts and Some Fictions.*
Children's Bureau Pub. 451–1967. U.S. Department of Health, Education, and Welfare, Washington, D.C., 1967.

Irelan, L. M., ed.: *Low-Income Life Styles.* Welfare Admin. Pub. 14. U.S. Department of Health, Education, and Welfare, Washington, D.C., 1968.

Jeffers, C.: "Hunger, Hustlin' and Homemaking," *J. Home Econ.*, **61**:755–61, 1969.

Mayer, J.: "Hospital's Role in Overcoming Malnutrition among Indigents," *Hospitals*, **43**:85–88, July 1969.

Moore, M. L.: "When Families Must Eat More for Less," *Nurs. Outlook*, **14**:66–69, April 1966.

O'Hagan, J. I., *et al.:* "Connecticut Hospital Sparks Supplemental Food Program," *J. Am. Diet. Assoc.*, **56**:419–21, 1970.

Nutrition Education (see also references at end of Chapter 28)

Hill, M. M.: "Nutrition Committees and Nutrition Education," *J. Nutr. Educ.*, **1**:14–15, Summer 1969.

Leong, Y.: "Nutrition Education for the Aged and Chronically Ill," *J. Nutr. Educ.*, **1**:18–20, Winter 1970.

Project Head Start—Nutrition Kit (a series of booklets for reference and training in the Head Start and Nutrition and Food Programs), Office of Child Development, U.S. Department of Health, Education, and Welfare, Washington, D.C., 1969.

Ritchie, J. A. S.: *Learning Better Nutrition. Second Study of Approaches and Techniques.* FAO Nutr. Studies No. 20, 1968.

Schild, D. T.: "A Converted Bus Takes Expanded Nutrition Program to the People," *J. Nutr. Educ.*, **1**:22–24, Winter 1970.

Sliepcevich, M., and Creswell, W. H.: "A Conceptual Approach to Health Education," *Am. J. Public Health*, **58**:684–92, 1968.

Spindler, E. B., *et al.:* "Action Programs to Improve Nutrition," *J. Home Econ.*, **61**:635–39, 1969.

Teaching Kit, FES Packet B. (Guides prepared by Consumer and Marketing Service for Program Aides; includes leaflets on Food for Thrifty Families) U.S. Government Printing Office, Washington, D.C.

Todhunter, E. N.: "Approaches to Nutrition Education," *J. Nutr. Educ.*, **1**:8–9, Summer 1969.

World Nutrition; Food Resources

Bengoa, J. M.: "Nutrition Activities of the World Health Organization," *J. Am. Diet. Assoc.*, **55**:228–32, 1969.

DeMaeyer, E. M.: "Food Supply and New Protein Resources," *WHO Chron.*, **22**:225–35, 1968.

Food for Us All—Yearbook of Agriculture 1969. U.S. Department of Agriculture, Washington, D.C., 1969, pp. 69–86.

Harrar, G. J.: *Strategy Toward the Conquest of Hunger.* The Rockefeller Foundation, New York, 1967.

Jansen, G. R.: "Total Protein Value of Protein- and Amino Acid-supplemented Bread," *Am. J. Clin. Nutr.*, **22**:38–43, 1969.

Munro, I. C., *et al.:* "Fish Protein Concentrate as a Supplement to Cereal Diets," *J. Am. Diet. Assoc.*, **54**:398–400, 1969.

Review: "Evaluation of High Protein Supplements Containing Oilseed Flours," *Nutr. Rev.*, **26**:333–35, 1968.

——: "The Green Revolution," *Nutr. Rev.*, **27**:133–36, 1969.

Roels, O. A.: "Marine Proteins," *Nutr. Rev.*, **27**:35–39, 1969.

Smith, V. E.: "Agricultural Planning and Nutrient Availability," *Nutr. Rev.*, **28**:143–50, 1970.

Swaminathan, M.: "Nutrition and the World Food Problem," *Bordens Rev. Nutr. Res.*, **28**:1–31, Jan. 1967.

Third World Food Survey: Freedom from Hunger Campaign. Basic Study No. 11, Food and Agriculture Organization, Rome, 1963.

Part Two
Therapeutic Nutrition

Unit VIII

Introduction to the Study of Therapeutic Nutrition

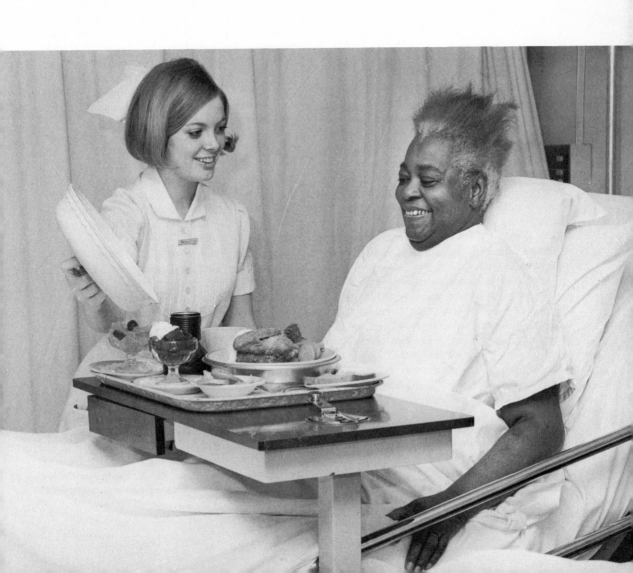

27 Therapeutic Nutrition: Factors in Patient Care

The best doctors in the world are Doctor Diet, Doctor Quiet, and Doctor Merryman.

JONATHAN SWIFT

Nutritional care of the patient. Man has probably always associated food, in one way or another, with health or illness. In fact, many of the ideas held by people for preventing or curing disease are based on food folklore. Some of these ideas are so firmly fixed that they may interfere with satisfactory food intake. Regardless of the diagnosis, the satisfactory intake of food by the patient is essential for the maintenance of tissue structures and body functions so that recovery from illness is not impeded.

The failure to ingest an adequate supply of the proper nutrients, or inability to digest, absorb, or metabolize foodstuffs, sooner or later leads to nutritional deficiency. This, in turn, may initiate or aggravate diseases of nonnutritional origin because of the body's lowered resistance. Many illnesses such as infections, injuries, and metabolic disturbances lead to deficiencies even in persons normally possessing good nutritional status because the individual is unable to ingest sufficient food or because the disease process imposes greatly increased demands for most, if not all, of the nutrients. Thus, a vicious cycle of disease, malnutrition, and prolonged convalescence is created.

The attributes of good nutrition and the principles and practices for achieving them have been discussed for all age categories in Part One of this text. The adaptation of the normal diet to the needs of individuals with some pathologic conditions is the objective of Part Two. For many patients no dietary modification is required. Good nutritional care for them consists in supplying a normal diet that furnishes the patient's nutritional, psychologic, and esthetic needs, and in taking appropriate measures to enable him to consume it. Modified diets are the principal therapeutic agents in some metabolic diseases such as diabetes mellitus and phenylketonuria. In other instances diet therapy serves in supporting the overall therapeutic program; for example, a sodium-restricted diet may be prescribed together with diuretics to maintain water balance. Modified diets are also used as preventive measures. One example of this is the fat-controlled diet believed to be beneficial to those individuals who have genetic, physical, and biochemical characteristics that predispose to coronary disease.

The purposes of diet therapy are (1) to maintain good nutritional status, (2) to correct deficiencies that may have occurred, (3) to afford rest to the whole body or to certain organs that may be affected, (4) to adjust the food intake to the body's ability to metabolize the nutrients, and (5) to bring about changes in body weight whenever necessary.

Team approach to nutritional care. Meeting the patient's nutritional needs involves the coordination of the medical, nursing, and dietary staff. (See Figure 27–1.) The physician prescribes the diet and should also give the patient some information concerning the reasons why a modified diet has been ordered. The dietitian is the specialist who is uniquely qualified to plan and direct the activities related to the patient's nutritional care. She interprets the physician's order in terms of daily meal patterns that have been individualized according to the patient's food habits as well as modified according to the therapeutic needs. The dietitian is responsible for the preparation and service of food to the patient, the evaluation of the patient's response to his diet, and the subsequent counseling

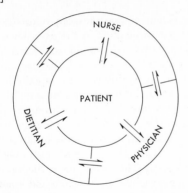

Figure 27–1. Lines of communication must be kept open between patient, dietitian, nurse, and physician.

of the patient and his family if a home diet is required. (See Figure 27–2.)

What, then, is the role of the nurse in meeting the patient's nutritional needs? Fundamentally, nutritional care is an integral part of—not apart from—nursing care of the patient. The nurse is the member of the health team who has the most constant and intimate association with the patient, and the direct services she gives to the patient differ from those of the physician and

the dietitian. In a large hospital the nurse maintains liaison between the patient, physician, and dietitian, gives assistance to the patient at mealtimes, observes the patient's response to his meals, and interprets the diet to the patient. The counseling of patients as well as the overall management of dietary services is provided by the dietary staff. In some small hospitals, nursing homes, and community nursing services the professional nurse may be responsible for planning modified diets, for supervising their use, and for patient counseling. Usually a dietitian is available for consultation in these situations.

The specific activities related to nutritional care that may be expected of the nurse include the following:

1. To maintain lines of communication with the physician and dietitian regarding the patient's dietary needs:
   a. Obtaining a diet prescription if there is none, and arranging for food service to the patient.
   b. Providing the dietitian and physician with information regarding the patient's response to his diet.

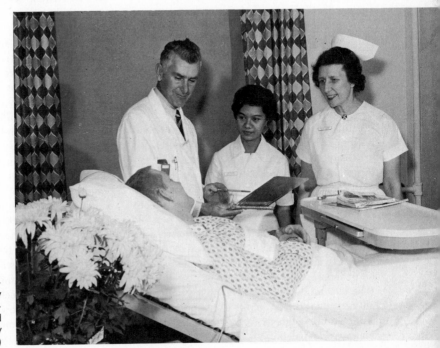

Figure 27–2. Physician, dietitian, and nurse discuss dietary changes with patient. (Courtesy, Miss Ruth Dickie and University Hospitals, University of Wisconsin Medical Center.)

c. Serving as liaison between the patient and the physician and dietitian.

2. To assist the patient at mealtimes:
   a. Providing a pleasant environment con-
   . ducive to eating.
   b. Preparing the patient for the meal.
   c. Giving assistance to the patient as needed, including feeding.
   d. Helping the handicapped to adjust to self-feeding.
   e. Giving encouragement and support to the patient.

3. To interpret the diet to the patient:
   a. Explaining the reasons for a modified diet and what may be expected of the diet.
   b. Answering questions about the diet.

4. To observe, record, and report the patient's response to diet:
   a. Eliciting information regarding food habits, likes and dislikes, and attitudes toward diet.
   b. Noting adequacy of food intake.
   c. Reporting patient's response to dietitian and physician.

5. To plan for home care:
   a. Identifying needs for outside assistance.
   b. Arranging for counseling regarding home diet with member of family as well as patient.
   c. Provided detailed counseling regarding the home diet. (This is given by the therapeutic or clinic dietitian in many hospitals.)

Factors to consider in the study of diet therapy. In order to assume the roles described above in patient care, it will be seen that certain understandings and abilities must be developed. An appreciation and knowledge are required of (1) the underlying disease conditions which require a change in diet, (2) the possible duration of the disease, (3) the factors in the dietary which must be altered to overcome these conditions, and (4) the patient's tolerance for food by mouth.

The planning of a modified diet implies the ability to adapt the principles of normal nutrition to the various regimens for adequacy, accuracy, economy, and palatability. This may necessitate

the calculation of one or more nutrients. Also essential is a recognition of the need for dietary supplements such as vitamin and mineral concentrates when the nature of the diet imposes severe restrictions, the patient's appetite is poor, or absorption and utilization are impaired.

A correctly planned diet is successful only if it is eaten. The dietitian and nurse must be able to apply the principles pertaining to the preparation and service of appealing, palatable, and nutritious food. They must have the necessary understanding of the psychologic and emotional factors influencing food acceptance.

Patient care includes planning for his full rehabilitation. For some patients a modified diet may be required for weeks, months, or even a lifetime; for others, guidance may be desirable in the improvement of a normal diet. Such planning necessitates consideration of social, religious, and cultural patterns, availability of foods, cost of food, suitable methods of food preparation, and so on. (See Chapter 28.)

EFFECT OF ILLNESS ON FOOD ACCEPTANCE AND UTILIZATION

The physiologic, psychologic, and emotional factors governing food acceptance have been discussed in Chapter 14. Likewise, a number of cultural food patterns have been presented in Chapter 15. Illness may modify or accentuate the influence of any of these factors.

The stress of illness. The sick person has many fears: those relating to the outcome of the illness itself; economic concerns for himself and his family; emotional adjustments to having to depend on others during the illness; anxiety about loss of love and self-esteem.

These problems are compounded when hospitalization becomes necessary. Some patients adjust easily to a hospital routine, but for others it is difficult. The patient is subjected to seemingly endless questions, physical examinations, laboratory tests, and ministrations of therapy by a parade of specialists and auxiliary workers who, too often, don't explain what is happening, thus causing much needless anxiety. On the other hand, the patient often experiences long delays when he requires attention to his personal needs. It is not surprising that patients feel that there is no specific person who has the primary concern and responsibility for his care. The loss of privacy is an especial embarrassment and even shock to an elderly individual who has never before been in a hospital. Likewise the loss of independence to eat when and what he wishes, to get out of bed or not, to come and go as he wishes, and so on, can be frustrating.

Nutritional stress. Immobilization is a stressful situation in which nitrogen and calcium excretions are elevated. In long-term illness, immobilization may be responsible for serious demineralization of bones.

Any trauma to the body such as bone fracture, wound injury, or infection increases the losses of nitrogen and various electrolytes. The secretion of several hormones is often increased, thereby elevating the needs for vitamins required to carry on metabolic processes.

Balance studies on healthy young people have shown that emotional stress, such as the taking of examinations or a pregnancy for an unmarried girl, leads to increased losses of nitrogen and calcium. In fact, persons under such stress may achieve balances only with considerable difficulty. One may reasonably assume that the anxiety concerning illness may also accentuate such losses.

Illness modifies food acceptance. The disease process itself may have a profound effect on food acceptance. Some foods may produce marked anorexia, others may be distending, and still others may be irritants to the gastrointestinal tract. According to Moore[1] and others, the illness may turn the preferences back to those of earlier years. These may be the bland foods of childhood, but they might be the special dishes associated with one's ethnic origin.

When illness takes the individual from the home to the hospital, food acceptance becomes much more difficult. When the patient most needs the comfort and companionship of family and friends, he is relegated to eating alone. Perhaps the meal hours are different from those to which he is accustomed; the foods appearing on his tray may be unlike those he usually eats with respect to choice, or flavoring, or size of portion; a single food to which he has a strong aversion may so upset him that he is unable to eat anything served with it; managing a tray and the utensils for eating may be awkward when one is in bed; his expressed needs are often minimized or brushed aside.

Modified diets impose additional problems. When a patient is confronted with the need for a therapeutic diet, he may respond with comments such as these: "I just can't get it down." "This food is tasteless." "I can't afford such food when I go home." "Who is going to prepare my food at home?" "I can't buy these foods at work." These reactions and many others must be met by the nurse or dietitian during instruction by providing help in budgeting, arrangements for preparation, suggestions for palatability, and other useful advice.

Babcock[2] has pointed out that remarks such as the above also imply many responses to the diet: unwillingness to accept change; anger at those associated with the diet—nurse, dietitian, physician, or even mother or wife who has nagged about the food habits at home; fear of having to eat disliked foods or those foods to which he has a strong aversion; sense of deprivation with respect to choice of foods; fear of loss of social status and self-esteem; and the feeling that diet is, in some way, a punishment of him.

Young[3] states that the patient may express fear by being angry, self-conscious, talkative or reticent, uneasy, depressed, indifferent, impatient, hostile, apologetic for his failure, or resentful. Some patients may use diet as a means of gaining the attention from hospital personnel and later from the family who must provide this food. They may insist upon meticulous attention to the minutest of details, in order to gain this attention. They may actually enjoy the trouble this may be to others, and the release of responsibility for their welfare to others. Occasionally, one may actually prefer not to get well!

INTERPERSONAL RELATIONSHIP WITH THE PATIENT

The needs of the patient. Each patient has physical, psychologic, social, and spiritual needs.

The pathophysiologic aspects of illness are the immediate reason for care by the health team, but too often patients are still treated as cases of pneumonia, cancer, and renal failure rather than as whole persons. The nursing profession constantly emphasizes the important role of the nurse in assessing the other needs of the patient and in helping to meet them. How nurses achieve this constitutes a major aspect of nursing education and has been well described in numerous publications, a few of which are listed among the references at the end of this chapter.

In a study of what patients want from nursing, Abdellah and Levine[4] identified five important needs. In listing them below some examples of their application to nutritional care have been included.

1. Each person wants to be treated as an individual. He has specific needs and values that are unique for him, and his care should be personalized rather than making him fit into a general mold.

Listening. She who cares for the patient must learn to listen carefully—not only to the words themselves but also to their tone and inflection. By taking time to listen, she may be made aware of a legitimate complaint about something wrong with the meals a patient receives—for example, cold coffee, an egg not cooked to his liking, or a vegetable he thoroughly dislikes. Such details are relatively easy to correct, and the patient is thereby made quite comfortable and satisfied. The seemingly casual conversation with the patient may bring to light that the past diet has been inadequate for a long period of time because of lack of teeth, poor health, inadequate income, or the inability to prepare food. Permitting the patient to talk about other things as well as the diet will often reveal that the problems encountered in food acceptance are actually a by-product of the deep anxieties caused by other problems; through understanding, the patient can often be helped.

2. Each person has a right to know what he should expect from the health team and what is expected of him. If a modified diet is prescribed, the patient should be given some understanding of the reasons for it and what he may expect by way of needed change in food habits. Reas-surance with respect to the diet is essential, but it must be realistic in terms of the difficulties of adjustment to it and its legitimate role in the total therapeutic program. To illustrate, appropriate diets for obesity and diabetes are basic to treatment, but some patients may find the adjustment to the restrictions extremely difficult; to minimize the problems involved is to invite failure. A low-fat diet may be helpful to the patient with gallstones, but it should never be held as a guarantee that surgery would not be required at a later time. Likewise, benefit may accrue to a patient with cardiovascular disease who is placed on a diet with modification of the amount and nature of the fat, but success is so variable that promises of marked improvement would be ill-advised and rash.

3. Each patient should be helped to participate in his own care. A selective menu can be a useful tool to help him make good choices for a normal as well as a modified diet. If instruction concerning a diet is begun early, each meal helps the patent to learn what changes he will need to make in his diet when he goes home. A patient who has a physical handicap should be helped to feed himself insofar as he is able, thereby increasing his independence.

4. Each person expects that his behavior during his illness will be accepted as part of his illness. The modification of food acceptance during illness as described on page 385 is an important expression of the change in behavior.

5. Each person expects to be treated with kindness, thoughtfulness, and firmness. The work of the dietitian, nurse, or homemaker is often more successful if she can place herself in the patient's role, although she must guard against overidentification; if she becomes too close to the patient, she may accept his reactions as being always so reasonable that she is unable to do anything about changing them.

Recognition of attitudes. How does the nurse or dietitian feel about the patient who doesn't eat his food, who eats too much, or who complains about his food a great deal? When the patient expresses resentment or hostility toward her, does she realize that this may be against the restrictions the diet puts upon him and not against her as an individual? It is important that she recognize her own attitudes toward the patient, lest she show him that she is pitying, superior, intolerant, resentful, or critical of him. Moreover, she must avoid an expression of any negative attitudes she may have toward food.

FEEDING THE PATIENT

Environment for meals. Time and effort directed toward creating an atmosphere conducive to the enjoyment of food are well spent. Such an environment implies that the surrounding areas are orderly and clean; that ventilation is good; and that distracting activities such as treatment of patients and doctors' rounds are not occurring at mealtime except as emergencies may arise.

Patients who are ambulatory enjoy eating with others. In some hospitals a dining room is provided for patients, and in others food service may be easily arranged at small tables set up in the patients' lounge.

Readiness of the patient. The patient should be ready for his meal whether he is in bed or ambulatory. This may entail mouth care, the washing of the hands, and the positioning of the patient so that he can eat with comfort. If tests or treatment unavoidably delay a meal,

arrangements must be made to hold trays so that the food can be fresh and appetizing when the patient is ready to eat.

The patient's tray. The appearance of the tray is of the utmost importance since the patient's consumption of the food presented to him is the goal to be achieved. It will be seen that some of the items listed below which describe standards for tray service are the primary responsibility of the dietary department, but that others require the maximum cooperation of nursing and medical staffs with the dietary department.

1. Variations in color, flavor, and texture for appeal to the senses would be expected as essentials in menu planning and food preparation. (See Chapter 16.)

2. The tray should be of a size suitable for the food to be served—small trays for liquid nourishment and large trays for full meals.

3. The tray cover and napkins should be of suitable size for the tray, immaculately clean, and unwrinkled.

4. Everything on the tray must reflect cleanliness—sparkling glassware, shining silver, clean china.

5. The tray should be set with the most attractive china available.

6. The tray should be symmetrically arranged

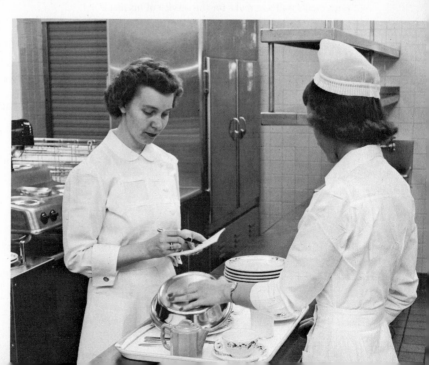

Figure 27–3. Dietitian and nurse work closely together to assure satisfactory meal service to the patient. (Courtesy, National Institutes of Health, U.S. Department of Health, Education, and Welfare.)

for the greatest convenience. All necessary silver and accessories should be included.

7. Foods should be attractively served, with the size of portions not being overlarge. Spilled liquid or sloppy serving of food is inexcusable. Garnishes help to make foods more appealing.

8. Meals should be served on time. This requires careful planning so that foods will be prepared in the proper sequence.

9. Foods should be served at the proper temperature. Hot foods should be served on hot plates, protected with a cover, and cold foods should be served on chilled dishes.

10. A final check of the tray should establish that it fully meets the requirements of the diet order, and that the patient's preferences have been implemented. (See Figure 27–3.)

Assistance in feeding. Some patients may require assistance in the cutting of meat or other foods, the pouring of a beverage, or the buttering of a piece of toast. Very ill or infirm patients must be fed. The nurse should sit down while she feeds the patient so that she can be at ease and avoid undue haste. Food will be enjoyed more if it can be eaten with reasonable leisure and if there is some conversation. Obviously, if the nurse is responsible for feeding several patients, she will make arrangements to delay tray service or to keep foods hot for those who must await their turn.

PROBLEMS AND REVIEW

1. What purposes are served by diet therapy?
2. Discuss the role of diet in total patient care.
3. How can you be sure that the diet prescribed for your patient is meeting his needs?
4. *Problem.* Keep a record of comments that your patients make about their meals.
   On the basis of these comments what can you do to ensure that your patients enjoy maximum comfort and optimum therapy insofar as their diets are concerned?
5. Discuss reasons why a patient's nutritional status may be unsatisfactory when he comes to the hospital.
6. A patient complains to you that his food is always cold. What steps can you take to correct this?
7. If a patient is having laboratory studies which will extend beyond the lunch hour, what arrangements will you make for the service of his meal?

CITED REFERENCES

1. Moore, H. B.: "Psychologic Facts and Dietary Fancies," *J. Am. Diet. Assoc.*, **28**:789–94, 1952.
2. Babcock, C. G.: "Problems in Sustaining the Nutritional Care of Patients," *J. Am. Diet. Assoc.*, **28**:222–26, 1952.
3. Young, C. M.: "Teaching the Patient Means Reaching the Patient," *J. Am. Diet. Assoc.*, **33**:52–54, 1957.
4. Abdellah, F., and Levine, E.: "What Patients Say About Their Nursing Care," *Hospitals*, **31**:44–48, Nov. 1, 1957.

ADDITIONAL REFERENCES

Ahart, H. E.: "Assessing Food Intake of Hospital Patients," *J. Am. Diet. Assoc.*, **40**:114–19, 1962.
Beland, I. L.: *Clinical Nursing. Pathophysiological and Psychosocial Approaches*, 2nd ed. The Macmillan Company, New York, 1970, pp. 1–23.

Brown, E. L.: *Newer Dimensions of Patient Care.* Part 1. The Use of Physical and Social En-
    vironment of the General Hospital for Therapeutic Purposes. Part 2. Improving Staff Motiva-
    tion and Competence in the General Hospital. Part 3. Patients as People. Russell Sage
    Foundation, New York, 1961, 1962, 1964.

Chiles, R. E.: "The Rights of Patients," *N. Engl. J. Med.*, **277**:409–11, 1967.

Dawson, M. J.: "New Patients Dine with the Nurse," *Am. J. Nurs.*, **66**:287–89, 1966.

Ewell, C. M., Jr.: "What Patients Really Think about Their Nursing Care," *Mod. Hosp.*,
    109:106–108, Dec. 1967.

Hall, B. L.: "Human Relations in the Hospital Setting," *Nurs. Outlook*, **16**:43–45, Mar. 1968.

Isch, C.: "A History of Hospital Fare," *J. Am. Diet. Assoc.*, **45**: 441–46, 1964.

Johnson, D.: "Present Concepts in Diet Therapy," *World Rev. Nutr. and Diet.*, Vol. 5, S. S.
    Karger, Basel/New York, 1965, pp. 79–131.

MacGregor, F. C.: "Uncooperative Patients. Some Cultural Interpretations," *Am. J. Nurs.*,
    67:88–91, 1967.

Manning, M. L.: "The Psychodynamics of Dietetics," *Nurs. Outlook*, **13**:57–59, April 1965.

Mussallem, H. K.: "The Changing Role of the Nurse," *Am. J. Nurs.*, **69**:514–17, 1969.

Smith, D. W.: "Patienthood and Its Threat to Privacy," *Am. J. Nurs.*, **69**:508–13, 1969.

Tarnower, W.: "Psychological Needs of the Hospitalized Patient," *Nurs. Outlook*, **13**:28–30,
    July 1965.

Wilson, N., and Wilson, R. H. L.: "You Can Lead a Patient to a Diet, But . . ." *Nutr. Today*,
    1:14–18, March 1966.

Wood, C. L.: "How the Chaplain and the Dietitian Can Cooperate," *J. Am. Diet. Assoc.*,
    35:821–22, 1959.

28 Coordinated Nutritional Services for Patients

Comprehensive care—a challenge. Chronic illnesses including cardiovascular diseases, neoplasms, diabetes, and arthritis are leading causes of illness in the United States. These diseases account for a large share of hospital admissions and place severe burdens of care, loss of income, and heavy medical costs on families who are often ill prepared to cope with these problems. The security and well-being of all members of the family may well be threatened.

Chronic diseases afflict the elderly more frequently, but younger people are not altogether immune to them. Many patients remain in hospitals longer than their therapy requires because there is no one in the home to adequately care for them, or because the other adult in the family is also the wage earner. Nursing homes sometimes provide for the transition from hospital to home. If single or multiple services are available within the home, the patient's rehabilitation is likely to be hastened in the happier environment of the home and the costs of care may be considerably reduced.

On a given day it has been estimated that 500 persons of each 100,000 are homebound because of illness or disability. Of these 500 persons, 20 could use some aspect of home care, and 40 would benefit most through coordinated home-care services. On the basis of a population

of over 200 million persons, the total number of homebound persons who could benefit by some home-care services is staggering.

Federal legislation has greatly expanded the opportunities for better health care of the population. Especially significant are Medicare, children and youth programs, and regional medical programs. Undoubtedly, during this decade, further legislation will be enacted for programs designed to promote the maintenance of health of the entire population as well as care during illness. As the expectations of people for better health care increase, so it will become necessary to develop new approaches in the health disciplines to meet these needs.

Nutritional care is an essential and dynamic component of comprehensive health care. In fact, the ability to deliver the needed nutritional services and the quality of nutrition that the patient can maintain are often the decisive factors in restoring health or in maintaining it. In a survey of 200 agencies[1] respondents were asked to list those subjects for which increased teaching-aid material would be required as a result of the Medicare legislation. Of more than 30 subjects listed, nutrition ranked second only to rehabilitation.

This chapter is concerned with (1) dietary counseling as a sound approach to patient rehabilitation, and (2) dietary aspects of home-care services.

DIETARY COUNSELING

The plan for rehabilitation of many patients includes counseling to effect improvement of a normal diet or adjustment to a modified diet. Brandt[2] has suggested that the term *home diet* is more appropriate than the term *discharge diet*, in that the former immediately establishes the setting of the diet.

Responsibility for counseling. Dietitians, nutritionists, nurses, and physicians share responsibility for dietary counseling. Within the hospital the dietitian may provide the formalized instruction for the patient's home diet or she may have supervisory responsibility for nurses who give instruction to selected patients. The physician has an obligation to the patient to discuss the reasons why he has ordered a given diet, and what the patient may expect in terms of health as a result of adherence to the diet.

Numerous opportunities arise within the hospital for informal instruction by the nurse. It goes without saying that all who provide guidance should be in common agreement about the essentials of the patient's diet. The nurse who doesn't know the answer to a question should seek the correct information from the dietitian or ask the dietitian to see the patient, if the problem is complex. Nothing is more confusing to the patient than to receive information from several sources which varies widely or is contradictory.

Counseling begins early. For the in-patient, dietary counseling should be planned well in advance, for little can be accomplished when the home diet is given just as the patient is ready to leave the hospital and is concerned about his trip home, the medicines he is to take, and his readjustment to normal activities. The process of instruction, in fact, is part of the daily care of the patient. For example, the diabetic tray becomes, at each meal, a lesson in the use of the meal exchange lists; a complaint about unsalted food may provide opportunity to tell about the use of other flavoring aids. Such informal instruction provided day by day gives the patient an opportunity to get used to the idea of the diet, to reflect on it, and to ask questions when they occur to him.

Establishing rapport. The nurse and dietitian have ample opportunity for establishing good rapport with the patient in the hospital, but in the clinic the patient may be seen for only a short time. The interviewer, then, must make every effort to make the patient feel comfortable and at ease before proceeding with the instruction. She must be cheerful, genuinely interested, and inspire confidence.

A quiet, pleasant room where privacy can be assured is essential. The patient and interviewer should be comfortably seated, preferably at a table or desk.

In establishing rapport, the interviewer gradually encourages the patient to talk about himself.[3] Initial questions may well be of a general nature, such as the patient's address, occupation, height, weight, or age. The conversation is then directed to the food habits and should bring out the home situation and possibly give some clues to the patient's emotional state.

Timing is important. According to Hildreth,[4] choosing the right time of day for the interview and counseling is important. Just before or during meals, the patient is directed to familiar foods which have satisfied his hunger in the past, and he will resist efforts to divert him from them. Immediately following the satisfaction of hunger, he will have little interest in, and may even be nauseated by, the further mention of food. Therefore, some time should elapse after the meal when food can be discussed objectively. Instruction should come at a time when the patient need not be interrupted for routine care, treatments, etc. The counselor must have sufficient time for calm, unhurried teaching.

The diet history. In order to individualize the nutritional services to the patient and to make the necessary adjustments for the home diet a good deal of information regarding the patient's food habits is essential. The nurse and dietitian will obtain as much information as possible from the patient's chart. They will also be alert to the comments the patient makes about his food from time to time and will record these. Nevertheless, an interview with the patient will usually be required to elicit further information. Effective dietary counseling requires a good deal of experience in communicating purposefully with people and much insight into the behavior of people. The interview will be more successful if the following points are observed.

1. For the patient in the hospital assess the patient's willingness to talk about his diet. A patient who is fatigued and uncomfortable may not be as cooperative as required. Some-

times a family member may supply some or all of the information.

2. Use a conversational and casual approach rather than one that is bound to a structured form. Note, however, that a form may be helpful to you in planning your interview.

3. Use open-ended questions that permit the patient to respond fully. Avoid questions answered "Yes" or "No," or that suggest a correct answer. For example, "Tell me what you usually eat for breakfast"—*not* "Do you eat eggs for breakfast?"

4. Ask only those questions that are relevant to success in dietary counseling. Patients generally resent questions that appear to have nothing to do with the diet and consider them to be an invasion of privacy. For example, although adequate income is essential, the nurse and dietitian can almost always obtain this information without direct questioning.

5. Give the patient time to think and to respond. Older people, especially, may be somewhat slow in responding.

The following items suggest the kinds of information that may be sought, but not every item will be required for every patient nor will direct questioning be necessary for all of them.

Socioeconomic History

Occupation: hours for work, travel time to and
   from work
Family relationships
Residence: house, apartment, room
Recreational activities: type, how often
Ethnic background
Religious beliefs regarding food

Medical History

Present illness: chief complaints, especially those
   relating to nutrition; diagnosis
Weight: any recent changes, comparison with
   desirable weight
Appetite: any recent changes
Digestion; ability to swallow, anorexia, vomiting,
   distention, cramps
Elimination: regular, constipation, diarrhea
Handicaps related to feeding: inability to chew,

need for self-help devices in eating, inability to prepare food

Dietary History

Meals: where eaten, when, with whom
Meals skipped: which, how often
Food preparation: by whom, facilities
Meals away from home: which, how often, type
   of facility (lunch counter, cafeteria, school
   lunch, restaurant)
Typical day's meals: 24-hour recall
Cross-check of day's meals: frequency of use of
   important food groups in a week, for example,
   milk, eggs, breakfast cereals
Snacks: how often, types, amounts
Mineral-vitamin supplements: type, how often,
   reasons for use
Food likes and dislikes: food intolerance, food
   allergies
Food budgeting: kinds of fruits, vegetables, meats
   purchased; sources of budget information;
   menu planning
Previous dietary restrictions: reasons for, type,
   how long, response to modified diet
Sources of nutrition information: use of advertising, popular publications, books

Dietary counseling based on patient needs. A fundamental tenet is to begin where the patient finds himself. Something good can be found in every diet, and every effort should be made to impose as few changes as necessary—not a complete discarding of the old pattern. The instruction should be in simple terms readily understood by the layman. Some judgment concerning the amount of detail which may be included is essential, for a weary patient may remember little when he gets home.

The patient will require guidance with respect to choice of foods, methods of preparation, kinds of seasonings which may be used, amounts of food allowed, the number of meals, and time for meals. A written meal pattern which has been developed with the patient is helpful. Printed menus that have little or no regard for individual preferences are of doubtful value.

Although the emphasis should always be directed to the foods the patient may have, in some instances, such as the sodium-restricted diets, it may be desirable also to provide a list of foods that are contraindicated. Printed aids such as the meal exchange lists are useful and time saving, but they should always be accompanied with appropriate explanation. Illustrations, posters, and food models are helpful in clarifying instruction; even films may be used where group instruction is used as for pregnant women, the obese, diabetics, and others.

Other members of the family must often be included in the instruction. The wife or mother of the patient may not understand the reasons for the diet, may feel that the diet is an imposition upon her, and may not understand the methods for preparing the necessary foods unless she is present at the time of instruction. For some patients it is necessary to plan a food budget, to make arrangements for meals carried to work, to make suggestions for a conference with the employer, or to provide guidelines for eating meals away from home.

Continuity of guidance. Dietary counseling is time consuming. The effort is often wasted when no opportunity is given for follow-up of the instruction given. The outpatient clinic and home visits serve to extend and clarify the instruction itself, to provide reassurance, to check progress, and to recognize any tensions which are building up in the patient.

Initial counseling may have been provided by a therapeutic dietitian or sometimes a nurse in the hospital, but it is quite likely that follow-up of the patient is the responsibility of a clinic dietitian, a nutritionist, or a public health nurse. Insofar as possible, each follow-up visit should be scheduled with the same person. Obviously, an important element of such continuing guidance is an adequate record of what has been presented to the patient initially.

Teaching machines have been used with some success for instruction of patients with diabetes mellitus.[5] Their use in hospitals, clinics, and health centers serves to reinforce the personalized instruction which has been given and to save instructional time. Programmed instruction through booklets pertaining to modified diets also merits attention. These aids allow the patient to progress at his own speed; they are not intended to replace individualized instruction, however.

Group instruction. In a food clinic or health center, classes may be held for groups with similar diet problems: pregnant women, mothers with preschool children, diabetic patients, those requiring sodium restriction, weight-control groups, and so on. Economy of time for the professional worker is an apparent advantage of using group instruction. Many patients are helped by this approach inasmuch as they learn to appreciate that others have similar problems and that they can share experiences with one another. The person who is given to much self-pity may receive encouragement toward a more positive outlook on his problems if proper guidance is provided in the group setting. Group instruction may be supplemented by individual teaching, particularly with respect to problems of finance and emotional reactions to the diet.

Group instruction must be a democratic process in which everyone feels free to participate. The nurse or dietitian cannot be authoritarian, the talkative patient should not monopolize all of the time, and the self-conscious, shy patient should not be made uncomfortable by having to respond when he is not ready. Verbal instruction should be coordinated with visual aids, including dietary lists, leaflets, posters, food models, and films as the occasion may warrant. The leader of the group cannot change the individual or the group; she can only help them to recognize their own goals and to make their own decisions for change.

COMPREHENSIVE CARE SERVICES

Concepts of comprehensive care. The provision of all necessary health services so that the patient can maintain or be restored to independent living is implied in the term *comprehensive care*. Although such a goal has long been held by professional health workers, its achievement through continuing services from hospital to home has been limited.

Piper[6] has described the concepts of comprehensive care programs as widening circles which surround the patient and his family as the focus. These include evaluation and referral; the setting of the care service; and the essential professional services.

Careful evaluation and reevaluation of the physical, psychologic, economic, and social dimensions are first required.[6] With each evaluation, and reevaluation as the needs change, the patient is referred to the essential service. The services may be provided on an in-patient basis, including hospital care for the acutely ill, a minimum-care facility within a hospital, or convalescent care in a nursing home. Care may be furnished through an out-patient clinic, utilizing a single service in a physician's office or multiple services provided by a clinic or health center. Home care, of course, implies services provided in the home, and can range from a single service such as nursing to coordinated services by many disciplines that could include medical, nursing, dental, dietetic, social, occupational therapy, physical therapy, and others.

Many home-care programs are now being developed in communities, some of which are sponsored by the hospital whereas others are directed by a public or voluntary health agency. Such services will require the assistance of a variety of technicians so that the services of the professional nurse, dietitian, and others may be most effectively used. A brief discussion of some elements of home care is given below.

Home-delivered meals. Many individuals or couples with physical limitations can remain in their own homes rather than be institutionalized if some provision can be made for their meals. Others who are temporarily disabled by illness but who are ambulatory and can feed themselves may find it possible to return to their homes at an earlier time if they can procure their meals.

A service described as "Meals-on-Wheels" was first offered by The Lighthouse in Philadelphia in 1954 and is now available in a number of communities though still on a limited basis. Most programs have been operated by women's clubs, church groups, family service organizations, and so on. Dietitians, nutritionists, or home economists usually serve as consultants, giving particular attention to menu planning, food purchasing, and food preparation. Paid employees and volunteers may share the responsibility for the actual purchase, preparation, packing, and delivery of meals.

Usually a hot noon meal and a packaged evening meal are delivered by a volunteer on a five-day basis. The recipient pays a fee for these meals, with gradations according to ability to pay. One important benefit of the service is the daily contact which the homebound person has with the volunteer who delivers the meals.

Homemaker services. The purpose of this service is to maintain the family in a healthful setting when no one in the family can fulfill the homemaking function. For example, the mother may be ill or convalescing from physical or mental illness; an aging person or couple is unable to perform the necessary tasks in the home, but could remain at home at less expense with homemaker assistance; death of the mother in a home with young children presents a major problem to the working father unless relatives help out or homemaker service is available.

The sponsoring organization may be a public or voluntary agency such as the welfare division, the family service organization, or the community nursing service. The organizations recruit, define duties, provide formalized training and in-service programs of education, and provide supervision on the job. Social workers, public health nurses, home economists, and others have participated in these duties.

The terms *homemaker, home health aide, housekeepers,* and *visiting homemakers* are used with some variations of duties depending upon the sponsoring agency. Generally speaking, homemakers are mature women who have had responsibility for raising their own families, who like to help other people, and who can follow instructions. Among the responsibilities pertaining to nutrition are meal planning, marketing, food preparation, and food service. (See Figure 28–1.) One of the problems may be that of getting children to eat regular meals; another may relate to a modified diet; a common problem is that of stretching the food dollar. The homemaker must be an adaptable individual who adjusts to the facilities within the home, whatever they may be. She must respect the wishes of the family and adhere to their socioeconomic and cultural values. She will accomplish little if in doing her job she creates antagonism and jealousy in any member of the family.

Physical Handicaps, Rehabilitation, and Nutrition

Physical handicaps. Millions of Americans have physical handicaps that restrict their ability to care for themselves and to work. Physical disabilities cover a wide range: the individual who has lost a hand or an arm, or who is hemiplegic and has the use of only one arm; arthritics with stiff, swollen, painful joints and who have a limited range of motion; those with cerebral palsy, Parkinson's disease, or multiple sclerosis and for whom incoordinated movements are a constant trial; those bound to a wheelchair; the blind; those who have limited cardiac and respiratory reserves such as patients with cardiac disease or emphysema; and many others.

Nutrition of the physically handicapped. Adequate nutrition is essential in restoring a patient to his potential capacity for independence, yet the handicap itself may be the principal factor that favors malnutrition even though the supply of food is plentiful.[7] The use of only one arm, or stiff, painful joints, or incoordinated movements present tremendous difficulties in feeding oneself and may limit the performance of simple kitchen tasks such as opening packages, cutting foods, peeling vegetables, and using appliances.

The energy balance is an important consideration. Some handicapped individuals have an increased energy requirement because they must

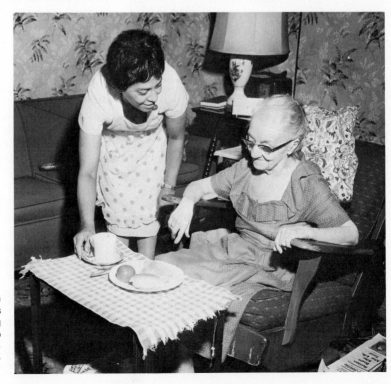

Figure 28–1. A home health aide adapts to the facilities within the home in providing meals that will be satisfying to the patient. (Courtesy, Community Nursing Service, Philadelphia.)

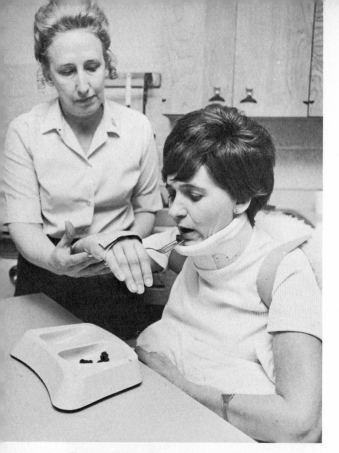

Figure 28–2. This patient is learning to use a universal cuff to become independent in self-feeding activities. A bowl with suction cups adheres to the table and prevents slipping. This will be used to make learning less difficult and will be replaced with regular utensils when the skill is perfected. (Courtesy, Allied Services for the Handicapped, Inc., Scranton, Pennsylvania.)

exert a tremendous effort to complete tasks. The increased requirement, on the one hand, and the difficulties experienced in eating, on the other hand, lead to excessive weight loss and to tissue depletion. Other individuals confined to wheelchairs and who exert little effort may become obese and require a low-calorie diet. (See Chapter 31.)

Good protein nutrition is essential for restoration of body tissues, to reduce the incidence of infection, and to maintain the integrity of the skin. For immobilized individuals decubitus ulcers are a frequent problem. During the early stages of immobilization the nitrogen losses from the body greatly exceed the intake. The accelerated catabolism of protein tissues appears to

run a time sequence that is not wholly reversed in the early stages even though a high-protein diet may be used. Nevertheless, the replacement of these losses requires a high-protein diet over an extended period of time. (See Chapter 32.)

Excessive losses of calcium from the bones may lead to urinary calculi. A liberal fluid intake is essential to facilitate the excretion of calcium, and some restriction of the calcium intake is often prescribed. (See Chapter 44.)

Constipation is a frequent complication of those who are immobilized. Its prevention or correction requires a liberal intake of fluids, a diet containing sufficient bulk, and regular habits of elimination. (See Chapter 35 for further details.)

The nature of rehabilitation. Rehabilitation is the return of a handicapped individual to his maximum potential—to what he will be able to do in the future. It is an individualized process in which therapy is designed specifically in terms of the patient's handicap, his psychologic problems, his family situation, and his economic circumstances. It is individualized in that each patient's progress is measured against his own possibilities, not against some normal standard.

Rehabilitation may occur in a rehabilitation center, in a school for handicapped children, or in the home. The economic consideration is important inasmuch as rehabilitation is costly in terms of weeks or months in a rehabilitation center, and the involvement of many specialists in the process. In addition, when the homemaker is handicapped, additional costs for her substitute in the home are likely to be appreciable.

The handicapped individual experiences helplessness, defeat, frustration, and even neglect. To surmount his difficulties becomes a constant uphill battle. Rehabilitation itself is usually slow, sometimes painful, and fatiguing both physically and emotionally. The patient needs the support of every member of the rehabilitation team.

The rehabilitation team. The skills and techniques in physical medicine, physical therapy, occupational therapy, nursing, home economics, nutrition, social work, and psychology are utilized in rehabilitation. The patient is not only the focus of these specialized skills but he is part of the team and participates in the plans for his restoration—as do members of his family. Each member of the team contributes his skills in a way that complements but does not overlap or duplicate the efforts of another. The nurse is usually the coordinator of these services in the rehabilitation center. For a full description of the specialized roles of the team members the student is referred to texts and articles listed in the references.

Self-help devices for eating. Numerous devices for daily activities have been designed at the Institute of Rehabilitation Medicine of the New York University Medical Center. In addition, publications such as the *Mealtime Manual for the Aged and Handicapped* are valuable.[8] Many of the devices can be made in the home, and others are available at moderate costs. A few of the devices that are helpful to those who have only one arm or who have difficulty in holding articles or bringing food to the mouth are described below. (See Figure 28–2.)

Jointed handles for spoons and forks. When the motions of the arm and wrist are restricted, the joints of the utensil permit an angle that can approach the mouth.

Knife for cutting. A knife needs a firm support, and cutting is difficult for persons with the use of only one arm. A cuff fitted over the hand permits the knife to be held firmly. A serrated edge is better than one with a smooth edge.

Plate guards. These are placed at the edge of the plate; they keep food from spilling and provide a surface against which food can be pushed. A deep dish with straight sides is also helpful. The plate can be kept from sliding by placing it in a support constructed to hold it, or by setting it on a sponge.

Buttering bread. A right-angle ledge affixed to the corner of the breadboard will hold a piece of bread in place while it is being buttered.

Drinking glass and tube. A drinking glass can be fitted with a holder that has a wide handle easily grasped by the hand. If it is difficult to bring the glass to the mouth, a wooden block into which a hole has been cut to hold a standard-size glass will hold the glass firmly on the table. A piece of plastic tubing bent at an angle for approach to the mouth can be used. To keep

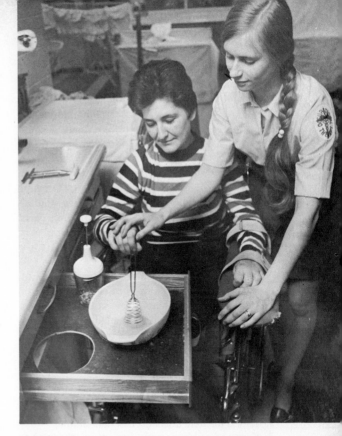

Figure 28–3. One-handed kitchen activities are learned in occupational therapy to enhance independence in the home. Illustrated are a one-handed egg beater, a one-handed nut chopper, and a simple method of holding the bowl steady. (Courtesy, Allied Service for the Handicapped, Inc., Scranton, Pennsylvania.)

the plastic tube from slipping a bulldog clip can be fastened to the edge of the glass and the tubing can be placed through the hole of the handle of the clip.

Aids in food preparation. Homemaking is the single most frequent occupation of the physically handicapped.[7] The rehabilitation of the homemaker in terms of food preparation skills and in overall homemaking activities benefits the entire family. Home economists, occupational therapists, and dietitians have specialized skills by which they are able to help the homemaker in simplification of procedures in food preparation and in more convenient kitchen arrangements.

The handicapped homemaker will find that each task requires a longer time to complete. As much food preparation should be completed in advance as possible so that there are few last-minute tasks. Arthritics fatigue easily and they should not attempt tasks that cannot be interrupted for a rest period. For many homemakers a list of things to be done is helpful.

Electric mixers, blenders, wedge-shape jar openers, electric can openers, long-handled tongs to reach packages and equipment out of reach, turntables in cupboards to hold supplies, sliding racks, magnetized equipment holders, and carts on wheels are among the pieces of equipment that facilitate work for the handicapped homemaker.

The person who has the use of only one arm needs firm support for devices. For example, a board with two stainless steel nails serves as a holder for vegetables to be peeled. (See Figure 28–3.) A sponge underneath a bowl helps to keep it from sliding. Boxes can be held firmly between the knees and a scissors can be used with one hand to cut off tops.

For those who will be confined to a wheelchair indefinitely or who must sit while working, a redesign of the kitchen is essential. Counter surfaces need to be lowered so that work can be done while sitting. Kneehole spaces are needed so that the chair or wheelchair can be partially underneath the work surface. Equipment and storage shelves must be within reach.

Dr. Howard Rusk has stated, "Rehabilitation, the fourth phase of medical care, can often be the most rewarding of all. Without wonder drugs, without scalpels, with only keen observation and a little ingenuity, millions of handicapped persons can resume relatively normal lives."*

*Rusk, H. A.: "Nutrition in the Fourth Phase of Medical Care," *Nutr. Today,* **5:** Autumn 1970, p. 31.

PROBLEMS AND REVIEW

1. Why is the term *discharge diet* undesirable?
2. Keep a record for a week of questions which relate to diet asked by patients under your care. How did you answer these questions?
3. *Problem.* Obtain a diet history from one of your patients who is receiving a normal diet. Use a form available in your hospital or develop one of your own. Evaluate the adequacy of the patient's diet according to the Four Food Groups. What recommendations can be made to the patient? How would you plan for this counseling?
4. Define these terms: coordinated home-care services; patient evaluation; homemaker service; programmed instruction; rehabilitation.
5. *Problem.* Determine the services available in your community for home care of patients. List the ways in which these services include nutritional care.
6. If you were asked to provide some guidelines for a group in your community which is setting up a meals-on-wheels service, what are the categories you would consider? What consultants would be desirable for this group?

CITED REFERENCES

1. "What 200 Agencies Are Saying about Medicare," *Nurs. Outlook,* **14:**30–32, June 1966.
2. Brandt, M. B.: "Perspective on Diet Manuals," *J. Am. Diet. Assoc.,* **47:**121–23, 1965.
3. Young, C. M.: "The Interview Itself," *J. Am. Diet. Assoc.,* **35:**677–81, 1959.
4. Hildreth, H. M.: "Hunger and Eating," *J. Am. Diet. Assoc.,* **31:**561–65, 1955.
5. McDonald, G. W., and Kaufman, M. B.: "Teaching Machines for Patients with Diabetes," *J. Am. Diet. Assoc.,* **42:**209–13, 1963.
6. Piper, G. M.: "Planning New Community Nutrition Services. Comprehensive Care Programs for the Aging," *J. Am. Diet. Assoc.,* **44:**461–64, 1965.
7. Rusk, H. A.: "Nutrition in the Fourth Phase of Medical Care," *Nutr. Today,* **5:**24–31, Autumn 1970.

8. Klinger, J. L., *et al.*: *Mealtime Manual for the Aged and Handicapped.* Simon and Schuster, Inc., New York, 1970.

ADDITIONAL REFERENCES

Barney, H. S., and Egan, M. C.: "Home Economists as Members of Health Teams," *J. Home Econ.*, **60**:427–31, 1968.

Coggeshall, L. T.: "Trends that Challenge Comprehensive Health Care," *J. Am. Diet. Assoc.*, **54**:191–93, 1969.

Coulter, P. P., and Brower, M. J.: "Parallel Experience: An Interview Technique," *Am. J. Nurs.*, **69**:1028–30, 1969.

Ford, C. S., *et al.*: "Home-delivered Meals Help Aged and Ill Live Independently," *Hospitals*, **42**:80–83, 1968, Aug. 1, 1968.

Hall, M. N.: "Home Health Aide Services Are Here to Stay," *Nurs. Outlook*, **14**:44–47, June 1966.

Johnson, D.: "Effective Diet Counseling Begins Early in Hospitalization," *Hospitals*, **41**:94–100, Jan. 16, 1967.

Knutson, A. L., and Newton, M. E.: "Behavioral Factors in Nutrition Education," *J. Am. Diet. Assoc.*, **37**:222–25, 1960.

Kornblueh, M., and Parke, H. C.: "Survey of the Use of Written Recipes," *J. Am. Diet. Assoc.*, **47**:113–15, 1965.

Matthews, L. I.: "Principles of Interviewing and Patient Counseling," *J. Am. Diet. Assoc.*, **50**:469–74, 1967.

May, E. E., *et al.*: *Homemaking for the Handicapped.* Dodd, Mead, and Company, Inc., New York, 1966.

Mohammed, M. F. B.: "Patients' Understanding of Written Health Information," *Nurs. Res.*, **13**:100–108, Spring 1964.

Moore, M. C., *et al.*: "Using Graduated Food Models in Taking Dietary Histories," *J. Am. Diet. Assoc.*, **51**:447–50, 1967.

Morris, E.: "How Does a Nurse Teach Nutrition to Patients?" *Am. J. Nurs.*, **60**:67–70, Jan. 1960.

Paynich, M. L.: "Cultural Barriers to Communication," *Am. J. Nurs.*, **64**:87–90, Feb. 1964.

Piper, G. M.: "Nutrition Services in Home Health Agencies," *J. Am. Diet. Assoc.*, **50**:23–25, 1967.

Rusk, H. A., *et al.*: *A Manual for Training the Disabled Homemaker.* Rehabilitation Monograph 8, Ed. 2. Institute of Rehabilitation Medicine, New York University Medical Center, New York, 1961.

———: *Rehabilitation Medicine.* C. V. Mosby Company, St. Louis, 1964.

Skiff, A. W.: "Programmed Instruction and Patient Teaching," *Am. J. Public Health*, **55**:409–15, 1965.

29 Therapeutic Adaptations of the Normal Diet

Normal, Soft, and Fluid Diets

Therapeutic nutrition begins with the normal diet. Normal and therapeutic diets are planned to maintain, or restore, good nutrition in the patient. In diet manuals the normal diet may be designated as *regular, house, normal,* or *full diet*. It may consist of any and all foods eaten by the person in health. Fried foods, pastries, strongly flavored vegetables, spices, and relishes are not taboo, but good menu planning means that these foods are used judiciously. The normal diet satisfies the nutritional needs for most patients and also serves as the basis for planning modified diets.

The nutritive contributions of a basic diet composed of recommended levels from each of the Four Food Groups were discussed in Unit II and are summarized in Table 13–2. One of the many ways by which such a foundation diet may be amplified to provide meal patterns that are typical in many hospitals is shown in Table 29–1. In the suggested additions to the basic list of foods an additional cup of milk is included because it provides important amounts of several nutrients that are likely to be needed in in-creased amounts by many patients. Contrary to the opinion held by some, milk is one of the best-accepted foods in the hospital dietary.

To use the normal diet as the basis for therapeutic diets is sound in that it emphasizes the similarity of psychologic and social needs of those who are ill with those who are well, even though there may be differences in quantitative or qualitative requirements. Insofar as possible the patient is provided a food allowance that avoids the connotation of a "special" diet that sets him apart from his family and friends. Moreover, in the home, food preparation is simplified when the modified diet is based upon the family pattern, and the number of items requiring special preparation is reduced to a minimum.

Although it is desirable that the normal diet provide the basis for planning modified diets, it must be remembered that the nutritional requirements of patients are likely to vary widely. The Recommended Dietary Allowances are designed to meet the nutritional needs for almost all healthy persons in the United States, and they should not be interpreted as being appropriate allowances during illness. For any given patient the nutritional requirements depend upon his nutritional status, modifications in activity, increased or decreased metabolic demands made by the illness, and the efficiency of digestive, absorptive, and excretory mechanisms.

Many adaptations to the plan presented in Table 29–1 could be devised for varying cultural and socoieconomic circumstances. The calculated values for the basic plan are useful in determining the effects of the omission or addition of foods to such a plan. For example, if a patient is allergic to milk, the plan shows that adjustment would need to be made especially for calcium, riboflavin, and protein. Or, if the intake of vegetables and fruits were to be curtailed, it is obvious that there would be a deficiency of vitamin A and ascorbic acid and that a supplement of vitamins should be prescribed.

REGULAR OR NORMAL DIET

Include these foods, or their nutritive equivalents, daily:
2–3 cups milk

4 ounces (cooked weight) meat, fish, or poultry; cheese, additional egg or milk, or legumes
    may substitute in part
1 egg
3–4 servings vegetables including:
    1 medium potato
    1 serving dark-green leafy or yellow vegetable
    1–2 servings other vegetable
    One of the above vegetables to be served raw
3 servings fruit including:
    1 serving citrus fruit, or other good source of ascorbic acid
    2 servings other fruit
1 serving enriched or whole-grain cereal
3 slices enriched or whole-grain bread
Additional foods such as butter or fortified margarine, soups, desserts, sweets, salad dressings,
or increased amounts of foods listed above will provide adequate calories. See calculation in
Table 29–1.

Meal Pattern	Sample Menu
BREAKFAST	
Fruit	Sliced banana in orange juice
Cereal, enriched or whole-grain	Oatmeal
Milk and sugar for cereal	Milk and sugar
Egg	Soft-cooked egg
Whole-grain or enriched roll or toast	Whole-wheat toast with butter
Butter or margarine	
Hot beverage with cream and sugar	Coffee with cream and sugar
LUNCHEON OR SUPPER	
Soup, if desired	
Egg or a substitute of cheese, meat, or fish	Cheese soufflé
Potato, rice, noodles, macaroni, spaghetti, or vegetable	Buttered peas
Salad	Lettuce and tomato salad
Enriched or whole-grain bread	Russian dressing
Butter or margarine	Hard roll with butter
Fruit	Royal Anne cherries
Milk	Milk
DINNER	
Meat, fish or poultry	Meat loaf with gravy
Potato	Mashed potato
Vegetable	Buttered carrots
Enriched or whole-grain bread	Enriched white, rye, or whole-wheat bread with butter
Butter or margarine	
Dessert	Apple Betty
Milk	Milk
Coffee or tea, if desired	

Therapeutic modifications of the normal diet. The normal diet may be modified (1) to provide change in consistency as in fluid and soft diets to be described below; (2) to increase or decrease the energy values; (3) to include greater of lesser amounts of one or more nutrients, for example, high protein, low sodium; (4) to increase or decrease bulk—high- and low-fiber diets; (5) to provide foods bland in flavor; (6) to include or exclude specific foods, as in allergic conditions; and (7) to modify the intervals of feeding.

Rationale for modified diets. The principles for diet therapy in many pathologic conditions are well established, and dietary regimens are based upon a sound rationale. In such regimens the food allowances may vary according to ethnic and socioeconomic factors. It is to be expected that differences in interpretation will be found in the detailed descriptions of diet that are presented in the diet manuals of hospitals. Some of these differences are caused by the fact that some modified diets have only an empiric basis. Research to establish the merits of a particular regimen as opposed to another is difficult to control because of the numerous physiologic and psychologic variables in human beings. Fortunately, a number of widely varying dietary programs may be equally effective because of the remarkable response of the human body.

Probably no diets are more subject to criticism than those modified for fiber and flavor. In order to reduce the fiber content of a diet, meats may be ground and vegetables and fruits strained. Yet, experience has shown that few patients consume such foods in satisfactory amounts, and the harm to nutritional status is likely to be greater than the possible insult to the mucosa of the gastrointestinal tract.

Some patients experience heartburn, abdominal distention, and flatulence following the ingestion of strongly flavored vegetables, dry beans or peas, and melons. Other patients refuse to eat these foods simply because they have been told that they are poorly digested. There is no evidence that justifies the omission of these foods for all patients.[1] Although dietitians and nurses have a responsibility to correct food misinformation whenever it is encountered, little is gained by coercing someone who is ill into eating a food that he dislikes intensely or against which he has a prejudice.

Diet manuals and dietary patterns. Numerous manuals are available as guides in the standardization of dietary procedures for a given hospital. The best of these manuals have been prepared by committees including representatives of the various medical specialties, nursing, and dietary departments. The manual generally includes statements concerning principles of diet, food allowances with detailed lists of foods to use and to avoid, typical meal patterns, and nutritive evaluations. They serve as a guide for the physician in prescribing a diet, a reference for the nurse, a procedural manual for the dietary department, and a teaching tool for professional personnel.

Although a manual achieves standardization in procedures, it does *not* mean that every patient on a given diet must have exactly the same food allowances as every other patient. In fact, within the guide ample opportunity is provided for individualization of a given patient's regimen. The diet manual is *not* an instructional guide for the patient for whom individualized and more detailed aids are necessary. It may, however, serve as the basis for the development of such teaching aids.

Through this text dietary regimens which are representative of those used in many hospitals are presented. Each description includes a statement of characteristics, lists of foods to include, detailed lists of foods permitted and contraindicated, a typical meal pattern, and a sample menu. The student will learn much by comparing one regimen with another and will begin to understand the rationale for diet therapy and how the goals may be achieved in a number of ways.

Nomenclature of diets. Insofar as possible, the nomenclature used in this text will describe the modification in consistency, in nutrients, or in flavor; thus *bland* diet, *1200-calorie* diet, etc. When the quantity of one or more nutrients is important to the success of the diet, it is essential that these quantities be specified in the diet prescription. Thus, the term *diabetic diet* has little meaning, but a prescription for 200 gm carbohydrate, 80 gm protein, and 90 gm fat can be accurately interpreted. Likewise, a *sodium-restricted* diet gives no indication of the exact level of restriction required, but the designation *500-mg sodium diet* leaves no room for misinterpretation.

Several undesirable practices have been, and still are, common in the naming of diets. The literature is replete with illustrations of diets named for their originators. The Sippy diet is a classic example, but there have been others from time to time. Unfortunately, such nomenclature tells nothing about the diet, and the practice should be discouraged.

Table 29–1. Nutritive Value of the Normal Diet Pattern as a Basis for Therapeutic Diets.*

Food	Measure	Weight gm	Energy calories	Protein gm	Fat gm	Carbohydrate gm	Minerals Ca mg	Fe mg	Vitamins A I.U.	Thiamine mg	Riboflavin mg	Niacin mg	Ascorbic Acid mg
Milk	2 cups	488	320	18	18	24	576	0.2	700	0.14	0.82	0.4	4
Meat Group													
Egg	1	50	80	6	6	tr	27	1.1	590	0.05	0.15	tr	0
Meat, fish, poultry (lean, cooked)	4 ounces	120	240	33	10	0	17	3.6	35	0.32	0.26	7.4	0
Vegetable-Fruit Group													
Leafy green or deep yellow	1/2–2/3 cup	100	30	2	tr	6	28	1.0	7400	0.06	0.08	0.6	28
Other vegetable	1/2–2/3 cup	100	30	2	tr	6	20	0.8	480	0.06	0.06	0.6	14
Potato	1 serving	122	80	2	tr	18	7	0.6	tr	0.11	0.04	1.4	20
Citrus fruit†	1 serving	100	40	1	tr	10	10	0.2	160	0.07	0.02	0.3	40
Other fruit	2 servings	200	120	2	tr	32	24	1.0	1200	0.08	0.08	0.8	18
Bread-Cereal Group													
Cereal, enriched or whole grain	3/4 cup	30 (dry)	105	3	tr	22	10	0.8	0	0.12	0.04	0.8	0
Bread, enriched or whole grain	3 slices	75	210	6	3	39	63	1.8	tr	0.18	0.15	1.8	tr
			1255	75	37	157	782	11.1	10,565	1.19	1.70	14.1‡	124
Additional Foods													
Milk	1 cup	244	160	9	9	12	288	0.1	350	0.07	0.41	0.2	2
Butter or margarine	4 pats	28	200	tr	24	tr	6	0	940	—			—
Sugars, sweets	3 tablespoons	33	120	0	0	33	0	0	0	0	0	0	0
Dessert§	1 serving	varies	190	4	6	30	70	0.3	190	0.03	0.10	0.1	tr
Bread	3 slices	75	210	6	3	39	63	1.8	tr	0.18	0.15	1.8	0
Total Nutritive Value			2135	94	79	271	1209	13.3	12,045	1.47	2.36	16.2	126

*The nutritive values of the foods listed for the normal diet, pages 400–401, have been calculated using Table A–1 in the Appendix. The additional foods listed at the bottom of the table suggest one of many ways to complete the diet.

†Other ascorbic-acid-rich foods such as cantaloupe and strawberries are also included.

‡The tryptophan content of this diet is about 750 mg, equivalent to 12.5 mg niacin, thus providing a niacin equivalent of 26.6 mg.

§ Desserts include plain gelatin, cake with icing, custard, ice cream, cookies, and plain pudding.

Others have used the name of a disease condition to specify a given diet, such as ulcer, ambulatory ulcer, ulcer discharge, cardiac, and gallbladder diets. Psychologically, this is not good practice, for the patient should not need to be reminded of his condition every time he looks at a diet list, or every time he notes the name of his diet on a tray card. Moreover, the diets used for many of these conditions have multiple uses, and the uninitiated may overlook the full usefulness of a given regimen with such disease-oriented terminology.

Frequency of feeding. Research on experimental animals and on humans has shown that more than three meals daily may be desirable for some patients. When the patient eats five, six, or more meals a day which are approximately balanced for protein, fat, and carbohydrate the metabolic load at a given time is less, and the nutrients can be more effectively utilized. It is well known that protein is inefficiently used if the day's allowance is more or less concentrated in one meal. Large amounts of carbohydrate at a given meal require the use of alternate metabolic pathways which favor the deposition of fat.

Norton[2] has described the principles for adapting home diets of patients to a six- or seven-meal program: breakfast, midmorning, luncheon, midafternoon, dinner, early evening, and late bedtime. She points out that the patient's daily food needs should be divided into the six or seven meals, with some protein, fat, and carbohydrate in each. Thus, milk or a protein sandwich may be useful for interval feedings, but juices or sweets alone do not satisfy the requirements. The interval between meals should be 1½ to 3 hours, with meals spread throughout the waking hours.

A bedtime snack is believed by some to enhance sleep, whereas others claim that it interferes with sleep. Hamilton and associates[3] recently studied the effects of snacks or their omission on 36 male subjects including students and patients with tuberculosis. The 275-calorie snack consisted of cereal with sugar and milk given at bedtime. A recorder was used to note the bed movements of the subject, and a psychologic rating scale concerning the subject's evaluation of his sleep was completed on the following morning. No measurable differences between snack and no-snack periods were found either in the patterns of body movements or in the psychologic evaluations.

On the basis of these studies any of the modified diets might be presented in more than three meals. A judicious choice of bedtime snacks apparently does not modify sleep.

Mechanical soft diet. Many persons require a soft diet simply because they have no teeth. It is neither desirable nor essential to restrict the patient to the selection allowed on the customary soft diet (page 405) employed for a postoperative patient or for a patient with a gastrointestinal disturbance. For example, stewed onions, baked beans, and apple pie are foods considered to be quite unsuitable for the latter patients but which may be enjoyed by those who simply require foods that are soft in texture. The terms *mechanical soft* and *dental soft* are used in some diet manuals to describe such a dietary modification. The following changes in the normal diet will usually suffice for individuals without teeth:

Meats should be finely minced or ground.

Soft breads are substituted for crusty breads.

Cooked vegetables may be used without restriction, but dicing or chopping may be desirable for some; for example, diced beets, chopped spinach, corn cut from cob.

Most raw vegetables are omitted; raw tomatoes, cut finely, may usually be used. Sometimes finely chopped lettuce in a sandwich may be accepted.

Many raw fruits may be used: banana, orange, grapefruit, soft berries, soft pear, apricots, peaches, grapes with tender skins.

Hard raw fruits such as pineapple and apple are usually avoided; but finely diced apple in fruit cup may be used.

Tough skins should be removed from fruits: raw, soft pear, or baked apple, etc.

Nuts and dried fruits, when used in desserts or other foods, are acceptable if finely chopped.

Soft diet. This diet represents the usual dietary step between the full fluid and normal diet. It may be used in acute infections, some gastrointestinal disturbances, and following surgery. The diet is soft in consistency, easy to chew, made up of simple, easily digestible food, and contains no harsh fiber, no rich or highly flavored food. It is nutritionally adequate when planned on the basis of the normal diet.

Soft Diet

Include these foods, or their nutritive equivalents, daily:

2–3 cups milk
   4 ounces (cooked weight) very tender or ground meat, fish, or poultry; soft cheese, or additional eggs or milk may substitute in part
   1 egg
3–4 servings vegetable including:
   1 medium potato
   1 serving dark-green or yellow vegetable—tender chopped or strained
   2 servings other vegetable—tender chopped or strained
   3 servings fruit including:
   2 servings citrus fruit or juice
   1 serving banana, cooked fruit without skin or seeds, or strained cooked fruit
   1 serving enriched or strained whole-grain cereal
   3 slices enriched or fine whole-grain bread
Additional foods such as butter or fortified margarine, soups, desserts, sweets, or increased amounts of the above will provide adequate calories.

Nutritive value. See calculation for the normal diet in Table 29–1.

Foods Allowed

All beverages

Bread—white, fine whole wheat, rye without seeds; white crackers

Cereal foods—dry, such as cornflakes, Puffed Rice, rice flakes; fine cooked, such as cornmeal, farina, hominy grits, macaroni, noodles, rice, spaghetti; strained coarse, such as oatmeal, Pettijohn's, whole-wheat

Cheese—mild, soft, such as cottage and cream; Cheddar; Swiss

Desserts—plain cake, cookies; custards; plain gelatin or with allowed fruit; Junket; plain ice cream, ices, sherbets; plain puddings, such as bread, cornstarch, rice, tapioca

Eggs—all except fried

Fats—butter, cream, margarine, vegetable oils and fats in cooking

Fruits—raw: ripe avocado, banana, grapefruit or orange sections without membrane; canned or cooked: apples, apricots, fruit cocktail, peaches, pears, plums—all without skins; Royal Anne cherries; strained prunes and other fruits with skins; all juices

Meat—very tender, minced, or ground; baked, broiled, creamed, roast, or stewed: beef, lamb, veal, poultry, fish, bacon, liver, sweetbreads

Foods to Avoid

Bread—coarse dark; whole-grain crackers; hot breads; pancakes; waffles

Cereals—bran; coarse unless strained

Cheese—sharp, such as Roquefort, Camembert, Limburger

Desserts—any made with dried fruit or nuts; pastries; rich puddings or cake

Eggs—fried

Fats—fried foods

Fruits—raw except as listed; stewed or canned berries; with tough skins

Meat—tough with gristle or fat; salted and smoked meat or fish, such as corned beef, smoked herring; cold cuts; frankfurter; pork

Milk—in any form

Soups—broth, strained cream or vegetable

Sweets—all sugars, syrup, jelly, honey, plain sugar
candy without fruit or nuts, molasses
Use in moderation.

Vegetables—white or sweet potato without skin, any
way except fried; young and tender asparagus,
beets, carrots, peas, pumpkin, squash without
seeds; tender chopped greens; strained cooked
vegetables if not tender; tomato juice

Miscellaneous—salt, seasonings and spices in moderation, gravy, cream sauces

Soups—fatty or highly seasoned

Sweets—jam, marmalade, rich candies with chocolate

Vegetables—raw; strongly flavored, such as broccoli,
Brussels sprouts, cabbage, cauliflower, cucumber,
onion, radish, sauerkraut, turnip; corn; dried beans
and peas; potato chips

Miscellaneous—pepper and other hot spices; fried
foods; nuts; olives; pickles; relishes

Meal Pattern

BREAKFAST

Fruit or fruit juice

Cereal—strained, if coarse

Milk and sugar for cereal

Egg

Soft roll or toast

Butter or fortified margarine

Hot beverage with cream and sugar

LUNCHEON OR SUPPER

Strained soup, if desired

Egg or substitute of mild cheese, tender or ground
meat, fish or poultry

Potato without skin, rice, noodles, macaroni, or
spaghetti; or

Cooked vegetable

Enriched bread

Butter or fortified margarine

Fruit

Milk

Coffee or tea, if desired

DINNER

Orange, grapefruit, or tomato juice

Tender or ground meat, fish, or poultry

Potato, any way except fried

Cooked vegetable

Enriched bread

Butter or fortified margarine

Dessert

Milk

Hot beverage with cream and sugar, if desired

Sample Menu

Orange sections and banana slices

Oatmeal

Milk and sugar for cereal

Soft-cooked egg

Buttered toast

Coffee

Cream of tomato soup

Cheese soufflé

Tender peas

Soft roll

Butter

Royal Anne cherries

Milk

Coffee or tea, if desired

Grapefruit juice

Meat loaf (no onion or pepper) with gravy

Mashed potato

Buttered carrots

Rye bread without seeds

Butter

Baked apple without skin; cream

Milk

Tea with sugar and lemon

Liquid diets. Fluid diets are used in febrile
states, postoperatively, or whenever the patient
is unable to tolerate solid foods. The degree to
which these diets are adequate will depend upon
the type of liquids permitted.

Clear-fluid diets. Whenever an acute illness
or surgery produces a marked intolerance for

food as may be evident by nausea, vomiting,
anorexia, distention, and diarrhea, it is advisable
to restrict the intake of nutrients. A clear-fluid
diet is usually used for one to two days, at the
end of which time the patient is usually able to
utilize a more liberal liquid diet.

Tea with lemon and sugar, coffee, fat-free

broth, carbonated beverages, and cereal waters are the usual liquids permitted. In addition, strained fruit juices, fruit ices, and plain gelatin are often included. A more liberal clear-fluid diet permits the addition of egg white, whole egg, and gelatin to strained fruit juices and other beverages.

The amount of fluid in a given feeding on the clear-fluid diet is usually restricted to 30 to 60 ml per hour at first, with gradually increasing amounts being given as the patient's tolerance improves. Obviously, such a diet can accomplish little beyond the replacement of fluids.

Full-fluid diet. This diet is indicated whenever a patient is acutely ill or is unable to chew or swallow solid food. It includes all foods liquid at room temperature and at body temperature. It is free from cellulose and irritating condiments. When properly planned, this diet can be used for relatively long periods of time. However, iron is provided at inadequate levels.

FULL-FLUID DIET

General rules
Give six or more feedings daily.

The protein content of the diet can be increased by incorporating nonfat dry milk in beverages and soups. Strained canned meats (used for infant feeding) may be added to broths.

The caloric value of the diet may be increased by: (1) substituting 10 per cent cream for part of the usual milk allowance; (2) adding butter to cereal gruels and soups; (3) including glucose in beverages; (4) using ice cream as dessert or in beverages.

If a decreased volume of fluid is desired, nonfat dry milk may be substituted for part of the fluid milk.

Include these foods, or their nutritive equivalents daily:
6 cups milk

2 eggs (in custards or pasteurized eggnog)

1–2 ounces strained meat

½ cup fine or strained whole-grain cooked cereal for gruel

¼ cup vegetable purée for cream soup

1 cup citrus fruit juices; plus other strained juices

½ cup tomato or vegetable juice

1 tablespoon cocoa

3 tablespoons sugar

1 tablespoon butter

2 servings plain gelatin dessert, Junket, soft or baked custard, ices, sherbets, plain ice cream, or plain cornstarch pudding

Broth, bouillon, or clear soups

Tea, coffee, carbonated beverages as desired

Flavoring extracts, salt

Nutritive values of foods listed in specified amounts: Calories, 1950; protein, 85 gm; calcium, 2.1 gm; iron, 7.7 mg; vitamin A, 7150 I.U.; thiamine, 1.1 mg; riboflavin, 3.2 mg; niacin equivalents, 19.1 mg; ascorbic acid, 160 mg.

Meal Pattern	Sample Menu
BREAKFAST	
Citrus juice	Orange juice
Cereal gruel with butter, sugar	Cream of wheat with milk, butter, and sugar
Milk	
Beverage with cream, sugar	Coffee with cream and sugar

MIDMORNING

Fruit juice with egg   Lemonade with egg white

     or

Milk, plain, malted, chocolate, or eggnog
  (pasteurized)

  LUNCHEON OR SUPPER

Strained soup   Beef broth with strained meat

Tomato juice   Tomato juice

Custard, Junket, ice cream, sherbet, ice, gelatin   Maple Junket
  dessert or plain pudding

Eggnog, milk, or cocoa   Milk

Tea with sugar, if desired   Tea with sugar and cream

  MIDAFTERNOON

Same as at midmorning   Pineapple eggnog (pasteurized)

  DINNER

Strained cream soup   Cream of carrot soup

Citrus juice   Grapefruit juice

Custard, Junket, ice cream, ice, sherbet, or gelatin   Vanilla ice cream
  dessert

Milk or cocoa   Cocoa

Tea, if desired   Tea with sugar and lemon

  EVENING NOURISHMENT

Same as at midmorning   Hot malted milk

Other methods of feeding. Food by mouth is the method of choice when the patient can eat, digest, and absorb sufficient food to meet his nutritive requirements. In illness, however, it is occasionally necessary to augment the oral intake by giving parenteral feedings of one type or another.

When the patient is unable to chew or swallow because of deformity or inflammation of the mouth or throat, corrosive poisoning, unconsciousness, paralysis of the throat muscles, etc., tube feeding is used (see page 498).

Intravenous feeding is used when it is necessary to rest the patient's stomach completely. Fluids given by such means include solutions of glucose, amino acids, salts, and vitamins. Transfusions of whole blood or of plasma are commonly used.

PROBLEMS AND REVIEW

1. What is meant by routine house diets?
2. Why is the normal diet used as a basis for planning therapeutic diets?
3. What are the advantages of using a diet manual for planning diets? What are the limitations?
4. What objections can you see to the following examples of dietary nomenclature: nephritic diet; Kempner diet; low-protein diet; ulcer discharge diet? Examine the nomenclature used for diets in your hospital, and suggest ways for improvement.
5. *Problem.* Write a menu for one day for a patient to receive a regular diet. Modify this pattern for a patient who is unable to chew foods well.
6. *Problem.* Prepare a table that shows the food intake for one day by a patient receiving a full-fluid diet. Calculate the protein, energy, and ascorbic acid intake.
7. *Problem.* Prepart a chart that shows the dietary orders for five patients. On this chart include a statement concerning the reasons for the diet order and the patient's acceptance of his diet.

CITED REFERENCES

1. Joint Committee, American Dietetic Association and American Medical Association: "Diet as Related to Gastrointestinal Function," *J. Am. Diet Assoc.*, **38**:425, 1961.
2. Norton, M.: "Practical Aspects of Serving Meals More Frequently," *J. Am. Diet. Assoc.*, **48**:505–509, 1966.
3. Hamilton, L. H., *et al.:* Effect of a Bedtime Snack on Sleep," *J. Am. Diet. Assoc.*, **48**:395–98, 1966.

ADDITIONAL REFERENCES

Balsley, M.: "A Look at Selected Diet Manuals," *J. Am. Diet. Assoc.*, **47**:123–26, 1965.
Barnes, R. H.: "Doctors' Dietary Antics," *Nutr. Today*, 3:21–25, Sept. 1968.
Brandt, M. B.: "Perspective on Diet Manuals," *J. Am. Diet. Assoc.*, **47**:121–23, 1965.
Robinson, C.: "Dietary Nomenclature," *J. Am. Diet. Assoc.*, **28**:640–44, 1952.
————: "Food Therapy Begins with the Normal Diet," *J. Clin. Nutr.*, **1**:150–53, 1953.

30 Dietary Calculation Using the Food Exchange Lists

Need for quick methods of dietary calculation. To provide for the nutritional needs of the patient the nurse and dietitian are frequently expected to make quick, yet reasonably accurate, estimations of nutritive values of diets. Some therapeutic diets must be planned within a stated maximum of one or more nutrients, for example, the low-fat diet. For other diets, such as that used for diabetic patients, carbohydrate, protein, and fat levels must be kept within relatively narrow allowances of the prescription. Sometimes a physician may request that the intake of protein or calories be charted from day to day for patients who are presenting nutritional problems.

The uses of Table A–1 have been described in Chapter 3, so that the student undoubtedly has had some experiences with dietary calculation on the basis of this table. It soon becomes evident that day-to-day calculations of all the listed nutrients—or even for selected nutrients—are much too time consuming for the nurse or dietitian with many responsibilities. Such detailed calculations are not justified unless great care is also taken in controlling the preparation procedures, and accurately measuring or weighing all food served to the patient and likewise all food which is returned on the tray. Moreover, the body itself varies from day to day in its net utilization of food, depending upon activity,

endocrine balance, and the proportions of nutrients presented to it. Thus, it is evident that dietary calculation should be directed to reasonable assurances of control without time-wasting paper work. To this end, a short method of dietary calculation will be discussed here.

FOOD EXCHANGE LISTS

Evolution of the food exchange lists. Probably the classic example requiring rapid dietary calculations is afforded by the diet used for the diabetic patient. At one time these calculations were time consuming. Far too much faith was placed on decimal point calculations, with too little understanding of the variability of food composition and of body utilization. Many short tables of food composition were developed for the calculation of diets, but to the patient the variations existing in them were confusing to say the least. Incorporating the best features of several methods in use, the food exchange lists (Table A–4) were evolved and published in 1950 by a joint committee of the American Dietetic Association, the American Diabetes Association, and the United States Public Health Service.[1]

These lists are now used for most diets for diabetic patients. With some experience the nurse and dietitian find that calculations can be made rapidly. Patients soon learn how to use the lists for planning a wide variety of menus within their daily food allowances. The wide use of the exchange method of dietary planning means that patients can move from one community to another without experiencing the frustrations of using different and often contradictory lists. The food exchange lists not only are used for calculating diets for diabetic patients, but have many applications in the planning of other diets that require control of calories, protein, fat, and/or carbohydrate.

More recently other lists have been developed for specialized needs such as the sodium-restricted diet (pages 564–70) and the fat-controlled diet (pages 552–53). The overall groupings of foods in these lists are similar but differences in food selection within the lists soon become obvious. The general procedure for dietary calculation described below is also applicable to these diets.

Six exchange lists. An exchange list is a grouping of foods in which specified amounts of all the foods listed are of approximately equal carbohydrate, protein, and fat value. Specific foods within the lists may differ slightly in their nutritive value from the averages stated for the group. (See Table 30–1.) These differences in composition tend to cancel out because of the variety of foods selected from day to day. Thus, any food within a given list can be substituted or exchanged for any other food in that list. In the fruit list, for example, 1 small apple, or ½ banana, or 2 prunes, or ½ cup orange juice would contain 10 gm carbohydrate.

Milk list. One cup of whole milk is the basis for this list. Evaporated milk or dry whole milk may be substituted in appropriate amounts. Skim milk, buttermilk, and nonfat dry milk contain no fat so that an adjustment must be made. For each cup of liquid nonfat milk used, two fat exchanges should be added to the diet; or, if nonfat milk is used on a daily basis the milk allowance would be calculated to provide 12 gm carbohydrate, 8 gm protein, and 0 gm fat per cupful.

Note that cheeses are listed with meat exchanges; cream, cream cheese, and butter are listed as fat exchanges; and ice cream is included with the bread exchanges.

Vegetable lists. Vegetables are listed in two groups, A and B. Some vegetables high in carbohydrate are included in the bread list. Group A vegetables are so low in carbohydrate and in calories that, for most diets, no calculation need be made for the first cupful used each day. When a second cupful is used, it would be calculated as one exchange of group B vegetable (7 gm carbohydrate, 2 gm protein).

Fruit list. Each fruit in the amount stated supplies 10 gm carbohydrate. Many of the fruits are in average-size servings, but some are not. For example, 2 prunes, 1 fig, and ¼ cup grape juice would be smaller-than-average servings. It is important, therefore, not to use the terms *exchange* and *serving* interchangeably.

Bread list. One slice of bread is the basis for the exchanges in this list. Included are biscuits, muffins, and rolls; dry and cooked breakfast cereals; grits, macaroni, noodles, spaghetti, and rice; crackers; and a number of vegetables— corn, Lima beans, baked beans, cooked dry beans and peas, white potato, and sweet potato. Ice cream and plain sponge cake also appear on this list.

Meat list. One ounce of cooked medium-fat meat, poultry, or fish is used as the basis for this list. On a raw-weight basis this is equivalent to about 1⅓ ounces of edible portion; thus, one would need to purchase 4 ounces of raw meat, edible portion, to equal a 3-ounce serving of cooked meat. It is assumed that the visible fat is trimmed off, but a wide selection of meat cuts including those marbled with fat is permissible.

Luncheon meats, canned fish, shellfish, Cheddar, American, Swiss, and cottage cheese, eggs, and peanut butter in the amounts listed are exchanges for meat.

Table 30–1. Composition of Food Exchange Lists*

Food Exchange	Measure	Weight gm	Carbohydrate gm	Protein gm	Fat gm	Calories
Milk, whole	1 cup	240	12	8	10	170
Milk, nonfat	1 cup	240	12	8	—	80
Vegetables—A	As desired	—	—	—	—	—
Vegetables—B	1/2 cup	100	7	2	—	35
Fruit	Varies		10	—	—	40
Bread	Varies		15	2	—	70
Meat	1 ounce	30	—	7	5	75
Fat	1 teaspoon	5	—	—	5	45

*Consult Table A–4 for food selections for each of the exchange lists.

Fat list. This list is based upon 1 teaspoon of butter. It includes margarine, solid fats and oils used in cooking, bacon, light and heavy cream, cream cheese, salad dressings, nuts, avocado, and olives.

Miscellaneous list. Coffee, tea, broth, spices, herbs, and some other items are insignificant for their nutritive values but they lend interest to the diet. They may be included in dietary plans without calculation.

Assuring mineral and vitamin adequacy. Since the exchange lists do not provide information on mineral and vitamin values it becomes evident that some degree of discretion must be used in establishing the daily food allowances and in selecting specific menus. For example, 2 cups of milk daily will supply sufficient calcium and riboflavin for the adult; 3 to 4 cups of milk would be included in the diet plan of children and pregnant or lactating women. At least two fruit exchanges are included daily, one of these being selected from those fruits rich in ascorbic acid. Fruits that are good sources of this vitamin are marked with an asterisk in the listing. Vegetables are often neglected in dietary planning or are restricted to a few choices. Those that are dark green or deep yellow are excellent sources of vitamin A, and one of these should be included daily. Note that vitamin-A-rich vegetables have been starred in the vegetable lists.

Procedure for calculation. The calculation of a diet requires only the nutritive values of Table 30–1. Let us suppose that the following diet prescription is to be calculated: carbohydrate, 185 gm; protein, 75 gm; and fat, 80 gm. A daily food allowance for this prescription is shown in Table 30–2, using the procedures described below.

1. Estimate the amounts of milk, vegetables, and fruits to be included. The allowances are dictated somewhat by the preferences of the patient, but the following amounts are minimum levels that should ordinarily be included:

Milk—2 cups for adults; 3 to 4 cups for children and
  for pregnant or lactating women
Vegetables, Group A—1 exchange
        Group B—1 exchange
Fruit—2 exchanges

2. Fill in the carbohydrate, protein, and fat values for the tentative amounts of milk, vegetables, and fruits.

3. To determine the number of bread exchanges: Total the carbohydrate value of the milk, vegetables, and fruit. Subtract this total from the total amount of carbohydrate prescribed. Divide the remainder by 15 (the carbohydrate value of one bread exchange). Use the nearest whole number of bread exchanges. Fill in the carbohydrate and protein values.

4. Total the carbohydrate column. If the total deviates more than 3 or 4 gm from the prescribed amount, adjust the amounts of vegetable, fruit, and bread. No diet should be planned with fractions of an exchange since awkward measures of food would sometimes be encountered.

5. To determine the number of meat exchanges: Total the protein value of the milk, vegetable, and bread. Subtract this total from the amount of protein prescribed. Divide the remainder by 7 (the protein value of one meat exchange). Use the nearest whole number of meat exchanges. Fill in the protein and fat values.

6. To determine the number of fat exchanges: Total the fat values for milk and meat. Subtract this total from the amount of fat prescribed. Divide the remainder by 5 (the fat content of one fat exchange). Fill in the fat value.

7. Check the entire diet for the accuracy of the computations. Divide the daily food allowance into a meal pattern suitable for the individual. For some diets the distribution of food may be specified in the prescription.

The following menu illustrates one way that the day's food allowance for the diet shown in Table 30–2 could be used. Another menu is shown on page 516 in the adaptation for a patient with diabetes.

BREAKFAST
Stewed prunes—2
Dry cereal—¾ cup
Milk—1 cup
Plain muffin—1
Butter—1 teaspoon
  LUNCHEON
Sandwich
  Rye bread—2 slices

Luncheon meat—1 slice
Swiss cheese—1 slice
Lettuce
Mayonnaise—2 teaspoons
Celery and radishes
Peach, fresh—1 medium
Milk—1 cup
  DINNER
Skewered lamb and vegetables
  Lamb—3 ounces
  Onions—4 small
  Tomato wedges
  Mushroom caps

Green-pepper strips
Oil—1 teaspoon for basting meat and vegetables
  while cooking
Rice—½ cup
Dinner roll—1
Butter—1 teaspoon
Fruit cup (2 exchanges fruit)
  Banana—½
  Blueberries—⅓ cup
  Grapes—6
  EVENING SNACK
Milk—1 cup
Graham crackers—2

Table 30–2. Calculation of Diet Using Food Exchange Lists
(Carbohydrate: 185 gm; Protein: 75 gm; Fat: 80 gm)

List	Food	Measure	Weight gm	Carbohydrate gm	Protein gm	Fat gm
1	Milk	3 cups	720	36	24	30
2	Vegetable					
	group A	Up to 1 cup		—	—	—
	group B	1/2 cup	100	7	2	—
3	Fruit	4 exchanges	Varies	40	—	—
				83		
4	Bread	7 exchanges	Varies	105	14	—
					40	
5	Meat	5 exchanges	Varies	—	35	25
						55
6	Fat	5 exchanges	Varies	—	—	25
				188	**75**	**80**

185 gm carbohydrate prescribed total
 83 gm carbohydrate from milk, vegetables, and fruit

102 gm carbohydrate to be supplied from bread exchanges
            102 ÷ 15 = 7 bread exchanges

 75 gm protein prescribed total
 40 gm protein from milk, vegetable, and bread exchanges

 35 gm protein to be supplied from meat exchanges
            35 ÷ 7 = 5 meat exchanges

 80 gm fat prescribed total
 55 gm fat from milk and meat exchanges

 25 gm fat to be supplied from fat exchanges
            25 ÷ 5 = 5 fat exchanges

PROBLEMS AND REVIEW

1. How do you explain the fact that Cheddar and cottage cheese are listed as meat exchanges, but that they are included in the milk group of the Four Food Groups (page 197)?
2. Which vegetables in the A group are especially rich in vitamin A? In iron? In ascorbic acid?
3. Explain the placement of potatoes, corn, Lima beans, and baked beans in the bread exchange list.
4. *Problem.* Plan a menu for a lunch that permits the following exchanges: one milk; two A vegetable; one fruit; three bread; two meat; three fat.
5. *Problem.* Write three breakfast menus based upon the following exchange requirements: one milk; one fruit; two bread; two meat; and three fat.
6. *Problem.* Keep a record of your food intake for one day and calculate the carbohydrate, protein, fat, and caloric value with the exchange lists.

CITED REFERENCE

1. Caso, E.: "Calculation of Diabetic Diets," *J. Am. Diet. Assoc.*, **26:**575, 1950.

Unit IX

Modification of the Normal Diet for Energy and Protein

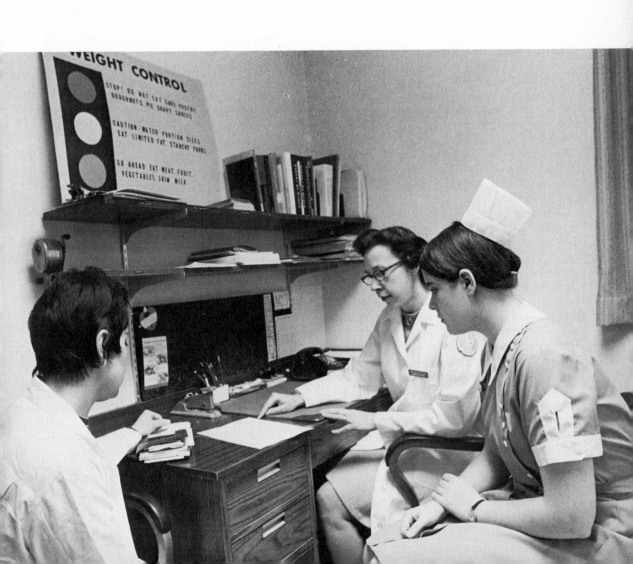

31 Overweight and Underweight

Low-Calorie and High-Calorie Diets

IMPORTANCE OF WEIGHT CONTROL

Hazards of obesity. The prevention and treatment of obesity are among the most perplexing problems facing the physician, the nutritionist, and, most especially, the patient himself. The incidence and mortality from degenerative diseases are significantly greater for those who are obese than those who are lean. The popular saying "The longer the belt, the shorter the life" is far too true.

Excessive weight is closely associated with cardiovascular and renal diseases, diabetes, degenerative arthritis, gout, and gallbladder disease. The obese frequently have elevated blood triglycerides and cholesterol, and a reduced carbohydrate tolerance. Obesity entails a respiratory cost in normal persons by increased work of breathing, a decrease in lung volume, and pulmonary hypertension. In any person with chronic pulmonary disorders such as emphysema and asthma obesity greatly increases the respiratory stress.[1] The hazards of surgery and of pregnancy and childbirth are multiplied in the presence of excessive adipose tissue.

Overweight is a physical handicap as well as a primary health hazard. Obese people are more uncomfortable during warm weather because the thick layers of fat serve as an insulator. More effort must be expended to do a given

amount of work because of the increase in body mass. Because of their lessened agility, obese people are more susceptible to accidents. Fatigue, backache, and foot troubles are common complaints of the obese.

Obesity is no longer fashionable, although in times past moderate overweight was considered a sign of health and beauty. Emotional and psychologic problems stem from obesity, just as these problems may indeed be the cause of obesity. The obese individual may be the butt of jokes, is sometimes looked upon as one who is greedy or who has no will power, or may experience social humiliation and inability to get a job. He may lose his self-esteem and may withdraw from others in order to avoid embarrassment. Such attitudes may serve to reinforce the conditions that led to the obesity.

Obesity and faddism. The preoccupation with slimness on the part of many young women is in itself—surprising as it may seem—a major problem. Too many people resort to fad diets, pills, and gadgets which result in nutritive inadequacy, economic loss, and sometimes serious effects on health. Medical supervision is bypassed and weight reduction is undertaken even though it might be contraindicated. Many people resort to one merry-go-round after another of reducing diets, losing a little only to gain it again, thus submitting themselves to repeated body stresses that accompany weight loss.

Reducing pills range from those that are nothing more than vitamin pills to those that are laxatives and diuretics, thus upsetting the water balance but being ineffective in loss of adipose tissue. So-called "reducing candies" are combinations of sugars, nonfat dry milk, some mineral salts, and vitamins.

Fad diets are numerous. The fact that a different one is held forth practically every month in some popular magazine as the answer to weight-losing problems is in itself an indication that the solution to obesity is poorly understood. Many of these diets include some bizarre food combinations, whereas others emphasize a single food or combination of foods. Some of the diets are nutritionally adequate but many are not. None possesses any magic qualities for weight loss, and seldom do they accomplish the essential lifetime change required to maintain a lower level of weight. Among the popular fad diets in recent years have been: "Drinking Man's Diet," "Ice Cream Diet," "Steak and Grapefruit Diet," "High-Fat Diet," and many others.

Problems of underweight. Much less attention has been directed to the problems of underweight although many people in all age categories are not enjoying optimum health because of the undernutrition associated with extreme underweight. The National Nutrition Survey[2] indicated that a significant number of children from low-income families had not achieved normal growth. Fatigue and lowered resistance to infections are corollaries of underweight. Tuberculosis, especially, is found more frequently among young people whose weight is considerably below normal. Underweight at the beginning of pregnancy and the failure to gain at a sufficient rate during pregnancy increases the likelihood of prematurity.[3]

EVALUATION OF WEIGHT STATUS AND BODY COMPOSITION

Desirable weight. The best weight for a given individual's height, age, bone structure, and muscular development is not exactly known. On the basis of life insurance statistics the most nearly ideal weight to maintain throughout life is that which is proper at age 25 for one's height and body build. More generally, the best weight is likely to be that at which one both looks and feels his best. Although a large number of people continue to gain weight until late middle life, this is not physiologically desirable nor need it be inevitable.

Height-weight tables (see Tables A-12, A-13) currently classify people as having a large, average, or small frame. Unfortunately, there is no simple guide by which an individual's body frame can be classified. The person who is stocky may be 5 to 10 per cent above the weight for average build without being considered overweight, whereas the individual who has a small frame should weigh 5 to 10 per cent less than the desirable weight for average build.

Recognizing the limitations of height-weight

tables, a deviation of not more than 10 per cent above or below the desirable weight for a given individual is not considered to be significant. The term *overweight* is applied to persons who are 10 to 20 per cent above desirable weight. *Obesity* is applied to persons 20 per cent or more over desirable weight. *Underweight* denotes those individuals who are more than 10 per cent below the established standards; those more than 20 per cent below these standards are considered to be seriously underweight.

Body composition. Gross obesity is easily identified by visual observation alone, but errors in making a diagnosis of moderate obesity are frequent by reference to height-weight tables. The concern in obesity, from a clinical point of view, is the excessive amount of adipose tissue and not overweight per se. A football player may be overweight by the usual height-weight standards but he has a well-developed musculature and does not have excessive fat deposits, and therefore is not to be classed as obese.

Many clinicians now measure body fatness by determining the thickness of subcutaneous tissues at designated body locations by means of calipers (see Figure 31-1). A number of anthropometric measurements may also be employed. These include the circumference of the chest, abdomen, buttocks, thigh, calf, ankle, biceps, forearm, and other body locations as measured with a flexible steel tape. Bony widths can be measured with a caliper, and the diameters of joints and the thickness of fat pads determined by x-ray.

Research centers employ precise measurements for the degree of adiposity but these tests are too complex for routine use in clinical practice. They include determination of the body density by underwater weighing, by measurement of total body water, by determination of lean body mass using a scintillation counter to assay body potassium, and by determination of the total body fat based upon the amounts of fat-soluble gases retained.

Estimation of weight gain or loss. Adipose tissue consists of about 72 per cent fat, 23 per cent water, and small amounts of protein and mineral salts.[4] Each pound of adipose tissue represents the storage of about 3500 calories.

Suppose an individual consumes an amount of food that provides 100 calories in excess of his energy requirements. In one month this excess of 3000 calories would result in a weight gain of 0.8 pound; in a year the gain is equivalent to about 10 pounds. If one were to overeat consistently by this relatively small amount, the gain over a 5-to-10-year period would indeed be impressive. The individual might well say that he "didn't eat such large amounts of food!" It requires about 3 teaspoons of butter, or two 1-inch squares of fudge, or an oatmeal cookie to supply the additional 100 calories each day.

Conversely, the loss of 1 pound of adipose tissue means that the diet would be deficient by 3500 calories for the total time period of the weight loss. Suppose a young woman requires 2000 calories a day to meet her energy needs, but she consumes a diet that supplies only 1200 calories. The weekly deficit would then be 5600 calories, and the adipose tissue loss would be 5600 ÷ 3500, or 1.6 pounds.

Weight gain and weight loss do not always follow the predicted straight line because of variations in water balance. Also, weight gain and weight loss are not explained solely on the basis of changes in adipose tissue; some changes in protein-rich tissues are likewise taking place.

OBESITY

Incidence. The exact incidence of obesity is not known, but it does not take much people-watching to become aware of the high numbers of most age groups who exceed their desirable weight. Based upon weight-height standards, it has been estimated that half of all men over age 30 are at least 10 per cent overweight and one fourth are obese. The incidence is even higher for women, with about 40 per cent being obese by the time they reach 40 years.

Increasing attention has been given to obesity in children and in adolescents, with estimates of 15 to 30 per cent in the obese category in various school populations. The incidence is higher in girls than in boys. Contrary to popular opinion, most children do not "grow out of" their overweight; they remain obese throughout life and are particularly refractory to treatment later in life.

Causes. Obesity is invariably caused by an intake of calories beyond the body's need for energy. Such a statement, however, tends to oversimplify the problem of obesity, for one might infer that its correction might be easily achieved by bringing the energy intake and expenditure into balance. The reasons for an

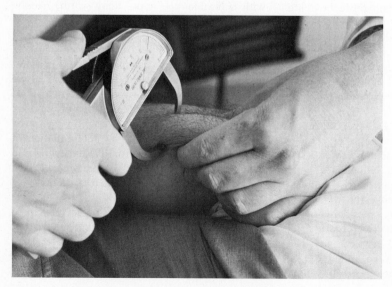

Figure 31–1. A skin-fold measurement is made by means of a caliper. This determines the amount of subcutaneous fat of an individual and is an indicator of total body fat. (Courtesy, *Roche Medical Image,* Hoffmann La Roche, Inc.)

existing imbalance are many and complex, and some understanding of the problems of the individual must be gained before therapy can be effectively instituted. A thorough physical examination, a dietary history, and an investigation of habits relating to activity, rest, and family and social relationships are indicated.

Food habits. Eating too much becomes a habit for many people. Sometimes this is the result of ignorance of the calorie value of food. The amounts of food are not necessarily excessive, but it is the extra foods, beyond the calorie need, that account for the gradual increase in weight, for example, the extra pats of butter, the spoonful of jelly, the second roll, the preference for a rich dessert, or the TV snack. Eating too much may result from having to maintain social relationships including rich party foods in addition to usual mealtime eating. Excessive amounts of carbohydrate-rich foods are sometimes eaten because they are cheaper than lower-calorie fruits and vegetables. (See Figure 31–2.)

Activity patterns. Numerous persons continue to gain weight throughout life because they fail to adjust their appetites to reduced energy requirements. The many laborsaving devices in the homes and in industry reduce the energy requirement. Most people enjoy sports as spectators rather than as participants. Riding rather than walking to school or work is common practice even for short distances. Other circumstances may further reduce the energy needs: (1) basal metabolism is gradually decreased from year to year (see Chapter 7); (2) changes in occupation may result in reduced activity; (3) the middle years of life sometimes bring about a repose and consequent reduction of muscle tension; (4) periods of quiet relaxation and sleep may be increased; and (5) disabling illness such as arthritis or cardiac disease may reduce markedly the need for calories.

Psychologic factors. Eating is a solace and a pleasure to the individual who is bored, feels lonely or unloved, has become discontented

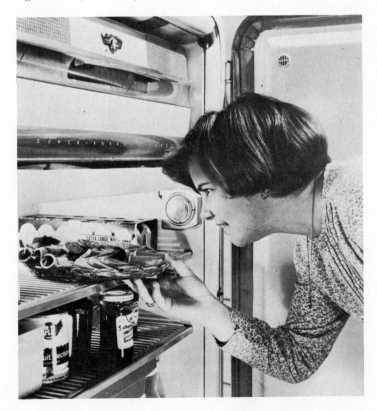

Figure 31–2. Almost everyone enjoys a snack from time to time. Do they provide a good balance of nutrients? Are they in line with calorie need? (Courtesy, U.S. Department of Agriculture.)

with his family, social, or financial standing, has experienced deep sorrow, or needs an excuse to avoid the realities of life. Such an individual often eats because he has nothing else to do or has no motivation to seek another outlet for his problems.

Genetic influences. Mayer[5] has noted that only 10 per cent of children with parents of normal weight are obese, 40 to 50 per cent of children with one obese parent are obese, and 80 per cent of children with two obese parents are overweight. His observations led him to conclude that food habits alone do not explain these differences.

Body build is genetically determined. The *endomorphic* or round, soft individual gains weight readily, whereas the *ectomorphic* or slender, wiry person rarely becomes overweight.[6] This does not mean that obesity is inevitable for the endomorph, but it does mean that constant vigilance is required to avoid it.

Metabolic abnormalities. Many people would like to lay the blame for their obesity on endocrine disorders, but only a small percentage of all obese individuals do have such disturbances. A deficiency of the thyroid gland can reduce the basal metabolism so that obesity results, but overweight from this cause can be prevented if the diet is sufficiently restricted in calories.

In experimental animals damage to the area of the hypothalamus that regulates feeding leads to excessive eating and obesity. Whether there is interference with the regulation of appetite by the hypothalamus in humans has not been proven. In fact, many obese persons actually have a lower intake of calories than those of normal weight, but they have become obese because of greatly decreased activity.[7]

Another explanation offered for obesity is that of overloading of the metabolic pathways for carbohydrate and fat so that lipogenesis is favored. When rats are restricted to forced feeding twice a day instead of being allowed to nibble they become obese.[8] According to this hypothesis, the individual who skips breakfast, eats little lunch, and then consumes a large dinner might be overloading the metabolic pathways at one time. Some grossly obese patients have shown alterations in blood lipids that suggest the possibility of increased formation of fatty tissue.[9]

PREVENTION OF OBESITY

Identifying those who are likely to become obese. The most vigorous efforts to prevent obesity should be directed to those individuals who are most susceptible, namely children of obese parents and children who have stocky frames. Certain periods of life are also likely to bring about obesity. Men of normal weight often begin to gain weight in the late 20's and early 30's, and women are more likely to gain in the 40's and 50's. Following pregnancy weight gain is common. If these trends are recognized the individual can elect to reduce his caloric intake, or increase his exercise, or both.

Education for prevention. The best hope for the prevention of obesity is through greatly expanded programs of nutrition education directed particularly to schoolchildren, teen-agers, and mothers. The pattern for obesity is often set in infancy when the mother overfeeds the baby in the erroneous belief that a "fat baby is a healthy baby." Sometimes overeating becomes a habit with a child following an illness because the mother keeps urging food upon the child through her concern for his state of nutrition. During adolescent years food is often used to submerge the many problems that face the boy and girl. By recognizing these trends, the mother can do much to redirect the food habits. The education of the mother in terms of weight control for her family and the education of the child in the elementary and secondary school can be effective.

Increased activity. In these times of affluence, mechanization, and automation many individuals become overweight because of lack of exercise. A pattern of activity is best taught during childhood and must also be emphasized during the school years. Too often competitive sports exclude the child who most needs the exercise. Physical education should be directed to those activities that are likely to carry over into adult life.

Public health approach. The Bureau of Nutrition of New York City since 1952 has used public health methodology in the control and treatment of obesity.[10] One project included 90 obese 13- and 14-year-old boys; 55 students were placed in an experimental group, and 35 boys served as the controls. During an 18-month period changes were observed in weight, height, skinfold thickness, and physical fitness. For the experimental group, short nutrition programs were given after school at biweekly intervals with attendance being voluntary. At these meetings diet histories were obtained, a physician talked of the relationship of body weight to physical fitness, and a nutritionist emphasized nutrient and calorie values of food. The boys were given a series of exercises during gym periods and were encouraged to continue to take them at home.

At the end of the 18-month period the boys in the experimental group had gained an average of 5.8 pounds as compared with 13.5 pounds by the control group. Thus, the experimental group at the end of this period had a noticeable decrease in the proportion of overweight, the grossly obese boys benefiting the most. The performance of physical fitness tests was much better for the experimental group than for the control group. For these teen-agers it is important to point out that correction of weight status was achieved by a proper diet pattern without a specific reducing regimen.

Treatment of Obesity

Two criteria must be satisfied if the treatment is to be considered successful: (1) weight loss must be such that desirable weight according to body frame and state of health is achieved; and (2) the desired weight must be maintained. The essential components of treatment are diet, activity, adequate dietary counseling, and psychologic support.

Assessment of the patient. The treatment of obesity is a frustrating problem to the physician, nutritionist, and nurse because failures are so frequent. To a patient a failure can be demoralizing. Therefore, it is important that each patient be evaluated in terms of his medical and dietary

history and his emotional stability. Weight reduction should be guided by a physician since the physiologic and psychologic stresses of weight loss are not equally tolerated by all.

Some persons, according to Young,[11] will lose weight satisfactorily when shown how to keep the caloric intake within prescribed limits; others need help in relieving their tensions before a dietary regimen will be effective; still others have such deep emotional problems that weight loss should not be attempted until these problems have been corrected by psychiatric help.

In the New York City antiobesity program,[10] a survey of almost 2600 obesity clinic patients has shown: (1) weight loss is more difficult to achieve as the duration of obesity and the degree of obesity increase; (2) married persons were more successful than single persons in effecting weight loss; (3) many women had onset of obesity associated with the first pregnancy; and (4) women over 40 years reduced more successfully than those who were younger. Men and women were equally able to reduce, level of education had no effect on success of reaching normal weight, and group methods supervised by the physician and nutritionist were more successful than individual instruction.

Low-calorie diets. The diets described below are representative of many widely accepted, nutritionally sound programs. They are intended to bring about steady weight loss, to establish good food habits, and to promote a sense of well-being. The diets are palatable, fit into the framework of family food habits, and do not require additional expense or long preparation time.

Energy. A diet that provides 800 to 1000 calories below the daily energy requirement leads to a loss of 6 to 8 pounds monthly. This gradual loss does not result in severe hunger, nervous exhaustion, and weakness that often accompany drastic reduction regimens. For most men 1400 to 1600 calories is a satisfactory level, and for women 1200 to 1400 calories are indicated. Diets that supply 1000 calories or less are rarely necessary except for individuals who are bedfast.

Protein. Although 1 gm protein per kilogram

desirable body weight is sufficient, an allowance of 1½ gm per kilogram improves the satiety value of the diet. Most dietary plans can include 70 to 100 gm protein daily.

Fat and carbohydrate. Many regimens drastically restrict the fat intake and thus allow a moderate intake of carbohydrates. (See the 1000-calorie diet in Table 31–1.) Some patients experience a greater sense of satisfaction when a somewhat more liberal intake of fat and reduced carbohydrate level are employed. In the high-protein moderate-fat 1500-calorie diet, Table 31–1, about half the calories are provided by fat.

Minerals and vitamins. A multivitamin preparation, iron salts, and possibly calcium are indicated for diets containing 1000 calories or less. Low-calorie diets for obese children and for pregnant women must be planned with the increased mineral and vitamin requirements in mind. For these reasons the diets used for them are usually less restricted.

Daily meal patterns. The diets in Table 31–1 have been calculated with the food exchange lists (Table A-4). A comparison with the basic diet on page 205 shows that the mineral and vitamin values will equal or exceed the recommended allowances.

These diets include 3 cups of milk, thus enhancing the calcium intake, and also providing a convenient bedtime snack, if desired. Some adults will prefer 2 cups of milk and more meat. This can be arranged by substituting one meat exchange for 1 cup of skim milk. The isocaloric exchange for 1 cup of whole milk would be two meat exchanges, thus giving a slightly higher protein intake.

A great deal of flexibility in food choices is possible with the exchange lists. One important consideration is the satiety value of the diet. Inasmuch as proteins and fats remain in the stomach longer, the protein and fat allowance should be divided approximately equally between the three meals. Thus, an egg and milk at breakfast, lean meat, cheese, or egg at lunch, and lean meat at dinner are desirable.

Some regimens employ six meals a day instead of three, stressing that some protein should be provided at each feeding.[12] Part of the success of a reducing diet depends upon learning to be content with smaller portions of food and less concentrated foods.

Table 31–1. Food Allowances for Low-Calorie Diets

	Normal Protein, Moderate Carbohydrate, Low to Moderate Fat			High Protein, Low Carbohydrate, Moderate Fat
Food for the Day	1000 Calories	1200 Calories	1500 Calories	1500 Calories
Milk, whole, cups	3 (skim)	3	3	3
Vegetable, group A	1 cup	1 cup	1 cup	1 cup
Group B	1/2 cup	1/2 cup	1/2 cup	1/2 cup
Fruit, unsweetened, exchanges	4	3	4	2
Bread, exchanges	2	2	4	2
Meat, exchanges	5	5	5	9
Fat, exchanges	1	1	3	2
Nutritive Value				
Protein, gm	65	65	69	93
Fat, gm	30	60	70	85
Carbohydrate, gm	113	103	143	93
Calories	980	1210	1480	1510

Sample Meal Patterns

Normal Protein, Moderate Carbohydrate, Moderate
  Fat
  1500 Calories
  BREAKFAST
Unsweetened citrus fruit—1 exchange
Egg—1
Bread—1 slice
Butter—1 teaspoon
Milk, whole—1 cup
Coffee or tea
  LUNCH
Meat, poultry, or fish—2 ounces
Vegetable, raw or cooked, group A—1 serving
Milk, whole—1 cup
Bread—1 slice
Butter—1 teaspoon
Unsweetened fruit—1 exchange
  DINNER
Meat, poultry, or fish—2 ounces
Potato—1 small
Vegetable, group B—½ cup
        group A—1 serving
Milk, whole—1 cup
Bread—1 slice
Butter—1 teaspoon
Unsweetened fruit—2 exchanges
Coffee or tea, if desired

High Protein, Low Carbohydrate, Moderate Fat
  1500 Calories

Unsweetened citrus fruit—1 exchange
Eggs—2
Bread—1 slice
Butter—1 teaspoon
Milk, whole—1 cup
Coffee or tea

Meat, poultry, or fish—4 ounces
Vegetable, raw or cooked, group A—1 serving
Milk, whole—1 cup

Meat, poultry, or fish—3 ounces
Potato—1 small
Vegetable, group B—½ cup
        group A—1 serving
Milk, whole—1 cup

Butter—1 teaspoon
Unsweetened fruit—1 exchange

Foods to restrict or avoid. The patient who learns to select his foods in appropriate amounts from the exchange lists does not require specific lists of foods to avoid. For some persons, however, it may help to create calorie consciousness if listings of concentrated foods are provided. Some of the foods listed below are permitted in specified amounts in the exchange lists, but others are best avoided altogether.

High-fat foods: butter, cheese, chocolate, cream, ice cream, fat meat, fatty fish, or fish canned
  in oil, fried foods of any kind such as doughnuts and potato chips, gravies, nuts, oil, pastries,
  and salad dressing
High-carbohydrate foods: breads of any kind, candy, cake, cookies, corn, cereal products such
  as macaroni, noodles, spaghetti, pancakes, waffles, sweetened or dried fruits, legumes such
  as Lima beans, navy beans, dried peas, potatoes, sweet potatoes, honey, molasses, sugar,
  syrup, rich puddings
Beverages: all fountain drinks, including malted milks and chocolate, carbonated beverages of
  all kinds, rich sundaes, alcoholic drinks

Other dietary regimens. *Formula diets* in liquid or powder form, as cookies, or as combination dishes continue to be popular. Generally, they are nutritionally adequate and possess the advantages of convenience and strict calorie control. Some patients find them useful for initiating the reduction regimen while they are learning the essentials of dietary planning. Other patients substitute these preparations for one meal a day.

The principal disadvantages of the formula diets are these: (1) they do not retrain the individual to a new pattern of food habits that must be followed once the weight is lost; (2)

they are monotonous if used for a long period of time; and (3) they may be constipating for some patients, whereas others occasionally experience diarrhea.

Starvation. Several clinicians have used total starvation for 30 or more days in the treatment of excessively obese individuals.[13] Patients were allowed water *ad libitum* and were given vitamin and mineral supplements. They must be carefully selected and must remain under constant supervision in a hospital since starvation is unphysiologic and there are a number of risks attached to this strenuous therapy. The regimen establishes rapid weight loss for the grossly obese; for example, during the first month weight losses for 12 patients were 24 to 63 pounds.[14]

The average nitrogen losses for 12 patients in the first month were equivalent to 1300 gm protein, and for 7 patients in the second month to 690 gm protein. This protein loss is the most critical deficiency encountered. It was noted that there was cessation of the growth of fingernails and hair; however, no changes were observed in the blood proteins. When patients were placed on 300- and 500-calorie diets, nitrogen equilibrium was rapidly established suggesting that nitrogen equilibrium can be achieved in the protein-depleted individual at low-calorie intakes when tissue fat is being metabolized for energy.

Duncan and his associates have used total starvation for periods up to two weeks and have then given the patients a moderately restricted calorie diet (1500 to 2300 calories) with the instructions that they were to fast one day a week.[15] The continued weight loss by most patients was found to be disappointing.

Exercise and weight loss. Moderate exercise on a consistent daily basis is an important aid in weight loss. It results in increased pulmonary and cardiovascular efficiency, better muscular tone, and a sense of well-being. It does not lead to increased appetite; conversely, a diminution of activity does not lead to a corresponding decrease in appetite. The exercise program should be determined by the physician on the basis of the patient's age, state of health and physical condition, and activity preferences.

The importance of exercise can be illustrated by calculating the energy equivalents of foods in terms of various kinds of activity. On the basis of a 70-kg man, Konishi has calculated the energy equivalents for 50 foods at five activity levels: reclining, walking, bicycle riding, swimming, and running.[16] Six of these foods shown in Figure 31–3 illustrate the wide ranges of time required to utilize the energy provided by various foods at sedentary to moderate activities.

Role of hormones and drugs. Most overweight persons have no deficiency of endocrine secre-

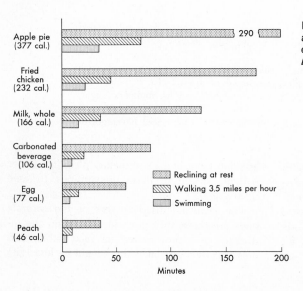

Figure 31–3. The energy value for foods expressed as number of minutes of activity for three levels of energy expenditure. (Data from F. Konishi, *J. Am. Diet. Assoc.,* **46**: 187, 1965.)

tions and should not be led to believe that they have glandular disturbances, nor should they be exposed to the increased nervousness and irritability that result from such medication. Thyroid deficiency should be treated only by a physician.

Anorexigenic drugs such as amphetamine sulfate are sometimes prescribed by a physician because of their ability to dull the appetite. They may produce insomnia, excitability, dryness of the mouth, gastrointestinal disturbances, and other toxic manifestations. For some patients they are a crutch and for others they have no effect on decreasing the appetite. If these agents are prescribed the patient must clearly understand that they do not eliminate the necessity for a controlled low-calorie diet. Usually these agents are effective for only a few weeks.

DIETARY COUNSELING

Leverton[17] has suggested that success in weight reduction is dependent upon effective motivation and suitable knowledge.

Motivation and psychologic support. A diet prescription is worthless unless the patient has some motivation for losing weight, such as the maintenance or recovery of health, the ability to win friendship, admiration, and affection, or the importance of normal weight in being able to earn one's livelihood or in being considered for occupational advancement, as the case may be. The patient must have the capacity for self-discipline, patience, and perseverance.

Although the motivation must come from within the patient, the physician, nurse, and dietitian can be of immeasurable help toward initiating this motivation, and subsequently by providing encouragement and guidance at frequent follow-up visits. The patient needs to understand that a calorie intake in excess of his needs is the cause of his overweight, and that weight loss is accomplished only when the calorie intake is reduced below his energy needs. But this explanation is not enough. He also needs to gain insights into the reasons why he is overeating, and to work at correcting these.

Obesity is not a moral issue but a clinical problem and it is important that all who work with obese patients keep this in mind. Threatening the patient with the dire consequences of failing to lose weight or chiding him because he has not adhered to his diet rarely accomplishes anything. On the contrary, each patient must be helped to maintain his self-esteem and deserves treatment with dignity.

Counseling and group sessions. Individual counseling is essential to determine the goals that are realistic for the patient and to initiate a dietary regimen that is appropriate for the patient's food habits and patterns of living. See also Chapter 28.

Group sessions are effective in that people compare their progress, share their problems in adhering to diets, and exchange ways to vary their diets. When groups are formed it is important that professional guidance be available from a physician, dietitian, or nurse. Each individual joining such a group should first be evaluated by his physician to determine his fitness for weight reduction.

Essential knowledge. Most people are quite ignorant of the calorie values of foods. Each of the food exchange lists (Table A-4) provides a variety of foods that have approximately equal calorie values, and their consistent use helps to develop awareness of nutritive values. Many other tables of calorie values of foods are also available. Keeping a record of the daily calorie intake is useful, at least for a period of time. However, it is important that clear distinctions be made between the calorie values of foods that also supply protein, minerals, and vitamins and those foods that are principally carbohydrate and fat.

Portion control, taught by means of measuring cups, spoons, food models, or actual foods, is essential. Although a given diet is planned for a specific calorie level it must be expected that the daily calorie intake may vary by as much as 200 to 300 calories because of variations in food composition as well as in the precision of measurements.

Few dietetic foods are necessary. When fresh fruits are expensive or unavailable, water-packed canned fruits may be used. Sweetening agents containing saccharin may be used if desired. Many low-calorie beverages currently available provide about half the calories contained in regular beverages. The calorie information on the label should be taken into account if these beverages are used.

Some patients ask about including cocktails and wine in their diets. If the physician permits these beverages, the patient needs to know that each gram of alcohol supplies 7 calories and that the calorie value of the beverage must be taken into consideration. A glass of dry table wine provides fewer calories than a cocktail. Usually an alcoholic beverage is restricted to one serving daily. (See Table A-7 for caloric values of alcoholic beverages.)

A single dinner in a restaurant can nullify careful adherence given to a diet for several days. Usually it is possible to select a clear soup, broiled or roasted meat without sauces, vegetables without sauces, and salad without dressing. Meat portions are likely to be larger than those allowed and the dieter will need to restrict his intake to that allowed. The diet will not be exceeded too much if one foregoes the rolls, butter, and dessert.

What does the dieter do when he has many dinner invitations? For every dieter there are occasions when the limitations of the diet are exceeded, and such breaks in the dieting pattern should be anticipated. Each day gives an opportunity to begin again toward the goal of desired weight. Nevertheless, the person who has many social engagements will find it difficult to make the progress he would like to make. Occasionally, when one knows that the social event will make it difficult to keep within dietary restrictions, the intake at the preceding meal can be kept especially light. Most hostesses are very understanding if the guest tells her that he is on a diet and is therefore restricting the size of portions or letting some of the foods pass by without partaking of them.

Maintenance of weight. To lose weight is by no means easy; to maintain the desirable level of weight is even more difficult. The low-calorie diet planned with regard for the patient's pattern of living also provides the basis upon which to build the diet for maintenance. The patient must learn that a change in food habits is essential not only for weight loss, but that such a change must also continue throughout life if desirable weight is to be maintained. Thus, additions of foods should be made judiciously until weight is being kept constant at the desired level. It is important for the patient to weigh himself at weekly intervals or so in order to be sure that the foods added are in appropriate amounts.

If foods added for maintenance are also selected from the Four Food Groups, the quality of the diet with respect to protein, minerals, and vitamins is thereby enhanced. On the other hand, the additions of concentrated high-calorie foods may be more difficult to control in amounts suitable for maintenance. For example, the sedentary person of middle age must continue to forego rich desserts and sweets except on rare occasions.

UNDERWEIGHT

Causes. Underweight results when the energy intake does not fully meet the energy requirements. Not infrequently this occurs in people who are very active, tense, and nervous, and who obtain too little rest. Sometimes irregular habits of eating and poor selection of foods are responsible for an inadequate caloric intake.

Just as psychologic factors have been noted as contributing to overeating, so they may contribute to eating too little food. Some patients with mental illness reject food to such an extent that severe weight loss results; this condition is referred to as *anorexia nervosa*.

Underweight also occurs in many pathologic

conditions such as fevers in which the appetite is poor but the energy requirements are increased; gastrointestinal disturbances characterized by nausea, vomiting, and diarrhea; and hyperthyroidism in which the metabolic rate is greatly accelerated.

Modifications of the diet. Before weight gain can be effected, the direct cause for the inadequate caloric intake must be sought. As in obesity, these causes in relation to the individual must be removed and a high-calorie diet provided.

Energy. Approximately 500 calories in excess of the daily needs will result in a weekly gain of about 1 pound. For moderately active individuals diets containing 3000 to 3500 calories will bring about effective weight gain. Somewhat higher levels are required when fever is high, or gastrointestinal disturbances are interfering with absorption, or metabolism is greatly increased.

Protein. A daily intake of 100 gm protein or more is usually desirable since body protein as well as body fat must be replaced.

Minerals and vitamins. If the quality of the diet resulting in weight loss was poor, considerable body deficits of minerals and vitamins may likewise have occurred. Usually the high-calorie diet will provide liberal levels of all these nutrients. When supplements are prescribed, it is important that the patient understand that they are in no way a substitute for the calories and protein provided by food.

Planning the daily diet. A patient cannot always adjust immediately to a higher caloric intake. It is better to begin with the patient's present intake and to improve the diet both qualitatively and quantitatively day by day until the desired caloric level is reached. Nothing is more conducive to loss of appetite than the appearance of an overloaded tray of food.

The caloric intake may be increased by using additional amounts of foods from the Four Food Groups, thus increasing the intake of protein, minerals, and vitamins. For example, 500 calories might be added to the patient's present intake as follows:

1 glass milk, ½ cup ice cream, 1 small potato, 1 small banana; *or*
2 slices bread, 2 ounces meat, 1 ounce cheese, ½ cup Lima beans.

The judicious use of cream, butter, jelly or jam, and sugars will quickly increase the caloric level, but excessive use may provoke nausea and loss of appetite.

Some patients make better progress if given small, frequent feedings; but for many patients midmorning and midafternoon feeding have been found to interfere with the appetite for the following meal. Bedtime snacks, however, may be planned to provide 300 to 800 calories, thus making it possible to follow a normal pattern for the three meals.

The following list of foods illustrates one way in which the Four Food Groups may be adapted to a high-calorie level. The meal patterns outlined for the high-protein diet (page 433) suggest suitable arrangements of these foods.

3 to 4 cups milk
1 cup light cream
4 to 6 ounces meat, fish, or poultry
2 eggs
4 servings vegetables including:
    1 serving green or yellow vegetable
    2 servings white or sweet potato, corn, or beans
    1 serving other vegetable
2 to 3 servings fruit, including one citrus fruit
1 serving whole-grain or enriched cereal
3 to 6 slices whole-grain or enriched bread
4 tablespoons or more butter or fortified margarine
High-calorie foods to complete the caloric requirement: cereals such as macaroni, rice, noodles, spaghetti; honey, molasses, syrups; hard candies; glucose; salad dressings; cakes; cookies, and pastry in moderation; ice cream, puddings, sauces

PROBLEMS AND REVIEW

1. What are the hazards of obesity to health?
2. List eight situations that may account for obesity.

3. *Problem.* As part of his weight reduction program Mr. Reese has increased his activity by walking each day. If he uses 285 calories per hour, how many hours will it take him to lose 1 pound of adipose tissue?

4. *Problem.* A man's daily calorie requirement is 2600, but he is restricting his diet to 1800 calories. How much weight might he expect to lose in a month?

5. A physician has indicated that a patient may include alcoholic beverages not to exceed 150 calories each day. By consulting Table A-7 prepare a list of several choices that come within this allowance. What adjustments would be necessary in the 1500-calorie diet in Table 31–1 to include the beverage?

6. What are some important factors to consider in order that maximum cooperation of the patient may be achieved?

7. *Problem.* Write menus for two days for the 1500-calorie moderate-fat diet listed in Table 31–1.

8. A young woman has adhered to her 1500-calorie diet for the last three weeks but has lost no weight. What possible explanations may there be for her failure to lose weight?

9. Mrs. Aston has brought her weight to the desired level. What measures are now important so that this weight level will be maintained?

10. *Problem.* A teen-age girl is 25 pounds underweight and needs some help in planning a diet to bring about weight gain. She is now averaging 55 gm protein and 1800 calories daily. Plan some additions to her diet that would increase calories to about 2600 with a minimum of bulk.

11. What are some factors that may contribute to underweight?

12. *Problem.* Using the food exchange lists, calculate the protein, fat, and carbohydrate value of the list of foods suggested for weight gain on page 427. How many calories are provided?

13. *Problem.* Plan three bedtime snacks that will each provide 500 calories.

CITED REFERENCES

1. Wilson, R. H. L., and Wilson, N. L.: "Obesity and Respiratory Stress," *J. Am. Diet. Assoc.,* **55**:465–69, 1969.

2. Schaefer, A. E., and Johnson, O. C.: "Are We Well Fed? The Search for the Answer," *Nutr. Today,* 4:2–11, Spring 1969.

3. Tompkins, W. T., and Wiehl, D. G.: "Nutritional Deficiencies as a Causal Factor in Toxemia and Premature Labor," *Am. J. Obstet. Gynecol.,* **62**:898–919, 1951.

4. West, E. S., *et al.: Textbook of Biochemistry,* 4th ed. The Macmillan Company, New York, 1966, p. 416.

5. Mayer, J.: "Obesity: Causes and Treatment," *Am. J. Nurs.,* **59**:1732–36, 1959.

6. ———: "Physical Activity and Anthropometric Measurements of Obese Adolescents," *Fed. Proc.,* **25**:11–14, 1966.

7. Bullen, B. A., *et al.:* "Physical Activity of Obese and Nonobese Adolescent Girls Appraised by Motion Picture Sampling," *Am. J. Clin. Nutr.,* **14**:211–23, 1964.

8. Cohn, C.: "Meal-Eating, Nibbling, and Body Metabolism," *J. Am. Diet. Assoc.,* **38**:433–36, 1961.

9. Goldberg, M., and Gordon, E. S.: "Energy Metabolism and Human Obesity," *J.A.M.A.,* **189**:616–23, 1964.

10. James, G., and Christakis, G.: "New York City's Bureau of Nutrition. Current Programs and Research Activities," *J. Am. Diet. Assoc.,* **48**:301–306, 1966.

11. Young, C. M., *et al.:* "The Problem of the Obese Patient," *J. Am. Diet. Assoc.,* **31**:1111–15, 1955.

12. Dietary Department: *Wisconsin Comprehensive Multi-Meal Weight Reduction Plans.* University Hospitals, University of Wisconsin, Madison.

13. Drenick, E. J., *et al.:* "Prolonged Starvation as Treatment for Severe Obesity," *J.A.M.A.*, **187:**100–105, 1964.
14. Swendseid, M. E., *et al.:* "Nitrogen and Weight Losses during Starvation and Realimentation in Obesity," *J. Am. Diet. Assoc.*, **46:**276–79, 1965.
15. Duncan, G. G., *et al.:* "Intermittent Fasts and the Correction and Control of Intractable Obesity," *Am. J. Med. Sci.*, **245:**515–20, 1963.
16. Konishi, F.: "Food Energy Equivalents of Various Activities," *J. Am. Diet. Assoc.*, **46:**186–88, 1965.
17. Leverton, R. M.: "Food Needs and Energy Use in Weight Reduction," *J. Am. Diet. Assoc.*, **49:**23–25, 1966.

ADDITIONAL REFERENCES

Albrink, M. J., ed.: "Symposium: Endocrine Aspects of Obesity," *Am. J. Clin. Nutr.*, **21:**1395–1485, 1968.
Bortz, W. M., *et al.:* "Fat, Carbohydrate, Salt, and Weight Loss," *Am. J. Clin. Nutr.*, **21:**1291–1301, 1968.
Dwyer, J. T., and Mayer, J.: "Potential Dieters: Who Are They?" *J. Am. Diet. Assoc.*, **56:**510–14, 1970.
Fineberg, S. K.: "Anorexigenic Drugs—Boon or Bust?" *Nutr. Today*, **2:**14–18, Dec. 1967.
Hashim, S. A., and Van Itallie, T. B.: "Clinical and Physiologic Aspects of Obesity. A Review," *J. Am. Diet. Assoc.*, **46:**15–19, 1965.
Krehl, W. H., *et al.:* "Some Metabolic Changes Induced by Low Carbohydrate Diets," *Am. J. Clin. Nutr.*, **20:**139–48, 1967.
Mayer, J.: "Some Aspects of the Problem of Regulation of Food Intake and Obesity," *N. Engl. J. Med.*, **274:**610–16; 662–73; 722–31, 1966.
Montagu, A.: "Obesity and the Evolution of Man," *J.A.M.A.*, **195:**105–107, 1966.
Nordsiek, F. W.: "An Epidemiological Approach to Obesity," *Am. J. Public Health*, **54:**1689–98, 1964.
Review: "Cues Affecting Eating Behavior and Obesity," *Nutr. Rev.*, **27:**11–14, 1969.
———: "Overfeeding Lean and Obese Individuals," *Nutr. Rev.*, **26:**202, 1968.
Ruffer, W. A.: "Two Simple Indexes for Identifying Obesity Compared," *J. Am. Diet. Assoc.*, **57:**326–30, 1970.
Schachter, S.: "Obesity and Eating," *Science*, **161:**751–56, 1968.
Seltzer, C. C., and Mayer, J.: "Body Build (Somatotype) Distinctiveness in Obese Women," *J. Am. Diet. Assoc.*, **55:**454–58, 1969.
Stokes, S. A.: "Fasting for Obesity," *Am. J. Nurs.*, **69:**796–99, 1969.
Weight Control Source Book. National Dairy Council, Chicago, 1966.

FOR PATIENT EDUCATION

Calories and Weight—the USDA Pocket Guide. Home and Garden Bull. 153, U.S. Department of Agriculture, Washington, D.C., 1968.
Leverton, R. M.: *A Girl and Her Figure.* National Dairy Council, Chicago, 1956.
Obesity and Health. Pub. Health Service Pub. 1485, U.S. Department of Health, Education, and Welfare, Washington, D.C., 1966.
Page, L., and Finch, L. J.: *Food and Your Weight.* Home and Garden Bull. 74, U.S. Department of Agriculture, Washington, D.C., 1960.
Washbon, M. B., and Harrison, G. G.: "Overweight, and What It Takes to Stay Trim," in *Food for Us All—Yearbook of Agriculture 1969,* U.S. Department of Agriculture, Washington, D.C., pp. 304–14.

32 Protein Deficiency

High-Protein Diets

Incidence and etiology. Protein deficiency resulting primarily from lack of dietary protein is extremely rare in the United States—at least in a degree of severity that it can be diagnosed. Moreover, dietary surveys provide little or no evidence that such deficiencies would be expected. (See Figure 1–3.) Under certain conditions the dietary intake of protein may be inadequate. An emphasis upon excessive thinness and ill-advised reduction regimens, especially by young women, can lead to gradual depletion of tissue proteins. Chronic alcoholism and drug addiction also interfere with a satisfactory food intake, in part because the cost of the habit often leaves insufficient money for the purchase of an adequate diet. Ignorance of the essentials of an adequate diet and child neglect are contributing factors to malnutrition in children. Protein-calorie malnutrition as a principal world health problem in children has been discussed in Chapter 25.

Protein undernutrition as a complication that requires attention during illness and injury is by no means unusual. Many pathologic conditions are aggravated by nutritional deficiency, and, conversely, an existing deficiency is likely to become more severe during illness.

1. Disturbances of the gastrointestinal tract frequently initiate nutritional deficiency because of interference with intake, digestion, or absorption of foods. Anorexia, nausea, vomiting, the discomfort of ulcers, the abdominal distention present in many illnesses, and the cramping associated with diarrhea preclude a satisfactory food intake. Many patients are afraid to eat and restrict their choice to a few foods that do not meet nutritional requirements.

Even though the food intake may be adequate under normal circumstances, increased motility that accompanies some disturbances does not permit sufficient time for digestion and absorption so that excessive amounts of nutrients are lost. In the malabsorption syndrome—sprue, for example—a reduction in the digestive enzymes and in the absorptive surfaces leads to great losses of all nutrients from the bowel.

2. Excessive protein losses result from proteinuria in certain renal diseases, from hemorrhage, from increased nitrogen losses in the urine during the catabolic phase accompanying injury and immobilization, and from exudates of burned surfaces or draining wounds. The increased catabolism that follows immobilization is not fully understood, but is related, at least in part, to an increased production of adrenocortical hormones. Following an injury healthy individuals show greater nitrogen losses than do persons who have more limited reserves. During the acute stage of catabolism high-protein high-calorie diets seem to have little effect on reducing the losses. Eventually, of course, such losses must be replaced.

3. An increased metabolic rate in fevers and in thyrotoxicosis is accompanied by increased destruction of tissue proteins.

4. In diseases of the liver the synthesis of plasma proteins may be reduced even though the supply of amino acids is satisfactory.

Clinical and biochemical signs of protein undernutrition. Fatigue, loss of weight, and lack of resistance to infection are among the symptoms presented by patients with protein deficiency. Because these are common to so many pathologic conditions they are of little diagnostic value. Nutritional edema, reduced levels of plasma proteins, a history of inadequate protein intake, and disorders of digestion, absorption, or metabolism help to establish the presence of protein malnutrition. None of these, however, is particularly useful in detecting deficiency in a mild stage when it can be easily corrected.

Underweight together with a history of weight loss is of particular concern in many disease conditions. The loss of weight has been at the expense of tissue proteins as well as adipose tissue. Recovery from illness is often slow, and wound healing is prolonged because the essential amino acids for tissue repair are lacking. Anemia is sometimes observed because of a reduced synthesis of the protein globin. Likewise antibodies are not manufactured in sufficient quantity and infections are more likely to occur.

The presence of nutritional edema supports a diagnosis of protein deficiency. When edema occurs it is necessary to rule out impaired circulation and excretion that occur in cardiac or renal failure. Nutritional edema does not become evident until the protein deficiency has advanced to a relatively severe level. Moreover, it is a rather inconstant finding that is not directly related to the plasma protein level. Thus, an individual may be severely depleted of proteins and show no signs of edema.

Following prolonged protein deficiency the concentration of the plasma proteins and the circulating blood volume are decreased. The principal deficit is in the plasma albumin fraction; the globulins are not appreciably reduced. Since plasma albumin is particularly important for the maintenance of osmotic pressure, the hypoalbuminemia has an adverse effect on the fluid balance between the extracellular and intracellular compartments. Sometimes the plasma protein concentration is essentially normal but a reduction in the total blood volume and hence the total circulating protein has taken place so that any stress could bring about circulatory failure.

Although the liver has an amazing ability to carry out its functions even under adverse conditions, a prolonged nutritional deficiency gradually reduces the regeneration of liver cells as well as the synthesis of many regulatory compounds. A deficit in the lipotropic factors and of the lipoproteins leads to a decreased mobilization of fats from the liver, and thus fatty infiltration reduces the efficiency of the organ. The liver is less able to neutralize the effects of toxic substances and its cells may be damaged—sometimes beyond repair.

Severity of tissue protein depletion. When the supply of amino acids from dietary sources is inadequate, tissues such as muscle, liver, and others are depleted in order to furnish amino acids for the synthesis of the vital regulatory proteins including the plasma proteins. The protein reserves of the tissues are seriously reduced before the concentration of plasma proteins is decreased. One estimate places the tissue protein loss at 30 gm for every gram by which the plasma proteins are reduced. For example, if the total plasma protein concentration has been reduced from 7 gm per 100 ml to 6 gm per 100 ml, and the total circulating plasma volume is 3000 ml, the reduction in circulating protein would be 30 gm. The tissue loss would be about 900 gm (30 × 30 gm). To replace these losses the diet would need to include 930 gm "ideal" protein over and above the maintenance requirement. If the efficiency of the protein in a typical diet is assumed to be 70 per cent,[1] the dietary requirement is increased to 1329 gm (930 ÷ 0.70). Suppose the patient consumes a diet that is adequate in calories and that supplies 25 gm of protein in excess of the daily maintenance level; about 57 days would be required at this level of intake for full repletion to occur (1329 ÷ 25).

Nitrogen balance studies have also shown that extensive depletion of tissue proteins takes place following immobilization, bone fractures, burns, or surgery. In one study the nitrogen loss following fracture of both legs was 137 gm in a 10-day period.[2] This is equivalent to 856 gm protein.

The above examples emphasize that protein repletion cannot be accomplished by giving a patient a high-protein diet for a few days, but that a diet adequate in calories and somewhat liberalized in protein is essential for several weeks to several months.

Just as the degree of protein deficiency is difficult to assess, so it is also hard to determine when full replacement of protein deficits has been made. The concentrations of the plasma protein fractions are poor indicators inasmuch as normal levels are reached long before tissue proteins are fully replaced. Weight gain is a useful, but not infallible, indicator that the protein and calorie deficits are being reversed. But the changes in body weight must be interpreted in relation to other findings. A sudden gain in weight could be caused by increased fluid retention. On the other hand, as improvement in the protein content of tissues is taking place, edema fluids are released and the patient shows weight loss rather than gain. If changes in fluid balance can be ruled out, any gain in weight suggests, at the very least, that protein tissue is not being further catabolized for energy. If the weight gain is correlated with a liberal protein intake, it is fairly safe to assume that it includes the replacement of protein as well as adipose tissue.

Modification of the diet. A high-protein diet furnishes 100 to 125 gm protein and includes at least 2500 calories. The calorie ratio from protein is about 16 to 20 per cent, thus permitting a selection of foods that is typical of American diets. When higher protein and calorie levels are necessary, the diet order should specify the amounts required.

Protein and calories. The levels of protein and calories are of equal importance in achieving satisfactory tissue synthesis. In a study of high-protein diets in 152 British hospitals Eddy and Pellett[3] concluded that there is too much concern about the patient's protein intake and not enough emphasis upon the calorie level. Too often a high-protein diet is ordered but the patient consumes such a low level of calories that the protein is used largely as a source of energy. These investigators believe that no advantage accrues to giving more than 14 per cent of the calories as protein until the patient's daily caloric intake is at least twice his daily basal metabolism. Thus, at 2500 calories an intake of 350 protein calories or about 90 gm protein would be just as satisfactory as a higher level of protein. When the caloric intake is more than twice the basal requirement, some advantage is realized with the protein as high as 18 per cent of the total calorie level.

Management of the diet. To consume a diet containing 100 to 125 gm protein and at least 2500 calories is not difficult for an individual with a good appetite. Most patients who require these liberal diets have had an impaired appetite for some time, and only the continuous and determined effort on the part of the nurse and others working with the patient can help the patient toward the goal of adequate intake. For some patients, small meals with between-meal feedings may be most suitable. Others may achieve a greater intake by eating three meals and an evening snack. High-protein beverages are effective in achieving maximum protein intake with a minimum increase in volume. They may be prepared by combining milk, nonfat dry milk, and eggs and using a variety of flavorings. A number of palatable, inexpensive, and convenient proprietary compounds using nonfat dry milk and casein as the principal sources of protein are also available.

For emaciated patients the amount of food and the concentration of protein are increased gradually until the gastrointestinal tract again becomes accustomed to handling more food, and until the heart and circulatory system can cope with the additional demands made on it. When the food intake by these patients is rapidly increased, circulatory failure and even death can occur.

HIGH-PROTEIN DIET

Characteristics and general rules

Select ½ to ⅔ of the day's protein allowance from complete protein foods. Include some
   complete protein at each meal.
Divide the protein allowance as evenly as practical among the meals of the day.

To increase the protein content of liquid milk add 2 to 4 tablespoons nonfat dry milk to each
cup of milk.

For a soft high-protein diet consult the list of foods for a soft diet, page 405.

Include these foods, or their nutritive equivalents, daily:
    4 cups (1 quart) milk
7–8 ounces (cooked weight) meat, fish, poultry, or cheese
    2 eggs
    4 servings vegetables including:
        1 serving green or yellow vegetable
        1 to 2 servings potato
        1 to 2 servings other vegetable
        One vegetable to be eaten raw daily
    2 servings fruit including:
        1 serving citrus fruit—or other good source of ascorbic acid
        1 serving other fruit
    1 serving whole-grain or enriched cereal
    5 slices whole-grain or enriched bread
Additional foods including butter or fortified margarine, sugars, desserts, or more of the listed
foods to meet caloric needs.

Nutritive value: On the basis of specified amounts of foods above: protein, 125 gm; calories, 2500.
All vitamins and minerals in excess of normal diet—see page 403.

Meal Pattern	Sample Menu
BREAKFAST	
Fruit	Half grapefruit
Cereal	Oatmeal
Eggs—2	Fried eggs
Bread, whole grain or enriched	Whole-wheat toast
Butter or margarine	Butter
Milk to drink and for cereal	Milk
Beverage	Coffee
LUNCHEON OR SUPPER	
Meat or substitute of egg, cheese, fish, or poultry—large serving	Chicken soufflé Mushroom sauce
Potato, macaroni, spaghetti, noodles, or vegetable	Buttered green beans
Salad with dressing	Shredded carrot and raisin salad
Bread with butter or margarine	Whole-wheat roll and butter
Fruit	Fresh peaches
Milk—1 glass	Milk
DINNER	
Meat, fish, or poultry—large serving	Broiled trout with parsley garnish
Potato	Creamed potato
Vegetable	Buttered spinach
Bread with butter or margarine	Rye bread with butter
Dessert	Lemon-flake ice cream Brownies
Milk	Milk
Beverage	Tea with lemon
EVENING NOURISHMENT	
Eggnog—1 glass	Chocolate eggnog
Sandwich with cheese or equivalent	American cheese and tomato sandwich

HIGH-PROTEIN FLUID DIET

Characteristics and general rules
From 2 to 4 tablespoons nonfat dry milk may be added to each cup of milk or it may be used in custards or cream soups.

Eggs are sometimes contaminated with *Salmonella*. Pasteurized eggnogs may be purchased and are preferable to those made with raw eggs.

The calorie intake is increased by adding butter to gruels and cream soups; adding sugar to beverages; and substituting light cream for part of the milk allowance.

Include these foods or their nutritive equivalents daily:
  6 cups milk
⅔ cup nonfat dry milk
  4 eggs
1–2 ounces strained meat
½ cup strained cereal for gruel
  1 cup citrus juice
½ cup tomato juice
¼ cup vegetable purée for cream soup
  2 servings plain dessert—gelatin, Junket, custard, cornstarch pudding, ice cream, sherbet
2–3 tablespoons sugar
1–2 tablespoons butter or margarine
Cream for coffee, for gruel, and in milk
Tea, coffee, decaffeinated coffee, cocoa powder, carbonated beverages
Flavoring extracts

    Nutritive value: Protein, 110 gm; calories, 2100.

Meal Pattern
  BREAKFAST
Citrus fruit juice
Cereal gruel with milk and sugar
Poached or soft-cooked egg
Hot beverage with cream, sugar
  MIDMORNING
Fruit juice with egg white
  LUNCHEON OR SUPPER
Cream soup with butter
Tomato juice
High-protein milk, plain or flavored
Fruit-juice gelatin, cornstarch pudding, ice cream, or custard
  MIDMORNING
Malted milk or eggnog
  DINNER
Broth with strained meat
Strained fruit juice
Milk, high-protein milk, or eggnog
Ice cream, Junket, custard, gelatin or plain pudding
  EVENING
Eggnog, milk shake, or plain milk
Ice cream, gelatin, or custard

DIETARY COUNSELING

Dietary counseling is initiated by an evaluation of the patient's present meal pattern and food intake. The patient needs to know why adequate calorie and protein intakes are essential. Practical suggestions are given for increasing the calorie intake (see page 427) and the protein intake. With a list of protein equivalents from which to choose, the patient is guided toward developing a meal pattern that more nearly meets his needs. (See Figure 32–1.)

Protein Equivalents (6–8 gm protein per unit)
1 cup milk or buttermilk
⅓ cup nonfat dry milk
1 ounce American type cheese
¼ cup cottage cheese
1 egg
1 ounce meat, fish, or poultry
2 tablespoons peanut butter
8 ounces ice cream
⅔ cup milk pudding

From such a list patients select a combination that will be acceptable to them. Some will prefer additional amounts of milk, whereas others find larger portions of meat to be more acceptable. A high-protein diet need not strain the food budget since nonfat dry milk can be used in substantial amounts. Most patients, and those who cook for them, need practical suggestions, including recipes, for incorporating dry milk into eggnogs, milk shakes, custards, puddings, cream soups, and other prepared foods.

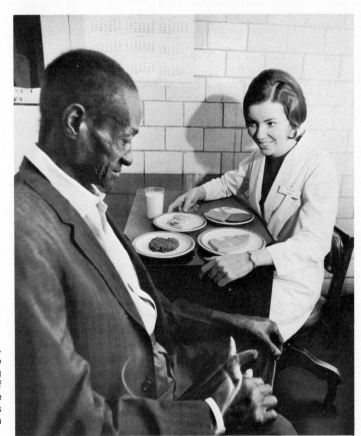

Figure 32–1. Protein equivalents. Dietetic intern gives instruction to undernourished patient pertaining to the selection of good sources of protein. (Courtesy, Medical College of Virginia, Health Sciences Division, Virginia Commonwealth University, Richmond.)

The individual who requires a high-protein high-calorie diet is likely to be one who finds it difficult to consume a large volume of food. One who has a daily intake of 55 gm protein and 1600 calories does not readily consume 120 gm protein and 2500 calories. The physician, nurse, and dietitian can help the patient to recognize his needs, but only the patient can set goals that are realistic for him. Perhaps a regular meal pattern requires emphasis; skipping breakfast, for example, makes it difficult to consume enough food for the rest of the day. Possibly a high-protein high-calorie beverage can be substituted for a low-calorie beverage, or an additional portion of dessert can be eaten at bedtime.

Patients need to know whether their efforts are, in fact, successful. Probably one of the better guides for the patient is gradual weight gain—1 to 2 pounds per week being a reasonable expectation. With improvement in the state of protein nutrition the patient will experience a greater sense of well-being.

PROBLEMS AND REVIEW

1. When the availability of protein for tissue synthesis is reduced, what functions of protein will be affected? What clinical and biochemical changes result?
2. In what pathologic conditions is protein deficiency likely to be a problem? Why?
3. Why is a liberal calorie intake essential for effective use of a high-protein diet?
4. *Problem.* The normal diet (page 403) furnishes about 94 gm protein and 2100 calories. Develop three plans whereby this pattern could be supplemented with 25 gm protein and 500 calories.
5. *Problem.* Plan a meal pattern for a 17-year-old boy who is allergic to eggs and who needs 150 gm protein and 4000 calories.
6. A patient's food intake averages 50 gm protein and 1700 calories. What are some things you need to know about this patient before you can give him guidance for a high-protein high-calorie diet?

CITED REFERENCES

1. Food and Nutrition Board: *Recommended Dietary Allowances,* 7th ed. National Academy of Sciences–National Research Council, Washington, D.C., 1968, p. 18.
2. Albanese, A. A., and Orto, L. A.: "The Proteins and Amino Acids," in Wohl, M. G., and Goodhart, R. S., eds.: *Modern Nutrition in Health and Disease,* 4th ed. Lea & Febiger Philadelphia, 1968, p. 140.
3. Eddy, T. P., and Pellett, P. L.: "Protein-Calorie Intakes of Hospital Patients," *Br. J. Nutr.,* 18:555–66, 1964.

ADDITIONAL REFERENCES

Brozek, J.: "Semistarvation and Nutritional Rehabilitation; Qualitative Case Study with Emphasis on Behavior," *J. Clin. Nutr.,* 1:107–18, 1953.
Chase, H. P., and Martin, H. P.: "Undernutrition and Child Development," *N. Engl. J. Med.,* 282:933–39, 1970.
Council on Foods and Nutrition: "Malnutrition and Hunger in the United States," *J.A.M.A.,* 213:272–75, 1970.

Downs, E. F.: "Nutritional Dwarfing. A Syndrome of Early Protein-Calorie Malnutrition," *Am. J. Clin. Nutr.*, **15:**275–81, 1965.

Mont, F. G.: "Undernutrition," in Wohl, M. G., and Goodhart, R. S., eds.: *Modern Nutrition in Health and Disease,* 4th ed. Lea & Febiger, Philadelphia, 1968, Chapter 33B.

Review: "Anorexia Nervosa," *Nutr. Rev.*, **26:**276–77, 1968.

Scrimshaw, N. S., and Behar, M.: "Malnutrition in Underdeveloped Countries," *N. Engl. J. Med.*, **272:**137–44; 193–98, 1965.

Sours, J. A.: "Clinical Studies in Anorexia Nervosa Syndrome," *N. Y. State J. Med.*, **68:**1363, 1968.

33 Diet in Fevers and Infections

Nutrition and infection. Resistance to infection is maintained by a number of mechanisms that may be adversely affected by poor nutrition. The skin and mucous membranes provide an important barrier to the invasion of bacteria. Deficiencies of vitamin A, niacin, riboflavin, vitamin B_6, and ascorbic acid lead to characteristic skin lesions which serve as entry points for bacteria and subsequent infections. A deficiency of protein and some of the B complex vitamins leads to reduced formation of antibodies. Nutritional deficiencies probably also interfere with phagocytosis and with the development of other mechanisms of resistance.

Persons who are chronically undernourished succumb to infections more readily than do the well nourished and have a longer period of recovery. In the United States the vulnerable groups are the elderly who are poor or who lack incentive to eat properly, the chronically ill who have a poor appetite, the young child living in a low-income area, and the teen-ager who follows a poor pattern of food intake. In the developing countries infants and preschool children are the most vulnerable. The effects of infection and malnutrition are synergistic. Infections are more severe in the poorly nourished, and the presence of an infection seriously aggravates an existing malnutrition. (See also page 357.)

Classification of fevers. Fever is an elevation of temperature above the normal and results from an imbalance between the heat produced in the body and the heat eliminated from the body. Fevers may be (1) acute or of short duration such as in colds, tonsillitis, influenza, pneumonia, measles, chickenpox, scarlet fever, and typhoid fever, or (2) chronic such as in tuberculosis lasting for years, or intermittent such as in malaria. Infectious hepatitis varies widely in that it is scarcely recognized in some and is severe in others, leading to permanent liver damage if nutrition is not rigorously maintained over a long period of time (see page 483). The acute phases of rheumatic fever and poliomyelitis are of short duration, but the nutritional problems may be prolonged. The high temperatures that accompany some fevers such as typhoid and malaria are extremely debilitating.

Metabolism in fevers. The metabolic effects of fevers are proportional to the elevation of the body temperature and the length of time the temperature remains elevated. Among these effects are:

1. An increase in the metabolic rate amounting to 7 per cent for every degree Fahrenheit rise in body temperature; an increase also in the restlessness and hence a greatly increased calorie need.

2. Decreased glycogen stores and decreased stores of adipose tissue.

3. Increased catabolism of proteins, especially in typhoid fever, malaria, typhus fever, poliomyelitis, and others; the increased nitrogen wastes place an additional burden upon the kidneys.

4. Accelerated loss of body water owing to increased perspiration and the excretion of body wastes.

5. Increased excretion of sodium and potassium.

6. Modified motility of the gastrointestinal tract. In some infections motility is reduced and nausea and vomiting may seriously interfere with the intake of food. In other infections the motility is increased and diarrhea interferes with the absorption of nutrients.

General dietary considerations. The diet in fevers and infections depends upon the nature and severity of the pathologic conditions and upon the length of the convalescence. In general it should meet the following requirements:

Energy. The caloric requirement may be increased as much as 50 per cent if the temperature is high and the tissue destruction is great. Restlessness also increases the caloric requirement. Initially, the patient may be able to ingest only 600 to 1200 calories daily, but this should be increased as rapidly as possible.

Protein. About 100 gm protein or more is prescribed for the adult when a fever is prolonged. This will be most efficiently utilized when the calorie intake is liberal (see Chapter 31). High-protein beverages may be used as supplements to the regular meals.

Carbohydrates. Glycogen stores are replenished by a liberal intake of carbohydrates. Any sugars such as glucose, corn syrup, and cane sugar may be used. However, glucose is less sweet than some other sugars and consequently more of it can be used. Furthermore, it is a simple sugar which is absorbed into the blood stream without the necessity for enzyme action. Lactose, used by some, is relatively expensive, dissolves poorly in cold solutions, and may increase fermentation in the small intestine resulting in diarrhea.

Fats. The energy intake may be rapidly increased through the judicious use of fats, but fried foods and rich pastries may retard digestion unduly.

Minerals. A sufficient intake of sodium chloride is accomplished by the use of salty broth and soups and by liberal sprinklings of salt on food. Generally speaking, foods are a good source of potassium, but a limited food intake might result in potassium depletion whenever fever is high and prolonged. Fruit juices and milk are relatively good sources of this element. Iron supplementation is often required to correct the anemia that results from some parasite infections.

Vitamins. Fevers apparently increase the requirements for vitamin A and ascorbic acid, just as the B complex vitamins are needed at increased levels proportionate to the increase in calories; that is, 0.5 mg thiamine, 0.6 mg riboflavin, and 6.6 mg niacin equivalents per 1000

additional calories. Oral therapy with antibiotics and drugs may interfere with intestinal synthesis of some B complex vitamins by intestinal bacteria, thus necessitating a prescription for vitamin supplements for a short time.

Fluid. The fluid intake must be liberal to compensate for the losses from the skin and to permit adequate volume of urine for excreting the wastes. From 2500 to 5000 ml daily are necessary, including beverages, soups, fruit juices, and water.

Ease of digestion. Bland, readily digested foods should be used to facilitate digestion and rapid absorption. The food may be soft or of regular consistency. Although fluid diets may be used initially there are some disadvantages: (1) most fluid diets occupy bulk out of all proportion to their caloric and nutrient values, so that reinforcement of liquids is essential; (2) a liquid diet may sometimes increase abdominal distention to the point of acute discomfort, whereas solid foods may be better tolerated; (3) many patients experience less anorexia, nausea, and vomiting when they are taking solid foods.

Intervals of feeding. Small quantities of food at intervals of two to three hours will permit adequate nutrition without overtaxing the digestive system at any one time. With improvement, many patients consume more food if given three meals and a bedtime feeding.

Diet in fevers of short duration. The duration of many fevers has been shortened by antibiotic and drug therapy, and nutritional needs are usually met without difficulty. During an acute fever the patient's appetite is often very poor, and small feedings of soft or liquid foods as desired should be offered at frequent intervals (see Chapter 29). Sufficient intake of fluids and salt is essential. If the illness persists for more than a few days, high-protein, high-calorie foods will need to be emphasized. See High-Protein Diet (Chapter 32).

Diet in typhoid fever. Improved sanitation has greatly reduced the incidence of typhoid fever, and antibiotic therapy has shortened the acute stage of the disease. Nevertheless, short and uneventful convalescence is determined to an important degree by adequate nutrition.

The febrile period may cause loss of tissue

protein amounting to as much as ½ to ¾ pound of muscle a day. The body store of glycogen is quickly depleted, and a probable upset in water balance occurs.

The intestinal tract becomes highly inflamed and irritable, and diarrhea, which is a frequent complication, interferes with the absorption of nutrients. The ulceration may be so severe that hemorrhage and even perforation of the intestines may occur.

The dietary considerations outlined on page 439 apply as in other fevers. Special emphasis must be placed upon a caloric intake of 3500 or more and a protein intake in excess of 100 gm. Because of the intestinal inflammation, great care must be exercised to eliminate all irritating fibers. The high-protein fluid diet may be used as a basis in dietary planning. In addition, low-fiber foods including white breads and crackers, refined cooked and dry cereals, eggs, cheese, tender meat, fish, and poultry, potato, and plain desserts may be used. A representative meal pattern is as follows:

BREAKFAST
Orange juice with glucose
Cream of Wheat with cream and sugar
Poached egg on
Buttered white toast
Cocoa
  MIDMORNING
Eggnog made with cream
  LUNCHEON OR SUPPER
Cream of tomato soup
Roast chicken
Baked potato (no skin) with butter
Buttered white toast
Vanilla ice cream
High-protein milk
  MIDAFTERNOON
Orange juice
Baked custard
  DINNER
Consommé with gelatin
Soft-cooked egg
Boiled rice with sugar and cream
Buttered white toast
Tapioca cream
Milk
  BEDTIME
Chocolate malted milk
Cream-cheese sandwich on white bread

Diet in rheumatic fever. Rheumatic fever is one of the leading causes of chronic illness in children. It will permanently damage the heart if it is not recognized early and treated promptly. Rheumatic fever follows Streptococcus infections and is more common among poorer classes of people. However, all attempts to correlate the incidence of the disease with specific nutrient deficiencies have so far failed.

The soft and liquid diets described in Chapter 29 are suitable during the acute phase of rheumatic fever. When cortisone or ACTH therapy is used, the diet must be mildly restricted in sodium to avoid sodium retention and edema formation (see Chapter 43).

The acute stage may last only a few weeks, but absolute bed rest is essential for many weeks or months. The chief problem in nutrition is that of maintaining an adequate intake of nutrients during the prolonged period of bed rest. Because the appetite may be poor, it has been suggested[1] that cereal foods and sweets be restricted as a means of ensuring adequate intake of milk, eggs, citrus fruits, and other essential foods. The diet is planned according to the principles of the normal diet described in Chapter 23.

Diet in poliomyelitis. The prophylactic use of Sabin or Salk vaccines has resulted in rare occurrence of poliomyelitis, except in countries that have not yet adopted this preventive measure. Spinal poliomyelitis requires essentially the same dietary attention during the acute phase as that for other acute fevers. However, convalescence is prolonged, and tissue destruction occurs. Immobilization leads to excessive excretion of calcium and the frequent incidence of urinary calculi (see Chapter 44).

Physical handicaps may interfere seriously with the ability to manage the foods served and may lead to discouragement and poor food intake. The nurse must assume responsibility not only for helping the patient through giving him foods he can manage or in feeding him, if required, but she must also give the necessary encouragement and psychologic support which brings the patient to make every effort to help himself, difficult though it may be.

The chief dietary problem in bulbar poliomyelitis is the difficulty or failure in swallowing food and the possibility of choking or aspiration. After the initial feedings by the parenteral route, a four-stage feeding program has been described by Seifert:*

Stage I. Tube feedings of 30 or 50 ml up to 150 or 200 ml are alternated every two hours with water. The tube feedings consist of skim-milk–egg–sugar formulas or milk–cream–orange-juice–sugar mixtures with or without added protein foods and oral fat emulsions.

Stage II. Tube feedings are continued. Ability to swallow is cautiously tested by giving 1 to 2 teaspoons of grape juice and noting whether the juice is seen in the tracheotomy opening. If swallowing is successful, broth, tea with sugar, apple juice, flavored gelatin, and diluted, strained juices are cautiously tried.

Stage III. A soft, low-fiber diet of easily digested foods is started. Tube feeding is continued until sufficient amounts of food can be swallowed. Sticky foods especially must be avoided. The foods which may be permitted include:

All foods from tube feedings in stages I and II
Beverages: tea with sugar, water, or coffee
Cereals: Cream of Wheat or farina with large amounts of sugar and a little milk
Desserts: custard, flavored gelatin, sherbet
Eggs: soft cooked or poached
Fats: butter
Fruits: puréed, cooked, or canned (without seeds, skin or fiber); strained fruit juices
Meats: strained
Soups: bouillon or strained meat soup
Vegetables: well cooked or puréed

Foods to avoid are fish; fried foods; milk; pastries; potatoes; raw fruits and vegetables; seeds as in berries, tomatoes; spicy or highly seasoned foods; starchy products: macaroni, rice, spaghetti; sticky foods: cheese dishes, ice cream, oatmeal; strongly flavored vegetables.

Stage IV. More solid foods, including ground meat, bread, and milk products, are introduced when the patient can take stage III without mishap. In addition to stage III, the following foods are permitted:

*Adapted from Seifert, M. H.: "Poliomyelitis and the Relation of Diet to Its Treatment," *J. Am. Diet. Assoc.*, 30:671, 1954.

Breads: soda crackers, white bread, or toast with butter
Desserts: plain cornstarch puddings and ice cream
Fruits: cooked or canned applesauce, apricots, peaches, or pears
Meats: ground beef, chicken, lamb, or turkey with light gravies or mayonnaise
Milk alone or with protein supplements
Vegetables: well-cooked but not puréed asparagus, French-cut green beans, carrots, canned peas, squash, or chopped spinach

Foods to avoid are fish; potatoes; starchy products; sticky foods—casserole dishes.

Diet in tuberculosis. One authority estimates that there are 50 million active cases of tuberculosis throughout the world and that three million die annually.[2] In the United States the morbidity and the mortality have declined but there is still some concern particularly in areas where poverty and poor sanitation prevail.

Pulmonary tuberculosis is an inflammatory disease of the lungs accompanied by a wasting of the tissues, exhaustion, cough, expectoration, and fever. In its acute form it resembles pneumonia, because the temperature is high and the circulation and respiration are increased. In the chronic phase of tuberculosis the fever is low grade and the metabolic rate is lower than in the acute fevers. Even in the chronic phase the wasting may be considerable because of the protracted illness. The following modifications of the normal diet are usually indicated:

Energy. Satisfactory weight is maintained, as a rule, at 2500 to 3000 calories. It is not desirable to gain weight beyond 10 per cent above the desirable weight for body frame.

Protein. From 80 to 120 gm protein help to regenerate the serum albumin levels, which are often low in cases of long standing.[3]

Minerals. Calcium requires particular emphasis to promote the healing of the tuberculous lesions. At least a quart of milk should be taken daily.[4] Iron supplementation may be necessary if there has been hemorrhage.

Vitamins. Carotene appears to be poorly converted to vitamin A so that the diet should provide as much preformed vitamin A as possible.[3] In addition, a vitamin A supplement may be necessary. Ascorbic acid deficiency is frequently present, and additional amounts of citrus fruits or ascorbic acid supplementation are essential.

Isoniazid has been found to be effective in the therapy of tuberculosis, but it is also an antagonist of vitamin B_6. Therefore, supplementation with vitamin B_6 is indicated to avoid the peripheral neuritis that is characteristic of vitamin B_6 deficiency.

Selection of foods. During the acute stage of the illness, a high-protein high-calorie fluid diet may be given as in other acute fevers, progressing to the soft and regular diets when improvement occurs. Most patients have very poor appetites. For some a six-meal routine is best, whereas others eat better if they receive three meals and a bedtime feeding. The individuals responsible for planning meals should respect the patient's food idiosyncrasies. To this end, a selective menu from which the patient chooses his foods each day is helpful. Other patients may eat better when they are not consulted in advance about their diets, thus introducing an element of surprise. Needless to say, every attention must be given to making meals as appetizing in appearance and taste as possible. The high-protein and high-calorie diets described in Chapters 31 and 32 may be adapted to the individual patient's needs.

DIETARY COUNSELING

Failure of the patient to secure the essentials of a normal diet leads to great increase in recurrence and repeated hospitalization.[5] The characteristics of a normal diet, with special emphasis on a liberal milk intake, protein-rich foods, fruits, and vegetables, must be pointed out. To increase the calcium and protein intake, 3 to 5 tablespoons of nonfat dry milk may be added to each 8 ounces of whole milk. If desired, fruit flavors or chocolate syrup may be added. This beverage supplementation is conveniently prepared, provides substantial nutritive value at minimum bulk, and is low in cost.

Because many of the patients with tuberculosis have low incomes, some assistance is necessary in providing practical measures to purchase the necessary foods. This entails not only additional welfare allowances in some instances but guidance in budgeting the food money. In families with low incomes it may not be practical to improve the diet of the patient alone, for additional allowances of money may be spent for the children's diet rather than for the patient. Moreover, in such situations the best prophylaxis may well be the improvement of the diet of all members of the family.

Emphysema. This is a pathologic enlargement or overdistention of the alveoli of the lung brought about by a number of causes, including bronchitis, asthma, infection, and cigarette smoking. Patients with emphysema often complain of abdominal distress, and peptic ulcers occur frequently. In early stages some patients may be obese, and the distress in breathing is further accentuated. Some improvement is noted when weight is brought within desirable levels.[6]

Shortness of breath places a severe limitation upon the ability to ingest an adequate diet, with the result that weight loss and tissue wasting are common. Not infrequently the purchase and preparation of food, or seeking a place to eat a meal, require more effort than the patient can expend. Because the patient is unable to work, there may be insufficient income to purchase adequate food. Chewing and swallowing require further effort and the patient often stops short of satisfactory intake.

A soft high-calorie diet is usually indicated. Patients are especially short of breath after a night's sleep and experience difficulty in eating breakfast.[7] Small, frequent feedings of concentrated foods should be used. Wilson found a high-protein commercial supplement to be useful because it was concentrated, palatable, easy to prepare, and easy to ingest. Too many fibrous fruits and vegetables or meats requiring much chewing may necessitate an energy expenditure beyond that justified by the nutrient values obtained. The patient will eat very slowly, and

should refrain from talking while eating since
the swallowing of air is responsible for much of
the discomfort.

For a discussion of infectious hepatitis see
page 483; for a discussion of infections from
food poisoning, see pages 262 to 265.

Problems and Review

1. What is the effect of nutritional status on the incidence of infections?
2. How great is the increase in energy metabolism brought about by fever? What other changes in metabolism of nutrients take place during fever? In view of these changes how do you view the widely held belief "Starve a fever."
3. Give examples of foods that can be used to reinforce the protein and calorie level of the diet.
4. *Problem.* Plan a fluid diet in six meals that eliminates milk. Calculate the calorie value.
5. *Problem.* Plan a full fluid diet in six meals to include 80 gm protein and 2500 calories.
6. *Problem.* Plan a diet for a 12-year-old boy with rheumatic fever. What techniques can you use to help the boy accept the diet?
7. What are the principles of dietary management in poliomyelitis?
8. Outline a plan of dietary counseling for a 34-year-old woman with healed tuberculosis. She has three children under the age of 10 years and is receiving welfare assistance. You will need to determine the amount of money available through welfare in your community to this family of four.
9. *Problem.* Keep a record of the food intake for two days by a patient with an infection. What factors enter into this patient's acceptance of food? Develop recommendations for any improvement that may be required.
10. What are the problems encountered in feeding a patient with emphysema? How would you try to solve them?

Cited References

1. Wilcox, E. B., and Galloway, L. S.: "Children With and Without Rheumatic Fever. II. Food Habits," *J. Am. Diet. Assoc.*, **30**:453–57, 1954.
2. Parry, W. H.: "Tuberculosis: A World Problem," *Nurs. Times*, **62**:1454–56, 1966.
3. Getz, H. R.: "Problems in Feeding the Tuberculosis Patient," *J. Am. Diet. Assoc.*, **30**:17–20, 1954.
4. Brewer, W. D. *et al.*: "Calcium and Phosphorus Metabolism of Women with Active Tuberculosis," *J. Am. Diet. Assoc.*, **30**:21–24, 1954.
5. Wilson, N. L., *et al.*: "Nutrition in Tuberculosis," *J. Am. Diet. Assoc.*, **33**:243–57, 1957.
6. Wilson, R. H. L., and Wilson, N. L.: "Obesity and Respiratory Distress," *J. Am. Diet. Assoc.*, **55**:465–69, 1969.
7. Wilson, N. L., *et al.*: "Protein Intakes in Pulmonary Emphysema and Tuberculosis," *J. Am. Diet. Assoc.*, **47**:194–97, 1965.

Additional References

Brewer, W. D., *et al.*: "Studies of Food Intake and Requirements of Women with Active and Arrested Tuberculosis," *Am. Rev. Tuberc.*, **60**:455–65, 1949.
Jackson, R. L., and Kelly, H. G.: "Nutrition in Rheumatic Fever," *J. Am. Diet. Assoc.*, **25**:392–97, 1949.

Johnston, R. F., and Hopewell, P. C.: "Chemotherapy of Pulmonary Tuberculosis," *Ann. Intern. Med.,* **70**:359–67, 1969.

Myers, J. A.: "Tuberculosis in the Aged," *Postgrad. Med.,* **41**:214–22, Feb. 1967.

Neva, F. A.: "Malaria—Recent Progress and Problems," *N. Engl. J. Med.,* **277**:1241–52, 1967.

Schwartz, W. S.: "Developments in Treatment of Tuberculosis and Other Pulmonary Diseases," *J.A.M.A.,* **178**:43–50, 1961.

Scrimshaw, N. S.: "Malnutrition and Infection," *Bordens Rev. Nutr. Res.,* **26** (No. 2): April–June 1965.

Secor, J.: "The Patient with Emphysema," *Am. J. Nurs.,* **65**:75–80, July 1965.

Unit X

Diet in Disturbances of the Gastrointestinal Tract

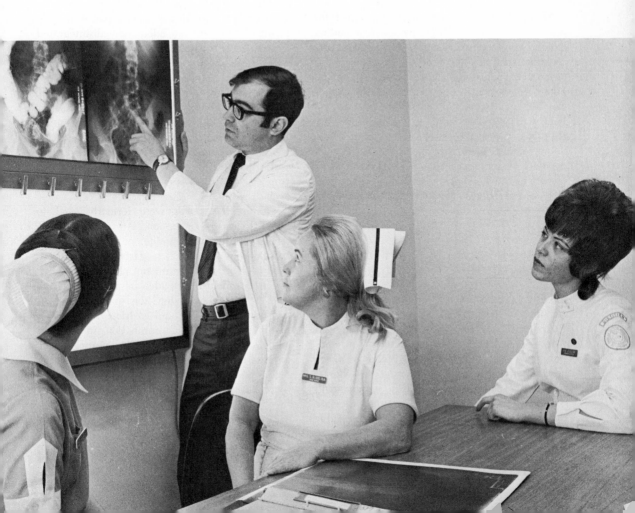

34 Diet in Diseases of the Esophagus, Stomach, and Duodenum

Bland Fiber-Restricted Diet in Three Stages

Modified diets are commonly prescribed for many disorders of the digestive tract, including hiatal hernia, peptic ulcer, gastritis, diarrhea, constipation, malabsorption syndrome, cirrhosis of the liver, cholecystitis, and pancreatitis, among others. Much controversy exists over the role of diet in the treatment of gastrointestinal disturbances. In certain conditions there is a physiologic basis for dietary modification; in others, a sound rationale is lacking and diets traditionally used are of unproven value. For the latter more objective evidence is needed before sound conclusions can be reached in regard to beneficial effects of dietary modification.

DIAGNOSTIC TESTS IN GASTROINTESTINAL DISEASE

Disorders of the gastrointestinal tract are classified as *functional* or *organic* in nature. Functional disturbances involve no alterations in structure. In organic diseases, on the other hand, pathologic lesions are seen in tissue, as in ulcers or carcinoma. Both types of disorders are characterized by changes in secretory activity and motility. A number of factors including diet are believed to influence these changes. (See Table 34–1.)

Studies of motility and secretion, together with radiologic evidence and, in some instances, biopsy specimens of the affected mucosa, are used in the diagnosis of gastrointestinal disease.

Measurement of motility. X-ray and fluoroscopic examinations are widely used to determine the emptying time and motility of the intestinal tract, and to locate the site of the disturbance. Following an overnight fast the patient is given a "barium swallow" consisting of a pint of buttermilk or malted milk in which barium sulfate has been mixed. The progress of this opaque "meal" along the intestinal tract can then be visualized by means of fluoroscopy. X-rays taken before and after the meal are studied for filling defects and other abnormalities.

In *gastric atony,* due to lack of normal muscle tone of the stomach, contractions are not of sufficient strength to move the food mass out of the stomach at a normal rate. Larger pieces or fragments of food are not adequately disintegrated and mixed with the stomach juices.

Increased action of the musculature of the stomach and intestine is known as *hyperperistalsis.* It may be brought on by excessive amounts of fibrous foods, psychologic factors such as worry or fear, or nervous stimulation.

Measurement of gastric acidity. Tests of gastric secretory function per se are of limited diagnostic value and are most useful in patients in whom a lesion has been demonstrated by x-ray or gastroscopy.

Various test meals were formerly used to stimulate gastric secretion. At present, drugs such as caffeine, histamine, or histalog, which are vigorous stimulants to gastric secretion, are used to determine the amount of acid produced.

Gastric analysis provides information on the rate of gastric emptying, the quantity of acid and pepsin secretion, and gastric cytology. Two methods are used: (1) intubation, in which a nasogastric tube is passed into the empty stomach and the contents are withdrawn for examination before a test "meal" and at specified intervals following the test "meal"; or (2) tubeless, which involves administration of a resin that exchanges a cation for hydrogen. The cation or dye is absorbed and excreted in the urine where its

Table 34–1. Factors That Modify Acid Secretion and Gastrointestinal Motility and Tone

Increased Flow of Acid and Enzyme Production	Decreased Flow of Acid and Enzyme Production
1. Chemical stimulation—meat extractives, seasonings, spices, alcohol, acid foods 2. Attractive, appetizing, well-liked foods 3. State of happiness and contentment 4. Pleasant surroundings for meals	1. Large amounts of fat, especially as fried foods, pastries, nuts, etc. 2. Large meals 3. Poor mastication of food 4. Foods of poor appearance, flavor, or texture 5. Foods acutely disliked 6. Worry, anger, fear, pain*

Increased Tone and Motility	Decreased Tone and Motility
1. Warm foods 2. Liquid and soft foods 3. Fibrous foods, as in certain fruits and vegetables 4. High-carbohydrate low-fat intake 5. Seasonings; concentrated sweets 6. Fear, anger, worry, nervous tension	1. Cold foods 2. Dry, solid foods 3. Low-fiber foods 4. High-fat intake, especially as fried foods, pastries, etc. 5. Vitamin B complex deficiency, especially thiamine 6. Sedentary habits 7. Fatigue 8. Worry, anger, fear, pain

*In certain individuals these emotional disturbances may stimulate the flow of gastric juice.

concentration indicates the amount of gastric acid exchanged.

The results of gastric analysis are usually described in terms of the "total" and "free" acid produced. Of the total acid secreted by the stomach, some combines with protein and that which remains uncombined is known as "free" hydrochloric acid. The total amount of acid secreted varies from one individual to another. Some persons continually secrete more gastric juice than normal without experiencing any discomfort. An excess secretion of acid is known as *hyperchlorhydria* and is often accompanied by gastric distress. It may be associated with emotional or nervous upsets, or it may accompany organic disease such as peptic ulcer or cholecystitis.

Hypochlorhydria denotes a diminished amount of free acid and may be present indefinitely in otherwise healthy persons. The cause should be determined, if possible, since hypochlorhydria also accompanies diseases such as pernicious anemia and is a common finding in sprue, chronic gastritis, and pellagra. It occurs occasionally in

cancer, nephritis, cholecystitis, and diabetes. In *achlorhydria* no free acid is present although there is some peptic activity; this finding suggests pernicious anemia and malignant gastric ulcer. *Achylia gastrica* refers to the absence of both free and combined acid and of enzyme activity.

GENERAL DIETARY CONSIDERATIONS IN DISEASES OF THE GASTROINTESTINAL TRACT

Factors in dietary management. Many dietary recommendations have been made for the management of gastrointestinal diseases; yet actual knowledge of the specific effects of various foods on the digestive tract is rather limited. Any proposed dietary modifications should take into consideration the possible effects of ingested food upon (1) the secretory activity of the stomach, small intestine, pancreas, liver, and gallbladder; (2) motility of the tract; (3) the bacterial flora; (4) the comfort and ease of digestion; and (5) the maintenance and repair of the mucosal structures. In addition, some disorders interfere with the completeness of digestion or the absorption of one or more nutrients so that the nutrient intake must be modified in order to meet the net requirements of the body.

Influence of foods on gastric acidity. Most foods have a pH between 5 and 7, thus are considerably less acid than gastric juice. No food is sufficiently acid to have any adverse effect on a gastric lesion, although citrus juices and fruits might cause some discomfort to a lesion of the mouth, esophagus, or the achlorhydric stomach.[1]

Gastric secretion is initiated by the sight, smell, and taste of food. As food enters the stomach, the secretion continues and reaches its height sometime later. Protein foods stimulate more acid secretion than do carbohydrates and fats.

Protein foods initially have a temporary buffering effect; hence there is less free acid immediately available to erode the lesion when protein is fed. Milk has some buffering effect, although other protein foods appear to be more effective. Nevertheless, most patients with peptic ulcer have progressed well on diets in which milk feedings were used for their neutralizing effect. Regardless of buffering activity, the amount of free acid again is high within ½ to 2 hours following a meal. No diet alone will maintain a 24-hour neutralization of gastric contents.

Fats inhibit gastric secretion. The entrance of fats into the duodenum stimulates the production of enterogastrone, a hormone, which in turn retards gastric secretion and likewise delays the emptying of the stomach. Dairy fats are not superior to other fats in this regard, but are useful as they are easily digested.

Meat extractives, tannins, caffeine, and alcohol are well known for their effect in stimulating the flow of acid. Spices are also commonly implicated in this respect, but experimental evidence on humans does not support this. Schneider and associates[2] tested the possible irritant effects of a number of spices and herbs on patients with active and healing ulcers. Subjective reactions by the patients, the rate of healing of the ulcer, and the gastroscopic appearance of the mucosa were not altered by all-

spice, caraway seeds, cinnamon, mace, paprika, thyme, or sage when given with foods. Slight reddening of the mucosa and some symptoms of gastric discomfort were noted with chili powder, cloves, mustard seeds, nutmeg, and black pepper. The elimination of most spices in favor of foods very bland in flavor therefore seems unnecessary.

Influence of foods on motility. Foods high in fiber are generally considered to increase peristaltic action, and low-fiber foods to reduce such motility. Evidence for or against these effects is meager.

The terms *fiber* and *residue,* although often used interchangeably, are not synonymous. *Fiber* refers to the skins, seeds, and structural parts of plant foods and to the connective tissue fibers of meats. Plant fibers include cellulose, hemicellulose, and lignins, and are not hydrolyzed by enzymes in the human intestinal tract; therefore, these fibers increase the bulk of the feces. *Residue* refers to the volume of the materials remaining after the digestive processes have been completed and includes not only indigestible fibers but also the bacterial residues and desquamated cells from the mucosa. Apples with skins, celery, cabbage, and whole-grain cereals are considered as high-residue foods because of their high fiber content. Milk is often cited as being a high-residue food, although studies have shown that it is more correctly termed a moderate-residue food.

The composition of the diet does not greatly influence the predominant type of intestinal organisms;[3,4] its effect on their production of gases is uncertain.

Foods and their effect on lesions. Fibrous foods have often been omitted from diets for diseases of the gastrointestinal tract in the belief that they might mechanically injure or retard the healing of a lesion such as an ulcer. Shull[5] has suggested that toleration for foods is best determined by trial with the individual. He states further:

It is highly improbable that "coarse" or "rough" foods, such as fruit skins, lettuce, cabbage, kale, nuts, celery, and endive when subjected to proper mastication or mixture with saliva could ever actually traumatize a peptic ulcer. The emphasis, therefore, should be placed upon the proper preparation of food for gastric digestion. Ordinarily this is done satisfactorily in the mouth by mastication and mixture with saliva. Only when the teeth are poor or absent is artificial grinding or puréeing necessary.*

Influence of foods upon digestive comfort. Ingestion of certain foods has long been associated with symptoms of belching, distention, epigastric distress, flatulence, constipation, or diarrhea in some persons with digestive disorders. Among these foods are baked beans, cabbage, fried foods, onions, and spicy foods. Tolerance to these and other foods has been shown to be a highly individual matter.[6] Not all patients react to foods in the same way, nor does the same patient always react to a specific food in the same way. It is now recognized that the emotional component in gastrointestinal disease may overshadow other contributing factors and may explain some of the differences in reaction to foods by patients. (See Figure 34–1.)

Traditional diets. Much of the present-day practice in dietary management of gastrointes-

*Shull, H. J.: "Diet in the Management of Peptic Ulcer," *J.A.M.A.,* **170:** 1068, 1959.

tinal disease is based upon recommendations made early in the century for treatment of peptic ulcer. The most widely used are diets based on regimens proposed by Sippy (1915) and Meulengracht (1935).[7,8] In contrast to the earlier practice of withholding food from ulcer patients, Sippy's program was designed to maintain continuous acid neutralization by means of antacids and small hourly feedings of milk and cream. A very limited variety of foods was gradually introduced over a period of several weeks. Meulengracht modified the Sippy plan somewhat by allowing a greater variety of foods at two-hour intervals in the treatment of bleeding ulcer.

Diets patterned after these regimens are based on the principle that the presence of some food in the stomach at all times will dilute and neutralize excess acid and consequently lessen pain. In most of these, milk forms the basis of the diet with small feedings of "bland" foods being given at frequent intervals. Generally speaking, foods allowed are limited to those considered to be *chemically, mechanically,* and *thermally* nonirritating; other foods are rigidly excluded.

Foods believed to be *chemically* irritating because of their stimulatory effect on gastric

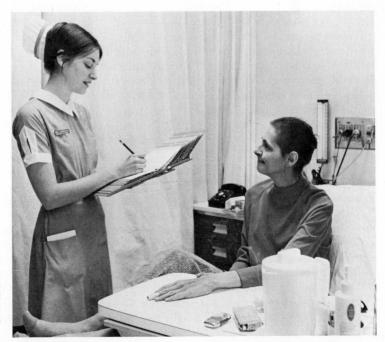

Figure 34–1. Tolerance for food is a highly individual matter. Patient is interviewed so that this can be taken into account in planning her modified diet. (Courtesy, Yale–New Haven Hospital.)

secretion include meat extractives, caffeine, alcohol, citrus fruits and juices, and spicy foods. *Mechanically* irritating foods include those with indigestible carbohydrate, such as most raw fruits and vegetables. Foods believed to be *thermally* irritating are those ordinarily served at extremes of temperature, such as very hot or iced liquids. In addition, certain foods traditionally forbidden include strongly flavored vegetables (Brussels sprouts, cabbage, cauliflower, onions, turnips, and others), baked beans, pork, and fried foods. Restriction of these foods is based on subjective evidence from patients who experienced distress following ingestion of these items.

Over the years, the practice of recommending or restricting certain foods in the management of ulcer disease has been carried over to treatment of other gastrointestinal disorders as well. Foods customarily allowed are described as bland, nonirritating, smooth, low fiber, or nonstimulating; those contraindicated are considered to be distending, gaseous, indigestible, stimulating, and so on. The soft diet, fiber-restricted diet, or stage 3 of the bland diet is appropriate for most gastrointestinal conditions; these diets are all very similar. The details of the soft diet are discussed in Chapter 29. The bland, fiber-restricted diet is on page 453.

Trends to more liberal diets. The rationale for diets in gastrointestinal diseases was reviewed in 1961 by a joint committee of the American Dietetic Association and the Council on Foods and Nutrition of the American Medical Association. The lack of objective evidence for many of the recommendations traditionally made in diet therapy of these disorders was pointed out by this committee.[1]

Increasing evidence that standard "ulcer" regimens have no beneficial value[9] and do not influence the rate of healing of the ulcer[10] has led many clinicians to recommend a more liberal approach to dietary management. Other evidence suggests that excessive use of milk and cream leads to elevated blood lipids, more rapid clotting time, and increased tendency to coronary thrombosis in ulcer patients.[11] A more flexible approach is further encouraged inasmuch as most traditional diets are nutritionally inade-

quate, are overly restrictive, and usually are not well accepted by patients. Much needed are objective studies of the effects of foods on the digestive tract and a greater appreciation of the many subjective factors at play in determining food tolerances.

DISORDERS OF THE ESOPHAGUS AND STOMACH

Esophagitis. This is an acute or chronic inflammation of the esophageal wall. *Acute* esophagitis is usually characterized by substernal pain brought on by swallowing. It may be a consequence of upper respiratory infections, extensive burns, prolonged gastric intubation, excessive vomiting, ingestion of poisonous substances such as lye, or diseases such as scarlet fever or diphtheria.

Most cases of *chronic* esophagitis are attributed to a sliding hernia that permits the reflux of gastric juice into the esophagus. Mucosal erosions and narrowing of the lumen occur. The disorder occurs most frequently in persons with high gastric acidity, many of whom have a history of duodenal ulcer.

Symptoms. Heartburn, intermittent at first, but becoming progressively worse, is often the chief complaint in esophagitis. Pain following ingestion of very hot or cold foods and spicy or acid foods and eventual dysphagia occur as the disease progresses.

Treatment. The objectives of therapy are to protect the esophagus, to reduce gastric acidity, and to reduce reflux of gastric contents into the esophagus. Antacid preparations are usually prescribed.

Dietary management consists of weight reduction (see Chapter 31) for obese individuals since excess abdominal fat is believed to increase gastric herniation and reflux. Large meals should be avoided in favor of more frequent small meals. A bland, fiber-restricted diet is desirable for most individuals (see page 453).

Hiatus hernia. A common disorder affecting the esophagus is the herniation of a portion of the stomach through the hiatus of the diaphragm. This disorder, known as *hiatal hernia,* occurs most frequently in persons over 45 years of age. The incidence is greater in persons of stocky build and in overweight persons. Loss of muscle tone weakens muscles around the diaphragm and increased abdominal pressure helps push the stomach through the diaphragm. Symptoms occur when the herniated portion is irritated or injured or is large enough to affect other organs. Tight garments or belts appear to provoke symptoms and should be avoided. Substernal pain, belching, or hiccoughing occur following meals or while lying down.

A bland, fiber-restricted diet with between-meal snacks is usually recommended (see page 453). Of equal importance are eating small amounts at any one time and omitting food for several hours before bedtime. Weight reduction is essential for obese individuals (see Chapter 31).

Achalasia. This is a disorder of esophageal motility in which the lower esophageal sphincter fails to relax normally upon swallowing so that food can enter the stomach. Loss or absence of ganglion cells is believed to be involved. Long-continued intraesophageal pressure may lead to dilatation above the point of stricture. The primary symptom is dysphagia with possible vomiting and eventual weight loss.

Treatment consists of dilatation of the stricture. Dietary considerations include avoidance of excessively hot or iced beverages and any foods that may be irritating to the esophagus. If weight loss has been considerable, increased calories and protein are needed (see Chapter 32). Some individuals tolerate several small feedings better than larger ones.

Esophageal obstruction. This may result from a number of causes including pressure from adjacent organs, hiatus hernia, scar tissue formation, foreign bodies, diverticula, and neoplasms. Swallowed foods do not progress beyond the point of stricture owing to narrowing of the lumen, and if the condition is untreated, death from starvation follows. Measures to restore the normal passageway include dilatation, irradiation, or surgical intervention, depending on the nature of the obstruction.

Dietary management is the same for obstruction from any cause. Efforts are directed toward providing foods in suitable form and sufficient amounts to meet the patient's needs. In partial obstruction, liquids should be offered with progression to low-fiber foods (see page 454) as tolerated. Small amounts of food at frequent intervals are preferable. When it is not possible or desirable for food to pass through the esophagus, the patient is fed by means of a gastrostomy. Food is administered through a tube inserted directly into the stomach. (See Chapter 38 for characteristics of tube feedings.)

Indigestion. Indigestion, or dyspepsia, is a functional or organic disease manifested by symptoms of heartburn, acid regurgitation, epigastric pain, "fullness" or bloating especially after meals, flatulence, nausea, or vomiting.

The majority of cases of indigestion are of functional origin and are usually due to faulty dietary habits or emotional factors. The organic type is associated with diseases affecting the digestive organs; it may also be a symptom of generalized disease as in uremia. Treatment in organic types consists of treating the underlying disease.

Persons with functional dyspepsia need individualized dietary counseling in the essentials of a nutritionally adequate diet. Specific instructions should be given with emphasis on selection of foods from each of the Four Food Groups and the importance of regular mealtimes, sufficient time to eat in a relaxed atmosphere, rest after meals, and avoidance of emotional tension.

Gastritis. This is an inflammation of the mucosa of the stomach, occurring as an acute or chronic lesion with atrophy or hypertrophy in some persons. Causes are toxins of bacterial or metabolic origin (*Salmonella, Staphylococcus,* uremia, syphilis); irritation of the gastric mucosa by ingestion of ethyl alcohol, certain drugs (digitalis, glucogenic steroids, salicylates, and others), heavy metals, strong alkali or acid; or faulty dietary habits. The latter may include excessive intake of fibrous, fried, or highly seasoned foods, very hot or very cold drinks, or rapid eating with poor mastication. Symptoms of indigestion usually occur.

Acute gastritis is characterized by a general inflammatory reaction of the mucosa with hyperemia, edema, and exudation; in more severe cases, erosion of localized areas and hemorrhages occur. Symptoms vary from anorexia, vague epigastric discomfort, or heartburn, to severe vomiting. The diagnosis of gastritis is based on biopsies of the gastric mucosa.

Since acute gastritis usually heals within three or four days, nutritional management is not the primary concern. Treatment is directed toward removal or neutralization of the offending agent by gastric lavage, antibiotics, withholding of food for 24 to 48 hours to allow the stomach to rest, and replacement of water and electrolyte losses due to severe vomiting. After one or two days small amounts of clear fluids (100 ml per hour) are administered with gradual progression to soft, easily digested foods (see page 405).

Chronic gastritis is characterized by recurrent inflammation of the gastric mucosa leading to glandular atrophy and changes in enzyme activities of the gastric mucosal cells. Complete atrophy results in the inability to absorb vitamin B_{12} and in pernicious anemia. Secretion of hydrochloric acid is impaired. Symptoms include epigastric distress, nausea, and vomiting. Chronic gastritis is often directly attributed to dietary indiscretion or indirectly to toxic substances; nevertheless, it may also occur in the absence of any known cause. Autoimmunologic factors, endocrine dysfunction, and nutritional deficiency, especially of iron, have been implicated.[12] Gastritis may be the cause of persistent symptoms in patients in whom peptic ulcer has seemingly healed.[13]

Dietary treatment of chronic gastritis consists in correcting faulty habits of eating or drinking, providing a relaxed atmosphere at mealtime, and emphasizing adequate caloric intake of soft or bland foods (see page 454). Arrangement of meals in four or six small feedings is sometimes preferred. Iron supplements may be desirable. Once symptoms have abated, progression to a normal diet may be made.

Carcinoma of the stomach. This usually occurs in persons over 50 years of age and rarely in younger age groups. However, the stomach is the second most common site of cancer of the gastrointestinal tract (the colon being first) in persons under 30 years of age.[14] Early diagnosis is essential for a complete cure. If the disease is

not too far advanced a gastrectomy is done. Unfortunately, the disease is often well advanced before symptoms of anorexia, weight loss, fatigue, abdominal discomfort and pain, nausea, and vomiting appear. Since these symptoms are common to many disorders, positive evidence as shown by x-ray examination or cytologic studies is needed to establish the presence of malignancy. Iron-deficiency anemia, hypoalbuminemia, achlorhydria, or hypochlorhydria may also occur.

Following gastrectomy, the postoperative regimen is used (see page 500). Small, frequent meals are given. For those patients who develop the dumping syndrome, foods should be high in protein and fat and low in carbohydrate (see page 502).

When surgical intervention is not feasible, every effort is made to promote the patient's comfort. Frequent small feedings of soft, low-fiber foods are provided (see Chapter 29). It is most important that the meals be attractive to coax the patient's appetite, and that efforts be made to accommodate the patient's requests. Unnecessary dietary restrictions should be avoided.

PEPTIC ULCER

The term *peptic ulcer* is used to describe any localized erosion of the mucosal lining of those portions of the alimentary tract that come in contact with gastric juice. The majority of ulcers are found in the duodenum, although they also occur in the esophagus, stomach, or jejunum. Similar symptoms are produced by the ulcer regardless of its location, and response to treatment is essentially the same. The same principles of dietary treatment apply to all regardless of etiology.

The incidence of peptic ulcer in the United States is approximately 10 per cent of the general population, occurring at any age, but particularly between the ages of 20 and 45. It occurs more frequently in males.

Etiology. In spite of extensive literature on the subject, the exact cause of peptic ulcer has not been determined. Multiple factors are probably involved. In duodenal ulcer, hypersecretion of acid is found, although tissue resistance is normal. In gastric ulcer, excess acid is seldom found, but there is decreased tissue resistance to the acid.

Repeated irritation of the mucosa by dietary indiscretion or alcohol may lower the tissue resistance to acid, thereby making the individual more susceptible to ulcer formation. Likewise, certain drugs, such as the adrenal steroids and salicylates, may induce gastric ulceration either by their irritating effect on the mucosa or by a stimulating effect on acid secretion.

Personality type plays a role—highly nervous and emotional individuals seem to be more susceptible to the disease. Anxiety, worry, and strain may cause hypersecretion of acid and hypermotility. A positive family history of recurrent pain is not uncommon.

Symptoms and clinical findings. Epigastric pain occurring as deep hunger contractions one to three hours after meals is often the chief complaint. The pain may be described as dull, piercing, burning, or gnawing and is usually relieved by the taking of food or alkalies. The basis for the pain may be the action of unneutralized hydrochloric acid on exposed nerve fibers at the site of the ulcer. Pain is also associated with hypermotility of the stomach or gastric distention following ingestion of large amounts of food or liquids.

Low plasma protein levels are often present and delay rapid and complete healing of the ulcer. Weight loss and iron-deficiency anemia are common. The intake of ascorbic acid, iron, and the B complex vitamins, particularly thiamine, may be less than desirable because of self-imposed limitation of leafy green vegetables and other food sources of these nutrients. (See Chapters 8, 11, and 12.)

In some instances, hemorrhage is the first indication of an ulcer and requires surgical intervention. Other complications such as intractability, obstruction, perforation, and carcinoma of gastric ulcer are treated surgically.

Rationale for treatment. Individualized attention to the whole person rather than to the ulcer per se is extremely important in the management of persons with ulcer disease. The patient must be taught to accept responsibility for his progress since medical and dietary therapies produce only symptomatic improvement. In general, treatment consists of drugs, rest, and diet therapy.

Drugs. *Antacid* preparations are prescribed to neutralize excess acid production. *Anticholinergic* drugs are used to inhibit acid secretion, and *antispasmodics* delay gastric emptying.

Rest. Good physical and mental hygiene is basic if the person is to learn to cope with his problems constructively. Mental and physical rest is important; modification of living and work habits is needed when overwork and physical stress cause exacerbations of the disease. Control of emotional stress is equally important.

Diet. Dietary management consists of providing a nutritionally adequate diet that includes frequent feedings. Such a diet is essential for persons with ulcers not only to promote rapid healing but to correct preexisting deficiencies. In some instances, intakes of nutrients in excess of the Recommended Dietary Allowances are desirable, with particular emphasis on high-quality protein, ascorbic acid, and iron. To help maintain neutrality of the gastric contents small feedings every two hours are often used initially with later progression to three meals plus snacks at midmorning, midafternoon, and bedtime. Establishing regularity of mealtimes is an important aspect of the diet. Some individuals experience fewer subjective symptoms if fiber is restricted (see page 454). Individualization of the diet to meet the patient's needs and preferences is essential.

BLAND FIBER-RESTRICTED DIET IN THREE STAGES

Characteristics and general rules
The stages of diet are set up for gradual progression in quantity of food eaten at a meal, in fiber content, and in selection of foods.

The selection of foods includes those mild in flavor, and which infrequently bring forth complaints of intolerance. The lists should not be considered as restrictive, inasmuch as food tolerance is a highly individual matter. Additions or subtractions should be made according to individual need.

For patients with peptic ulcer, frequent feedings are essential. The six-meal sample menus listed below could be rearranged for two-hourly feedings of smaller size, if the physician believes this to be necessary.

FOOD SELECTION FOR THREE STAGES OF DIET

Stages I and II

Beverages—milk and fruit juices

Breads—enriched white bread or toast; saltines; soda crackers; Melba toast; zwieback

Cereals—cornflakes, cornmeal, farina, hominy grits, oatmeal, Puffed Rice, rice flakes; macaroni, noodles, rice, spaghetti

Cheese—mild American in sauces; cream; cottage

Desserts—plain cake and cookies; custard; fruit whip; gelatin; plain ice cream; bread, cornstarch, rice, or tapioca puddings without raisins or nuts

Eggs—any way except fried

Fats—butter, cream, margarine, smooth peanut butter, cooking fat, vegetable oils

Fruits—fruit juices; avocado, banana, grapefruit and orange sections; baked apple without skin, applesauce; canned apricots, cherries, peaches, pears

Meat—tender or ground. Baked, broiled, creamed, roasted, stewed: beef, chicken, fish, lamb, liver, pork, sweetbreads, turkey, veal

Milk—in all forms

Seasonings—salt, sugar, flavoring extracts

Soups—cream

Vegetables—cooked; asparagus tips, green and wax beans, beets, carrots, white potato, winter squash, spinach, sweet potato

Stage III

All foods of stages I and II plus the following:

Beverages—decaffeinated coffee; 1 cup regular coffee with half milk, if desired; weak tea

Breads—rye without seeds; fine whole wheat

Cereals—all except coarse bran

Cheeses—all

Eggs—including fried

Fats—mayonnaise and salad dressings

Fruits—raw apple, cherries, peaches, pears, plums; stewed apricots and prunes

Seasonings—allspice, cinnamon, mace, paprika, sage, thyme

Soups—fish chowders

Vegetables—lettuce and other tender salad greens; celery; tomatoes; any others as tolerated

MEAL PATTERNS FOR STAGES I AND II

Stage I
(10–12 oz per meal)
ON AWAKING
Milk—8 oz
BREAKFAST
Cereal—4 oz
Milk—4 oz
Sugar
Egg—1

Stage II
(approximately 12–16 oz)

Milk—8 oz

Cooked or dry cereal
Milk
Sugar
Egg

Stage I (Cont.)
White toast—1 slice
Butter

MIDMORNING
Milk beverage—8 oz
Crackers, custard, plain pudding, gelatin—3 oz
LUNCHEON
Cream soup—4 oz
Crackers—2
Egg—1; or mild cheese—1 oz; or tender meat—1 oz
White bread or toast—1 slice
Butter
Dessert—3 to 4 oz
Citrus juice—3 oz

MIDAFTERNOON
Milk beverage—8 oz
Crackers, custard, plain pudding, gelatin—3 oz
DINNER
Egg, soft cheese, or tender meat—1 oz
Potato or substitute—3 oz
Toast or bread—1 slice
Butter
Fruit—3 oz
Milk or cream soup—4 oz

EVENING
Milk beverage—8 oz
Crackers or dessert—3 oz

Stage II (Cont.)
Enriched toast
Butter
Fruit juice or fruit

Milk beverage—8 oz
Crackers, custard, plain pudding, gelatin

Cream soup
Crackers
Meat, fish, poultry, eggs, or cheese—2 to 3 oz
Potato or substitute
White bread or toast
Butter
Dessert
Fruit
Milk

Milk beverage or small meat sandwich
Plain dessert

Meat, fish, poultry, eggs, or cheese—3 oz
Potato or substitute
Cooked vegetable
Bread or roll
Butter
Fruit or dessert
Milk

Milk beverage or small meat sandwich
Crackers or plain dessert

A TYPICAL DAY'S MENU FOR STAGE III

BREAKFAST
Stewed apricots
Oatmeal with milk and sugar
Soft-cooked egg
Enriched toast with butter
Coffee with half milk—1 cup
MIDMORNING
Milk—8 oz
Saltines—4
LUNCHEON
Cream of asparagus soup
Baked rice with cheese
Buttered peas
Lettuce and sliced tomatoes with mayonnaise
Rye bread and butter

Vanilla ice cream
Milk
MIDAFTERNOON
Chicken sandwich
Jello
DINNER
Broiled lamb chop
Mashed potato
Diced buttered beets
Dinner roll with butter
Sliced peaches (fresh, frozen, or canned)
Milk
EVENING NOURISHMENT
Malted milk
Sugar cookies

Modification of diet in bleeding ulcer. The degree of dietary modification in bleeding ulcer depends on the peculiarities of the individual case. In severe hemorrhage, it is customary to give no food until the bleeding has been controlled and the patient's condition is stabilized.

If hemorrhage is not severe, and if nausea and vomiting are not a problem, the patient may desire food and tolerate it well. Initial dietary treatment usually consists of milk alternated at two-hour intervals with small feedings of easily digested foods, such as egg, custards or simple puddings, toast, crackers, and tender cooked fruits and vegetables. Gradual progression in amounts and types of foods is made as the patient improves.

Dietary Counseling

The patient with an ulcer needs careful counseling about his diet with emphasis on positive rather than negative aspects of the diet. He needs to know which foods are needed for a nutritionally adequate diet and the importance of including these daily. He should be taught to select an essentially normal diet from a wide variety of foods, omitting those foods which he knows to be distressing to him. Moderate use of seasonings is permitted and may greatly enhance the flavor of foods. The patient should be instructed to establish regularity of mealtimes, to include between-meal snacks—preferably of some protein foods, and to use moderation in amounts eaten. If the diet to be used at home is planned with the patient, giving consideration to his cultural pattern, he is more likely to follow recommendations made. Meals eaten in restaurants should pose no particular problems if the individual uses good judgment in food selection.

The nurse should stress the importance of eating meals in a relaxed atmosphere with a happy frame of mind and advise the patient to try to forget personal or family problems while eating. A short rest before and after meals may be conducive to greater enjoyment of meals.

Ulcers frequently recur even after complete healing is believed to have taken place. To prevent recurrence of symptoms prompt treatment is advisable following great stress. The stomach tends to be empty of foods but full of highly acid gastric juice throughout the night and it is likely that this is the period when the greatest part of the injury to the gastric and duodenal mucosa occurs. In periods of great emotional strain, taking of food every few hours from dinnertime until 2 or 3 o'clock in the morning is recommended.

Problems and Review

1. List some of the nutritional disturbances which may develop when the stomach and intestinal tract are impaired.
2. Miss B. is a 28-year-old file clerk who is about 20 pounds overweight and has a hiatal hernia. Her physician has recommended a bland diet for her but she is afraid she will gain weight if she follows the diet. What suggestions could you offer to assist her in planning her diet?
3. Mrs. D. is a 33-year-old housewife who complains of indigestion. Name five dietary factors which could lead to development of this condition. What recommendations would you make concerning her diet?
4. Mrs. G. and Mrs. F. are discussing their husbands' recent hospitalizations for peptic ulcer. Mr. G.'s physician recommended a traditional bland diet; Mr. F. was advised to follow a liberal diet.
   a. In what respects would you expect their diets to be similar? How would you expect them to differ?
   b. Mr. G. will soon return to his teaching position and he plans to carry his lunch to school. Plan a day's menu for him.
   c. List five food combinations suitable for between-meal feedings for Mr. G.
   d. Mr. F. eats lunch in a restaurant. Plan a day's menu for him.

5. Mrs. G. does not understand the reasons for some of the recommendations made concerning her husband's diet. Explain the principle involved in each of the following:
   a. Milk and cream.
   b. Orange juice at the end of the meal, but not between meals.
   c. Tender meat, fish, poultry.
   d. Feedings at two-hour intervals.
   e. Omission of coffee and tea.
6. Mrs. F. has asked whether it makes any difference what foods her husband eats as long as he takes antacids. What would you tell her in regard to:
   a. Foods that are most likely to stimulate acid secretion.
   b. Those foods that depress acid secretion.
   c. Foods that are most effective in acid neutralization.
   d. Foods that increase motility of the gastrointestinal tract.
7. Mr. F. is concerned that his ulcer will recur when he returns to his job and his very demanding boss. What prophylactic measures can he take to prevent recurrence?
8. What possible role may diet play in causing or relieving the emotional stress to which some patients with peptic ulcer may be subjected?

CITED REFERENCES

1. Weinstein, L., *et al.:* "Diet as Related to Gastrointestinal Function," *J.A.M.A.,* **176**:935–41, 1961.
2. Schneider, M. A., *et al.:* "The Effect of Spice Ingestion upon the Stomach," *Am. J. Gastroenterol.,* **26**:722–32, 1956.
3. Haenel, H.: "Human Normal and Abnormal Gastrointestinal Flora," *Am. J. Clin. Nutr.,* **23**:1433–39, 1970.
4. Speck, R. S., *et al.:* "Human Fecal Flora under Controlled Diet Intake," *Am. J. Clin. Nutr.,* **23**:1488–94, 1970.
5. Shull, H. J.: "Diet in the Management of Peptic Ulcer," *J.A.M.A.,* **170**:1068–71, 1959.
6. Koch, J. P., and Donaldson, R. M.: "A Survey of Food Intolerances in Hospitalized Patients," *N. Engl. J. Med.,* **271**:657–60, 1964.
7. Sippy, B. W.: "Gastric and Duodenal Ulcers. Medical Cure by an Efficient Removal of Gastric Juice Corrosion," *J.A.M.A.,* **64**:1625–30, 1915.
8. Meulengracht, E.: "Treatment of Haematemesis and Melaena with Food," *Lancet,* **2**:1220–22, 1935.
9. Doll, R., *et al.:* "Dietetic Treatment of Peptic Ulcer," *Lancet,* **1**:5–9, 1956.
10. Buchman, E., *et al.:* "Unrestricted Diet in the Treatment of Duodenal Ulcer," *Gastroenterology,* **56**:1016–20, 1969.
11. Hartroft, W. S.: "The Incidence of Coronary Artery Disease in Patients Treated with the Sippy Diet," *Am. J. Clin. Nutr.,* **15**:205–10, 1964.
12. Taylor, K. B.: "Gastritis," *N. Engl. J. Med.,* **280**:818–20, 1969.
13. Edwards, F. C., and Coghill, N. F.: "Clinical Manifestations in Patients with Chronic Atrophic Gastritis, Gastric Ulcer, and Duodenal Ulcer," *Q. J. Med.,* **37**:337–60, 1968.
14. Janower, M. L., *et al.:* "Cancer of the Gastrointestinal Tract in Young People," *Radiol. Clin. North Am.,* **7**:121–30, 1969.

ADDITIONAL REFERENCES

"Bland Diet in the Treatment of Chronic Duodenal Ulcer Disease," Position Paper. *J. Am. Diet. Assoc.,* **59**:244–45, 1971.
Bralow, S. P.: "Current Concepts of Peptic Ulceration," *Am. J. Dig. Dis.,* **14**:655–77, 1969.

Donaldson, R. M., Jr.: "Diet and Gastrointestinal Disorders," *Gastroenterology,* **52**:897–900, 1967.

Dragstedt, L. R.: "Peptic Ulcer. An Abnormality in Gastric Secretion," *Am. J. Surg.,* **117**:143–56, 1969.

Jay, A. N.: "Is It Indigestion?" *Am. J. Nurs.,* **58**:1552–54, 1958.

Kirsner, J. B.: "Peptic Ulcer: A Review of the Recent Literature on Various Clinical Aspects," *Gastroenterology,* **54**:611–41, 1968 (Part I); *Gastroenterology,* **54**:945–75, 1968 (Part II).

Kramer, P., and Caso, E. K.: "Is the Rationale for Gastrointestinal Diet Therapy Sound?" *J. Am. Diet. Assoc.,* **42**:505–10, 1963.

Odell, A. C.: "Ulcer Dietotherapy—Past and Present," *J. Am. Diet. Assoc.,* **58**:447–50, 1971.

Review: "Diet Therapy of Gastrointestinal Diseases," *Nutr. Rev.,* **27**:49–51, 1969.

Roth, H. P., and Caron, H. S.: "Patients' Misconceptions About Their Peptic Ulcer Diets. Potential Obstacles to Cooperation," *J. Chronic Dis.,* **20**:5–11, 1967.

Schuster, M. M.: "Functional Gastrointestinal Disorders," *GP,* **35**:131–39, March 1967.

35 Diet in Disturbances of the Small Intestine and Colon

Very Low-Residue Diet

The functions of the small intestine may be unfavorably influenced by diseases affecting the tract itself or those organs closely related to the digestive process—the liver, gallbladder, and pancreas. In addition, many seemingly unrelated pathologic conditions to be discussed in chapters that follow have profound effects on the functioning of the gastrointestinal tract, for example, renal diseases. Depending upon the nature of the disease, there may be disturbances in motility, adequacy of enzyme production or release, hydrolytic activity, integrity of the mucosal surfaces, transport mechanisms, and so on. Any of these abnormalities interferes with the efficiency and completeness of absorption and hence the nutritional status of the individual. This chapter includes a discussion of alterations in bowel motility, inflammatory diseases of the mucosa, and carcinoma of the bowel. The malabsorption syndrome will be discussed in the chapter that follows, and diseases of the liver, gallbladder, and pancreas in Chapter 37.

ALTERATIONS IN BOWEL MOTILITY

Diarrhea. Diarrhea is the passage of stools of liquid to semisolid consistency at frequent intervals. The number of stools may vary from several per day to one every few minutes. Diarrhea is a symptom of underlying functional or organic disease and is acute or chronic in nature. Some causes of diarrhea are shown in Table 35–1.

Acute diarrhea is characterized by the sudden onset of frequent stools of watery consistency, abdominal pain, cramping, weakness, and sometimes fever and vomiting. Since the duration is usually 24 to 48 hours, nutritional losses are not a prime concern. Acute diarrhea may be the presenting symptom of systemic infection or chronic gastrointestinal disease such as regional enteritis or ulcerative colitis.

In chronic diarrhea, nutritional deficiencies eventually develop because the rapid passage of the intestinal contents does not allow sufficient time for absorption.

Nutritional considerations in diarrheas. Fluid, electrolyte, and tissue protein losses may be severe if diarrhea is prolonged.

Fluids. Losses of fluids should be replaced by

Table 35–1. Causes of Diarrhea

Acute Types	Chronic Types
1. Chemical toxins, such as arsenic, lead, mercury, or cadmium	1. Malabsorptive lesions of anatomic, mucosal, or enzymatic origin
2. Bacterial toxins, such as *Salmonella* or staphylococcal food poisoning	2. Metabolic diseases, such as diabetic neuropathy, uremia, or Addison's disease
3. Bacterial infections, such as *Streptococcus*, *E. coli,* or *Shigella*	3. Alcoholism
4. Drugs, such as quinidine, colchicine, or neomycin	4. Carcinoma of small bowel or colon
5. Psychogenic factors, such as emotional instability	5. Postirradiation to small bowel or colon
6. Dietary factors, such as food sensitivity or allergy	6. Cirrhosis

a liberal intake to prevent dehydration, especially in susceptible age groups such as the very young or elderly persons. Parenteral fluids are often administered to these individuals.

Electrolytes. Losses of sodium, potassium, and other electrolytes may account for the profound weakness associated with severe diarrhea. Potassium loss, in particular, is detrimental as potassium is necessary for normal muscle tone of the gastrointestinal tract. Anorexia, vomiting, listlessness, and muscle weakness may occur unless losses are replaced by a liberal intake of fluids such as fruit juices that are high in potassium (see Chapter 44).

Nutrient malabsorption. Long-continued diarrhea may result in depletion of tissue proteins and decreased serum protein levels. Fat losses are considerable in certain disorders with consequent loss of calories and fat-soluble vitamins. Intake of calories must be great enough to replace losses and may need to be as high as 3000, with 100 to 150 gm protein, 100 to 120 gm fat, and the remainder as carbohydrate (see Chapter 32).

Vitamin deficiencies frequently seen in chronic diarrheas are related to the decreased intake of vitamins and the increased requirements because of losses in the stools. A temporary reduction of synthesis of some B complex vitamins also occurs when antibiotic therapy is used. Vitamin B_{12}, folic acid, and niacin deficiencies have been observed in various diarrheas.

Iron deficiency is a prominent finding in patients with chronic diarrhea owing to the increased losses of iron in the feces, the occasional blood losses, and the reduced intake of iron-rich foods because of fear that some foods may aggravate an existing lesion. Patients often show remarkable improvement when given supplemental iron therapy.

Diet in diarrheal states. Any dietary modification in diarrheal states depends on the nature of the underlying defect. In acute diarrhea, clear liquids are usually tolerated best until the bowel has a chance to rest, usually 12 to 24 hours, after which progression to a soft (see Chapter 29) or regular diet is made.

Many patients with chronic diarrhea of functional or organic nature do not tolerate milk or foods high in fat or fiber content. Generally speaking, however, the need is for a diet high in protein (see Chapter 32) and calories, with adequate amounts of vitamins and minerals, and liberal amounts of fluids.

Constipation. This is a condition in which there is infrequent or difficult evacuation of feces from the intestine. An accurate definition is related to personal habits since the frequency of bowel movements varies greatly among individuals. For some, daily elimination is normal; in other equally healthy persons, regular evacuation occurs every second or third day.

Infrequent or insufficient emptying of the bowel may lead to malaise, headache, coated tongue, foul breath, and lack of appetite. These symptoms usually disappear after satisfactory evacuation has taken place.

Temporary or chronic constipation may be due to any one of a number of factors such as: (1) failure to establish regular times for eating, adequate rest, and elimination; (2) faulty dietary habits, such as inadequate fluid intake or use of highly refined and concentrated foods that leave little residue in the colon; (3) interference with the urge to defecate brought on by poor personal hygiene or injury to the nervous mechanism; (4) changes in one's usual routine brought on by illness, nervous tension, or a trip away from home; (5) chronic use of laxatives and cathartics; (6) difficult or painful defecation due to hemorrhoids or fissures; (7) poor muscle tone of the intestine and stasis due to lack of exercise occurring especially in bedridden patients, invalids such as arthritics, the aged, and others; (8) organic disorders, such as diverticulosis or obstruction from adhesions or neoplasms; (9) ingestion of drugs, large amounts of sedatives, ganglionic blocking agents, or opiates; and (10) spasm of the intestine due to presence of irritating material, psychogenic influences, or others.

Determination of the cause is important so that proper treatment can be given. Correction of constipation depends in large measure on establishing regularity in habits—eating, rest, exercise, and elimination.

The inflammatory reaction extends through the entire intestinal wall causing edema and fibrosis. It may be confined to one segment or involve multiple segments with normal areas in between.

Characteristic symptoms include abdominal pain, cramping, diarrhea, steatorrhea, weight loss, fever, and weakness. Systemic complications, malnutrition, and fistula formation are common.

Conservative management is used unless obstruction or other complications make surgical intervention (ileal resection) necessary.

Dietary considerations. The diet should provide at least 125 gm protein and 2500 calories to overcome losses due to exudation and malab-

Very Low-Residue Diet

Characteristics and general rules
This diet is essentially fiber-free and leaves a minim discussion on page 448.

If the diet is used for more than a few days, it should multivitamin concentrates.

As improvement takes place, the diet is liberalized b fruits, and milk.

Foods Allowed
Beverages—coffee in limited amounts, tea

Breads—enriched bread or toast, crackers, plain rolls, Melba toast, zwieback

Cereals—cornmeal, farina, strained oatmeal; cornflakes, Puffed Rice, rice flakes; macaroni, noodles, rice, spaghetti

Cheese—cottage, cream, mild American in sauces

Desserts—plain cake, cookies, custard, gelatin, ice cream, puddings, rennet desserts

Eggs—cooked any way except fried

Fats—butter, cream, margarine, vegetable oils

Fruits—strained juices only. Occasionally applesauce is given to patients with diarrhea because of its pectin content

Meats—tender or minced lean meat, fish, or poultry

Soups—clear: bouillon or broth without fat

Sweets—hard candy, honey, jelly, syrup, sugar in moderation

Vegetables—tomato juice; white potato

Miscellaneous—salt; spices in moderation

verticulitis should continue to use a diet moderately restricted in fiber (see Chapter 34). In recurrent or persistent attacks, surgical resection of the involved portion of colon may be necessary. Complications, such as obstruction, perforation, or fistula formation, also necessitate surgical intervention.

Ulcerative colitis. This is a diffuse inflammatory and ulcerative disease of unknown etiology involving the mucosa and submucosa of the large intestine. No single etiologic factor has been identified, although genetic, psychiatric, and autoimmune factors are thought to be involved. Much attention has been directed toward the role of psychologic factors since many individuals with this disease are nervous, introspective, apprehensive, and emotionally unstable. However, it is not known whether these are predisposing factors, part of the disease, or secondary to the physical state.

Symptoms and clinical findings. Ulcerative colitis may occur at any age but predominates in young adults. The onset is insidious in the majority of cases with mild abdominal discomfort, an urgent need to defecate several times a day, and diarrhea accompanied by rectal bleeding. Loss of water, electrolytes, blood, and protein from the colon produces systemic symptoms such as weight loss, dehydration, fever, anemia, and general debility. In early stages the mucosa is edematous and hyperemic. In more severe disease, necrosis and frank ulceration of the mucosa occur. The severity of the symptoms does not necessarily correlate with the extent of the disease. Patients with localized disease can be very seriously ill; on the other hand, persons with very troublesome symptoms may have mild disease.

The seriousness of this disease was pointed out by Morowitz and Kirsner in a study of causes of death in 137 patients. In this study, one third of deaths were directly attributable to the disease process, another third were due to complications of the disease, and the remainder of deaths were unrelated to ulcerative colitis. The average age at death was 43 years for the first two groups, and 54 years in the third group. The average duration of the disease was 10.7 years.[4]

Dietary considerations. One of the most important factors in the dietary management of this disorder is the individual attention given to the patient. Frequent visits by the dietitian and the nurse can do much toward convincing the patient of a sincere interest in his welfare. Many individuals with this disease are extremely apprehensive about what they can eat and seem to need constant reassurance. Mealtime visits provide an excellent opportunity to give encouragement and support.

Much patience and understanding are needed in helping ulcerative colitis patients with dietary problems. The diet must be highly individualized and yet be nutritionally adequate. Genuine efforts to meet the patient's requests must be

Figure 35–1. The patient's chart provides important information that must be considered in planning for nutritional care. The chart should include progress notes concerning the patient's acceptance of his diet and any problems of nutritional adequacy that may be present. Sometimes the intake of specific nutrients is calculated and charted. (Courtesy, Yale–New Haven Hospital.)

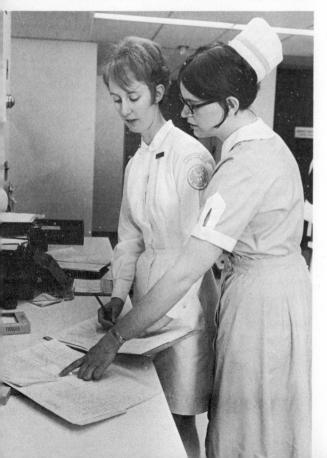

made; he must never be made to feel that his numerous questions and frequent demands are troublesome. On the other hand, gentle, but firm guidance must be given in helping the patient select a nutritionally adequate diet. He must understand he is expected to eat his entire meal. Many patients have poor appetites, and it may be preferable to provide six or eight small feedings; for others, however, having less frequent meal intervals is a more satisfactory approach. (See Figure 35–1.)

Liberal amounts of high-quality protein (up to 150 gm daily) are needed since nitrogen losses from the bowel may be considerable (see Chapter 32). Emphasis should be on tender meats, fish, poultry, and eggs for those patients who are allergic or intolerant to milk. Intakes of 3000 calories, or more, are necessary to replace losses due to steatorrhea, and to promote weight gain. The very low-residue diet may be used at first; thereafter, some degree of fiber restriction is usually needed as many ulcerative colitis patients do not tolerate raw fruits or vegetables, and further damage to an already inflamed mucosa must be prevented. The bland, fiber-restricted diet (Chapter 34) is usually suitable. Supplementary vitamins and minerals are usually indicated to compensate for gastrointestinal losses and inadequate dietary intake. Especially important are iron salts when anemia is present, and calcium salts if milk is not tolerated.

CARCINOMA OF THE INTESTINE

Cancer of the intestine is rarely symptomatic until the disease is well advanced. Pain, diarrhea or constipation, and weight loss are common symptoms.

Cancer of the colon is the leading cause of death among all types of cancer in the United States.[5] This type of cancer progresses rapidly. The incidence of carcinoma in ulcerative colitis is related to the duration and extent of the disease, but increases to 25 per cent in cases of 20 years' duration.

Dietary treatment. When tumors can be excised, dietary management following operation is the same as that following any intestinal surgery (see Chapter 38). For inoperable tumors, the comfort of the patient is of prime concern. Most such patients are more comfortable if fiber is restricted and small, frequent meals are provided.

PROBLEMS AND REVIEW

1. Discuss the role of diet in the incidence of diseases of the small intestine and colon.
2. What is the relationship of psychologic factors to the occurrence of gastrointestinal disorders? Cite examples.
3. What do the terms *fiber* and *residue* mean?
4. Mrs. K. is troubled with chronic diarrhea, although her physician has ruled out organic disease. What other factors might provoke diarrhea? In what ways would you expect her diet to be modified? What are the reasons for each modification?
5. Mrs. L. complains of constipation. List five possible causes.
   a. What type of person is likely to develop atonic constipation?
   b. What factors should be considered in treating constipation?
   c. What dietary recommendations would you make for Mrs. L.?
6. Plan a day's menu with emphasis on fiber. Show how you would modify this menu for a soft diet; for a very low-residue diet.
7. List the recommendations you would make for a person with irritable colon.
8. Mr. P., a 16-year-old student, is hospitalized with ulcerative colitis. His doctor has ordered a 3500-calorie, 150-gm protein diet for him.
   a. Plan a day's menu for him. He has many food intolerances, does not eat raw fruits or vegetables, and dislikes milk. He is especially fond of pizza and carbonated beverages.
   b. Mr. P. will be going home soon but is somewhat apprehensive about this as he does not get along well with his parents. What advice would you give him concerning his diet?
   c. What suggestions could you offer Mr. P.'s mother to help her win her son's cooperation at mealtime?

CITED REFERENCES

1. Law, D. H.: "Regional Enteritis," *Gastroenterology,* **56**:1086–1110, 1969.
2. Tamvakopoulos, S. K., *et al.:* "Nutritional Implications of Regional Enteritis," *R.I. Med. J.,* **52**:221–23, 1969.
3. Colcock, B. P.: "Diverticulitis in the Elderly," *Geriatrics,* **23**:122–27, Nov. 1968.
4. Morowitz, D. A., and Kirsner, J. B.: "Mortality in Ulcerative Colitis: 1930 to 1966," *Gastroenterology,* **57**:481–90, 1969.
5. Janower, M. L., *et al.:* "Cancer of the Gastrointestinal Tract in Young People," *Radiol. Clin. North Am.,* **7**:121–30, 1969.

ADDITIONAL REFERENCES

Albacete, R. A.: "Nonspecific Inflammatory Diseases of the Intestines," *Med. Clin. North Am.,* **52**:1387–96, 1968.

Cohn, E. M., *et al.:* "Regional Enteritis and Its Relation to Emotional Disorders," *Am. J. Gastroenterol.* **54**:378–87, 1970.

Crane, R. K.: "A Perspective of Digestive-Absorptive Function," *Am. J. Clin. Nutr.,* **22**:242–49, 1969.

Fordtran, J. S.: "Speculations on the Pathogenesis of Diarrhea," *Fed. Proc.,* **26**:1405–14, 1967.

Jackman, K. V., and Douglas, E. W.: "Crohn's Disease of the Large Bowel," *Surgery,* **66**:980–85, 1969.

Roy, J. H. B.: "Diarrhoea of Nutritional Origin," *Proc. Nutr. Soc.,* **28**:160–70, 1969.

36 Malabsorption Syndrome

Medium-Chain-Triglyceride Diet;
Lactose-Restricted Diet;
Sucrose-Restricted Diet;
Gluten-Restricted Diet

General Characteristics and Treatment

The term *malabsorption syndrome* is used to describe a number of disorders that are characterized by steatorrhea and multiple abnormalities in absorption of nutrients. Malabsorption in these disorders may be due to defects in (1) the intestinal lumen, resulting in inadequate fat hydrolysis or altered bile salt metabolism; (2) the mucosal epithelial cells, affecting absorbing surfaces and interfering with transport functions; or (3) intestinal lymphatics. (See Table 36–1.)

Symptoms and laboratory findings. Symptoms present to a variable degree in most persons with this syndrome include (1) pale, bulky, frothy, and offensive stools due to abnormally high fat content; (2) muscle wasting and progressive weight loss due to steatorrhea, diarrhea, and anorexia; (3) abdominal distention in children, less marked in adults; (4) evidence of vitamin and mineral deficiencies, such as macrocytic anemia due to inadequate absorption of folic acid and vitamin B_{12}, iron-deficiency anemia, hypocalcemic tetany, glossitis, and so on.

Laboratory findings include decreases in serum concentrations of electrolytes, albumin, and carotene; impaired absorption of d-xylose, glucose, folic acid, and vitamin B_{12}; and increased fecal fat and nitrogen.

Diagnostic tests. The diagnosis of malabsorption syndrome is based upon findings from absorption tests, intestinal mucosal biopsy, and radiologic studies.

Direct tests of absorption involve measurement of *fecal fat*. The balance study method is widely used and involves the chemical analysis of a 72-hour stool collection. The patient is fed a diet containing a known amount of fat, usually 50 to 100 gm, for several days before and during the collection period. Stools are then analyzed for fat. Normal excretion is less than 5 gm per 24 hours. Stool collections are also used to measure fecal radioactivity following administration of a test dose of ^{131}I-labeled triolein. The triolein is mixed with a marker and stools are collected until the marker is no longer visible. Normal fecal radioactivity is less than 7 per cent of the test dose.

The *serum carotene* level is a useful screening test, and malabsorption is suspected if levels of less than 60 micrograms per 100 ml are found.

Oral tolerance tests provide indirect evidence of malabsorption. Most commonly used are d-*xylose* and *lactose*. Urinary excretion of d-xylose following ingestion of a 25-gm load is used as an indication of carbohydrate absorption. Excretion of less than 4.5 gm in five hours in patients with normal renal function indicates decreased absorptive capacity. The *lactose tolerance test* is used in suspected lactase deficiency. Administration of 50 or 100 gm lactose is followed by determination of blood glucose levels for two hours. Lactase deficiency is indicated if the blood glucose fails to rise above the fasting level. Symptoms of abdominal distention, cramping, and diarrhea may occur following ingestion of the lactose in persons with malabsorption.

The *Schilling test* is frequently used as an index of vitamin B_{12} absorption; an oral dose of radioactive vitamin B_{12} is administered followed at two hours by an intramuscular injection of nonradioactive B_{12}. Urinary excretion of less than 5 to 8 per cent of the radioactive dose indicates malabsorption.

The *folic acid test* consists of assaying urine

Table 36–1. Some Malabsorptive Disorders Responsive to Dietary Modification

Abnormalities in the Intestinal Lumen	Abnormalities in the Mucosa

Inadequate lipid hydrolysis
  1. Pancreatic insufficiency
  2. Gastric resection
	Specific defects
	  1. Lactase insufficiency
	  2. Sucrase-isomaltase deficiency
	  3. Glucose-galactose deficiency
	  4. A-beta-lipoproteinemia

Alteration of bile salt metabolism
  1. Hepatobiliary disease
  2. Intestinal resection
  3. Bacterial overgrowth
	Nonspecific defects
	  1. Short-bowel syndrome
	  2. Gluten enteropathy
	  3. Tropical sprue
	Intestinal lymphatic obstruction
	  Lymphangiectasia

for 24 hours following injection of the vitamin and again after it is given orally 48 hours later. In malabsorption, excretion of folic acid is less after an oral dose than after injection.

Biopsy specimens of the jejunal mucosa showing villous atrophy provide nonspecific evidence of disturbances in absorptive function. Radiologic evidence of intestinal dilatation, altered motility, and bone demineralization may also be seen in malabsorption.

Treatment. Therapy is directed toward alleviation of symptoms by correction of the basic defect insofar as possible, dietary modification in accordance with the nature of the defect, vitamin and mineral supplements, and prevention or correction of complications by administration of appropriate agents.

Dietary modification. Generally speaking, the diet in malabsorption syndrome should be high in protein and calories (see Chapters 31 and 32). Modification of fat intake is often indicated. In some disorders elimination of specific carbohydrates or proteins is necessary. Vitamin and mineral supplementation is usually needed. A soft or fiber-restricted diet is useful for patients with persistent diarrhea (see Chapter 29).

Fat absorption can be improved in some malabsorptive disorders by changing the type of fat ingested. Food fats are composed principally of fatty acids containing 12 to 18 carbon atoms (long-chain triglycerides). In contrast, fats composed almost entirely of fatty acids containing 8 and 10 carbon atoms (medium-chain triglycer-

ides) have been synthesized. Substitution of medium-chain triglycerides (MCT) for longer-chain fats (LCT) is associated with reduced steatorrhea and decreased losses of calcium, sodium, and potassium in many of the disorders comprising the malabsorption syndrome.

The effectiveness of MCT over long-chain fats appears to be due to differences in the rate of hydrolysis, absorption, and route of transport. Medium-chain fats are hydrolyzed much more rapidly than long-chain fats in the intestinal lumen. The presence of pancreatic enzymes and bile salts is not required for absorption of the fats of medium-chain length. A mucosal enzyme system, specific for medium-chain-triglyceride hydrolysis, has been described. Medium-chain triglycerides are transported by way of the portal vein as free fatty acids bound to albumin whereas long-chain fats must undergo esterification and chylomicron formation and are transported by way of the lymph.[1]

Greenberger[2] has suggested that the primary indications for MCT therapy in patients with malabsorption include

. . . patients with malabsorption not responding to other measures; and those with disorders such as pancreatic insufficiency, bile-salt deficiency and bacterial overgrowth of the small bowel. In such circumstances conventional therapy may be only partially or temporarily effective, and these patients may benefit from supplemental treatment with MCT. On the other hand, MCT are of minor therapeutic importance in diseases for which effective therapy is available. Thus, in disorders such as nontropical sprue and Whipple's disease, MCT should be used as a nutritional adjunct and not as a substitute for established specific treatment.*

Side effects of nausea, abdominal distention or cramps, and diarrhea have been noted in about 10 per cent of patients receiving MCT supplements. Symptoms are attributed to the hyperosmolar load produced by rapid hydrolysis of MCT and possible irritating effects of high levels of free fatty acids in the stomach and intestine. These symptoms can be overcome by slow ingestion of small amounts of the supplement.

Medium-chain triglycerides are available commercially as an oil preparation† or as a powdered formula.‡ A number of recipes have been developed for incorporating these products into the diet.§ The oil has greater usefulness in that

it does not contain lactose as the powder does, provides a more concentrated source of calories, and can be used in frying and a greater number of recipes such as salad dressings, hot breads, and desserts. It is a clear, odorless oil with a bland taste. The powder, on the other hand, is useful as a calorie-protein supplement to an otherwise very low-fat diet.

Dietary management. From 50 to 70 per cent of the fat is supplied as MCT and the remainder as long-chain fats. To maintain this ratio, foods containing LCT are limited to

4 ounces meat, fish, or poultry
1 egg
3 teaspoons butter

This provides about 25 gm LCT daily.

The following diet is adapted from the plan described by Schizas et al.[3]

---

*Greenberger, N. J., and Skillman, T. G.: "Medium-Chain Triglycerides. Physiologic Considerations and Clinical Implications," *N. Engl. J. Med.*, 280:1051, 1969.

†MCT® from fractionated coconut oil, by Mead Johnson & Co., Evansville, Indiana. Provides 8.3 calories per gram, or approximately 225 calories per 30 ml.

†Portagen by Mead Johnson & Co., Evansville, Indiana. An 8-ounce glass of the product reconstituted to 30 calories per ounce provides 9.6 gm protein from milk, 26.4 gm carbohydrate (a mixture of lactose and sucrose), 11.0 gm MCT, and 0.5 gm safflower oil.

§Available from Mead Johnson & Co., Evansville, Indiana.

MEDIUM-CHAIN-TRIGLYCERIDE (MCT) DIET

Characteristics and general rules

This diet provides for a reduction in long-chain triglycerides by substituting an oil containing medium-chain triglycerides as a source of fat. The diet may be adjusted to provide 50 to 70 per cent of the fat calories as MCT.

The protein intake may be increased by adding nonfat dry milk to fluid skim milk, skim cottage cheese, egg whites, and cereal products.

The caloric level may be increased by adding high-carbohydrate foods such as fruits, sugar, jelly, and fat-free desserts.

Modifications in fiber and consistency may be made by applying restrictions concerning the soft diet (see Chapter 29) to the foods listed below.

Initially, small amounts of MCT should be taken with meals and gradually increased according to individual tolerance. Between-meal feedings may be desirable if large amounts of food are not tolerated.

Include these foods daily:

2 or more cups skim milk
4 ounces (cooked weight) lean meat, poultry, or fish
1 egg
3 or more fruits including
    1–2 servings citrus fruit or other good source of ascorbic acid
    1–2 other fruits

3–4 servings vegetables including
    1 dark green or deep yellow
    1 potato
    1–2 other vegetables, raw or cooked, as tolerated
  5 servings bread and cereals
  3 teaspoons butter
MCT oil in amounts prescribed (usually 2 ounces)

Nutritive value: On the basis of specified amounts of foods above: protein, 75 gm (13 per cent of calories); fat, 35 gm (13 per cent of calories); carbohydrate, 315 gm (53 per cent of calories); MCT, 60 gm (21 per cent of calories); 2400 calories.

Foods Allowed

Beverages—cereal beverages, coffee, tea, soft drinks
Breads and substitutes—hamburger rolls, hard rolls, white enriched, whole-wheat, pumpernickel, or rye bread. Bread products contain some LCT but are permitted to add palatability and variety to the diet.
  Cooked or dry cereals, macaroni, noodles, rice, spaghetti
Cheese—skim cottage cheese
Desserts—angel cake, gelatin, meringues, any made from MCT special recipes

Egg—egg whites as desired; whole eggs and egg yolks only in prescribed amounts
Fats—butter in prescribed amounts, gravies made from clear soups and MCT oil
Fruits—all except avocado
Meats—lean meat, fish, and poultry only in prescribed amounts
Milk—skim milk

Soups—fat-free broth, bouillon, consommé
Sweets—jelly, syrups, sugars
Vegetables—all to which no fat is added except MCT

Miscellaneous—any special recipe in which MCT is substituted for long-chain fats

Foods to Avoid

Commercial biscuits, coffeecake, cornbread, crackers, doughnuts, muffins, sweet rolls

Cheese made from whole milk
Commercial cakes, pies, cookies, pastries, puddings and custards; mixes allowed only if they contain no LCT
Whole eggs and egg yolks except as prescribed

Oils and shortenings of all types, sauces and gravies except those made with MCT oil
Avocado
Fatty meats, fish, frankfurters, cold cuts, sausages

Buttermilk, partially skim milk, whole milk, light, heavy, or sour cream
Cream soups, others
Butter, chocolate, coconut, or cream candies
Creamed vegetables, or those with fats other than MCT added
Creamed dishes; commercial popcorn; frozen dinners; homemade products containing eggs, whole milk, and fats; mixes for biscuits, muffins, and cakes; olives

---

Sample Menu

BREAKFAST
Fresh grapefruit—1 half
MCT waffle—1
Butter—1 teaspoon
Maple syrup—2 tablespoons
Sugar—1 teaspoon

Coffee or tea
LUNCHEON OR SUPPER
Chicken sandwich
  Chicken—2 ounces
  MCT mayonnaise—1 tablespoon
  Whole-wheat bread—2 slices
  Lettuce and tomato

Fresh fruit cup—½ cup
MCT brownie—1
Skim milk—1 cup
  DINNER
Veal chop—2 ounces
MCT scalloped potatoes—½ cup
Carrots—½ cup
  With lemon butter—2 teaspoons
Mixed green salad—1 serving
MCT Italian dressing—2 teaspoons
Angel cake—$\frac{1}{16}$ of 8 inch diameter
Fresh strawberries—1 cup
Coffee or tea
  EVENING SNACK
Skim milk—1 cup
MCT sugar cookies—2

DIETARY COUNSELING

Careful counseling is needed to ensure that the patient understands the importance of using the recommended amounts of MCT in the diet. He should be cautioned to take the oil slowly in small amounts; no more than 1 tablespoon of MCT should be taken at any given feeding. The diet to be used at home should be planned with consideration given to the individual's cultural background and usual meal pattern. He must be taught to use cuts of meat that are low in fat and to select only lean meats. Suggestions for incorporating the MCT oil into meals should be offered and suitable recipes supplied. Some persons prefer to take the oil mixed in fruit juice or as a "milkshake" composed of skim milk, fruit ice, and the oil. Others prefer to add the oil to solid foods such as cooked cereals, mashed potatoes, or sauces. The oil imparts a golden color to foods when used in frying; care should be taken to see that all the oil is removed from the frying pan, however, and actually consumed. Meals eaten away from home need not be a problem if the individual orders clear soups, lean meats trimmed of all visible fat, vegetables without cream sauces or other added fat, and so on. Desserts such as fruits, angel cake, and gelatin are suitable and usually available.

ABNORMALITIES IN THE INTESTINAL LUMEN

Inadequate digestion. Any condition that interferes with normal secretion or activity of pancreatic lipase causes inadequate hydrolysis of lipids in the intestinal lumen and results in malabsorption.

Pancreatic insufficiency. Inadequate production of lipase occurs in pancreatic insufficiency. This disorder may result from chronic pancreatitis, cystic fibrosis, carcinoma, pancreatectomy, or destruction of exocrine function by ligation of the duct. Steatorrhea and symptoms of generalized malabsorption occur due to poor utilization of fats and protein. Weight loss may be significant in spite of a good appetite.

The diet is designed to prevent further weight loss and to control gastrointestinal symptoms. Intakes should provide 2500 to 4000 calories daily, 80 to 150 gm protein, 60 to 200 gm fat, and 400 gm carbohydrate. Pancreatic extract is administered with meals to aid in fat absorption. If these supplements are not effective, MCT are sometimes used.

Gastric resection. Steatorrhea sometimes follows gastric resection because of inadequate mixing of food with pancreatic juice and bile or bacterial overgrowth in an afferent loop of intestine. In addition anemia is frequently seen because of limited intake or impaired absorption of iron, vitamin B_{12}, and folic acid. Weight loss is common and persistent. Improved absorption of fats may be achieved by supplementing the diet with MCT. Other dietary considerations are described on page 500.

Altered bile salt metabolism. Steatorrhea occurs if adequate amounts of conjugated bile salts are not available for micelle formation and is frequently associated with the following conditions.

Hepatobiliary disease. Decreased amounts of bile salts in the lumen in hepatobiliary disease are due to impaired synthesis of bile acids or biliary stasis.

Ileal resection. Removal of the ileum reduces the bile salt pool thereby lowering the concentration of conjugated bile salts in the jejunum available for hydrolysis of fats. Unabsorbed fatty acids and bile salts may provoke diarrhea.

Bacterial overgrowth (blind loop syndrome). Intestinal stasis is associated with changes in the bacterial flora. Deconjugation of bile salts by bacteria prevents adequate micelle formation. In some instances steatorrhea can be corrected by feeding conjugated bile salts.

Supplements of MCT are useful in all the above disorders.

ABNORMALITIES IN MUCOSAL CELL TRANSPORT—SPECIFIC DISORDERS

A deficiency or absence of specific enzymes in the cell interferes with the absorption of certain nutrients and produces symptoms of malabsorption.

Lactase deficiency. Primary lactase deficiency occurs as a congenital abnormality in the intestinal mucosa, whereas secondary deficiency accompanies diseases that produce alterations in absorptive surfaces. In the absence of lactase, lactose is not hydrolyzed to glucose and galactose. The accumulation of lactose in the intestine causes fermentation, abdominal pain, cramping, and diarrhea. Failure to gain weight is an important symptom in infants.

In primary lactase deficiency symptoms occur following ingestion of milk by the infant. A strict lactose-free formula is used, several commercial products being available.* All products containing lactose in any form whatsoever are rigidly excluded.

Acquired lactase deficiency has been reported in healthy adults who have no history of gastrointestinal disease or childhood intolerance to milk. The onset occurs in the late teens and early twenties and is manifested by abdominal bloating, cramps, and diarrhea following excessive milk ingestion. For these persons a controlled lactose diet which restricts only obvious sources of lactose may be used to keep the patient asymptomatic. The quantity of lactose allowed is a matter of individual tolerance. Many persons remain symptom free simply by limiting their intake of milk to one glass per day. Calcium supplements should be prescribed to replace that ordinarily supplied by milk.

Secondary lactose intolerance is often observed in celiac disease, sprue, kwashiorkor, cystic fibrosis, enteritis, colitis, and malnutrition.[4]

Some individuals are not lactase deficient yet are intolerant to lactose, as shown by symptoms produced by a lactose tolerance test.[5] The mechanism for this is unknown. These individuals usually get along quite well by limiting their intake of milk products.

*CHO-free Formula Base by the Borden Company, New York, New York. MBF (Meat-base Formula) by Gerber Products Company, Fremont, Michigan. Mul-Soy® by the Borden Company, New York, New York. Nutramigen® and Sobee® by Mead Johnson & Co., Evansville, Indiana.

LACTOSE-FREE DIET

Characteristics and general rules

This diet is designed to eliminate all sources of lactose.

All milk and milk products must be eliminated.

Lactose is used in the manufacture of many foods and medicines. It is essential to read labels of commercial products before use.

The diet is inadequate in calcium and riboflavin. Supplements of these nutrients should be prescribed.

The protein intake may be increased by adding meat, fish, poultry, or eggs, lactose-free milk substitutes, or breads and cereals from those allowed.

The caloric level may be increased by adding high-carbohydrate foods such as fruits, sugar, jelly, and desserts free of lactose.

Modifications in fiber and consistency may be made by applying restrictions concerning the soft diet (see Chapter 29) to the foods listed below.

Include the following foods daily:

7 ounces meat, fish, or poultry
1 egg
3 or more fruits including
   1–2 servings citrus fruit or other good source of ascorbic acid
   1–2 other fruits
3–4 servings vegetables including
   1 dark green or deep yellow
   1 potato
   1–2 other vegetables, raw or cooked, as tolerated
6 servings enriched bread or cereals
6 teaspoons fortified milk-free margarine
Other foods as needed to provide calories

Foods Allowed	Foods to Avoid
Beverages—carbonated drinks, fruit drinks, coffee, tea	Cereal beverages, cocoa, instant coffee
Breads and cereals—breads and rolls made without milk, cooked cereals, some prepared cereals (check labels), macaroni, spaghetti, soda crackers	Bread with milk added, crackers made with butter or margarine, Cream of Rice or Cream of Wheat cereal, French toast, mixes of all types, pancakes, some dry cereals, waffles, zwieback.
Cheese—none	All types
Desserts—angel cake, cakes made with vegetable oils, gelatin, puddings made with fruit juices, water, or allowed milk substitutes, water ices	Cakes, cookies, pies, puddings or other desserts made with milk and butter or margarine, commercial fruit fillings, commercial sweet rolls, custards, custard and cream pies, ice cream, pie crust made with butter or margarine, sherbets
Eggs—prepared any way except with milk or cheese	Any prepared with milk or cheese
Fats—lard, peanut butter, pure mayonnaise, vegetable oils, margarines without milk or butter added, some cream substitutes (check labels)	Butter, cream substitutes, cream, sweet and sour, margarine with butter or milk added, salad dressings
Fruits—all except canned and frozen to which lactose is added	Canned or frozen prepared with lactose
Milk—none	All types, infant food formulas, simulated mother's milk, yogurt
Meat, fish, or poultry—all kinds, cold cuts (check labels for added nonfat dry milk), kosher frankfurters	Brain, breaded or creamed dishes, cold cuts and frankfurters containing nonfat dry milk, liver, liver sausage, sweetbreads
Vegetables—fresh, canned, or frozen—plain or with milk-free margarine (check labels of canned or frozen)	Canned or frozen vegetables prepared with lactose, commercial French-fried potatoes, corn curls, creamed vegetables, instant or mashed potatoes, any seasoned with butter or margarine
Soups—meat and vegetable only (check labels)	All others
Miscellaneous—corn syrup, honey, nuts, nut butters, olives, pickles, pure seasonings and spices, pure jams and jellies, pure sugar candies, some cream substitutes, sugar	Ascorbic acid and citric acid mixtures, butterscotch, caramels, chewing gum, chocolate candy, cordials and liqueurs, cream sauces, cream soups, diabetic and dietetic preparations, dried soups, frozen cultures, frozen desserts, gravy, health and geriatric foods, molasses, monosodium glutamate extender, party dips, peppermints, powdered soft drinks, spice blends, starter cultures, sweetness reducers in candies, fruit pie fillings, icings, and preserves, toffee

Meal Pattern

BREAKFAST

Fruit

Cereal with milk substitute and sugar

Egg

Bread or roll made without milk—2 slices

Margarine, milk free—2 teaspoons

Beverage with cream substitute and sugar

LUNCHEON OR SUPPER

Lean meat, fish, or poultry—3 ounces

Potato or substitute

Cooked vegetable

Salad

Bread made without milk—2 slices

Margarine, milk free—2 teaspoons

Jelly

Fruit

Beverage

DINNER

Lean meat, fish, or fowl—4 ounces

Potato

Vegetable

Bread or roll made without milk—2 slices

Margarine, milk free—2 teaspoons

Jelly

Fruit or dessert

Beverage

Sample Menu

Orange juice

Cornflakes with cream substitute and sugar

Soft-cooked egg

French bread, toasted enriched

Margarine—milk free

Coffee with cream substitute and sugar

Baked chicken breast

Parslied potato

Asparagus tips

Sliced tomato and lettuce

French or Italian bread, enriched

Margarine—milk free

Grape jelly

Canned peach halves

Tea with lemon and sugar

Roast beef sirloin

Baked potato

Diced carrots

French or Italian bread, enriched

Margarine—milk free

Apple jelly

Fresh fruit cup

Tea with lemon and sugar

Controlled lactose diet. When patients with acquired lactose intolerance have responded well to a lactose-free diet, small amounts of lactose-containing foods may be allowed. A regular diet is used except that all milk and foods containing milk such as cottage cheese, custards, cream soups, ice creams, puddings, and so on are omitted. Hard cheeses, butter, and many foods that contain lactose as an additive in minute amounts may be included, for example, cold cuts, commercial breads, and prepared mixes.

DIETARY COUNSELING

Persons on lactose-free diets should be advised to carefully check labels on all commercial products. Foods containing milk in any form, butter, or margarine are to be avoided. Typical sources of lactose include breads, candies, cold cuts, mixes of all types, powdered soft drinks, preserves, soups, and so on. Fruit juices or water can be substituted for milk in many recipes. Meals eaten away from home should include foods prepared without breading, cream sauces, gravies, and so on. Broiled or roasted meats, baked potato, vegetables without added fat, salads, and desserts such as plain angel cake, fresh fruit, and gelatin are good choices. Kosher-style foods are suitable.

Sucrase-isomaltase deficiency. Deficiencies of these enzymes lead to symptoms similar to those seen in lactase insufficiency following ingestion of significant amounts of sucrose and isomaltose. A sucrose tolerance test is used to confirm the diagnosis.

Sucrose is added to many foods during processing and preparation. In addition, naturally occurring sucrose is present in a number of foods, making a strict sucrose-free diet impractical. Nevertheless, elimination of foods containing relatively large amounts of sucrose should be made (see Table 36–2). Glucose is substituted as a sweetening agent. Products containing wheat and potato starches should be avoided as these yield more isomaltose upon hydrolysis than do other starches such as rice and corn.

Glucose-galactase deficiency. In this rare disease, there is inability to absorb any carbohydrate that yields glucose or galactose upon hydrolysis. Substitution of fructose as the sole source of carbohydrate in the diet leads to improvement in symptoms. A special formula containing 4 to 8 per cent fructose has been devised for infants.[4] This formula is used almost exclusively for the first few months, after which it is gradually decreased and addition of foods low in starch is begun. By the age of three, a regular diet for age is usually tolerated with limited amounts of milk and starch-containing foods. Some degree of dietary restriction is necessary throughout life in order to prevent recurrence of symptoms of diarrhea. If a galactose-free diet is ordered, the lactose-free diet (see page 472) is used with omission of sugar beets, peas, and Lima beans.

A-beta-lipoproteinemia. This is a rare congenital disorder which is believed to involve a defect in the release or synthesis of β-lipoprotein. As a result fat is not transported from the intestinal cells into the lacteals. Total β-lipoprotein deficiency is manifested by steatorrhea and failure to thrive in infants among other symptoms. The malabsorption of fats is associated with extremely low serum concentrations of β-lipopro-

tein, cholesterol, vitamin A, and phospholipids.

Substitution of medium-chain triglycerides for long-chain fats in the diet results in improved fat absorption since the shorter-chain fats are absorbed via the portal vein rather than by lymph.

ABNORMALITIES IN MUCOSAL CELL TRANSPORT—NONSPECIFIC DISORDERS

Reduction in the absorptive surface area by massive intestinal resection or by damage to the villi produced by disease may have profound effects on nutrient uptake and absorption.

Short-bowel syndrome. This term is used to describe those patients who are in metabolic imbalance as a consequence of massive resection of the small intestine. Removal of large portions of the bowel shortens the transit time of the contents through the intestine, thereby reducing the time for absorption. In this syndrome, the length of the remaining bowel is generally less than 8 feet. The amount of bowel left intact and the site of resection have an important bearing on the patient's nutritional status.

Nutrients normally absorbed in the proximal intestine are shown in Figure 36–1. Following removal of the jejunum, some absorption of these nutrients may take place in the ileum by virtue of its ability to act as a functional intestinal reserve. On the other hand, the jejunum has a limited capacity to absorb water and electrolytes and cannot compensate for the massive losses

Table 36–2. Foods Containing More Then 5 gm Sucrose per 100 gm Edible Portion*

Apricots	Jams and jellies	Puddings
Bananas	Macadamia nuts	Syrups
Candy	Mangoes	Sorghum
Cane sugar	Milk chocolate	Soybeans
Cake	Molasses	Soybean flour or meal
Chestnuts, Va.	Oranges	Sugar beets
Chocolate, sweet	Pastries	Sweet breads and rolls
Condensed milk	Peaches	Sweet pickles
Cookies	Peanuts	Sweet potatoes
Dates	Peas	Tangerine
Honeydew melon	Pineapple	Watermelon
Ice cream	Prune plums, Italian	Wheat germ

*Adapted from Hardinge, M. G., *et al.*: "Carbohydrates in Foods," *J. Am. Diet. Assoc.,* **46** : 197–204, 1965.

Figure 36–1. Sites of absorption in the small bowel. Most nutrients are absorbed from the proximal portion of the small intestine. (Adapted from Booth, C. C.: "Effect of Location Along Small Intestine on Absorption of Nutrients," Chapter 76 in *Handbook of Physiology. Alimentary Canal.* Vol. I. American Physiological Society, Washington, D. C. 1967.)

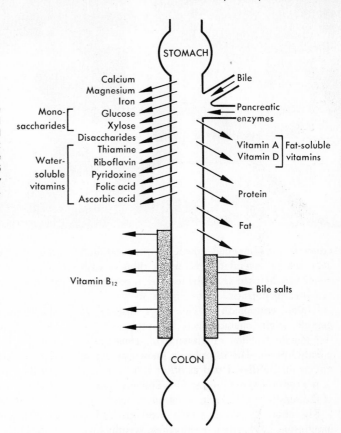

that occur when the ileum is removed. Following ileal resection, steatorrhea occurs because of bile salt deficiency.

Typically, the patient goes through three stages after massive resection of the bowel. In the immediate postoperative period, diarrhea and fluid and electrolyte imbalance may be so severe as to be life threatening. The patient surviving this period enters the second stage when nutritional concerns are of prime importance. Steady weight loss occurs as a result of anorexia, diarrhea, and steatorrhea. Osteomalacia may develop. Finally, after two or three months, the patient's condition stabilizes, usually at a substantially lower weight.

Attempts to increase absorption by delaying transit time include surgical measures, such as small bowel reversal, drug therapy, and dietary modification.

The extreme losses of all nutrients in this syndrome require greatly increased intakes of calories, protein, vitamins, and minerals. Up to 5000 calories and 175 gm of protein may be needed to prevent further weight loss. Substitution of medium-chain triglycerides for long-chain fats has led to decreased diarrhea and electrolyte losses and improvement in nutritional status.[6]

Recently, use of chemically defined synthetic diets has been shown to have beneficial effects in this and other malabsorptive disorders.[7] These diets are designed to provide complete nutritional support for extended periods in patients in whom it is desirable to reduce gastrointestinal residue to a minimum. Synthetic diets, composed of purified amino acids, simple carbohydrates, fats, vitamins, and minerals, have no indigestible bulk, hence require minimum digestion, and are rapidly absorbed from the upper intestinal tract. Both frequency and volume of stools are de-

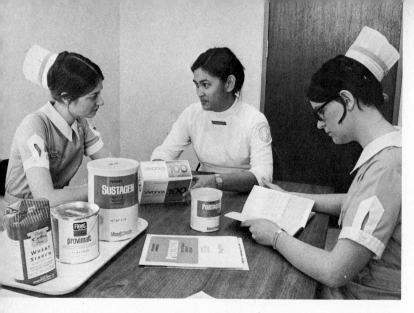

creased. A commercial powdered preparation,* available in several flavors, when diluted with water may be used as a tube feeding, a beverage, or frozen as popsicles. (See Figure 36–2.)

Gluten enteropathy. This is a disease of genetic origin characterized by intolerance to the gliadin fraction of gluten with consequent malabsorption. The disorder is known as *celiac disease* in childhood and as *adult celiac disease* or *nontropical sprue* in later life. The mechanism of the sensitivity to gluten is not understood.

The onset of this disease is insidious and is manifested by diarrhea, steatorrhea, weight loss, and other symptoms of the malabsorption syndrome. Stools are characteristically loose, pale, and frothy (due to fermentation of undigested carbohydrate) and contain excessive amounts of fat. Biopsy specimens of the mucosal surface have a flattened appearance; the villi may become shorter and club shaped and appear to be fused. A marked decrease in the number of microvilli in the brush border drastically reduces

the absorptive surface. Laboratory findings are consistent with those of the malabsorption syndrome (see page 466).

Exacerbations and remissions are common in this disorder. Symptoms are provoked by ingestion of gluten from wheat, rye, barley, buckwheat, and, in some instances, oats. Gluten from rice and potato has no deleterious effect.

Elimination of gluten from the diet (below) should be given a trial of at least six weeks. Regeneration of villi and return of enzyme activity occur in most cases following strict adherence to a gluten-restricted diet. Lack of response to the diet in some cases may be due to failure to follow the diet or to secondary lactose intolerance resulting from mucosal damage. In this case, a gluten-restricted, lactose-free diet leads to improved fat and carbohydrate absorption.

The diet should provide 100 gm or more protein to replace wasted tissue. Some moderation in fiber content and fat intake may be needed initially as these are usually poorly tolerated. Improved fat absorption may be achieved through the use of MCT. Supplementary vitamins and minerals are needed to overcome nutritional deficiencies resulting from excessive losses in the stools.

---

*Vivonex-100, from Eton Laboratories, Division of Norwich Pharmacal Company. Contains 8.5 per cent amino acids, 0.7 per cent fat, and 90.8 per cent carbohydrates. Normal dilution provides 1 calorie per milliliter. Six packets supply 5.88 gm nitrogen, 1.33 gm fat, 406.8 gm carbohydrate, and 1800 calories.

GLUTEN-RESTRICTED DIET

Characteristics and general rules

This diet excludes all products containing wheat, rye, oats, and barley. Read all labels carefully.

Aqueous multivitamins are usually prescribed in addition to the diet.

The diet may be progressed gradually; that is, small amounts of unsaturated fats may be used at first, adding harder fats later. Fiber may be reduced initially by using only cooked fruits and vegetables. Strongly flavored vegetables may be poorly tolerated at first.

Include these foods, or their nutritive equivalents, daily:

  4 cups milk
6–8 ounces (cooked weight) lean meat, fish, or poultry
  1 egg
  4 vegetables including:
     1 dark green or deep yellow
     1 potato
     2 other vegetables
     Other to be served raw, if tolerated
  3 fruits including:
     1–2 servings citrus fruit or other good source ascorbic acid
     1–2 other fruits
  4 servings bread and cereals: corn, rice, soybean
     NO WHEAT, RYE, OATS, BARLEY
  2 tablespoons fat

Additional calories are provided by using more of the foods listed, desserts, soups, sweets

Nutritive value of listed foods: Protein, 105 gm; fat, 110 gm; carbohydrate, 200 gm; calories, 2200. Minerals and vitamins in excess of recommended allowances.

Foods Allowed

Beverages—carbonated, cocoa, coffee, fruit juices, milk, tea

Breads—cornbread, muffins, and pone with no wheat flour; breads made with cornmeal, cornstarch, potato, rice, soybean, wheat starch flour

Cereals—cooked cornmeal, Cream of Rice, hominy or grits, rice; ready to eat: corn or rice cereals such as cornflakes, rice flakes, Puffed Rice

Cheese—cottage; later, cream cheese

Desserts—custard, fruit ice, fruit whips, plain or fruit ice cream (homemade), plain or fruit gelatin, meringues; homemade puddings—cornstarch, rice, tapioca; rennet desserts; sherbet; cakes and cookies made with allowed flours

Eggs—as desired

Fats—oil: corn, cottonseed, olive, sesame, soybean; French dressing, pure mayonnaise, salad dressing with cornstarch thickening

Later addition: butter, cream, margarine, peanut oil, vegetable shortening

Flour—cornmeal, potato, rice, soybean

Fruits—all cooked, canned, and juices; fresh and frozen as tolerated, avoiding skin and seeds initially

Foods to Avoid

Beverages—ale, beer, instant coffee containing cereal, malted milk, Postum, products containing cereal

Breads—all containing any wheat, rye, oats, or barley; bread crumbs, muffins, pancakes, rolls, rusks, waffles, zwieback; all commercial yeast and quick bread mixes; all crackers, pretzels, Ry-Krisp

Cereals—cooked or ready-to-eat breakfast cereals containing wheat, oats; barley, macaroni, noodles, pasta, spaghetti, wheat germ

Desserts—cake, cookies, doughnuts, pastries, pie; bisques, commercial ice cream, ice cream cones; prepared mixes containing wheat, rye, oats, or barley; puddings thickened with wheat flour

Fats—bacon, lard, suet, salad dressing with flour thickening

Flour—barley, oat, rye, wheat—bread, cake, entire wheat, graham, self-rising, whole wheat, wheat germ

Fruits—prunes, plums, and their juices; those with skins and seeds at first

Meat—all lean meats, poultry, fish: baked, broiled, roasted, stewed

Milk—all kinds

Soups—broth, bouillon, cream if thickened with cornstarch, vegetable

Sweets—candy, honey, jam, jelly, marmalade, marshmallows, molasses, syrup, sugar

Vegetables—cooked or canned: buttered; fresh as tolerated

Miscellaneous—gravy and sauces thickened with cornstarch; olives, peanut butter, pickles, popcorn, potato chips

Meat—breaded, creamed, croquettes, luncheon meats unless pure meat, meat loaf, stuffings with bread, scrapple, thickened stew
Fat meats such as corned beef, duck, frankfurters, goose, ham, luncheon meats, pork, sausage
Fatty fish such as herring, mackerel, sardines, swordfish, or canned in heavy oil

Soups—thickened with flour; containing barley, noodles, etc.

Sweets—candies with high fat content, nuts; candies containing wheat products

Vegetables—creamed if thickened with wheat, oat, rye, or barley products. Strongly flavored if they produce discomfort: baked beans, broccoli, Brussels sprouts, cabbage, cauliflower, corn, cucumber, lentils, onions, peppers, radishes, turnips

Miscellaneous—gravies and sauces thickened with flours not permitted

Meal Pattern

BREAKFAST

Fruit, preferably citrus or good source of ascorbic acid
Rice or corn cereal
Milk, sugar
Bread: rice or corn
Butter or margarine
Jelly, if desired
Eggs
Beverage

LUNCHEON OR SUPPER

Meat, poultry, or fish; or cheese; eggs (no thickened casserole dishes)
Potato, or substitute, or vegetable

Salad—vegetable or fruit, if tolerated

Bread: rice or corn
Butter or margarine
Milk
Dessert or fruit

DINNER

Meat, poultry, or fish

Potato or rice
Cooked vegetable
Salad, if tolerated
Bread, corn or rice, if desired
Butter
Milk

Sample Menu

Tomato juice

Rice Krispies
Milk, sugar
Southern corn muffins
Butter or margarine
Currant jelly
Scrambled eggs
Coffee, with cream, sugar

Beef stew (not thickened)
    Beef cubes
    Potato
    Carrots
    Onions
Tossed green salad
French dressing
Rice-flour bread
Butter or margarine
Milk
Vanilla cornstarch pudding with sliced frozen peaches

Broiled lamb patties (all meat)
Mint jelly
Rice with saffron seasoning
Buttered asparagus
Celery and olives

Milk

Dessert or fruit

Tea or coffee

Lemon meringue pudding (thickened with cornstarch)
Coffee with cream, sugar

DIETARY COUNSELING

Proteins from lean meats, poultry, fish, cottage cheese, egg white, and skim milk are
well utilized and should be encouraged. Individual tolerance for fibrous foods and
strongly flavored vegetables should determine
whether or not these foods are included. The
patient should be advised to read labels on all
commercial food products in order to avoid
any foods containing wheat, rye, oats, or
barley. Besides cereals and breads as obvious
sources, many other foods contain wheat or
other flour as a thickener or stabilizer. Canned
soups, cheese spreads, cooked salad dressings,
cold cuts, breaded meats, mixes of all kinds,
catsup, ice cream, and pastries are but a few
of the many foods that may contain cereal
products. Information on prepared and packaged foods known to be gluten free is available for patients.* Many standard cookbooks
contain suitable recipes utilizing cornstarch,
cornmeal, potato, rice, or tapioca instead of
flour. Sources of special recipes utilizing ar-
rowroot starch or wheat starch (from which
the gluten is removed) should be supplied
to the patient.* However, patients should be
cautioned that mere substitution of other
flours for wheat will not produce satisfactory
results; other adjustments in mixing technique, baking time, and temperature are also
needed. When meals are eaten away from
home, plain foods, without breading, gravies,
cream sauces, and so on, should be selected.

*Available from Clinical Research Unit, University
Hospital, Ann Arbor, Michigan.

Tropical sprue. This disorder is a form of the
malabsorption syndrome that occurs chiefly in
the West Indies, Central America, and the Far
East. In some respects it is similar to nontropical
sprue, but the onset is more acute and it responds to different therapy. Both disorders are
characterized by steatorrhea and secondary enzyme deficiencies in the intestinal mucosa. In
tropical sprue there is also ileal involvement.
Hypocalcemia with tetany and osteomalacia do
not occur as commonly as in nontropical sprue;
however, nutritional deficiencies of folic acid
and vitamin B_{12} do occur and are manifested as
macrocytic anemia. Dramatic improvement in
symptoms is often shown following administration of folic acid and vitamin B_{12}.

The diet in tropical sprue should be high in
protein and calories and restricted in fiber and in
fat. The substitution of medium-chain triglycerides for some of the fat has resulted in weight
gain and disappearance of steatorrhea. The restriction of gluten for patients with tropical sprue
does not usually lead to further improvement.

ABNORMALITY OF INTESTINAL LYM-PHATICS

Intestinal lymphangiectasia. This is a congenital defect in which obstruction of intestinal
lymphatics is associated with leakage of chylomicron fat and plasma proteins into the intestinal lumen. In addition to decreased serum protein levels and associated edema and ascites
formation, steatorrhea occurs. Protein losses are
reduced considerably by use of medium-chain
triglycerides or a fat-restricted diet (see page
489).

PROBLEMS AND REVIEW

1. What symptoms are characteristic of the malabsorption syndrome? In what ways is the diet
modified?
2. What information is provided by each of the following tests:

a. Serum carotene level
b. Schilling test
c. *d*-Xylose test

3. Plan a lactose-free diet for Mr. R., a single graduate student, who lives alone in an apartment with adequate cooking facilities. He enjoys Italian and Mexican foods. His caloric needs are estimated to be 2500 per day.
    a. List at least 10 foods that may contain lactose.
    b. Give suggestions for increasing calories in this diet.
    c. In which nutrients would this diet be inadequate?
    d. Which foods could be added if the diet is changed to controlled lactose?
    e. Mr. R. sometimes eats his lunch in a cafeteria. Give suggestions for suitable food choices.

4. Mrs. W. is a 45-year-old housewife and mother of four who was recently diagnosed as having adult celiac disease. The doctor prescribed a gluten-restricted diet for her.
    a. Explain what gluten is, and why it must be restricted in her diet.
    b. What are typical sources of gluten in the diet? Name some other less obvious foods that may contain gluten. What cereal grains can be substituted for those containing gluten?
    c. Mrs. W. is quite apprehensive about her diet. She states that she does not have time to bake special products for herself because her husband is a diabetic and one child has severe asthma. Give suggestions to help her in planning her diet. She wants to gain 10 pounds.

5. How could you change the diet you ate yesterday to make it free of gluten? To make it lactose free? To eliminate both lactose and gluten?

6. Mr. N. had a massive bowel resection. Which nutrients are likely to be poorly absorbed? Would MCT be useful in this disorder? Why?

7. Compare the dietary modifications used in nontropical and tropical sprue.

CITED REFERENCES

1. Isselbacher, K. J.: "Mechanisms of Absorption of Long and Medium Chain Triglycerides," in Senior, J. R., ed.: *Medium Chain Triglycerides.* University of Pennsylvania Press, Philadelphia, 1968, Chapter 3.
2. Greenberger, N. J., and Skillman, T. G.: "Medium-Chain Triglycerides. Physiologic Considerations and Clinical Implications," *N. Engl. J. Med.,* **280:**1045–58, 1969.
3. Schizas, A. A., *et al.:* "Medium-Chain Triglycerides—Use in Food Preparation," *J. Am. Diet. Assoc.,* **51:**228–32, 1967.
4. Lindquist, B., and Meeuwisse, G.: "Diets in Disaccharidase Deficiency and Defective Monosaccharide Absorption," *J. Am. Diet. Assoc.,* **48:**307–10, 1966.
5. Bayless, T. M., and Christopher, N. L.: "Disaccharide Deficiency," *Am. J. Clin. Nutr.,* **22:**181–90, 1969.
6. Bochenek, W., Rodgers, J. B., and Balint, J. A.: "Effects of Changes in Dietary Lipids on Intestinal Fluid Loss in the Short Bowel Syndrome," *Ann. Intern. Med.,* **72:**205–13, 1970.
7. Thompson, W. R., *et al.:* "Use of the 'Space' Diet in the Management of a Patient with Extreme Short Bowel Syndrome," *Am. J. Surg.,* **117:**449–59, 1969.

ADDITIONAL REFERENCES

Jeffries, G. H., *et al.:* "Malabsorption," *Gastroneterology,* **56:**777–97, 1969.
Pinter, K. G., *et al.:* "Fat and Nitrogen Balance with Medium Chain Triglycerides After Massive Intestinal Resection," *Am. J. Clin. Nutr.,* **22:**14–20, 1969.
Senior, J. R.: "The Place of Medium Chain Triglycerides," *Am. J. Med. Sci.,* **257:**75–80, 1969.
Sleisenger, M. H.: "Malabsorption Syndrome," *N. Engl. J. Med.,* **281:**1111–17, 1969.

Welsh, J. D., *et al.:* "Intestinal Disaccharidase Activity in Celiac Sprue (Gluten Sensitive Enteropathy)," *Arch. Intern. Med.,* **123**:33–38, 1969.

Sources of Special Recipes

Medium-Chain-Triglyceride Diet

Mead Johnson Laboratories: *Recipes Using MCT Oil and Portagen.* Mead Johnson & Company, Evansville, Indiana.

Schizas, A. A., *et al.:* "Medium-Chain Triglycerides—Use in Food Preparation," *J. Am. Diet Assoc.,* **51**:228–32, 1967.

Gluten-Restricted Diet

Allergy Recipes. American Dietetic Association, 620 North Michigan Ave., Chicago, $0.50.

Celiac Disease Recipes. Hospital for Sick Children, Toronto, 1968.

French, A. B.: *Low Gluten Diet with Tested Recipes.* Clinical Research Unit, University Hospital, Ann Arbor, Michigan. $1.00.

125 Great Recipes for Allergy Diets. Good Housekeeping Institute, 959 Eighth Ave. New York, $0.50.

Sheedy, C. M., and Keifetz, N.: *Cooking for Your Celiac Child.* Dial Press, New York, 1969.

Lactose-Free Diet

Allergy Recipes. American Dietetic Association, Chicago, $0.50.

Koch, R., *et al.:* "Nutrition in the Treatment of Galactosemia," *J. Am. Diet. Assoc.,* **43**:216–22, 1963.

125 Great Recipes for Allergy Diets. Good Housekeeping Institute, New York, $0.50.

37 Diet in Disturbances of the Liver, Gallbladder, and Pancreas

High-Protein, High-Carbohydrate, Moderate-Fat Diet; Fat-Restricted Diet

DISEASES OF THE LIVER—GENERAL CONSIDERATIONS

The liver is the largest and most complex organ in the body. It performs many functions that have an important bearing on one's nutritional state. Diseases of this organ may therefore markedly affect health.

Functions. The role of the liver in intermediary metabolism with reference to proteins, fats, and carbohydrates has been described in Chapters 4, 5, and 6 and is briefly summarized as follows:

1. Protein metabolism (Chapter 4)—synthesis of plasma proteins; deaminization of amino acids; formation of urea.

2. Carbohydrate metabolism (Chapter 5)—synthesis, storage, and release of glycogen; synthesis of heparin.

3. Lipid metabolism (Chapter 6)—synthesis of lipoproteins, phospholipids, cholesterol; formation of bile; conjugation of bile salts; oxidation of fatty acids.

4. Mineral metabolism (Chapter 8)—storage of iron, copper, and other minerals.

5. Vitamin metabolism (Chapter 10)—storage of vitamins A and D; some conversion of carotene to vitamin A, and of vitamin K to prothrombin.

6. Detoxification of bacterial decomposition products, mineral poisons, and certain drugs and dyes.

Etiology. Liver diseases may have a number of causes: infectious agents, toxins, metabolic or nutritional factors, biliary obstruction, and carcinoma. The pathologic changes in the liver parenchymal cells are similar regardless of the etiology of the disease. Basic changes include atrophy, fatty infiltration, fibrosis, and necrosis.

Symptoms and clinical findings. *Jaundice* is a symptom common to many diseases of the liver and biliary tract and consists of a yellow pigmentation of the skin and body tissues because of the accumulation of bile pigments in the blood. *Obstructive jaundice* results from the interference of the flow of bile by stones, tumors, or inflammation of the mucosa of the ducts. *Hemolytic jaundice* results from an abnormally large destruction of blood cells such as occurs in yellow fever, pernicious anemia, etc. *Toxic jaundice* originates from poisons, drugs, or virus infections.

Other symptoms commonly seen in liver diseases include lassitude, weakness, fatigue, fever, anorexia, and weight loss; abdominal pain, flatulence, nausea, and vomiting; hepatomegaly; ascites and edema; and portal hypertension.

Nutritional considerations in liver disease. Protection of the parenchymal cells is the foremost consideration in all types of liver injury. Since the liver is so intimately involved in the metabolism of foodstuffs, a nutritious diet is an important part of therapy and should be designed to protect the liver from stress and to enable it to function as efficiently as possible. With the exception of hepatic coma, generous amounts of high-quality protein should be provided for tissue repair and for prevention of fatty infiltration and degeneration of liver cells. A high-carbohydrate intake ensures an adequate reserve of glycogen, which, together with adequate protein stores, has a protective effect. Moderate amounts of fat are indicated for many persons. Signs of nutritional deficiency such as glossitis, nutritional anemia, or peripheral neuropathy are not uncommon in patients with liver disease. Generous amounts of vitamins, especially of the B complex, must be provided to compensate for deficiencies. If edema and ascites are present, sodium restriction may be necessary.

HEPATITIS

Etiology and symptoms. This is an infectious disease characterized by inflammatory and degenerative changes of the liver. Two types are recognized, *viral* and *drug induced*. The viral type is more common and occurs as either *infectious* or *serum hepatitis*. Infectious hepatitis is due to an unidentified virus transmitted either by fecal contamination of water or food or parenterally. Epidemics occur from time to time in young people and are usually traced to a breakdown in sanitation. On the other hand, serum hepatitis is transmitted only by the parenteral route in blood products containing the specific virus or through improperly sterilized needles. Drug-induced hepatitis may be due to hypersensitivity to certain drugs, such as sulfa or penicillin, or to a direct toxic effect on the liver by agents such as carbon tetrachloride.

Aside from mode of transmission and period of incubation, the two types of hepatitis are similar. Nonspecific symptoms such as anorexia, fatigue, nausea and vomiting, diarrhea, fever, weight loss, and abdominal discomfort usually precede the development of jaundice, which ordinarily subsides after one or two weeks. Complete recovery may take several months. Treatment consists of adequate rest, nutritious diet, and avoidance of further damage to the liver.

Dietary modification. The objectives of dietary treatment are to aid in the regeneration of liver tissue and to prevent further liver damage.

Calories. A high caloric intake, 3000 to 4000 daily, is needed to promote weight gain and to ensure maximum protein utilization.

Protein. An intake of 1½ to 2 gm protein per kilogram of body weight, or 100 to 150 gm protein daily, is needed to overcome negative nitrogen balance, to promote regeneration of parenchymal cells, and to prevent fatty infiltration of the liver.

Fat. Diets restricted in fats are not necessary in the majority of patients with hepatitis; in fact, their use may retard recovery if calories are thereby limited. Weight gain is more rapid and liver function tests revert to normal sooner when patients receive up to 150 gm fat daily.[1,2] Fats from dairy products, salad dressings, and cooking fats are easily utilized and add palatability to the diet without large amounts of bulk. If there is anorexia, fats may cause nausea and should be limited to amounts tolerated by the patient.

Carbohydrate. An intake of 300 to 400 gm carbohydrate ensures adequate glycogen reserves needed for the maintenance of liver function, for protection against further injury to the liver, and for its protein-sparing action.

Consistency. Foods of liquid to soft consistency (see Chapter 29) may be preferable if there is anorexia in the acute stages of the illness, progressing to a wider selection of foods with convalescence.

Dietary management. The patient must be convinced of the importance of the diet in promoting recovery and preventing relapses. Anorexia is frequently a problem; hence every effort

Figure 37–1. Patients who are weak and debilitated need some assistance at mealtime. The nurse also provides encouragement to the patient. (Courtesy, Yale–New Haven Hospital.)

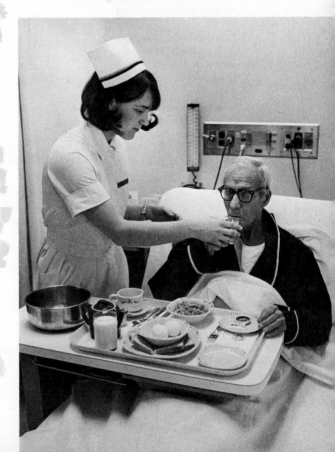

must be made to encourage the patient to eat. Foods served must be well prepared and attractively served with consideration given to the individual's food preferences. Judicious use of spices and condiments may help to stimulate the appetite. Small to moderate portions at mealtime with between-meal supplements of high-protein beverages are frequently more acceptable than larger meals. Some individuals need assistance in feeding themselves and should be allowed adequate time to eat at a leisurely pace. (See Figure 37–1.)

HIGH-PROTEIN, MODERATE-FAT, HIGH-CARBOHYDRATE DIET

Characteristics and general rules
The caloric level may be increased by adding high-carbohydrate foods. Small amounts of cream and ice cream may be used when tolerated.
The protein intake may be increased by adding nonfat dry milk to liquid milk.
Modifications in fiber and consistency may be made by applying restrictions concerning the soft diet (Chapter 29) to the foods listed below.
Six or more small feedings may be preferred when there is lack of appetite.
When sodium restriction is ordered, all food must be prepared without salt. Low-sodium milk should replace part or all of the prescribed milk. See Sodium-Restricted Diets, Chapter 43.

Include these foods daily:
1 quart milk
8 ounces lean meat, poultry, or fish
1 egg
4 servings vegetables including:
  2 servings potato or substitute
  1 serving green leafy or yellow vegetable
  1–2 servings other vegetable
  One vegetable to be raw each day
3 servings fruit including:
  1 serving citrus fruit or other good source of ascorbic acid
  2 servings other fruit
1 serving enriched or whole-grain cereal
6 slices enriched or whole-grain bread
2 tablespoons butter or fortified margarine
4 tablespoons sugar, jelly, marmalade, or jam
Additional foods to further increase the carbohydrate as the patient is able to take them

Nutritive value of basic pattern above: Protein, 135 gm; fat, 106 gm; carbohydrate, 236 gm; calories, 2590; calcium, 2.53 gm; iron, 18.3 mg; vitamin A, 18,770 I.U.; thiamine, 2.11 mg; riboflavin, 3.39 mg; niacin, 27.6 mg; ascorbic acid, 159 mg.

Typical Food Selection
Beverages—carbonated beverages, milk and milk drinks, coffee, tea, fruit juices, cocoa flavoring
Breads and cereals—all kinds
Cheese—cottage, cream, mild Cheddar
Desserts—angel cake, plain cake and cookies, custard, plain or fruit gelatin, fruit whip, fruit pudding, Junket, milk and cereal desserts, sherbets, ices, plain ice cream
Eggs—any way
Fat—butter, fortified margarine, cream, cooking fat, vegetable oils
Fruits—all

Meat—lean beef, chicken, fish, lamb, liver, pork, turkey
Potato or substitute—hominy, macaroni, noodles, rice, spaghetti, sweet potato
Seasonings—salt, spices, vinegar (in moderation)
Soups—clear and cream
Sweets—honey, jam, jelly, sugar, sugar candy, syrups
Vegetables—all

Foods to Avoid

No foods are specifically contraindicated. Many patients complain of intolerance to the following groups of foods: strongly flavored vegetables; rich desserts; fried and fatty foods; chocolate; nuts; and highly seasoned foods. Although such complaints cannot always be explained on a physiologic basis, nothing is gained by giving the offending foods to the patient.

Meal Pattern	Sample Menu
BREAKFAST	
Fruit	Half grapefruit
Cereal with milk and sugar	Wheatena with milk and sugar
Egg	Scrambled egg
Whole-grain or enriched toast—2 slices	Whole-wheat toast
Butter or margarine—2 teaspoons	Butter
Marmalade—1 tablespoon	Orange marmalade
Beverage with cream and sugar	Coffee with cream and sugar
LUNCHEON OR SUPPER	
Lean meat, fish, or poultry—4 ounces	Broiled whitefish
Potato or substitute	Escalloped potatoes
Cooked vegetable	Buttered asparagus
Salad	Celery and carrot strips
Whole-grain or enriched bread—2 slices	Whole-wheat bread
Butter or margarine—2 teaspoons	Butter
Jelly—1 tablespoon	Grape jelly
Fruit	Sliced banana
Milk	Milk
MIDAFTERNOON	
Milk with nonfat dry milk	High-protein milk with strawberry flavor
DINNER	
Lean meat, fish, or fowl—4 ounces	Roast beef
Potato	Mashed potato
Vegetable	Baked acorn squash
Whole-grain or enriched bread—2 slices	Dinner rolls
Butter or margarine—2 teaspoons	Butter
Jelly—1 tablespoon	Apple jelly
Fruit, or dessert	Raspberry sherbet
Milk—1 glass	Milk
Tea, if desired	
EVENING NOURISHMENT	
Milk beverage	High-protein milk flavored with caramel
	Bread-and-jelly sandwich

CIRRHOSIS

Etiology. This chronic disease of the liver is characterized by diffuse degenerative changes, fibrosis, and nodular regeneration of the remaining cells. The causes include infectious hepatitis in a small percentage of patients, chronic alcoholism in association with malnutrition, underlying metabolic disturbances such as hemochromatosis or Wilson's disease, hepatotoxins derived from certain plants and fungi, and prolonged biliary stasis. The mortality from this disease appears to be increasing, and it presently ranks among the five most frequent causes of death in persons over 40 years of age in the United States.[3]

Laennec's cirrhosis. The most common type of cirrhosis in the United States is Laennec's (*alcoholic, portal*) cirrhosis. The exact etiology has not been established although alcohol and relative or absolute malnutrition are implicated in the majority of patients. Whether alcohol per se has a direct toxic effect on the liver is still a matter of controversy.[4,5] Pathologic changes include fatty infiltration, necrosis, and proliferation of fibrous tissue.

Symptoms and clinical findings. The onset of cirrhosis may be gradual with gastrointestinal disturbances such as anorexia, nausea, vomiting, pain, and distention. As the disease progresses, jaundice and other serious changes occur.

Ascites. Ascites is the accumulation of abnormal amounts of fluid in the abdomen. It may develop as a consequence of portal vein hypertension, obstruction of the hepatic vein, a fall in plasma colloid osmotic pressure due to impaired albumin synthesis, increased sodium retention, or impaired water excretion.

Esophageal varices (varicose veins). Varices in the esophagus and upper part of the stomach may develop as a complication of portal hypertension. Hemorrhage is then an ever-present danger and may be provoked by roughage of any kind. The hemorrhage itself may be fatal, or the blood may provide for the accumulation of ammonia and subsequent hepatic coma.

Modification of the diet. Regeneration of parenchymal cells occurs if appropriate diet therapy is initiated before the disease is well advanced. The high-protein, high-carbohydrate diet outlined for infectious hepatitis is satisfactory. In advanced cirrhosis, however, further dietary modification is needed.

Protein. Individual requirements for protein must be considered and intake must be adjusted as the disease progresses or improves. The optimal level of protein intake in advanced cirrhosis

is not clear. Liberal intakes are advocated by some,[6] whereas others recommend an initial protein intake high enough to maintain nitrogen equilibrium, but low enough to prevent hepatic coma (approximately 50 gm per day).[7] Gradual increments to a maximal level of 1 gm protein per kilogram of body weight per day, or 65 to 85 gm daily, are associated with improved liver function and nutritional status. Intakes greater than this risk hepatic coma. Protein intake is restricted to less than 35 gm daily if signs of impending coma develop.

Fats. Malabsorption of fats occurs in many cirrhotics. For some patients the substitution of medium-chain triglycerides for part of the dietary fat is effective in reducing steatorrhea[8] (see Chapter 36).

Vitamins and minerals. Malabsorption of fat-soluble and B complex vitamins occurs in alcoholic and biliary cirrhosis. Serum calcium and magnesium are decreased. Vitamin supplements may be advisable to replenish liver stores and repair tissue damage, especially if there is anorexia.

Sodium. Sodium restriction is prescribed if edema and ascites are present. Severe restriction of sodium for many months is often necessary for effective removal of excess fluid accumulation. Diets restricted to 250 mg sodium daily are not uncommon in this disorder. On such very low-sodium diets, all food used must be naturally low in sodium and prepared without sodium-containing compounds. Low-sodium milk is substituted for regular milk. Close attention to food selection is needed in order to provide an adequate protein intake without exceeding the sodium allowance (see Chapter 43).

Consistency. Reduction in fiber content of the diet is necessary in advanced cirrhosis when there is danger of hemorrhage from esophageal varices. A liquid or soft diet is used (see Chapter 29).

HEPATIC COMA

Etiology. This is a complex syndrome characterized by neurological disturbances which may develop as a complication of severe liver disease. It usually results from entrance of certain nitrogen-containing substances such as ammonia into the cerebral circulation without being metabolized by the liver. It may be a consequence of shunting of the portal blood into the systemic circulation in cirrhosis, or of severe damage to liver cells in hepatitis. Precipitating factors include gastrointestinal bleeding, severe infections, surgical procedures, excessive dietary protein, and sedatives.

Symptoms. Signs of impending coma include confusion, restlessness, irritability, inappropriate behavior, delirium, and drowsiness. There may also be incoordination and a flapping tremor of the arms and legs when extended. Electrolyte imbalance occurs. The patient may go into coma and may have convulsions. The breath has a fecal odor (*fetor hepaticus*). Prompt treatment is imperative or death occurs.

Dietary modification. The fundamental principle in the dietary management of hepatic coma is to reduce the protein intake to a minimum, thus decreasing the amount of ammonia produced. Catabolism of tissue proteins must also be avoided.

Calories. About 1500 to 2000 calories are needed to prevent breakdown of tissue proteins for energy and are provided chiefly in the form of carbohydrates and fats. Although anorexia may occur, attempts should be made to keep the caloric intake as high as is practical to minimize tissue breakdown.

Protein. Some clinicians omit protein completely for two or three days and others permit 20 to 30 gm daily. As the patient improves, the protein intake is gradually increased by 10 to 15 gm at a time until a maximum of 1 gm per kilogram of body weight is reached. The patient must be carefully watched following each increment lest signs of coma recur.

Levels of 40 to 50 gm protein daily may be used for long periods of time without detriment to nutritional status provided the diet is otherwise adequate. Nitrogen balance can be achieved on protein intakes as low as 35 gm daily[7] if high-quality protein is used and caloric intake is adequate.

Dietary management. These patients pose problems in feeding because of anorexia and behavioral patterns ranging from apathy, drowsiness, and confusion to irritability and hyperexcitability. The protein-free diet consisting of commercial sugar-fat emulsions, a butter-sugar mixture, or glucose in beverages or fruit juices may be used initially through oral or tube feeding. (See Chapter 44.) With improvements, the diets providing 20, 40, and 60 gm protein (see page 587) may be gradually introduced.

DISEASES OF THE GALLBLADDER

Function of the gallbladder. The gallbladder concentrates bile formed in the liver and stores it until needed for digestion of fats. The entrance of fat into the duodenum stimulates secretion of the hormone *cholecystokinin* by the intestinal mucosa. The hormone is carried by way of the bloodstream to the gallbladder and forces it to contract, thus releasing bile into the common duct, and then into the small intestine where it is needed for the emulsification of fats. Interference with the flow of bile occurring in gallbladder disease may cause impaired fat digestion. From 5 to 10 per cent of the adult population have symptoms of gallbladder disease.

Inflammation of the gallbladder is known as *cholecystitis.* Gallstone formation, or *cholelithiasis,* occurs when cholesterol, bile pigments, bile salts, calcium, and other substances precipitate out of the bile. The etiology of gallstone formation is obscure although stasis, infection, and metabolic or chemical changes are all believed to play a role. *Choledocholithiasis* refers to stones lodged in the common duct.

Symptoms and clinical findings. Mere presence of gallstones does not always produce symptoms; however, inflammation of the gallbladder or obstruction of the ducts by stones may cause severe pain whenever the gallbladder contracts. Ingestion of fatty foods may thus cause discomfort, and fat digestion may be impaired because of the diminished flow of bile. Intolerance to certain strongly flavored vegetables, legumes, melons, and berries occurs in many persons with gallbladder disease but the reason for this is not known. A recent study by Breneman also revealed intolerance to eggs in 63 of 69 patients studied.[9]

Acute cholecystitis is usually associated with a gallstone lodged in the cystic duct and is accompanied by mild to severe pain, abdominal distention, nausea and vomiting, and fever.

Modification of the diet. The principal aim of dietary management in gallbladder disease is to reduce discomfort by providing a diet restricted in fat. Reduction of fibrous foods may be desirable.

Calories. Many persons with gallbladder disease are overweight and should be given a low-calorie diet (see Chapter 31). Sarles and co-workers suggest that excessive intake of calories from any source is associated with increases in the biliary cholesterol composition and favors formation of cholesterol gallstones.[10] With restriction of fats, carbohydrates are used more liberally to furnish the needed calories.

Fat. The patient receives no food initially during acute attacks of cholecystitis. Progression to a 20- to 30-gm fat diet is then made. If this is tolerated, the fat can then be increased to 50 to 60-gm daily, thus improving palatability of the diet. In chronic cholecystitis some degree of fat restriction is usually necessary.

Cholesterol. The chief component of most gallstones is cholesterol. Although some cholesterol is supplied by the diet, much more is synthesized in the body from fragments of carbohydrates, amino acids, and fat metabolism. Dietary restriction of cholesterol, therefore, is probably not very effective in prevention of gallstones. If a reduction in cholesterol content of the diet is ordered, egg yolks, liver, and other organ meats are omitted, and skim milk and margarine are substituted for whole milk and butter. See Table A-6 for cholesterol content of foods. Food allowances for two levels of fat restriction are shown in Table 37–1.

Table 37–1. Food Allowances for Two Levels of Fat Restriction
(Approximately 1500 Calories)

	20 gm Fat	50 gm Fat
Milk, skim	2 cups	2 cups
Meat, fish, poultry (lean)	6 ounces*	6 ounces*
Eggs (3 per week)	1/2	1/2
Vegetables		
Dark-green leafy or deep yellow	1 serving	1 serving
Potato	1 serving	1 serving
Other	1 or more servings	1 or more servings
Fruits		
Citrus	1 serving	1 serving
Other	3 servings	3 servings
Breads and cereals		
Cereals	1 serving	1 serving
Breads	6 slices	3 slices
Fats, vegetable	none	6 teaspoons
Sweets	3 tablespoons	2 tablespoons
Total fat, gm	20	50
Cholesterol, mg	270†	270†
Protein, gm	85	80
Calories (approximate)	1500	1500

*Only lean cuts of meat, fish, poultry may be used. Each ounce is equivalent to 8 gm protein and 3 gm fat.

†Cholesterol level would be reduced to about half this level if eggs were not used. If butter is used instead of vegetable fat, the cholesterol level would be increased.

FAT-RESTRICTED DIET

Foods Allowed

Beverages—whole milk, only 2 cups; skim milk as desired; coffee, coffee substitute, tea; fruit juices

Breads—all kinds except those with added fat

Cereals—all cooked or dry breakfast cereals, except possibly bran; macaroni, noodles, rice, spaghetti

Cheese—cottage only

Desserts—angel cake; fruit whip; fruit pudding; gelatin, ices and sherbets; milk and cereal puddings using part of milk allowance

Eggs—3 per week

Fats—vegetable oil or margarine

Fruits—all kinds when tolerated

Meats—broiled, baked, roasted, or stewed without fat: lean beef, chicken, lamb, pork, veal, fish

Seasonings—in moderation: salt, pepper, spices, herbs, flavoring extracts

Soups—clear

Sweets—all kinds: hard candy, jam, jelly, marmalade, sugars

Vegetables—all kinds when well tolerated; cooked without added butter, or cream

Foods to Avoid

Beverages—with cream; soda-fountain beverages with milk, cream, or ice cream

Breads—griddle cakes; sweet rolls with fat; French toast

Cheese—all whole-milk cheeses, both hard and soft

Desserts—any containing chocolate, cream, nuts, or fats: cookies, cake, doughnuts, ice cream, pastries, pies, rich puddings

Eggs—fried

Fats—cooking fats, cream, salad dressings

Fruits—avocado; raw apple, berries, melons may not be tolerated

Meats—fatty meats, poultry, or fish: bacon, corned beef, duck, goose, ham, fish canned in oil, mackerel, pork, sausage; organ meats
Smoked and spiced meats if they are poorly tolerated

Seasonings—sometimes not tolerated: pepper; curries; meat sauces; excessive spices; vinegar

Soups—cream, unless made with milk and fat allowance

Sweets—candy with chocolate and nuts

Vegetables—strongly flavored may be poorly tolerated: broccoli, Brussels sprouts, cabbage, cauliflower, cucumber, onion, peppers, radish, turnips; dried cooked peas and beans

Miscellaneous—fried foods; gravies; nuts; olives; peanut butter; pickles; popcorn; relishes

Meal Pattern (20 gm fat)

BREAKFAST

Fruit

Cereal with skim milk and sugar

Egg—1 only (3 per week)

Enriched or whole-grain toast

Jelly

Beverage with milk and sugar

LUNCHEON OR SUPPER

Lean meat, fish, poultry, or cottage cheese

Potato or substitute

Vegetable

Salad; no oil dressing

Enriched or whole-grain bread

Sample Menu

Stewed apricots

Cornflakes with skim milk and sugar

Poached egg

Whole-wheat toast with jelly

Coffee with milk and sugar

Tomato bouillon

Fruit salad plate:
    Cottage cheese
    Sliced orange
    Tokay grapes
    Pear
    Romaine

Sliced chicken sandwich

Dessert or fruit
Milk, skim—½ cup
  DINNER
Lean meat, poultry, or fish
Potato or substitute
Vegetable
Enriched or whole-grain bread
Jelly
Dessert or fruit
Milk, skim—1 glass

Vanilla blanc mange (using milk allowance)
Tea with milk, sugar

Roast lamb, trimmed of fat
Boiled new potatoes; no added fat
Zucchini squash
Parkerhouse roll
Jelly
Angel cake with sliced peaches
Milk, skim—1 glass

Diet following cholecystectomy. A fat-restricted diet may be used for some months following removal of the gallbladder. Thereafter, most individuals can tolerate a regular diet.

DIETARY COUNSELING

Restriction of dietary fat influences the methods of food preparation permitted. The patient should be advised to prepare meats by baking, broiling, roasting, or stewing, and to use only lean meats trimmed of all visible fats. Meat drippings, cream sauces, and so on are not allowed, but spices and herbs in moderation can be used to enhance flavor of foods. Use of fortified skim milk and inclusion of green leafy or yellow vegetables is needed to help ensure adequate intake of vitamin A. The small amounts of fat permitted should be taken as butter or fortified margarine. Any foods known to cause distention should be omitted. Most individuals need guidance in selecting suitable substitutes for desserts that are high in fat.

PANCREATIC DISORDERS

Disorders of the pancreas usually involve inadequate production of enzymes needed for normal digestive processes. Interference with this process leads to impaired digestion and is manifested by the presence of excess fat and undigested protein in the stools. Some starch may also be present. Dietary treatment of pancreatic disorders depends on the nature and extent of digestive impairment rather than on the disease itself. Pancreatic disease may be due to congenital or inflammatory diseases, trauma, or tumors. The dietary treatment is similar in all of these.

Acute pancreatitis. Acute inflammatory disease of the pancreas may result from interference with the blood supply to the organ or from obstruction to the outflow of pancreatic juice. The usual causes are alcoholism and biliary tract disease; however, acute pancreatitis may also be due to trauma, virus infections, tumors, nutritional deficiency, certain vascular diseases, and a number of metabolic diseases.

Acute pancreatitis may range from a mild inflammatory reaction to severe illness. The most predominant symptom is severe upper-abdominal pain radiating to the back and is aggravated by eating. Epigastric tenderness, distention, constipation, nausea, and vomiting occur.

Increased pressure in the ducts causes the activated pancreatic enzymes to escape into the interstitial tissues, thus leading to elevations in the serum concentrations of amylase and lipase. Alteration of structure or function of the pancreas or adjacent organs may be demonstrated radiographically. The islets of Langerhans are not necessarily involved.

Treatment. Conservative management is used. Aims are to alleviate pain, to keep pancreatic secretory activity at a minimum, and to replace fluids and electrolytes. Dietary management usually consists of giving the patient nothing by mouth during acute attacks. Progression from clear liquids to a soft (see Chapter 29) or bland (Chapter 34) diet is made as tolerated.

Chronic pancreatitis. This disease may be described as relapsing, recurrent, or continuous in nature. As in acute pancreatitis, alcoholism is the most common cause of attacks by virtue of its stimulating effect on gastric secretion, which, in turn, enhances release of pancreatic secretin.

The chronic form is characterized by recurrent attacks of burning epigastric pain, especially after meals containing alcohol and fat. Other symptoms include flatulence, anorexia, weight loss, nausea, and vomiting. Chronic changes lead to destruction of the islets of Langerhans in some patients, fibrosis, pseudocyst, and pancreatic calcification. Impaired digestion due to interference with enzyme activity leads to steatorrhea, creatorrhea, and deficiency of the B complex and fat-soluble vitamins.

Treatment. Conservative management is used unless the patient has unremitting pain or complications necessitating partial or complete pancreatectomy. Medications to alleviate pain and to inhibit pancreatic secretion are used.

The aim of dietary treatment is to minimize gastric secretion because of its stimulating effect on secretin output. Diet during attacks is the same as in acute pancreatitis. Thereafter, a soft diet, high in protein and calories, and low in fat, should be used. Six small meals are better tolerated than large meals. Pancreatic extract is used to aid in fat absorption.

Cystic fibrosis. This is a congenital disorder of unknown etiology in which there is generalized dysfunction of exocrine glands (glands that excrete to the outside of the body).

Characteristics of the disease include mucus secretion and abnormally high sweat sodium and chloride levels. Secretion of abnormally thick mucus by exocrine glands obstructs ducts in the pancreas, lungs, and liver. Blockage of the ducts in the pancreas leads to fibrosis and cyst formation, and pancreatic enzymes are not released into the duodenum, interfering seriously with the utilization of proteins, fat, and carbohydrates. As much as 50 per cent of the protein and fat of the diet may be present in the feces. Recent interest has focused on the possibility of vitamin E deficiency in this disorder based on tissue changes similar to those seen in vitamin-E-deficient animals. The significance of this finding is not known.[11] Impaired absorption of all nutrients occurs in many cases. Chronic pulmonary disease and bronchial obstruction develop, and in some instances, obstruction of hepatic biliary ducts leads to portal hypertension and cirrhosis. Osteoporosis may be demonstrated radiologically. Elevated levels of sodium and chloride—up to 2½ times normal—are found in sweat. Massive salt loss in hot weather may cause heat stroke.

Symptoms. In the neonatal period, cystic fibrosis may present as meconium ileus, or there may be insidious onset of malnutrition in infants with good appetite but who nevertheless fail to grow and gain weight. Passage of foul-smelling, bulky, soft stools, haggard appearance, marked enlargement of the abdomen, and tissue wasting, especially about the buttocks, occur.

Treatment. General treatment consists of controlling pulmonary complications, maintaining good nutrition, and preventing abnormal salt loss. Measures designed to liquefy mucus, to minimize its formation, and to prevent obstruction are taken. Daily administration of pancreatin is prescribed.

Optimum nutrition should be maintained by careful attention to diet. A diet high in protein and calories with moderation in fat intake is needed in cases where fat is poorly tolerated. The protein intake must be great enough to compensate for that lost in the stools. Protein hydrolysates may be useful in place of whole or evaporated milk in treating infants who show severe intestinal involvement. Calorie allowances must be sufficient to enable the individual to achieve desirable weight. Medium-chain triglycerides have been found to be useful in this disorder. Additional B complex vitamins, ascorbic acid, and aqueous preparations of vitamins A and D should be prescribed. Distribution of foods into six small feedings may be advisable for some persons, especially in the younger age groups.

PROBLEMS AND REVIEW

1. Mr. T. is a 70-year-old retired bricklayer whose physician has recommended a soft, fat-restricted diet. Mr. T. lives alone since the recent death of his wife. He does some light

cooking but usually eats his evening meal in a restaurant. He states that he does not have much of an appetite. Plan a day's menu for him. What recommendations would you make for foods eaten away from home?

2. Mr. J. is a 20-year-old unemployed laborer who has infectious hepatitis. Ordinarily, he eats all foods, but has lost 18 pounds due to marked anorexia. He still enjoys milkshakes, however.
  a. What type of diet would you expect his doctor to order for him?
  b. Plan two days' menus for him.
  c. He has a history of very irregular eating habits. Will this affect the course of his disease at present?

3. Mrs. V. has cirrhosis of the liver and her physician has prescribed a 2500-calorie diet to help her regain some of the 22 pounds she has lost. The diet is to provide 100 gm protein, 80 gm fat, and 350 gm carbohydrate.
  a. Plan a day's menu for her.
  b. Show how you would modify this menu to reduce the sodium to 250 mg.
  c. Mrs. V.'s husband deserted her and she depends on state aid for financial assistance. Because of her limited resources, she is accustomed to buying salt pork and other less expensive cuts of meat. How would you advise her in this regard?
  d. Mrs. V.'s physician wants her to learn to adjust her protein intake at home so that she can adapt her diet upon his recommendation when signs of impending coma appear. How would you go about teaching her to do this?
  e. Mrs. V. was later readmitted to the hospital in hepatic coma. The doctor has ordered a protein-free diet for her. Plan a day's menu that supplies 2000 calories. Adjust this menu to provide 10, 20, 30, and 40 gm protein.

4. Mrs. M. is a 56-year-old woman with cholelithiasis whose physician has ordered a 1200-calorie fat-restricted diet. What factors are important in the dietary management of this woman?
  a. What problems might she face in preparing meals if fat is limited to 25 gm per day?
  b. Plan a day's menu for her with 25 gm fat; adjust to provide 50 gm fat.

5. Mr. H. has chronic pancreatitis. What type of diet would you expect his doctor to order? Plan a day's menu. Should he take vitamin supplements?

Cited References

1. Sherlock, S.: "The Treatment of Hepatitis," *Bull. N.Y. Acad. Med.*, **45**:189–200, 1969.
2. Silverberg, M., *et al.:* "An Evaluation of Rest and Low Fat Diets in the Management of Acute Infectious Hepatitis," *J. Pediatr.*, **74**:260–64, 1969.
3. Popper, H., *et al.:* "The Social Impact of Liver Disease," *N. Engl. J. Med.*, **281**:1455–58, 1969.
4. Rubin, E., and Lieber, C. S.: "Alcohol Induced Hepatic Injury in Nonalcoholic Volunteers," *N. Engl. J. Med.*, **278**:869–76, 1968.
5. Davidson, C. S.: "Nutrition, Geography, and Liver Diseases," *Am. J. Clin. Nutr.*, **23**:427–36, 1970.
6. Bielski, M. T., and Molander, D. W.: "Laennec's Cirrhosis," *Am. J. Nurs.*, **65**:82–86, 1965.
7. Gabuzda, G. J., and Shear, L.: "Metabolism of Dietary Protein in Hepatic Cirrhosis. Nutritional and Clinical Considerations," *Am. J. Clin. Nutr.*, **23**:479–87, 1970.
8. Linscheer, W. G.: "Malabsorption in Cirrhosis," *Am. J. Clin. Nutr.*, **23**:488–92, 1970.
9. Breneman, J.C.: "Allergy Elimination Diet as the Most Effective Gallbladder Diet," *Ann. Allergy*, **26**:83–87, 1968.
10. Sarles, H., *et al.:* "Diet, Cholesterol Gallstones, and Composition of the Bile," *Am. J. Dig. Dis.*, **15**:251–60, 1970.

11. Di Sant' Agnese, P. A., and Talamo, R. C.: "Pathogenesis and Physiopathology of Cystic Fibrosis of the Pancreas," *N. Engl. J. Med.*, **277**:1399–1408, 1967.

ADDITIONAL REFERENCES

Anderson, M. C.: "Review of Pancreatic Disease," *Surgery*, **66**:434–49, 1969.
Barker, L. F., *et al.:* "Transmission of Serum Hepatitis," *J.A.M.A.*, **211**:1509–12, 1970.
Bolt, R. J.: "Medical Treatment of Cholecystitis," *Mod. Treat.*, **5**:514–27, 1968.
Carper, J.: "Cirrhosis: A Growing Threat to Life," *Today's Health*, **48**:26–27, 1970.
Henderson, L. M.: "Nursing Care in Acute Cholecystitis," *Am. J. Nurs.*, **64**:93–96, 1964.
Illingworth, C.: "Gallstones," *Nurs. Times*, **66**:167–68, 1970.
Leevy, C. M., *et al.:* "Vitamins and Liver Injury," *Am. J. Clin. Nutr.*, **23**:493–99, 1970.
Paton, A.: "Hepatic Coma," *Nurs. Times*, **65**:1351–52, 1969.
Sherlock, S.: "Nutritional Complications of Biliary Cirrhosis," *Am. J. Clin. Nutr.*, **23**:640–44, 1970.
Zieve, L.: "Pathogenesis of Hepatic Coma," *Arch. Intern. Med.*, **118**:211–23, 1966.

Unit XI

Dietary Modification for Surgical Conditions

Chapter

38 Nutrition in Surgical Conditions
Tube Feedings; High-Protein, High-Fat, Low-Carbohydrate Diet (for Dumping Syndrome)

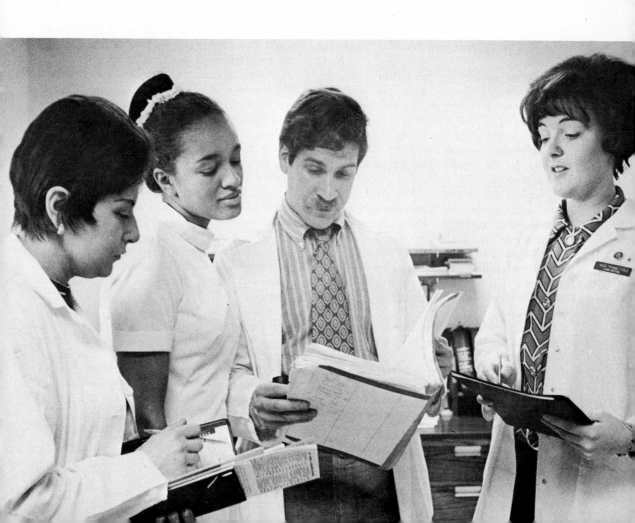

38 Nutrition in Surgical Conditions

*Tube Feedings;
High-Protein, High-Fat,
Low-Carbohydrate Diet*

Good nutrition prior to and following surgery assures fewer postoperative complications, better wound healing, shorter convalescence, and lower mortality.

Effects of surgery on the nutritive requirements. Surgery or injury brings about a greatly increased need for nutrients as a result of loss of blood, plasma, or pus from the wound surface; hemorrhage from the gastrointestinal or pulmonary tract; vomiting; and fever. During immobilization, the loss of some nutrients such as protein is accelerated.

A fairly simple operation often involves moderate deficiency in food intake for a few days following the operation. Even though some nutrients may be supplied by parenteral fluids, the full needs of the body usually cannot be met by that means alone. Moreover, when foods are permitted following surgery, the choice and amount are sometimes too limited to permit nutritive balance.

Far more serious is the problem of the patient whose poor nutritional state prior to surgery imposes a severe additional strain. Chronic infection as in bronchiectasis or heightened metabolism as in hyperthyroidism may lead to increased requirements. Poor appetite and inadequate intake of nutrients are the rule in many diseases. Especially in liver diseases and in sprue absorp-

tive failure may be serious. Extensive losses of nutrients and fluids may have occurred through hemorrhage, vomiting or diarrhea. The extent of the deficiency is manifested by weight loss, poor wound healing, decreased intestinal motility, anemia, edema, or dehydration, and the presence of decubitus ulcers. The circulating blood volume and the concentration of the serum proteins, hemoglobin, and electrolytes may be reduced.

Nutritional considerations. The objectives in the dietary management of surgical conditions are (1) to improve the preoperative nutrition whenever the operation is not of an emergency nature, (2) to maintain correct nutrition after operation or injury insofar as possible, and (3) to avoid harm from injudicious choice of foods.

Protein. A satisfactory state of protein nutrition ensures rapid wound healing by providing the correct assortment and quantity of essential amino acids, increases the resistance to infection, exerts a protective action upon the liver against the toxic effects of anesthesia, and reduces the possibility of edema at the site of the wound. The presence of edema is a hindrance to wound healing and, in operations on the gastrointestinal tract, may reduce motility thus leading to distention.

It is not always realistic to fully replace protein losses prior to surgery because the disease process itself may be such as to preclude a satisfactory intake of food. Improved surgical results of recent years have come about through adequate replacement of blood volume and better operative techniques rather than preoperative protein replacement. The extent to which surgery should be delayed in order to improve the nutritional state is obviously a highly individual matter.

Protein catabolism is increased for several days immediately following surgery or injury; patients are characteristically in negative nitrogen balance even though the protein intake may be appreciable. Well-nourished persons lose more nitrogen than poorly nourished persons whose labile protein stores are already depleted.[1]

The level of protein to be used in preoperative

and postoperative diets depends upon the previous state of nutrition, the nature of the operation, and the extent of the postoperative losses. Intakes of 100 gm protein, and frequently much more, are necessary as a rule.

Energy. The weight status is an important pre- and postoperative consideration, for it serves as a guide to the caloric level to be recommended. Without sufficient caloric intake, tissue proteins cannot be synthesized. Excessive metabolism of body fat may lead to acidosis, whereas depletion of the liver glycogen may increase the likelihood of damage to the liver.

In hyperthyroidism or fever, as much as 4000 calories daily may be essential to bring about weight gain. Other patients will make satisfactory progress at 2500 to 3000 calories.

Obesity constitutes a hazard in surgery. Whenever possible, it should be corrected, at least in part, by using one of the low-calorie diets (see page 422).

Minerals. Phosphorus and potassium are lost in proportion to the breakdown of body tissue. In addition, derangements of sodium and chloride metabolism may occur subsequent to vomiting, diarrhea, perspiration, drainage, anorexia, and diuresis or renal failure. The detection of electrolyte imbalance and appropriate parenteral fluid therapy requires careful study of clinical signs and biochemical evaluation.

Iron-deficiency anemia may occur in association with malabsorption or excessive blood loss. Diet alone is ineffective in correction of anemia, but a liberal intake of protein and ascorbic acid, together with administration of iron salts, is of value in convalescence. Transfusions are usually required to overcome severe reduction in hemoglobin level.

Fluids. A review of the maintenance of water balance (see page 126) will bring to the attention of the student the large amounts of fluid lost daily by the normal individual and the several sources of water to the body. The fluid balance may be upset prior to and following surgery owing to failure to ingest normal quantities of fluids and to increased losses from vomiting, exudates, hemorrhage, diuresis, and fever. A patient should not go to operation in a state of dehydra-

tion since the subsequent dangers of acidosis are great. When dehydration exists prior to operation, parenteral fluids are administered if the patient is unable to ingest sufficient liquid by mouth. Following major surgery the fluid balance is maintained by parenteral fluids until satisfactory oral intake can be established.

Vitamins. Ascorbic acid is especially important for wound healing and should be provided in increased amounts prior to and following surgery. Vitamin K is of concern to the surgeon since the failure to synthesize vitamin K in the small intestine, the inability to absorb it, or the defect in conversion to prothrombin is likely to result in bleeding. Hemorrhage is especially likely to occur in patients who have diseases of the liver.

Planning the preoperative diet. Patients who have lost much weight prior to surgery may benefit considerably by ingesting a high-protein, high-calorie diet (see page 432) for even a week or two prior to surgery. The diet may be of liquid, soft, or regular consistency depending upon the nature of the pathologic condition. Certain patients may benefit from parenteral hyperalimentation.[2] In addition, the maintenance of metabolic equilibrium as in diabetes or other diseases must not be overlooked.

When surgery is delayed in order to improve the nutritional status, each day's intake should represent such improvement in nutrition that the delay is justified. This necessitates constant encouragement by the nurse and dietitian; it likewise requires imagination in varying the foods offered to the patient and ingenuity in getting the patient to eat. Foods which provide a maximum amount of nutrients in a minimum volume are essential. Small feedings at frequent intervals are likely to be more effective than large meals which cannot be fully consumed.

For additional protein, milk beverages may be fortified with nonfat dry milk, whole egg, and egg whites. Strained meat in broth may be used when patients are unable to eat other meats. Fruit juices fortified with glucose, high-carbohydrate lemonade, jelly with crackers and bread, and hard candy may be used to increase the carbohydrate intake and to facilitate storage of glycogen. Butter incorporated into foods and light cream mixed with equal amounts of milk are also useful for increasing the caloric intake. The excessive use of sugars and fats may provoke nausea, however.

Food and fluids are generally allowed until midnight just preceding the day of operation, although a light breakfast may be given when the operation is scheduled for afternoon and local anesthesia is to be used. It is essential that the stomach be empty prior to administering the anesthesia so as to reduce the incidence of vomiting and the subsequent danger of aspiration of vomitus. When an operation is to be performed on the gastrointestinal tract, a diet very low in residue (page 462) may be ordered two to three days prior to operation. Chemically defined liquid diets (see Chapter 36) are useful for such cases.[3] In acute abdominal conditions such as appendicitis and cholecystitis, no food is allowed by mouth until nausea, vomiting, pain, and distention have passed in order to prevent the danger of peritonitis.

Planning the postoperative diet. The patient enters a catabolic phase during the first few days following surgery and remains in negative nitrogen balance regardless of his intake of protein and calories. The degree of negative balance can be reduced at higher intakes of protein and calories.

Parenteral feedings. The maintenance or restoration of fluid and electrolyte balance is of paramount importance during the interval when the patient is unable to ingest food or fluid by mouth. In addition to furnishing fluid and salts, the intravenous fluid often contains glucose, which serves to prevent ketosis and to minimize tissue catabolism. For selected patients parenteral hyperalimentation is useful in maintaining nutrition for extended periods. By means of an indwelling catheter passed into the superior vena cava, a hypertonic solution consisting of glucose, protein hydrolysate, vitamins, minerals, and electrolytes is administered continuously. The ratio of nonprotein calories to nitrogen is approximately 150 to 1.[1] Dudrick and coworkers have shown that up to 4000 calories daily can be supplied using this technique.[4]

Intravenous fat emulsions make possible a substantial increase in caloric intake and may thus aid in reducing nitrogen losses.[5] These emulsions, though widely used abroad, have had limited use in this country because of undesirable side effects.[6]

Parenteral nutrition requires a careful consideration of the nature of the illness, physical examination to evaluate subjective changes, and laboratory analyses for blood electrolytes, pH, and blood proteins. The student should be aware of the nutritional contributions made by such feedings although the details of management are beyond the scope of this text.

Progression of oral feeding. Oral feeding is begun when gastrointestinal secretions are being produced and peristalsis resumes. Feeding should not be delayed once such function has returned. The accumulation of gastrointestinal secretions may result in a feeling of fullness. Moreover, the wound strength is sufficient to permit digestion of food.

Patients usually respond better if they are given solid foods rather than liquid foods. Initially, the feedings are small and may be restricted to a low-residue diet. (See also Chapter 34.) Foods which are high in protein and fat are believed to be less distending than those which are high in carbohydrate.[7] Perhaps of greater importance is the emphasis upon eating slowly and in small amounts to reduce the amount of air which is swallowed. As the patient improves, the selection of foods is that of a soft or regular diet, depending upon the nature of the surgery.

TUBE FEEDINGS

Feeding by tube may be required for a short period of time or indefinitely in a variety of circumstances: surgery of the mouth; esophageal obstruction; gastrointestinal surgery; in severe burns; in anorexia nervosa; and in the comatose patient. Ordinarily, the feedings are given by nasogastric tube, but if the esophagus is obstructed they are given through a tube inserted into an opening in the abdominal wall.

Characteristics of tube feedings. A satisfactory tube feeding must be (1) nutritionally adequate; (2) well tolerated by the patient so that vomiting is not induced; (3) easily digested with no unfavorable reactions such as distention, diarrhea, or constipation; (4) easily prepared; and (5) inexpensive.

The concentration of the feeding may be adjusted from about ⅔ to 1⅓ calories per milliliter; likewise, the protein level may be increased if needed. A concentration of about 1 calorie per milliliter is satisfactory and is less likely to produce diarrhea than feedings of higher concentration. About 2 liters per 24 hours is a customary volume.

Tube feedings prepared from the ordinary foods of a normal diet by using a high-speed blender are generally preferred to other types of formulas. Patients accept these feedings more readily because they see that they are receiving foods that other people normally consume and are modified only in consistency. The blenderized feedings are well tolerated and are only infrequently associated with diarrhea.

Numerous commercial feedings are available to meet specific needs in terms of protein, fat, and calorie content. Likewise, recipes are available for the preparation of feedings within the hospital or home. Most of these feedings use whole or skim milk, eggs, and vitamin supplements together with some form of carbohydrate such as strained cooked cereals, sugar, or molasses. Vegetable oil or cream and nonfat dry

milk are also incorporated to increase the calorie and protein levels, respectively. Commercial formulas ensure constancy of composition and simplicity of preparation. They may be preferred for short-term use, but blenderized feedings are more likely to be used for longer periods of time.

Blenderized feedings. Any foods which lend themselves to liquefaction in a high-speed blender may be used. The following procedure is recommended.[8]

1. Food is mixed with sufficient liquid in a blender to facilitate homogenization and liquefaction.

2. Homogenized milk should be used since plain milk will form butter.

3. About four to five minutes is usually required for homogenization.

4. The homogenate must be strained several times through a fine-mesh wire sieve to remove all fibers that would clog the tube.

Alternate procedure. The straining of the formula may be avoided by using only those foods already in a fine state of division. These include strained baby foods such as meats, fruits, and vegetables; strained fruit juices; nonfat dry milk, or homogenized milk; cream, or vegetable oil; brewers' yeast or vitamin supplements. A formula providing 1 calorie per milliliter is given in Table 38–1. Normal daily intake would be about 2 liters.

Table 38–1. Blenderized Formula

Ingredients	Weight gm	Protein gm	Fat gm	Carbohydrate gm
Orange juice, frozen concentrate	70	1.7	0.2	25.7
Milk, skim, 2% nonfat milk solids added	360	15.1	7.2	21.6
Egg, whole, frozen or hard cooked	50	6.5	5.8	0.5
Farina, cooked, enriched	100	1.3	0.1	8.7
Nonfat dry milk	15	5.4	0.1	7.9
Liver, strained*	100	13.9	3.2	2.0
Peaches, strained*	100	0.6	0.1	19.1
Vegetable oil	20	—	20.0	—
Bread, whole wheat	60	6.3	1.8	28.6
Water to 1000 ml				
		50.8	38.5	114.1

*Nutritional composition based on Gerber's brand.

Administration of tube feedings. Depending upon its nature, the feeding may be heated over hot water to body temperature, taking care that curdling does not occur with certain mixtures. Initially, small amounts of a dilute formula (50 ml) are given at hourly intervals. It is important that the feeding be given at a slow constant rate. Barron[8] recommends the use of a food pump with blenderized feedings. In patients who do not have an adequate swallowing mechanism or who are comatose, special care must be taken to avoid vomiting and aspiration of the vomitus. The patient should be positioned to prevent aspiration, and suction should be readily available at the bedside if vomiting occurs.[9] Close attention to individual water needs is essential to prevent salt or protein overload.

When the small feedings are satisfactorily tolerated, the concentration and amount of the formula is gradually increased, with feedings not exceeding 12 ounces per three- to four-hour interval.

DIET IN SPECIFIED SURGICAL CONDITIONS

Diet following operations on the mouth, throat, or esophagus. The extraction of teeth, the period of waiting for dentures, and the time required to become accustomed to new dentures could result in nutritive inadequacy if suggestions for adequate diet are not given to the patient. For one or two days following the extraction of teeth, it may be necessary to restrict the diet to liquids taken through a drinking tube. Thereafter, any soft foods which require little if any chewing may be used for three weeks or longer.

Radical surgery of the mouth necessitates the use of a full fluid diet, but immediately after surgery one of the regimens for tube feeding described in the previous section may be used. Tube feeding is likewise required for an operation on the esophagus, the tube being inserted directly into the stomach.

Following tonsillectomy the patient may be given cold fluids including milk, bland fruit juices, ginger ale, plain ice cream, and sherbets. Tart fruit juices and fibrous foods must be avoided. On the second day, soft foods such as custard, plain puddings, soft eggs, warm but not hot cereals, strained cream soups, mashed potatoes, and fruit and vegetable purées may be tolerated. As a rule, the regular diet is swallowed without difficulty within the week.

Diet following gastrectomy. A number of problems arise following gastrectomy, and their treatment should be anticipated. Weight loss is common, and studies undertaken up to 10 years following surgery indicate that about one third of patients fail to regain weight to desirable levels.[10] The loss of a reservoir for food means that small feedings given at frequent intervals must be used if sufficient nutrients are to be ingested. Moreover, the absence of pepsin and hydrochloric acid entails the entire digestion of protein by the enzymes of the small intestine. Fat utilization is often impaired because of inadequate biliary and pancreatic secretions or defective mixing of food with the digestive juices. Intestinal motility is frequently increased.

Iron is less readily absorbed and hypochromic microcytic anemia is common. In the absence of gastric juice and its intrinsic factor vitamin B_{12} cannot be absorbed from the intestine, thereby leading to macrocytic anemia in two to five years after operation unless injections of vitamin B_{12} are given.

Dietary progression. Oral feedings vary widely from one patient to another. The usual sequence consists of hourly feedings of 60 to 90 ml fluids for several days with progression from water to full liquids by the third day. Thereafter, the diet increases from day to day according to the individual's tolerance for food. By the fourth or fifth day, soft low-fiber foods are used. Eggs, custards, thickened soups, cereals, crackers, milk, and fruit purées are suitable. Tender chicken, cottage cheese, and puréed vegetables are the next foods added. Meals are divided into five or six small feedings daily with emphasis on foods high in protein and fat; carbohydrate is kept relatively low. The selection of foods allowed for the first stage of the Bland Low-Fiber Diet (Chapter 34) or the Very Low-Residue Diet (Chapter 35) may be used initially. Many patients progress more satisfactorily if no liquids are taken with meals, and if the diet continues to be low in carbohydrate, especially the simple sugars.

Diet following intestinal surgery. Obstruction, persistent ileitis or diverticulitis, perforation, and malignancy are among the reasons for removal of a section of the ileum (ileectomy) or colon (colectomy). A permanent opening in the abdominal wall is provided through which the digestive wastes are eliminated. Following removal of part of the ileum and colon, the proximal end of the ileum is attached to the opening (*ileostomy*). Because the absorptive function of the colon has been eliminated by the surgery, the waste material is fluid and continuous. Fluid, sodium, and potassium losses may be considerable, fat absorption is often poor, and vitamin B_{12} absorption is reduced or absent.

A *colostomy* consists in attaching the proximal end of the resected colon to the opening in the abdominal wall. Some ability to absorb water is retained so that feces are more or less formed, and bowel regularity can be reestablished.

Following any operation upon the small intestine or colon, the initial intake is restricted to clear fluids and followed with a low-residue diet as a rule. Patients with an ileostomy are usually young and require a good deal of guidance and support from the nurse and dietitian. Gradually, they may add foods moderately low in fiber, but each food should be tested for tolerance before introducing a second. Weight loss may be considerable, and a high-protein, high-calorie diet is generally required. Vitamin B_{12} injections are required to prevent the occurrence of macrocytic anemia in later years.

Colostomy is performed more frequently on elderly persons. In time they may resume an essentially normal diet, but usually they require some counseling concerning the foods required for nutritive adequacy. They too require emotional support, as well as assurance that foods will not be harmful.

Diet following other abdominal operations. The principles outlined on page 496 pertain to the planning of diet following appendectomy, cholecystectomy, and other abdominal operations. Adynamic ileus is present longer following cholecystectomy and hysterectomy than after

removal of the appendix. Patients who have had the gallbladder removed may require a low-fat diet for three months or longer, after which a regular diet is used.

Following peritonitis and intestinal obstruction, nothing whatever is given by mouth until gastrointestinal function has been resumed. Drainage of the stomach and upper intestine is essential until there is reduction of distention and passage of gas. This may require four to six days, during which time nutrition is maintained by complete intravenous therapy. When the patient shows tolerance for water, broth, and weak tea, a very low-residue diet may be introduced cautiously.

Diet following burns. Tremendous losses of protein, salts, and fluid take place when large areas of the body have been burned. Greatly increased nutritive requirements exist for weeks or months following burns. Severe hypoproteinemia, edema at the site of injury, failure to obtain satisfactory skin growth, and gastric atony are among the nutritional problems encountered.

When vomiting and diarrhea are severe, reliance must be placed primarily on complete intravenous therapy. Tube feeding may precede oral feeding and is continued until the high nutritive requirements can be met by the usual feeding procedures. At least 150 gm protein, and often as much as 300 gm protein, is required daily together with 3500 to 5000 calories. High-protein meals supplemented with high-protein beverages are used (see Chapter 32). Oral fat emulsions taken as a beverage or given by tube are useful in maintaining a high-caloric intake. The need for as much as 1.0 gm ascorbic acid has been definitely established, and additional B complex vitamins are also considered essential.

Diet following fractures. Following fractures there is a tremendous catabolism of protein, which may not be reversed for several weeks. Nitrogen loss is accompanied by loss of phosphorus, potassium, and sulfur. Fever and infection may further accentuate such losses.

Calcium loss is also great but is not corrected by the administration of calcium. In fact, calcium therapy may lead to the formation of renal calculi and should not be attempted until the cast is removed and some mobilization is possible.

A liberal intake of protein is essential to permit restoration of the protein matrix of the bone so that calcium can be deposited. Sufficient calories to permit maximum use of the protein for synthesis should be provided.

DUMPING SYNDROME

Nature of the dumping syndrome. Following convalescence from gastric surgery a relatively high proportion of patients experience distressing symptoms about 10 to 15 minutes after eating. There is a sense of fullness in the epigastrium with weakness, nausea, pallor, sweating, and dizziness. The pulse rate increases and the patient seeks to obtain relief by lying down for a few minutes. Vomiting and diarrhea are infrequently present. Failure to gain weight is commonly observed because the patient eats less food.

The exact etiology of the dumping has not been established, but may be partly explained as follows: When a high proportion of easily hydrolyzed carbohydrate is introduced into the small intestine, a hyperosmolar mixture is produced. This is made isotonic by the withdrawal of water from the blood into the intestine. The withdrawal of fluid from the blood leads to a reduction in the blood volume and blood pressure, and signs of cardiac insufficiency appear—rapid pulse rate, weakness, and sweating. The presence of large amounts of fluid in the intestine leads to the feeling of fullness.

Modification of the diet. Dietary regimens developed to alleviate the symptoms of the dumping syndrome emphasize the following: (1) avoidance of sugar and concentrated forms of carbohydrate, (2) liberal protein, (3) small frequent feedings, and (4) dry meals with fluids taken only between meals.[11]

Initially, calories from carbohydrates, proteins, and fats are supplied in a ratio of 1:1.5:5. The diet may have several stages, each providing for more liberalization in the foods allowed. The patient should be stabilized at a given stage before progressing to the next. Many persons who adhere to such dietary plans have achieved satisfactory weight status without marked nutritional deficiencies. Some are able to tolerate buttermilk, evaporated milk, nonfat dry milk, and simmered or boiled milk in modest quantities when taken between meals. Although a few individuals eventually progress to a near regular diet, stage II below has been found to be the most satisfactory on a long-term basis.[12]

HIGH-PROTEIN, HIGH-FAT, LOW-CARBOHYDRATE DIET*

Characteristics and general rules

1. Three routines are employed, with progression from one to another as the patient's condition warrants. The composition of the three routines is approximately:

	ROUTINE I	ROUTINE II	ROUTINE III
Carbohydrate, gm	0	100	100
Protein, gm	115	150	150
Fat, gm	170	225	225
Calories	2000	3000	3000
Calorie ratio:			
Carbohydrate	0	1	1
Fat	5	5	5
Protein	1.5	1.5	1.5

2. Multiple vitamin supplements are prescribed; iron may be necessary.
3. Six small dry meals are given daily; meals must be eaten regularly without omissions.

*Adapted from Pittman, A. C., and Robinson, F. W.: "Dumping Syndrome—Control by Diet," *J. Am. Diet Assoc.,* **34:**596–602, 1958.

4. Liquids are taken 30 to 45 minutes after meals.
5. Carbohydrate foods are severely restricted. Those allowed must be measured accurately.
6. Liberal portions of meat are used; 1 pat margarine or butter should be eaten with each ounce of meat.
7. Foods to avoid include: milk, ice cream and other frozen desserts; sugars, sweets, candy, syrup, chocolate; gravies and rich sauces.
8. Rest before meals, eating slowly and chewing well, and relaxation are essential.

Foods allowed for three routines

ROUTINE I

Meat, fish, poultry—all kinds: broiled, baked, poached, stewed, grilled. Luncheon meats without cereal filler

Eggs—2 to 3: poached, scrambled, coddled, shirred, hard cooked

Fats—1 pat margarine or butter per ounce meat; 2 to 3 strips crisp bacon

Beverages—never at meals, but 30 to 45 minutes *after* meals: small amounts of cool water, or coffee, tea, limeade or lemonade without sugar. Use artificial sweetener

Miscellaneous—salt; lemon or lime juice on fish, etc.

ROUTINE II. All foods of routine I plus

Bread—enriched day-old white toast, zwieback, soda crackers, Melba toast. Only 1 slice with each feeding

Bread substitutes—fresh Lima beans, sweet corn, cooked dried beans and peas, saltines, soda crackers, grits, noodles, macaroni, rice, spaghetti, parsnips, boiled potato, mashed potato, sweet potato. See Table A–4, Bread List, for equivalents

Cereals—thick, cooked. Only 1 serving

Fats—1 ounce whipping cream; cream cheese

Nuts, when tolerated—plain or salted; chew thoroughly

Vegetables—all kinds. Not more than one serving per meal

Miscellaneous—olives, pimiento

ROUTINE III. All foods of routines I and II plus

Fruits, fresh, canned, or frozen; *no sugar.* Drained of all liquid. Fruit juices may be taken only 30 to 40 minutes after meals.

SAMPLE MENU PLANS FOR PATIENTS WITH DUMPING SYNDROME

Routine I	Routine II	Routine III
MORNING		
2 eggs with	2 scrambled eggs with	2 scrambled eggs with
2–3 pats margarine or butter (or more)	3 pats margarine or butter	3 pats margarine or butter
2 or more strips crisp bacon	2 slices crisp bacon	2 strips crisp bacon
	1 average slice bread	½ slice bread
	1 pat margarine or butter	1 pat margarine or butter
		½ cup orange sections (no liquid)
MIDMORNING		
3 oz meat with	2 oz meat with	2 oz meat with
3 pats margarine or butter, if possible	1 pat margarine or butter	1 pat margarine or butter
	2 thin slices of bread for sandwich	2 thin slices bread for sandwich
NOON		
2 beef patties or hamburger, steak, chops, roast with	4 oz chicken with	4 oz chicken with
3 pats margarine or butter (or more)	2 pats margarine or butter	3 pats margarine or butter
	½ cup string beans with	½ cup string beans with
	1 pat margarine or butter	1 pat margarine or butter
	1 slice bread with	½ slice bread with
	2 pats margarine or butter	1 pat margarine or butter
		½ small banana

Routine I (Cont.)	Routine II (Cont.)	Routine III (Cont.)
MIDAFTERNOON		
Meat or eggs with 3 pats margarine or butter	2 oz meat or 4 tbsp peanut butter with 1 pat margarine or butter 2 thin slices bread for sandwich	2 oz meat or 4 tbsp peanut butter 1 pat margarine or butter 2 thin slices bread for sandwich
EVENING		
Same as at noon	4 oz broiled fish with 2 pats margarine or butter Asparagus tips with 1 pat margarine or butter 1 average slice bread 1 pat margarine or butter	4 oz broiled fish with 3 pats margarine or butter Asparagus tips with 1 pat margarine or butter ½ slice bread ½ cup applesauce
BEDTIME		
Same as midafternoon	Same as midafternoon	Same as midafternoon

PROBLEMS AND REVIEW

1. Mrs. N. needs to undergo major surgery but her physician has recommended that the surgery be delayed for two weeks in order to improve her nutritional status.
   a. List some symptoms and laboratory findings that indicate the need for specific attention to dietary management before surgery.
   b. Which nutrients will be especially important in Mrs. N.'s diet?
   c. Is a high-carbohydrate diet advantageous prior to surgery? Why?
   d. List several high-protein beverages which could be used to supplement Mrs. N.'s protein intake.
   e. Which fluids should be emphasized in the diet if a high potassium intake is ordered?
2. Study the charts of six postoperative patients and prepare a chart showing the following: nature of the surgery; orders for parenteral fluids; orders for diet. Indicate the length of time each diet was used, and explain the variations which were found.
3. Prepare a list of parenteral feedings used in your hospital and enumerate the chief nutritive contributions made by each.
4. Mr. E.'s physician ordered a tube feeding for him following surgery.
   a. Compare advantages and disadvantages of blenderized and commercial formula feedings.
   b. What adjustments might be made to correct diarrhea in patients receiving tube feedings?
   c. List several precautions that must be considered in administration of tube feedings.
5. List the factors important to consider in the dietary management of persons with a gastrostomy; an ileostomy; a colostomy.
6. Mrs. Q. recently underwent a subtotal gastrectomy.
   a. List some of the nutritional problems she may develop.
   b. What type of diet would you expect Mrs. Q.'s physician to order?
   c. Mrs. Q. has symptoms of the dumping syndrome; list some of these. What steps can she take to prevent occurrence of symptoms?
   d. What dietary modifications should be made for persons with this condition? Explain the rationale for each change. Plan a day's menu for Mrs. Q.

CITED REFERENCES

1. Doolas, A.: "Planning Intravenous Alimentation of Surgical Patients," *Surg. Clin. North Am.*, **50**:103–12, 1970.

2. Sherman, J. O., Egan, T., and Macalad, F. V.: "Parenteral Hyperalimentation. A Useful Surgical Adjunct," *Surg. Clin. North Am.*, **51**:37–47, 1971.
3. Winitz, M., Seedman, D. A., and Graff, J.: "Studies in Metabolic Nutrition Employing Chemically Defined Diets. I. Extended Feeding of Normal Human Adult Males," *Am. J. Clin. Nutr.*, **23**:525–45, 1970.
4. Dudrick, S. J., *et al.:* "Long Term Total Parenteral Nutrition with Growth, Development, and Positive Nitrogen Balance," *Surgery*, **64**:134–42, 1968.
5. Levey, S.: "Reduction of Nitrogen Deficits in Surgical Patients Maintained by Intravenous Alimentation," *Nutr. Rev.*, **24**:193–95, 1966.
6. Jones, R. J.: "Present Knowledge of Intravenous Fat Emulsions," *Nutr. Rev.*, **24**:225–28, 1966.
7. "Postoperative Distention and Fruit Juices," Questions and Answers, *J.A.M.A.*, **194**:476, 1965.
8. Barron, J.: "Preparation of Natural Foods for Tube Feeding," *Henry Ford Hosp. Med. Bull.*, **4**:18–21, March 1956.
9. Krehl, W. A.: "Tube Feeding," *J.A.M.A.*, **169**:1153–55, 1959.
10. Biggar, B. L., *et al.:* "Nutrition Following Gastric Resection," *J. Am. Diet. Assoc.*, **37**:344–47, 1960.
11. Pittman, A. C., and Robinson, F. W.: "Dumping Syndrome—Control by Diet," *J. Am. Diet. Assoc.*, **34**:596–602, 1958.
12. Pittman, A. C., and Robinson, F. W.: "Dietary Management of the 'Dumping' Syndrome," *J. Am. Diet. Assoc.*, **40**:108–10, 1962.

ADDITIONAL REFERENCES

Berk, J. L.: "The Dumping Syndrome," *Arch. Surg.*, **102**:88–89, 1971.
Campbell, E. B.: "Nursing Problems Associated with Prolonged Recovery Following Trauma," *Nurs. Clin. North Am.*, **5**:551–62, 1970.
"Diet with Ileostomy," *Br. Med. J.*, **4**:634, 1970.
Dudrick, S. J.: "Intravenous Hyperalimentation," *Surgery*, **68**:726–27, 1970.
Gault, M. H., *et al.:* "Hypernatremia, Azotemia, and Dehydration Due to High-Protein Tube Feeding," *Ann. Intern. Med.*, **68**:778–91, 1968.
Grant, J. A. N., Moir, E., and Fago, M.: "Parenteral Hyperalimentation," *Am. J. Nurs.*, **69**:2392–95, 1969.
Hanngren, A., Hedenstedt, S., and Reizenstein, P.: "Nutritional Studies in Patients with Dumping Syndrome. I. Subjects with Postcibal Symptoms," *Am. J. Dig. Dis.*, **12**:71–80, 1967.
Kirksey, T. D., *et al.:* "Gastrointestinal Complications in Burns," *Am. J. Surg.*, **116**:627–33, 1968.
Larsen, R. B.: "Dietary Needs of Patients Following General Surgery," *Hospitals*, **39**:133–36, July 16, 1965.
Lenneberg, E., and Mendelssohn, A. N.: "Colostomies: A Guide for the Patient," *Dis. Colon Rectum*, **12**:201–17, 1969.
Morgan, A., Filler, R. M., and Moore, F. D.: "Surgical Nutrition," *Med. Clin. North Am.*, **54**:1367–81, 1970.
Peaston, M. J.: "Nasogastric Feeding and Metabolic Balance," *Nurs. Times*, **63**:372–74, 1967.
Randall, H. T.: "Nutrition in Surgical Patients," *Am. J. Surg.*, **119**:530–33, 1970.
Thomson, T. J., Runcie, J., and Khan, A.: "The Effect of Diet on Ileostomy Function," *Gut*, **11**:482–85, 1970.
Willis, M. T., and Postlewait, R. W.: "Dietary Problems After Gastric Resection," *J. Am. Diet. Assoc.*, **40**:111–13, 1962.

Unit XII
Diet in Metabolic and Nervous Disorders

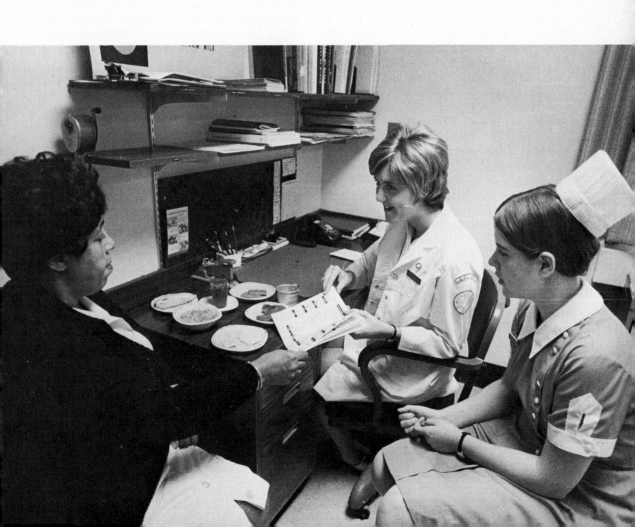

39 Diabetes Mellitus

Diabetes mellitus is a chronic disease that has affected mankind throughout the world. The records of the ancient civilizations of Egypt, India, Japan, Greece, and Rome describe the symptoms of the disease and usually include recommendations for treatment. The wasting away of flesh, copious urination, and the sweet taste of the urine were frequently noted by the ancient medical writers. Aretaeus of Cappadocia, who lived between A.D. 30 and 90, not only named the disease *diabetes*, which means "to run through or to siphon," but also recommended, "The food is to be milk and with it the cereals, starch, autumn fruits and sweet wines."*
The term *mellitus*, which means honeylike, was added by a London physician, Willis, in 1675.

THE NATURE OF DIABETES

Insulin and metabolic defects. Diabetes mellitus is a genetic disease of metabolism in which there is a partial or total lack of functioning insulin; it is characterized by the lessened ability or complete inability of the tissues to utilize carbohydrate. The metabolism of fat and of protein is also altered. Hyperglycemia, glycosuria, and excessive urination are cardinal findings.

*Stowers, J. M.: "Nutrition in Diabetes," *Nutr. Abstr. Rev.*, 33:1, 1963.

The insulin defect may be a failure in its formation, liberation, or action. Since insulin is produced by the beta cells of the islands of Langerhans, any reduction in the number of functioning cells will decrease the amount of insulin that can be synthesized. Many diabetics can produce sufficient insulin, but some stimulus to the islet tissue is needed in order that secretion can take place. Especially in the early stages of the disease the insulinlike activity (ILA) of the blood is often increased, but most of this insulin appears to be bound to protein and is not available for transport across the cell membrane and action within the cell.

The hormones of the anterior pituitary, adrenal cortex, thyroid, and alpha cells of the islands of Langerhans are glucogenic; that is, they increase the supply of glucose. Just how these hormones are involved in the etiology of diabetes is not fully understood. Possibly they could increase the demand, decrease the secretion, or antagonize and inhibit the action of insulin.

Scope of the problem. Diabetes mellitus is a major public health problem for it affects about 4.4 million persons in the United States of whom about 1.6 million do not know that they have the disease.[1] Each year about 325,000 new cases are diagnosed, most of whom are over 40 years of age and who are also affected by one or more chronic conditions of the vascular system including heart disease, high blood pressure, neuropathy, nephropathy, and retinopathy. Diabetes ranks third as a cause of blindness with about 45,000 diabetics being blind.

About 35,000 deaths from diabetes are reported annually in the United States, placing diabetes eighth as a cause of death. In addition, an equal number of diabetics are estimated to die each year from the complications associated with the disease, principally ailments of the cardiovascular system.

The rate of diabetes among persons under 25 years is 2.3 per 1000; for persons over 45 years the rate is 62 per 1000, with the highest incidence occurring in the two decades 55 to 74 years.[1]

Diabetes is a major socioeconomic ill that costs more than two billion dollars annually in terms

Figure 39–1. Diabetes rate increases as weight increases. (Data from diabetic screening of federal employees reported in *Diabetes Source Book,* U.S. Department of Health, Education, and Welfare, 1968, p. 31.)

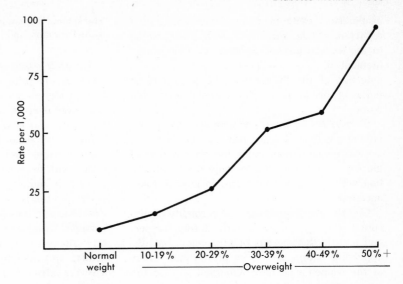

of loss of earnings and costs of hospitalization, physicians' fees, medication, and rehabilitation. The disease is much more prevalent in lower economic groups, with the rate in families with annual incomes below $4000 being more than double that in families with incomes over $4000.

Factors influencing the incidence of diabetes. The high-risk individuals include (1) those who are blood relatives of diabetics; (2) those over 40 years of age; (3) those who are obese; (4) women who have some carbohydrate intolerance during pregnancy; and (5) women who give birth to babies weighing 9 pounds or more.

Diabetes occurs with striking frequency among blood relatives. It has been widely held that the predisposition was inherited as a mendelian recessive character, but this explanation is now in doubt. A number of genetic factors are probably involved, but the mechanism is not fully understood.

The incidence of diabetes increases with overweight, being 12 times as prevalent among those who are 50 per cent overweight as it is among persons of normal weight. (See Figure 39–1.) About 80 per cent of the adults in Joslin's diabetic clinic have previously been overweight by 5 per cent or more. By contrast, young diabetics are rarely obese. Although obesity and diabetes are highly associated, this does not mean that obesity is a cause of diabetes. It has been sug-

gested by some that obesity may be a stress that uncovers the diabetic condition, and by others that obesity and diabetes are different manifestations of a common metabolic defect.

Women are somewhat more susceptible to diabetes than are men. Some women show abnormal glucose tolerance curves during pregnancy but return to normal once the baby has been born, only to become diabetic 10 or 20 years later. Women who give birth to large babies are much more likely to become diabetic in later years than are women who bear babies of normal weight. These heavy babies are also likely to become diabetic in later years.

Stages of diabetes. Diabetes is presumed to be present at birth, but detectable chemical and clinical manifestations of the disease may not be apparent for many years. The disease is often classified according to stages of development.

Prediabetes has been defined as "that period in a patient's life from birth until recognition of carbohydrate intolerance by the latest available technique."* Studies on the high-risk individuals described in the preceding section have shown a higher incidence than normal of microscopic changes in blood vessels of the conjunctiva, ear lobe, and kidney; an increase in the

*Review: "Coronary Disease and Preclinical Diabetes," *Nutr. Rev.,* 23:323, 1965.

insulinlike activity of the blood serum; and a reduction of the release of complexed insulin to the active form.[2] It is hoped that the measurement of such changes can lead to earlier detection of the disease and the possibility of reducing or avoiding the complications that ensue.

Chemical diabetes is characterized by an abnormal glucose tolerance test but no symptoms are yet evident. Sometimes the abnormality of glucose tolerance is evident only upon stimulation with cortisone (the cortisone glucose tolerance test).

Gestational diabetes is the abnormality of glucose tolerance seen particularly during the second and third trimesters of pregnancy, but disappearing within six weeks postpartum. Many of the women who have abnormal glucose tolerance curves produce large babies.[3]

Clinical diabetes is characterized by typical symptoms such as thirst, excessive urination, and increased appetite as well as an abnormal glucose tolerance curve.

Symptoms of juvenile and adult diabetes. Two types of diabetes are recognized, namely growth onset or juvenile diabetes, and maturity onset or adult diabetes.

Growth onset diabetes occurs relatively infrequently and, as a rule, is seen prior to age 20 but occasionally it occurs up to age 40. The onset is usually acute, the abnormality of carbohydrate metabolism is severe, and insulin production is minimal or lacking. The patients are sensitive to insulin, unstable, difficult to manage, and fluctuate from diabetic coma on the one hand to hypoglycemia on the other. Most juvenile diabetics are of normal weight or have lost some weight. Most or all of the classic symptoms of diabetes are present in growth onset diabetes.

Polyuria, or frequent urination and an abnormally large volume of urine

Polydipsia, or excessive thirst

Polyphagia, or increased appetite

Loss of weight

Ketosis is sometimes the abnormality that brings the patient to the physician. It is a condition in which the accumulation of lower fatty acids in the blood leads to the excretion of ketones in the urine.

The ketonuria is accompanied by loss of base, acidosis, dehydration, and eventually coma.

Maturity onset diabetes. The adult-type diabetes occurs primarily after age 30 years but has its highest incidence in the 50's and 60's. The onset is insidious and often does not present any of the classic symptoms. These patients may consult a physician because of a continued feeling of fatigue and because of symptoms associated with degenerative changes in the vascular system including high blood pressure, heart disease, retinitis, and peripheral neuritis. Sometimes they complain of increased thirst, more frequent urination, and itching. These patients are usually obese, have only a mild hyperglycemia, and seldom have ketosis except after a severe infection. They are not dependent upon insulin and can be controlled by diet alone or by diet and one of the oral hypoglycemic agents.

Laboratory studies. The diagnosis of diabetes is based upon the above-listed symptoms together with the results of several laboratory tests.

Glycosuria, or the presence of an abnormal amount of sugar in the urine, should be regarded as evidence of diabetes until proved otherwise. Sugar is present in the urine in many other conditions including pentosuria as a result of the body's failure to use the 5-carbon sugars; lactosuria in nursing mothers; alimentary glycosuria from excessive dietary loads of carbohydrate; fructosuria and galactosuria, resulting from enzyme deficiencies; and renal glycosuria because of a reduced ability of the tubules to reabsorb glucose.

Hyperglycemia, a high blood sugar, may be detected after a fast of 12 hours. A fasting blood sugar of more than 140 mg per 100 ml is suggestive of diabetes. Many older persons have slightly elevated blood sugar levels without having diabetes.

The *glucose tolerance test* is a measure of the ability of the body to utilize a known amount of glucose. At least three days prior to the test the patient is instructed to consume a diet containing 200 to 300 gm carbohydrate each day. The test is performed 12 to 14 hours after the evening meal of the third day. A fasting blood sample is drawn and then a solution containing a weighed amount of glucose is given. Usually 100 gm glucose dissolved in 300 ml water and flavored with lemon juice is given to the adult. Blood samples are taken at ½, 1, 2, and 3 hours after the ingestion of the glucose. The urine is also collected at each of these time intervals and tested for glucose. Under the conditions of the test, according to Public Health Service criteria,[4] diabetes is present if the fasting and 3-hour sugar levels exceed the following levels, or if any three of the stated levels are exceeded:

Fasting	110 mg per 100 ml
1 hour	170 mg
2 hours	120 mg
3 hours	110 mg

(See Figure 39–2.)

Ketonuria, or excretion of ketones, occurs when fatty acids are incompletely oxidized in the body.

Metabolism in diabetes. To understand the changes in metabolism that occur in diabetes, the student should first review the normal metabolism of proteins, carbohydrates, and fats (see Chapters 4, 5, and 6). A deficient supply of functioning insulin affects the metabolism of carbohydrates, fats, proteins, electrolytes, and water, and the consequences of the impairments are complex.

When insulin is not being produced or is ineffective, the formation of glycogen is decreased, and the utilization of glucose in the peripheral tissues is reduced. As a consequence

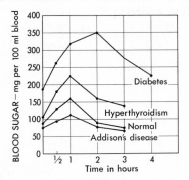

Figure 39–2. Glucose tolerance curves in various metabolic disorders.

the glucose that enters the circulation from various sources is removed more slowly and hyperglycemia follows. This is further accentuated by gluconeogenesis through which about 58 per cent of the protein molecule and 10 per cent of the fat molecule can yield glucose. When the blood glucose level exceeds the renal threshold (about 160 to 180 mg per 100 ml), glycosuria occurs. The loss of glucose in the urine represents a wastage of energy and entails an increased elimination of water and sodium. Ordinarily thirst and the increased ingestion of liquids compensates for the water loss, but interference with the intake such as occurs in nausea or through vomiting could lead to rapid dehydration.

With a deficiency of insulin lipogenesis decreases and lipolysis is greatly increased, these effects being of both immediate and long-range consequence. The fatty acids released from adipose tissue or available by absorption from the intestinal tract are oxidized by the liver to form "ketone bodies" including acetoacetic acid, β-hydroxybutyric acid, and acetone. The liver utilizes only limited quantities of the ketones and releases them to the circulation. Normally the peripheral tissues metabolize the ketones at a rate equal to their production by the liver so that the blood level at any given time is minimal. In diabetes mellitus the ketones are produced at a rate that far exceeds the ability of the tissues to utilize them and the concentration in the blood is greatly increased (ketonemia). Acetone is excreted by the lungs and gives the characteristic fruity odor to the breath. Acetoacetic acid and β-hydroxybutyric acid are excreted in the urine (ketonuria). Being fairly strong organic acids, these ketones combine with base so that the alkaline reserve is depleted, and acidosis results. The accompanying dehydration leads to circulatory failure, renal failure, and coma if not corrected. (See page 519.)

The rapid release of fatty acids into the blood circulation often results in a hyperlipemia and the blood serum may have a milky opalescent appearance. The blood levels of cholesterol are usually increased either because of increased synthesis or because of decreased destruction by the liver. The development of atherosclerosis in diabetic individuals occurs at an earlier age than in the nondiabetic and is more pronounced. (See page 544.)

The accelerated breakdown of protein tissues that occurs in uncontrolled diabetes not only adds to the glucose level of the blood, but increases the amount of nitrogen that must be excreted as a result of deaminization. The catabolism of protein tissues is accompanied by the release of cellular potassium and its excretion in the urine.

TREATMENT FOR DIABETES MELLITUS

Objectives for therapy. The goal of therapy in diabetes mellitus is to maintain and prolong a healthy, productive, satisfying life. This goal involves such specific aims as (1) optimum nutrition, (2) achieving normal weight, (3) a normal blood sugar level, (4) minimum glycosuria, (5) absence of ketoacidosis, and (6) minimum chronic degenerative complications. In planning the program of therapy the patient must always be considered with respect to his individual needs and desires; he must be fully involved in all aspects of the plans for his welfare. What constitutes a realistic goal for an 80-year-old with stable diabetes would be quite unsatisfactory for the adolescent diabetic who has his life ahead of him. For example, a level of control to reduce the degree of atherosclerosis may be important for the young diabetic, but is likely to be of limited value to the elderly person. On the other hand, the psychosocial problems of the adolescent may require primary consideration.

Dietary control is central to success. It is accompanied, when necessary, by insulin or oral hypoglycemic drugs. A regulated program of exercise and attention to personal hygiene are important to the total program. The many aspects of therapy require a continuing program of education for the patient together with periodic evaluation by the physician, nutritionist, and other specialists in health care.

Insulin. When the islands of Langerhans are unable to produce insulin, typically in growth onset diabetes, insulin must be supplied by injection. Insulin cannot be taken orally because the insulin molecule, being protein in nature, would be hydrolyzed in the digestive tract and thus inactivated.

Insulin is measured in units, 1 unit being the activity of 0.125 mg of the international standard. Insulin is generally supplied in solution of 40 units per milliliter (U-40) or 80 units per milliliter (U-80); thus, U-80 is twice as strong as U-40. Specific circumstances vary the insulin requirement considerably. Exercise reduces the need and infections increase the need. Emotional upsets may also modify the utilization of insulin. The types of insulin and their action are listed in Table 39–1.

Table 39–1. Types of Insulin and Their Action*

Types	Onset Hours	Peak Action Hours	Duration Hours
Short acting Regular (crystalline) Semilente	1 or less	3–4	6–8
Intermediate acting Globin NPH (isophane) Lente	2	9	24
Long acting PZI (protamine zinc insulin) Ultralente	6	18	36–48

*Adapted from *Diabetes Guide for Nurses.* U.S. Public Health Service Pub. No. 861, U.S. Department of Health, Education, and Welfare, Washington, D.C., revised 1969, p. 20.

Oral hypoglycemic drugs. Two groups of oral compounds are now in use, namely, the sulfonylureas and the biguanides. These compounds do not have the same action as insulin and are of value only when the islands of Langerhans are able to produce some insulin.

Among the sulfonylurea compounds are tolbutamide (Orinase*), chlorpropamide (Diabinese†), acetohexamide (Dymelor‡), and tolazamide (Tolinase§). These drugs appear to stimulate the production or release of insulin by the beta cells of the islands of Langerhans.

Phenformin (DBI[II]) is a phenethylbiguanide that has hypoglycemic activity. It appears to increase the uptake of glucose in the peripheral tissues but does not influence insulin production by the pancreas.

The oral compounds are useful in the management of maturity onset diabetes which cannot be controlled by diet alone. Oral compounds may produce a hypoglycemia if food intake is delayed or inadequate. They should never be regarded as a substitute for a controlled diet, and they should not be used in complications of diabetes such as acidosis and coma. They are not satisfactory for the juvenile, unstable, severe diabetic.

Rationale for dietary management. Three points of view concerning the degree of dietary control have been summarized by Cohen.[5]

Chemical control. A measured diet and insulin dosage are carefully regulated so that the blood sugar is kept within normal limits and the urine is free or nearly free of sugar at all times. Such control is believed to reduce the incidence and severity of degenerative complications. One criticism sometimes leveled against it is that the treatment may tend to be directed to the diabetes and not to the person as a whole.

Clinical control. Hyperglycemia and glycosuria are disregarded, and insulin is used to control ketosis. The diet differs little if any from that of normal persons and is controlled only to the point of maintenance of normal weight. Some physicians use these so-called "free" diets in the most liberal sense, but others restrict concentrated carbohydrate foods, especially those from sources contributing no other nutrients. Those who favor clinical control believe that the patient has an increased sense of well-being and that the degenerative complications are not more frequent.

Intermediate control. The majority of physicians adopt a regimen that falls between the preceding two. The objectives are: (1) to treat the patient as an individual and not on the basis of his diabetes alone; (2) to provide adequate nutrition for the maintenance of normal weight, a sense of well-being, and a life of usefulness; (3) to keep the blood sugar almost at normal levels for a large part of the day by using insulin as needed by avoiding hypoglycemia; (4) to keep the urine sugar free or with only traces of sugar for most of the day.

Daughaday[6] cites three arguments for a controlled diabetic diet: (1) it has educational value in helping the patient to understand his disease and the need for optimum nutrition; (2) 30 to 40 per cent of all diabetic patients do not need insulin if their diets are controlled; and (3) dietary control with insulin permits correlation of the diet with the type of insulin so that a normal blood sugar is achieved without too much risk of insulin shock.

Nutritional needs. The diabetic patient must observe dietary control for the remainder of his life. Great care must be taken that the diet always provides the essentials for good nutrition and that adjustments are made from time to time for changing metabolic needs, for example, during growth, pregnancy, or modified activity.

Energy. The caloric allowance is essentially the same as that for normal individuals of the same activity, size, and sex. Obese individuals should be placed on a low-calorie diet until the desirable weight for height and age is attained. Such weight loss in middle-aged obese patients very often leads to return of normal glucose tolerance.

One approach to planning the calorie level

---

*Orinase, The Upjohn Company, Kalamazoo, Michigan.

†Diabinese, Chas. Pfizer & Co., Inc., New York, New York.

‡Dymelor®, Eli Lilly Company, Indianapolis, Indiana.

§Tolinase, The Upjohn Company, Kalamazoo, Michigan.

II DBI, U.S. Vitamin Pharmaceutical Corporation, New York, New York.

is to determine the patients' present food intake and to use it as a guide for the calculated diet. The patient's continuing weight status determines whether the diet, in fact, is satisfactory in its calorie level—assuming, of course, that the patient is adhering to it. A convenient guide for planning the energy level is as follows:

	Calories per Pound (Desirable Weight)
For weight loss	8 to 12
For a bed patient	12
For light work	14
For medium work	16
For heavy work	18

Protein. The Recommended Dietary Allowance for protein for each age and sex category is satisfactory for the diabetic individual. Diets usually include 1 to 1½ gm protein per kilogram (½ to ⅔ gm per pound) of desirable body weight. The higher allowance is typical of American diets and lends satiety value to the diet.

Carbohydrate. Although a level of 100 gm carbohydrate is satisfactory for preventing ketosis, typical diets for adult diabetic patients usually contain 200 gm carbohydrate or more. The diet plans prepared by a committee of the American Dietetic Association[7] range in carbohydrate levels from 125 to 370 gm.

The insulin requirement is not proportionately increased when the carbohydrate level of the diet is increased, but is more directly correlated with the total calorie requirement. Thus, to restrict carbohydrate on the basis of the insulin requirement scarcely seems justified.

Fat. Most diets allow a fat intake that is typical of American diets, that is, 35 to 45 per cent of the calories. After protein and carbohydrate levels have been established, the fat allowance makes up the remaining calories.

Many clinicians now recommend that the type of fat in the diet be controlled, giving emphasis to fats rich in linoleic acid and sharply restricting those foods that are rich in saturated fatty acids. When such modification is prescribed, the food lists for fat-controlled diets (pages 552 to 553) would be used for calculating the diet and planning the daily meals.

Calculation of the diabetic diet prescription. A number of procedures may be used to arrive at the diet prescription. This is the responsibility of the physician, but the nurse and dietitian should have an understanding of the basis for the calculation. One of the methods often used is described below.

Let us assume that a diet is to be planned for a secretary who is 25 years old and 66 inches tall. According to the table of heights and weights (Table A-13), her desirable weight is 128 pounds (medium frame).

1. *Calories:* 14 calories per pound of desirable body weight
   $128 \times 14 = 1792$ calories per day.
2. *Protein:* 0.5 to 0.67 gm per pound of desirable body weight
   $128 \times 0.6 = 77$ gm protein per day.
3. *Nonprotein calories:* $1792 - 308 = 1484$ calories to be divided between carbohydrate and fat.
4. *Carbohydrate:* allow 40 to 60 per cent of nonprotein calories
   50 per cent of 1484 calories $= 742$ calories
   $742 \div 4 = 185.5$ gm carbohydrate per day.
5. *Fat calories:* total calories − calories from protein and carbohydrate
   $1792 - (308 + 742) = 742$ calories
6. *Fat:* fat calories $\div 9$
   $742 \div 9 = 82.4$ gm fat per day.

By rounding off the numbers the prescription becomes: carbohydrate, 185 gm; protein, 75 gm; and fat, 80 gm.

Distribution of carbohydrate. The meal distribution of carbohydrate is determined according to the type of insulin being used and is modified according to each patient's needs in order to achieve the best possible regulation of carbohydrate utilization. When moderate- or slow-acting insulins are used, a portion of the carbohydrate—usually 20 to 40 gm—is reserved for a midafternoon or bedtime feeding or both. This carbohydrate must be in slowly available form and should be accompanied by a portion of the day's protein. After the bedtime carbohydrate has been subtracted from the day's allowance, the remainder of the carbohydrate is distributed to correspond to the peak activity and the duration of the activity of the insulin that is being used (see Table 39–2).

Table 39–2. Typical Meal Distribution of Carbohydrate*

Type of Insulin	Breakfast	Noon	Mid-afternoon	Evening	Bedtime* gm
None	1/3	1/3		1/3	Usually none
	1/5	2/5		2/5	
Short acting (before breakfast and dinner)	2/5	1/5		2/5	Usually none
Intermediate acting	1/5	2/5		2/5	20–40
Globin	2/10	3/10	1/10	4/10	
Long acting	1/5	2/5		2/5	20–40
With regular insulin at breakfast	1/3	1/3		1/3	20–40

*When a bedtime feeding is prescribed, the carbohydrate is first subtracted from the day's total allowance. Then the meal fractions are applied to the remainder of the carbohydrate.

Planning the meal pattern. The dietitian and the nurse must translate the prescription into terms of common foods, keeping the following points especially in mind.

1. The diet should be planned with the patient so that it can be adjusted to his pattern of living. This requires consideration of the patient's economic status, the availability and cost of food, national, religious, and social customs, personal idiosyncrasies, occupation, facilities for preparing or obtaining meals, and so on.

The diabetic diet need not be an expensive one, and, ideally, it should be so planned that it fits in with the menus of the rest of the family. However, if the family diet is a poor one, the entire family will benefit when the basic food groups become the center about which meals are planned. Every effort should be made to regard the patient as a normal individual who does not require many special foods and who does not deprive other members of the family.

2. The adequacy of the diet for minerals and vitamins is most easily assured if one includes minimum amounts of the Four Food Groups.

3. Including some of the protein and fat into each meal helps to provide satiety and balance of food selection.

4. The food exchange lists (Table A-4) permit reasonable dietary constancy from day to day and considerable flexibility in meal planning. The method for dietary calculation using these lists has been described in Chapter 30 and is illustrated in Table 30–2.

5. The meal distribution of the carbohydrate can be adjusted to within 7 or 8 gm without using fractions of exchanges. The protein and fat should be adjusted within meals so that maximum flexibility is possible in meal planning. For example, the inclusion of milk at breakfast permits either cereal or bread to be selected from the bread exchanges; meat exchanges are wisely divided among the three meals with somewhat larger amounts being allocated to dinner. An example of the distribution of food exchanges into meal patterns is shown in Table 39–3 for the diet calculation illustrated on page 413.

DIETARY COUNSELING

Essential knowledge. The diabetic patient needs to know about (1) the nature of diabetes and the reasons for the measures that will be recommended, (2) the importance of weight control, (3) the details of his dietary program, (4) the amounts, time intervals, and method of administration of insulin or oral drugs, if needed, (5) skin care and personal hygiene, (6) procedures for testing the urine, (7) signs of hypoglycemia or acidosis and what steps to take in the event they occur, (8) emergency measures to take during infection and illness until medical help is available, and (9) the importance of periodic visits to his physician. (See Figure 39–3.)

Table 39–3. Meal Pattern and Sample Menu*

Carbohydrate division: breakfast, 55 gm; luncheon, 55 gm; dinner, 55 gm; bedtime, 25 gm

Meal Pattern	Exchanges	Carbohydrate gm	Sample Menu	Measure	Weight† gm
Breakfast			*Breakfast*		
Fruit, list 3	1	10	Orange	1 small	100
Meat, list 5	1	—	Egg, poached	1	
Bread, list 4	2	30	Whole-wheat toast	1 slice	25
			Wheat flakes	3/4 cup	20
Milk, list 1	1	12	Milk	1 cup	240
Fat, list 6	1	—	Butter	1 teaspoon	5
Coffee or tea			Coffee: no sugar		
		52			
Luncheon			*Luncheon*		
Meat, list 5	1	—	Cheese sandwich		
Bread, list 4	2	30	Cheese	1 ounce	30
Fat, list 6	2	—	Rye bread	2 slices	50
			Butter	1 teaspoon	5
Vegetable, group A, list 2		—	Sliced tomatoes on lettuce	medium salad	
			French dressing	1 tablespoon	15
Milk, list 1	1	12	Milk	1 cup	240
Fruit, list 3	1	10	Fresh blackberries	1 cup	150
		52			
Dinner			*Dinner*		
Meat, list 5	2	—	Chopped round steak	2 ounces	60
Bread, list 4	2	30	Potato, mashed	1/2 cup	100
			Roll	1, 2 inch diameter	30
Fat, list 6	1	—	Butter	1 teaspoon	5
Vegetable, group B, list 2	1	7	Parsley carrots	1/2 cup	100
Fruit, list 3	2	20	Cantaloupe	1/4, 6 inch diameter	200
Coffee or tea			Tea with lemon		
		57			
Bedtime			*Bedtime*		
Milk, list 1	1	12	Milk	1 cup	240
Bread, list 4	1	15	Saltines	5	20
Meat, list 5	1	—	Peanut butter	2 tablespoons	30
Fat, list 6	1	—	Butter	1 teaspoon	5
		27			
Total Carbohydrate		**188**			

*The calculation for this diet is shown on page 413.

†In practice diabetic diets are rarely weighed. The weights indicated here are a guide to portion control.

Figure 39–3. Nurse teaching patient how to administer insulin. (Courtesy, Medical College of Virginia, Health Sciences Division, Virginia Commonwealth University, Richmond.)

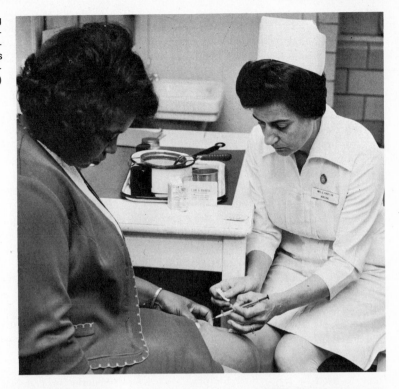

Insofar as diet is concerned, the patient needs to be taught the amount of food exchanges he is to use at each meal, how to use the food exchange lists in daily meal planning, how to interpret labels when purchasing food, and how to prepare food for his meals.

Responsibility for education. The physician, nurse, and dietitian share the responsibility for counseling the patient. The physician explains the nature of diabetes and the factors of importance in maintaining control. He also makes referrals to the dietitian and nurse for detailed aspects of education. In the hospital or outpatient clinic the dietitian usually initiates dietary instruction and arranges for a continuing program of education. The nurse instructs the patient regarding insulin administration, urine testing, and hygiene. She is a valuable assistant for dietary counseling and may be fully responsible for dietary instruction in some situations where no dietitian is available.

Satisfactory counseling of the patient includes individualized instruction which may be supplemented by group instruction. The patient must be involved throughout in order that he fully understand and adopt the program necessary for him. Periodic visits with the dietitian or public health nurse are essential to reinforce motivation, to answer questions, and to give added information.

Not only the patient but members of his family must be included in the counseling sessions. Each member of the family needs to understand that the diet for the diabetic patient is essentially a normal one, but that a regulated routine of meals and of the quantities of food is a vital aspect of the program. Members of the family also need to be aware of the complications that could arise and should know what to do in emergencies.

Teaching aids. Many books and pamphlets pertaining to diabetes have been prepared by health agencies, pharmaceutical firms, and physicians for the guidance of the patient. When these are selected at a reading level appropriate for the patient, these printed materials are useful for further study and reference. They should never be regarded as a substitute for personal counseling.

The patient's tray at each meal constitutes one of the best visual aids if the dietitian and nurse take the opportunity to so use it. If the patient has been introduced to the food exchange lists, the foods on the tray can be located in these lists and the amounts served identified in number of exchanges. Needless to say, careful checking of the tray before it is brought to the patient is important to emphasize dietary control. Measuring cups, measuring spoons, and various sizes of glasses and cups used for table service should be demonstrated during the instruction of the patient. Paper and plastic food models are useful in demonstrating menu planning and may be used by the patient for practice sessions in planning his own diet. In a relatively short time most patients can learn to estimate the portion sizes allowed on their diets.

Programmed instruction, when available, can be an important teaching aid. Slides, filmstrips, and movies pertaining to the many aspects of diabetic care are especially useful for group instruction. Each patient should be encouraged to participate in some group events not only for their instructional value, but to afford him opportunity to share experiences with others.

Some problems in education of the diabetic patient. Lack of education, inability to read English, and failing vision are among the problems encountered in the use of printed materials. Sometimes a member of the family can assist in using printed materials. Posters, films, and food models may be used. The nurse and dietitian must expect to spend more time with patients who present these problems, but repeated verbal instruction can be successful.

About half the diabetic patients are from families with very limited incomes. Although the diabetic diet need not be more expensive than a normal diet, the daily meal pattern must be carefully planned to make the best use of inexpensive foods. Most patients and their families can profit by advice in the wise purchase of foods.

Patients often ask about the use of dietetic foods. Water-packed fruits are available in most supermarkets at costs only slightly above that of regular packs and are useful when fresh fruits are out of season. Many water-packed fruits are sweetened with artificial sweeteners.

Dietetic foods such as cookies, candies, and gluten breads are not needed since most diabetic diets are sufficiently liberal to include a wide choice of foods. Some of the specialty products are expensive. Although low in carbohydrate, most of them contain protein and fat, thus contributing available glucose and calories. The patient who wishes to use such products should be advised about the specific changes he needs to make in his meal pattern.

Some patients ask about the use of alcoholic beverages. If the physician permits their use, the caloric content of the beverage is first subtracted from the day's allowance, and the balance of the diet is calculated accordingly.

Initially the patient should become thoroughly familiar with the kinds and amounts of foods allowed from the exchange lists. Once he has developed confidence in the use of these lists, he needs to be given some assistance in the use of food mixtures. A number of cookbooks have been prepared specifically for diabetic patients and include calculations of nutritive values. Some food processors have developed tables showing how their products can fit into the food exchanges. Patients usually need some assistance in the interpretation of these printed materials.

COMPLICATIONS OF DIABETES

Hypoglycemia. Insulin shock or hypoglycemia is caused by an overdose of insulin, a decrease in the available glucose because of delay in eating, omission of food, or loss of food by vomiting and diarrhea, or an increase in exercise without accompanying modification of the insulin dosage.

The patient going into insulin shock becomes uneasy, nervous, weak, and hungry. He is pale, his skin is moist, and he perspires excessively. He may complain of trembling, dizziness, faintness, headache, and double vision. His movements may be uncoordinated. Emotional instability may be indicated by crying, by hilarious behavior, or by belligerency. Occasionally, there may be nausea and vomiting or convulsions. Without treatment coma follows and death is impending. Laboratory studies show a blood sugar below 70 mg per 100 ml for mild symptoms and below 50 mg for coma. The second urine specimen is negative for sugar and acetone.

Orange juice or other fruit juices, sugar, candy, syrup, honey, a carbonated beverage, or any readily available carbohydrate may be given. If absorption is normal, recovery follows in a few minutes. If there is stupor, intravenous glucose is necessary. Most patients are now using one or another of the slowly acting insulins, in which case reactions may recur after a few hours. To avoid such subsequent reactions, it is necessary to follow the initial carbohydrate therapy in one or two hours and at later intervals with foods containing carbohydrate which is slowly absorbed—such as in milk and bread.

The patient must be impressed with the importance of balance between his diet and insulin dosage and the importance of close adherence to the physician's orders. He should always carry some sugar or hard candy to avert symptoms when they are still mild.

Diabetic acidosis and coma. A dreaded complication in diabetes is the state of coma which is brought about by acidosis. Diabetic coma often originates because the patient consumed additional foods for which his insulin did not provide, or because he failed to take the correct amount of insulin or omitted it entirely. The presence of diabetes is first detected in some persons who were not aware of the disease until coma occurred. Infection is an especially sinister influence since even a mild infection reduces the carbohydrate tolerance and severe acidosis may sometimes occur before the insulin dosage has been appropriately increased. Trauma of any kind, whether an injury or surgery, aggravates the diabetes so that acidosis is more likely.

Some of the signs of diabetic acidosis and coma are similar to those of insulin shock, and a differentiation cannot be made without information concerning the patient prior to the onset of the symptoms, together with blood and urine studies. The patient complains of feeling ill and weak; he may have a headache, anorexia, nausea and vomiting, abdominal pain, and aches and pains elsewhere. His skin is hot, flushed, and dry; his mouth is dry and he is thirsty. An acetone odor on the breath, painful, rapid breathing, and drowsiness are typical signs. Symptoms of shock, unconsciousness, and death follow unless prompt measures are taken. Sugar, acetone, and acetoacetic acid are present in the urine, the blood glucose is elevated to very high levels, and the blood carbon dioxide content is decreased.

When early signs of ketosis are present, small repeated doses of insulin are given together with small carbohydrate feedings. Diabetic coma, however, is a medical emergency best treated in a hospital where close nursing care can be given. The physician directs the therapy which includes large doses of regular insulin with smaller doses repeated as needed every hour or so until the urine sugar is reduced and the blood sugar is lowered to less than 200 mg per 100 ml; saline infusions for the correction of dehydration; gastric lavage if the patient has been vomiting; and alkali therapy for the correction of the severe acidosis.

When the urine sugar decreases and the blood sugar begins to fall, glucose is given by infusion in order to avoid subsequent hypoglycemic reactions. As soon as fluids can be taken orally, the patient is given fruit juices, gruels, ginger ale, tea, and broth. All of these are useful for their fluid content; fruit juice, ginger ale, and gruels provide carbohydrate; broth and gruels contain sodium chloride; and fruit juices, broth and gruels contribute potassium. These fluids may be given in amounts of 100 ml, more or less, every hour or so during the first day. By the second day, the patient is usually able to take a soft diet which is calculated to contain 100 to 200 gm carbohydrate, and by the third day he may take the diet which meets his particular requirements.

Surgery. Ideally, the diabetic patient who is having surgery should have a normal blood sugar, no glycosuria, and no ketosis. A glycogen reserve is essential and can be assured only if sufficient carbohydrate is included up to 12 hours prior to the operation and if insulin is supplied in great enough amounts for the utilization of the carbohydrate. Fluids in abundance are indicated. When emergency surgery is needed, parenteral glucose is usually ordered.

Carbohydrate feedings should begin within three hours after operation, as a rule. Initially glucose may be given parenterally. When liquids can be taken by mouth, tea with sugar, orange juice, and ginger ale may be used. When a full fluid or soft diet can be tolerated the diet can be calculated to provide the protein and fat as well as the carbohydrate allowances.

Infection. The guidance of a physician is important when a diabetic patient has an infection. An infection lowers the carbohydrate tolerance and increases the insulin requirement. A mild diabetic may become a severe case, and infections may precipitate coma. The physician sometimes orders insulin for patients who are not ordinarily required to use insulin.

Pregnancy. Diabetes increases the hazards of pregnancy because of the dangers of glycogen depletion, hypoglycemia, acidosis, and infection. Despite the increased hazards the diabetic woman can have an uneventful pregnancy and a healthy baby. She should have medical guidance throughout her pregnancy with emphasis on control of the rate of weight gain and the prevention of edema. The nutritional requirements are similar to those of the nondiabetic pregnant woman. The insulin requirements are usually increased. Most diabetic women are unable to produce enough milk for the baby and should not be encouraged to nurse their infants.

PROBLEMS AND REVIEW

1. What are the important predisposing factors in diabetes mellitus?
2. How does a deficiency of functioning insulin affect the metabolism of carbohydrate; protein; fat; sodium; potassium; water?
3. Explain the typical symptoms of diabetes on the basis of the metabolic changes.
4. State the important objectives to be achieved in the therapy of a diabetic patient. What factors may influence the realization of these objectives?
5. What information do you need in order to plan a satisfactory dietary program for a patient?
6. *Problem.* Calculate the following dietary prescription for an overweight 45-year-old man working in a factory who must carry his lunch: carbohydrate, 160 gm; protein, 75 gm; fat, 80 gm. He is taking tolbutamide and the carbohydrate should be distributed in thirds.
7. *Problem.* Show how each of the following combinations could be used in the dinner pattern you planned in problem 6:
   Macaroni and cheese
   Beef stew with carrots, onions, potatoes, and celery
   A picnic lunch including cold cuts, potato salad
   Baked custard
8. *Problem.* A patient has refused to eat the following foods on his tray: ½ slice bread, ½ cup peas, 1½ ounces meat, and 1 small potato. He has agreed to take a carbohydrate replacement as orange juice.
   a. On the basis of the carbohydrate content of the foods refused, how much orange juice would be required?

b. If the amount of orange juice given was kept to ½ cup, how much sugar would you need to add to the juice to cover the carbohydrate replacement?

c. If the replacement were based on the total glucose available from the foods refused, what changes would you need to make in items a and b?

9. *Problem.* Calculate a full fluid diet that provides for lunch: carbohydrate, 45 gm; protein, 20 gm; fat, 25 gm.

10. A 50-year-old woman with mild diabetes believes that she can eat as she pleases because the oral hypoglycemic drug that she is taking will control her diabetes. Explain why this thinking is erroneous.

11. What is the basis for using a diet high in polyunsaturated fats and low in saturated fats?

12. What advice might be appropriate for the relatives of a diabetic patient to delay or avoid the onset of diabetes mellitus?

Cited References

1. Vavra, H. M.: *Diabetes Source Book.* Public Health Service Pub. 1168. U.S. Department of Health, Education, and Welfare, Washington, D.C., 1969.
2. Sharkey, T. P.: "Recent Research Developments in Diabetes Mellitus—Part I," *J. Am. Diet. Assoc.,* **48**:281–87, 1966.
3. Walker, E.: *Diabetes Guide for Nurses.* Public Health Service Pub. 861. U.S. Department of Health, Education, and Welfare, Washington, D.C., 1969.
4. *Diabetes Control—A Public Health Program Guide.* Public Health Service Pub. 506, U.S. Department of Health, Education, and Welfare, Washington, D.C., 1969.
5. Cohen, A. S.: "Current Concepts in Diabetes Mellitus," *J. Am. Diet. Assoc.,* **32**:102–109, 1956.
6. Daughaday, W. H.: "Dietary Treatment of Adults with Diabetes Mellitus," *J.A.M.A.,* **167**:859–62, 1958.
7. *ADA Meal Plans Nos. 1 Through 9.* The American Dietetic Association, Chicago, 1956.

Additional References

Beigelman, P. M., *et al.*: "Severe Diabetic Ketoacidosis," *J.A.M.A.,* **210**:1082–86, 1969.
Danowski, T. S.: "Therapies of Diabetes Mellitus," *Postgrad Med.,* **45**:137–41, April 1969.
"The Diagnosis of Diabetes," (Programmed Instruction), *GP,* **39**:132–49, Jan. 1969; 133–54, Feb. 1969; 141–60, March 1969; 141–59, April 1969; 133–55, May 1969; 141–60, June 1969.
Etzwiler, D. D.: "Developing a Regional Program to Help Patients with Diabetes," *J. Am. Diet. Assoc.,* **52**:394–400, 1968.
Goodman, S. J., and Gaffney, P. M.: "Restaurants Cater to Persons with Diabetes," *J. Am. Diet. Assoc.,* **49**:513–15, 1966.
Hinkle, L. E.: "Customs, Emotions, and Behavior in the Dietary Treatment of Diabetes," *J. Am. Diet. Assoc.,* **41**:341–44, 1962.
Holland, W. M.: "The Diabetes Supplement of the National Health Survey. III. The Patient Reports on His Diet," *J. Am. Diet. Assoc.,* **52**:387–90, 1968.
Kahn, C. B., *et al.*: "Clinical and Chemical Diabetes in Offspring of Diabetic Couples," *N. Engl. J. Med.,* **281**:343–47, 1969.
Krysan, G. S.: "How Do We Teach Four Million Diabetics?" *Am. J. Nurs.,* **65**:105–107, Nov. 1965.
Levine, R.: "Nutritional Aspects of Diabetes Mellitus," *Bordens Rev. Nutr. Res.,* **29**:15–22, 1968.
Martin, M. M.: "Diabetes Mellitus: Current Concepts," *Am. J. Nurs.,* **66**:510–14, 1966.
———: "Insulin Reactions," *Am. J. Nurs.,* **67**:328–31, 1967.

Podolsky, S.: "Special Needs of the Diabetic Undergoing Surgery," *Postgrad. Med.*, **45**:128–31, Feb. 1969.

Reardon, E.: "Can Sub-Professionals Assist in Teaching Patients with Diabetes?" *J. Am. Diet. Assoc.*, **52**:405–406, 1968.

Sharkey, T. P.: "Diabetes Mellitus—Present Problems and New Research," *J. Am. Diet. Assoc.*, **58**:201–209, 1971.

———: "Recent Research in Diabetes Mellitus," *J. Am. Diet. Assoc.*, **52**:103–107; 108–17, 1968.

Stulb, S. C.: "The Diabetes Supplement of the National Health Survey. IV. The Patient's Knowledge of the Food Exchanges," *J. Am. Diet. Assoc.*, **52**:391–93, 1968.

Watkins, J. D., and Moss, F. T.: "Confusion in the Management of Diabetes," *Am. J. Nurs.*, **69**:521–24, 1969.

Wilder, R. M.: "Adventures Among the Islands of Langerhans," *J. Am. Diet. Assoc.*, **36**:309–12, 1960.

Williams, T. F., *et al.:* "Dietary Errors Made at Home by Patients with Diabetes," *J. Am. Diet. Assoc.*, **51**:19–25, 1967.

Zitnik, R.: "First, You Take a Grapefruit," *Am. J. Nurs.*, **68**:1285-86, 1968.

INSTRUCTIONAL MATERIALS FOR THE PATIENT

American Diabetes Association, New York
  Facts about Diabetes, 1966.
  Forecast (bimonthly magazine).
American Dietetic Association, Chicago
  ADA Meal Plans Nos. 1 Through 9.
  Meal Planning with Exchange Lists.
Behrman, Sister M.: *A Cookbook for Diabetics.* American Diabetes Association, New York, 1959.
Duncan, G. G., and Duncan, T. G.: *A Modern Pilgrim's Progress with Further Revelations for Diabetics,* 2nd ed. W. B. Saunders Company, Philadelphia, 1967.
Strachan, C. B.: *The Diabetic's Cookbook.* University of Texas Press, Austin, 1967.
U.S. Public Health Service
  Answers to Questions That Are Often Asked about Diabetic Diets, Pub. 1847.
  Diabetes and You, Pub. 567.
Weller, C.: *The New Way to Live with Diabetes.* Doubleday and Company, Inc., Garden City, N.Y., 1966.

40 Various Metabolic Disorders

Low-Purine Diet

Many diseases for which dietary modification is an effective part of treatment are deviations of normal metabolic pathways in the body. They occur because of abnormal production of one or more hormones, a deficiency of an enzyme, or a modification of excretion. Those which are discussed in this chapter fall into one or another of these categories but otherwise bear little, if any, relation to each other.

SPONTANEOUS HYPOGLYCEMIA

Types of hypoglycemia. Spontaneous hypoglycemia is a symptom of disordered carbohydrate metabolism which may be of functional or organic origin. The symptoms are characteristic of those described for insulin shock (see page 519). The patient becomes weak, nervous, extremely hungry, perspires freely, trembles, and may even lose consciousness. Convulsions occur occasionally.

On the basis of dietary management, hypoglycemias fall into two groups, namely, (1) stimulative and (2) fasting. Tumors of the islet cells of Langerhans also lead to overproduction of insulin, but surgery rather than dietary management is essential.

FUNCTIONAL HYPERINSULINISM

Nature of hypoglycemia. Functional hyperinsulinism is a stimulative type of hypoglycemia in which there is no known organic lesion. Under the stimulus of carbohydrate the islet cells respond to a greater than normal degree with the following characteristics of the blood sugar: (1) a normal fasting blood sugar; (2) hypoglycemia two to four hours after meals, especially in the forenoon and late afternoon; (3) no hypoglycemia following fasting or the omission of meals; and (4) a glucose tolerance curve (see Figure 39–2) which shows a normal fasting sugar, initially elevated glucose level after taking the glucose, and a sharp fall to very low sugar levels.

A condition similar to functional hyperinsulinism occurs when nutrients are absorbed at an extremely rapid rate, for example, following gastroenterostomy or gastrectomy. In such situations the food reaches the small intestine much more rapidly than is normal, is very quickly absorbed, and the sudden elevation of the blood sugar serves as an extra stimulus to the islet cells and a subsequent hypoglycemia. See Chapter 38 for description of the dumping syndrome.

Modification of the diet. A diet prescription to meet each patient's needs is calculated according to the following principles.

Carbohydrate. Because the carbohydrate serves as a stimulus to further insulin secretion and is provocative of the hypoglycemic attack, it is usually restricted to levels below 100 gm. The initial diet may be planned to contain 75 gm carbohydrate with further reduction to 50 gm if the patient shows no improvement.

Protein. A high-protein diet, 120 to 140 gm, is essential, since there is no appreciable increase in the blood sugar level following high-protein meals even though protein furnishes approximately 50 per cent of its weight in available glucose. This available glucose is released to the bloodstream so gradually that there is little stimulation to the islands of Langerhans.

Fat. When the levels of carbohydrate and protein have been established, the remaining calories are obtained from fat. Because the carbohydrate is so severely restricted, the fat level is, of necessity, high.

Planning the diet. The exchange lists (see Table A-4) may be used for calculation of the diet prescription. Since carbohydrates are drastically restricted, it becomes apparent that the bread exchanges will usually be omitted. In order to include adequate amounts of fruits and vegetables, milk is limited to 2 or 3 cups; children should receive calcium supplements. Vegetables from the 2A list are calculated to provide 2 gm protein and 3 gm carbohydrate per 100 gm.

In order that absorption from the intestine will be gradual, the daily allowances of protein and fat, as well as carbohydrate, are divided into three approximately equal parts. Midmorning, midafternoon, and bedtime feedings are often desirable, in which case part of the food planned for the preceding meal can be used for the interval feeding. Carbohydrate-containing foods must be carefully measured.

ADRENOCORTICAL INSUFFICIENCY

Addison's disease is a comparatively rare condition resulting from an impairment of the functioning of the adrenal cortex because of atrophy of unknown origin, or, in some instances, because of tuberculosis.[2] Sometimes adrenalectomy is necessary because of cancer, in which event the resultant metabolic effects are those of Addison's disease. Since the pituitary governs the activity of the adrenal cortex, hypophysectomy will also lead to characteristic symptoms of adrenal insufficiency.

Metabolic effects and related symptoms. The symptoms of insufficiency are directly related to the absence of hormones produced by the adrenal cortex.

Glucocorticoids. The principal action of these hormones, chiefly cortisol, is upon the regulation of the metabolism of carbohydrate, protein, and fat. Upon stimulation of cortisol, the liver forms glycogen from the amino acids supplied by the tissues. The hormone increases the rate of protein catabolism and decreases the permeability of the muscle cells to amino acids. On the other hand, the permeability of the liver

cells is increased and liver proteins increase. The glucocorticoids also influence the deposition of fatty tissue or the mobilization of fats.

In the absence of glucocorticoids rapid glycogen depletion occurs, followed by hypoglycemia a few hours after meals. Such hypoglycemia may be severe in a patient who has had no food for 10 or 12 hours. A glucose tolerance test shows a lower maximum blood sugar and a more rapid return to normal fasting levels than is obtained in normal individuals (see Figure 39–2).

The production of glucocorticoids by the adrenal gland is governed by the adrenocorticotropic hormone (ACTH) of the pituitary. In the event hypophysectomy is performed, the adrenal cortex atrophies and glucocorticoids are not produced, just as they are not elaborated in Addison's disease.

Mineralocorticoids. Mineralocorticoids, of which aldosterone is of primary importance, are concerned with maintaining electrolyte homeostasis, especially for sodium and potassium. The production is regulated by the levels of sodium and potassium in the circulation. Aldosterone production leads to increased retention of sodium and greater excretion of potassium. Unlike the glucocorticoids, aldosterone production is not influenced by the pituitary. A deficiency of aldosterone, as seen in Addison's disease, leads to excessive excretion of sodium and increased retention of potassium. With the large salt loss much water is also excreted, thus leading to dehydration, hemoconcentration, reduced blood volume, and hypotension. In severe deficiency the patient experiences profound weakness and may have a craving for salt.

Androgenic hormones. These stimulate protein synthesis. In their absence tissue wasting, weight loss, reduction of muscle strength, and fatigue are present.

Patients with adrenal insufficiency frequently experience anorexia, nausea, vomiting, abdominal discomfort, and diarrhea. Most of the patients have an increased pigmentation of the skin, often that of a deep tan or bronze. This results from the excessive production of *melanophore-stimulating hormone* by the pituitary when the adrenal steroids are lacking to exert an inhibitory effect.

Modification of the diet. Mild degrees of insufficiency are often satisfactorily treated by giving a higher salt intake, and by increasing the number of meals to five or six a day.[2] As the deficiency becomes more severe cortisone may be given to control the hypoglycemia, and, to some extent, to increase sodium retention. An increase in the salt intake is usually needed.[2]

Patients with severe insufficiency are treated with injections of deoxycorticosterone (DOCA) or by implantation of pellets of the synthetic hormone. The mineral metabolism is thereby controlled so that no change is usually required in the sodium and potassium levels of the diet.

A diet high in protein and relatively low in carbohydrate reduces the stimulation of insulin and helps to avoid the episodes of hypoglycemia. Meals should be given at frequent intervals—allowing between-meal feedings and a late bedtime feeding. Each of the feedings should include protein in order to reduce the rate of carbohydrate absorption. Simple carbohydrates—candy, sugar, and other sweets—are best avoided because of their rapid digestion and absorption and their stimulation of excessive insulin production.

METABOLIC EFFECTS OF ADRENOCORTICAL THERAPY

The adrenocorticotropic hormone of the anterior pituitary gland (ACTH) and the steroids of the adrenal cortex are used for the treatment of a wide variety of diseases such as arthritis, allergies, skin disturbances, adrenal insufficiency, many gastrointestinal diseases, and others. Although the various products used may vary somewhat in the degree of their effects on metabolism, it is important to be aware of possible nutritional implications of long-continued use of these hormones.

Water and electrolyte metabolism. Adrenocortical steroids in excess lead to retention of sodium and water and loss of potassium. Some sodium restriction is necessary for many patients. Usually, it is sufficient to avoid salty foods and to use no salt at the table, but a 1000-mg-sodium diet may occasionally be required (see Chapter 43). When the patient is eating well, the amounts of potassium in the diet are liberal. Foods especially high in potassium include broth, fruit juices, vegetables, whole-grain cereals, and meats.

Protein metabolism. A negative nitrogen balance may result when large doses of cortisone are used. This can be prevented when the diet is sufficiently liberal in carbohydrate to exert maximum protein-sparing effect and when high protein intakes are emphasized.

Carbohydrate metabolism. Cortisone therapy increases the storage of glycogen by increasing the amount of glycogen formation from protein. There also appears to be an insensitivity to insulin, as indicated by hyperglycemia and glycosuria. In diabetic patients who are also receiving cortisone, additional insulin may be required.

Gastrointestinal system. Hydrochloric acid secretion is increased following adrenocortical steroid therapy, and peptic ulceration may develop. In such a situation, the dietary modification described for peptic ulcer should be used (see Chapter 34).

HYPERTHYROIDISM

Symptoms and clinical findings. Hyperthyroidism is a disturbance in which there is an excessive secretion of the thyroid gland with a consequent increase in the metabolic rate. The disease is also known as exophthalmic goiter, thyrotoxicosis, Graves' disease, or Basedow's disease. The chief symptoms are weight loss sometimes to the point of emaciation, excessive nervousness, prominence of the eyes, and a generally enlarged thyroid gland. The appetite is often increased, weakness may be marked, and signs of cardiac failure may be present.

Metabolism. All of the metabolic processes in the body are accelerated in hyperthyroidism. Serum protein-bound iodine values are elevated. The basal metabolic rate may be increased 50 per cent or more in severe cases. Moreover, the patient tends to be restless so that the total energy metabolism is further increased. When the level of calories is insufficient, the liver store of glycogen is rapidly depleted. This is especially serious just prior to surgery since postoperative shock is more likely.

The increased level of nitrogen metabolism leads to destruction of tissue proteins. Unless both protein and caloric levels are adequate, loss of weight may be rapid.

The excretion of calcium and phosphorus is greatly increased in hyperthyroidism. Osteoporosis and bone fractures are associated with severe losses. The increased level of energy metabolism increases the requirement for B complex vitamins. For reasons not fully understood, the utilization of vitamin A and ascorbic acid is also speeded up.

Modification of the diet. Antithyroid compounds are now widely used to relieve the symptoms of hyperthyroidism, and in more severe instances to prepare the patient for surgery. These drugs reduce the basal metabolic rate to normal, but a liberal diet is still indicated because patients have usually experienced severe malnutrition prior to therapy.

Until normal nutrition is restored, approximately 4000 to 5000 calories and 100 to 125 gm protein should be allowed (see High-Calorie Diet, Chapter 31). Calcium intakes of 2 to 3 gm daily are desirable together with supplements of Vitamin D.[3] The calcium may be provided as calcium salts in addition to the liberal use of milk. The diet itself will include generous allowances of vitamin A, the B complex, and ascorbic acid, but supplements are often prescribed.

HYPOTHYROIDISM

Hypothyroidism, or decreased production of the thyroid hormone, is known as myxedema when severe in the adult, or cretinism when its symptoms become apparent shortly after birth (see Chapter 8). Myxedema is characterized by a lowered rate of energy metabolism—often 30 to 40 per cent below normal, muscular flabbiness, puffy face, eyelids, and hands, sensitivity to cold, marked fatigue with slight exertion, and a personality change including apathy and dullness. The patient frequently responds to therapy with desiccated thyroid.

Obesity is an occasional problem in patients with hypothyroidism since they may continue in their earlier patterns of eating even though the energy metabolism has been significantly reduced. In other patients, the appetite may be so poor that undernutrition results.

JOINT DISEASES

Incidence. Arthritis is the principal crippler in the United States. It affects about 16 million Americans, of whom some 3 million persons are limited in their usual activity. The incidence is higher in women, in people with low incomes, in the later years of life, and among residents of rural areas. Eighty-five per cent of all cases of arthritis occur in persons over 45 years of age.[4]

Symptoms and clinical findings. The terms *arthritis* and *rheumatism* are applied to many joint diseases. Rheumatic fever is a special threat to the child or young adult because inadequate treatment may permanently damage the heart (see page 440). Gout, another of the joint diseases, is an error of uric acid metabolism and is discussed on page 527.

Osteoarthritis or *degenerative arthritis* is the most common form of arthritis and is usually associated with advancing age. It seems to be caused by mechanical factors such as constant strain to a joint, for example, "housemaid's knee." The joints of the fingers, knees, shoulders, and lumbar and cervical spines are most frequently affected. The onset is slow and noninflammatory. Gradual changes occur in the cartilages of the joints and new bone spurs grow at the edges. The joint stiffness is characteristic and pain is often severe.

Rheumatoid arthritis is a highly inflammatory and very painful condition having its onset in young adults, especially women. Among the theories to explain its cause are infection, hypersensitivity, heredity, and some metabolic derangement. It is characterized by fatigue, pain, stiffness, deformity which may be severe, and limited function. The disease is progressive but the symptoms may spontaneously disappear only to reappear again at a later time. With early diagnosis the disabling effects can be delayed but there is no known cure.

Treatment. Probably few diseases have had more theories offered concerning therapy. Arthritics spend over $300 million annually on phony diets and devices. None of the claims made by promoters have been supported by research. Over the years numerous diets have been tried by clinicians, but none has been effective in modifying the course of the disease. These trials have included diets high or low in protein, fat, and carbohydrate; modified for acid or alkaline ash; or supplemented with vitamins, especially ascorbic acid and vitamin D.

A number of drugs beginning with aspirin bring relief to the arthritic patient. Steroid therapy and gold salts have been effective for many. Since these drugs may bring about undesirable side effects, their use for each patient must be carefully evaluated.

Patients whose deformities limit their activities can be helped by physical and occupational therapy. The occupational therapist, home economist, dietitian, and nurse can help patients to greater independence by teaching them how to use many self-help devices that have been designed. (See Figure 40–1.) Homemakers need counseling on ways to accomplish their housekeeping activities with less effort. Sometimes a rearrangement of kitchen equipment is sufficient; in other instances some modification of the design of the kitchen itself is needed. (See also pages 397 to 398.)

The supportive role of diet. Arthritic patients require the same foods for health that other persons need. When patients are of normal weight and in good nutritional status, the normal diet is suitable.

Obesity is a common problem in osteoarthritis, and weight loss should be brought about in order to reduce the added stress on weight-bearing joints. (See Chapter 31 for low-calorie diets.)

Many patients with rheumatoid arthritis have lost weight and are in poor nutritional status. For them a high-calorie high-protein diet is indicated until good nutritional status has been achieved. (See pages 427 and 432.)

Steroid therapy leads to sodium retention in some in which case mild sodium restriction is

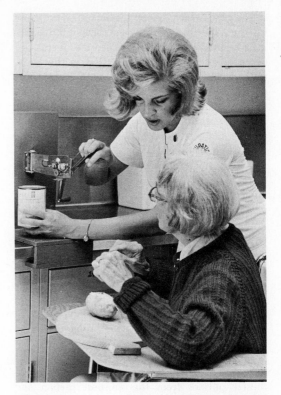

Figure 40–1. An occupational therapist shows a handicapped homemaker how to modify food preparation procedures for her physical limitations. (Courtesy, The Arthritis Foundation.)

indicated. Usually it is sufficient to omit salty foods and the use of salt at the table; sometimes, a 1000-mg-sodium diet may be required. Continued steroid therapy adversely affects the calcium balance, leading to gradual bone demineralization. A liberal intake of milk, contrary to popular opinion, is desirable.

GOUT

Incidence and etiology. Gout accounts for about 3 to 5 of every 100 persons afflicted with joint diseases. It is a hereditary disease occurring principally in males after 30 years of age. Women are more susceptible after the menopause. Hyperuricemia (high blood level of uric acid) is transmitted by a single dominant autosomal gene which is not sex linked. The cause for the hyperuricemia has not been fully established but various theories ascribe it to (1) decreased destruction of uric acid in the body, (2) increased production of uric acid in the body, or (3) decreased excretion of uric acid.

Overeating and excessive drinking of alcoholic beverages are not primary etiologic agents, but alcohol, high-fat diets, and obesity can aggravate an existing condition.

Nature and occurrence of uric acid. Cellular material of both plant and animal origin contains *nucleoproteins.* Glandular organs such as liver, pancreas, and kidney are among the richest sources; meats and the embryo or germ of grains and legumes, together with the growing parts of young plants, also furnish appreciable amounts. During digestion nucleoproteins are first split into proteins and nucleic acid. Further cleavage of nucleic acid leads to several products, one group of which are the purines. The latter in turn are oxidized to uric acid, probably by the liver.

In addition to the uric acid available from the metabolism of nucleic acid, the body can synthesize purines from the simplest carbon and nitrogen compounds such as carbon dioxide, acetic acid, and glycine. Thus any substances from which these materials originate, namely carbohydrate, fat, and protein, give rise to a considerable production of uric acid. Even in the fasting state there is a constant production of uric acid from cellular breakdown.

The liver and tissues store uric acid and its precursors for variable lengths of time and release them later. As a normal constituent of urine, uric acid represents a part of the daily nitrogenous excretion. Some uric acid is also excreted via the bile into the intestinal tract.

Symptoms and clinical findings. The range of plasma uric acid in normal individuals is 2 to 5 mg per cent, whereas in those with susceptibility to gout the concentration is above 7 mg per cent and may reach as high as 20 mg per cent. A large percentage of individuals with hyperuricemia sooner or later will have acute attacks of gout characterized by sudden inflammation and swelling accompanied by severe pain of the joints, especially the metatarsal, knee, and toe joints. The acute attack usually responds dramatically in 24 to 48 hours to treatment with colchicine.

Many patients have only occasional acute attacks of gout with moderate hyperuricemia and the disease does not progress. Others have attacks with greater and greater frequency, and deposits of sodium urate (tophi) in the tendon, cartilage, and kidneys lead to permanent damage of the joints and other tissues and increasing invalidism. Renal impairment is often present.

Treatment. A number of drugs are effective in the treatment of gout, and diet is considered to be an adjunct to drug therapy. Colchicine and a number of other drugs provide effective relief from the pain that accompanies the acute attack. In addition, these drugs reduce the frequency of attacks when they are also used as interval therapy.

Uricosuric drugs (probenecid and others) increase the excretion of uric acid, thereby bringing plasma levels within a normal range. With the lowering of the plasma uric acid levels, sodium urate deposits in the joints are gradually dissolved out. These drugs are not effective in reducing the pain of the acute attack and may exacerbate the symptoms during an attack. Therefore, they are used during the quiescent periods of the disease.

More recently *allopurinol* has been found to be effective.[5] It is a drug that inhibits the action of the enzyme *xanthine oxidase,* which is responsible for the formation of uric acid from xanthine and hypoxanthine. Therefore, the excretion of uric acid is diminished and that of xanthine is increased. Inasmuch as xanthine can precipitate out to form kidney stones, it is essential that the patient have a liberal fluid intake and excrete a urine that is neutral or slightly alkaline.

Modification of the diet. During acute attacks a low-purine diet is often ordered in addition to drug therapy. Some physicians also recommend moderate restriction of purines as interval therapy. Data on the purine content of foods are limited. Foods have been grouped in three categories in Table 40–1. As may be seen from this classification, all flesh foods and extractives from them such as gravies and soups must be

Table 40–1. Purine Content of Foods per 100 Grams*

Group I (0–15 mg)	Group II (50–150 mg)	Group III (150 mg and over)
Vegetables	Meats	Sweetbreads
Fruits	Poultry*	Anchovies
Milk	Fish	Sardines
Cheese	Sea food	Liver
Eggs	Beans, dry	Kidney
Breads and cereals	Peas, dry	Meat extracts
Fish roe*	Lentils	Gravies*
Caviar*	Spinach	Brains*
Gelatin*	Oatmeal*	
Butter and other fats*		
Nuts*		
Sugar, sweets*		

*Adapted from Turner, D.: *Handbook of Diet Therapy,* 3rd ed. University of Chicago Press, Chicago, 1959, p. 100. Starred items are additions to Turner's list.

eliminated for the low-purine diet. If purine restriction is also prescribed for interval therapy, the allowance of meat, poultry, and fish is limited to 2 to 3 ounces on each of three to five days.

Energy. Since obesity has adverse effects on general health as well as on gout, the overweight individual should gradually lose weight. Patients should not be placed on low-calorie diets during acute attacks of gout since the catabolism of adipose tissue reduces the excretion of uric acid. Rapid weight loss effected by starvation or by extremely low-calorie diets can precipitate an attack of gout. Usually, men can lose weight satisfactorily when their diets are restricted to 1200 to 1600 calories. (See Chapter 31.)

Protein, fat, and carbohydrate. Because the nitrogen of the purine nucleus is supplied by protein, the intake is restricted to about 1 gm per kilogram. Fat is often restricted to about 60 gm daily. When the food intake is poor because of illness, it is essential that high-carbohydrate fluids be given so that adipose tissue is not excessively catabolized.

Fluid. The daily intake of fluids should be at least 3 liters. Coffee and tea may be used in moderate amounts. These beverages contain methylated purines, which are oxidized to methyl uric acid. The latter is excreted in the urine and is not deposited in the tissues. Hence, the customary omission of coffee and tea may impose an unnecessary hardship. Alcohol is contraindicated.

To effect a neutral or slightly alkaline urine when allopurinol is prescribed, the diet should be liberal in its content of fruits and vegetables. In addition, the physician usually prescribes small amounts of sodium bicarbonate or sodium citrate.

LOW-PURINE DIET

General rules

For a diet essentially free of exogenous purines, use foods only from group I, Table 40–1.

For a low-purine level, allow 3 to 5 small servings of lean meat, poultry, and fish from group II each week.

If a low-fat regimen is ordered, the butter is omitted, and skim milk is substituted for the whole milk.

Include these foods daily:

3–4 cups milk

  2 eggs
1–2 ounces cheese; allow 2 to 3 ounces lean beef, veal, lamb, poultry, or fish 3 to 5 times a
    week during interval therapy
3–4 servings vegetables including:
      1 medium potato
      1–2 servings green leafy or yellow vegetable
      1 serving other vegetable
2–3 servings fruit including:
      1 serving citrus fruit
      1–2 servings other fruits
  1 serving enriched cereal
4–6 slices enriched bread
  2 tablespoons butter or fortified margarine
Additional calories are provided as needed by increasing the amount of potato, potato substi-
    tutes such as macaroni, rice, noodles, bread, sugars, sweets, fruits, and vegetables.

Nutritive value of basic foods above: Calories, 1850; protein, 68 gm; fat, 80 gm; carbohydrate,
220 gm; calcium, 1400 mg; iron, 11.3 mg; vitamin A, 11,350 I.U.; thiamine, 1.3 mg; riboflavin, 2.3
mg; niacin, 10 mg; ascorbic acid, 145 mg.

Foods to Avoid
All foods high in purines (see group III, Table 40–1)
Condiments and excessive seasoning
Alcohol
For low-fat diets:
    Pastries and rich desserts
    Cream and ice cream
    Fried foods
    Eggs not to exceed 2 daily; hard cheese not to exceed 1 ounce. Severe restriction may require
      the omission of eggs, whole milk, cheese, and butter. Skim milk and cottage cheese must
      then be used in ample amounts to provide the necessary protein.

Sample Menu
  BREAKFAST
Half grapefruit
Rice Krispies with milk and sugar
Buttered toast
Scrambled egg
Coffee with milk and sugar
  LUNCHEON OR SUPPER
Jelly omelet
Boiled rice
Broiled tomato
Half peach with cottage cheese on lettuce

Bread with 1 teaspoon butter
Milk—1 glass
  DINNER
Cheese soufflé
Baked potato
Beets
Green celery strips
Bread with 1 teaspoon butter
Apple snow
Milk—1 glass
  BEDTIME
Milk—1 glass

OSTEOPOROSIS

Osteoporosis is a bone disease of frequent
occurrence in middle age, yet its etiology and
its treatment are poorly understood. Various
surveys of populations in homes for the aged
and of other patients receiving ambulatory care
have shown 15 to 50 per cent of the population
over age 65 to be affected. A minimum of four

million noninstitutionalized persons are believed to have severe osteoporosis. The disease occurs four times as frequently in women as in men.

Etiology. Osteoporosis is a deficiency disease, but it would be erroneous to assume that a deficit in dietary intake is primarily responsible. Rather, the aspects of deficiency are the result of many factors, among which are the following: endocrine disorders such as hyperthyroidism, hyperparathyroidism, hyperadrenocorticism, and acromegaly; immobilization; rheumatoid arthritis; sickle-cell anemia; nutritional deficiencies such as of calcium, protein, ascorbic acid, and others.[6]

Some authorities consider osteoporosis to be a disease of the protein matrix and have associated this with the frequent occurrence of a low protein intake. Others have shown a close correlation between the degree of mineralization of the bone and the intake of calcium. Osteoporosis occurs far more frequently in women who have had a lifetime history of low calcium intake than it does in women who have always had a liberal calcium intake.

Metabolic changes and their effects. The principal symptoms of osteoporosis are low-back pain, sometimes severe, and often a history of vertebral fractures. Over a period of years the individual may have lost height—sometimes several inches. Roentgenographic changes are not diagnosed until as much as 30 per cent of the bone mass has been lost.

Osteoporosis is characterized by a reduction in the total bone mass, but with no known change in the structure or chemical composition of the bone. Because of the reduction in the number of cells, there is a decrease in the thickness of the cortex, a thinning of the trabeculae, and an increased porosity of the bone. As a result, fractures occur with greater frequency.

Blood levels of calcium, phosphorus, and alkaline phosphatase are normal, as are also the serum protein and lipoprotein levels. Calcium, phosphorus, and nitrogen balances are frequently negative. Inadequate dietary intake, defective absorption from the gastrointestinal tract, or excessive bone resorption could explain such negative balances. It is well to keep in mind that older individuals may require more calcium to achieve balance than those who are younger.

Treatment. The factors which may have initiated the osteoporosis must be determined before effective therapy can be instituted. Estrogens and androgens have been used advantageously in many patients, since the hormones exert an anabolic effect on proteins and also play a role in better retention of minerals in bone. Physiotherapy is required to relieve pain and to prevent immobilization.

A diet liberal in calcium is generally recommended. The inclusion of at least 1 quart of milk, some hard cheese, and a normal allowance of other foods would bring the daily intake of calcium to about 1.5 gm. A calcium supplement may also be used in the form of calcium gluconate or calcium lactate. In some instances a supplement of vitamin D has appeared to improve the absorption of calcium and the mineralization of bone. The resorption of bone is less in those areas where the water is fluoridated with 1 ppm of fluoride. At best, the treatment of osteoporosis is likely to inhibit the progression of the disease; reversal of the disease is not likely.

The primary effort should be directed early in life to the prevention of bone loss. A diet adequate in calcium and protein is important for maintenance of bone structure; however, until more is known of the etiology of this disease the most effective prophylaxis as well as treatment cannot be prescribed.

PROBLEMS AND REVIEW

1. Differentiate between the hypoglycemia in functional hyperinsulinism, Addison's disease, and liver disease. What modification of carbohydrate level of the diet is required for each?
2. What is the advantage of a high protein and high fat intake in hyperinsulinism?

3. *Problem.* Calculate a diet for a patient with functional hyperinsulinism who requires 2400 calories, 130 gm protein, and 75 gm carbohydrate. Use the exchange lists for the calculation. Divide the day's allowance into three equal meals.

4. What modifications of mineral and water metabolism are present in Addison's disease? In what way is this corrected by hormone therapy?

5. Why is a sodium-restricted diet occasionally ordered for a patient receiving hormone therapy in Addison's disease? Under what circumstances would an increase in sodium intake be used?

6. On the basis of your understanding of the metabolism in Addison's disease, what are some of the functions of the adrenal gland in the normal individual? What is the effect of the activity of the pituitary?

7. What are the characteristic symptoms of hyperthyroidism?

8. Compare the diet which might be used in a hyperthyroid patient who is well controlled with antithyroid drugs, and one who has an elevated metabolic rate.

9. Suggest five ways in which the calories of a diet for a patient with hyperthyroidism might be increased.

10. Why does a surgeon so frequently insist that a patient gain weight before an operation on the thyroid?

11. What is myxedema? What is its chief cause? How can you explain the frequent occurrence of overweight?

12. Diet is neither causative nor curative in arthritis. On this basis, outline briefly the principles of dietary consideration in arthritis.

13. What are the dietary implications of long-term use of cortisone in arthritis or other diseases?

14. What are the sources of uric acid to the body? In what ways is uric acid metabolism disturbed in gout?

15. How can you explain the fact that a person who has gout may have an acute attack following surgery or during an acute infection?

16. What is the basis for restricting the protein intake to 1 gm per kilogram in the dietary planning for a patient with gout?

17. What problems are entailed when a purine-free diet is ordered for a patient, insofar as nutritional adequacy is concerned?

18. *Problem.* Plan a menu for one day for a low-purine diet.

19. What is the role of each of these hormones on protein and mineral metabolism: thyroxine; parathormone; androgen; cortisone?

20. On the basis of current research related to osteoporosis, what dietary measures may be instrumental in preventing the disease?

21. What modifications of the normal diet may be helpful in the treatment of osteoporosis?

CITED REFERENCES

1. Beeuwkes, A. M.: "The Dietary Treatment of Functional Hyperinsulinism," *J. Am. Diet. Assoc.,* **18**:731, 1942.

2. Greenblatt, R. B., and Metts, J. C., Jr.: "Addison's Disease," *Am. J. Nurs.,* **60**:1249, 1960.

3. Puppel, I. D.: "Some Metabolic Factors in the Treatment of Hyperthyroidism," *Ann. Intern. Med.,* **48**:1300, 1958.

4. *Arthritis Source Book.* Pub. 1431, Public Health Service, U.S. Department of Health, Education, and Welfare, Washington, D.C., 1966.

5. *Gout. Diagnosis and Treatment.* Pub. 1606, Public Health Service, National Institutes of Arthritis and Metabolic Diseases, Bethesda, Md., 1967.

6. Lutwak, L., and Whedon, G. D.: "Osteoporosis—A Disorder of Mineral Nutrition," *Bordens Rev. Nutr. Res.,* **23**:45, 1962.

ADDITIONAL REFERENCES

Anderson, J. W., and Herman, R. H.: "Classification of Reactive Hypoglycemia," *Am. J. Clin. Nutr.*, **22**:646–50, 1969.

Berkowitz, D.: "Blood Lipids and Uric Acid Relationships," *J.A.M.A.*, **190**:856–58, 1964.

Cohn, S. H., *et al.*: "High Calcium Diet and the Parameters of Calcium Metabolism in Osteoporosis," *Am. J. Clin. Nutr.*, **21**:1246–53, 1968.

Gutman, A. B.: "A View of Gout as an Inborn Error of Metabolism," *Am. J. Med.*, **29**:545–53, 1960.

Hamwi, G. J., and Tzagournis, M.: "Nutrition and Diseases of the Endocrine Glands," *Am. J. Clin. Nutr.*, **23**:311–29, 1970.

Hegsted, D. M.: "Nutrition, Bone and Calcified Tissue," *J. Am. Diet. Assoc.*, **50**:105–11, 1967.

Herman, I., and Smith, R.: "Gout and Gouty Arthritis," *Am. J. Nurs.*, **64**:111–13, Dec. 1964.

Iskrant, A. P.: "The Etiology of Fractured Hips in Females," *Am. J. Public Health*, **58**:485–90, 1968.

Jay, A. N.: "Hypoglycemia," *Am. J. Nurs.*, **62**:77, Jan. 1962.

Lutwak, L.: "Nutritional Aspects of Osteoporosis," *J. Am. Geriatr. Soc.*, **17**:115–19, 1969.

McCormick, E. W.: "Gout in the Elderly," *Geriatrics*, **20**:756–58, 1965.

Rich, C., and Ensinck, J.: "Effect of Sodium Fluoride on Calcium Metabolism in Human Beings," *Nature*, **191**:184–85, 1961.

Smith, R. W., Jr.: "Dietary and Hormonal Factors in Bone Loss," *Fed. Proc.*, **26**:1737–46, 1967.

Sorenson, L. B.: "Recent Advances in the Study of Uric Acid Metabolism," *Postgrad. Med.*, **37**:659–66, 1965.

Stein, I., and Beller, M. L.: "Therapeutic Progress in Osteoporosis," *Geriatrics*, **25**:159–63, 1970.

Traut, E. F., and Thrift, C. B.: "Obesity in Arthritis: Related Factors: Dietary Therapy," *J. Am. Geriatr. Soc.*, **17**:710–17, 1969.

Walike, B. C., *et al.*: "Rheumatoid Arthritis," *Am. J. Nurs.*, **67**:1420–26, 1967.

PUBLICATIONS FOR THE LAYMAN

Diet and Arthritis. Pub. 1857, Public Health Service, Diabetes and Arthritis Control Program, U.S. Department of Health, Education, and Welfare, Washington, D.C., 1969.

Hamilton, A.: "Good News about Gout," *Today's Health*, **45**:16, Dec. 1967.

Maddox, G.: *Food and Arthritis.* Taplinger Publishing Company, New York, 1969.

41 Nutrition in Nervous Disturbances

Ketogenic Diet

Nutrition and the nervous system. The nervous tissues, like other tissues of the body, require energy for metabolic functions, protein for cell synthesis, vitamins as components of the enzyme systems, and mineral elements as activators of metabolic reactions and to maintain homeostasis of the fluid environment. The role of these nutrients and the effects of deficiency have been described especially in Unit II. The following discussion presents a brief summary of the principal effects of nutrient lack upon the functioning of the nervous system.

Energy. The brain utilizes glucose exclusively as its source of energy. To shut off the supply of glucose and oxygen from the brain for even a few minutes leads to irreversible damage. The body at rest utilizes up to 25 per cent of its total oxygen consumption for the brain alone.[1]

Protein. The influence of amino acid imbalances on mental development are dramatically illustrated by the severe mental retardation that accompanies inborn errors of metabolism. These are fully discussed in Chapter 48.

In recent years much research on experimental animals and on humans has shown that severe protein deficiency during pregnancy and during the first year of life especially can lead to irreversible mental retardation. Children with kwashiorkor or marasmus were found to have psychologic, neuromuscular, and intellectual capacities 10 to 25 per cent below normal.[2] The ability of these children to catch up is uncertain. The retardation of development is accentuated when infection is also present. Although much evidence has been presented that implicates nutrition, it is exceedingly difficult to separate the effects of malnutrition from the economic, educational, emotional, and social deprivation that are simultaneously present. See also pages 356 to 358 for further discussion of protein-calorie malnutrition.

Vitamins. Deficiencies of the water-soluble vitamins bring about serious changes in functioning of the nervous system. (See Chapter 12.) Thiamine deficiency is characterized by reduced tendon reflexes, peripheral neuritis, incoordination of gait, muscle pains; irritability, inability to concentrate, lack of interest in affairs, and personality deterioration including hypochondriasis, depression and hysteria.[3-5]

Classic niacin deficiency, pellagra, is rarely seen in the United States. Its neurologic signs include poor memory, irritability, dizziness, hallucinations, delusions of persecution, and finally dementia.

Vitamin B_6 deficiency is characterized by weakness, ataxia, and convulsions. Pantothenic acid lack leads to mental depression, peripheral neuritis, sullenness, cramping pains in the arms and legs, and burning sensations of the feet. The inability to absorb vitamin B_{12} because of lack of intrinsic factor is the condition known as pernicious anemia and which presents such symptoms as unsteady gait, depression, and mental deterioration. (See Chapter 45.)

NUTRITION FOR THE MENTALLY ILL

Feeding older persons in nursing homes. Weiner[6] has described four categories of pathologic-psychologic reactions in aging persons in nursing homes: anxiety, depression, suspicion, and confusion. In some individuals all of these may be present to a varying degree or they may appear one after the other. Each type of reaction requires specific measures in feeding.

The anxious person requires assurance that everything is all right. He worries about the effects that foods may have on bowel function and often asks questions about which foods are constipating. Worry about his food may increase gastrointestinal motility so that he has cramps or may reduce motility so that he becomes distended. The anxious person needs to be comforted, to have someone around him, to be made to feel secure, and to be given special consideration by being served his favorite foods as often as possible.

The depressed individual feels that his situation is hopeless and has a conscious or unconscious desire to die. Reassurance only frightens him more and he will continue to demand more and more of it until there seems to be no end to his demands. He needs external control and should be told firmly exactly what he must do, that he must eat, that he will be taken care of, and that he will be helped to eat what he needs for his nourishment. Sometimes spoon feeding is needed to get him started. It is not advisable for him to choose his own menu.

The suspicious person is afraid that he will be hurt and often suspects that his food is poisoned. He feels that he must constantly be on watch unless something happens to his security. Efforts to reassure him to the contrary only increase his suspicions. Matter-of-factly he should be told that there is nothing wrong with his food, but it may be necessary for the attendant to taste the food in his presence to show that it is not poisoned. The suspicious person, unlike the depressed person, must not be forced to eat. He should be allowed to eat or not to eat what is presented to him.

The confused person has usually had some brain damage as in a stroke, from diabetic or hepatic coma, or from head injury. He doesn't know what is happening around him and he often becomes anxious, depressed, or suspicious. He may not know where he is, and regardless of what he is told he believes himself to be in his own home as an adult or in his childhood home. He needs help in understanding what is going on around him. With respect to feeding, he needs to be told that it is mealtime, what meal it is, and what foods are on his tray. When a favorite food is served, it is a good idea to specially identify it.

Diet for patients in the mental hospital. Diet is an important part of the total program of rehabilitation for the psychiatric patient. Aside from its nutritional necessity, food provides basic security and pleasurable satisfaction. The patient needs to feel that someone is genuinely concerned about his welfare and cares for him. The dietitian and nurse—through the care shown in meal planning, preparation, and service, and through their expressions of interest to the individual—are participants in the therapy.

To plan a nutritionally adequate diet is obviously not enough. The service of food which is attractive to the eye, tempting of odor, and satisfying to the palate is just as important in the psychiatric hospital as in any other feeding situation. The mentally ill may express marked irritability when given foods they dislike. Food service in a cafeteria permits the patient to exercise some choice in his food selection, and thus helps to eliminate some of the irritations.

Patients react favorably and are less destructive when an attractive dining environment is provided. A well-planned dining room with a cheerful color scheme, curtains or draperies at the windows, small attractive tables, and suitable background music is conducive to food acceptance and contributes to the therapy of the patient. Attention to birthdays, holidays, and other special events provides additional evidence that the patient is cared for.

Psychiatric patients frequently eat inadequate or excessive amounts of food. A regular schedule of weighing of patients—about once a month—will help to detect such changes, and correction can be started before marked weight change has occurred. Marked weight gain is not uncommon. It would seem easy to control this in a hospital by providing a diet designed for weight maintenance. However, the privileges of food purchases from a canteen and food gifts from relatives and friends must be taken into consideration. Patients are often known to eat food left by other patients.

Refusal to eat is a problem presented by other psychiatric patients. Hussar[7] recommends that the nurse or attendant should note any patient who refuses more than half of a meal. A four- or five-day simple checklist helps to identify whether the refusal follows a pattern with respect to a particular food or meal. Refusal of food sometimes denotes an underlying physical illness about which the patient who is withdrawn or mute does not complain. Those who need to gain weight may require close supervision in taking small, frequent feedings; some may be helped if butter is spread on the bread, milk and sugar are put on the cereal, the milk container is opened, the meat is cut, and so on; sincere words of encouragement should be offered when progress is made. Tube feeding (see Chapter 38) may be resorted to when all attempts to achieve satisfactory intake of food fail.

Feeding the mentally retarded presents many problems which may be especially acute in the child. The management of the diet for these patients is discussed in Chapter 47.

ALCOHOLISM

For about 9 million Americans chronic alcoholism severely affects health, job security, and family life.[8] Only about one fourth of these seek any kind of treatment. At least 20,000 hospital admissions annually, accounting for half a million hospital days, are for major illnesses that result from the problems of malnutrition associated with alcoholism. Clearly, this is a major public health problem that must be considered in its physiologic, psychologic, and social aspects.

Alcohol and metabolism. Alcohol is looked upon as a foodstuff in the sense that it yields 7 calories per gram. But, unlike almost all foodstuffs, there are few if any nutrients associated with these calories. A pint of bourbon, for example, furnishes 1350 calories, but it contains no nutrients whatsoever. Some claims are made for the nutritional properties of beer, but a 1-ounce slice of bread is a better source of nutrition than one 12-ounce bottle of beer.[8]

Alcohol is rapidly and almost completely absorbed. The presence of food in the stomach, as is well known, delays gastric absorption. However, from the small intestine absorption is rapid

regardless of whether food is present or not.

Upon absorption alcohol is dispersed rapidly throughout the body water. The liver accounts for about 90 per cent of the total oxidation of alcohol. The first step in oxidation is to acetaldehyde, a reaction that is limited in rate by the level of alcohol dehydrogenase that is present. The liver of the average-size adult can oxidize 8 to 15 ml alcohol per hour.[9] Acetaldehyde is further oxidized to acetyl coenzyme A and enters the citric acid cycle where the oxidation is completed to yield energy, carbon dioxide, and water. (See page 70.)

Effects of alcohol upon nutrition. Alcohol reduces the appetite so that the heavy drinker eats poorly. Moreover, the chronic alcoholic often does not have the money to purchase an adequate diet inasmuch as he may be out of a job and he spends what money he has for alcohol. The incidence of malnutrition is not high according to Olson,[9] who claims that no more than 20 per cent of alcoholics show biochemical changes suggestive of mild deficiency and that only 3 per cent have frank deficiency symptoms. On the other hand, Iber[8] has emphasized the relationship of major illnesses to alcoholic malnutrition.

Formerly it was believed that alcohol was directly toxic to the liver; this view is now generally disputed. On the other hand, the liver is impaired because of the interfering effects of alcohol upon normal metabolic processes. Fatty infiltration of the liver results from one of several causes: increased synthesis of triglycerides; reduced synthesis of lipoproteins that are required for transport of fats; and possibly an increased mobilization of fat from adipose tissue during periods of starvation. In fatty infiltration there is little damage to the liver cells, but subsequently the hepatic cells are damaged, leading first to alcoholic hepatitis and then to cirrhosis. Even the early stages of cirrhosis can be reversed when a nutritious diet is given.

The urinary losses of amino acids, magnesium, potassium, and zinc are increased during periods of drinking. According to Flink,[10] the associated hypomagnesemia helps to explain the symptoms of *delirium tremens* and is relieved by intravenous or intramuscular administration of magnesium sulfate.

Diet for alcoholics. A diet that meets normal nutritional requirements will restore the nutritional status of the alcoholic. When there is evidence of vitamin deficiencies, a supplement, especially of water-soluble factors, is indicated. It is a fallacy, however, that vitamin deficiencies are an etiologic factor in alcoholism, or that the correction of these deficiencies will cure the alcoholic.

When hepatitis or cirrhosis is present, the dietary modifications described on pages 483 to 485 should be considered. The possibility of hepatic coma and the need for drastic protein restriction when it occurs must always be kept in mind.

Nurses and dietitians can help the alcoholic return to better health by considering his food habits, by encouraging him to eat, and by providing dietary counseling. No useful purpose is served by assuming a critical, moralizing posture either by what one says or by one's attitude.

Wernicke's—Korsakoff's syndrome. Wernicke's syndrome and Korsakoff's psychoses are highly associated with alcoholism and appear to be different phases of the same disease. Wernicke's syndrome has an abrupt onset characterized by ophthalmoplegia (paralysis of the eye muscles), nystagmus (rapid movement of the eyeballs), and ataxia (uncoordinated gait).[11] The patient is often unable to stand or walk without support. The eye changes and the gait are dramatically corrected, often within hours, by the administration of thiamine.

Korsakoff's syndrome may not be apparent until several weeks after the changes in the eye and gait have become evident. The chief defect is the disturbance in memory and the inability to learn new things so that only the most routine tasks can be performed. Moreover, there is failure to associate past events in their proper sequence. Patients may be confused, anxious, fearful, and even delirious. Vitamin therapy has produced marked effects in restoring the patient to being responsive, alert, and attentive. However, when memory defects are present, they appear to persist despite therapy, suggesting that structural changes in the brain may be irreversible.

EPILEPSY

The nature of epilepsy. Epilepsy is a disease of the central nervous system characterized by loss of consciousness which may last for only a few seconds, as in petit mal attacks, or which may be accompanied by convulsions, as in grand mal attacks. It occurs more frequently in children than in adults. The disease in no way affects the individual's mental ability, but unthinking relatives and friends sometimes attach an entirely unwarranted stigma to the disease and thus may increase the tension states in the individual.

Treatment. Various drugs such as phenobarbital or diphenylhydantoin sodium or others have been employed with considerable success in the treatment of epilepsy and have largely replaced the ketogenic diet once so widely used.[12,13] As a rule, a normal diet for the individual's age and activity is prescribed when drug therapy is used. Some fluid restriction is considered to be effective by several clinicians.

Mike[14] has described the use of the ketogenic diet for selected children, especially of preschool age, who have petit mal epilepsy. The purpose of the diet is to produce an acidosis by curtailing very severely the amount of available glucose and increasing markedly the intake of fat so that complete combustion of fats cannot take place. The accumulation of acetone bodies (acetone, acetoacetic acid, and beta-hydroxybutyric acid) has a favorable effect on the irritability and restlessness of the child and does not dull the mental function as some drugs do. In fact, children thought to be mentally retarded were found to be alert and bright when their seizures were controlled by diet.[14] The maintenance of a continuous state of acidosis is essential, for even small amounts of carbohydrate lead to seizures.

Mike has emphasized the difficulties of dietary management inasmuch as the diet is severely restricted in carbohydrate, is unpalatable, lacks bulk, and deviates sharply from customary food patterns. The diet requires greater care in its planning and preparation than other metabolic diets. A careful evaluation of the probable success of the diet for each patient and the ability of the parents to understand and adhere to the regulations is essential.

Modification of the diet. Sufficient calories for normal weight and for the maintenance of normal growth are necessary. The allowances recommended by Mike[14] are

Age (years)	Calories per kg
2–3	100 to 80
3–5	80 to 60
5–10	79 to 55

Protein. An allowance of 1 gm protein per kilogram of body weight is sufficient, but may be increased to 1.5 gm per kilogram for the older child.

Carbohydrate and fat. The nonprotein calories are so divided that a ketogenic to antiketogenic ratio of approximately 3 to 1 or 4 to 1 is maintained. Ketogenic factors (fatty acids) in the diet include 90 per cent of the fat, and

about 50 per cent of the protein. The antiketogenic factors in the diet (available glucose) are derived from 100 per cent of the carbohydrate, plus approximately 50 per cent of the protein and 10 per cent of the fat. Obviously, to achieve a 3-to-1 or 4-to-1 ratio, the carbohydrate must be sharply restricted and the fat intake greatly increased. The level of carbohydrate usually needs to be less than 30 gm if ketosis is to be produced, but should never be less than 10 gm daily.

The diet for a five-year-old child weighing 25 kg illustrates the calculation of a diet prescription.

1. Calories: $25 \times 70 = 1750$
2. Protein: $25 \times 1 = 25$ gm
3. Calories from protein $= 25 \times 4 = 100$
4. Calories from carbohydrate and fat: $1750 - 100 = 1650$

If we allow 25 gm carbohydrate, the fat intake would need to be 172 gm as noted in the following calculations:

5. Calories from carbohydrate: $25 \times 4 = 100$
6. Calories from fat: $1650 - 100 = 1550$
7. Grams of fat: $1550 \div 9 = 172$

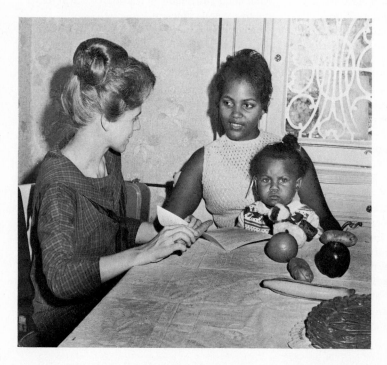

Figure 41–1. A nutritionist discusses problems of dietary management within the home. She makes such visits upon the request of the public health nurse when problems of diet may be somewhat complex. (Courtesy, Community Nursing Services, Philadelphia.)

The fatty acid to glucose ratio of this diet is as follows:

$$\frac{\text{Fatty acids}}{\text{Available glucose}} =$$

$$\frac{0.50\ (25) + 0.9\ (172)}{0.50\ (25) + 0.1\ (172) + 1.0\ (25)} = \frac{167}{55} = \frac{3}{1}$$

The maintenance of a constant acidosis requires that the protein, fat, and carbohydrate for the day be divided in three equal meals. The urine shows a positive test for acetoacetic acid when acidosis is being maintained.

Minerals and vitamins. Calcium gluconate or lactate is prescribed to furnish calcium. An iron supplement providing 7 to 10 mg elemental iron is also given. The vitamin needs are met by giving an aqueous multivitamin preparation.

Management of the diet. For the first 24 to 72 hours the child is given nothing but water, usually restricted to 500 to 1000 ml. Hunger disappears as ketosis increases. When ketosis is marked the diet is initiated, but is not forced until the transition has been accomplished. During this period nausea and vomiting may occur.

The diet may be calculated by using the values for individual foods as in Table A-1, or by using food groupings such as those developed by Mike. The meal exchange lists are not satisfactory for the calculation.[14] The predominant foods in the diet are carefully restricted amounts of meat, cheese, and eggs; cream, butter, bacon, mayonnaise; restricted amounts of low-carbohydrate vegetables and fruits. (See Figure 41–1.) Other foods are avoided: sugar-containing beverages; breads and cereals; desserts such as cake, cookies, ice cream, pastries, pie, puddings; milk; all sweets including sugar, jellies, candy, preserves; vegetables and fruits high in carbohydrate.

The diet must be weighed on a gram scale and all food must be consumed at each meal.

Table 41–1. Sample Calculation for Ketogenic Diet

Food	Household Measure	Weight gm	Protein gm	Fat gm	Carbohydrate gm
Breakfast					
Egg, whole	1	50	6	6	—
Butter	2 teaspoons	10	—	8	—
Cream, whipping	1/2 cup	120	3	45	4
Fruit (orange)	1/3	60	1	—	5
			10	59	9
Luncheon or Supper					
Beef, lean	2/3 ounce	20	6	2	—
Tomato, canned	1/2 cup	120	1	—	5
Cream, whipping	1/2 cup	120	3	45	4
Butter	2 teaspoons	10	—	8	—
Cellu wafers					
			10	55	9
Dinner					
Cheddar cheese	2/3 ounce	20	4	6	—
Cream, whipping	1/2 cup	120	3	45	4
Grapes, seedless	1/4 cup	40	1	—	6
Butter	2 teaspoons	10	—	8	—
Cellu wafers					
			8	59	10
Total for the Day			28	173	28

$$\frac{\text{Ketogenic factors}}{\text{Antiketogenic factors}} = \frac{170}{59} = 2.9$$

Foods may not be saved for later consumption. If no improvement occurs within six weeks, there is nothing to be gained by further continuance of the diet. If improvement does occur, the diet must be continued for a year or longer.

Gradually the diet is liberalized with very small increases in the carbohydrate and corresponding caloric decreases in the fat. Table 41–1 illustrates a sample calculation for the ketogenic diet.

PROBLEMS AND REVIEW

1. Describe the development of the nervous system in relation to other factors in growth and development of the young child.
2. What is the principal source of energy for the brain? What proportion of oxygen consumption is required by the brain?
3. Why would you expect vitamin deficiencies to have an adverse effect on the functioning of the nervous system? Describe the changes that take place in deficiency of thiamine; of vitamin B_6.
4. What is the effect of alcoholism on the nutritional state of the individual? How can you explain some of the symptoms characteristic of Wernicke's syndrome?
5. What are some of the meanings of food that may have special relevance to the mentally ill? What recommendations could you make for the feeding of the mentally ill?
6. What is epilepsy? What is the rationale for a ketogenic diet for the treatment of epilepsy? Why is the diet seldom used?
7. *Problem.* Modify the diet calculated in Table 41–1 so that it provides a ketogenic-antiketogenic ratio of 3.5 to 1.
8. *Problem.* List some ways in which the whipping cream and butter may be used in the ketogenic diet. What purpose is served by the Cellu wafers?

CITED REFERENCES

1. Horwitt, M. K.: "Nutrition in Mental Health," *Nutr. Rev.,* **23**:289, 1965.
2. Coursin, D. B.: "Effects of Undernutrition on Central Nervous System Function," *Nutr. Rev.,* **23**:65, 1965.
3. Brozek, J.: "Psychologic Effects of Thiamine Restriction and Deprivation in Normal Young Men," *Am. J. Clin. Nutr.,* **5**:109, 1957.
4. Jolliffe, N., *et al.:* "The Experimental Production of Vitamin B_1 Deficiency in Normal Subjects," *Am. J. Med. Sci.,* **198**:198, 1939.
5. Williams, R. R., *et. al.:* "Observations on Induced Thiamine Deficiency in Man," *Arch. Intern. Med.,* **66**:785, 1940.
6. Weiner, M. F.: "A Practical Approach to Encouraging Geriatric Patients to Eat," *J. Am. Diet. Assoc.,* **55**:384–86, 1969.
7. Hussar, A. E., and Sturdevant, J. E.: "An Advisory Committee Considers Dietetic Problems in a Psychiatric Hospital," *J. Am. Diet. Assoc.,* **32**:1188, 1956.
8. Iber, F. L.: "In Alcoholism, the Liver Sets the Pace," *Nutr. Today,* **6**:2–9, Jan. 1971.
9. Olson, R. E.: "Nutrition and Alcoholism," in Wohl, M. G., and Goodhart, R. S., eds.: *Modern Nutrition in Health and Disease,* 4th ed. Lea & Febiger, Philadelphia, 1968, Chapter 25.
10. Flink, E. B.: "Magnesium Deficiency Syndrome in Man," *J.A.M.A.,* **160**:1406–1409, 1956.
11. Victor, M.: "Alcohol and the Nutritional Diseases of the Nervous System," *J.A.M.A.,* **167**:65–71, 1958.
12. Peterman, M. G.: "Epilepsy in Childhood; Newer Methods of Diagnosis and Treatment," *J.A.M.A.,* **138**:1012, 1948.

13. Hughes, J. G., and Jabbour, J. T.: "The Treatment of the Epileptic Child," *J. Pediatr.*, **53**:66, 1958.
14. Mike, E. M.: "Practical Guide and Dietary Management of Children with Seizures Using the Ketogenic Diet," *Am. J. Clin. Nutr.*, **17**:399–405, 1965.

ADDITIONAL REFERENCES

Barnes, R. H.: "Effects of Malnutrition on Mental Development," *J. Home Econ.*, **61**:67–76, 1969.
Coursin, D. B.: "Undernutrition and Brain Function," *Bordens Rev. Nutr. Res.*, **26**:1–16, Jan. 1965.
Donahue, H. H., and Fowler, P. A.: "Some Problems of Feeding Mental Patients," *Am. J. Clin. Nutr.*, **5**:180, 1957.
Gee, D. A.: "Effects of Psychiatric Services on the Hospital Dietary Department," *J. Am. Diet. Assoc.*, **41**:345, 1962.
Mayer, J.: "Vitamins and Mental Disorders," *Postgrad. Med.*, **45**:268–69, April 1969.
Neville, J. N., *et al.*: "Nutritional Status of Alcoholics," *Am. J. Clin. Nutr.*, **21**:1329–40, 1968.
Owens, L., and White, G. S.: "Observations on Food Acceptance during Mental Illness," *J. Am. Diet. Assoc.*, **30**:1110, 1954.
Review: "Undernutrition in Children and Subsequent Brain Growth and Intellectual Development," *Nutr. Rev.*, **26**:197–99, 1968.
Ross, M.: "Food in the Mental Hospital," *J. Am. Diet. Assoc.*, **40**:318, 1962.
Rupp, C.: "Management of Epilepsy," *J.A.M.A.*, **166**:1967, 1958.
Sullivan, J. F., and Lankford, H. G.: "Zinc Metabolism and Chronic Alcoholism," *Am. J. Clin. Nutr.*, **17**:57–63, 1965.

Unit XIII

Diet in Cardiovascular and Renal Disorders

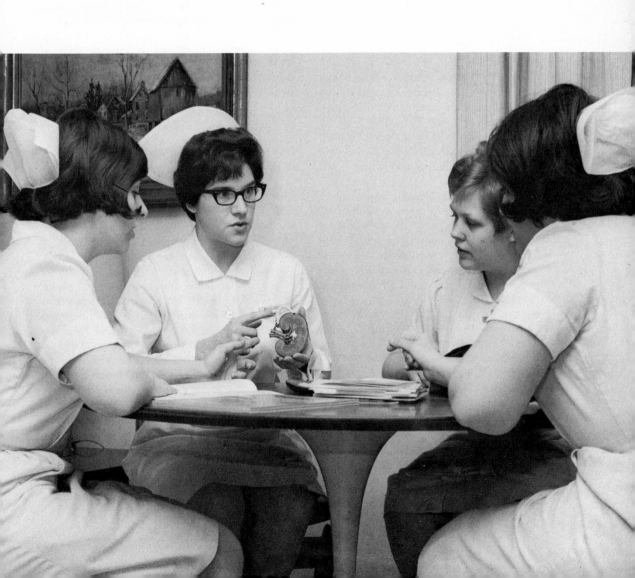

42 Hyperlipidemia and Atherosclerosis

Fat-Controlled Diets

Cardiovascular disease, a major public health problem. About a million persons in the United States die each year from cardiovascular diseases, a number that is greater than that from all other causes combined.[1] Of these deaths 560,000 are caused by arteriosclerotic heart disease and some 200,000 by cerebrovascular disease. Almost 15 million adults have some heart disorders and another 13 million are suspected of having some defects. In a given year approximately 600,000 new cases of coronary disease will be added to the number who are ill. The morbidity and mortality rates are not exceeded in any country of the world, and it almost seems that this is a kind of penalty paid for an affluent, often indulgent, but also stressful way of life. The costs are exhorbitant in terms of time and talents lost from productive work, the financial burdens of medical care, the losses of earnings, the psychologic cost of fear, and the anxiety and modified life style imposed upon the family.

Coronary heart disease may occur at any age, but it is not common until middle age at which time it practically assumes epidemic proportions. Males over 40 years of age are highly susceptible. Except for those who have hypertension or diabetes mellitus, coronary heart disease is not common in women until after the menopause.

Multiple risk factors in coronary disease. No single factor is an absolute cause either of atherosclerosis or of coronary disease. Many factors are interrelated and to the extent that they are present they increase the risk of disease. A committee of the American Heart Association has listed the following factors that affect the rate of development of disease.

Overt problems and personal attributes: familial occurrence of coronary disease at an early age; hypertension; electrocardiographic abnormalities; diabetes mellitus; lipid abnormalities involving serum cholesterol and triglycerides and their lipoprotein vehicles; obesity; gout (hyperuricemia); certain personality-behavior patterns

Environmental factors: cigarette smoking; lack of physical activity; emotionally stressful situations.*

If a single abnormality is present there is about a twofold risk of coronary disease. An individual with several abnormalities is 10 times as likely to have coronary disease as one who has no abnormalities. (See Figure 42–1)

CORONARY DISEASE AND THE ROLE OF DIET

The discussion in this chapter is concerned with (1) the rationale for dietary modification to reduce the incidence of atherosclerosis and coronary disease, (2) the fat-controlled diet, and (3) diets for five types of hyperlipoproteinemia. The dietary management of acute episodes of illness is discussed in the chapter that follows. The student should review normal fat and carbohydrate metabolism in order to understand the effects of altered physiology and biochemistry in coronary disease. (See Chapters 5 and 6.)

Coronary heart disease. *Myocardial ischemia* is a cardiac disability resulting from an inadequacy of the coronary arterial system to meet the needs of the heart muscle for oxygen and nutrients. It may be manifested as sudden death, myocardial infarction, or angina pectoris.

An *infarct* is a localized area of necrosis that

---

*"Risk Factors and Coronary Disease. A Statement for Physicians." Leaflet, American Heart Association, New York, 1968.

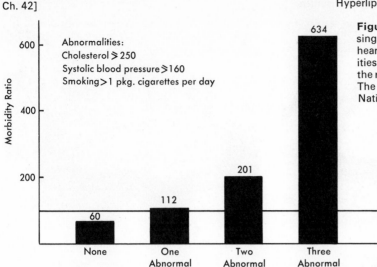

634

Figure 42–1. The presence of a single risk factor doubles the risk of heart disease. If the three abnormalities listed in this chart are present, the risk is ten times as high. (Courtesy, The Framingham Heart Study and National Heart Institute.)

results when the supply of blood to that area is inadequate for cellular survival. An infarct of the heart is known as a *myocardial infarction,* and one in the brain as a *cerebrovascular accident* (stroke). If the infarct is small, the remainder of the organ can function and healing takes place with the formation of scar tissue. The functional capacity of the organ is curtailed to the extent that tissue has been lost. Thus, repeated myocardial infarctions continue to reduce the functional capacity of the heart.

Angina pectoris literally means "sore throat of the chest." It refers to the tight, pressing, burning, and sometimes severe pain across the chest that follows exertion and that is a result of inadequate oxygen to the myocardium. As the coronary arteries become increasingly occluded, the pain develops with less and less exertion.

Atherosclerosis. This is a disease of the blood vessels resulting from the interaction of multiple factors such as heredity and the individual's environment (diet, activity, smoking, life style, etc.). Atheromatous plaques begin as soft, mushy accumulations of lipid material in the intima of the blood vessels. These plaques consist of a proliferation in the blood vessel wall of connective tissue into which lipids are deposited. The lipids include free cholesterol, cholesterol esters, and triglycerides in proportions that approximate those of the circulating blood lipids.

Atherosclerosis begins in the first decades of life and is almost universally present in people who live in affluent, highly developed countries. It develops gradually with increasing thickening of the arterial wall, loss of elasticity, and narrowing of the lumen. Finally, some event brings about occlusion of the vessel and ischemia of the affected part. (See Figure 42–2.)

Unquestionably, atherosclerosis sets the stage for coronary heart disease, but many people with atherosclerosis do not develop clinical disease.[2] The conditions that bring about occlusion are not well understood. In some instances ulceration of the atheroma and hemorrhage into the lumen with clot formation may occur. The anatomic location of the atheroma, the extent to which the lumen has been narrowed, the changes in the clearing of the blood lipids, and decrease in fibrinolytic activity are probably involved in the process.

Blood studies related to coronary disease. Measurements of various blood constituents can be used not only to determine the presence of abnormal concentrations but also to evaluate the effects of changes in diet and other therapy on the levels of these components. *Hyperlipidemia* is a general term that denotes an elevation of one or more lipids in the blood. *Hypercholesterolemia* is a serum cholesterol in excess of 260 mg per 100 ml[3]; many clinicians believe that a serum cholesterol of 200 mg per 100 ml

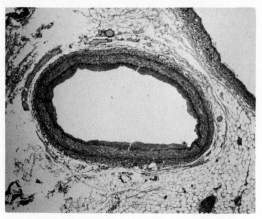

A. Normal artery

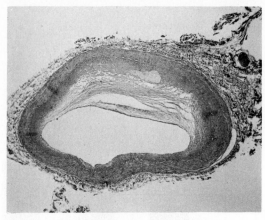

B. Deposits formed in inner lining of artery

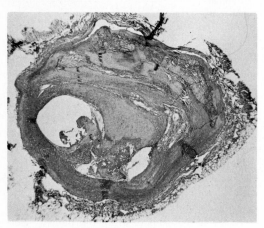

C. Deposits harden

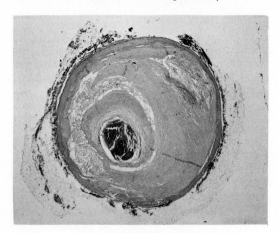

D. Normal channel is blocked by a blood clot

Figure 42–2. Gradual development of atherosclerosis in a coronary artery, leading to a heart attack. (Courtesy, American Heart Association.)

is preferable and that levels above this become increasingly undesirable. *Hypertriglyceridemia* is present when the fasting triglyceride level exceeds 250 mg per cent.[3]

Elevated levels of cholesterol and/or triglyceride in the blood are believed to result in more rapid and severe development of atherosclerosis and in turn of coronary disease. On the other hand, a reduction in the concentrations of these lipids in the blood is presumed to reduce the rate of atherosclerosis and with it to lower the incidence of clinical disease. A change in blood lipid levels must be interpreted with caution. Statis-

tically, the likelihood of coronary disease is greater in persons with a consistent hypercholesterolemia than in those with a normocholesterolemia. Not all persons with increased levels of blood cholesterol will develop heart disease. On the other hand, a lowering of a high blood cholesterol level reduces the risk of disease, but it is no guarantee that a given person will not have a heart attack.

In some individuals hyperlipidemia results from carbohydrate intolerance. When this is suspected it is useful to determine the fasting blood glucose and a glucose tolerance test. Glycosuria may also be present in such persons. A history of gout and a blood uric acid level above 7.5 mg per cent is another risk factor that should be evaluated.[3]

Fredrickson and his associates have described five types of hyperlipoproteinemia.[4] The differentiation is based upon the appearance of the serum, the concentrations of cholesterol and triglyceride, and the classes of lipoproteins that serve as the vehicles for the lipids. The distinctions are important in determining whether the disorders are fat induced or carbohydrate induced so that appropriate diet therapy can be instituted. See pages 549 to 551.

Long-term studies on modified diets. A tremendous number of studies have established that the serum cholesterol can be lowered in a short period of time by dietary modification. Short-term studies, however, do not establish that the lowering of the serum cholesterol also reduces the incidence of coronary heart disease. Several studies have now been reported on the effects of a cholesterol-lowering diet after five to seven years. The ages and health characteristics of men assigned to the control and experimental groups were similar. The experimental groups consumed diets in which the polyunsaturated fats replaced part of the saturated fats and that were reduced in cholesterol, whereas the control groups ate their customary diets.

Men free of coronary heart disease between the ages of 40 and 59 in the Anti-coronary Club Project of New York City were observed up to seven years.[5] The serum cholesterol in the experimental group was significantly lowered within the first year, but during the first two years there was no difference between experimental and control groups in the incidence of clinical disease. After two years, however, the experimental group had a significantly lower rate of disease.

In a Norwegian study 412 men who had survived a coronary infarction were assigned to control and experimental diets.[6] The relapse rate of myocardial infarction and of new cases of angina pectoris was significantly less for men under 60 years of age who consumed the cholesterol-lowering diet, but at 60 years and after the experimental and control groups did not differ. The rate of sudden death was identical in the two groups.

The results of an investigation on men living in a Veterans Administration hospital in Los Angeles also showed that a diet reduced in saturated fat, increased in polyunsaturated fat, and lower in cholesterol was effective in lowering the blood lipids and had a favorable influence on reducing the complications of atherosclerosis.[7] Of special interest in this study was the finding that the linoleic acid content of adipose tissue increased from 10 per cent at the beginning of the study to 30 per cent at the end of seven years. During the study postmortem examinations were made on the arteries of 34 men in the experimental group and about 40 men in the control group. The atherosclerotic plaques were not substantially different in the two groups, indicating that the experimental diet had not brought about any regression in atherosclerosis.

Dietary adjustments for hyperlipidemias. Important changes in the typical American diet must be made if hyperlipidemia is to be avoided and the incidence of heart disease is to be reduced.

Calorie balance. Obesity has long been recognized as one of the risk factors in cardiovascular disease. In the Framingham Heart Study overweight alone constituted only a slight risk; when obesity was associated with increased serum lipid levels, the risk was considerably greater.[8] When overweight is associated with diabetes mellitus, the serum cholesterol and triglyceride levels are customarily high. A reduction in calories together with a relatively high proportion of polyunsaturated fats is quite effective in reducing the lipid levels as well as the weight.

Increased body weight probably has its greatest effect on the increased work load of the heart. A mild stenosis associated with obesity can be critical in a situation of added stress.

Normal weight is maintained only when energy intake and output are equal. Therefore, early in life it is important to develop a program of regular exercise that can be continued throughout the years. (See Chapter 31.)

Fat. Dietary fat is the single most important factor requiring adjustment in programs of pre-

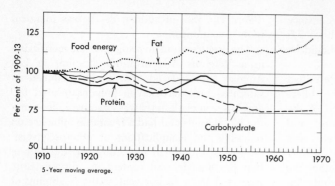

Figure 42–3. Per capita civilian consumption of food energy, protein, fat, and carbohydrate since 1909. Note that the fat level has increased almost 25 per cent, and the carbohydrate level has decreased about 25 per cent. Most of the decrease in carbohydrate has resulted from reduced intakes of grain foods and potatoes. (Courtesy, Agricultural Research Service, U.S. Department of Agriculture.)

vention and control. (See also Figure 42–3.) The typical American diet furnishes about 40 per cent of the calories from fat. Moreover, the saturated fat in the diet is about four times as high as the polyunsaturated fat.

For the prevention of hyperlipidemia the total fat content should be kept below 40 per cent of the calories; a level of 30 to 35 per cent may be preferable. The content of polyunsaturated fat should be increased and that of saturated fat strictly limited. Ratios of polyunsaturated fat to saturated fat (P-S ratio) may range from 1:1 to 2:1.

Cholesterol. The cholesterol content of American diets may range from 500 to 1000 mg daily, depending largely upon the number of eggs that are consumed. (See Table 6–2.) Increasing the dietary cholesterol from 0 to 800 mg daily without other dietary change results in a progressive increase in the blood cholesterol.[9] Thus, even the addition of one or two eggs a day can in part nullify the effects of a diet high in polyunsaturated fat. Most dietary regimens now restrict the cholesterol intake to 300 mg daily when hypercholesterolemia is present.

Carbohydrate. In the United States a marked decline has taken place in the consumption of breads and cereals, and the use of sugars and sugar-containing foods has increased considerably. Some investigators believe that the increase in sugars in the diet is as important in the elevation of blood lipids as is the increase in saturated fats.[10,11] A high-carbohydrate low-fat diet brings about an elevation in serum triglycerides even in normal individuals, although the effect is a temporary one.

Some hyperglyceridemias are carbohydrate in-

duced and the most important adjustment in diet is a reduction of the total carbohydrate and an elimination, insofar as possible, of sugars. This entails not only the elimination of sugar and sugar-containing foods, but control of the amounts of fruits and vegetables that are sources of fructose and sucrose. See also pages 63 and 474.

Other dietary factors. The mortality rate from cardiovascular diseases has been found to be significantly lower in areas where the drinking water is hard than in those areas where the water is soft. The higher levels of calcium in the hard water appeared to correlate well with the reduced death rate.[12] Pectins, gums, and hemicellulose as well as plant sterols interfere with the absorption of dietary cholesterol and therefore have a serum-cholesterol-lowering effect.[13]

FAT-CONTROLLED DIETS

Diet plans. The plans for fat-controlled meals at 1200 and 1800 calories and for 2000 to 2600 calories have been presented in two booklets prepared by a committee of dietitians and published by the American Heart Association.[14] The principal characteristics of these diets are summarized below.

1. About 30 to 35 per cent of the calories are supplied by fat.

2. Less than 10 per cent of the calories are furnished by saturated fat. Only skim milk and very lean meats, fish, and poultry may be used. Beef, lamb, and pork are restricted to three 3-ounce portions per week. Butter, cream, and whole-milk cheeses are not used.

3. From 11 to 14 per cent of the calories are supplied by polyunsaturated fats. The P/S ratio of the diets ranges from 2:1 to 2.8:1. The polyunsaturated fat content is increased principally by the use of safflower, corn, soy, or cottonseed oils. Limited amounts of special margarines may be included. (See Figure 42–4.)

4. Cholesterol is restricted to 300 mg daily or less. No more than 3 egg yolks per week may be used. Liver and shellfish are used only as a substitute for egg yolk.

5. Calorie adjustments may be made in the diet plans by including some sweets and desserts. These lists are not used when the hyperlipidemia is carbohydrate induced.

The dietary plans are adequate for men in all nutritional essentials, but for women the level of iron does not meet the recommended allowances.

Food lists. The food lists for fat-controlled diets are similar but not identical to the food exchange lists used for diabetic and other calculated diets. (See Table A-4.) The composition

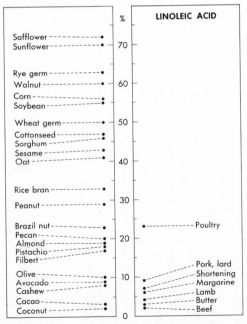

Figure 42–4. Percentage of linoleic acid in fats and oils of plant and animal origin. (Courtesy, Dr. Callie M. Coons and the *Journal of the American Dietetic Association*.)

of food groups for fat-controlled diets is shown in Table 42–1, the daily food allowances at varying calorie levels are listed in Table 42–2, and the detailed listings of foods appear in Table 42–3.

HYPERLIPOPROTEINEMIA

Types 1 to 5. Some hyperlipoproteinemias are induced by an excess of endogenous or exogenous fat, others by an intolerance to carbohydrates, especially sugars, and still others are influenced by dietary cholesterol.[15] These disorders of lipid metabolism may be hereditary or they may be caused by an intake of an abnormal diet. They are frequently associated with diabetes mellitus. Some types predispose to early atherosclerosis. Xanthomas are frequent, and in types 1 and 5 abdominal pain and acute pancreatitis may occur.

Type 1. An extremely high triglyceride concentration in the serum is characteristic of this type, with the serum cholesterol being normal to high. There is an inability to clear chylomicrons (dietary fat) from the blood, probably as a result of a genetic deficiency of lipoprotein lipase. The condition is rare, usually familial, and seen early in life. It may be associated with diabetes mellitus.

The diet must be very low in fat—25 to 30 gm daily for adults and about 15 gm for children. Cholesterol restriction is not essential. The carbohydrate is necessarily high in order to supply the needed calories. Alcohol is contraindicated because it increases the serum triglyceride levels when it is metabolized. The elimination of table spreads, cooking fats, and oils results in a dry diet. Medium-chain triglycerides are sometimes prescribed by the physician since they increase the calorie intake and may be used in food preparation.

Type 2. The beta-lipoprotein fraction and the serum cholesterol are increased, with triglycerides usually being normal. This type is a common hereditary disorder, often detectable as early as the first year of life. It may also be associated with an excessive cholesterol intake or with nephrosis, myxedema, or liver disease. Xan-

Table 42–1. Nutritive Composition of Food Groups for Fat-Controlled Diets*

Food	Measure	Calories	Carbohydrate gm	Protein gm	Total Fat gm	Saturated Fat gm	Linoleic Acid gm	Cholesterol mg
Skim milk	8 ounces	80	12	8	tr	—	—	7
Vegetables, group A	1/2 cup	—	—	2	—	—	—	—
Vegetables, group B	1/2 cup	35	7	2	—	—	—	—
Fruit, unsweetened	Varies	40	10	—	—	—	—	—
Breads, cereals	Varies	70	15	2	—	—	—	—
Meat, fish, poultry (lean, weighted average)†	1 ounce	50	—	8	2	0.6	0.1	21
Beef, lamb, pork, and ham, lean	1 ounce	65	—	9	3	1.3	—	21
Egg	1 whole	80	—	6	6	2.0	0.5	275
Vegetable oils								
Corn	1 tablespoon	125	—	—	14	1.0	7.0	—
Cottonseed	1 tablespoon	125	—	—	14	4.0	7.0	—
Safflower	1 tablespoon	125	—	—	14	1.0	10.0	—
Soybean	1 tablespoon	125	—	—	14	2.0	7.0	—
Margarine, soft, safflower	1 tablespoon	100	—	—	11	1.9	6.3	—
Other soft	1 tablespoon	100	—	—	11	2.5	3.7	—
Sugar	1 tablespoon	50	12	—	—	—	—	—

*Adapted from Zukel, M. C.: "Revising Booklets on Fat-controlled Meals," Tables 5 and 6, *J. Am. Diet. Assoc.*, 54: 23, 1969.

†Weighted average assumes weekly consumption to be: beef, lamb, pork, ham, three servings; poultry, four servings; veal, two servings; fish, five servings.

thomas and vascular disease are often seen early in adult life.

The cholesterol content of the diet is restricted to 300 mg or less, and polyunsaturated fats are emphasized with a sharp restriction of saturated fats so that a P/S ratio of 2 is achieved. Carbohydrate and protein are not restricted and alcohol may be used with discretion.

Type 3. This relatively rare disorder is characterized by an abnormal form of beta-lipoproteins with an elevation of the serum cholesterol and triglycerides. The incidence of vascular diseases is increased. Lesions on the elbows, knees, and buttocks are common.

Overweight is frequent, and a low-calorie diet is indicated until the desirable weight is attained. The fat and carbohydrate are restricted to not more than 40 per cent of the calories. Concentrated sweets are eliminated and polyunsaturated fats are substituted for saturated fats. Cholesterol is restricted to 300 mg per day. Alcohol may be substituted for up to two servings bread or cereal.

Type 4. This is a very common pattern characterized by an increase in endogenous triglycerides. The pre-beta-lipoproteins and the triglycerides are elevated, but the serum cholesterol is often normal. Many patients in this group have an abnormal glucose tolerance and some have

hyperuricemia. This disorder may be hereditary or associated with diabetes mellitus or another metabolic disorder. Obesity and the complications of atherosclerosis are frequent.

Initially the calories are restricted until desirable weight is achieved. Weight loss alone usually lowers the serum lipids, sometimes to normal. The maintenance diet provides not more than 40 per cent of the calories from carbohydrates and eliminates concentrated sweets. A P/S ratio of about 1 is maintained by substituting polyunsaturated fats for saturated fats. Cholesterol is restricted to 300 to 500 mg daily. Alcohol may be used at the physician's discretion.

Type 5. Chylomicrons and pre-beta-lipoproteins are elevated in this type, indicating intolerance to both endogenous and exogenous sources of fat. As with type 4, glucose tolerance and blood uric acid levels are often abnormal. This disorder is commonly associated with diabetic acidosis, nephrosis, alcoholism, and obesity. The liver and spleen may be enlarged, and abdominal pain is relatively common.

Calorie restriction is emphasized until the desired weight is achieved. The fat in the maintenance diet is kept as low as practical, but not more than 25 to 30 per cent of the calories. The P/S ratio, although not important, is somewhat

Table 42–2. Diet Plans for Fat-Controlled Diets*

	1200 Calories	1800 Calories	2000–2600 Calories
Milk, skim	2 cups	2 cups	2 cups
Vegetables	3 or more servings	3 or more servings	As desired
1 dark green or deep yellow			
Fruits—1 citrus	3 servings	3 servings	3 or more servings
Breads and cereals	4 servings	7 servings	As desired
Meat, fish, or poultry, cooked	5 ounces	6 ounces	6 ounces
Eggs	3 yolks/week	3 yolks/week	3 yolks/week
Oils	5 teaspoons	3 tablespoons	3–4 tablespoons
Special margarine	1 teaspoon	1 tablespoon	1–2 tablespoons
Sugars and sweets	1 serving if substituted for 1 serving bread	2 servings	As desired

*Adapted from *Planning Fat-Controlled Meals for 1200 and 1800 Calories,* revised 1966, and *Planning Fat-Controlled Meals for 2000 to 2600 Calories,* revised 1967.   American Heart Association, New York City.

Table 42–3. Food Lists for Fat-Controlled Diets*

Foods to Use	Foods to Avoid
Milk List	
Skim milk	Whole milk, homogenized milk, canned milk
Nonfat dry milk	Sweet cream, powdered cream
Buttermilk	Ice cream unless homemade with nonfat dry milk
	Sour cream
	Whole-milk buttermilk and whole-milk yogurt
	Cheese made from whole milk
Vegetables	
See list 2, Table A–4	
Fruits	
See list 3, Table A–4	Avocados
	Olives
Breads, Cereals List	
1 slice bread	Commercial biscuits, muffins, cornbreads, waffles,
1 roll (2–3 inches across)	griddle cakes, cookies, crackers
1 homemade biscuit or muffin (2–3 inches across)	Mixes for biscuits, muffins, and cakes
1 square homemade cornbread (1 1/2 inches square)	Coffee cakes, cakes (except angel food), pies, sweet
1 griddlecake (4 inches across) made with skim milk	rolls, doughnuts, and pastries
and fat from day's allowance	
4 pieces melba toast (3 1/2 by 1 1/2 by 1/8 inches)	
1 piece matso (5 inches square)	
3/4 ounce bread sticks, rye wafers, or pretzels	
1 1/2 cups popcorn (popped at home with fat or oil	
from day's allowance)	
1/2 cup cooked cereal	
3/4 cup dry cereal	
1/2 cup cooked rice, grits, hominy, barley, or	
buckwheat groats	
1/2 cup cooked spaghetti, noodles, or macaroni	
1/4 cup dry bread crumbs	
3 tablespoons flour	
2 1/2 tablespoons cornmeal	
Vegetables	
1/2 cup cooked dried beans, peas, lentils, or chickpeas	Potato chips
1/3 cup corn, kernels or cream style	French-fried potatoes
1 ear corn on the cob (4 inches long)	
1 small white potato	
1/4 cup sweet potato, cooked	
Meat, Fish, and Poultry List	
Make selections from this group for 11 of the 14 main meals	
Poultry without skin—chicken, turkey, Cornish hens,	Skin of chicken or turkey
squab	Duck or goose
Fish—any kind except shellfish	Fish roe; caviar
Veal—any lean cut	Fish canned in olive oil
Meat substitute	Shellfish (shrimp, crab, lobster, clams)
Cottage cheese (preferably uncreamed)	Note: 2 ounces may be used in place of 1 egg
Yogurt from partially skimmed milk	Coconut
Dried peas or beans	Macadamia nuts
Peanut butter, nuts (especially walnuts)	
Make selections from this group for 3 of the 14 main meals	
Beef:	
Hamburger—ground round or chuck	Beef high in fat or marbled
Roasts, pot roasts, stew meats—sirloin tip, round,	Lamb high in fat
rump, chuck, arm	Pork high in fat
Steaks—flank, sirloin, T bone, porterhouse, tender-	Bacon, salt pork, spareribs
loin, round, cube	Frankfurters, sausage, cold cuts
Soup meats—shank or shin	Canned meats and meat mixtures: stew, hash
Other—dried chipped beef	Organ meats such as kidney, brain, sweetbread, liver
Lamb:	Note: 2 ounces liver, sweetbreads, or heart may be
Roast or steak—leg	substituted for one egg
Chops, loin, rib, shoulder	Any visible fat on meat

*Adapted from food lists and text in *Planning Fat-Controlled Meals for 1200 and 1800 Calories*, revised 1966, and *Planning Fat-Controlled Meals for Approximately 2000–2600 Calories*, revised 1967, American Heart Association, New York City.

Table 42–3. (Cont.)

Foods to Use	Foods to Avoid
Pork:	Commercially fried meats, chicken, or fish
Roast—loin, center cut ham	Frozen or packaged casseroles or dinners
Chops—loin	
Tenderloin	
Ham:	
Baked, center cut steaks, picnic, butt, Canadian bacon	

Fat List

Foods to Use	Foods to Avoid
Corn oil	Butter
Cottonseed oil	Ordinary margarines
Safflower oil	Ordinary solid shortenings
Sesame seed oil	Lard
Soybean oil	Salt pork
Sunflower oil	Chicken fat
Mayonnaise (1 tsp mayonnaise equals 1 tsp oil)	Coconut oil
French dressing made with allowed oil (1 1/2 tsp	Olive oil
dressing equals 1 tsp oil)	Chocolate
Special margarine	

Sugars and Sweet List

Corn syrup or maple syrup
White, brown, or maple sugar
Honey
Molasses
Jelly, jam, or marmalade

Dessert List
(Each serving listed equals the calorie value of 1 tablespoon sugar—about 50 calories. All desserts except sugar cookies are fat free)

Foods to Use	Foods to Avoid
1/4 cup tapioca or cornstarch pudding made with fruit and fruit juice or with skim milk	Puddings, custards, and ice creams unless made with skim milk or nonfat dry milk
1/4 cup fruit whip such as prune or apricot	Whipped-cream desserts
1/3 cup gelatin dessert	Cookies unless made with allowed fat or oil and egg
1/4 cup sherbet, preferably water ice	
1/3 cup sweetened canned or frozen fruit (equals 1 portion fruit plus 1 tablespoon sugar)	
1 small slice angel food cake	
2 sugar cookies	
3 nut meringues	
3/4 cup (6 ounces) carbonated beverage	
2/3 cup cocoa (not chocolate) made with skim milk from allowance	
Candies—3 medium or 14 small gum drops; 3 marshmallows; 4 hard fruit drops; or 2 mint patties (no chocolate)	Candies made with chocolate, butter, cream, or coconut
When calories are not restricted, and if allowed fat, skim milk, and eggs are used in preparation:	
Sugar cookies	
Chiffon cake	
Quick yellow cake	
Quick white cake	
Fruit pies	

Miscellaneous—as Desired

Foods to Use	Foods to Avoid
Coffee	Sauces and gravies unless made with allowed fat or oil or made with skimmed milk
Coffee substitutes	
Tea	Cream soups; creamed dishes (may be used if prepared with skim milk and allowed oil)
Unsweetened carbonated beverages	
Artificial sweeteners	Foods containing egg yolk except from day's allowance
Egg white	
Unsweetened gelatin	Commercial popcorn
Lemons and lemon juice	Substitutes for coffee cream
Fat-free consommé and bouillon	
Pickles	
Relishes, catsup	
Vinegar	
Prepared mustard	
Herbs	
Spices	

Table 42–4. Food Allowances for 1800-Calorie Diets for Types 1 to 5 Hyperlipoproteinemia

Food	Type 1	Type 2	Type 3	Type 4	Type 5
Skim milk, cups	4	2	2	2	4
Lean meat, poultry, fish, ounces	5	6–9	6	Ad lib.	6
Egg yolks as substitute for 1 ounce meat	3/week	None	None	3/week	3/week
Bread, cereals	6+	7+	7	8	9
Potato or other starchy vegetable	1+	1+	1	1	1
Vegetables			Ad lib.	Ad lib.	Ad lib.
Dark green or yellow, daily	5	5			
Fruit, servings			3	3	3
Citrus, daily					
Fat, teaspoons	None	6–9	12	Ad lib.	6
Sugars, sweets	Ad lib.	Ad lib.	None	None	None
Low-fat dessert	Ad lib.	Ad lib.	None	None	None
Alcohol	None	With discretion	Subst.*	Subst.*	None

*In these diets up to two servings of alcoholic beverage may be substituted for 2 slices bread. One slice of bread is equal to 1 ounce gin, rum, vodka, or whiskey; 1 1/2 ounces sweet or dessert wine; 2 1/2 ounces dry wine; or 5 ounces beer.

higher than in typical diets because polyunsaturated fats are substituted for saturated fats. Cholesterol is restricted to 300 to 500 mg daily. The carbohydrate intake is not more than 50 per cent of the calories, thus necessitating a protein intake of 20 to 25 per cent of calories. Concentrated sweets and alcohol are contraindicated.

Dietary plans. A committee of the Heart and Lung Institute, National Institutes of Health, has developed detailed dietary plans for the five types of hyperlipoproteinemia described above. These are available in separate booklets for the patient, including individualized dietary plans for the patient, food lists, guidelines for the purchase and preparation of food, and suggestions for eating out. The daily food allowances for the five diets at 1800 calories are summarized in Table 42–4. Although the food lists for these diet plans differ in some details, the lists for the fat-controlled diet in Table 42–3 may be used with complete confidence. The sample menu for the fat-controlled diet and for diets for type 1 and type 4 hyperlipoproteinemia are shown in Table 42–5 to illustrate the variations that are applicable for a given menu.

DIETARY COUNSELING

The National Diet Heart Study established that dietary modification for the correction of hyperlipidemia is feasible for people living in a free-living society.[16] The diet is a palatable one that fits into family menus, the foods are selected from ordinary supplies in any food market, the cost is not greater than that of conventional diets, and the program can be followed indefinitely.

Food lists. The food lists must be meticulously followed with respect to the kinds and amounts of food that may be used and also those that must be avoided. Once the patient is familiar with the lists a great deal of flexibility is both possible and desirable. The food habits must be permanently changed and the connotation of a "special" diet should be avoided. Rather, it is a choice of foods for a more healthful way of living. The nurse and dietitian must recognize that even the most conscientious patient will break his diet once in a while, and he should not be made to feel guilty about an occasional indiscretion.

Table 42–5. Sample Menus for Three 1800-Calorie Diets

Fat-Controlled Diet	Very Low-Fat Diet (Type 1)	Carbohydrate-Restricted Diet (Type 4)
Breakfast		
Orange and grapefruit slices	Same	Same
Whole-wheat cooked cereal	Same	Same
Brown sugar—1 teaspoon	Same	None
Skim milk—1 cup	Same	Same
Egg fried in oil (only 3 times in a week)	None	None
Homemade muffin—2	Toast	Toast
Special margarine—2 teaspoons	None; use jelly	Margarine—2 teaspoons
Coffee	Coffee	Coffee
Sugar for coffee—2 teaspoons	Sugar	No sugar
Luncheon or Supper		
Broiled chicken—3 ounces brushed with oil	Roast chicken—2 ounces; no fat	Broiled chicken brushed with oil
	Mashed potato without fat	Mashed potato with special margarine
Ripe tomato slices fried in 1 teaspoon oil	Tomato wedges on salad; no fat	Ripe tomato slices, fried
Tossed green salad	Same	Same
French dressing—1 tablespoon	None	French dressing
Rye bread—1 slice	Bread—2 slices	Bread—2 slices
Special margarine—1 teaspoon	None; use jelly	Special margarine
Skim milk—1 cup	Skim milk	Skim milk
Baked apple with 1 tablespoon sugar	Same	Fresh apple
Dinner		
Veal baked in tomato sauce with oil	Veal baked in sauce; no oil	Veal baked in sauce with oil
Rice	Same; no fat	Same
Asparagus with pimento and oil	Same but no oil	Asparagus with pimento and oil
Dinner roll	Hard roll	Dinner roll
Special margarine—1 teaspoon	None; use jelly	Special margarine
Skim milk—1 cup	Skim milk—1 cup	Skim milk—1 cup
Sliced peaches	Jello	Sliced peaches
Angel cake, small slice	Angel cake	No cake
Tea or coffee	Tea or coffee with sugar	Tea or coffee, no sugar
Snack		
	Skim milk	
	Sliced peach	
	Bread with jam	

Motivation. Because the serum lipids generally respond within a few weeks following dietary modification, the lowering of lipid levels usually encourages dietary adherence. On the other hand, the patient needs to know that the full benefits of diet on the incidence of clinical disease may not become apparent for up to two or even three years. Although the risk of disease is reduced with appropriate modification of diet, the nurse or dietitian of course would not guarantee that a heart attack will not occur.

Usually the patient who has had a heart attack is more highly motivated to adhere to a modified diet than is the coronary-prone individual. Periodic visits to the physician and the dietitian or nurse are helpful in giving support to the patient as well as in giving greater depth to the level of instruction.

Some special problems. Some patients find it difficult for one reason or another to restrict beef, lamb, and pork to three meals a week. The market supply of fish and veal in some locations is limited, and some people dislike fish and poultry. When beef, lamb, and pork are used more often, the use of safflower oil in preference to other oils helps to counteract the effect of the higher saturated fatty acid content of these meats. (See Table 42–1.)

Food preparation. More food preparation "from scratch" is a key rule for these modified diets. Frozen dinners, casseroles, baked foods, and cake, bread, and pudding mixes usually contain more saturated fat than is permitted. Although home preparation implies that more time must be spent in the kitchen, the results can be rewarding in terms of creating numerous dishes that are delicious and lower in cost than the convenience foods of comparable quality. The person responsible for food preparation often needs some guidance in adapting recipes to the needs of the diet. Home economists for processors of fats and oils have developed many excellent recipes, and the dietitian or nurse should give the homemaker guidance in using those that are appropriate for the diet prescription. The following guidelines may be helpful:

1. Select only lean cuts of meat. Cut off any visible fat. Use only skim milk. (See Figure 42–5.)

2. Meat, fish, and poultry may be cooked in any way. If calories are restricted, frying should not be used. Part of the daily oil allowance may be used in meat preparation.

3. When including soups or stews prepare them a day before use. Chill them thoroughly and remove the fat when it is hardened.

4. The oil allowance may be used in these ways:
   a. Substitute oil for an equivalent amount of solid fat in recipes for muffins, griddle cakes, waffles, yeast breads. Special recipes are also available for pie crust, cake, and cookies made with oil.
   b. Brush meat, poultry, or fish with oil before broiling. Put drippings as a sauce over the food before serving.
   c. Make cream sauces by using oil instead of solid fat, flour, and skim milk; season with herbs.
   d. Marinate meat, poultry, or fish in a mixture of oil, lemon juice or vinegar, and herb seasonings. Use the marinade for basting meat when broiling.
   e. Cook vegetables in a tightly covered pan, using a minimum amount of water, and adding oil and seasonings for flavor. Remove the vegetable when cooked; reduce the volume of liquid and pour over the vegetable as a sauce.
   f. Oil may be blended with skim milk in a blender and flavored for a beverage. It should be consumed immediately after blending.

5. Special margarines may be substituted for part of the oil allowance as stated in Table 42–2.

Eating away from home. Adhering to a fat- or carbohydrate-controlled diet is more difficult in a restaurant, partly because the composition of foods is unknown and partly because the varied menu may be too tempting for the dieter. Nevertheless, an occasional meal away from home should be enjoyed. Those who must eat all their meals in a restaurant will need to determine which ones can best meet their dietary requirements. Some restaurants may be able to give a regular customer some special consideration if his needs are made known. The dieter can safely choose from these foods: fruit, fruit juice, or clear soup; roasted or broiled meat, fish or

Figure 42–5. These cuts of meat show extremely lean portions and those that are lean with some marbling of fat. Some fat is easily separable from the meat. The individual who requires a fat-controlled diet would use the extremely lean portion of the cut. (Courtesy, National Live Stock and Meat Board.)

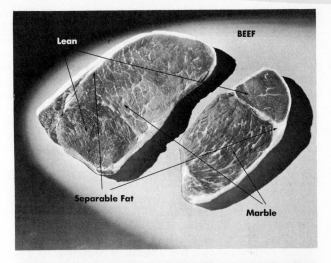

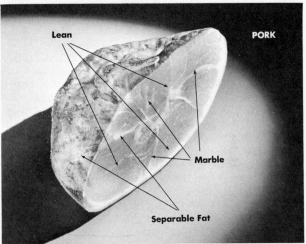

poultry without gravy; plain vegetables (many restaurants do not add much seasoning); tossed or fruit salad with or without dressing (no cheese dressing); hard rolls; fruit, plain gelatin, or fruit ice. Sauces, cream soups, butter, cream, ice cream, pastries, and puddings should be avoided.

PROBLEMS AND REVIEW

1. List at least eight factors that have a bearing on the serum cholesterol level.
2. What relationship exists between the amount and nature of the dietary fat and the serum cholesterol level?
3. In what circumstances is a carbohydrate-restricted diet recommended?

4. *Problem.* Plan a normal diet for one day. Calculate the total fat, the saturated fat, and the linoleic acid content. Revise the diet so that the linoleic acid level is two times as high as the saturated fat. What measures can you suggest for making such a change acceptable to the patient?
5. Examine several pieces of advertising for food fats. Evaluate the statements made according to your understanding of the relationship of fat to the change in blood lipid levels.
6. *Problem.* Look up recipes for escalloped potatoes; fish chowder; waffles. How could you adjust these so that they are suitable for a fat-controlled diet?
7. What are some of the problems that the patient might encounter when restricted to a very low-fat diet for type 1 hyperlipoproteinemia?

CITED REFERENCES

1. Hundley, J. M.: "Heart Disease: Recent Trends in Morbidity and Mortality," *J. Am. Diet. Assoc.,* **52**:195–97, 1968.
2. Review: "The Geographic Pathology of Atherosclerosis," *Nutr. Rev.,* **26**:327–30, 1968.
3. *Risk Factors and Coronary Disease. A Statement for Physicians.* Leaflet. The American Heart Association, New York, 1968.
4. Fredrickson, D. S., *et al.:* "Fat Transport in Lipoproteins—An Integrated Approach to Mechanisms and Disorders," *N. Engl. J. Med.,* **276**:34–44; 94–103; 148–56; 215–26; 273–81, 1967.
5. Christakis, G., *et al.:* "The Anti-coronary Club. A Dietary Approach to the Prevention of Coronary Heart Disease—A Seven-Year Report," *Am. J. Public Health,* **56**:299–314, 1966.
6. Leren, P.: "Effect of Plasma Cholesterol Lowering Diet in Male Survivors of Myocardial Infarction," *Bull. N.Y. Acad. Med.,* **44**:1012–20, 1968.
7. Review: "Los Angeles Veterans Administration Diet Study," *Nutr. Rev.,* **27**:311–16, 1969.
8. Dawber, T. R., and Kannel, W. B.: "Atherosclerosis and You: Pathogenetic Implications from Epidemiologic Observations," *J. Am. Geriatr. Soc.,* **10**:805–21, 1962.
9. Food and Nutrition Board: *Dietary Fat and Human Health.* Pub. 1147. National Academy of Sciences–National Research Council, Washington, D.C., 1966, p. 34.
10. Groen, J. J. *et al.:* "Effect of Interchanging Bread and Sucrose as Main Source of Carbohydrate in a Low Fat Diet on the Serum Cholesterol Levels of Healthy Volunteer Subjects," *Am. J. Clin. Nutr.,* **19**:46–58, 1966.
11. Hodges, R. E., and Krehl, W. A.: "The Role of Carbohydrate in Lipid Metabolism," *Am. J. Clin. Nutr.,* **17**:334–46, 1965.
12. Review: "Cardiovascular Mortality and Soft Drinking Water," *Nutr. Rev.,* **26**:295–97, 1968.
13. Hodges, R. E.: "Dietary and Other Factors Which Influence Serum Lipids," *J. Am. Diet. Assoc.,* **52**:198–201, 1968.
14. Zukel, M. C.: "Revising Booklets on Fat-controlled Meals," *J. Am. Diet. Assoc.,* **54**:20–24, 1969.
15. *Dietary Management of Hyperlipoproteinemia. A Handbook for Physicians.* National Heart and Lung Institute, Bethesda, Md., 1970.
16. Remmell, P. S., *et al.:* "A Dietary Program to Lower Serum Cholesterol," *J. Am. Diet. Assoc.,* **54**:13–19, 1969.

ADDITIONAL REFERENCES

American Heart Association: "The National Diet-Heart Study. Final Report," Monograph No. 18, March 1968, pp. 1–428.

Brown, H. B.: "The National Diet-Heart Study. Implications for Dietitians and Nutritionists," *J. Am. Diet. Assoc.,* **52**:279–87, 1968.

Dayton, S., and Pearce, M. L.: "Prevention of Coronary Heart Disease and Other Complications of Atherosclerosis by Modified Diet," *Am. J. Med.,* **46**:751–62, 1969.

Jernigan, A. K.: "Ideas for Fat-Restricted Diets," *Hospitals,* **43**:121–24, May 1, 1969.

Kaufman, N. A., *et al.:* "Comparison of Effects of Fructose, Sucrose, Glucose, and Starch on Serum Lipids in Patients with Hypertriglyceridemia and Normal Subjects," *Am. J. Clin. Nutr.* **20**:131–32, 1967.

Keys, A.: "Official Collective Recommendations on Diet in the Scandinavian Countries," *Nutr. Rev.,* **26**:259–63, 1968.

Kuo, P. T., *et al.:* "Dietary Carbohydrates in Hyperlipidemia (Hyperglyceridemia); Hepatic and Adipose Tissue Lipogenic Activities," *Am. J. Clin. Nutr.,* **20**:116–25, 1967.

Levy, R. I., and Glueck, C. J.: "Hypertriglyceridemia, Diabetes Mellitus, and Coronary Vessel Disease," *Arch. Intern. Med.,* **123**:220–28, 1969.

Mojonnier, L., and Hall, Y.: "The National Diet-Heart Study—Assessment of Dietary Adherence," *J. Am. Diet. Assoc.,* **52**:288–92, 1968.

Moore, M. C., *et al.:* "Dietary-Atherosclerosis Study on Deceased Persons, Methodology," *J. Am. Diet. Assoc.,* **56**:13–22, 1970.

Remmell, P. S., *et al.:* "A Dietary Program to Lower Serum Cholesterol," *J. Am. Diet. Assoc.,* **54**:13–19, 1969.

Review: "Physical Training and Cardiovascular Status," *Nutr. Rev.,* **27**:103–108, 1969.

Shaffer, C. F.: "Ascorbic Acid and Atherosclerosis," *Am. J. Clin. Nutr.,* **23**:27–30, 1970.

Stamler, J., *et al.:* "Coronary Proneness and Approaches to Preventing Heart Attacks," *Am. J. Nurs.,* **66**:1788–93, 1966.

Stare, F. J.: "Nutritional Suggestions for the Primary Prevention of Coronary Heart Disease," *J. Am. Diet. Assoc.,* **48**:88–94, 1966.

Vavra, C. E., *et al.:* "Meeting the Challenge of Educational Care in Heart Disease," *Am. J. Public Health,* **56**:1507–11, 1966.

INSTRUCTIONAL MATERIALS FOR THE PATIENT

American Heart Association, New York (or local chapters)
  Eat Well But Eat Wisely, leaflet, 1969.
  Planning Fat-Controlled Meals for Approximately 2000–2600 Calories (revised), 1967.
  Planning Fat-Controlled Meals for 1200 and 1800 Calories (revised), 1966.
  Programmed Instruction for Fat-Controlled Diet, 1800 Calories, 1969.
  Recipes for Fat-Controlled, Low Cholesterol Meals, Leaflet, 1968.
  Reduce Your Risk of Heart Attack, leaflet, 1966.
  The Way to a Man's Heart, 1968.

Blakeslee, A., and Stamler, J.: *Your Heart Has Nine Lives,* condensed ed., Corn Products Co., New York, 1966.

Dietary Management of Hyperlipoproteinemia. Booklets for Type I, Type II, Type III, Type IV, and Type V. National Heart and Lung Institute, National Institutes of Health, Bethesda, Md., 1970.

Keys, A., and Keys, M.: *Eat Well and Stay Well,* 2nd ed. Doubleday & Co., Garden City, N.Y., 1963.

A Low Cholesterol Diet Manual. The University of Iowa, Iowa City, 1968.

The Prudent Diet. Bureau of Nutrition, Department of Health, New York, 1969.

Stead, E. S., and Warren, G. K.: *Low Fat Cookery.* McGraw-Hill Book Co., New York, 1959.

43 Dietary Management of Acute and Chronic Diseases of the Heart

Sodium-Restricted Diet

Role of nutrition in cardiac efficiency. The heart muscle, like any other body tissue, is dependent upon an adequate supply of all the essential nutrients. The markedly malnourished peoples of the world frequently manifest cardiac impairment such as dyspnea and palpitation on exertion, enlargement of the heart and systolic murmurs. Severe thiamine deficiency has been shown to be especially responsible for these conditions which are common manifestations of beriberi.

Semistarvation diets given to 36 young men in controlled studies at the University of Minnesota[1] resulted in loss of weight, lower metabolic rate, decrease in blood pressure, pulse rate, and heart size. There was a general depression of circulatory function in these previously normal individuals which must not be confused with circulatory failure. When these men were again given normal diets, the blood pressure returned to normal. The increase in body weight and the total daily metabolism placed a temporary strain on the cardiovascular system which resulted in the frequent occurrence of moderate tachycardia and dyspnea.

Similar observations were made in a survey of the population in Leningrad during and following the siege of World War II. During the period of semistarvation the incidence of hypertension and of associated cardiac disease decreased very markedly, but the rate and severity of hypertensive disease increased so alarmingly during recovery as to constitute a major medical problem.

Clinical findings related to dietary management. Heart disease affects people of all ages, but it is most frequent in those of middle age and is most often caused by atherosclerosis. (See Chapter 42.) Diseases of the heart may affect (1) the pericardium or outer covering of the organ, (2) the endocardium or membranes lining the heart, or (3) the myocardium or the heart muscle. In addition, the blood vessels within the heart or those leaving the heart or the heart valves may be diseased. Heart disease may be acute with no prior warning, as in a coronary occlusion, or chronic with progressively decreasing ability to maintain the circulation.

The heart may be only slightly damaged so that nearly normal circulation is maintained to all parts of the body; this is a period of "compensation." The patient is able to continue normal activities with perhaps some restriction of vigorous activity. On the other hand, in severe damage, or "decompensation," the heart is no longer able to maintain the normal circulation to supply nutrients and oxygen to the tissues, or to dispose of carbon dioxide and other wastes. Prompt measures including bed rest, oxygen, and drug therapy are essential to relieve the strain.

Impairment of the heart may be manifested by dyspnea on exertion, weakness, and pain in the chest. In severe failure there is a marked dilatation of the heart with enlargement of the liver. The circulation to the tissues and through the kidney is so impaired that sodium and water are held in the tissue spaces. Edema fluid collects first in the extremities and, with increasing failure, in the abdominal and chest cavities. This is referred to as congestive heart failure.

Infections, obesity, hypertension, and constipation complicate and make the treatment of diseases of the heart more difficult. Moreover, the heart is located close to several other organs, especially the stomach and intestines, and distention taking place in either of these organs is likely to press against and interfere with the functioning of the heart. Loss of appetite, nausea, vomiting, and other digestive disorders are common symptoms of heart disease.

Modification of the diet. Objectives in the dietary management of cardiac patients include (1) maximum rest for the heart, (2) prevention or elimination of edema, (3) maintenance of good nutrition, and (4) acceptability of the program by the patient. The following modifications of the diet are necessary to achieve these goals.

Energy. Loss of weight by the obese leads to considerable reduction in the work of the heart because the imbalance between body mass and strength of the heart muscle is corrected. There are a slowing of the heart rate, a drop in blood pressure, and thereby improved cardiac efficiency. Some physicians recommend a mild degree of weight loss even for the cardiac patient of normal weight. Usually a 1000- to 1200-calorie diet is suitable for an obese patient in bed; rarely is it necessary to reduce calories to a level below this.

Those patients whose weight is at a desirable level are permitted a maintenance level of calories during convalescence and their return to activity. Usually 1600 to 2000 calories will suffice, with slight increases as the activity becomes greater.

Nutritive adequacy. Normal allowances of protein, minerals, and vitamins are recommended. The proportions and kinds of fat and carbohydrate may be modified so that polyunsaturated fatty acids and/or complex carbohydrates predominate (see Chapter 42). When sodium is restricted, other sources of iodine should be prescribed especially for pregnant women and children. A severe restriction of sodium also reduces the intake of vitamin A because carrots and some of the deep-green leafy vegetables that are high in sodium must be omitted.

Sodium. A sodium-restricted diet is indicated when there is retention of fluid and sodium. Usually a restriction of sodium to 500 mg is satisfactory in congestive heart failure, but occasionally sodium may need to be reduced further. Some patients who have associated renal disease are unable to reabsorb sodium in a normal fashion; these "salt wasters" may become depleted of sodium on a severely restricted diet.

Once edema has disappeared, a moderately-restricted sodium diet—about 1000 mg—is likely to be satisfactory. Many patients require only a mild restriction of sodium, or none at all.

Fluid. The restriction of fluid is not required so long as the sodium is restricted. Less work is required by the kidney when ample fluid is available for the excretion of wastes. Because of the homeostatic mechanisms afforded by adrenal and pituitary hormones, water is retained only when there is sufficient sodium to maintain physiologic concentrations. (See also page 132.) An intake of 2 liters of fluid daily has been found to be less work for the kidney than the ingestion of 1 or 3 liters.[2]

In advanced congestive failure, especially with excessive use of diuretics, water may be retained even though the sodium intake is low. The hormonal controls are no longer balanced, and the sodium concentration of extracellular fluid is lower even though the total body content of sodium may be high. Such a circumstance necessitates the restriction of fluid as well as sodium.

Amount of food. Small amounts of food given in five or six meals are preferable to bulky, large meals that place an excessive burden upon the heart during digestion. Part of the food normally allowed at mealtime may be saved for between-meal feedings.

Consistency. When decompensation occurs, liquid or soft, bland, easily digested foods that require little chewing should be used. During the early stages of illness, the patient must be fed. When his condition improves, he may be given foods that are not strained, but that are easy to chew and to digest.

Choice of food. Abdominal distention must be avoided. Until the patient's food tolerances are known, it is best to omit vegetables of the cabbage family, onions, turnips, legumes, and melons. Occasionally a patient may complain that milk is distending to him. Because of its relaxing effect, the physician may prescribe small amounts of alcohol.

Constipation must be avoided by the judicious

use of fruits and vegetables, prune juice, and a sufficient fluid intake.

Progression of the diet. During severe decompensation, as in coronary occlusion, rest is the primary consideration, and all attempts to feed the patient are avoided for the first few days. Then small feedings of bland, easily digested foods are given as tolerated. At this stage, sodium is restricted to 500 mg or less daily. The foods may be selected from those permitted for the Soft Diet, page 404, giving only small amounts at each of five or six feedings. Initially, the foods may be puréed to eliminate the need for chewing.

The *Karell* diet has been prescribed by many physicians for more than 100 years during the initial stages of treatment. It consists of only 800 ml of milk daily in four feedings of 200 ml each given at four-hour intervals. This amount of milk provides 32 gm protein, 680 calories, and 480 mg sodium. After three or four days this routine is liberalized to include toast, eggs, cream soups, and fruit. A diet of regular consistency is allowed only when the patient is able to feed himself and can chew without too much strain on the heart.

Dangers of sodium restriction. Diets that are very low in sodium must be used with caution since there is occasional danger of depletion of body sodium. Hot weather may bring about great losses of sodium through the skin, and vomiting, diarrhea, surgery, renal damage, or the use of mercurial diuretics also increases the amounts of sodium lost from the body. Sodium depletion is characterized by weakness, abdominal cramps, lethargy, oliguria, azotemia, and disturbances in the acid-base balance. Patients must be instructed to recognize the symptoms of danger and to consult a physician immediately when they occur.

SODIUM-RESTRICTED DIETS

Levels of sodium restriction. Sodium-restricted diets are used for the prevention, control, and elimination of edema in many pathologic conditions, and occasionally for the alleviation of hypertension. Since sodium is the ion of importance, it is incorrect to designate a diet as salt free, salt poor, or low salt. Moreover, to call a diet low sodium or sodium restricted is misleading, since any amount of sodium below the normal sodium intake would satisfy such a description, but would not necessarily be at therapeutic levels. Sodium-restricted diets should be prescribed in terms of milligrams of sodium, e.g., 500-mg-sodium diet.

The normal diet contains about 3 to 6 gm of sodium daily, although a liberal intake of salty food results in considerably higher sodium levels. The normal diet may be modified for its sodium content as described in the following paragraphs.

250-mg-sodium diet (11 mEq[*]; very low sodium). No salt used in cooking; careful selection of foods low in sodium; low-sodium milk substituted for regular milk. This diet is used in conditions such as cirrhosis of the liver with ascites; very occasionally in hypertension; for congestive heart failure if the 500-mg level is ineffective.

500-mg-sodium diet (22 mEq; strict sodium restriction). No salt used in cooking; careful selection of foods in measured amounts; regular milk. This level may be used for congestive heart failure; occasionally in renal diseases with edema, or cirrhosis with ascites.

1000-mg sodium diet (43mEq; moderate sodium restriction). No salt in cooking; permits slightly higher protein level if needed, as in pregnancy; may include measured amount of salt, or salted bread and butter.

Mild sodium restriction. Some salt may be used in cooking, but no salty foods are permitted; no salt is used at the table. Sodium content may vary from 2400 to 4500 mg. This level is used as a maintenance diet in cardiac and renal diseases.

Sources of sodium. The sodium-restricted diet must be planned with respect to the amount of naturally occurring sodium in foods and the sodium added in food preparation and processing. Sodium values for common foods are given in Table A-2. Most prepared foods show wide variations in sodium content, depending upon conditions of growth and processing of the food, so-

[*]1 milliequivalent of sodium is 23 mg; thus, $250 \div 23 = 11$ mEq.

dium content of water used in preparation, and others.[3] The values listed in any table should not be considered absolute, but they do give reasonable approximations of foods which may be used and which should be avoided.

Naturally occurring sodium in foods. The natural sodium content of animal foods is relatively high and reasonably constant. Thus, meat, poultry, fish, eggs, milk, and cheese are the foods which, although nutritionally essential, must be used in measured amounts. Organ meats contain somewhat more sodium than muscle meats. Shellfish of all kinds are especially high in sodium, but other saltwater fish contain no more sodium than freshwater fish. A few plant foods, especially greens like spinach, chard, and kale, contain significant amounts of sodium and are omitted in the more severely restricted diets.

Fruits, cereals, and most vegetables are insignificant sources of sodium. Likewise, sugars, oils, shortenings, and unsalted butter and margarine are negligible sources of sodium.

The drinking water in many localities contains appreciable quantities of sodium, either naturally or through the use of water softeners. When the sodium content is in excess of 20 mg per liter, the daily intake from water alone may be appreciable.[4]

Sodium added to foods. Table salt is by far the most important source of sodium in the diet. Each gram of salt contains about 400 mg sodium; thus, a teaspoon of salt would furnish 2000 mg sodium. Salt is not only used in cooking and at the table but it also finds its way into many products through manufacturing processes: as in the preservation of ham, bacon, frozen and dried fish; in the brining of pickles, corned beef, and sauerkraut; in koshering of meat; as a rinse to prevent discoloration of fruits in canning; as a means of separating peas and lima beans for quality before freezing or canning. Canned foods (except fruits), frozen casseroles, dinners, and baked foods, biscuit, bread, cookie, dessert, and sauce mixes contain high levels of salt.

Baking powder and baking soda are widely used in food preparation. Potassium bicarbonate may be used in place of sodium bicarbonate, and sodium-free baking powder may be substituted for regular baking powder.

Numerous sodium compounds other than sodium chloride, baking soda, and baking powder are used in food manufacture: sodium benzoate as a preservative in relishes, sauces, margarine; disodium phosphate to shorten the cooking time of cereals; sodium citrate to enhance the flavor of gelatin desserts and beverages; monosodium glutamate (MSG) as a widely used seasoning in restaurants and in food processing; sodium propionate in cheeses, breads, and cakes to retard mold growth; sodium alginate for smooth texture in chocolate milk and ice cream; and sodium sulfite as a bleach in the preparation of maraschino cherries and to prevent discoloration of dried fruits. (See Figure 43–1.)

Sodium in drugs. Many laxatives, antibiotics, alkalizers, cough medicines, and sedatives contain sodium, and the physician needs to determine whether the amount of a given drug may nullify the effects of a prescribed diet. Patients need to be especially warned against self-medication with sodium bicarbonate or antacids.

Unit lists for sodium-restricted diets. A joint committee of the American Dietetic Association, the American Heart Association, and the United States Public Health Service has grouped foods for sodium-restricted diets in *Unit Lists*. Each list corresponds closely to the meal exchange lists (Table A-4, Appendix), but foods which are not to be used are also listed. It will be noted that the group C vegetables of the unit lists are those included in the bread exchange lists. In addition, a "Free Choice" list providing 75 calories per unit permits somewhat more flexibility in menu planning.

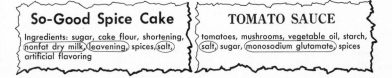

Figure 43–1. Watch for the words *salt* and *sodium* on labels when selecting foods for sodium-restricted diets. Leavenings and nonfat dry milk also contribute significant amounts of sodium.

So-Good Spice Cake
Ingredients: sugar, cake flour, shortening, nonfat dry milk, leavening, spices, salt, artificial flavoring

TOMATO SAUCE
tomatoes, mushrooms, vegetable oil, starch, salt, sugar, monosodium glutamate, spices

Table 43–1. Nutritive Values of Food Lists for Planning Sodium-Restricted Diets*

List	Amount	Energy calories	Protein gm	Fat gm	Carbo-hydrate gm	Sodium mg
1. Milk, whole	1 cup, regular	170	8	10	12	120
	1 cup, low-sodium	170	8	10	12	7
Milk, nonfat	1 cup, regular	85	8	—	12	120
	1 cup, low-sodium	85	8	—	12	7
2. Vegetables						
Group A	1/2 cup	—	—	—	—	9
Group B	1/2 cup	35	2	—	7	9
Group C	Varies with choice	70	2	—	15	5
3. Fruits	Varies with choice	40	—	—	10	2
4. Low-sodium breads, cereals	Varies with choice	70	2	—	15	5
5. Meat, poultry, fish, eggs, or cheese	1 ounce meat or equivalent	75	7	5	—	25
6. Fats	1 teaspoon butter or equivalent	45	—	5	—	tr
7. Free choice	Varies with choice	75	See list; depends on selection made			

*Arranged from *Your 500 Milligram Sodium Diet,* American Heart Association, New York, 1958.

LIST 1. MILK UNITS

Each unit whole milk: sodium 120 mg (7 mg when low-sodium milk is used); calories, 170; protein, 8 gm; fat, 10 gm; carbohydrate, 12 gm.

Each unit fresh skim milk or nonfat dry milk: sodium 120 mg (7 mg when low-sodium milk is used); calories, 85; protein, 8 gm; fat, negligible; carbohydrate, 12 gm.

Milk, whole — 1 cup
Milk, evaporated whole — 1 cup reconstituted
Milk, nonfat dry — 3 to 4 tablespoons (Read label for exact amount to make 1 cup)
Milk, fresh skim, evaporated skim reconstituted, or nonfat dry reconstituted — 1 cup

Foods to Avoid

Commercial foods made with milk: ice cream, sherbet, milk shakes, chocolate milk, malted milk, milk mixes, condensed milk.

Note: Nonfat dry or fresh skim milk are equal to whole milk in caloric and fat value when 2 fat units are added to each milk unit.

LIST 2. VEGETABLES

Fresh, Frozen, or Dietetic Canned Vegetables Only

Group A, each unit: sodium, 9 mg; calories, protein, fat, and carbohydrate, negligible. Each unit is a ½ cup serving.

Asparagus
Broccoli
Brussels sprouts
Cabbage
Cauliflower
Chicory
Cucumber
Eggplant
Endive
Escarole
Green beans
Lettuce
Mushrooms
Okra
Peppers, green or red
Radishes
Squash, summer (yellow, zucchini, etc.)
Tomato juice (low-sodium dietetic)
Tomatoes
Turnip greens
Wax beans

Food to Avoid

Canned vegetables or juices except low-sodium dietetic
Artichoke
Beet greens
Celery
Chard, Swiss
Dandelion greens
Kale
Mustard greens
Sauerkraut
Spinach

Group B, each unit: sodium, 9 mg; calories, 35; protein, 2 gm; fat, negligible; carbohydrate, 7 gm. Each unit is a ½ cup serving.

Onions
Peas (fresh or low-sodium dietetic canned)
Pumpkin
Rutabaga (yellow turnip)
Squash, winter (acorn, butternut, Hubbard, etc.)

Foods to Avoid

Beets
Carrots
White turnips
Frozen peas if processed with salt
Canned vegetables except dietetic

Note: Two units of vegetables from group A may be substituted for one unit from group B.

Group C, each unit: sodium, 5 mg; calories, 70; protein, 2 gm; fat, negligible; carbohydrate, 15 gm.

Beans, dried, Lima or navy	½ cup cooked	**Foods to Avoid**
Beans, Lima, fresh	⅓ cup cooked	Frozen Lima beans if processed with salt
Beans, baked (no pork)	¼ cup	Canned vegetables except dietetic low-sodium
Corn	⅓ cup or ½ small ear	Hominy
Lentils, dried	½ cup cooked	Potato chips
Parsnips	⅔ cup	
Peas, split green or yellow or cowpeas	½ cup cooked	
Potato, white	1 small or ½ cup mashed	
Potato, sweet	¼ cup or ½ small	

Note: One unit from the bread list may be substituted for one unit of group C vegetable.

LIST 3. FRUITS

Unsweetened: Fresh, Frozen, Canned, or Dried

Each unit fruit: sodium, 2 mg; calories, 40; protein, negligible; fat, negligible; carbohydrate, 10 gm.

Apple	1 small	
Apple juice or apple cider	⅓ cup	
Applesauce	½ cup	
Apricots, dried	4 halves	
Apricots, fresh	2 medium	
Apricot nectar	¼ cup	
Banana	½ small	
Blackberries	1 cup	
Blueberries	⅔ cup	
Cantaloupe	¼ small	
Cherries	10 large	
Cranberries, sweetened	1 tablespoon	
Cranberry juice	⅓ cup	
Dates	2	
Fig	1 medium	
Fruit cup or mixed fruit	½ cup	
Grapefruit	½ small	
Grapefruit juice	½ cup	
Grapes	12	
Grape juice	¼ cup	
Honeydew melon	⅛ medium	
Mango	½ small	
Orange	1 small	
Orange juice	½ cup	
Papaya	⅓ medium	
Peach	1 medium	
Pear	1 small	
Pineapple	2 slices	
Pineapple	½ cup diced	
Pineapple juice	⅓ cup	
Plums	2 medium	
Prunes	2 medium	
Prune juice	¼ cup	
Raisins	2 tablespoons	
Raspberries	1 cup	
Rhubarb, sweetened	2 tablespoons	
Strawberries	1 cup	
Tangerine	1 large	
Tangerine juice	½ cup	
Watermelon	1 cup	

Foods to Avoid

Crystallized or glazed fruit
Maraschino cherries
Dried fruit with sodium sulfite added

Note: Use as desired: fresh lemons and limes and their juices; unsweetened cranberries and cranberry juice; unsweetened rhubarb.

LIST 4. BREAD

Low-Sodium Breads, Cereals, and Cereal Products

Each bread unit: sodium, 5 mg; calories, 70; protein, 2 gm; fat, negligible; carbohydrate, 15 gm.

Breads and rolls (yeast) made without salt

Bread	1 slice	**Foods to Avoid**
Melba toast, unsalted	4 pieces (3½″ × 1½″ × ⅛″)	Yeast bread, rolls, or Melba toast made with salt or from commercial mixes
Roll	1 medium	

Breads (quick) made with sodium-free baking powder or potassium bicarbonate and without salt, or made from low-sodium dietetic mix

Biscuit	1 medium	**Foods to Avoid**
Corn bread	1 cube (1½″)	Quick breads made with baking powder, baking soda, salt or MSG or made from commercial mixes
Griddle cakes	2 three-inch	
Muffin	1 medium	

Cereals, cooked, unsalted

Farina	½ cup cooked	**Foods to Avoid**
Grits	½ cup cooked	Quick-cooking and enriched cereals which contain a sodium compound. Read the label.
Oatmeal	½ cup cooked	
Rolled wheat	½ cup cooked	
Wheat meal	½ cup cooked	

Cereals, dry

Puffed Rice	¾ cup	**Foods to Avoid**
Puffed Wheat	¾ cup	Dry cereals except as listed
Shredded Wheat	1 biscuit	

Any for which the label indicates the sodium content is less than 6 mg sodium per 100 gm cereal.

Barley	1½ tablespoons, uncooked	**Foods to Avoid**
		Self-rising cornmeal
Cornmeal	2 tablespoons	Graham crackers or any other except low-sodium dietetic
Cornstarch	2½ tablespoons	
Crackers, low sodium	5 two-inch squares	Salted popcorn
Flour	2½ tablespoons	Pretzels
Macaroni	½ cup cooked	Waffles containing salt, baking powder, baking soda, or egg white
Matzo, plain, unsalted	1 five-inch square	
Noodles	½ cup cooked	
Popcorn, unsalted	1½ cups	
Rice, brown or white	½ cup cooked	
Spaghetti	½ cup cooked	
Tapioca	2 tablespoons uncooked	
Waffle, yeast	1 three-inch square	

Note: One unit from the vegetable list, group C, may be substituted for one bread unit.

LIST 5. MEAT

Meat, Poultry, Fish, Eggs, and Low-Sodium Cheese and Peanut Butter
  Each meat unit: sodium, 25 mg; calories, 75; protein, 7 gm; fat, 5 gm; carbohydrate, negligible.

Meat or poultry: fresh, frozen, or canned low-sodium. One ounce cooked is a unit.

Beef	**Foods to Avoid**
Chicken	Brains or kidneys
Duck	Canned, salted, or smoked meat: bacon, bologna,
Lamb	chipped or corned beef, frankfurters, ham, kosher
Liver (only once in 2 weeks)	meats, luncheon meat, salt pork, sausage, smoked
Pork	tongue, etc.
Quail	
Rabbit	
Tongue, fresh	
Turkey	
Veal	

Fish or fish fillets, fresh only. One ounce cooked is one unit.

Bass		**Foods to Avoid**
Bluefish		Frozen fish fillets
Catfish		Canned, salted, or smoked fish: anchovies, caviar,
Cod		salted and dried cod, herring, canned salmon
Eels		(except dietetic low-sodium), sardines, canned
Flounder		tuna (except dietetic low-sodium)
Halibut		Shellfish: clams, crabs, lobsters, oysters, scallops,
Rockfish		shrimp, etc.
Salmon		
Sole		
Trout		
Tuna		
Salmon, canned low-sodium dietetic	1 ounce	
Tuna, canned low-sodium dietetic	1 ounce	
Cheese, cottage, unsalted	¼ cup	**Foods to Avoid**
Cheese, processed, low-sodium dietetic	1 ounce	Cheese, except low-sodium dietetic
Egg (limit, 1 per day)	1	Peanut butter unless low-sodium dietetic
Peanut butter, low-sodium dietetic	2 tablespoons	

LIST 6. FAT

Each fat unit: negligible sodium; calories, 45; fat, 5 gm.

Avocado	⅓ of four-inch	**Foods to Avoid**
Butter, unsalted	1 teaspoon	Salted butter
Cream, heavy, sweet or sour	1 tablespoon	Bacon and bacon fat
Cream, light, sweet or sour	2 tablespoons	Salt pork
Fat or oil, cooking, unsalted	1 teaspoon	Olives
French dressing, unsalted	1 tablespoon	Commercial French or other dressing except low
		sodium
Margarine, unsalted	1 teaspoon	Salted margarine
Mayonnaise, unsalted	1 teaspoon	Commercial mayonnaise, except low sodium
Nuts, unsalted	6 small	Salted nuts

LIST 7. FREE CHOICE

Each free choice unit: 75 calories, and small amount of sodium. Other nutrients depend upon the choice which is made.

Bread list	1 unit
Candy, homemade, salt free, or special low sodium	75 calories
Fat list	2 units
Fruit list	2 units
Sugar, white or brown	4 teaspoons
Syrup, honey, jelly, jam, or marmalade	4 teaspoons
Vegetable list, group C.	1 unit

MISCELLANEOUS FOODS

Beverages
Alcoholic with doctor's permission
Cocoa made with milk from diet
Coffee, instant or regular
Coffee substitute
Fruit juices (but count as fruit units)
Lemonade, using sugar from diet, or calcium cycla-
  mate, or saccharin
Milk (but count as milk units)
Postum
Tea

Foods to Avoid
Instant cocoa mixes
Prepared beverage mixes, including fruit-flavored
  powders
Fountain beverages
Malted milk and other milk preparations

Candy, homemade, salt free, or special low sodium
Cornstarch
Gelatin, plain, unflavored (use fruit allowance)

Foods to Avoid
Commercial candies
Commercial sweetened gelatin desserts

Leavening agents
Cream of tartar
Sodium-free baking powder
Potassium bicarbonate
Yeast

Foods to Avoid
Regular baking powder
Baking soda (sodium bicarbonate)

Rennet dessert powder (not tablets)
Tapioca (count as bread unit)

Foods to Avoid
Rennet tablets
Pudding mixes
Molasses

FLAVORING AIDS

Allspice
Almond extract
Anise seed
Basil
Bay leaf

Bouillon cube (low so-
  dium)
Caraway seed
Cardamom
Chives

Avoid These Flavoring Aids
Barbecue sauce
Bouillon cube, regular
Catsup
Celery salt, seed, leaves

Cinnamon
Cloves
Cocoa (1–2 teaspoons)
Cumin
Curry
Dill
Fennel
Garlic
Ginger
Horseradish (prepared without salt)
Juniper
Lemon juice or extract
Mace
Maple extract
Marjoram
Mint
Mustard, dry
Nutmeg
Onion, fresh, juice or sliced
Orange extract
Oregano
Paprika
Parsley
Pepper

Peppermint extract
Pimento
Poppy seed
Poultry seasoning
Purslane
Rosemary
Saccharin
Sucaryl (calcium salt only)
Saffron
Sage
Salt substitutes (with physician's approval)
Savory
Sesame seeds
Sorrel
Sugar
Tarragon
Thyme
Turmeric
Vanilla extract
Vinegar
Wine, if allowed by physician
Walnut extract

Foods to Avoid
Chili sauce
Cyclamates
Garlic salt
Horse radish prepared with salt
Meat extracts, sauces, tenderizers
Monosodium glutamate
Mustard, prepared
Olives
Onion salt
Pickles
Relishes
Salt
Soy sauce
Worcestershire sauce

Meal planning with unit lists. The 500-mg-sodium diet at three caloric levels is shown in Table 43–2.

Table 43–2. Food Allowances for 500-Milligram-Sodium Diet*

Food List	1200 Calories units	1800 Calories units	Unrestricted Calories units
Milk	2 (skim)	2 (whole)	2 (whole)
Vegetables, A	1	1	1 or more
B	1	1	1 or more
C	1	1	1 or more
Fruit	4	4	2 or more
Bread	5	7	4 or more
Meat	5	5	5 only
Fat	0	4	as desired
Free choice	1	2	as desired

*The 500-mg-sodium diet may be adjusted for lower or higher levels of sodium as follows:

250 mg sodium: substitute low-sodium milk for regular milk

1000 mg sodium: substitute 2 slices ordinary salted bread (contains 400 mg sodium) and 2 teaspoons salted butter (contains 100 mg sodium) for 2 slices unsalted bread and 2 teaspoons unsalted butter; *or* use 1/4 teaspoon salt each day at the table to salt the food.

Mild sodium restriction: use foods lightly salted and allow ordinary salted bread and butter, regular milk. Omit the salting of food at the table; salty foods such as potato chips, salted popcorn and nuts, olives, pickles, relishes, meat sauces, smoked and salted meats.

Meal Pattern (500 mg sodium, 1800 calories)

BREAKFAST

Fruit—1 unit
Egg—1 only

Bread—2 units
Butter—1 unit
Milk—½ cup whole
Coffee or tea
Sugar—4 teaspoons

LUNCHEON OR SUPPER

Meat, fish, or poultry—2 ounces
Vegetable, A group
Bread—3 units

Butter, unsalted—1 unit
Jelly—2 teaspoons
Milk—1 cup
Fruit—1 unit

DINNER

Meat, fish, or poultry—2 ounces
Vegetable, B group—½ cup
Vegetable, C group—½ cup
Bread, unsalted—2 units
Butter, unsalted—2 units
Jelly—2 teaspoons
Fruit—2 units
Milk—½ cup

Sample Menu

Baked apple with sugar
Soft-cooked egg
Puffed Wheat
Low-sodium toast—1 slice
Butter, unsalted—1 teaspoon
Milk—½ cup
Coffee with sugar (Note: 3 teaspoons sugar used in apple)

Broiled fresh flounder
Stewed tomatoes
Baked potato—1 small
Low-sodium muffins—2 medium
Butter, unsalted—1 teaspoon
Grape jelly—2 teaspoons
Milk, whole—1 cup
Bing cherries

Broiled breast of chicken
Fresh green peas
Steamed rice (from bread list)
Low-sodium rolls—2
Butter, unsalted—2 teaspoons
Currant jelly—2 teaspoons
Sliced banana
Milk—½ cup
Tea with lemon

DIETARY COUNSELING

Perhaps no diet provides greater obstacles with respect to acceptance for taste appeal, and understanding of the permissible food choices than does the sodium-restricted diet. Skilled counseling of the patient by dietitian, nurse, and physician is essential from the time the diet is first prescribed. Far too many patients have assumed that the omission of salt merely represented poor cookery and have eaten forbidden foods brought in by well-meaning but uninformed relatives and friends. (See Figure 43–2.)

When a sodium-restricted diet is to be continued in the home, the patient should be given some understanding of the purposes of the diet and some indication regarding the length of time he may need to use the diet.

He needs information on the foods that are permitted on the diet, what foods are contraindicated, where foods may be purchased, and how to prepare palatable foods with flavoring aids. He should not expect foods to taste the same as those that are salted, but in time most patients learn to adjust to the change in flavors.

The individual responsible for meal preparation must be included in all phases of dietary counseling so that she understands the importance of the diet and learns what modifications in planning, purchasing, and preparation are required.

The American Heart Association has published detailed booklets concerning three levels of sodium restriction and low-calorie and maintenance energy allowances. For patients who find the details confusing, concise leaflets have also been prepared. Neither of these teaching aids should take the place of individualized instruction, nor should the patient be expected to comprehend all the information in one or two counseling sessions.

Cultural patterns must be considered, inasmuch as favorite dishes are often high in sodium. Usually, these dishes may be adapted within the sodium restriction rather than omitting them entirely.

Label information. The patient and the homemaker must be taught to read labels of food products, looking especially for the words *salt* and *sodium*. (See Figure 43–1.) Standards of identity have been established for many food products by the Food and Drug Administration. Such products do not need to carry a listing of ingredients. Thus, the fact that salt is not listed is no guarantee that it is a low-sodium product. Mayonnaise, catsup, and canned vegetables are examples of foods ordinarily prepared with salt but which belong in the category of foods for which a standard of identity has been set up.

Foods specially produced for sodium-restricted diets must be labeled according to regulations set up by the Food and Drug Administration. The label must indicate the sodium content in an average serving and also in 100 gm of the food. (See Figure 43–3.) Although foods may have been processed without added sodium compounds, some of them may exceed the limits allowed for a given category. For example, a vegetable that contains 50 mg sodium per serving is much higher than the average sodium content of vegetables in lists 2A, B, and C.

Preparation of food. Ingenuity is required in the preparation of foods for sodium-restricted diets so that they may be accepted by the patient. A number of salt substitutes are available, but they should be used only upon the recommendation of the physician since some of them contain potassium which may be contraindicated when there is renal damage.

Numerous flavoring aids are available (see page 569 for list) to provide taste appeal. Herbs and spices are especially useful, but they should be used with a light touch.

Delicious yeast breads, muffins, waffles, and doughnuts may be prepared using part of the milk and egg allowance of the diet. Low-sodium baking powder must be substituted for regular baking powder. Low-sodium milk is prepared by passing milk through an ion exchange resin in the cold. The sodium is replaced by an equivalent amount of potassium, and the resultant milk is similar in flavor to whole milk. The calcium value of low-sodium milk is about 80 per cent of that

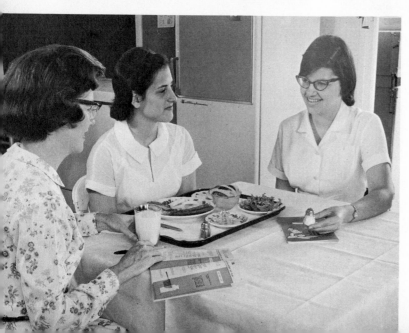

Figure 43–2. Students evaluate appearance and flavor of a sodium-restricted diet. Essential characteristics are reviewed with the 500-mg sodium-restricted diet booklet of the American Heart Association. (Courtesy, College of Home Economics, Drexel University.)

Figure 43–3. Foods intended for use in therapeutic diets must be labeled with information concerning their nutritive values. The sodium content per 100 gm and per average serving is included.

Dietetic Peaches
Packed in water without added sugar

PROXIMATE ANALYSIS
(including liquid in this can)

Protein	0.6%	Milligrams sodium per	
Fat	0.03%	100 grams	6
Crude fiber	0.4%	Milligrams sodium per	
Ash	0.3%	4 ounce serving	7
Moisture	92%	Calories per 100 grams	31
Available carbohydrate	6.7%	Calories per ounce	9

of whole milk, the thiamine content is about half as great, and the potassium level is almost twice as high. In other nutrients low-sodium milk compares favorably with whole milk.[5] When diets are restricted to low-sodium milk, recipes requiring milk may be prepared successfully by substituting low-sodium milk.

The sodium content of kosher meats is too high for sodium-restricted diets. Orthodox Jewish patients should salt their meats lightly and allow them to stand for a minimum length of time to draw out the blood. Thoroughly washing with water will remove much of the salt. Then meats are simmered in a large volume of water, and the cooking liquid is discarded. The leaching is more effective if the meat is cut into pieces before cookery.

HYPERTENSION

Hypertension, or elevation of the blood pressure above normal, is a symptom which accompanies many cardiovascular and renal diseases. It may occur at any age but is found most frequently in people over 40 years of age. Hypertension may be caused temporarily by emotional disturbances or by excessive smoking. Certain kidney disturbances or tumor of the adrenal are responsible for a small proportion of cases. However, about 85 to 90 per cent of patients belong to the group known as essential hypertension, for which the cause is unknown. Dahl[7] and others have suggested that a high salt intake over long periods of time is accompanied by an increased probability of high blood pressure.

Dietary modification. Hypertension is often reduced if weight loss is brought about in the obese patient. In 1945 Kempner described the success he had with a rice-fruit diet in lowering blood pressure.[8] This diet includes each day 200 to 300 gm rice (dry weight), fruits, fruit juices, and sugars to provide 2000 calories, 15 to 20 gm protein, 5 gm fat, and 100 to 150 mg sodium. Other diets restricted to about 200 mg sodium, but allowing a wider choice of foods, have also been successful in lowering the blood pressure. These regimens are helpful only if they are used for a long period of time. Not only is it difficult to counsel patients regarding the rigid restrictions, but most patients find the diet to be monotonous and unpalatable. Today antihypertensive drugs have replaced the very low-sodium diets, but mild restriction of sodium is often ordered.

PROBLEMS AND REVIEW

1. For a patient with congestive heart failure, what are the dietary modifications with respect to calorie level; protein; fluid intake; frequency of feeding; selection of foods?
2. When is a 250-mg-sodium diet likely to be ordered? A 500-mg-sodium diet? A 1000-mg-sodium diet? A mildly-restricted-sodium diet? Outline the important differences in food allowances for each of these levels.
3. *Problem.* Plan a menu for one day that furnishes 500 mg sodium and 1800 calories.

4. Suppose a 1000-mg-sodium diet has been ordered for a man who is going home. What are some of the questions that you should anticipate during the counseling?
5. Compare the sodium content of 1 slice (25 gm) regular bread and 1 slice low-sodium bread; 2 teaspoons (10 gm) regular butter and 2 teaspoons low-sodium butter; and ½ cup fresh peas and ½ cup canned peas.
6. Examine the labeling on five food products to find examples of different sodium compounds used in processing.
7. *Problem.* A 1000-mg-sodium-restricted diet has been ordered for a 60-year-old man. Neither he nor his wife has had much education and they read with difficulty. Their income is low. What steps would you take to provide guidance for them in the management of the diet at home?
8. *Problem.* Determine the sodium content of the local water supply? If a patient drinks 2 quarts of this water daily, how much sodium will be ingested? If the sodium content of the water is high, what recommendations would you make to a patient?
9. How does low-sodium milk compare with regular milk in nutritive value? Under what circumstances should it be used?
10. What foods may present problems in salt restrictions for the Jewish patient? The Chinese patient? The Puerto Rican? The Italian?

CITED REFERENCES

1. Brozek, J., *et al.:* "Drastic Food Restriction. Effect on Cardiovascular Dynamics in Normotensive and Hypertensive Conditions," *J.A.M.A.,* **137**:1569–74, 1948.
2. Newburgh, L. H., and Reimer, A.: "The Rationale and Administration of Low-Sodium Diets," *J. Am. Diet. Assoc.,* **23**:1047, 1947.
3. Holinger, B. W., *et al.:* "Analyzed Sodium Values in Foods Ready to Serve," *J. Am. Diet. Assoc.,* **48**:501–504, 1966.
4. White, J. M., *et al.:* "Sodium Ion in Drinking Water," *J. Am. Diet. Assoc.,* **50**:32–36, 1967.
5. Council on Foods and Nutrition: "Low-Sodium Milk," *J.A.M.A.,* **163**:739, 1957.
6. Kaufman, M.: "Adapting Therapeutic Diets to Jewish Food Customs," *Am. J. Clin. Nutr.,* **5**:676–81, 1957.
7. Dahl, L. K.: "Role of Dietary Sodium in Essential Hypertension," *J. Am. Diet. Assoc.,* **34**:585–90, 1958.
8. Kempner, W.: "Treatment of Kidney Disease and Hypertensive Vascular Disease with Rice Diet," *N. C. Med. J.,* **5**:125–33, 1944; **6**:61–87; 117–61, 1945.

ADDITIONAL REFERENCES

Bruce, T. A., and Bing, R. J.: "Clinical Management of Myocardial Infarction," *J.A.M.A.,* **191**:124–26, 1965.
Cooper, G. R., and Heap, B.: "Sodium Ion in Drinking Water," *J. Am. Diet. Assoc.,* **50**:37–41, 1967.
Danowski, T. S.: "Low-Sodium Diets—Physiological Adaptation and Clinical Usefulness," *J.A.M.A.,* **168**:1886–90, 1958.
Davidson, C. S., *et al.: Sodium Restricted Diets. The Rationale, Complications, and Practical Aspects of Their Use.* Pub. 325, Food and Nutrition Board, National Academy of Sciences–National Research Council, Washington, D.C., 1954.
Farag, S. A., and Mozer, H. N.: "Preventing Recurring Congestive Heart Failure," *J. Am. Diet. Assoc.,* **51**:26–28, 1967.
Frank, R. L., and Mickelsen, O.: "Sodium-Potassium Chloride Mixtures as Table Salt," *Am. J. Clin. Nutr.,* **22**:464–70, 1969.

Hartroft, W. S.: "The Nutritional Aspects of Hypertension and Its Reversibility," *Am. J. Public Health*, **56**:462–68, 1966.

Heap, B.: "Low-Sodium Milk—Current Status," *J. Am. Diet. Assoc.*, **53**:43–44, 1968.

Heap, B., *et al.*: "Simplifying the Sodium-Restricted Diets," *J. Am. Diet. Assoc.*, **49**:327–30, 1966.

Johnson, D.: "Planning a Restricted Sodium Diet and Bland, Low-Fiber Diet for Diabetic Patients," *Am. J. Clin. Nutr.*, **5**:569–74, 1957.

Metzger, R. A., *et al.*: "Renal Excretion of Sodium during Oral Water Administration in Patients with Systemic Hypertension," *Circulation*, **38**:955–64, 1968.

Newborg, B.: "Sodium-Restricted Diet. Sodium Content of Various Wines and Other Alcoholic Beverages," *Arch. Intern. Med.*, **123**:692–93, 1969.

Searight, M. W.: "A Low-Sodium Potluck Luncheon," *Nurs. Outlook,* **16**:30–32, Aug. 1968.

INSTRUCTIONAL AIDS FOR THE PATIENT

American Heart Association (or local chapters):
    Your Sodium Restricted Diet: 500 mg, 1000 mg, Mild Restriction, 1958.
    Fold-out charts: *Sodium-Restricted Diet, 500 mg, 1965.*
                  Sodium-Restricted Diet, Mild Restriction, 1967.
                  Sodium-Restricted Diet, 1000 mg, 1966.
Payne, A. S., and Callahan, D.: *The Low-Sodium, Fat-Controlled Cookbook.* Little Brown & Co., Boston, 1965.

44 Diet in Diseases of the Kidney

Controlled Protein, Potassium, and Sodium Diet; Calcium- and Phosphorus-Restricted Diet

Renal function and disease. The important function of the kidneys is to maintain the normal composition and volume of the blood. They accomplish this by the excretion of nitrogenous and other metabolic wastes, by regulation of electrolyte and fluid excretion so that water balance is maintained, by making the final adjustment of acid-base balance, and by the synthesis of enzymes and other substances that influence metabolic activities. In view of the central role of the kidneys in maintaining the constant internal environment it is not surprising that renal disease and eventually renal failure affect every system and tissue in the body. A review of the functions of the normal kidney (see pages 132 to 133) is recommended before the student begins the study of dietary management in renal diseases.

Disease may affect the glomeruli, the tubules, or both. Nephritis means literally an inflammation of the nephrons. Although glomerulonephritis indicates that the glomeruli are particularly affected, the functioning of the tubules will also be disturbed. Renal disease may be acute, subacute or latent, or chronic. (See Figure 44–1.) The majority of patients with acute glomerulonephritis recover completely but a small group progress to chronic nephritis. In some patients disease may be in a latent stage for months or even years during which the individual is asymptomatic. Obviously, for each patient a careful evaluation must be made of the etiology, the presenting symptoms, and the level of renal function before any treatment including dietary control can be initiated.

ACUTE GLOMERULONEPHRITIS

Symptoms and clinical findings. Acute glomerulonephritis, also known as hemorrhagic nephritis, is primarily confined to the glomeruli. It occurs mostly in children and young adults as a frequent sequel to streptococcic infections such as scarlet fever, tonsillitis, pneumonia, and respiratory infections. In some patients the renal infection is so mild that there is no awareness of the disease until symptoms resulting from permanent damage appear much later. Others notice some swelling of the ankles and puffiness around the eyes and complain of headache, anorexia, nausea, and vomiting. Varying degrees of hypertension, dimness of vision, and even convulsions may occur. Usually there is a diminished urinary volume (oliguria), hematuria, some albuminuria, and some nitrogen retention (azotemia).

The acute phase of the illness lasts from several days to a week, but renal function returns to normal much more slowly. Full recovery is the rule, provided that treatment is prompt and appropriate. The recovery time may vary from two or three weeks to several months, as determined by renal function tests rather than subjective impressions.

Modification of the diet. During the acute phase of illness when nausea and vomiting are present it is unrealistic to provide a diet that fully meets nutritional requirements. An effort should be made to maintain fluid balance and to provide nonprotein calories, either orally or parentally, to minimize the catabolism of tissue proteins. Fruit juices sweetened with glucose, sweetened tea, ginger ale, fruit ices, and hard candy contribute to the carbohydrate intake. Excessive amounts of sweet foods, however, may contribute to the nausea.

As the patient improves and the appetite returns, the following dietary modifications are appropriate:

Figure 44–1. Alternate courses for acute nephritis. (Courtesy, Duncan, G. G.: *Diseases of Metabolism.* W. B. Saunders Company, Philadelphia.)

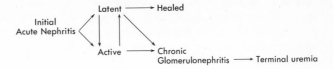

Energy. The Recommended Dietary Allowances (page 31) provide a general guide to the caloric requirement for persons of various ages and body size. In the absence of fever and at bed rest, these allowances can be reduced somewhat if there is not a previous condition of malnutrition.

Protein. Some clinicians restrict protein only when there is nitrogen retention, whereas others prescribe low-protein diets until healing has taken place.[1] The protein restriction for adults may be 0.5 gm per kilogram or less and 0.75 gm per kilogram for children. When there is marked albuminuria, the protein intake should be increased by the amount of protein lost in the urine.

Sodium. If there is edema or hypertension, sodium restriction to 500 or 1000 mg may be prescribed. Danowski[2] recommends some sodium restriction for all patients because of the dangers of hypertension, congestive failure, and pulmonary edema.

Fluid. In the presence of oliguria, fluids are usually limited to the losses from the skin, in the feces, and by the lungs—about 500 to 700 ml daily. Larger amounts of fluid are given to replace losses by vomiting, diarrhea, or excessive perspiration.

Selection of foods. The food allowances for 20 gm-, or 40 gm-, and 60-gm-protein diets listed in Table 44–2 are used as the basis for meal planning. The emphasis is upon protein foods of high biologic value, especially eggs and milk; however, the amounts of each must be carefully controlled. Peas, Lima beans, dried beans and peas, nuts, peanut butter, and gelatin are high in protein of poor biologic value and they should be omitted.

Achieving a satisfactory caloric intake is doubly difficult; the limitations placed upon protein intake necessitate restrictions of breads, cereals, potatoes, and similar foods that are good sources of calories, and poor appetite often in-

terferes with food intake. The caloric intake can be increased by emphasizing sugars, jellies, hard candy, butter or margarine, vegetable oils, and carbonated beverages. Cream may be substituted for part of the milk allowance.

When sodium restriction is ordered, the food lists on pages 564 to 567 should be consulted. Regular milk can be used in the amounts listed, but all foods must be prepared without salt or other sodium-containing compounds for any restriction of 1000 mg or less.

CHRONIC GLOMERULONEPHRITIS

Clinical findings. Patients with chronic glomerulonephritis may be asymptomatic for months or even years. The nephritis may be detected only by laboratory studies. As the disease progresses there is gradually increasing involvement: proteinuria, hematuria, hypertension, and vascular changes in the retina. The kidneys are unable to concentrate urine and there are both frequent urination and nocturia. Although the specific gravity of the urine is low, the large volume of urine makes possible the excretion of the metabolic wastes. In some patients the nephrotic syndrome (see page 578) characterized by massive edema and severe proteinuria develops. Hypoproteinemia and anemia are sometimes encountered. Eventually the symptoms of renal failure occur (see page 578).

Modification of the diet. The objectives of dietary management are (1) to maintain a state of good nutrition; (2) to control or correct protein deficiency; (3) to prevent edema; and (4) to provide palatable, easily digested meals adjusted to the individual patient's needs.

During the period when the kidneys are able to excrete wastes adequately it is doubtful that protein restriction serves any useful purpose. In fact, protein restriction may result in failure to maintain satisfactory levels of blood proteins and in progressive weakness and susceptibility to infection. The normal daily allowance of protein—60 to 70 gm for the adult—plus the amount of protein lost in the urine is usually allowed.

Sufficient carbohydrate and fat should be provided so that the energy needs of the body can be met without the breakdown of body protein. The daily caloric needs for the adult will usually range from 2000 to 3000 calories.

Sodium restriction to 500 or 1000 mg is indicated only when edema is present. Some clinicians recommend a mild level of sodium restriction (see page 562) even when there is no edema. During the diuretic phase of nephritis increased amounts of sodium may be excreted because of the kidneys' inability to reabsorb the ion. Thus, a markedly restricted sodium diet could lead to body depletion with its attendant weakness, nausea, and symptoms of shock.

DEGENERATIVE BRIGHT'S DISEASE (NEPHROSIS)

Degenerative Bright's disease is distinguished clinically from glomerulonephritis by the consistent absence of hypertension and hematuria and the usual absence of anemia and nitrogen retention. Like glomerulonephritis, it is characterized by proteinuria, but to an even more marked degree. The serum proteins are more seriously depleted than in glomerulonephritis, and this characteristic, which often results in massive edema, presents a primary problem in treatment. There is usually no associated cardiovascular disease.

The primary dietary factor requiring consideration is the replacement of protein, since urinary losses may be very large. A high-protein diet with sodium restriction is suitable.

NEPHROSCLEROSIS (ARTERIOSCLEROTIC BRIGHT'S DISEASE)

Nephrosclerosis, or hardening of the renal arteries, occurs in adults after 35 years of age,

as a rule, and is associated with arteriosclerosis. The disease may run a benign course for many years. During late stages some albuminuria, nitrogen retention, and retinal changes develop. Death usually results from circulatory failure. In a small number of younger persons nephrosclerosis runs a stormy, rapid course leading to uremia and death. This is called malignant hypertension.

Modification of the diet. Weight reduction of the obese is desirable. A 200-mg-sodium diet has been used successfully in some instances. The protein intake may be kept at a normal level until marked nitrogen retention indicates that the kidney is no longer able to eliminate wastes satisfactorily. The diet on page 587, Table 44–2, may be used with or without sodium restriction when a lower level of protein becomes necessary.

RENAL FAILURE

Symptoms and biochemical findings. Chronic glomerulonephritis, nephrosclerosis, and chronic pyelonephritis are the principal diseases of the kidney leading to renal failure.[3] This is a condition in which the kidneys are no longer able to maintain the normal composition of the blood. *Uremia*, a term applied to the condition arising from the failing function of the kidney, means literally "urine in the blood." *Azotemia*, a more specific term, refers to the accumulation of nitrogenous constituents in the blood. *Oliguria* denotes a scanty output of urine (less than 500 ml), and *anuria* is the minimal production or absence of urine (less than 100 ml per day).

Renal failure may be acute or chronic. Acute renal failure may occur in severe acute glomerulonephritis or following inhalation or ingestion of poisons such as carbon tetrachloride or mercury, crushing injuries, or shock from surgery. Dialysis is often employed until the kidney again resumes its function.

The symptoms of chronic renal failure appear when the glomerular filtration rate (GFR) is inadequate to excrete nitrogenous wastes. Gastrointestinal symptoms are usually present and are especially trying because of the discomfort associated with them and the constant interference with food intake. The sight or smell of food may bring about nausea or vomiting. The breath has an ammoniacal odor that interferes with the taste of food. Ulcerations of the mouth and hiccups also interfere with food intake.

The nervous system is usually affected. Patients may be irritable or may become drowsy and eventually sink into coma. Headache, dizziness, muscular twitchings, neuritis, and even failing vision occur, especially if there is also hypertension.

The functioning of the heart is seriously disturbed. Congestive failure occurs when the heart failure is associated with retention of sodium and water. Death results when hyperpotassemia blocks the contraction of the heart.

Patients with terminal uremia have a progressively worsening anemia. There is interference with the clotting mechanism, the capillaries are fragile, ulcerations in the gastrointestinal tract may lead to bleeding, the life-span of the red cells is reduced, hemolysis occurs readily, and hematopoiesis is reduced. Because the anemia reduces the effective exchange of oxygen and carbon dioxide at the tissues and in the lungs, fatigue and weakness are ever present.

The reduced ability to excrete phosphate interferes with calcium and phosphorus metabolism. Many patients complain of bone and joint pains. Hypocalcemia is common in renal failure, and osteomalacia and bone deformities may result from calcium wastage in tubular disorders.

As the function of the kidneys further deteriorates, the potassium level in the blood increases, the acidosis becomes increasingly severe, and edema is marked. Drowsiness, mental disorientation, severe gastrointestinal symptoms, bleeding, and a sense of doom are characteristic of the final stages.[4]

The development of controlled dietary regimens. Early in this century diets containing 30 gm protein or less were recommended for chronic nephritis, but these diets, of course, did not have the benefit of the present-day knowledge of the essential amino acid requirements. However, the diets described by Koehne[5] in 1925 were based upon food groupings according to "protein points" with emphasis upon protein quality and adequacy of minerals and vitamins as these needs were then understood. In 1945 Kempner reported that a rice-fruit diet supplying only 20 gm protein and 2000 calories was beneficial in treating patients with hypertension and renal disease.[6] These diets were later shown to maintain nitrogen balance, but they have been used infrequently because of the lack of palatability.

A protein-free electrolyte-free diet consisting of sugar and fat and supplying 2000 calories was described by Borst in 1948.[7] It consisted of

¾ cup sugar
¾ cup butter
2 tablespoons flour
2 cups water

and was prepared as a "soup." Another variation was a mixture of butter and sugar rolled into balls and frozen. Patients who were able to consume the full amount of butter and sugar improved because tissue catabolism was greatly reduced and the consequent accumulations of nitrogenous substances and potassium in the blood were likewise reduced. However, the protein-free diet is only temporarily beneficial because some catabolism always occurs when there is no exogenous source of essential amino acids.

In 1963 Giordano reported that uremic patients who were fed a semisynthetic diet which supplied about 3 gm nitrogen daily in the form of essential amino acids were able to maintain nitrogen balance and improved remarkably.[8] Giovanetti and Maggiore in 1964 achieved similar results with a diet based upon the principles of the Giordano diet but which employed natural foods with proteins of high biologic value.[9] Since that time the Giordano-Giovanetti diet (G-G diet) has been adapted in many clinical centers with equally successful results.[10–12] In patients on the diet within a few weeks the blood urea levels dropped to almost normal levels, and anorexia, nausea, vomiting, and other distressing symptoms disappeared.

The G-G diet is based upon the principle that the large urea pool in uremic patients can be utilized for the synthesis of the nonessential amino acids. When the urea is so utilized, the blood level drops and the accompanying gastrointestinal symptoms disappear. In order to prevent tissue catabolism the essential amino acid requirement is met by using protein foods of high biologic value, and the calorie intake is maintained at 2000 to 3000 calories. Sodium is restricted to 600 to 900 mg and potassium to 1400 to 2000 mg. A multivitamin-and-iron supplement is prescribed.

Dietary modification in renal failure. As many as 100,000 patients in the United States who have advanced renal insufficiency might benefit by diets controlled for protein, potassium, and sodium.[13] An individualized regimen can maintain patients in relative comfort if the GFR is 3 ml per minute or more. The controlled diet is also useful for maintenance of patients who are awaiting dialysis equipment or kidney transplants. When the GFR falls to 1 to 1.5 ml per minute, diet alone cannot maintain the patient and deterioration is rapid unless dialysis is initiated. Dietary control is also necessary for patients who are being kept on dialysis.

Energy. Sufficient calories are of first importance, for without an adequate calorie intake body tissues will be rapidly catabolized, thus increasing the blood urea and potassium levels beyond the capacity of the kidney to excrete them. Berlyne states that in his experience with more than 300 patients in four years the major reason for failure of the diet was an inadequate calorie intake, usually because the patients disliked the low-protein bread.[10] Tissue depletion is often difficult to assess because even moderate edema can mask muscle wasting.

Protein. The principles of protein restriction are generally accepted, but the exact level of restriction that is desirable has not been determined. Individuals vary in their amino acid requirements, and a level suitable for one person may be too high or too low for another.

Patients with a GFR of 3 to 5 ml per minute respond well to diets restricted to 18 to 20 gm per day, of which the essential amino acid requirement is met by 1 egg and ¾ cup milk (13 to 14 gm protein). The blood urea pool is depended upon as a source of nitrogen for the synthesis of the nonessential amino acids. When the blood urea level has dropped to well below 100 mg per 100 ml and when the disturbing symptoms have disappeared, Berlyne suggests that the protein may be increased to a daily intake of 25 to 30 gm. He cautions, however, that an excess of even 5 gm protein can lead to serious deterioration.[10] On the other hand, Kopple found that diets containing 40 gm protein resulted in only modest elevation of blood urea and that these diets were more acceptable than those restricted to 20 gm protein.[13]

Potassium. Restriction of potassium from 1000 to 2000 mg is generally recommended. Since potassium is so widely distributed in foods, even a level of 2000 mg places severe limitations upon food choice. Potassium becomes the principal factor that limits the choice of foods and the palatability of the diet.

Sodium. Overhydration is more likely to occur in renal failure than is dehydration. The accumulation of fluid is particularly hazardous because of the possibility of congestive heart failure. The excretion of sodium may be only 10 mEq or less when the GFR is 2 ml per minute or less. This would necessitate a dietary restriction between 250 and 500 mg, allowing for small losses from the skin and the feces. Patients who are not retaining sodium and who have a mild hypertension can be maintained at sodium intakes ranging from 500 to 2000 mg.

Other minerals. Blood levels of phosphorus gradually increase in the uremic patients, thus contributing to the acidosis and also to metastatic calcification. Aluminum hydroxide gel is often prescribed to bind some of the phosphate in the intestinal tract, thereby reducing the absorption. The diets are low in calcium and a supplement is usually prescribed. Diet alone cannot meet the iron requirements, and a supplement should be prescribed.

Vitamins. Because raw fruits and vegetables are restricted and because foods may be cooked in large volumes of water to reduce the potassium content, the water-soluble vitamin intake is likely to be low. A multivitamin supplement should be prescribed.

Some patients with terminal uremia have a resistance to vitamin D, in which case therapeutic doses as high as 50,000 I.U. are prescribed.[14]

DIALYSIS

Hemodialysis. The artificial kidney was first described by Dr. Willem J. Kolff[15] and has since been developed to the point where it can be used in the hospital or the home without the constant supervision of the physician or nurse. In hemodialysis the patient's blood circulates outside his body through coils or sheets of semipermeable membranes that are constantly bathed by a hypotonic dialyzing fluid so that the nitrogenous wastes are removed into the dialysate. The membranes do not permit bacteria to enter the blood nor can proteins escape from the blood. However, some amino acids are lost into the dialysate.

With dialysis for 12 to 14 hours twice weekly, blood urea levels that range from 100 to 170 mg per 100 ml fall to 20 to 40 mg per 100 ml.[14] Between each dialysis nitrogenous end products, potassium, and sodium accumulate. If the diet is uncontrolled, dialysis will need to be more frequent.

Dialysis is often used in acute renal failure until the kidney can take over its functions again. For patients with chronic renal failure who cannot be maintained on the low-protein diet alone, dialysis is used, when the equipment is available, on a permanent basis. Although it is a lifesaving measure, the patient does not return to a full normal life.[15] He must be attached to a dialyzer for perhaps 24 hours each week. Most of the patients have severe anemia and hypertensive disease because the artificial kidney does not correct the endocrine failure of the kidneys. Dialysis and the associated diet require a great deal of the patient in terms of emotional stability, motivation, and intelligence. Those who are under 21 years especially resent the program, and those between 21 and 41 years seem to adapt best to the program. Finally, the scarcity of the equipment and the great cost limit the program to only a small number of those who could benefit. The husband or wife, father or mother, or other relative or friend must provide moral support to the patient; they may also be trained to operate the dialyzer within the home.

Peritoneal dialysis. This is used when hemodialysis is not available. It consists in introducing 1 to 2 liters of dialysis fluid into the peritoneal cavity and 30 to 90 minutes later withdrawing the fluid. The process is repeated until the blood urea level drops to tolerable levels.

Some blood proteins (10 to 44 gm per dialysis period) as well as amino acids are lost through peritoneal dialysis and compensation must be made for this loss in order to avoid severe hypoproteinemia.

Dietary modification for dialysis. The dietary modification for patients on permanent dialysis follows the overall principles of diet in renal failure (see page 580). Without the restriction of protein, potassium, and sodium the blood levels would increase rapidly and necessitate more frequent dialysis. Sodium retention leads to edema, and hyperkalemia could be life threatening by resulting in cardiac arrest. Rapid increase in the blood urea level makes comfortable living impossible. Needless to say, each aspect of diet must be individualized for each patient so that he is maintained at the desired levels of biochemical control.

Protein. The best level of protein restriction with dialysis is not known. A diet restricted to 20 to 30 gm protein is recommended by some.[10,16] Each 28 to 32 hours of dialysis removes amino acids equivalent to about 20 gm protein. To compensate for this loss, 3 eggs should be given immediately following dialysis,[16] or the daily protein allowance may be increased by 3 gm.

Other clinicians allow 40 to 60 gm protein because the diets are more palatable, the caloric intake is more likely to be adequate, and there is less cheating on the diets.[12,13,14,17] On such diets some regular bread (low sodium if needed) can replace the low-protein low-electrolyte bread to which many patients object. According to these physicians, the increases in blood urea have not been a serious problem.

CONTROLLED PROTEIN, POTASSIUM, AND SODIUM DIET

Food lists. A number of dietary regimens have been described for the control of protein, potassium, and sodium.[17–20] Each of these is based upon food groupings in which the foods within a given list are of approximately the same protein, potassium, and sodium value. Food choices for daily menus can therefore be made from a given group in the amounts specified. Generally speaking, the broad food groupings used in the various regimens are similar, but they differ in the specific foods included and the portion sizes, depending upon the criteria used in setting them up. For example, oranges are relatively high in potassium and are omitted from some lists; they are included in other lists in controlled amounts because of their popular appeal, their relatively low cost, and their content of ascorbic acid. Potatoes are excluded in some lists but included in others, provided that they are prepared by methods to minimize their potassium content. When the directions for the use of any of these regimens are explicitly followed any one of them will lead to satisfactory results.

Dietitians, nurses, and physicians must be aware of the many factors that modify the sodium and potassium content of foods. The calculation of sodium and potassium values to decimal fractions of a milligram fails to take into account that actual diet contents may be higher or lower than published values. The methods of food preparation significantly modify the electrolyte levels. Those factors that enter into the sodium content of foods have been discussed in Chapter 43. With respect to potassium, considerable leaching out occurs when foods are cooked in large volumes of water. The amount lost to the water is greater if food is cut into small pieces.

One dietary regimen for these controlled diets is described in detail in the pages that follow. Table 44–1 lists the composition of the food groups that follow. Table 44–2 indicates the food allowances for three levels of protein. Each of these plans must be individualized according to the patient's caloric requirement, the nutritional status, and the level of biochemical control. The 20-gm-protein level furnishes 1800 calories and 1200 ml fluid, including the water content of the solid foods. These diets should be supplemented with B complex vitamins, calcium, iron, and sometimes vitamin D.

The 20-gm- and 40-gm-protein diets are used only for patients whose renal function has deteriorated so much that they are no longer able to avoid the gastrointestinal and other symptoms of renal failure. The patient who has blood urea levels well below 100 mg per cent and who is asymptomatic is not well served by being placed upon too restricted a diet. He does not have the motivation to adhere to it, and by the time he really needs it he is likely to have lost patience with the diet. Moreover, there is no indication that the rigid regimen will in any way prolong his life. Until the blood urea levels can no longer be maintained at reasonable levels the dietary regimen should be somewhat more liberal. This does not mean lack of any control, but it does permit sufficient protein for a palatable diet.

DIETARY COUNSELING

Importance of adequate guidance. Dietary treatment in renal failure, without or with dialysis, is a primary aspect of therapy and its success is dependent upon the degree of adherence to the diet. Although the diet does not improve kidney function, it helps to maintain nearly normal levels of nitrogen, sodium, and potassium in the blood so that the patient can live comfortably rather than in misery. The rigid controls required make this as complex as any diet that can be prescribed. Moreover, the diet lacks much in palatability, especially if sodium restriction is also severe, and the level of motivation of the patient and those who care for him must be high.

Many hours of dietary instruction are required for the patient and for those who will prepare the food for him at home. The counseling started in the hospital must be con-

Table 44–1. Protein, Sodium, and Potassium Values for Food Lists

Food List	Household Measure	Weight gm	Protein gm	Sodium* mg	Potassium mg
Milk, whole or nonfat	1 cup	240	8	120	335
Milk, low sodium	1 cup	240	8	7	600
Meat, poultry, fish, cooked	1 ounce	30	7	25	100
Egg	1	50	7	60	65
Cheese, American, salted	1 ounce	30	7	210	25
Cheese, cottage, salted	1 ounce	30	7	85	25
Fruits, list I	1/2 cup	100	Less than 0.5	2	85
Fruits, list II	1/2 cup	100	1	2	135
Vegetables, list I	1/2 cup	100	0.5	9	110
List II	1/2 cup	100	1	9	125
List III	1/2 cup	100	2	9	160
Bread, low sodium	1 slice	30	2	5	30
Bread, regular	1 slice	30	2	160	30
Bread, low-protein, low-electrolyte	1 slice	30	0.1	9	3
Butter, unsalted	1 teaspoon	5	tr	tr	tr
Butter, salted	1 teaspoon	5	tr	50	tr

*Except for cheese, regular bread, and salted butter, the values listed for sodium are those that apply when no salt is used in processing or preparation of the food. Also, certain high-sodium items in the meat and vegetable lists would be omitted if the diet is restricted in sodium.

FOOD LISTS FOR CONTROLLED PROTEIN, SODIUM, AND POTASSIUM DIETS*

Milk List
1 cup equals 8 gm protein, 335 mg potassium

Buttermilk, unsalted
Evaporated milk, reconstituted
Low sodium milk
Nonfat dry milk, reconstituted
Skim milk
Whole milk

Foods to Avoid
Commercial foods made of milk:
    Chocolate milk
    Condensed milk
    Ice cream
    Malted milk
    Milkshake
    Milk mixes
    Sherbet

Meat or Substitute List
1 ounce cooked equals 7 gm protein, 100 mg potassium

Beef, chicken, duck, lamb, liver, pork, tongue (unsalted), turkey, veal

*Adapted from *Manual of Diets*, Departments of Dietetics, Hospital of St. Raphael, Veterans Administration Hospital, and Yale–New Haven Hospital, New Haven, Conn., 1968.

Foods to Avoid
Brains, kidneys
Canned, salted, or smoked meats as: bacon, bologna, chipped beef, corned beef, frankfurters, ham, kosher meats, luncheon meats, salt pork, sausage, smoked tongue

Cod, flatfish (flounder and sole), kingfish (whiting), haddock, perch; canned salmon and tuna (omit on sodium-restricted diet)

Clams, crab, lobster, oysters, scallops, shrimp (all omitted on sodium-restricted diet)

Egg (1 egg equals 7 gm protein, 65 mg potassium)

Cheese (1 ounce equals 7 gm protein, 25 mg potassium) Cheddar, cottage, American, Swiss

Foods to Avoid

Frozen fish fillets

Canned, salted, or smoked fish: anchovies, caviar, cod (dried and salted), herring, halibut, sardines salmon, tuna

Omit on sodium-restricted diets

Fruit List, Group I

Less than 0.5 gm protein, 85 mg potassium per serving

Apple, raw   1 small
Grapes, European   12
½ cup servings of: canned applesauce, pears, pineapple; watermelon (diced)
½ cup of these juices: apple, grape, peach nectar, pear nectar, orange-apricot, pineapple-grapefruit, pineapple-orange

Foods to Avoid

All dried and frozen fruits with sodium sulfite added
Apricots, fresh
Avocado
Bananas
Glazed fruits
Maraschino cherries
Nectarines
Prunes
Raisins

The following may be used for diets with liberal potassium allowance:
Less than 0.5 gm protein, 145 mg potassium per serving

½ cup servings of apricot nectar, pineapple juice; canned fruit cocktail, peaches, purple plums

Fruit List, Group II

1 gm protein, 135 mg potassium per serving

Pear, raw   1 small
Tangerine   1 small
½ cup servings of fresh or frozen blackberries, blueberries, boysenberries; canned cherries, figs; canned or fresh grapefruit; frozen red raspberries

The following may be used for diets with liberal potassium allowance:
1 gm protein, 200 mg potassium per serving

Orange   1 small
Peach, raw   1 small
Plums, fresh   2 medium
Strawberries, fresh   ⅔ cup
½ cup servings of cantaloupe, honeydew, frozen melon balls, fresh or frozen rhubarb
½ cup of these juices: grapefruit, grapefruit-orange, orange, tomato

Avoid tomato juice if diet is sodium restricted

Vegetable List, Group I

0.5 gm protein, 110 mg potassium per serving

½ cup servings of raw cabbage, cucumber, lettuce, onion, tomato

The following may be used for diets with liberal potassium allowance:

0.5 gm protein, 165 mg potassium per serving

Carrot, raw	1 small (+)
Celery, raw	1 stalk (+)
Endive, raw	½ cup

Vegetable List, Group II

1 gm protein, 125 mg potassium per serving

½ cup servings of canned green or wax beans, carrots (+), spinach (+); fresh cooked cabbage, eggplant, mustard greens, onion, summer squash

The following may be used for diets with liberal potassium allowance:

1 gm protein, 190 mg potassium per serving

½ cup servings of: canned beets (+), rutabagas, tomatoes; fresh cooked carrots (+), turnips (+); frozen summer squash, winter squash

Vegetable List, Group III

2 gm protein, 160 mg potassium per serving

½ cup servings of canned asparagus; fresh or frozen green or wax beans, okra

The following may be used for diets with liberal potassium allowance:

2 gm protein, 245 mg potassium per serving

½ cup servings of: fresh or frozen cauliflower; cooked dandelion greens (+); potato, boiled (pared before cooking), or mashed

Vegetable List, Group IV

3 gm protein, 210 mg potassium per serving

½ cup servings of kale (+); frozen asparagus, broccoli, collards (+), mixed vegetables (+), whole kernel corn

Foods to Avoid

All items marked (+) if diet is sodium restricted
Artichokes
Beans, baked
Beans, dried
Beans, Lima
Beet greens
Broccoli, fresh
Brussels sprouts
Chard
Parsnips
Peas
Potato in skin, or frozen
Sauerkraut
Spinach, fresh or frozen
Squash, baked

Breads and Substitutes
2 gm protein, 30 mg potassium per serving

Bread	1 slice
Cereals, dry	1 cup
Cornflakes, Puffed Rice, Puffed Wheat, shredded wheat	
Cereals, cooked	½ cup
cornmeal, farina, oatmeal, rice, rolled wheat	
Crackers, soda	3 squares
Flour	2 tablespoons
Grits	1 cup
Macaroni, noodles, or spaghetti	¼ cup
Rice	½ cup

Fats
Negligible protein and potassium

Butter
Cream, light or heavy (1 ounce contains 35 mg potassium)
Fat or cooking oil
Margarine
Salad dressings: French or mayonnaise

Miscellaneous
Cornstarch
Flavoring extracts (see list, page 569)
Ginger ale
Hard candies
Herbs (see list, page 569)
Honey
Jam or jelly
Jellybeans
Rice starch
Spices (see list, page 569)
Sugar, white, confectioners'
Syrup
Tapioca, granulated
Vinegar
Wheat starch

Foods to Avoid
Yeast breads or rolls or melba toast made with salt or from commercial mixes
Quick breads made with baking powder, baking soda, or salt, or made from commercial mixes
Commercial baked products
Dry cereals except as listed
Self-rising cornmeal
Graham or other crackers except low-sodium dietetic
Self-rising flour
Salted popcorn
Potato chips
Pretzels
Waffles containing salt, baking powder, baking soda, or egg white

Foods to Avoid
Salted fats on sodium-restricted diets
Avocado
Bacon, bacon fat
Olives
Nuts
Salt pork

Foods to Avoid
Antacids, laxatives
Bouillon, broth
Canned, dried, frozen soups
Chocolate
Cocoa, instant cocoa mixes
Coconut
Consommé
Fruit-flavored powders and prepared beverage mixes
Fountain beverages
Commercial candies except as listed
Commercial gelatin desserts
Regular baking powder and soda
Rennet tablets
Molasses
Pudding mixes
Peanut butter
Most carbonated beverages

Seasonings to Avoid
Catsup, celery leaves, celery salt, chili sauce, garlic salt, prepared horseradish, meat extracts, meat sauces, meat tenderizers, monosodium glutamate, prepared mustard, onion salt, pickles, relishes, salt, and salt substitutes, soy sauce, Worcestershire sauce

Table 44–2. Suggested Daily Meal Pattern for Controlled Protein, Sodium, and Potassium Diet*

		Protein		
	Measure	20 gm	40 gm	60 gm
Breakfast				
Fruit, group I	1 exchange	1	1	1
Egg	1	—	1	1
Cereal	1 exchange	1	1	1
Low-protein bread	1 slice	2	—	—
Bread, enriched	1 slice	—	1	1
Milk	cup	1/4	1/4	1/4
Lunch				
Egg	1	1	—	—
Meat of equivalent	1 ounce	—	1	2
Bread or substitute	1 exchange	—	1	2
Low-protein bread	1 slice	2	—	—
Vegetable, group I	1 exchange	—	1	1
Milk	cup	—	1/2	1/2
Low-protein dessert	1 serving	1	1	1
Fruit, group I	1 exchange	1	1	1
Dinner				
Meat or equivalent	1 ounce	—	1	2
Bread or substitute	1 exchange	1	1	2
Low-protein bread	1 slice	2	—	—
Vegetable, group I	1 exchange	1	—	—
Vegetable, group II	1 exchange	—	1	1
Fruit, group II	1 exchange	—	1	2
Milk	cup	1/2	—	—
Low-protein dessert	1 serving	1	—	—

*Manual of Diets. Departments of Dietetics, Hospital of St. Raphael, Veterans Administration Hospital, Yale–New Haven Hospital, New Haven, Conn., 1968, page 90.

tinued either in the out-patient clinic or by home visitation. (See Figure 44–2.)

What the patient needs to know. Each patient needs to know why the diet is important, and what risks he encounters if he fails to follow the diet. He must understand that it is important to include the exact amounts of high-quality protein foods that have been prescribed. Likewise he needs to know the importance of eating sufficient quantities of low-protein low-electrolyte foods so that body weight is maintained and tissue catabolism does not take place.

There must be a thorough familiarity with the food lists and the amounts of foods that may be used from each. Some practice in planning the daily meals from these lists is essential. If special products such as wheat starch are needed, the patient must be told where he can purchase them, and how much they will cost. Recipes for the use of these special products are needed together with precautions to take in food preparation.

Food preparation. The extraction of gluten from wheat flour yields a low-protein wheat starch that is also practically electrolyte free.*

*Dietetic Paygel-P Wheat Starch T.M., General Mills, Minneapolis. Wheatstarch Flour, Chicago Dietetic Supply House, Inc., Chicago. Resource® Baking Mix, The Doyle Pharmaceutical Company, Minneapolis.

yeast must be used as a leavening agent; regular leavening agents are too high in sodium, and low-sodium leavening agents are too high in potassium. Breads and other products made from wheat starch do not have the same texture as those made from wheat flour because of the absence of the elastic gluten. Some patients find the bread more acceptable when toasted, or served with butter and jelly or jam, or prepared as cinnamon toast or French toast.

If potatoes are allowed they should be cut into small pieces and boiled in a large volume of water.[21] Following this they may be pan fried with some of the fat or mashed with part of the milk and fat allowance. Meats that are simmered in a large volume of water also lose some of their potassium to the cooking liquid. Of course, these cooking procedures also result in greater losses of the water-soluble vitamins and of some other mineral elements.

Canned fruits are used, for the most part, instead of fresh raw fruits. Since part of the potassium has leached out into the syrup, only the solid fruit should be used.

HYPOKALEMIA

Occurrence. Although the emphasis in the preceding discussion has been upon the problems of elevated levels of blood potassium, there are renal and extrarenal circumstances in which the plasma or serum level of potassium is below 3.3 mEq per liter. One situation in which this occurs is by dilution of the extracellular fluid volume. This results when the fluid intake exceeds the ability of the kidney to excrete it as in oliguria and anuria. The total amount of the ion in the extracellular fluid remains the same, but the concentration is lowered because of the expanded volume.

In the diuretic stage of nephritis, the kidneys do not conserve potassium as effectively as normal, and potassium depletion occurs, especially if the intake is low because of a poor appetite. Adrenocortical steroids and mercurial diuretics

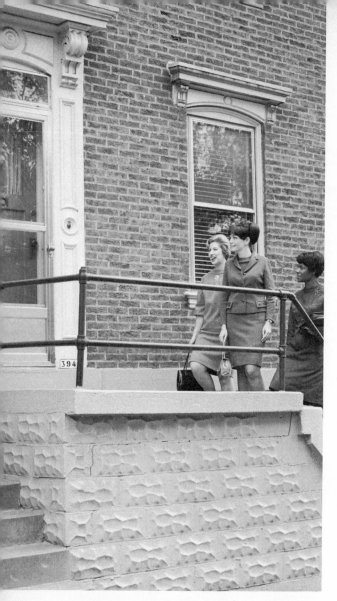

Figure 44–2. The nutritionist, public health nurse, and dietary technician are important members of the nutritional care team. After consultation with the nutritionist the dietary technician and the public health nurse provide direct services to the patient. For complex dietary problems, as in dietary control for renal failure, visits to the home may be required. (Courtesy, Pittsburgh Dietetic Association and Pittsburgh Hospital Association.)

Several sources of recipes using wheat starch are listed at the end of this chapter. One recipe for low-protein bread is given on page 589. With sodium and potassium restriction

LOW-PROTEIN, LOW-ELECTROLYTE BREAD*

	Measure	Weight
		gm
Margarine, unsalted	⅔ cup	120
Water, distilled	1⅞ cups	450
Methyl cellulose (Dow Chemical Methocel)	3 teaspoons	5
Yeast, active dry	1½ teaspoons	4
Water, lukewarm (105° F)	2 tablespoons	30
Sugar	2 tablespoons	25
Wheat starch (Cellu)	4⅔ cups	630

Procedure. Melt margarine and heat to a rapid boil. Cool to about 100° F. Separate fat from the sediment and discard sediment. Heat distilled water to boiling; blend in methyl cellulose with a wire whip. Pour mixture into bowl of electric mixer. Cool until it begins to form a colloidal solution, stirring frequently.

Mix yeast, ½ teaspoon of the sugar, and lukewarm water. Let stand for 10 minutes.

With a spoon blend wheat starch and remaining sugar into the water-cellulose mixture. Add margarine and mix. Add yeast mixture. Blend dough with electric mixer at low speed for six to eight minutes. Scrape sides and bottom of bowl frequently.

Grease two loaf pans (8 × 4 × 2¼ inches) with margarine fat. Pour batter into the two pans, smooth the top, and spread 1 teaspoon liquid margarine over each. Cover pans with foil or plastic wrap and let rise in warm place (90° F) until batter reaches top edge of pan—about 1½ to 2 hours. Remove covering.

Preheat oven to 350° F. Bake bread for five minutes; then turn temperature to 525° F and bake for 25 minutes. Remove bread from pans and cool on wire rack.

are likely to accentuate the renal losses of potassium.

Hypokalemia also occurs when there is rapid uptake of potassium by the cells. Growth, cellular repair, cellular dehydration, glycogen formation, and administration of glucose and insulin in diabetic acidosis promote entrance of potassium into the cell. In dehydration and in the correction of diabetic acidosis emergency measures are required to replace the extracellular potassium.

Excessive losses of potassium occur with vomiting, diarrhea, and gastrointestinal drainage. Unless these losses are replaced the plasma levels are often lowered to dangerous levels.

Treatment. If hypokalemia is severe, the correction will require the parenteral administration of potassium-containing fluids. This is followed

*Recipe and directions adapted from procedure by Sorensen, M. K.: "A Yeast-leavened, Low-Protein, Low-Electrolyte Bread," *J. Am. Diet. Assoc.,* **56:**521–23, 1970.

by emphasis upon foods that are rich in potassium. When the appetite is good, any varied diet will supply a considerable amount of potassium. A few foods that are especially good sources of potassium include orange juice, tomato juice, milk, baked potato, and banana.

URINARY CALCULI

Nature of calculi. Urinary calculi (kidney stones) may be found in the kidney, ureter, bladder, or urethra. They consist of an organic matrix with interspersed crystals and may vary in size from fine gravel to large stones.

About 90 per cent of all stones contain calcium as the chief cation. More than half the stones are mixtures of calcium oxalate and magnesium ammonium phosphate. Uric acid stones occur rarely, and xanthine stones are extremely rare.[22] Cystine stones are unique in that they are often pure and are a hereditary defect.

Incidence and etiology. Lonsdale reports that about 1 person in every 1000 in the United States is admitted to a hospital each year for renal calculi.[22] In the southeastern United States the rate is 2 per 1000 persons, and in Wyoming and Missouri the rate is only one fourth as high. About 54 per cent of admissions are male.

In Thailand, India, and Turkey (known as stone belts) bladder stones are a common occurrence in children, especially small boys. Most of these are urate and oxalate stones and their cause is unknown. The incidence of bladder stones in adults is high in Syria, Bulgaria, India, China, Madagascar, and Turkey, but low in Africa. The reasons for these geographic variations are not known.

Lonsdale found that renal calculi are more prevalent in sedentary people than in those who are active, with administrative workers being 20 times as susceptible as farmworkers. No dietary relationship has been established, but kidney dehydration may be a factor and more fluid intake and exercise are urged as prophylaxis.

The formation of stones is more probable in the presence of urinary tract infections, during periods of high urinary excretion of calcium, and in disorders of cystine or uric acid metabolism. High urinary excretion of calcium occurs in hyperparathyroidism, following overdosage with vitamin D, in long periods of immobilization, in osteoporosis, or following excessive ingestion of calcium and of absorbable alkalies as in the Sippy regimen for peptic ulcer. Even though vitamin A deficiency has been cited as contributing to the formation of calculi, it is not believed to be an important factor in the United States.

Rationale of treatment. When the cause of urinary calculi is known, the physician can effectively direct treatment toward the correction of the disorder. For example, this might entail the treatment of an infection, or modification of the regimen for peptic ulcer, or avoidance of long immobilization. However, in a large percentage of urinary calculi, the cause is not known or the disorder is not easily corrected.

The solubility of salts may be increased and the tendency to stone formation minimized by means of acidifying or alkalinizing agents which increase or decrease the pH of the urine. Such treatment implies that the nature of the stones has been determined by laboratory analyses of the stones themselves or by appropriate urine and blood studies.

A liberal fluid intake is essential—3000 ml or more daily—to prevent the production of a urine at a concentration where the salts precipitate out. The patient should be impressed with the importance of taking fluids throughout the day, so that the urine dilution is maintained.

Binding agents are often used to reduce the absorption of calcium and phosphorus from the gastrointestinal tract. One study has shown that patients who form calcium oxalate stones and their relatives had significantly higher urinary calcium excretion than normal individuals and that this excretion was enhanced following the ingestion of glucose or sucrose.[23] The authors suggest that patients with a history of stone formation might avoid a large intake of carbohydrate-rich foods and beverages especially when the urine is more concentrated.

Modification of the diet. No diet of itself is effective in bringing about solution of stones already formed. However, for the predisposed individual it is thought that diet may be of some value in retarding the growth of stones or preventing their recurrence, although the effectiveness of such prophylaxis has not been fully established.

Calcium and phosphorus restriction. The diet on page 591 is planned to provide maintenance levels of calcium and phosphorus. Such a diet serves as the starting point for the prevention of calcium phosphate stones. Aluminum hydroxide gel is sometimes prescribed since it combines with phosphate to form an insoluble aluminum phosphate and thus diminishes the absorption of phosphorus and the subsequent formation of insoluble precipitates in the urinary tract. Sodium acid phosphate or sodium phytate similarly reduces the absorption of calcium

Modification of urine pH. When stones are composed of calcium and magnesium phosphates and carbonates, therapy is directed toward maintaining an acid urine. On the other hand, if oxalate and uric acid stones are being formed, the urine should be kept alkaline. Acidifying or alkalinizing agents are more effective than dietary

Table 44–3. Acid-Producing, Alkali-Producing, and Neutral Foods

Acid-Producing	Alkali-Producing	Neutral
Bread, especially whole wheat	Milk	Butter
Cereals	Fruits	Candy, not chocolate
Cheese	Vegetables	Coffee
Corn		Cornstarch
Crackers	**Especially these**	Fats, cooking
Cranberries	Almonds	Honey
Eggs	Apricots, dried	Lard
Lentils	Beans, Lima, navy	Salad oils
Macaroni, spaghetti, noodles	Beet greens	Sugar
Meat, fish, poultry	Chard	Tapioca
Pastries	Dandelion greens	Tea
Peanuts	Dates	
Plums	Figs	
Prunes	Molasses	
Rice	Olives	
Walnuts	Peas, dried	
	Parsnips	
	Raisins	
	Spinach	
	Watercress	
	Foods prepared with baking powder or baking soda	

modification, although the diet should support the therapy by medications.

When an acid-ash diet is prescribed, acid-producing foods (see Table 44–3) would be emphasized. Only 1 pint of milk, two servings of fruit, and two servings of vegetables would be permitted.

On the other hand, for an alkaline-ash diet fruits and vegetables are used liberally, and the acid-producing foods are restricted to the amounts necessary for satisfactory nutrition.

Oxalate restriction. Some oxalate is produced in the body during the metabolism of foodstuffs. Dietary restriction of oxalates may be tried when calculi contain oxalate, but such restriction has not been shown conclusively to be of value. Oxalate-rich foods include green and wax beans, beets and beet greens, chard, endive, okra, spinach, sweet potatoes; currants, figs, gooseberries, Concord grapes, plums, rhubarb, raspberries; almonds, cashew nuts; chocolate, cocoa, tea.

Reduction of uric acid metabolism. The formation of uric acid stones may be minimized by using a Low-Purine Diet (see Chapter 40) and restricting the protein intake to 1 gm per kilogram body weight.

Cystine stones. A low-protein diet reduces the intake of sulfur-containing amino acids but has not been shown to be effective in the prevention of cystine stones.

CALCIUM- AND PHOSPHORUS-RESTRICTED DIET*

Characteristics and general rules

The diet provides maintenance levels of calcium and phosphorus. Milk constitutes the main source of calcium in the diet, and milk, eggs, and meat are the principal sources of phosphorus. (See Table 44-4.)

*Modification of regimen described by Mary Alice White, unpublished report, Drexel Institute of Technology, 1958.

Table 44–4. Calcium- and Phosphorus-Restricted Diet

Include These Foods Daily*		Protein gm	Fat gm	Carbohydrate gm	Ca mg	P mg
Milk	1 1/2 cups	12	15	18	430	340
Egg	1 whole	7	5	—	25	105
Meat, fish, or poultry	6 ounces	42	30	—	20	375
Vegetables:						
Potato	1 small	2	—	15	15	65
Leafy or yellow	1/2 cup	2	—	7	25	35
Other	1/2 cup	2	—	7	25	45
Fruits:						
Citrus	1/2 cup	—	—	10	30	20
Other	2 servings	—	—	20	25	40
Cereal, refined, without added calcium	2 servings	4	—	30	5	30
Bread, refined, without added calcium	6 slices	12	—	90	20	115
Fats	2 tablespoons	—	30	—	—	—
Sugars, sweets	2 tablespoons	—	—	30	—	—
		83	80	227	620	1170

*Protein, fat, and carbohydrate values on the basis of Meal Exchange Lists, Table A–4. Calcium and phosphorus values have been rounded off to the nearest 5 mg. Values for vegetables, fruits, cereals, and breads are averages of those permitted. Individual selections vary somewhat from these averages.

When further restrictions of calcium and phosphorus are desired, the milk and egg may be eliminated. The calcium level is then reduced to 170 mg, the phosphorus level to 740 mg, and the protein level to 64 gm.

Foods Allowed

Beverages—milk in allowed amounts; coffee, tea

Breads—French or Italian without added milk; pretzels; saltines, matzoth; water rolls

Cereals—cornflakes, corn grits, farina, rice, rice flakes, Puffed Rice; macaroni, noodles, spaghetti; cornmeal, cornstarch, tapioca, white flour

Cheese—½ ounce Cheddar or Swiss cheese may be used instead of ½ cup milk

Desserts—angel cake, white sugar cookies, gelatin, fruit pies, fruit tapioca, fruit whip, pudding with allowed milk and egg, shortbread, water ices

Eggs—1 whole. Whites as desired

Fats—butter, cooking oils and fats, lard, margarine, French dressing

Fruits—all, but restricting dried fruits to dates (3), prunes (2), raisins (1 tbsp.)

Foods to Avoid

Beverages—chocolate; cocoa; fountain beverages; proprietary beverages containing milk powder

Breads—biscuits; breads: brown, corn, cracked wheat, raisin, rye, white with nonfat dry milk, whole wheat; rye wafers; muffins; pancakes; waffles

Cereals—bran, bran flakes, corn and soy grits, oatmeal, wheat flakes, wheat germ, Puffed Wheat, Shredded Wheat; rye flour, soybean flour, self-rising flour, whole-wheat flour

Desserts—cakes and cake mixes, custard, doughnuts, ice cream, Junket, pies with cream filling or milk and eggs, milk puddings—except when daily allowance is used

Fats—mayonnaise, sweet and sour cream

Meats—beef, ham, lamb, pork, veal; chicken, duck, turkey; bluefish, cod, haddock, halibut, scallops, shad, swordfish, tuna

Milk—1½ cups daily

Soups—broth of allowed meats; consommé; cream soups using allowed milk

Sweets—sugar, syrup, jam, jelly, preserves, hard candy, marshmallows, mints without chocolate

Vegetables—artichokes, asparagus, beans—green or wax, Brussels sprouts, cabbage, carrots, cauliflower, corn, cucumber, eggplant, escarole, lettuce, onions, peppers, potatoes—white and sweet, pumpkin, radishes, romaine, squash, tomatoes, turnips

Miscellaneous—pickles, mustard, salt, spices

Meats—clams, crab, herring, lobster, mackerel, oyster, fish roe, salmon, sardines, shrimp; brains, heart, kidney, liver, sweetbreads

Soups—cream in excess of milk allowance; bean, lentil, split pea

Sweets—caramels, fudge, milk chocolate, molasses, dark brown sugar

Vegetables—dry beans—kidney, Lima, navy, pea, soybean; beet greens, broccoli, chard, collards, chickpeas, dandelion greens, kale, okra, parsnips, peas—fresh and dried, rutabagas, soybeans, soybean sprouts, spinach, turnip greens, watercress

Miscellaneous—chocolate, cocoa, nuts, olives, brewers' yeast

Sample Menu

Breakfast

Fresh raspberries
Cornflakes
Milk—½ cup
Soft-cooked egg
Toasted Italian bread
Butter or margarine
Apple jelly
Coffee

Lunch or Supper

Cold sliced turkey
Potato salad (potato, diced cucumber, minced green pepper and onion, French dressing) on lettuce; tomato wedges

Italian bread
Butter or margarine
Angel cake with fresh strawberries
Milk—1 cup only

Dinner

Roast pork
Buttered noodles
Zucchini squash
Hard rolls, made without milk
Butter or margarine
Fruit gelatin
Tea with lemon

Problems and Review

1. What are the parts of the nephron? How do these parts function?
2. What are the chief wastes excreted by the kidney?
3. In addition to excreting wastes, what other functions are performed by the kidney?
4. What are the characteristic symptoms of acute glomerulonephritis? In what way do these symptoms affect dietary planning?
5. In what way do the abnormal excretion products in renal diseases affect dietary planning?
6. *Problem.* Outline the principles for a dietary regimen for a patient with acute glomerulonephritis, showing the progression of diet from time to time.
7. *Problem.* On the basis of the principles outlined in problem 6, write a menu for a patient for one day. Assume that the diet order restricts protein to 40 gm and sodium to 1000 mg.
8. What reasons can you give for using a protein-free, high-carbohydrate, high-fat diet in acute renal failure? Why are frequent small feedings preferable to three meals?
9. What is accomplished by dialysis with an artificial kidney? Why is a diet restricted in protein and potassium necessary?
10. What problems are you likely to encounter in planning a potassium-restricted diet?
11. *Problem.* Write a menu for one day for a 20-gm controlled protein, sodium, and potassium diet, using the plan in Table 44–2 and the food lists on pages 583 to 587. What foods can

you suggest that would increase the caloric intake without increasing the protein and potassium levels?

12. What is meant by hypokalemia? Under what circumstances is it likely to occur? What foods could you suggest for increasing the potassium intake of a patient who has a poor appetite?

13. Why is a calcium-and-phosphorus-restricted diet often prescribed for certain patients with urinary calculi? What is the purpose of using a binding agent with such a diet?

14. Under what circumstances would an acid-ash diet be used? An alkaline-ash diet?

CITED REFERENCES

1. Zimmerman, H. J.: "Nutritional Aspects of Acute Glomerulonephritis," *Am. J. Clin. Nutr.,* **4**:482, 1956.

2. Danowski, T. S.: "Low-Sodium Diets—Physiological Adaptation and Clinical Usefulness," *J.A.M.A.,* **168**:1886–90, 1958.

3. Winters, R. W.: "Nutrition and Renal Disease," *Bordens Rev. Nutr. Res.,* **19**:75–90; 91–108, 1958.

4. Burton, B. T.: "Diet Therapy in Uremia," *J. Am. Diet. Assoc.,* **54**:475–80, 1969.

5. Koehne, M.: "Dietary Control of Nephritis," *J.A.M.A.,* **84**:1103, 1925.

6. Kempner, W.: "Treatment of Kidney Disease and Hypertensive Vascular Disease with Rice Diet," *N.C. Med. J.,* **5**:125–33, 1944; **6**:61–87; 117–61, 1945.

7. Borst, J. C. G.: "Protein Katabolism in Uraemia. Effects of Protein-Free Diet, Infections and Blood Transfusions," *Lancet,* **1**:824–28, 1948.

8. Giordano, C.: "Use of Exogenous and Endogenous Urea for Protein Synthesis in Normal and Uremic Subjects," *J. Lab. Clin. Med.,* **62**:231–46, 1963.

9. Giovanetti, S., and Maggiore, Q.: "A Low Nitrogen Diet with Proteins of High Biological Value for Severe Chronic Uremia," **1**:1000–1003, 1964.

10. Berlyne, G. M., *et al.:* "Dietary Treatment of Chronic Renal Failure," *Am. J. Clin. Nutr.,* **21**:547–52, 1968.

11. Franklin, S. S., *et al.:* "Use of a Balanced Low-Protein Diet in Chronic Renal Failure," *J.A.M.A.,* **202**:477–84, 1967.

12. Kopple, J. D., *et al.:* "Controlled Comparison of 20 gm and 40 gm Protein Diets in the Treatment of Chronic Uremia," *Am. J. Clin. Nutr.,* **21**:553–64, 1968.

13. Kopple, J. D., *et al.:* "Evaluating Modified Protein Diets for Uremia," *J. Am. Diet. Assoc.,* **54**:481–85, 1969.

14. Comty, C. M.: "Long Term Dietary Management of Dialysis Patients. I. Pathologic Problems and Dietary Requirements," *J. Am. Diet. Assoc.,* **53**:439–44, 1968.

15. Kiley, J. E.: "Comments on the Past, Present, and Future of the Artificial Kidney," *J. Am. Diet. Assoc.,* **54**:469–74, 1969.

16. Lonergan, E. T., and Lange, K.: "Use of a Special Protein-Restricted Diet in Uremia," *Am. J. Clin. Nutr.,* **21**:595–602, 1968.

17. de St. Jeor, S. T., *et al.:* "Planning Low-Protein Diets for Use in Chronic Renal Failure," *J. Am. Diet. Assoc.,* **54**:34–38, 1969.

18. Jordan, W. L., *et al.:* "Basic Pattern for a Controlled Protein, Sodium, and Potassium Diet," *J. Am. Diet. Assoc.,* **50**:137–41, 1967.

19. Bailey, G. L., and Sullivan, N. R.: "Selected-Protein Diet in Terminal Uremia," *J. Am. Diet. Assoc.,* **52**:125–29, 1968.

20. Mitchell, M. C., and Smith, E. J.: "Dietary Care of the Patient with Chronic Oliguria," *Am. J. Clin. Nutr.,* **19**:163–69, 1966.

21. Tsaltas, T. T.: "Dietetic Management of Uremic Patients. I. Extraction of Potassium from Foods for Uremic Patients," *Am. J. Clin. Nutr.,* **22**:490–93, 1969.

22. Lonsdale, K.: "Human Stones," *Science,* **159**:1199–1207, 1968.
23. Lemann, J., *et al.:* "Possible Role of Carbohydrate-Induced Calciuria in Calcium Oxalate Kidney-Stone Formation," *N. Engl. J. Med.,* **280**:232–37, 1969.

ADDITIONAL REFERENCES

Berlyne, G. M., ed.: *Nutrition in Renal Disease.* The Williams & Wilkins Company, Baltimore, 1968.
Brand, L., and Komorita, N. I.: "Adapting to Long-Term Hemodialysis," *Am. J. Nurs.,* **66**:1778–81, 1966.
Downing, S. R.: "Nursing Support in Early Renal Failure," *Am. J. Nurs.,* **69**:1212–16, 1969.
Fellows, B. J.: "Hemodialysis at Home," *Am. J. Nurs.,* **66**:1775–78, 1966.
Freeman, R. M., and Bulechek, G. M.: "Programmed Instruction: An Approach to Dietary Management of Dialysis Patients," *Am. J. Clin. Nutr.,* **21**:613–17, 1968.
Merrill, J. P., and Hampers, C. L.: "Uremia," *N. Engl. J. Med.,* **282**:953–61; 1014–21, 1970.
"Programmed Instruction: Potassium Imbalance," *Am. J. Nurs.,* **67**:343–66, 1967.

INSTRUCTIONAL AIDS FOR THE PATIENT

de St. Jeor, S. T., *et al.: Low Protein Diets for the Treatment of Chronic Renal Failure.* University of Utah Press, Salt Lake City, 1970 ($4.50).
More Good Things Made with Dietetic Paygel-P Wheat Starch. Nutrition Services, General Mills, Inc., Minneapolis.
Recipes for Protein-Restricted Diets. The Doyle Pharmaceutical Company, Minneapolis.
Renal Failure Diet Manual. University of Alabama Hospitals and Clinics. Available from University of Alabama Book Store, Birmingham ($3.13).

45 Anemias

Blood is a constantly changing, highly complex tissue which is concerned with the transport of cell nutrients, the elimination of wastes, and the maintenance of chemical equilibrium. Its intricate function and composition suggest the need for a considerable variety of nutrients, and these have been discussed especially in Unit II. This chapter is concerned with those deficiencies that arise in the framework of the red blood cells and in the hemoglobin within these cells.

Synthesis of erythrocytes and hemoglobin. The red blood cells are synthesized in the bone marrow and proceed through a number of stages before they are released into the circulation as nonnucleated fully mature cells. For their synthesis many nutrients are required, including the amino acids. Vitamin B_{12} and folinic acid are required for the synthesis of DNA, which is essential for the growth and normal division of cells. When either or both of these vitamins are deficient, fewer cells can be produced, and they are released into the circulation as large, nucleated cells called megaloblasts. (See also Chapter 12, pages 182 and 183.)

Hemoglobin synthesis requires a constant source of iron for the formation of heme and of protein for the formation of globin. The rate of synthesis can be no more rapid than the supply of iron. The iron is made available to the erythroid marrow by the plasma, which in turn is supplied by the reserves held in the liver and by the absorption from the intestinal tract. (See page 113 for discussion of iron metabolism.)

The normal red cell count is about 5 million per cubic millimeter for males and 4.5 million for females. Normal hemoglobin levels for males range from 14 to 17 gm per 100 ml, and from 12 to 15 gm per 100 ml for females. The normal packed-cell volume (hematocrit) is about 45 per cent; for men the lower limit of normal is 42 per cent, for women, 36 per cent, and for pregnant women, 33 per cent.[1]

Anemia. Anemia is a condition in which there is a reduction in the total circulating hemoglobin. Anemias may be described biochemically in terms of lowered hemoglobin levels, number of red blood cells, and hematocrit. They are also differentiated on the basis of appearance of red cells: normocytic, macrocytic, or microcytic; nucleated or nonnucleated; normochromic, hyperchromic, or hypochromic. It is also possible to measure the iron reserves and the changes in the level of plasma iron and of transferrin.

According to Elwood,[2] mild anemias diagnosed by laboratory studies are not closely associated with clinical symptoms or with changes in cardiorespiratory functions. When anemias become more severe, the symptoms are more consistent. They include skin pallor, weakness, easy fatigability, headaches, dizziness, sensitivity to cold, and paresthesia. Cheilosis, glossitis, loss of appetite, and loss of gastrointestinal tone with accompanying symptoms of distress are seen in severe anemias. Concave "spoon" fingernails (koilonychia) with longitudinal ridging of the nails is sometimes present. With increasing severity of anemia, the oxygenation of tissues is reduced—hence the feeling of fatigue. The heart rate increases, palpitation occurs, and there is shortness of breath.

Etiology. Anemias may be caused by blood loss, decreased production of blood, or increased destruction of blood. Faulty nutrition occasioned either by failure to provide the essential nutrients, such as iron and protein, or by poor utilization of dietary constituents (for example, failure to absorb vitamin B_{12}) may lead to anemia, the type being dependent upon the initiating defect. Exposure to x-ray or radium, bone tumors, cirrhosis of the liver, carcinoma, and leukemias are examples of conditions that may interfere with red cell formation within the bone marrow. Increased destruction of the blood may be the result of the action of intestinal parasites, hemolytic bacteria, chemical agents such as coal tar products and sulfonamide compounds, or abnormal red cell structure (sickle cells).

The treatment of anemias is dependent upon a determination of the cause and eliminating it whenever possible. Nutritionally, specific supplements may be required to improve the formation of red cells and hemoglobin. A normal diet to restore good nutrition is usually emphasized to support the specific therapy.

Iron-Deficiency Anemia

Incidence. Iron deficiency follows a specific sequence.[3] First, the iron reserves drop to lower levels, the transferrin level of the blood increases slightly, and the hematocrit and plasma iron levels remain normal. Then the iron reserves are used up, the transferrin level increases further, the hematocrit and plasma iron are reduced, and fewer red blood cells are produced. Finally, with no remaining iron reserves, the hematocrit and plasma iron continue to fall, and the cells are pale and reduced in size. Thus, the designation for the anemia is microcytic, hypochromic.

The term *nutritional* anemia is sometimes applied to iron-deficiency anemia, but this can be misleading inasmuch as some of the macrocytic anemias are also of nutritional origin.

Iron-deficiency anemias are widely prevalent throughout the world, but the exact incidence is not known. In four studies on pregnant women, the percentage that had hemoglobin levels below 11 gm per 100 ml ranged from 15 to 58; in four studies on infants the percentage of anemic babies ranged from 8 to 64.[1] These wide variations are explained, in part, by the differing socioeconomic groups studied. (See Figure 45–1.) Generally, the incidence is high in infants and pregnant women of low economic status, and higher in black than in white individuals. In better economic circumstances, the incidence is lower.

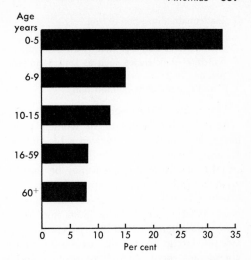

Figure 45–1. The National Nutrition Survey showed that low levels of hemoglobin were present in all age categories. Infants and preschool children had an especially high incidence. (Courtesy, Drs. A. E. Schaefer and O. C. Johnson. Reprinted from *Nutrition Today,* **4:** 6 [Spring], 1969.)

According to Elwood, the incidence of iron-deficiency anemia is relatively high if one accepts the WHO criteria for anemia: below 12 gm hemoglobin per 100 ml for women, and below 14 gm for men, and a hematocrit below 34 per cent. On the other hand, Elwood states that anemia is not so common if one also includes the symptoms and cardiorespiratory changes clearly attributable to the changes in blood cells and hemoglobin.[2]

Etiology. Among the factors to be considered as initiating iron-deficiency anemia are these:

1. Blood loss (most common cause in adults)
    a. Accidental hemorrhage
    b. Chronic diseases, such as tuberculosis, ulcers or intestinal disorders, when accompanied by hemorrhage
    c. Excessive menstrual losses
    d. Excessive blood donation
    e. Parasites such as hookworm
2. Deficiency of iron in the diet during period of accelerated demand
    a. Infancy—rapidly expanding blood volume
    b. Adolescent girls—rapid growth and onset of menses
    c. Pregnancy and lactation

3. Inadequate absorption of iron
   a. Diarrhea, as in sprue, pellagra
   b. Lack of acid secretion by the stomach
4. Nutrition deficiencies such as severe protein depletion
   a. Protein-calorie malnutrition

Blood loss. Whenever hypochromic anemia occurs in adult males or in women past the menopause, blood loss, as from a bleeding ulcer or other cause, must always be suspected. Menstrual losses by some women may be sufficiently great to result in anemia, especially if the diet is poorly selected. The range of such losses has been found to be 2.28 to 78.96 mg.[4] The repeated donation of blood likewise could be a significant factor in anemia causation unless a liberal diet relatively rich in protein and iron were taken.

Whenever there is a loss of blood, fluid is quickly drawn in from the tissues to maintain the blood volume. The hemoglobin level and red cells are thus reduced in concentration, but the individual with adequate stores quickly replenishes the levels so that anemia is not evident unless hemorrhage is prolonged or repeated. From three weeks to three months may be required to replenish the losses from the donation of 1 pint of blood.

Infants and preschool children. The full-term infant born of a well-nourished mother has a sufficient hemoglobin supply for the first two or three months of life, after which iron-rich foods should be added to the milk diet. Many babies, however, are not born with this endowment of hemoglobin. Infants of low birth weight, those who are multiple births, and those whose mothers have had several previous pregnancies are least likely to have adequate reserves.

Iron-fortified cereals should be given to the infant as early as six weeks of life. When they are discontinued after six months of age, the foods substituted are likely to supply too little iron and thus an anemia follows. Many infants from low socioeconomic groups are anemic because mothers are unaware of the importance of using iron-fortified cereals or because they cannot afford to purchase them.

A cause of anemia in certain infants has been gastrointestinal bleeding resulting from the ingestion of homogenized milk. Heat-labile proteins in milk are believed to be responsible inasmuch as heat-processed cow's milk formulas do not produce the blood loss.[5,6]

Anemia in adolescent girls and women. Because of the lower calorie requirements of women the iron intake is likely to be no more than 10 to 12 mg per day, even though the other aspects of the diet may be fully adequate. With absorption at 5 to 10 per cent, these intakes are not adequate to cover fully the losses entailed by menstruation and to build up reserves. Adolescent girls, in addition, must have iron to meet their growth requirements; yet, during these years their diets are often of generally poor quality.

Pregnancy imposes substantial additional demands upon the iron supply. The woman who has had repeated pregnancies and the young girl who is still maturing are most likely to become anemic and to bear infants who have little or no reserves.

Treatment. For iron-deficiency anemia the primary emphasis in treatment is a supplement of iron salts such as ferrous sulfate, gluconate, or fumarate. Oral therapy is as effective as parenteral therapy except where there is severe interference with absorption as in ulcerative colitis or regional enteritis. Some individuals have an initial intolerance to iron salts, but usually become adjusted to the medication. It is helpful to take the salts after meals.

DIETARY COUNSELING

Although the specific therapy for iron-deficiency anemia is iron medication, the patient needs specific guidance in the selection of an adequate diet. The diet history will establish the previous pattern of food intake and will indicate the corrections that are to be recommended. Frequently, the choice of foods has been poor with respect to sources of iron. With special emphasis on the inclusion of liver every week, if possible, and on the liberal use of dried fruits, dark-green leafy vegetables, and enriched breads and cereals, the daily iron intake for women will be approximately 12 to 15 mg. Some animal foods at each meal help to improve the absorption of iron from the plant sources as well. Ascorbic-acid-rich juices also improve iron absorption and should be used generously. For many women, the importance of continuing to use a prophylactic supplement even after the anemia has been corrected may need to be emphasized.

In moderately severe anemias the regeneration of hemoglobin is improved if protein intakes are increased to 80 to 100 gm daily. The diets of many women and girls are low in protein, and specific suggestions for increasing the protein content of the diet should be given. When cost is an important factor, simple recipes for dishes that use nonfat dry milk, poultry, fish, and less expensive cuts of meat are useful if food is prepared in the home.

PERNICIOUS ANEMIA

Characteristics. Pernicious anemia is caused by a lack of intrinsic factor in the gastric juice, and therefore vitamin B_{12} cannot be absorbed. With the absence of vitamin B_{12} the synthesis and maturation of the red blood cells are arrested. The anemia occurs chiefly in middle-aged to elderly persons and may be a genetic defect. Pernicious anemia also occurs following surgical removal of the portion of the stomach that produces the intrinsic factor, or the portion of the ileum where absorption of vitamin B_{12} takes place. These effects of surgery do not become evident until three to five years after surgery, indicating the reserves of vitamin B_{12} ordinarily held in the body.

In pernicious anemia the red cell count is often less than 2.5 million per cubic millimeter, with a large proportion of these cells being macrocytic. Patients have a lemon-yellow pallor, anorexia, glossitis, achlorhydria, abdominal discomfort, frequent diarrhea, weight loss, and general weakness. Numbness of the limbs, coldness of the extremities, and difficulty in walking are manifestations of neurologic changes in the untreated patient.

Treatment. Until Minot and Murphy introduced liver therapy in 1926, pernicious anemia was invariably fatal.[7] Their use of large amounts of liver started the search for the factor that was responsible for improvement. Liver extract replaced the liver diet and was in turn superseded by vitamin B_{12}.

When given parenterally, vitamin B_{12} produces marked hematopoietic response in dosages as small as 1 mcg daily. The vitamin is ineffective when given orally because of the absence of intrinsic factor.

Although folic acid brings about correction of the hematologic picture in pernicious anemia, it has no effect on the associated neurologic symptoms. Folic acid should never be used in place of vitamin B_{12} for the treatment of these patients, lest the neurologic symptoms become progressively worse. Because of this danger, multivitamin preparations may not contain more than 0.1 mg folic acid in a daily dosage.

DIETARY COUNSELING

Poor appetite, sore mouth, and gastrointestinal discomfort seriously interfere with an adequate food intake so that patients often present a picture of general nutritional deficiency. Their diets must be corrected for adequate calories and for protein. Because of the achlorhydria, the rate of digestion is retarded. Hence, the fat content of the diet should be kept to moderate levels, restricting especially fried foods that may further delay gastric emptying.

A soft, or even liquid, diet is preferable until the glossitis disappears. Tart and spicy foods should especially be avoided. (See Soft Diet, page 404, and Full-Fluid Diet, page 407.) Supplementation with ascorbic acid is essential if citrus fruits and other rich sources of the vitamin are not ingested. One practical way to supplement the usual diet is to use high-protein high-calorie beverages two or three times daily. They may be prepared from milk, nonfat dry milk, and flavorings, or one of several relatively inexpensive proprietary preparations may be used.

FOLIC ACID DEFICIENCY

A deficiency of folic acid leads to arrest of the synthesis and maturation of the red blood cells thus leading to megaloblastic anemia. Although the blood picture from folic acid lack resembles that occurring with vitamin B_{12} deficiency, it must be emphasized that one vitamin does not replace the other but that they are interrelated in function. Folic acid deficiency is observed in a variety of circumstances.

1. Elderly patients. A high incidence of folic acid deficiency has been noted in elderly patients, correlated with a poor intake of milk, fresh fruits, and vegetables.[8] The dietary fault results from lack of knowledge concerning the needs for foods in later life, insufficient income to purchase the essential foods, and organic diseases that interfere with food intake and further aggravate the deficiency. Malignancies, malabsorption, loss of blood, and certain drug therapies also reduce

the serum folate levels. Additional folate therapy is recommended especially during acute stages of illness, but the blood levels of vitamin B_{12} should also be monitored.

2. Pregnancy. Megaloblastic anemia occurs with lesser frequency than iron-deficiency anemia. It is usually caused by inadequate diet and is corrected by folic acid therapy.

3. Infancy. Macrocytic anemia in babies is more frequent in those born to mothers who also have a folic acid deficiency. Anemia is present in infants who have scurvy, because lack of ascorbic acid reduces the conversion of folic acid to its active form folinic acid.

4. Disorders of absorption. Macrocytic anemia, often severe in tropical sprue, improves dramatically with folic acid therapy. Some improvement is often seen in the anemia of nontropical sprue and celiac disease with folic acid therapy. (See Chapter 36.)

5. Prolonged use of contraceptives. A preliminary report of women who had used oral contraceptives for a long time indicated a suppression of a rise of serum folates from dietary folic acid. The women had complaints of fatigue and nausea, and laboratory studies established the presence of megaloblastic anemia. Folic acid therapy reversed these findings.[9]

PROBLEMS AND REVIEW

1. What nutrients are essential for the production of hemoglobin and red blood cells?
2. What are some of the etiologic agents that cause anemia? Which anemias originate because of a faulty diet? Which anemias may be classed as secondary nutritional deficiencies?
3. What are the laboratory findings and clinical symptoms of iron-deficiency anemia? Which groups are especially vulnerable?
4. What factors may interfere with the efficient use of iron in the body? Why is a so-called "high-iron" diet impractical in the treatment of iron-deficiency anemia?
5. What iron preparations are commonly provided for patients with iron-deficiency anemia? What dietary modification may be indicated?
6. List important steps that can be taken to prevent iron-deficiency anemia.
7. Why is vitamin B_{12} given parenterally to patients with pernicious anemia?
8. What problems may be encountered in the dietary intake by patients with pernicious anemia? How can these be controlled?
9. *Problem.* Plan a diet for a young woman who has iron-deficiency anemia to include 80 gm protein, 15 mg iron, and not more than 2000 calories.

CITED REFERENCES

1. Committee on Iron Deficiency, Council on Foods and Nutrition: "Iron Deficiency in the United States," *J.A.M.A.*, **203**:407–14, 1968.
2. Elwood, Peter C., and Waters, W. E.: "The Vital Distinction," *Nutr. Today*, **4**:14–19, Summer 1969.
3. Finch, C. A.: "Iron Metabolism," *Nutr. Today*, **4**:2–7, Summer 1969.
4. Frenchman, R., and Johnston, F. A.: "Relation of Menstrual Losses to Iron Requirement," *J. Am. Diet. Assoc.*, **25**:217–20, 1949.
5. Wilson, J. F., *et al.*: "Studies on Iron Metabolism. IV. Milk-Induced Gastrointestinal Bleeding in Infants with Hypochromic Microcytic Anemia," *J.A.M.A.*, **189**:568–72, 1964.
6. Woodruff, C.: "Nutritional Anemias in Early Childhood," *Am. J. Clin. Nutr.*, **22**:504–11, 1969.
7. Minot, G. R., and Murphy, W. P.: "Treatment of Pernicious Anemia by a Special Diet," *J.A.M.A.*, **87**:470–76, 1926.
8. Meindok, H., and Dvorsky, R.: "Serum Folate and Vitamin B_{12} Levels in the Elderly," *J. Am. Geriatr. Soc.*, **18**:317–26, 1970.
9. Necheles, T. F., and Snyder, L. M.: "Malabsorption of Folate Polyglutamates Associated with Oral Contraceptive Therapy," *N. Engl. J. Med.*, **282**:858–59, 1970.

ADDITIONAL REFERENCES

Bainton, D. F., and Finch, C. A.: "The Diagnosis of Iron Deficiency Anemia," *Am. J. Med.*, **37**:62–70, 1964.
Bianchi, A., *et al.*: "Nutritional Folic Acid Deficiency with Megaloblastic Changes in the Small-Bowel Epithelium," *N. Engl. J. Med.*, **282**:859–61, 1970.
Jacobs, A: "Pernicious Anemia—1822–1929," *Arch. Intern. Med.*, **103**:329–33, 1959.
Moore, C. V.: "The Importance of Nutritional Factors in the Pathogenesis of Iron Deficiency Anemia," *Am. J. Clin. Nutr.*, **3**:3–10, 1955.
Patwardhan, V. N.: "Nutritional Anemias—WHO Research Program," *Am. J. Clin. Nutr.*, **19**:63–71, 1966.
Review: "Folacin and Megaloblastic Anemia," *Nutr. Rev.*, **22**:3–5, 1964.
———: "Iron Deficiency Anemia due to Hookworm Infection in Man," *Nutr. Rev.*, **26**:47–49, 1968.
———: "The Prevalence of Iron Deficiency Anemia," *Nutr. Rev.*, **26**:263–65, 1968.
———: "Secondary Effects of Iron Deficiency," *Nutr. Rev.*, **27**:41–43, 1969.
West, R.: "Activity of Vitamin B_{12} in Addisonian Pernicious Anemia," *Science*, **107**:398, 1948.
Wintrobe, M. M.: *Clinical Hematology*, 6th ed. Lea & Febiger, Philadelphia, 1967.

Unit XIV
Diet in Miscellaneous Disorders

Chapter

46 Diet in Allergic and Skin Disturbances
Elimination Diets

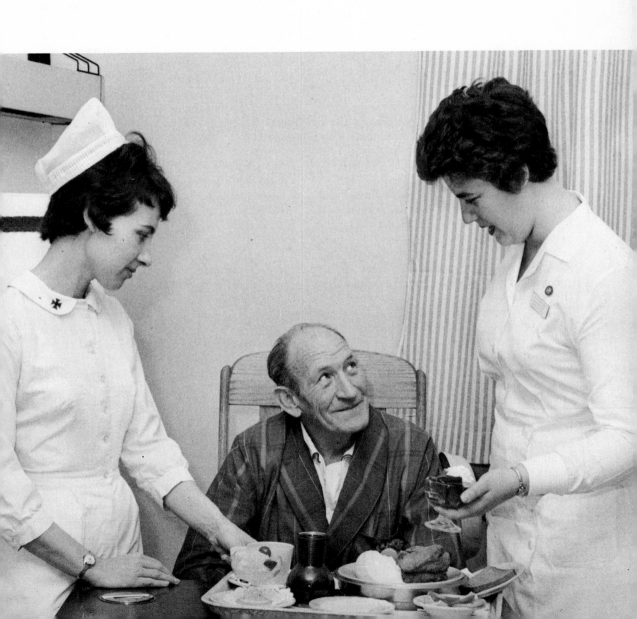

46 Diet in Allergic and Skin Disturbances

Elimination Diets

Incidence. The Allergy Foundation of America estimates that about 22 million Americans (1 in 10 persons) suffer from some form of allergy; about 16 million of these have hay fever, asthma, or both.[1] This high incidence places allergy as an important public health problem exceeded only by heart disease, arthritis, and high blood pressure. For example, the time lost from work because of allergies totaled 25 million man-days in 1969.[1] Food allergies account for a relatively small proportion of all allergies, but allergies to major food groups present serious problems in meal planning and in adequate nutrition. Moreover, many people who suffer from nonfood allergies find it difficult to ingest an adequate diet—the individual with severe asthma, for example.

The allergic reaction. *Allergies* are the abnormal reactions of an individual to the food he eats, the air he breathes, or the substances he touches. An *allergen* is any substance that sets off the allergic reaction. It is usually a protein, but it may be a polysaccharide or a complex of protein and polysaccharide. Simple substances such as aspirin that produce allergic reactions do not fit into these groups of compounds, but it is believed that they attach to body proteins and form a complex that becomes the active allergen.[1]

The *antibody-antigen* complex is the body's normal protective mechanism against foreign substances such as bacteria and viruses; thus, when bacteria (antigens) gain entrance to the body, they are complexed with antibodies to provide the immune reaction. In allergic persons this mechanism has in some way gone awry; that is, the antibodies react with substances that are normally harmless and set off a chain of damaging reactions. The details of the mechanisms involved are beyond the scope of this text; a comprehensive report published in 1970 describes the many approaches to the study.[1]

Allergic reactions may be brought about by (1) ingestion of food or drugs; (2) contact with foods, pesticides, drugs, adhesive, fur, hair, feathers, molds, fungi, and so on; (3) inhalation of pollens, dust, molds, fungi, cosmetics, perfumes; and (4) injection of vaccines, serums, antibiotics, and hormones.

The allergic reaction may be immediate, that is within four hours, or delayed, that is 4 to 72 hours following exposure.[2] An individual may have an immediate reaction to one substance, for example oysters, and a delayed reaction to another substance, such as eggs. The time at which the reaction occurs varies from one individual to another, but it is always the same in a given individual. For example, if the reaction to oysters is immediate, it will always be so and not delayed.

Some individuals are only mildly sensitive and can eat a particular food for several days before characteristic symptoms develop, whereas others have violent reactions within minutes after ingesting only minute traces of the offending substance. The tiny amount of egg adhering to a poorly washed fork or the trace of shrimp remaining in an unwashed pan used for another food preparation is enough to cause immediate, violent symptoms in highly sensitive persons.

Heredity plays an important role in allergy. The incidence is higher in families where one parent has an allergy than in families in which neither parent is affected; when both parents are affected, the incidence among children is still higher. The child does not inherit a sensitivity to a specific substance or an identical manifestation of the allergy. The parent may be sensitive to wheat, for example, and the child to pollens. The parent may have eczema or a gastrointestinal disturbance whereas the child suffers from asthma.

Any kind of physical or emotional stress increases the severity of allergic reactions. However, the stress situation is not the cause of allergy, and too often the genuinely allergic individual is regarded by his family and friends as well as professional health personnel as reacting because of his emotions.

Food allergens. Any food may produce reactions but the most frequent offenders are eggs, milk, wheat, grapefruit, oranges, strawberries, corn, tomatoes, potatoes, nuts, fish, shellfish, chocolate, and some spices.

Foods unlike in flavor and structure but belonging to the same botanic group may result in allergic manifestations. For example, buckwheat is not of the cereal family but in a group which includes rhubarb. The sweet potato is not related to the white potato but is a member of the morning-glory family. Spinach, a frequent reactor, is in the same family with beets. The following botanic classification of a few common foods illustrates the relation of foods which at first thought appear to be dissimilar.

Cereal—wheat, rye, barley, rice, oats, malt, corn, sorghum, cane sugar
Lily—onion, garlic, asparagus, chives, leeks, shallots
Gourd—squash, pumpkin, cucumber, cantaloupe, watermelon
Cabbage and mustard—turnips, cabbage, collards, cauliflower, broccoli, kale, radish, horseradish, watercress, Brussels sprouts

Symptoms of food allergies. Manifestations of allergy may occur in any part of the body. The tissues of these systems are frequently involved, singly or in combination: respiratory, cutaneous, neural, gastrointestinal, cardiovascular, genitourinary, and articular.[2] The symptoms are consequently varied depending upon the parts affected.

1. Skin lesions may include dermatitis, canker sores, fever blisters, pruritus, and edema.

2. Nausea, vomiting, stomatitis, bad breath, diarrhea, constipation, and abdominal distention are common gastrointestinal manifestations. The symptoms are often suggestive of colitis, appendicitis, ulcers, or even gallbladder disease, and there may be confusion in diagnosis.

3. Redness, swelling, burning, and itching of the eyes may accompany irritation of the nasal passages or be independent of it.

4. Head colds, asthma, and migraine headaches are often caused by allergy.

Diagnosis of food allergies. The procedures used include a careful diet history, skin testing, and testing with restricted diets.

History. A complete history is the single most important diagnostic tool. When a severe reaction occurs immediately, the patient is usually aware of the circumstances leading up to it. However, when reactions are delayed or when allergies are multiple in nature, the elucidation of the offending factors is often exceedingly difficult. The history must include a complete evaluation of the physical status and the conditions and events preceding the attack.

The patient is asked to keep a rigorous diary of all foods ingested and of the occurrence of any symptoms. Individual likes and dislikes must be taken into consideration. One patient may dislike an important food and claim to be allergic to it in order not to be called upon to eat it. Another may like a food sufficiently well to risk an attack in order to eat it.

Skin tests. Fully half of all food allergies do not produce skin reactions.[2] A skin test is potentially dangerous when an allergen to which the person is highly sensitive is injected. Therefore, skin tests are ordinarily administered subsequent to a careful diet history.

Skin tests include (1) the *scratch test,* in which a bit of suspected solution is dropped onto a scratch made on the back or arm of the patient; (2) the *intradermal test,* in which the suspected solution is injected underneath the skin; and (3) the *patch test,* in which the suspected powder or liquid is put on a filter paper which is placed on the skin, covered with cellophane, and held in place with adhesive. Readings are made at the end of 10 to 20 minutes, except in the patch test, where readings are made after 48 hours or more. If a red inflammation or hivelike wheal appears at the site of the scratch or point of contact, the material is suspected as an allergen. The tests are suggestive but not conclusive. A positive skin test does not necessarily mean that the patient is sensitive at the time to the material; it may represent a past sensitivity.

Restricted diets. Many variants of restricted diets have been proposed as diagnostic aids. One of these is the substitution of a synthetic formula consisting of amino acids, sugar, emulsified fats, salt mixtures, vitamin concentrates, and water for the typical dietary intake.[3,4] Individuals who are allergic to foods will show marked improvement after a few days' restriction to the formula. If they are sensitive to nonfood items, no improvement will take place. When improvement occurs, the formula may be continued with the addition of one food item at a time to determine which ones may be safely included and which ones must be excluded. The formula is accepted poorly by adults and therefore is seldom used for them, but the procedure is much more acceptable to infants.

Another approach is to restrict the patient to a list of foods to which no skin reactions were shown. The restricted diet may be tested for one to three weeks, after which new foods are added, one at a time, at three-day intervals. This procedure is not infallible inasmuch as persons often react to foods without showing any skin reactions.

A number of elimination diets have been developed, based upon the principle that only those foods that are seldom responsible for allergy are included in the trial diet. One of the most widely used of these regimens is the Rowe Elimination Diet, reproduced in part on pages 607 to 608.

The patient is first placed on the diet which, on the basis of skin tests and a dietary history, is least likely to produce allergic reactions. The diet will be used from one to three weeks, unless severe reactions have occurred in the meantime. A second diet is then tried for a similar period. Two to three weeks are usually necessary to give time for previous allergic manifestations to wear off and for any possible new reactions to appear. If there has been no adverse reaction to two or more diets, all foods on the combined lists may be used. On the other hand, when untoward symptoms appear, another diet is used until all diets have been tried. If the patient shows no improvement on any of the diets of a given regimen, the allergy is probably not of food origin.

Dietary treatment. If a single food such as strawberries or grapefruit is implicated, it is easy to omit this food from the diet. If allergy involves more than one food, the beginning diet is one that contains only those foods that produce no reactions. Thus, if improvement has occurred on an elimination diet, simple, not mixed, foods are added, one at a time, to the allowed list of foods. Several days to a week must elapse between the addition of each new food. Moreover, a given food should be tested on at least two, preferably three, occasions before it is permanently added to, or eliminated from, the diet. Because wheat, eggs, and milk are frequent allergens, these foods are added last.

Dietary adequacy becomes a matter of great concern when important foods are eliminated for a long period of time. For example, if milk cannot be used, additional amounts of meat should be included to provide the required allowance of protein, and calcium salts will need to be prescribed.

Desensitization consists in decreasing the sensitivity to a given substance by giving minute doses of the allergen in gradually increasing amounts. No hard-and-fast rule can be given for the amount of the allergen initially introduced, but it is very minute. For example, if a child is sensitive to milk he may be given a few drops of a dilution in which a drop of milk is mixed with a pint of water. If his progress is satisfactory on such a dilution, he is given gradually increasing amounts from time to time. If severe reactions occur at any time during the period of desensitization, the next dose is not increased and the progression must be more gradual. Two or three years may be required before a normal amount of the food can be tolerated.

Desensitization is a very tedious procedure and is employed only when a major food group is involved.

Dietary management for asthmatic patients. Those who have severe asthma often find it difficult to consume an adequate diet. The meals should be small and eaten slowly in an environment free from stress. Interval feedings are

ELIMINATION DIETS*

Diet 1	Diet 2	Diet 3	Diet 4
Rice	Corn	Tapioca	Milk†
Tapioca	Rye	White potato	Tapioca
Rice biscuit	Corn pone	Breads made of any com-	Cane sugar
Rice bread	Corn-rye muffins	bination of soy, Lima	
	Rye bread	bean, and potato starch	
	Ry-Krisp	and tapioca flours	
Lettuce	Beets	Tomato	
Chard	Squash	Carrot	
Spinach	Asparagus	Lima beans	
Carrot	Artichoke	String beans	
Sweet potato or yam		Peas	
Lamb	Chicken (no hens)	Beef	
	Bacon	Bacon	
Lemon	Pineapple	Lemon	
Grapefruit	Peach	Grapefruit	
Pears	Prunes	Peach	
	Apricot	Apricot	
Cane sugar	Cane or beet sugar	Cane sugar	
Sesame oil	Mazola oil	Sesame oil	
Olive oil‡	Sesame oil	Soybean oil	
Salt	Salt	Salt	
Gelatin, plain or fla-	Gelatin, plain or fla-	Gelatin, plain or flavored	
vored with lime or	vored with pine-	with lime or lemon	
lemon	apple		
Maple syrup or syrup	Karo corn syrup	Maple syrup or syrup	
made with cane	White vinegar	made with cane sugar	
sugar flavored with		flavored with maple	
maple			
Royal baking powder	Royal baking powder	Royal baking powder	
Baking soda	Baking soda	Baking soda	
Cream of tartar	Cream of tartar	Cream of tartar	
Vanilla extract	Vanilla extract	Vanilla extract	
Lemon extract		Lemon extract	

*Rowe, A. H.: *Elimination Diets and the Patient's Allergies,* 2nd ed. Lea & Febiger, Philadelphia, 1944.

† Milk should be taken up to 2 to 3 quarts a day. Plain cottage cheese and cream may be used. Tapioca cooked with milk and milk sugar may be taken.

‡Allergy to it may occur with or without allergy to olive pollen. Mazola oil may be used if corn allergy is not present.

SAMPLE MENUS FOR ELIMINATION DIETS

Diet 1

BREAKFAST
Half grapefruit with or
without sugar
Rice Krispies with pear juice
or maple syrup
Lamb patties
Lemonade, hot or cold; or
grapefruit juice*

LUNCHEON OR SUPPER
Sautéed lamb liver (using
sesame oil)
Boiled rice
Carrots
Rice bread or biscuits
Grapefruit marmalade or
maple syrup
Molded pear in lemon
gelatin
Grapefruit juice or lemonade

DINNER
Lamb chop or roast lamb
Baked sweet potato or yam
Spinach
Lettuce with French dressing
(sesame oil, lemon juice,
salt)
Rice bread or biscuit
Grapefruit marmalade or
maple syrup
Fresh pear
Lemonade or grapefruit juice

Diet 2

BREAKFAST
Sliced peaches on cornflakes
or cornmeal mush
Bacon
Rye toast or rye muffins
(whole rye flour only)
Pineapple or apricot jam
Prune, pineapple, or apricot
juice*

LUNCHEON OR SUPPER
Baked or fried chicken
(using Mazola)
Harvard beets (white
vinegar, sugar, cornstarch)
Rye-corn muffins
Pineapple or apricot jam
Sliced pineapple
Pineapple, apricot, or prune
juice

DINNER
Sliced chicken
Baked squash
Asparagus
Ry-Krisp or rye bread
Pineapple or apricot
preserves
Stewed apricots or prunes
Pineapple, apricot, or prune
juice

Diet 3

BREAKFAST
Half grapefruit with or
without sugar
Bacon
Muffins, using soybean, Lima
bean, or potato flour
Apricot, peach, or grapefruit
marmalade or maple
syrup
Tomato juice, grapefruit
juice or lemonade*

LUNCHEON OR SUPPER
Beef broth
Beef patties
Baked white potato
Sliced tomatoes
French dressing (soybean
oil, lemon juice, salt)
Biscuits made of Lima bean,
potato, or soybean flour
Apricot or peach preserves
Tomato juice, grapefruit
juice or lemonade

DINNER
Roast beef
Carrots and peas (no cream
sauce)
String beans
Grapefruit with French
dressing (no lettuce)
Lima bean, soybean, or
potato bread
Grapefruit marmalade
Apricot tapioca
Tomato, grapefruit, or
apricot juice, or lemonade

*If the patient remains symptom free on the diet being used for five to seven days, tea may be added as a beverage. In the same manner coffee may be added.

necessary to bolster the caloric intake. Usually breakfast and lunch are the best meals of the day, and particular attention should be paid to their nutritional quality and attractiveness. A rest period after meals is helpful. Ordinarily, late-evening feedings are not advisable.[2]

DIETARY COUNSELING

Labeling. Patients who are allergic to important foods such as milk, eggs, and wheat must be constantly on guard lest they inadvertently ingest a mixture that contains the offending allergen. The first rule that the patient and those who cook for him must learn is to read *all* labels on food products *every* time that purchases are made. Because formulations change from time to time, there is no guarantee that a food that did not contain the allergen at one time will continue to be free of the offending substance.

Foods for which a standard of identity has been established by the Food and Drug Administration need not be labeled with a complete listing of ingredients; only optional ingredients need be listed for such products. Therefore, the label is not an adequate protection for those individuals with food allergies. For example, mayonnaise contains small amounts of egg, but this is not indicated on the label. A number of breads have been included under standards of identity, and thus the label would not indicate that milk is an ingredient.

Lists of foods to avoid for diets without eggs, wheat, or milk are given below. The patient should be encouraged to add foods to these lists as he discovers from his label reading that they contain the allergen.

Diet Without Eggs—Foods to Avoid

Eggs in any form

Beverages—Cocomalt, eggnog, malted beverages, Ovaltine, root beer

Breads and rolls containing eggs—crust glazed with egg, French toast, sweet rolls, griddle cakes, muffins, waffles, pretzels, zwieback

Desserts—cake, cookies, custard, doughnuts, ice cream, meringue, cream-filled pies—coconut, cream, custard, lemon, pumpkin, puddings

Meats—meat loaf; breaded meats dipped in egg

Noodles

Salad dressings—mayonnaise, cooked dressing

Sauces—Hollandaise

Soups: broth, consommé

Sweets—many cake icings, candies: cream, chocolate, fondant, marshmallow, nougat

Diet Without Wheat—Foods to Avoid

Beverages—Cocomalt, malted milk, instant coffee unless 100 per cent coffee, coffee substitutes; beer, gin, whiskey

Breads, crackers, and rolls—all breads including rye, oatmeal, and corn; hot breads and muffins; baking-powder biscuits; gluten bread; matzoth, pretzels, zwieback; crackers; griddle cakes, waffles

Note: bread, crackers, or wafers made of 100 per cent rye, corn, rice, soy, or potato flours may be used.

Cereals

All-bran	Pablum
Beemax	Pep
Bran flakes	Pettijohn's
Cheerios	Puffed Wheat
Crackels	Ralston cereals
Cream of Wheat	Shredded Wheat
Farina	Special K
Grape-Nuts	Total
Grape-Nuts flakes	Wheatena
Kix	Wheat flakes
Krumbles	Wheat germ
Maltex	Wheaties
Mello-wheat	Wheatsworth
Muffets	Wheat Chex
New oats	

Desserts—cake or cookies, homemade, from mixes, or bakery; doughnuts, ice cream, ice-cream cones, pies, puddings

Flour—white, whole wheat, graham

Gravies and sauces thickened with flour

Meats—prepared with flour, bread, or cracker crumbs such as croquettes and meat loaf; stews thickened with flour or made with dumplings; frankfurters, luncheon meats, or sausage in which wheat has been used as a filler; canned meat dishes such as stews, chili

Pastas—macaroni, noodles, spaghetti, vermicelli, and so on

Salad dressings—thickened with flour

Soups—commercially canned

Diet Without Milk—Foods to Avoid

Milk—all forms—fresh whole or skim; buttermilk; dry; evaporated; malted; yogurt

Beverages—Cocomalt, cocoa, chocolate, Ovaltine

Breads and rolls—any made with milk (most breads contain milk); sweet rolls; bread mixes; griddle cakes; waffles; zwieback

Cereals—Cream of Rice, Instant Cream of Wheat, Special K, Total

Cheese—all kinds

Desserts—cakes, cookies, custard, ice cream, pie crust made with butter or margarine, pies with cream fillings such as chocolate, coconut, cream, custard, lemon, pumpkin; puddings with milk, sherbets

Fats—butter, cream, margarine

Meat—frankfurters, luncheon meats, meat loaf—unless 100 per cent meat

Sauces—cream; any made with butter, margarine, milk, or cream

Soups—cream

Sweets—caramels, chocolate candy

Vegetables—seasoned with butter or margarine; with cream sauces; mashed potatoes

Food preparation. Cookery for milk-free, egg-free, or wheat-free diets is quite a challenge. A list of sources for recipes is given at the end of this chapter. In recipes using milk, water or fruit juices can usually be substituted. Quick breads can be made from soy, rice, potato, corn, rye, or other flours, but the proportion of baking powder is increased because of the lack of gluten in these flours. The finished products differ in texture from those prepared from wheat. They dry out rapidly and should be stored in a freezer rather than in the refrigerator.

DISEASES OF THE SKIN

The quality of the diet is a determining factor in skin health. Deficiencies of one or more nutrients are known to produce various cutaneous disorders. For example, there are the dermatitis associated with pellagra and resulting from lack of niacin (see page 176), the eruptions which accompany severe vitamin A deficiency (see page 150), the cheilosis of riboflavin lack (see page 173), and the eczema that occurs in infants with essential fatty acid deficiency (see page 82).

Some individuals may be allergic to certain substances and thus manifest skin disorders such as eczema or urticaria. Whenever allergy is suspected, it is essential to determine the offending agent as described in the preceding part of this chapter. No single food or food group predominates in producing allergic skin disorders.

Acne vulgaris is a particular problem during adolescence, and many boys and girls try bizarre diets in an effort to correct the situation. High-fat and concentrated carbohydrate diets have been considered to be undesirable. A study on 65 persons with acne vulgaris who consumed large amounts of chocolate showed that the course of the acne was not adversely affected nor were the output and composition of sebum changed.[5] The authors of this study state that the "effect of dietary fats and carbohydrates on acne and sebaceous secretion is singularly confusing, contradictory, and controversial."[*] They further state that the stimulation of sebaceous secretion by diets high in carbohydrate or in fat remains to be proven.

Dietary emphasis in skin disorders should be placed on nutritional adequacy; that is, the diet should contain sufficient milk, meat, eggs, fruits, vegetables, and whole-grain or enriched cereals and breads. Attention should be directed to improving the general hygiene, including skin cleanliness, regular meal hours, sufficient fluid intake, adequate rest, proper elimination, and psychologic support. There is no harm in excluding candies and sweets, fried foods, chocolate, and rich desserts, but such exclusion probably is most useful in that these foods are replaced by others that are more nutritionally satisfactory.

[*]Fulton, J. E., Jr., *et al.*: "Effect of Chocolate on Acne Vulgaris," *J.A.M.A.*, **210**:2071–74, 1969.

PROBLEMS AND REVIEW

1. Name some of the characteristic symptoms of allergy.
2. Name five foods to which a great number of allergies are due. Name some foods which rarely cause sensitivity.
3. What is meant by skin test? Elimination diet?
4. What are the principles for the construction of elimination diets? What are some of the shortcomings of many of these diets?
5. *Problem.* Plan a day's menu for a patient who is sensitive to wheat, potatoes, and grapefruit.
6. *Problem.* Prepare a list of foods which a patient should avoid if he is allergic to corn.

7. What recommendation could you make to a 15-year-old girl who has acne vulgaris?
8. *Problem.* Prepare a table which shows the nature of skin disorders when a diet is markedly deficient in each of the following: protein, essential fatty acids, vitamin A, riboflavin, niacin, ascorbic acid. Under what circumstances would you ˙expect these changes in the skin to become apparent? What is the incidence of these disorders in the United States?

CITED REFERENCES

1. Sanders, H. I.: "Allergy. A Protective Mechanism Out of Control," *Chem. Eng. News,* **48**:84–135, May 11, 1970.
2. Fontana, V. J., and Strauss, M. B.: "Nutrition in the Allergies," in Wohl, M. G., and Goodhart, R. S., eds.: *Modern Nutrition in Health and Disease,* 4th ed. Lea & Febiger, Philadelphia, 1968, Chapter 30.
3. Olmstead, W. H., *et al.:* "Use of Synthetic Diets for Food Allergy and Typhoid," *Arch. Intern. Med.,* **73**:341, 1944.
4. Rowe, P., and Sheldon, J. M.: "Synthetic Diets—Their Use as a Diagnostic Procedure in Allergic Disease," *J. Lab. Clin. Med.,* **33**:1059, 1948.
5. Fulton, J. E., *et al.:* "Effects of Chocolate on Acne Vulgaris," *J.A.M.A.,* **210**:2071–74, 1969.

ADDITIONAL REFERENCES

Alvarez, W. C.: "The Production of Food Allergy," *Gastroenterology,* **30**:325, 1956.
Derlacki, E.: "Food Sensitization as a Cause of Perennial Nasal Allergy," *Ann. Allergy,* **13**:82, 1956.
Heiner, D. C., *et al.:* "Sensitivity to Cow's Milk," *J.A.M.A.* **189**:536–67, 1964.
Krehl, W. A.: "Skin Disease and Nutritional Therapy," *J. Am. Diet. Assoc.,* **35**:923–28, 1959.
Kingery, F. A.: "Why Psoriasis Looks That Way," *J.A.M.A.,* **195**:953, 1966.
Lorincz, A. L.: "Nutrition in Relation to Dermatology," *J.A.M.A.,* **166**:1862–67, 1958.
Markow, H.: "Food Allergy," *N.Y. State J. Med.* **56**:3735, 1956.
Roe, D. A.: "Nutrient Requirements in Psoriasis," *N.Y. State J. Med.,* **65**:1319, 1965.
Roe, D. A.: "Taurine Intolerance in Psoriasis," *J. Invest. Dermatol.,* **46**:420–30, 1966.
Rowe, A. H., *et al.:* "Diarrhea Caused by Food Allergy," *J. Allergy,* **27**:424, 1956.
Rowe, A. H., *et al.:* "Bronchial Asthma Due to Food Allergy Alone in Ninety-five Patients," *J.A.M.A.,* **169**:1158, 1959.
Sheldon, J. M., *et al.:* A *Manual of Clinical Allergy,* 2nd ed. W. B. Saunders Company, Philadelphia, 1967.
Waldmann, T. A., *et al.:* "Allergic Gastroenteropathy," *N. Engl. J. Med.,* **276**:761–69, 1967.

SOURCES OF ALLERGY RECIPES

Allergy Diets. Ralston Purina Company, Checkerboard Square, St. Louis.
Allergy Recipes. The American Dietetic Association, 620 North Michigan Avenue, Chicago, 1969 ($1.00).
Baking for People with Food Allergies. HG 147, Government Printing Office, Washington, D.C., 1968 (10 cents).
Good Recipes to Brighten the Allergy Diet. Best Foods, Division Corn Products Company, 717 Fifth Avenue, New York, 1966.
125 Great Recipes for Allergy Diets. Good Housekeeping, 959 Fifth Avenue, New York (50 cents).

Unit XV

Diet in Children's Diseases

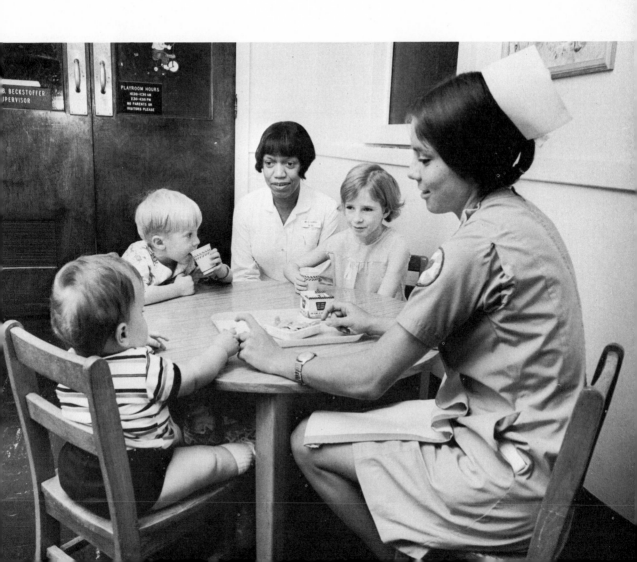

47 Nutrition in Children's Diseases

Although the principles of normal and therapeutic nutrition that apply to the adult are also applicable to the sick child, additional factors that must be carefully considered for the child are (1) growth needs; (2) stage of physical, emotional, and social development; (3) the presence of physical handicaps in some; and (4) the more rapid nutritional deterioration which occurs.

The essentials of normal nutrition provide the base line for planning meals for the sick child (see Chapters 22 and 23). The factors affecting food acceptance must be considered (see Chapter 14), and the principles of nutritional care and counseling are similar to those for adults (see Chapters 27 and 28). The principles of dietary modification for many conditions are similar for adults and for children, and the preceding chapters pertaining to therapeutic nutrition should be consulted for specific regimens. The discussion that follows supplements the descriptive material set forth in the earlier chapters.

Feeding problems of the sick child. Like adults, children face many obstacles in illness. Eating a satisfactory diet may be difficult because of fatigue, nausea, lack of appetite occasioned by the illness and by drugs, and pain. Children often regress to an earlier stage of feeding; for example, the child who has learned to accept chopped foods may refuse them, or the child who can feed himself may refuse to eat unless someone feeds him. Older children especially may experience a sense of failure and express it by excessive eating or refusal to eat. Illness produces emotional tensions in the child as well as in the adult. When the child must be placed in a hospital, he is also faced with the separation from his home and his parents. The principles of feeding the normal child apply in even greater degree to the child who is ill.

Insofar as possible the feeding program should establish a pattern of continuity with that to which the child is accustomed. A record of the child's feeding history is a first requisite so that the normal or therapeutic diet makes allowances for individual likes and dislikes. The period of a child's illness is no time in which to introduce new foods or to provide equipment that the child does not know how to handle. (See Figure 47–1.)

Even though careful menu planning takes into consideration the usual likes and dislikes of children and includes variations in both flavor and textures, foods may be refused. The illness itself and the strange environment are sufficient cause for such refusal; sometimes portions are a bit too large, or there may be a slight change in the flavoring or texture of a familiar food. Regardless of the reason for refusal, nothing can be gained by trying to force a child to eat.

Nurses and nutritionists must like children and must enjoy working with them if they expect to achieve good results in nutritional care. They must be observant of the child's behavior, of the acceptance or rejection of food, and of what the child says about his food. They have a special responsibility to communicate with the parents. From the parents they learn about the child's food habits at home, and about his attitudes toward food. In turn the parents are kept informed about the child's progress in food acceptance while in the hospital, and about changes that may be required after discharge.

Children often eat better when they are fed in groups. Family-style service in the pediatric ward to children who are well enough to sit up is more successful than individual tray service. Older children enjoy selecting their foods from a cafeteria arrangement whenever that is pos-

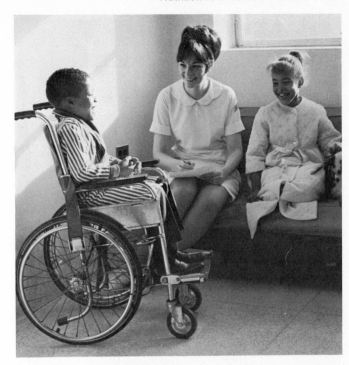

Figure 47–1. "Tell me what you like to eat." By learning something about the patients' food habits, the dietary technician can help to make their hospital stay more pleasant. Sometimes nutrition education can also be given on an informal basis. (Courtesy, Pittsburgh Dietetic Association and Pittsburgh Hospital Association.)

sible. Every advantage should be taken of birthdays and holidays to provide favorite foods and special treats. Many children are encouraged to eat when the mother can bring a favorite food, provided that it does not contradict the dietary regimen that has been ordered. Most hospitals now encourage parents to visit at any time they wish, and a young child fed by his mother may respond better than one who is fed by someone strange to him. (See Figure 47–2.)

DIETARY COUNSELING

Parents and children who are old enough to understand are jointly counseled regarding dietary modifications that will be required at home. Much less friction is likely to occur at home when the child is included in the interview. Parents assume the primary responsibility for nutritional care of the young child, but the child needs to know what is expected of him. As early as possible the child should

begin to assume some responsibility for his care. Older children under parental guidance gradually assume full responsibility for their own diets. In counseling it is important to direct the interview and the instructions to the child rather than to the parent.

One important aspect of counseling is to determine the attitudes of the parent toward the development of food habits, and likewise the child's attitudes not only toward his food but also toward his parents. Not infrequently the child uses food to achieve various ends.

If a modified diet will be required indefinitely as for diabetes mellitus, every effort must be made to plan this within the framework of the normal life pattern of the child; the diet must not become the dominating factor that interferes with the child's psychosocial development. Being like his peers is very important to the child, and for many reasons he may be reluctant to disclose that he is in any way different. Insofar as possible the diet should be planned so that it can in-

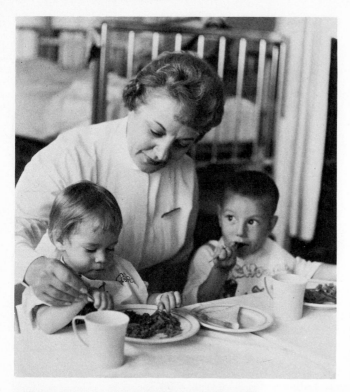

Figure 47–2. A guiding hand and a little encouragement will improve food intake greatly. Sick children away from home need the security of familiar foods and the understanding and affection of nurses, dietitians, and others. (Courtesy, Mrs. Elizabeth Wilcox and The Babies Hospital, New York City.)

clude foods that are popular with other children. The child must be helped to understand that his condition does not make him abnormal in his relations with others of his group. Selecting foods from those offered by the school lunch would be better for the diabetic child, for example, than carrying a lunch.

Sometimes the hospital stay is sufficiently long that some nutrition education can be included in a group situation.[1,2] (See Figure 47–3.) Movies appropriate for young children are available from the National Dairy Council and other sources. Older children often view movies with interest in the hospital playroom that they might consider to be boring in the school situation. The teacher assigned to the hospital schoolroom may also be involved in the dietary instruction. For example, children can learn to keep records, to score their diets, and to learn about their needs for basic foods. The calculation of a diet with meal ex-

changes may be used as an arithmetic assignment. Eye-catching fliers on patient's trays have been used to introduce new ideas about foods such as a food custom of an ethnic group or a simple recipe.

WEIGHT CONTROL

Obesity. Excessive weight is found in 10 to 20 per cent of all children and teen-agers and poses a problem for later years. If obesity is not corrected in childhood, the chances are very slim for successful weight loss later in life.

Like adults, children eat too much because an abundance of rich, high-calorie foods is readily available and becomes part of the family pattern. They use food to cover up loneliness, failure in schoolwork, or lack of social relationships. Some children overeat because a pattern of overfeeding has been established since infancy. But many

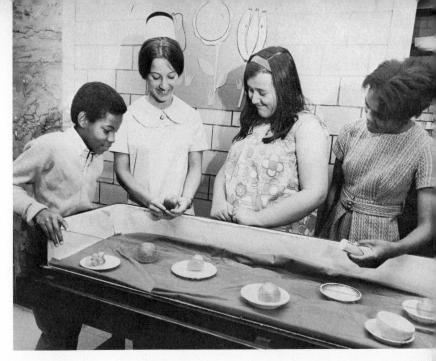

Figure 47–3. Nurse demonstrates nutritive equivalents of fruits to three teen-agers. (Courtesy, Medical College of Virginia, Health Sciences Division, Virginia Commonwealth University, Richmond.)

obese children do not eat any more food than normal-weight children; in fact, they may eat less. The difference lies in an appreciably lesser expenditure of energy by the obese.[3,4] They avoid active sports, and even when they are engaged in activities they manage to become involved as little as possible. (See also page 424.)

Because the energy requirements of children are relatively high, their diet is usually less restricted than that for adults. About 1200 to 1800 calories may be included, depending upon the stature and activity of the child. Liberal protein, mineral, and vitamin allowances are essential so that tissue and stature development are not adversely affected. The low-calorie diets described on page 422 may be used as a basis for planning the child's diet. To this diet should be added 1 cup of milk daily so that the child receives his quota of 1 quart. Vitamin D concentrates are prescribed if the milk is not fortified.

It is vital that the child (and his mother) realize what a loss of weight may mean to him. For some children this means emphasis on good appearance, poise, and gracefulness; for others it means greater participation in sports; and for still others it implies the approbation of fellow playmates and schoolmates. The physician, nurse, and dietitian who are guiding the child's weight-reduction program must show understanding of the child's problems and must maintain interest through a careful follow-up of the progress being made.

Underweight. The child who fails to show normal gains in weight and height usually tires easily, is irritable and restless, and is more susceptible to infections. As in the correction of obesity, the cause for underweight must first be sought so that treatment may be properly directed. The diet is corrected with respect to its adequacy of the essential nutrients, after which increases in the caloric level may be made gradually. A reasonable amount of outdoor exercise and regulated rest are important elements of the weight-gaining program. For high-calorie diets see Chapter 31.

Growth failure. It has been frequently observed that infants fail to thrive when placed in institutions because they are deprived of the normal emotional environment of the home. Such growth failure also occurs in the home when parents reject their children, neglect them, or provide an otherwise hostile environment. In 1967 Powell and his associates[5] reported that children from such environments begin to thrive when placed in an institution. The children they studied had voracious appetites on admission, presented symptoms not unlike those of the celiac syndrome, and had subnormal production of growth hormone. With feeding these children gained weight and their pituitary and adrenal function returned to normal. These observers suggested that the emotional trauma had an adverse effect on hormonal function leading to the growth failure and that removal from the home climate resulted in normal food utilization.

In 1969 Whitten and his associates[6] reported on 16 infants who were from emotionally deprived homes, and who were all below the third percentile for both weight and height. Thirteen of these infants were confined for two weeks in a room without windows and were visited infrequently. They were given adequate diet and physical care. Although such a situation can scarcely be considered to be emotionally appropriate, 10 of the infants grew at a rate greater than normal as if they were "catching up" in growth.

Subsequently six of these infants were mothered and given all the attention expected for babies. Their weight gain continued unchanged from that observed in the preceding period of emotional deprivation. Several infants were also fed in their own homes in the presence of an observer who made sure that they actually consumed the amounts of food the mothers claimed they had been eating. Under observation, the infants gained satisfactorily whereas earlier they had failed to do so.

Whitten and his coworkers do not believe that emotional deprivation produced a malfunction in metabolism and the utilization of food. They believed that the caloric intake was simply too low to support the needs for growth, and that the infants had not been consuming the foods the mothers claimed they were receiving. They did not believe the mothers were deliberately deceitful, but that their own emotional problems made it impossible for them to accurately determine the intake.

GASTROINTESTINAL DISTURBANCES IN INFANTS AND CHILDREN

Infant feeding problems. Many babies regurgitate small amounts of food, and this is no cause for concern. Usually it can be avoided by more frequent "burping" of the infant. Vomiting is more serious and should receive the attention of the physician.

Some babies cry loudly and for long intervals following feeding. Usually they have swallowed excessive amounts of air and have been inadequately "burped." However, some babies continue to cry even with "burping" and parents are likely to become quite distraught. These "colicky" babies usually grow well, and the parents need reassurance that they are progressing satisfactorily. Colic sometimes occurs because the baby is overfed, is tired, or is cold.

Constipation. Formula-fed infants usually have but one bowel movement daily, whereas breast-fed infants have two or three. Only when the stools are hard and dry and eliminated with difficulty does constipation exist. Prune juice or strained prunes given daily usually suffice to correct the constipation.

The causes for constipation in older children are similar to those in adults, and corrective treatment includes emphasis upon regularity of habits, increased fluid intake, and a diet that includes raw and cooked vegetables and fruits and some whole-grain cereals and breads. (See Chapter 35.)

Diarrhea. Diarrhea occurring in infants and children may be functional or organic and is caused by the same factors as in adults. (See Chapters 35 and 36.) Probably most acute diarrhea is accounted for by improper handling of the food supply, especially milk. The incidence is several times as high in bottle-fed as in breast-fed infants and is greatly increased during the summer months when it is traceable to unsanitary preparation or inadequate refrigeration of food, including infant formulas. Greater emphasis on education of parents in the preparation, sterilization, and storage of formulas has resulted in a markedly decreased incidence and mortality.

Serious consequences follow diarrhea in infants under one year of age if treatment is not prompt. The large loss of fluids and electrolytes quickly leads to dehydration, fever, loss of kidney function, and severe acidosis if electrolyte loss is chiefly through the intestinal tract. There may also be marked vomiting with loss of acid, in which case there may be no acidosis but a lowering of the total body anions and cations.

Modification of the diet. When mild diarrhea occurs in breast-fed infants, breast feeding may be continued but the baby is likely to take less milk for a few days. A 5 per cent glucose solution may also be offered at three- or four-hour intervals. Bottle-fed babies may be given a half-strength formula of skim milk or skim lactic acid milk. Both the volume of formula given and the concentration of the formula are increased gradually. Since it is important to maintain fluid balance, the formula may be supplemented with 5 per cent oral glucose solution.

When diarrhea in infants is severe, it is essential to correct the dehydration and acidosis by the intravenous administration of glucose and electrolyte solutions. Initially only glucose and electrolyte solutions are offered. Then a dilute formula consisting of boiled skim milk, skim lactic acid milk, or high-protein milk is offered. Convalescence may be prolonged and the increases in concentration and in volume of the formula must be made cautiously.

Scraped apple or apple powder has been useful in the treatment of diarrhea in infants and older children. The apple powder may be mixed with water or with milk, if milk is tolerated. A thick paste is prepared using 4 level teaspoons of apple powder and a small quantity of boiled and cooled water. When the paste is smooth, it is gradually diluted with liquid until the volume equals 8 ounces. This quantity is taken every three to four hours, as directed by the physician.

The treatment of diarrhea in older children is similar to that for adults, namely, the omission of food during the first day or two, the gradual introduction of low-residue foods (Chapter 35), and progression to a soft diet.

Celiac disturbances. The celiac syndrome includes several disturbances in which the symptoms, the disorders of absorption, and the nutritional deficiencies are similar. They are gluten-induced enteropathy also known as primary idiopathic steatorrhea, celiac disease (in children), or nontropical sprue (in adults); cystic fibrosis of the pancreas; and kwashiorkor. The symptoms, metabolic alterations, and dietary management for gluten enteropathy have been discussed in Chapter 36, and for cystic fibrosis in Chapter 37. However, some adaptations of the diet will need to be made for the infant and toddler according to their food requirements for growth and development.

Modification of the diet. A high caloric intake is mandatory in these diseases because up to 50 per cent of the calories may be excreted in the stools. The intake should be increased by 50 to 75 per cent above normal levels. For infants during the acute phase of illness this necessitates 120 to 200 calories per kilogram. A high protein intake—6 to 8 gm per kilogram—is also recommended initially.[7] As improvement occurs the protein intake is gradually reduced to normal levels. Supplements of the fat-soluble and water-soluble vitamins are always indicated, and iron supplementation may also be needed.

In celiac disease and in cystic fibrosis large amounts of fat are excreted. This may persist for a long time after subjective improvement occurs. Some pediatricians severely restrict fat in these conditions in order to reduce the amount of fat excreted. Others maintain that it is better to allow a moderate fat intake.[8] Although an increased intake of fat leads to greater quantities of fat in the stool, the total amount of fat absorbed is also increased, thereby increasing the caloric intake. Pancreatin is prescribed for patients with cystic fibrosis of the pancreas and is taken with each meal. In hot weather the salt intake needs to be increased for patients with cystic fibrosis, but this is not necessary for celiac disease.

Weihofer and Pringle found that children with cystic fibrosis varied widely in their tolerance to foods, and they suggest that a single diet cannot be recommended for all patients.[9] The levels of calories, protein, fat, and carbohydrate must be adjusted individually for each child. Some foods increase abdominal distention, pain, and steatorrhea in some children but not others.

For the young infant a formula of *Probana, Hi-Pro,* or *Protein Milk** supplies two thirds to three fourths of all the calories.[7] The remaining

*Probana and *Protein Milk* by Mead Johnson and Company, Evansville, Indiana; *Hi Pro* by Jackson-Mitchell Pharmaceuticals, Inc., Santa Barbara, California.

calories are furnished by glucose and/or banana flakes or banana powder added to the formula. At two to four months these foods are gradually introduced: cottage cheese, egg yolk, strained beef or liver, scraped raw apple, apple juice, or applesauce, and banana or banana flakes.

With improvement, other foods are gradually added to include a wider variety of strained and then chopped meats, mild cheese, puréed and then chopped cooked vegetables and fruits, and plain gelatin. Wheat, oats, rye, and barley products must be rigorously excluded for the patient with gluten enteropathy, but these cereals may be gradually introduced into the diet of the patient with cystic fibrosis. See also pages 476 to 479. The additions of food are made more gradually than for normal infants and children. Strained foods are used for a somewhat longer period of time, and raw fruits and vegetables are introduced at a later time.

DIABETES

The first patient treated with insulin prepared by Banting and Best in January 1922 was a 14-year-old diabetic boy. Approximately 1 in every 2000 children under 15 years is diabetic.

Comparison with adult diabetes. The disease in children differs in a number of important respects from that in adults. The onset of symptoms is usually more sudden and violent, and the disease usually increases in severity during the period of growth. In contrast to the adult, obesity is uncommon; in fact, when first seen the diabetic child is likely to be underweight and not growing because he has not been metabolizing his food adequately.

All diabetic children need insulin, since there appear to be few if any functioning cells of the islands of Langerhans. The maintenance of control between acidosis on the one hand and hypoglycemia on the other is often difficult because of the greater frequency of infections and the erratic physical activity and emotional control.

Psychologic considerations. Too often the child and his parents as well feel that he is somehow different from other children and that there

is a certain stigma attached to the diabetic state. If the child experiences insulin reactions, he will be afraid to participate in the activities of other children, and he may become more dependent upon his parents. The diabetic adolescent is likely to be especially difficult to control. Like other adolescents he may rebel against authority, and one of the ways in which he may show his independence is through breaking his diet.

The guidance of the child in all aspects of his development, not only in the treatment of the diabetes, requires great patience, forbearance, and understanding on the part of the parent and physician. The child and the parent must recognize the interrelationship of diet, insulin, and activity and the importance of regulation. It is equally important that the child learn—and his parents understand—that he can take his place in the family and society just as does the non-diabetic child. Nelson states: "The child who is not physically, mentally and socially able to compete with his colleagues cannot be considered an adequately treated diabetic child."*

Modification of the diet. The principles of dietary modification for the diabetic child are similar to those for the adult (see Chapter 39). The nutritive requirements are the same as those for the normal child of the same age, size, and activity (see Chapter 23). Briefly, these needs are as follows:

Calories: to maintain desirable rate of growth; usually about 35 to 40 calories per pound desirable weight.

Protein: 1.5 gm per pound if under three years of age; 1 gm per pound for older children.

Carbohydrate and fat: 40 to 45 per cent of the calories from carbohydrate with the remaining calories from fat. Some clinicians restrict carbohydrate to 225 or 250 gm per day, or even less, in which case the fat level is proportionately higher to ensure adequate caloric intake.

The additional calcium requirements are easily met when 3 to 4 cups of milk are included daily. Other minerals and vitamins are provided in satisfactory amounts when the exchange lists

---

*Nelson, W. E.: *Textbook of Pediatrics,* 8th ed. W. B. Saunders Company, Philadelphia, 1964, p. 1324.

are used as the basis of meal planning. Children should receive vitamin D either in milk or as a supplement.

The diet prescription should be adjusted periodically to make allowances for satisfactory growth. A reasonable meal constancy from day to day is desirable. Between-meal snacks should be included. It is better that a child receive a snack before activity to forestall the possibility of insulin reaction.

Dietary control. Although the life-span of diabetic children has improved greatly, the incidence of degenerative diseases is unusually high after 10 to 20 years. The possibilities of diminished vision and even blindness, of coronary artery disease, and of kidney disease during the prime of life are serious, and as yet unsolved, problems. Jackson believes that these changes can be put off at least 30 to 40 years if the diabetes is well controlled.[10] Under such control the blood sugar is kept as nearly normal as possible and glycosuria is avoided for the most part.

Some pediatricians use a so-called *free diet*, allowing the child to eat all family foods but usually restricting concentrated sweets and high-carbohydrate desserts. Enough insulin is given to metabolize food for normal growth and to avoid ketosis, but hyperglycemia and glycosuria are disregarded. At the other extreme are those pediatricians who maintain rigid chemical control and require weighed or carefully measured diets.

Insulin. In early stages of juvenile diabetes the pancreas sometimes produces small amounts of insulin, but this rapidly diminishes. As growth accelerates the insulin requirement increases greatly and control becomes much more difficult.

Jackson recommends at least two doses of intermediate-acting insulin for the desirable three-meal-plus-snack pattern. The morning dose could be a mixture of regular and globin or NPH insulin. A second dose of intermediate-acting insulin is given late in the afternoon (about 4:30 P.M.). With this program the blood sugar is maintained as nearly normal as possible throughout the 24-hour day. This regimen is intended to avoid glycosuria or insulin reactions.[10]

DIETARY COUNSELING

Whenever possible, initial hospitalization is desirable not only to stabilize the diabetes in

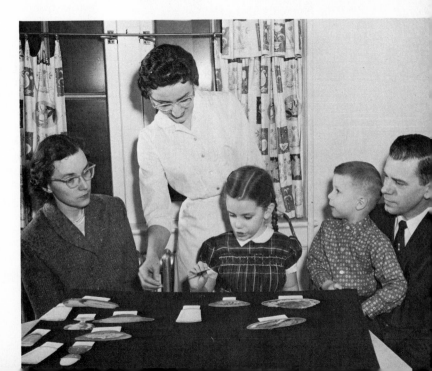

Figure 47–4. The child and her parents learn together about the important essentials of the diet through the use of food models and setting up examples of meals. Although the parents assume responsibility for supervision of the dietary regimen, the child must be an active participant in making menu decisions. (Courtesy, Dietary Department, University Hospitals, University of Wisconsin Medical Center.)

the child but especially to set up an adequate program of education. The child and his parents must face the issue of diabetes squarely, but also recognize that the child can live a happy, useful life.[10] Regardless of the opinions regarding chemical or clinical control, pediatricians agree that close adherence to the diet at the beginning provides security and guidance for the child and parent during the period of adjustment to the disease. The initial diet could be one that provides few substitutions until the patient is thoroughly accustomed to it; then gradually the diet is liberalized with respect to the food choice until the meal exchange lists are used with ease.

Children, like adults, need to be taught the nature of the disease, how to administer insulin, how to select the daily diet from the plan set up, how to test the urine, and how to keep records. The importance of cleanliness and personal hygiene must be emphasized. The recognition of the signs of insulin reactions or of acidosis and what to do when these signs appear must be learned. See also pages 615 to 616 for further details on dietary counseling.

Diabetic camps provide an unusual educational opportunity for children to learn more about the care of themselves and also to learn the important social adjustments with other children. Such camps are well staffed with recreational leaders, nurses, dietitians, physicians, and laboratory technicians.[11,12]

Nephrotic Syndrome

Symptoms and clinical findings. The nephrotic syndrome includes so-called lipoid nephrosis and the nephrotic phase of glomerulonephritis. This rare syndrome occurs in young children at an average age of 2½ years. Its onset is usually insidious and is characterized by marked edema, heavy proteinuria (2 to 10 gm or more), serious depletion of plasma proteins, especially the albumin fraction, and elevated blood cholesterol. The edema is often so marked that it seems as if the skin would burst. When diuresis occurs the severe depletion of tissue proteins and the accompanying undernutrition become fully apparent.

Excessive wastage in the urine also occurs of ceruloplasmin, protein-bound iodine, iron-binding proteins, prothrombin, and complement. Because of the loss of complement, the incidence of infections is high and is an important cause of death. Hematuria, hypertension, and azotemia are minimal or absent in lipoid nephrosis.

The aims of therapy include control of infections and edema and establishment of good nutrition. Corticosteroid therapy results in remission of clinical and biochemical aspects of the disease in over 80 per cent of patients.[13] Although some children recover completely, others progress to terminal stages of nephritis or succumb to infections.

Modification of the diet. Patients with nephrosis have a particularly poor appetite, and the high-calorie high-protein diets that are often ordered are not necessarily consumed. Much attention must be given to the selection of foods that are acceptable to the child. With the loss of edema fluid the appetite usually improves.

The caloric intake should be based upon the child's desirable weight for his height and body build. Unless the caloric intake is adequate, effective tissue regeneration cannot take place. The protein intake is generally a little higher than normal; about 3 to 4 gm per kilogram is suitable for the preschool child and 2 to 3 gm per kilogram for school-age children.

Sodium restriction is prescribed in the presence of edema. Since unsalted foods are poorly accepted, prolonged restriction is undesirable. Diuretics may bring about such rapid diuresis that the blood levels of both sodium and potassium are reduced. In such instances the sodium content of the diet should be increased, and juices rich in potassium offered. See Chapter 43 for planning of sodium-restricted diets.

Allergy

The designation of allergy has been used frequently for those conditions resulting from a

sensitivity to a food. With the increased understanding of hereditary diseases, it is now apparent that many so-called allergies are, in fact,
the failure to metabolize a given nutrient because of the congenital deficiency of one or more
enzymes. There remain, however, many diseases
which are not yet explained on any such basis
and which are classified as allergies.

Foods are responsible for the majority of allergies in children under three years of age. The
chief offending foods are milk, eggs, wheat,
white potatoes, chocolate, and oranges. When
the child is young, it is relatively simple to determine which food is responsible by allowing only
milk and crystalline vitamins. If a food other
than milk is responsible, the symptoms, such as
eczema, will be relieved in a few days; but if
milk or nonfood allergy is responsible for the
disturbance, no improvement will take place.

When the symptoms of allergy are mild, it is
always necessary to consider the relative importance of the allergic disturbance in relation
to the diet of the child. It is better management,
for example, to treat a mild case of eczema locally
than to subject the child to the dangers of an
inadequate diet with its far more serious consequences.

For older children, the diagnosis of allergy is
accomplished by means of skin tests and the
usual elimination diet, and the treatment is
planned as for adults (see Chapter 46).

Milk sensitivity. From 0.3 to 7 per cent of all
children are sensitive to milk, according to various estimates.[14] In many instances this may be
associated with infection and emotional stress; in
others genetic factors may be a cause (see
Galactose Disease, Chapter 48, and Lactose Intolerance, Chapter 36).

The response to the ingestion of milk is almost
immediate in some and may lead to colic, spitting
up of the feeding, irritability, diarrhea, and
respiratory disorders. A delayed reaction may occur hours to days following the ingestion of milk,
and thus it becomes difficult to determine the
exact cause. Recently, the incidence of hypochromic anemia in some infants has been attributed to sensitivity to milk.[14] Following the
ingestion of milk by these sensitive infants, some
blood is lost from the gastrointestinal tract. This

may average several milliliters per day and may
go unnoticed until the anemia becomes apparent
months later. Some infants may have a sufficiently high intake of other iron-rich foods so
that the anemic tendency is counteracted.

Dietary treatment. Sometimes it is only necessary to change the form of the milk to improve
tolerance—that is, boiled, powdered, acidulated,
or evaporated milk may be satisfactory when
fresh cow's milk is not. In other instances goat's
milk may be an effective substitute for cow's
milk, but occasionally the child will tolerate
no milk whatsoever.

A number of formulas containing no milk
have been found to be satisfactory. One of these
is a formula containing cooked rice, strained
beef, Dextrimaltose, lard, salt mixture, and vitamins.[15] The tolerance to milk improves in many
infants, but others need to continue a milk-free
diet indefinitely.

FEEDING HANDICAPPED CHILDREN

Cerebral palsy. Various crippling conditions
occur as the result of brain damage. The feeding
problems depend upon the type of crippling
present.[16]

Reverse swallowing wave. When the motor
system of the tongue and throat is affected, food
is not pushed back to the throat, but the tongue
motion pushes the food forward. Initially such
children must be tube fed, but in time they learn
to put food at the back of the tongue and by tilt-
ing the head backward learn to swallow. These
children often become severely undernourished
because feeding is such a prolonged process.
Concentrated foods with maximum protein and
calorie value should be emphasized to keep the
volume to a minimum. Vitamin and mineral supplements are usually required.

Athetoids are those who are constantly in motion and who thus burn up a great deal of energy. Although they require a high-calorie
high-protein diet, the ingestion of the necessary
amounts of food is difficult because of the constant motion. Feeding is quite time consuming
and emphasis should be placed upon concentrated foods of high caloric value. Children

should be encouraged to feed themselves by giving them foods that they can pick up with their fingers such as pieces of fruit and sandwiches. Many devices have been developed as aids in feeding. (See page 397.)

Spastics are very limited in their activity, and they may also be indulged in eating by their parents. Consequently they gain excessive amounts of weight, and the obesity in turn further restricts their ability to get around. These individuals require marked restriction of caloric intake without jeopardizing the intake of protein, minerals, and vitamins.

Cleft palate. Surgery for cleft palate is often not completed for several years. In addition to the needs for normal development, the infant and child must build up reserves for surgery, the promotion of healing, and the development of normal healthy gums and teeth. According to Zickefoose,[17] the major problems of feeding these children may be met in the following ways:

1. Infants may have difficulty in sucking, but most of them learn to use chewing movements to get the milk out of the nipple. An enlarged nipple opening is helpful. Some babies may be fed with a medicine dropper or a Brecht feeder.

2. To counteract the tendency to choke, liquids should be taken in small amounts and swallowed slowly.

3. More frequent "burpings" are necessary because of the large amount of air which may be swallowed.

4. Spicy and acid foods often irritate the mouth and nose and should be avoided. If orange juice is not well taken, ascorbic acid supplement should be prescribed.

5. Among the foods which may get into the opening of the palate are peanut butter, peelings of raw fruit, nuts, leafy vegetables, and creamed dishes. Some children have no difficulty with any foods.

6. Puréed foods may be diluted with milk, fruit juice, or broth and given from a bottle with a large nipple opening. Some babies accept purées well if they are thickened with vanilla wafer or graham-cracker crumbs.

7. The time required for feeding may be long and requires much patience on the part of parent and nurse. For the older child, five or six small meals may be better than three.

When surgery has been performed, a liquid or puréed diet is offered until healing is complete.

Mental retardation. Some five million persons in the United States are estimated to be mentally retarded. Of these, about 75 per cent have an I.Q. between 51 and 75 (educable) and are designated as "high grade." Approximately 20 per cent of the mentally retarded are "middle grade" that is, they have an I.Q. between 21 and 50 (trainable). The "low-grade" individual with an I.Q. below 20 is believed to account for 5 per cent of the mentally retarded and presents the problems in feeding.

The nutritional requirements of the mentally retarded child and adult are like those of the individual of normal mental development. The nurse can help parents to understand the problems of feeding by giving encouragement and support.

The mentally retarded child may be kept on the bottle too long, thus increasing the difficulties of introducing other foods. The child may eat very slowly, and feeding may be messy. Hand sucking and vomiting are not uncommon.[18] To obtain adequate food intake for growth may require frequent, small feedings, and certainly an abundance of patience and ingenuity. One must strike a balance between overprotectiveness and lack of caring.

The retarded individual, like the normal person, has an active emotional life. He feels the shunning of others and his failure to achieve, but will respond to loving attention.[19] He resists new foods, has definite likes and dislikes, and finds it difficult to manage eating. He responds to the color of foods and like all children is fond of sweets.

When the individual is able to feed himself, he should be permitted to do so even though feeding may be messy. Food must be presented in a form that can be easily managed. Foods may be eaten with the fingers for a long time until simple utensils can be managed. The child unable to support himself should be held in a sitting position while he is being fed.

PROBLEMS AND REVIEW

1. What dietary problems may be anticipated in children who must be hospitalized? How can these problems be overcome?
2. How can a schoolchild be helped to adjust to a prolonged therapeutic diet?
3. *Problem.* Adjust a 1500-calorie diet of an adult so that it will be suitable for a 12-year-old boy. In what ways would you try to effect acceptance of this diet?
4. What dietary considerations would apply for a seven-year-old child with scarlet fever?
5. *Problem.* List a number of ways in which you could encourage a boy with rheumatic fever to take an adequate diet.
6. *Problem.* Plan six high-calorie after-school and bedtime snacks which could be added to the regular diet of a teen-age girl who is 20 pounds underweight.
7. What changes in diet might be indicated for an infant who is constipated? A four-year-old child?
8. What are the similarities between celiac disease and cystic fibrosis? What differences are there?
9. *Problem.* Plan a day's meals for a three-year-old child with celiac disease for whom a gluten-restricted diet has been ordered. He is 34 inches tall and weighs 24 pounds; he appears to be somewhat undernourished.
10. List the differences between diabetes in children and in adults.
11. What arguments can you give for, and against, chemical control in childhood diabetes?
12. Enumerate the essential points in the instruction of the child and/or his parent with respect to diabetes.
13. What is the effect of physical activity on the control of diabetes in the child?
14. Prepare a plan for the organization of a diabetic club for children. Include suggestions for meetings for such a group.
15. A diabetic child is invited to a birthday party. What plans can be made so that the child may eat at this party?
16. *Problem.* For a two-year-old child with nephrosis plan a suitable diet containing 50 gm protein and 1200 calories. How would you modify the diet for 500 mg sodium?
17. List several ways in which milk intolerance may be manifested. What substances in milk have been shown to produce such sensitivity? List three products that may be used satisfactorily in place of a milk formula.

CITED REFERENCES

1. Dodds, J.: "A New Audience for Nutrition Education," *J. Nutr. Educ.,* 1:23–24, Fall 1969.
2. Corrado, C.: "Nutrition Education and the Hospitalized Child," *J. Nutr. Educ.,* 1:24–25, Fall 1969.
3. Bullen, B., *et al.:* "Physical Activity of Obese and Nonobese Adolescent Girls Appraised by Motion Picture Sampling," *Am. J. Clin. Nutr.,* 14:211–23, 1964.
4. Mayer, J.: "Physical Activity and Anthropometric Measurements of Obese Adolescents," *Fed. Proc.,* 25:11–14, 1966.
5. Powell, G. F., *et al.:* "Emotional Deprivation and Growth Retardation Simulating Idiopathic Hypopituitarism," *N. Engl. J. Med.,* 276:1271–78; 1279–83, 1967.
6. Whitten, C. F., *et al.:* "Evidence That Growth Failure from Maternal Deprivation Is Secondary to Undereating," *J.A.M.A.,* 209:1675–82, 1969.
7. Mike, E. M.: "Practical Management of Patients with the Celiac Syndrome," *Am. J. Clin. Nutr.,* 7:463–76, 1959.

8. Holt, L. E., Jr., and Snyderman, S. E.: "Nutrition in Infancy and Adolescence," in Wohl, M. G., and Goodhart, R. S., eds. *Modern Nutrition in Health and Disease*, 4th ed. Lea & Febiger, Philadelphia, 1968, pp. 1107–30.
9. Weihofer, D. M., and Pringle, D. J.: "Dietary Intake and Food Tolerances of Children with Cystic Fibrosis," *J. Am. Diet. Assoc.*, **54:**206–209, 1969.
10. Jackson, R. L.: "The Child with Diabetes," *Nutr. Today*, **6:**2–9, March/April 1971.
11. Parker, J. A.: "Camping for Children with Diabetes—A Diet Therapy Section Project," *J. Am. Diet. Assoc.*, **53:**486–88, 1968.
12. Prater, B. M.: "Why Diabetic Children Go to Summer Camp," *J. Am. Diet. Assoc.*, **55:**584–87, 1969.
13. Nelson, W. E.: *Textbook of Pediatrics*, 8th ed. W. B. Saunders Company, 1964, p. 1128.
14. Heiner, D. C.: "Sensitivity to Cow's Milk," *J.A.M.A.*, **189:**563–67, 1964.
15. Ziegler, M. R.: "Mineral-enriched Meats for Diets of Infants Requiring a Milk Substitute," *J. Am. Diet. Assoc.*, **29:**660–65, 1953.
16. Phelps, W. M.: "Dietary Requirements in Cerebral Palsy," *J. Am. Diet. Assoc.*, **27:**869–70, 1951.
17. Zickefoose, M.: "Feeding the Child with a Cleft Palate," *J. Am. Diet. Assoc.*, **36:**129–31, 1960.
18. Walker, G. A.: "Nutrition in Mentally Deficient Children," *J. Am. Diet. Assoc.*, **31:**494–97, 1955.
19. Adair, R.: "Home Care and Feeding of a Mentally Retarded Child," *J. Am. Diet. Assoc.*, **36:**133–34, 1960.

ADDITIONAL REFERENCES

General References

Amend, E. L.: "A Parent Education Program in a Children's Hospital," *Nurs. Outlook*, **14:**53–56, April 1966.
Getty, G., and Hollensworth, M.: "Through a Child's Eye Seeing," *Nutr. Today*, **2:**17, 1967.
Jernigan, A. K.: "Suggestions for Feeding of Hospitalized Children," *Hospitals*, **44:**86–89, May 16, 1970.
Mason, E. A.: "The Hospitalized Child: His Emotional Needs," *N. Engl. J. Med.*, **272:**406–14, 1965.
Nelson, W. E.: *Textbook of Pediatrics*, 9th ed. W. B. Saunders Company, Philadelphia, 1970.
Weinberg, S., *et al.*: "Seminars in Nursing Care of the Adolescent," *Nurs. Outlook*, **16:**18–23, Dec. 1968.

Obesity

Christakis, G., *et al.*: "Effect of a Combined Nutrition Education and Physical Fitness Program on the Weight Status of Obese High School Boys," *Fed. Proc.*, **25:**15–19, 1966.
Goldbloom, R. G.: "Obesity in Childhood," *Bordens Rev. Nutr. Res.*, **29:**1–13, 1968.
Heald, F. P.: "Natural History and Physiological Basis of Adolescent Obesity," *Fed. Proc.*, **25:**1–3, 1966.
Huenemann, R. L., *et al.*: "Adolescent Food Practices Associated with Obesity," *Fed. Proc.*, **25:**4–10, 1966.
Peckos, P. S., and Spargo, J. A.: "For Overweight Teenage Girls," *Am. J. Nurs.*, **64:**85–87, May 1964.
Rauh, J. L., and Schumsky, D. A.: "Relative Accuracy of Visual Assessment of Juvenile Obesity," *J. Am. Diet. Assoc.*, **55:**459–64, 1969.
Spargo, J. A., *et al.*: "Adolescent Obesity," *Nutr. Today*, **1:**2, Dec. 1966.

Diabetes Mellitus

Appelman, D. H.: "Juvenile Diabetes," *N.Y. State J. Med.*, **65**:399–402, 1965.

Bailey, C. C.: "Diabetes in Adolescence," *Med. Clin. North Am.*, **49**:451–66, Mar. 1965.

Davis, D. M., *et al.:* "Attitudes of Diabetic Boys and Girls Towards Diabetes," *Diabetes,* **14:** 106–108, 1965.

Gaspard, N. J.: "Summer Camp for Diabetic Children," *Am. J. Nurs.*, **63**:108–109, June 1963.

Knowles, H. C., Jr., *et al.:* "The Course of Juvenile Diabetes Treated with Unmeasured Diet. Clinical Monograph," *Diabetes,* **14**:239–73, 1965.

Leiner, M. S., and Rahmer, A. E.: "The Juvenile Diabetic and the Visiting Nurse," *Am. J. Nurs.*, **68**:106–108, Jan. 1968.

Long, P. J.: "The Diabetic Child at Home," *Nurs. Outlook*, **12**:55–56, Dec. 1964.

Moore, M. L.: "Diabetes in Children," *Am. J. Nurs.*, **67**:104–107, 1967.

O'Sullivan, J. B., and Mahan, C. M.: "Prospective Study of 352 Young Patients with Chemical Diabetes," *N. Engl. J. Med.*, **278**:1038–41, 1968.

Weil, W. B., Jr.: "Juvenile Diabetes Mellitus. Current Concepts," *N. Engl. J. Med.*, **278**:829–31, 1968.

Celiac Disturbances

Anderson, D. M.: "History of Celiac Disease," *J. Am. Diet. Assoc.*, **35**:1158–62, 1959.

Di Sant'Agnese, P. A., and Talano, R. C.: "Pathogenesis and Physiopathology of Cystic Fibrosis of the Pancreas. Fibrocystic Disease of the Pancreas," *N. Engl. J. Med.*, **277**:1287–94; 1344–52; 1399–1408, 1967.

Milio, M.: "Family Centered Care for Cystic Fibrosis," *Nurs. Outlook*, **11**:718–21, 1963.

Review: "The Celiac Syndrome (Malabsorption) in Pediatrics," *Nutr. Rev.*, **21**:195–98, 1963.

Schwab, L., *et al.:* "Cystic Fibrosis," *Am.. J. Nurs.*, **63**:62–69, Feb. 1963.

Sheldon, W.: "Prognosis in Early Adult Life of Coeliac Children Treated with a Gluten-Free Diet," *Br. Med. J.*, **2**:401–404, 1969.

Weijers, H. A., and van de Kamer, J. H.: "Some Considerations of Celiac Disease," *Am. J. Clin. Nutr.*, **17**:51–54, 1965.

Other Childhood Diseases

Gordon, J. E.: "Weanling Diarrhea. A Synergism of Nutrition and Infection," *Nutr. Rev.*, **22:** 161–63, 1964.

Korsch, G., and Barnett, H. L.: "The Physician, the Family and the Child with Nephrosis," *J. Pediatr.*, **58**:707–15, 1961.

Rapaport, H. G.: "Psychosomatic Aspects of Allergy in Childhood," *J.A.M.A.*, **165**:812–15, 1957.

Saxena, K. M., and Crawford, J. D.: "Current Concepts. The Treatment of Nephrosis," *N. Engl. J. Med.*, **272**:522–26, 1965.

Soyka, L. F., and Saxena, K. M.: "Alternate-Day Steroid Therapy for Nephrotic Children," *J.A.M.A.*, **192**:225–30, 1965.

Wilson, J. F., *et al.:* "Milk-Induced Gastrointestinal Bleeding in Infants with Hypochromic Microcytic Anemia," *J.A.M.A.*, **189**:568–72, 1964.

Feeding the Handicapped

Feeding the Child with a Handicap. Children's Bureau Pub. 450, U.S. Department of Health, Education, and Welfare, Washington, D.C., 1967.

Flory, M. C.: "Training the Mentally Retarded Child," *Nurs. Outlook*, **5**:344–47, 1957.

Leamy, C. M.: "A Study of the Food Intake of a Group of Children with Cerebral Palsy in the Lakeville Sanatorium," *Am. J. Public Health*, **43**:1310–17, 1953.

MacCollum, D. W., and Richardson, S. O.: "Care of the Child with Cleft Lip and Cleft Palate," *Am. J. Nurs.*, **58**:211–16, 1958.

48 Inborn Errors of Metabolism

Phenylalanine-Restricted Diet; Galactose-Free Diet

Many professional and lay groups have united in their efforts to understand the nature of the ever-growing number of inborn errors of metabolism and to seek methods of prevention and treatment. To the physician, the problems are those of diagnosis, of early detection before damage has occurred, and of effective treatment. To the biochemist falls the task of identifying the metabolic defect so that a possible rationale of therapy can be developed. To the nurse and dietitian fall the practical aspects of nursing care and of dietary planning and implementation. The problem of control through genetic counseling belongs to the geneticist. Most of all, to the parent of a child affected the problem is immediate and urgent; in some disorders treatment is effective, but in others no remedy is available.

Nature of inborn errors. The term *inborn error* was coined at the beginning of this century by Sir Archibald E. Garrod who wrote a book in which he described four diseases of a hereditary nature.[1] These were alkaptonuria, a defect of phenylalanine metabolism in which a metabolite excreted into the urine becomes dark upon standing; albinism, also a defect in phenylalanine metabolism characterized by a lack of pigmentation; cystinuria, or an excessive excretion of cystine because of a defect in the renal tubules which prevents the reabsorption of the amino acid cystine; and pentosuria, characterized by the presence of pentose in the urine owing to the lack of an enzyme in metabolism.

Inborn errors of metabolism include well over 100 disorders that originate in one or more mutations of the gene so that normal function is disrupted. These diseases are also referred to as *genetic diseases* or as *hereditary molecular diseases*. The effects of genetic mutation vary widely and may alter the metabolism of specific amino acids, carbohydrates, lipids, or minerals. They may affect the synthesis of a body product; they may interfere with the transport of materials across a cell membrane; they may produce toxic effects on tissues because of the accumulation of intermediate products.

Some errors of metabolism result in no serious limitations upon the individual; others lead to rapid changes in the central nervous system so that mental retardation is severe; still others may be lethal shortly after birth. Some become evident a few days after birth, whereas other hereditary diseases such as diabetes mellitus and gout may show no signs until adult life. Dietary management is effective in the control of many disorders but no known therapy is yet available for others.

Some of the inborn errors of metabolism are characterized by serious mental retardation if the condition is not treated promptly. During the first years of life the brain is developing so rapidly that any interference with its growth cannot be fully corrected at a later time. Thus, diagnosis at a very early age is important if effective treatment is to take place before serious damage has occurred. Inexpensive screening tests may be applied to some conditions during the first weeks of life. Several conditions for which dietary treatment has been successful are discussed in this chapter.

PHENYLKETONURIA

Phenylketonuria (often abbreviated PKU) was first diagnosed by Asbjörn Fölling, a Norwegian biochemist, in 1934, and has been successfully treated with a low-phenylalanine diet since 1952. When the disorder is discovered early in infancy and is treated with the low-phenylalanine diet, the child is not doomed to a life of mental retardation.

Incidence. About 1 child in each 10,000 births has phenylketonuria, although 1 person in 50 is a carrier of the trait. About 1 per cent of all patients in mental institutions are estimated to be phenylketonurics.

Phenylketonuria is transmitted by an autosomal recessive gene. Thus, each of the parents would have one defective gene and would be clinically normal. Each birth from the mating of two heterozygotes involves a one in four chance that the child will be phenylketonuric, two chances that he will be a heterozygote but clinically normal, and one chance that he will be entirely normal.

Biochemical defect. An enzyme, *phenylalanine hydroxylase,* is missing in the phenylketonuric individual. As a consequence the hydroxyl (OH) grouping cannot be incorporated into the phenylalanine molecule to form tyrosine. Several products accumulate in the blood circulation and are excreted in the urine. One of these, phenylpyruvic acid, is a ketone which accounts for the naming of the condition. It reacts with ferric chloride to give a vivid green color, thus forming the basis for the widely used "diaper" tests. Another intermediate product is phenylacetic acid, which accounts for the characteristic "wild," "gamey," or "mousy" odor from the skin and urine of these patients. (See Figure 48–1.)

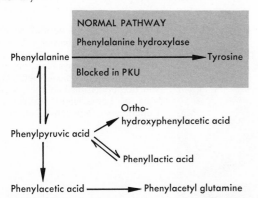

Figure 48–1. In the absence of phenylalanine hydroxylase, the normal pathway of phenylalanine to tyrosine is blocked, and a number of alternate by-products are excreted in the urine.

Testing for phenylketonuria. Most states require the testing of newborn infants, using the "diaper" tests. To avoid false interpretations these should be followed by blood tests in four to six weeks. The acceptable range of phenylalanine in the blood serum is 3 to 7 mg per cent. In phenylketonuric infants the initial blood level is usually above 15 mg per cent and as high as 30 mg per cent by 10 days of age. In untreated persons with PKU, the serum level reaches as high as 75 mg per cent.[2]

Occasionally infants have an initial elevation of serum phenylalanine that later returns to normal; this has been attributed to PKU in the mother. Other infants, especially prematures, show a slight elevation of serum phenylalanine because there is a delayed maturation of the tyrosine-oxidizing system. Usually this is corrected by the administration of ascorbic acid.[2] It is important that these conditions not be mistaken for true PKU so that they are not subjected to the low-phenylalanine diet.

Clinical changes. Mental retardation in untreated subjects is usually severe with most patients having an intelligence quotient below 50. The child appears to be normal at birth but within the first few days or weeks of life the various intermediate products of faulty phenylalanine metabolism accumulate and can be detected in the blood and urine. If treatment is not initiated promptly progressive irreversible brain damage occurs. Although the faulty phenylalanine metabolism is clearly understood as the cause of the brain damage, it is not yet known just how this change takes place.

Because of the block in tyrosine formation, the production of pigments is reduced. Consequently, these children are usually blond, blue eyed, and have a fair skin, even though their parents may be of darker skin, eye, and hair coloring. Eczema is a common finding.

The behavior of untreated children is considerably altered. They are hyperactive, wave their arms, rock back and forth, and grind their teeth. They show poor coordination, are irritable, immature, and overdependent. At times they may have seizures. Their behavior can be extremely trying even to the most loving parents.

Treatment. The successful treatment of PKU

depends upon (1) early diagnosis; (2) restriction of phenylalanine intake to maintain an acceptable range of serum phenylalanine; (3) a nutritionally adequate diet adjusted from time to time to meet the requirements for normal growth and development; (4) continuing clinical and biochemical monitoring; and (5) a comprehensive program of education of the parents. The team approach is essential, including the physician, nurse, clinical chemist, social workers, dietitian, parents, and sometimes others. (See Figure 48–2.)

Children for whom such treatment was begun within the first few weeks or months of life show apparently normal mental and physical development.[3] One boy who has been successfully treated with a low-phenylalanine diet since 3½ weeks of age is shown in Figure 48–3. According to a progress report by Dr. Robert Warner,[4] the boy at six years of age is slightly tall for his age, well developed, and well nourished. His health has been good, and his parents and teacher have been well pleased with his progress in school; his report card has been good.

Although there are many foods this boy does not like, he has been "very good about staying on his diet. The neighbors have remarked about his willpower and his ability to give it up [foods that he must avoid], and he simply will not eat that which is bad for him." The parents are very proud of him and how well he has done, and their cooperation has been excellent.

A delay in the initiation of the diet reduces the likelihood of satisfactory mental development. Once brain damage has occurred reversal does not take place. After three years of age, little improvement in mental development can be expected. However, even for the older child the phenylalanine-restricted diet is believed to be of some benefit in modifying the behavior characteristics.

Modification of the diet. The allowances for protein and for calories are essentially the same as those for normal children. Some clinicians allow slightly more protein and calories initially since the source of protein is casein hydrolysate rather than natural protein. The allowances for protein, energy, and phenylalanine are summarized in Table 48–1.

Sutherland and her associates[5] emphasize that a balance must be maintained between the amount of low-phenylalanine formula and the amount of natural foods that are fed. The formula supplies most of the energy, protein, and other nutrients, and if inadequate amounts are fed, the amino acid and other nutritional requirements of the child will not be met. On the other hand, if inadequate amounts of natural foods are given, the phenylalanine intake will be too low to meet the requirements. Although the phenylalanine intake is restricted, it must always be remembered that this is one of the essential amino acids.

When the phenylalanine intake is inadequate,

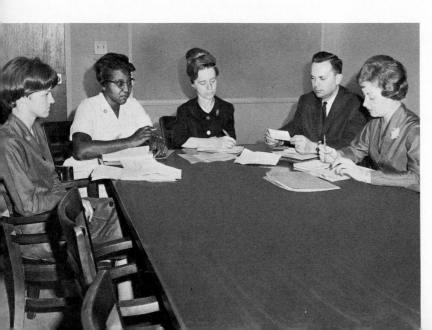

Figure 48–2. Successful treatment of many diseases requires coordinated services to the patient in the home. A physician, public health nurse, physical therapist, and nutritionist discuss the problems of home care. (Courtesy, Community Nursing Services, Philadelphia.)

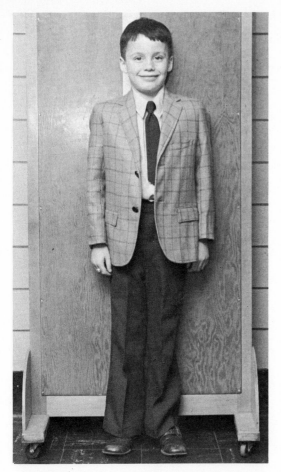

Figure 48–3. This six-year-old boy has been successfully treated with a low-phenylalanine diet since the age of 3 1/2 weeks. (Courtesy, Children's Rehabilitation Center, Buffalo, New York.)

the signs of deficiency include anorexia, vomiting, listlessness, inconsistent growth or failure to grow, pallor, and skin rash. The serum level of phenylalanine is low, but it may be temporarily increased because of the breakdown of tissue proteins.

The low-phenylalanine formula (Lofenalac*) is nutritionally complete except for phenylalanine and thus supplies the necessary amounts of minerals and vitamins.

___

*Lofenalac®, Mead Johnson & Company, Evansville, Indiana.

Management of the diet. The diet is so unlike a normal diet that many problems are encountered in its administration. A skillful approach by physician, nurses, and nutritionist is required to achieve acceptance on the part of the parent as well as the child.

Lofenalac. Proteins contain 4 to 6 per cent phenylalanine, which is far in excess of that tolerated by children with phenylketonuria. Lofenalac, a casein hydrolysate from which 95 per cent of the phenylalanine has been removed, is the basis for the dietary regimen. This preparation contains unsaturated fat, carbohydrate, vitamins, and minerals. It is a completely satisfactory substitute for milk and other protein foods from a nutritional point of view.

Lofenalac is the only source of protein for the infant not yet receiving other foods and continues to provide 85 per cent of the protein needs of the older child.

Milk. Milk contains about 55 mg phenylalanine per ounce and is used as a source of this essential amino acid for the first few months until other phenylalanine-containing foods are introduced. From 1 to 2 ounces of milk are used, always incorporated into the Lofenalac formula lest the child acquire a taste for milk.

Diet lists. Serving lists have been developed in which all foods within a given group will provide the same amount of phenylalanine, protein, and calories when given in the specified amounts. (See Table 48–2.)

Once the child's daily protein, calorie, and phenylalanine requirements are established according to his age and weight, the amount of Lofenalac required to meet the protein and calorie need can be calculated. The day's allowance for phenylalanine is completed by adding the necessary amount of milk for the young infant, or the appropriate amounts of foods from the serving lists for the older child. (See Table 48–3.)

The diet should be progressed as for a normal infant and child. (See Table 48–4.) That is, fruits, vegetables, and cereal foods from the allowed lists are introduced as the child grows. Lofenalac may be incorporated with other foods as the child grows. A variety of recipes have been developed for such use.

Table 48–1. Phenylalanine, Protein, and Calories Recommended for Various Age Groups of Phenylketonuric Patients*

Age	Phenylalanine mg per pound	Protein gm per pound	Calories per pound
0–3 months	20–22	1.75–2.0	60–65
4–12 months	18–20	1.5	55–60
1–3 years	16–18	32 gm total	50–55
4–7 years	10–16	40 gm total	40–50

*Acosta, P. B.: "Nutritional Aspects of Phenylketonuria," in *The Clinical Team Looks at Phenylketonuria,* Revised. Children's Bureau, U.S. Department of Health, Education, and Welfare, Washington, D.C., 1964, p. 45.

DIETARY COUNSELING

Eating problems are encountered frequently in phenylketonuric children. These may be the result of great parental anxiety and feelings of guilt. The parent may overemphasize diet and allow it to dominate the relationships with the child. Initially, the acceptance of Lofenalac may be poor. If it is forced at first, or if the parent or brothers and sisters indicate dislike for the diet, the child may continue to refuse the formula. It is best to offer the formula at the beginning of the feeding when the child is hungry, and to avoid any show of concern if it is not fully accepted. When parents begin to see the improvement in the child, encouragement is provided for the considerable effort needed to maintain careful vigilance in its preparation.

Both parents must receive detailed information concerning the amounts of phenylalanine permitted daily and the amounts of foods that will provide them. They should be asked to demonstrate the measurement and preparation of the formula. A program of home services is invaluable in assuring that the diet is being used as planned. (See Figure 48–4.) The public health nurse often supervises the home care and also consults with the dietitian or nutritionist in the planning and in problems of dietary management. Printed recipe materials should be carefully explained to the parent.

Table 48–2. Phenylalanine, Protein, and Caloric Content of Serving Lists Used on Restricted Phenylalanine Diets*

	Phenylalanine mg	Protein gm	Calories
Lofenalac, 1 measure (1 tablespoon)	7.5	1.5	43
Vegetables	15	0.3	5
Fruits	15	0.2	80
Breads	30	0.5	20
Fats	5	0.1	45
Desserts (special recipes required)	30	2.0	270
Free foods	0	0.0	varies
Milk (per ounce)	55	1.1	20

*Acosta, P. B.: "Nutritional Aspects of Phenylketonuria," in *The Clinical Team Looks at Phenylketonuria,* revised. Children's Bureau, U.S. Department of Health, Education, and Welfare, 1964, p. 40.

Table 48–3. Serving Lists for Phenylalanine-Restricted Diet*

Food	Amount	Food	Amount
Vegetables—15 mg phenylalanine per serving		Grapefruit, sections or juice	1/3 cup
Asparagus	1 stalk	Grapes, green, seedless	20 medium
Beans, green, cooked	3 tbsp	Guava, raw	1/3 medium
junior	2 tbsp	Grape juice	1/3 cup
strained	2 tbsp	Lemon or lime juice	3 tbsp
Beets, cooked	3 tbsp	frozen, diluted	1/2 cup
strained	2 tbsp	Mango	1/2 small
Cabbage, raw, shredded	4 tbsp	Orange	1 medium†
Carrots, raw	1/2 large	Papaya, cubed	1/4 cup
canned	4 tbsp	juice	1/2 cup
junior	3 tbsp	Peach, raw	1 medium†
strained	3 tbsp	canned in syrup	1 1/2 halves
Cauliflower	2 tbsp	junior	7 tbsp
Celery, raw, 5-in. stalks	2 stalks	strained	5 tbsp
Cucumber, raw	1/3 medium	Pear, raw	1 1/3 medium†
Lettuce, head	2 leaves	canned in syrup	3 halves
Mushrooms, cooked	2 tbsp	junior	10 tbsp
Okra, pod, cooked	1 pod	strained	10 tbsp
Onion, green	2 medium	Pear-pineapple, junior	
mature	1/4 medium	and strained	7 tbsp
Parsley	2 sprigs	Pineapple, raw	1/3 cup
Pumpkin, cooked	2 tbsp	canned in syrup	1 1/2 small slices
Radish	3 small	juice	1/2 cup
Spinach, cooked	1 tbsp	Plums, canned	1 medium
creamed, junior and strained	2 tbsp	with tapioca, junior	7 tbsp
Squash, summer cooked	4 tbsp	with tapioca, strained	5 tbsp
Squash, winter, cooked	2 tbsp	Popsicle with fruit juice	2 medium
junior	6 tbsp	Prunes, dried	2 large†
strained	3 tbsp	juice	1/3 cup
Tomato, raw	1/4 small	strained	3 tbsp
canned	2 tbsp	Raisins, dried	2 tbsp†
juice	2 tbsp	Strawberries	3 large
Turnip	4 tbsp	Tangerine	2/3 small
Yam or sweet potato, strained	2 tbsp	Watermelon	1/3 cup
Fruits—15 mg phenylalanine per serving		*Breads and Cereals*—30 mg phenylalanine per serving	
Apple, raw	2 medium†	Barley cereal, Gerber's dry	2 tbsp
Apricots, canned	2 halves	Biscuit‡	1 small
dried, halves	4 large†	Cereal food, Gerber's, dry	2 tbsp
juice	1/4 cup	Corn, cooked	2 tbsp
Apricot-applesauce,		Cornflakes	1/3 cup
junior	10 tbsp	Crackers, Barnum animal	6
strained	10 tbsp	Crackers, graham	1
Avocado	2 tbsp	Crackers, soda	1
Banana, 6 in. long	1/2†	Crackers, saltines	2
Cantaloupe, diced	1/2 cup†	Cream of Rice, cooked	2 tbsp
Dates, dried	2	Cream of Wheat, cooked	2 tbsp
Fruit cocktail, canned	2 tbsp	Hominy	3 tbsp

*Arranged from Acosta, P. B.: "Nutritional Aspects of Phenylketonuria," in *The Clinical Team Looks at Phenylketonuria,* revised 1964. Children's Bureau, U.S. Department of Health, Education, and Welfare Washington, D.C., 1964, pp. 40–44.

Table 48–3. (Cont.)

Food	Amount	Food	Amount
Hominy grits, cooked	3 tbsp	Candy	
Mixed cereal, Pablum, dry	3 tbsp	butterscotch	
Muffin, pineapple‡	2	cream mints	
Oatmeal, Gerber's, strained	2 tbsp	fondant	
Pablum, dry	2 tbsp	gum drops	
Popcorn, popped	1/3 cup	hard	
Potato, white	2 tbsp	jelly beans	
Rice, cooked	2 tbsp	lollipops	
Rice Flakes, Quaker	1/3 cup	Cornstarch	
Rice Krispies, Kellogg's	1/3 cup	Gingerbread‡	
Rice Pablum	4 tbsp	Guava butter	
Rice, Puffed, Quaker	1/3 cup	Honey	
Sugar Crisps	1/4 cup	Jams, jellies, marmalades	
Wheat, Puffed, Quaker	1/3 cup	Margarine	
Yam, sweet potato, cooked	2 tbsp	Molasses	
Fats—5 mg phenylalanine per serving		Oil	
Cream, heavy	1 tsp	Pepper	
Mayonnaise	2 tsp	Popsicle (with fruit flavor only)	
Olives, ripe	1 large	Rich's topping	
		Salt	
Desserts—30 mg phenylalanine per serving		Sauces	
Cake‡	1/2 of cake	lemon‡	
Cookies—rice flour‡	2	white‡	
corn starch‡	2	Sugar, brown or white	
Cookies, Arrowroot	1 1/2	Syrups, corn, maple	
Ice cream—chocolate‡	2/3 cup	Tapioca	
pineapple‡	2/3 cup	*Foods to Avoid*—very high in phenylalanine	
strawberry‡	2/3 cup	Breads	
Jello	1/3 cup	Cheese, all kinds	
Puddings‡	1/2 cup	Eggs	
Sauce, Hershey	2 tbsp	Flour, all kinds	
Wafers, sugar, Nabisco	6	Meat, poultry, fish	
Free Foods—negligible phenylalanine; may be used as		Legumes (dried peas, beans and seeds)	
desired		Nuts	
Apple juice ⎫		Nut butters	
Applesauce ⎬ Count as fruit if more than 1 cup		Milk (55 mg phenylalanine per ounce)	
Butter ⎭		except as calculated for formula	

†Miller, G. T., *et al.*: "Phenylalanine Content of Fruit," *J. Am. Diet. Assoc.,* **46**: 43, 1965.
‡Special recipes required.

Maple Syrup Urine Disease

This inborn error of metabolism derives its name from the maple syrup odor of urine, a valuable clue in the diagnosis. The disease is also known as *branched-chain ketoaciduria*, a term which relates to the biochemical defect. It was first recognized in the United States in 1954 and since then has been described in several European countries and in Japan. It is believed to be transmitted as an autosomal recessive trait. The incidence is not known.

Biochemical defect and clinical changes. Three branched-chain amino acids, namely, leucine, isoleucine, and valine, are normally metabolized to keto acids and then further degraded through decarboxylation to simple acids.

Table 48–4. Restricted Phenylalanine Diets for Infants and Children*

Age	1 Month	8 Months	2 Years	4 Years
Weight, pounds	8	18	26	36
Diet prescription				
Phenylalanine, mg	160–176	324–360	416–468	360–576
Protein, gm	14–16	27	32	40
Calories	440	810	1300	1700
Lofenalac, measures†	10	18	19	23
Water to make	24 oz	32 oz	24 oz	24 oz
Milk as necessary	1 1/2 oz	1 oz	—	—
Vegetables, servings	—	2	4	4
Fruits, servings	1	1	4	4
Breads, servings	—	3	5	4
Fats, servings	—	—	1	1
Desserts,‡ servings	—	—	—	1
Free foods§	—	—	as desired	as desired
Nutritive values				
Phenylalanine, mg	172	325	417	447
Protein, gm	16.8	30.4	33.1	40.6
Calories	540	944	1302	1724

*Acosta, P. B.: "Nutritional Aspects of Phenylketonuria," in *The Clinical Team Looks at Phenylketonuria,* 1964. Children's Bureau, U.S. Department of Health, Education, and Welfare, Washington, D.C., p. 52.
†One measure = 1 tablespoon
‡Special recipes are required for desserts.
§If free foods are given in excessive amounts child may not consume proper amounts of other foods.

Figure   48–4. Nutritionist counsels boy with PKU and his mother about the kinds and amounts of foods that may be included in his diet. (Courtesy, Children's Rehabilitation Center, Buffalo, New York.)

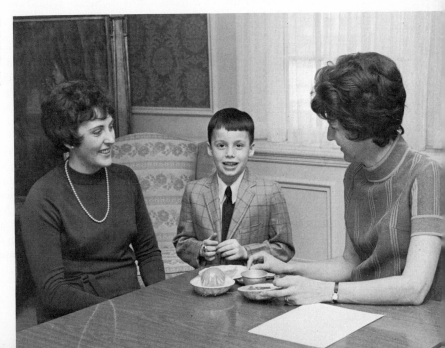

In maple syrup urine disease an *oxidative decarboxylase* in the white blood cells is missing. Because the carboxyl group cannot be removed, the amino acids and their keto acids accumulate in the blood and are excreted in excessive amounts in the urine. A metabolite related to isoleucine is believed to be responsible for the odor of the urine and of the sweat.

Infants appear normal at birth but begin to show symptoms within the first few days. They are unable to suck and swallow satisfactorily, respiration is irregular, and there are intermittent periods of rigidity and flaccidity. Seizures of the grand mal type may occur. If the infants survive, mental retardation is severe. Hypoglycemia has been observed in several patients and may be related to leucine sensitivity. Frequent infections lead to increased tissue catabolism and thus to a further accumulation of the offending metabolites in the circulation.

Dietary treatment. A diet restricted in leucine, isoleucine, and valine has given some encouraging results. After the synthetic formula has reduced the high blood levels of leucine, isoleucine, and valine together with their incompletely metabolized products, small amounts of milk are added to provide for the growth requirements of the infant. Weight gain will not proceed without some supply of the branched-chain amino acids. Puréed carrots, applesauce, and brewers' yeast are among the other foods which have been used with the formula.[6]

HOMOCYSTINURIA

Biochemical and clinical findings. *Cystathionine synthetase* is an enzyme normally present in the brain and liver. It is essential for the conversion of homocysteine to cystathionine, which are intermediate products formed in the metabolism of methionine. When the enzyme is lacking, increased amounts of methionine and homocystine are found in the plasma, and large amounts of homocystine are excreted in the urine. Lack of the enzyme is an autosomal recessive trait.

Homocystinuria occurs almost as frequently as phenylketonuria. Severe mental retardation is present in almost all patients. The optic lens is dislocated in all patients, and glaucoma and cataracts occur in some. There is a weakness of the muscles of the pelvic girdle and a shuffling gait. Skeletal abnormalities include long extremities, osteoporosis, and curvature of the spine. Pulmonary embolism, thrombosis, and cerebral accidents are common.

Dietary modification. A low-methionine high-cystine diet has been used successfully with normal physical and mental development.[7,8] The methionine is restricted to 18 to 20 mg per kilogram and the cystine is increased to 116 mg per kilogram.[7] Gelatin is used as a source of protein because it is low in methionine. This is supplemented with synthetic amino acids—leucine, isoleucine, phenylalanine, tryptophan, and valine—to meet the requirements for growth. (See Table 4–2.)

LEUCINE-INDUCED HYPOGLYCEMIA

A relatively rare inborn error of metabolism, leucine-induced hypoglycemia becomes apparent after about the fourth month of life. Convulsions may be the first indication of an abnormality. Infants with this disorder fail to thrive and show some evidence of delayed mental development. Signs typical of Cushing's syndrome—acne, hirsutism, obesity, and osteoporosis—are often present.

When L-leucine is given in a test dose to the infant, a profound lowering of the blood glucose occurs in the leucine-sensitive infant. The exact reason for the increased sensitivity is not known. Among the several theories suggested, the most likely one appears to be that leucine may act as a stimulus to insulin production or as an enhancement of insulin utilization.

Dietary management. A diet low in leucine is used,[9] but the minimum leucine requirement of 150 to 230 mg per kilogram must be included. Since all protein foods are sources of leucine, a restriction of this amino acid places restrictions upon the inclusion of protein-rich foods. The diet is planned to furnish the minimum requirements of protein for normal development. Fruits and vegetables are added to the diet according to the infant's normal feeding schedule. To counteract the hypoglycemic effects of the leucine, a carbohydrate feeding (equivalent to 10 gm) is given 30 to 40 minutes after each meal. By the age of five to six years the disease has run its course, and from that time on the child is able to tolerate a normal diet.

TYROSINOSIS

Clinical and biochemical findings. Tyrosinosis is an error of metabolism transmitted as an autosomal recessive gene. A deficiency of *para-hydroxyphenylpyruvic acid oxidase* places a block upon the conversion of tyrosine to homogentisic acid. Consequently, the tyrosine levels of the blood are elevated, and increased amounts of tyrosine, p-hydroxyphenylpyruvic acid, other amino acids, and phosphates are excreted in the urine.

Patients with this deficiency show extensive liver and renal damage. Abdominal distention is present because of the enlarged liver and spleen. Liver disease may progress so rapidly that death results from liver failure. The reduced levels of blood phosphate are associated with vitamin-D-resistant rickets. Mental retardation is present.

Dietary modification. A diet low in phenylalanine and in tyrosine has been described, but the ultimate success of the regimen has yet to be determined. A formula, not yet commercially available, has been tested on a 13-year-old mentally retarded girl with tyrosinosis.[10] This product* supplies sufficient quantities of other essential amino acids, minerals, and vitamins. The girl has remained in good health over a period of three months, and her weight status has been satisfactory, but no change has occurred in her behavior or mental development. The synthetic product has been supplemented with restricted amounts of vegetables and breads and cereals together with generous amounts of fruits, sugar, jelly, hard candy, and butter.

*Investigational product 3200AB, Mead Johnson Laboratories, Evansville, Indiana.

TRANSIENT TYROSINEMIA

Newborn infants sometimes have a transient form of tyrosinemia and tyrosyluria.[11] These abnormalities occur especially in premature infants and are directly correlated with the level of protein intake. This appears to be a benign condition and is not associated with specific symptoms. The increased tyrosine levels in the blood and in the urine return to normal as the infant matures. The blood levels are reduced if adequate ascorbic acid is given early.

GALACTOSE DISEASE

Biochemical defect. Galactose disease is caused by the absence of an enzyme (galactose-1-phosphate uridyl transferase, sometimes abbreviated P-Gal-transferase) which is needed in the liver for the conversion of galactose to glucose. Galactose is derived from the hydrolysis of lactose in the intestine. It is absorbed normally in this inborn error, but in the absence of transferase, galactose, galactose-1-phosphate, and galactitol accumulate in the blood and tissues. Analysis of the red blood cells shows little or no transferase in those who have the disease, and only half the normal levels in carriers of the defect.[12] Urine tests show the presence of galactose, albumin, and amino acids. A galactose tolerance test helps to establish the diagnosis. Mothers of galactosemic infants have a diminished ability to metabolize galactose. If they drink unlimited amounts of milk during pregnancy, the possibility of damage to the fetus exists since galactose may pass the placenta.[12] The enzyme defect is inherited as an autosomal recessive trait.

Clinical changes. The disease becomes apparent within a few days after birth by such symptoms as anorexia, vomiting, occasional diarrhea, drowsiness, jaundice, puffiness of the face, edema of the lower extremities, and weight loss. The spleen and liver enlarge, and in some there may be evidences of liver failure within a short time leading to ascites, bleeding, and early death. Mental retardation becomes evident very early in the course of the disease, and cataracts develop within the first year.

Dietary treatment. Milk is the important dietary source of lactose which in turn yields galactose. Human milk is especially high in galactose, and thus the breast-fed infant who lacks the necessary enzyme shows symptoms very early. The substitution of a nonmilk formula leads to rapid improvement as a rule. All of the symptoms disappear except that mental retardation which has already occurred is not reversible. Damage to the central nervous system is greatest during the first few weeks and months of life when growth is rapid. Therefore, the prompt initiation of therapy can scarcely be overemphasized.

A number of nonmilk formula products are available. These include Nutramigen,* Sobee,* and Mul-Soy,† and a meat-base formula.‡ Some pediatricians do not use the soybean preparations since stachyose, a tetrasaccharide in soybeans, is believed to be hydrolyzed to galactose. Others have used such formulas with success. The maintenance of a galactose-free diet is monitored by testing red blood cells for their content of galactose-1-phosphate transferase.

The formulas are supplemented with calcium gluconate or chloride, iron, and vitamins. Since milk is the only food which supplies lactose, other foods may be introduced into the infant's diet at the appropriate times. These include breads, crackers, and cereals made without milk, eggs, meat, poultry, fish, fruits, vegetables, and gelatin desserts. All foods that contain milk must be rigidly excluded: most commercial breads, cookies, cakes, puddings, pudding mixes, some ready-to-eat cereals, all cheeses, cream, ice cream, butter, margarine churned with milk, chocolate, cold cuts, and others. See the list of foods to avoid in allergy to milk, page 609. Liver, brains, and pancreas store galactose and are usually avoided. The question remains whether

---

*Nutramigen and Sobee by Mead Johnson & Co., Evansville, Indiana.

†Mul-Soy by the Borden Company, New York, New York.

‡Meat-base formula by Gerber Products Company, Fremont, Michigan.

the stachyose present in soybeans, beets, Lima beans, and peas is hydrolyzed to galactose. (See also Lactose-Free Diet, Chapter 36.)

As with phenylketonuria, dietary counseling is of paramount importance. Infants accept the substitute formulas quite well, but older children may refuse them for a time. Parents must avoid showing too much anxiety about refusal of food. They need to become thoroughly familiar with lists of foods that contain milk and must learn to read labels with care. The diet is successful only when repeated opportunities are available for follow-up, whether in the clinic or in the home. Such follow-up visits not only reinforce dietary instruction but provide encouragement to the parents. Blood galactose determinations are essential to establish that normal limits are not being exceeded.

FRUCTOSEMIA

Fructosemia is an inborn error in which the introduction of fructose in the infant's diet before six months of age results in anorexia, vomiting, failure to thrive, hypoglycemic convulsions, and dysfunction of the liver and kidney.[13] Older children with the defect are often asymptomatic or they may have spontaneous hypoglycemia. When an oral dose of fructose is given, the blood fructose and magnesium levels rise, but the levels of glucose and phosphate fall. The hypoglycemia that occurs is believed to be caused by reduced glycogenolysis and gluconeogenesis.

Treatment. This condition is controlled by a diet that eliminates all sources of fructose from the diet. Most fruits contain some fructose,[14] and the intestinal hydrolysis of sucrose also yields fructose. Glucose should be used in place of sucrose, and starches are utilized normally. For the infant a formula is calculated to meet normal requirements, using glucose as the source of carbohydrate. Unsweetened cereals, egg yolk, strained meats, and strained vegetables are added at intervals as in normal infant feeding. Sugar beets, sweet potatoes, and peas contain appreciable amounts of cucrose.[14] (See also Table 36–2.)

Wilson's Disease

Hepatolenticular degeneration, or Wilson's disease, is a hereditary disorder transmitted by an autosomal recessive gene. The characteristic defect is a low serum level of ceruloplasmin, a copper-containing protein of the blood. The consequence of this defect is an increased absorption of copper from the intestinal tract and an increased deposit of copper in the brain, liver, and kidney. Because of renal intoxication by the copper, there is a marked aminoaciduria and a negative phosphate balance.

Clinical findings. The onset of symptoms is correlated with the time required for sufficient copper to accumulate in the tissues to produce damage. They may appear as early as four or five years of age, or as late as the thirties. In some patients ascites, jaundice, liver enlargement, and neurologic involvement are observed. The common neurologic signs include indistinct speech, a fixed unblinking stare, hypertonus or rigidity, tremor, seizures, and dementia. The most important physical sign is the Kayser-Fleischer ring, a greenish-brown discoloration seen in the eye.

Treatment. An agent which chelates with cop-per of the diet is used, thereby reducing the amount of copper absorbed. The normal range of copper intake is about 2 or 3 mg, with the traces of copper being distributed in most foods. A low-copper diet should contain 1 mg copper or less.

Foods especially rich in copper include organ meats, shellfish, mushrooms, legumes, whole-grain cereals, bran, chocolate, and nuts. Canned foods and most commercial products must be omitted. If the water supply contains more than 1 ppm of copper, distilled water must be used. Cooking utensils made of copper cannot be used. A paucity of data on the copper content of foods introduces difficulty in planning a diet that is reliably low in copper. Because of the presence of copper in most foods, it is difficult to maintain a sufficiently high caloric intake. Ten recipes for low-copper high-calorie desserts have been developed by Lawler and Jelenc.[15] When these desserts are included at a level of 10 per cent of the day's copper allowance, the caloric intake can be increased by 500 calories.

See Chapter 36 for discussion of the following genetic errors characterized by malabsorption: lactose intolerance; invertase-isomaltase deficiency; glucose-galactose malabsorption.

Problems and Review

1. What is phenylalanine? In what way is its function modified in phenylketonuria?
2. What is Lofenalac? Why is it necessary to include some source of phenylalanine in the diet of the infant with phenylketonuria? What food source may be used?
3. Why is prompt diet therapy essential for the treatment of phenylketonuria and other errors of metabolism?
4. *Problem.* Plan a diet appropriate for an infant with phenylketonuria who is five months old and who weighs 14 pounds. Calculate the phenylalanine, protein, and calorie content of the diet.
5. Outline the essential points to be covered in the counseling of the parents of a patient with phenylketonuria or galactosemia.
6. Examine the labels of proprietary compounds such as Nutramigen, Sobee, Mul-Soy, and Lofenalac. What supplements, if any, to these formulas are required? What is the cost of a formula for one day for a four-month-old infant weighing 12 pounds?
7. Examine the labels of a variety of packaged foods in a market, and prepare a list of those which contain milk.
8. What is the principal defect in galactose disease?
9. Why is carbohydrate given after meals to infants who are sensitive to leucine? What class of foods must be restricted when a low-leucine diet is to be used?

CITED REFERENCES

1. Garrod, A. E.: *Inborn Errors of Metabolism.* Frowde, Hodder & Stoughton, London, 1909.
2. *Phenylketonuria—Low-Phenylalanine Dietary Management with Lofenalac.*® Mead Johnson Laboratories, Evansville, Ind., 1969.
3. Koch, R., *et al.: Clinical Observations on Phenylketonuria,* for Los Angeles Childrens Hospital by Mead Johnson Laboratories, Evansville, Ind.
4. Warner, R.: Personal communication, April 1971.
5. Sutherland, B. S., *et al.:* "Growth and Nutrition in Treated Phenylketonuric Patients," *J.A.M.A.,* **211:**270–76, 1970.
6. Snyderman, S. E., *et al.:* "Maple Syrup Urine Disease with Particular Reference to Dietotherapy," *Pediatrics,* **34:**454–72, 1964.
7. Komrower, G. M.: "Dietary Treatment of Homocystinuria," *Am. J. Dis. Child.,* **113:**98–100, 1967.
8. Sardharwalla, I. B., *et al.:* "Homocystinuria. A Study with Low-Methionine Diet in Three Patients," *Can. Med. Assoc. J.,* **99:**731–40, 1968.
9. Roth, H., and Segal, S.: "The Dietary Management of Leucine Sensitive Hypoglycemia with Report of a Case," *Pediatrics,* **34:**831–38, 1964.
10. Hill, A. *et al.:* "Dietary Treatment of Tyrosinosis," *J. Am. Diet. Assoc.,* **56:**308–12, 1970.
11. Avery, M. E., *et al.:* "Transient Tyrosinemia of the Newborn: Dietary and Clinical Aspects," *Pediatrics,* **39:**378–84, 1967.
12. Hansen, R. G.: "Hereditary Galactosemia," *J.A.M.A.,* **208:**2077–82, 1969.
13. Levin, B., *et al.:* "Fructosemia. Observations on Seven Cases," *Am. J. Med.,* **45:**826–38, 1968.
14. Hardinge, M. G., *et al.:* "Carbohydrates in Foods," *J. Am. Diet. Assoc.,* **46:**197–204, 1965.
15. Lawler, M. R., and Jelenc, M. A.: "Recipes for Low-Copper Diets," *J. Am. Diet. Assoc.,* **57:**420–22, 1970.

ADDITIONAL REFERENCES

Phenylketonuria
Children's Bureau: *The Clinical Team Looks at Phenylketonuria.* U.S. Department of Health, Education, and Welfare, Washington, D.C., 1964.
Davis, L.: "Practical Points in PKU Testing," *Nurs. Outlook,* **14:**46–48, Jan. 1966.
Forbes, N. P., *et al.:* "Maternal Phenylketonuria," *Nurs. Outlook,* **14:**40, Jan. 1966.
Koch, R., *et al.:* "Nutrition in the Treatment of Phenylketonuria," *J. Am. Diet. Assoc.,* **43:**212–15, 1963.
O'Flynn, M. E.: "Diet Therapy in Phenylketonuria. How Long Should It Continue?" *Am. J. Nurs.,* **67:**1658–60, 1967.
Ragsdale, N., and Koch, R.: "Phenylketonuria. Detection and Therapy," *Am. J. Nurs.,* **64:**90–95, Jan. 1964.
Review: "Atypical Phenylketonuria," *Nutr. Rev.,* **27:**110–11, 1969.
———: "Growth and Nutrition in Treated Phenylketonuric Patients," *Nutr. Rev.,* **28:**151–53, 1970.
Rincie, M. M., and Rogers, P. J.: "A Low-Protein Low-Phenylalanine Vegetable Casserole," *J. Am. Diet. Assoc.,* **55:**353–56, 1969.
Saunders, C.: "Phenylketonuria 1969," *Postgrad. Med.,* **46:**159–62, Oct. 1969.
Umbarger, B. J.: "Phenylketonuria. Dietary Treatment," *Am. J. Nurs.,* **64:**96–99, 1964.
Wong, R., *et al.:* "Mineral Balance in Treated Phenylketonuric Children," *J. Am. Diet. Assoc.,* **57:**229–33, 1970.

Maple Syrup Urine Disease

Blattner, R. J.: "Inborn Errors of Metabolism. A Variant of Maple Syrup Urine Disease," *J. Pediatr.*, **66**:139–42, 1965.

Lin-Fu, J. S.: *Maple Syrup Urine Disease.* Children's Bureau, U.S. Department of Health, Education, and Welfare, Washington, D.C., 1964.

Review: "Dietary Treatment of Maple Syrup Urine Disease," *Nutr. Rev.*, **23**:260–62, 1965.

Snyderman, S. E.: "The Therapy of Maple Syrup Urine Disease," *Am. J. Dis. Child*, **113**:68–73, 1967.

Westall, R. G.: "Dietary Treatment of a Child with Maple Syrup Urine Disease (Branched-chain Ketoaciduria)," *Arch. Dis. Child*, **38**:485–91, 1963.

Leucine-Induced Hypoglycemia

DiGeorge, A. M., and Auerbach, V. H.: "Leucine Induced Hypoglycemia. A Review and Speculations," *Am. J. Med. Sci.* **240**:792–801, 1960.

Haddad, W. C., *et al.*: "Leucine-Induced Hypoglycemia," *N. Engl. J. Med.*, **267**:1057–60, 1962.

Snyder, R. D., and Robinson, A.: "Leucine-Induced Hypoglycemia," *Am. J. Dis. Child.*, **113**:566–70, 1967.

Other Metabolic Errors

Halvorsen, S.: "Dietary Treatment of Tyrosinosis," *Am. J. Dis. Child*, **113**:38–40, 1967.

Hillsman, G. M.: "Genetics and the Nurse," *Nurs. Outlook*, **14**:34–39, Jan. 1966.

Juberg, R. C.: "Heredity Counseling," *Nurs. Outlook*, **14**:28–30, Jan. 1966.

Koch, R., *et al.*: "Nutrition in the Treatment of Galactosemia," *J. Am. Diet. Assoc.*, **43**:216–22, 1963.

Scheinberg, I. H., and Sternlieb, I.: "Wilson's Disease," *Ann. Rev. Med.*, **16**:119–34, 1965.

Schimke, K. N., *et al.*: "Homocystinuria. Studies of Twenty Families with Thirty-eight Affected Members," *J.A.M.A.*, **193**:711–19, 1965.

Appendices

Tabular Materials

FOREWORD

Included in this section are 7 tables of the nutritive values of foods; 6 weight-height tables for age-sex categories; and 2 tables of blood and urine constituents.

The student should take time to review the arrangement and content of each of the tables so that he is able to refer to them rapidly and use them with skill. Probably more questions asked by the public pertain to the composition of foods than to any other aspect of nutrition. Tables of food values provide an invaluable reference source to answer such questions. Moreover, the quantitation of diets is possible only when nutritive values are known.

The uses of tables of food composition, as well as their limitations, have been described in Chapter 3. Tables A-1 and A-4 are for specific household measures of food. Other tables of nutritive values are stated for 100 gm of food. If a student, for example, wishes to determine the sodium content of 1 cup of milk, he will follow this procedure:

1 cup milk weighs 244 gm (see Table A–1)

100 gm milk contains 50 mg sodium (see Table A–2)

$\dfrac{244 \times 50}{100} = 122$ mg sodium in 1 cup milk

TABLE A-1 EXPLANATION

Table A-1 is an alphabetic arrangement of items listed in the publication of the Consumer and Food Economics Research Division in 1970 *Nutritive Value of Foods*. A few additional items from Agriculture Handbook 8 *Composition of Foods—Raw, Processed, Prepared* are also included. The explanation provided in the bulletin for this table is reproduced here in part:*

Weight in grams—rounded to the nearest whole gram—is shown for an approximate measure of each food as it is described; if inedible parts are included in the description, both measure and weight include these parts.

The approximate measure shown for each food is in cups, ounces, pounds, some other well-known unit, or a piece of certain size. Usually, the measure shown can be calculated to larger or smaller amounts by multiplying or dividing. Because the measures are approximate (some are rounded for convenient use), calculated nutritive values for larger quantities of some food items may be less representative than those calculated for smaller quantities.

The cup measure refers to the standard measuring cup of 8 fluid ounces or ½ liquid pint. The ounce refers to 1/16 of a pound avoirdupois, unless fluid ounce is indicated. The weight of a fluid ounce varies according to the food measured. . . .

The values for food energy (calories) and nutri-

*Consumer and Food Economics Research Division, Agricultural Research Service: *Nutritive Value of Foods*. Home and Garden Bull. 72, U.S. Department of Agriculture, Washington, D.C., 1970.

ents shown in Table A-1 are the amounts present in the edible part of the item, that is, in only that portion of the weight of the item customarily eaten —corn without cob, meat without bone, potatoes without skin, European-type grapes without seeds. If additional parts are eaten—the skin of the potato, for example—amounts of some nutrients obtained will be somewhat greater than those shown.

For many of the prepared items, values have been calculated from the ingredients in typical recipes. Examples of such items are biscuits, corn muffins, oyster stew, macaroni and cheese, custard, and a number of other dessert-type items.

For toast and for vegetables, values are without fat added, either during preparation or at the table. Values for the thiamine content of toast are about 20 per cent lower than for fresh bread; it was impossible to show this loss adequately because of the small amount of thiamine present in a slice of bread. Some destruction of vitamins in vegetables, especially of ascorbic acid, may occur when foods are cut or shredded. Such losses are variable, and no deduction for these losses has been made.

For meat, values are for meat as cooked, drained, and without drippings. For many cuts, two sets of values are shown: Meat including the fat, and meat from which the fat has been trimmed off in the kitchen or on the plate.

A variety of manufactured items, such as some of the milk products, ready-to-eat breakfast cereals, imitation cream products, fruit drinks, and various mixes are included in Table A-1. Frequently these foods are fortified with one or more nutrients. If nutrients are added, this information is on the label. Values shown in this bulletin for these foods are usually based on products from several manufacturers and may differ somewhat from the values provided by any one source.

Table A–1. Nutritive Values of the Edible Part of Foods*

[Dashes in the columns for nutrients show that no suitable value could be found although there is reason to believe that a measurable amount of the nutrient may be present]

Milk, Cheese, Cream, Imitation Cream; Related Products

	Food, Approximate Measure, and Weight	(in grams) gm	Water per cent	Food Energy calories	Protein gm	Fat gm	Fatty Acids Saturated (total) gm	Unsaturated Oleic gm	Unsaturated Linoleic gm	Carbohydrate gm	Calcium mg	Iron mg	Vitamin A Value I.U.	Thiamine mg	Riboflavin mg	Niacin mg	Ascorbic Acid mg
	Milk:																
	Fluid:																
1	Whole, 3.5% fat	1 cup 244	87	160	9	9	5	3	Trace	12	288	0.1	350	0.07	0.41	0.2	2
2	Nonfat (skim)	1 cup 245	90	90	9	Trace	—	—	—	12	296	0.1	10	0.09	0.44	0.2	2
3	Partly skimmed, 2% nonfat milk solids added	1 cup 246	87	145	10	5	3	2	Trace	15	352	0.1	200	0.10	0.52	0.2	2
	Canned, concentrated, undiluted:																
4	Evaporated, unsweetened	1 cup 252	74	345	18	20	11	7	1	24	635	0.3	810	0.10	0.86	0.5	3
5	Condensed, sweetened	1 cup 306	27	980	25	27	15	9	1	166	802	0.3	1,100	0.24	1.16	0.6	3
	Dry, nonfat instant:																
6	Low-density (1 1/3 cups needed for reconstitution to 1 qt)	1 cup 68	4	245	24	Trace	—	—	—	35	879	0.4	120	0.24	1.21	0.6	5
7	High-density (7/8 cup needed for reconstitution to 1 qt)	1 cup 104	4	375	37	1	—	—	—	54	1,345	0.6	130	0.36	1.85	0.9	7
	Buttermilk:																
8	Fluid, cultured, made from skim milk	1 cup 245	90	90	9	Trace	—	—	—	12	296	0.1	10	0.10	0.44	0.2	2
9	Dried, packaged	1 cup 120	3	465	41	6	3	2	Trace	60	1,498	0.7	260	0.31	2.06	1.1	—
	Cheese:																
	Natural:																
	Blue or Roquefort type:																
10	Ounce	1 oz. 28	40	105	6	9	5	3	Trace	1	89	0.1	350	0.01	0.17	0.3	0
11	Cubic inch	1 cu. in. 17	40	65	4	5	3	2	Trace	Trace	54	0.1	210	0.01	0.11	0.2	0
12	Camembert, packaged in 4-oz pkg. with 3 wedges per pkg.	1 wedge 38	52	115	7	9	5	3	Trace	1	40	0.2	380	0.02	0.29	0.3	0
	Cheddar:																
13	Ounce	1 oz 28	37	115	7	9	5	3	Trace	1	213	0.3	370	0.01	0.13	Trace	0
14	Cubic inch	1 cu in 17	37	70	4	6	3	2	Trace	Trace	129	0.2	230	0.01	0.08	Trace	0
	Cottage, large or small curd:																
	Creamed:																
15	Package of 12 oz, net wt.	1 pkg 340	78	360	46	14	8	5	Trace	10	320	1.0	580	0.10	0.85	0.3	0
16	Cup, curd pressed down	1 cup 245	78	260	33	10	6	3	Trace	7	230	0.7	420	0.07	0.61	0.2	0
	Uncreamed:																
17	Package of 12 oz, net wt.	1 pkg 340	79	290	58	1	1	Trace	Trace	9	306	1.4	30	0.10	0.95	0.3	0
18	Cup, curd pressed down	1 cup 200	79	170	34	1	Trace	Trace	Trace	5	180	0.8	20	0.06	0.56	0.2	0

No.	Food, approximate measure	Measure	Grams	Water (%)	Food energy (Cal.)	Protein (g)	Fat (g)	Saturated (total) (g)	Unsaturated Oleic (g)	Unsaturated Linoleic (g)	Carbohydrate (g)	Calcium (mg)	Iron (mg)	Vitamin A value (I.U.)	Thiamin (mg)	Riboflavin (mg)	Niacin (mg)	Ascorbic acid (mg)
	Cream:																	
19	Package of 8 oz, net wt.	1 pkg	227	51	850	18	86	48	28	3	5	141	0.5	3,500	0.05	0.54	0.2	0
20	Package of 3 oz, net wt.	1 pkg	85	51	320	7	32	18	11	1	2	53	0.2	1,310	0.02	0.20	0.1	0
21	Cubic inch	1 cu in	16	51	60	1	6	3	2	Trace	Trace	10	Trace	250	Trace	0.04	Trace	0
	Parmesan, grated:																	
22	Cup, pressed down	1 cup	140	17	655	60	43	24	14	1	5	1,893	0.7	1,760	0.03	1.22	0.3	0
23	Tablespoon	1 tbsp	5	17	25	2	2	1	Trace	Trace	Trace	68	Trace	60	Trace	0.04	Trace	0
24	Ounce	1 oz	28	17	130	12	9	5	3	Trace	1	383	0.1	360	0.01	0.25	0.1	0
	Swiss:																	
25	Ounce	1 oz	28	39	105	8	8	5	3	Trace	1	262	0.3	320	Trace	0.11	Trace	0
26	Cubic inch	1 cu in	15	39	55	4	4	3	1	Trace	Trace	139	0.1	170	Trace	0.06	Trace	0
	Pasteurized processed cheese:																	
	American:																	
27	Ounce	1 oz	28	40	105	7	9	5	3	Trace	1	198	0.3	350	0.01	0.12	Trace	0
28	Cubic inch	1 cu in	18	40	65	4	5	3	2	Trace	Trace	122	0.2	210	Trace	0.07	Trace	0
	Swiss:																	
29	Ounce	1 oz	28	40	100	8	8	4	3	Trace	1	251	0.3	310	Trace	0.11	Trace	0
30	Cubic inch	1 cu in	18	40	65	5	5	3	2	Trace	Trace	159	0.2	200	Trace	0.07	Trace	0
	Pasteurized process cheese food, American:																	
31	Tablespoon	1 tbsp	14	43	45	3	3	2	Trace	Trace	1	80	0.1	140	Trace	0.08	Trace	0
32	Cubic inch	1 cu in	18	43	60	4	4	2	1	Trace	1	100	0.1	170	Trace	0.10	Trace	0
33	Pasteurized process cheese spread, American	1 oz	28	49	80	5	6	3	2	Trace	2	160	0.2	250	Trace	0.15	Trace	0
	Cream:																	
34	Half-and-half (cream and milk)	1 cup	242	80	325	8	28	15	9	1	11	261	0.1	1,160	0.07	0.39	0.1	2
35		1 tbsp	15	80	20	Trace	2	1	1	Trace	1	16	Trace	70	Trace	0.02	Trace	Trace
	Light, coffee or table:																	
36		1 cup	240	72	505	7	49	27	16	1	10	245	0.1	2,020	0.07	0.36	0.1	2
		1 tbsp	15	72	30	Trace	3	2	1	Trace	1	15	Trace	130	Trace	0.02	Trace	Trace
	Sour:																	
38		1 cup	230	72	485	7	47	26	16	1	10	235	0.1	1,930	0.07	0.35	0.1	2
		1 tbsp	12	72	25	Trace	2	1	1	Trace	1	12	Trace	100	Trace	0.02	Trace	Trace
	Whipped topping (pressurized)																	
40		1 cup	60	62	155	1	14	8	5	Trace	6	67	Trace	570	—	0.04	—	—
		1 tbsp	3	62	10	Trace	Trace	Trace	Trace	Trace	Trace	3	—	30	—	Trace	—	—
	Whipping, unwhipped (volume about double when whipped):																	
	Light:																	
42		1 cup	239	62	715	6	75	41	25	2	9	203	0.1	3,060	0.05	0.29	0.1	2
43		1 tbsp	15	62	45	Trace	5	3	2	Trace	1	13	Trace	190	Trace	0.02	Trace	Trace
	Heavy:																	
44		1 cup	238	57	840	5	90	50	30	3	7	179	0.1	3,670	0.05	0.26	0.1	2
45		1 tbsp	15	57	55	Trace	6	3	2	Trace	1	11	Trace	230	Trace	0.02	Trace	Trace
	Imitation cream products (made with vegetable fat):																	
	Creamers:																	
46	Powdered	1 cup	94	2	505	2	33	31	1	0	52	21	0.6	2,200[2]	—	—	—	—
47		1 tsp	2	2	10	Trace	1	Trace	Trace	0	1	1	Trace	Trace[2]	—	—	—	—
48	Liquid (frozen)	1 cup	245	77	345	2	27	25	Trace	0	25	29	—	2,100[2]	0	0	—	—
49		1 tbsp	15	77	20	Trace	2	2	Trace	0	2	2	—	210	0	0	—	—
50	Sour dressing (imitation sour cream) made with nonfat dry milk	1 cup	235	72	440	8	38	35	1	Trace	17	277	0.1	10	0.07	0.38	0.2	1
51		1 tbsp	12	72	20	Trace	2	2	Trace	Trace	1	14	Trace	Trace	Trace	Trace	Trace	Trace
	Whipped topping:																	
52	Pressurized	1 cup	70	61	190	1	17	15	1	0	9	5	—	2,340[2]	—	0	—	—
53		1 tbsp	4	61	10	Trace	1	1	Trace	0	Trace	Trace	—	220	—	0	—	—

*Nutritive Value of Foods, Home and Garden Bulletin No. 72. U.S. Department of Agriculture, Washington, D.C., 1970.

[1] Value applies to unfortified product; value for fortified low-density product would be 1500 I.U. and the fortified high-density product would be 2290 I.U.

[2] Contributed largely from beta-carotene used for coloring.

Table A-1. (Cont.)

No.	Food, Approximate Measure, and Weight		(in grams) gm	Water per cent	Food Energy calories	Pro-tein gm	Fat gm	Fatty Acids — Satu-rated (total) gm	Unsaturated Oleic gm	Unsaturated Lin-oleic gm	Carbo-hy-drate gm	Cal-cium mg	Iron mg	Vita-min A Value I.U.	Thia-mine mg	Ribo-flavin mg	Niacin mg	Ascor-bic Acid mg
	Whipped topping (cont.)																	
54	Frozen	1 cup	75	52	230	1	20	18	Trace	0	15	5	—	2560	—	0	—	—
55	Powdered, made with	1 tbsp	4	52	10	Trace	1	1	Trace	0	1	Trace	—	230	—	0	—	—
56	whole milk	1 cup	75	58	175	3	12	10	1	Trace	15	62	Trace	2330	0.02	0.08	0.1	Trace
	Milk beverages:																	
57		1 tbsp	4	58	10	Trace	1	1	Trace	Trace	1	3	Trace	220	Trace	Trace	Trace	Trace
58	Cocoa, homemade	1 cup	250	79	245	10	12	7	4	Trace	27	295	1.0	400	0.10	0.45	0.5	3
59	Chocolate-flavored drink made with skim milk and 2% added butterfat	1 cup	250	83	190	8	6	3	2	Trace	27	270	0.5	210	0.10	0.40	0.3	3
	Malted milk:																	
60	Dry powder, approx. 3 heaping teaspoons per ounce	1 oz	28	3	115	4	2	—	—	—	20	82	0.6	290	0.09	0.15	0.1	0
61	Beverage	1 cup	235	78	245	11	10	—	—	—	28	317	0.7	590	0.14	0.49	0.2	2
	Milk desserts:																	
62	Custard	1 cup	265	77	305	14	15	7	5	1	29	297	1.1	930	0.11	0.50	0.3	1
	Ice cream:																	
	Regular (approx. 10% fat)																	
63		1/2 gal	1,064	63	2,055	48	113	62	37	3	221	1,553	0.5	4,680	0.43	2.23	1.1	11
64		1 cup	133	63	255	6	14	8	5	Trace	28	194	0.1	590	0.05	0.28	0.1	1
65		3-fl-oz cup	50	63	95	2	5	3	2	Trace	10	73	Trace	220	0.02	0.11	0.1	1
	Rich (approx. 16% fat)																	
66		1/2 gal	1,188	63	2,635	31	191	105	63	6	214	927	0.2	7,840	0.24	1.31	1.2	12
67		1 cup	148	63	330	4	24	13	8	1	27	115	Trace	980	0.03	0.16	0.1	1
	Ice milk:																	
68	Hardened	1/2 gal	1,048	67	1,595	50	53	29	17	2	235	1,635	1.0	2,200	0.52	2.31	1.0	10
69		1 cup	131	67	200	6	7	4	2	Trace	29	204	0.1	280	0.07	0.29	0.1	1
70	Soft-serve	1 cup	175	67	265	8	9	5	3	Trace	39	273	0.2	370	0.09	0.39	0.2	2
	Yoghurt:																	
71	Made from partially skimmed milk	1 cup	245	89	125	8	4	2	1	Trace	13	294	0.1	170	0.10	0.44	0.2	2
72	Made from whole milk	1 cup	245	88	150	7	8	5	3	Trace	12	272	0.1	340	0.07	0.39	0.2	2
	Eggs																	
	Eggs, large, 24 ounces per dozen:																	
	Raw or cooked in shell or with nothing added:																	
73	Whole, without shell	1 egg	50	74	80	6	6	2	3	Trace	Trace	27	1.1	590	0.05	0.15	Trace	0
74	White of egg	1 white	33	88	15	4	Trace	Trace	—	—	Trace	3	Trace	0	Trace	0.09	Trace	0
75	Yolk of egg	1 yolk	17	51	60	3	5	2	2	Trace	Trace	24	0.9	580	0.04	0.07	Trace	0
76	Scrambled with milk and fat	1 egg	64	72	110	7	8	3	3	Trace	1	51	1.1	690	0.05	0.18	Trace	0
	Meat, Poultry, Fish, Shellfish; Related Products																	
77	Bacon (20 slices per lb raw), broiled or fried crisp	2 slices	15	8	90	5	8	3	4	1	1	2	0.5	0	0.08	0.05	0.8	—
	Beef,[3] cooked:																	
	Cuts braised, simmered, or pot-roasted:																	
78	Lean and fat	3 ounces	85	53	245	23	16	8	7	Trace	0	10	2.9	30	0.04	0.18	3.5	—

No.	Food, approximate measure, and weight	Weight (g)	Water (%)	Food energy (cal)	Protein (g)	Fat (g)	Saturated (g)	Oleic (g)	Linoleic (g)	Carbohydrate (g)	Calcium (mg)	Iron (mg)	Vitamin A (IU)	Thiamin (mg)	Riboflavin (mg)	Niacin (mg)	Ascorbic acid (mg)
79	Lean only — 2.5 ounces	72	62	140	22	5	2	2	Trace	0	10	2.7	10	0.04	0.16	3.3	—
	Hamburger (ground beef), broiled:																
80	Lean — 3 ounces	85	60	185	23	10	5	4	Trace	0	10	3.0	20	0.08	0.20	5.1	—
81	Regular — 3 ounces	85	54	245	21	17	8	8	Trace	0	9	2.7	30	0.07	0.18	4.6	—
	Roast, oven-cooked, no liquid added: Relatively fat, such as rib:																
82	Lean and fat — 3 ounces	85	40	375	17	34	16	15	1	0	8	2.2	70	0.05	0.13	3.1	—
83	Lean only — 1.8 ounces	51	57	125	14	7	3	3	Trace	0	6	1.8	10	0.04	0.11	2.6	—
	Relatively lean, such as heel of round:																
84	Lean and fat — 3 ounces	85	62	165	25	7	3	3	Trace	0	11	3.2	10	0.06	0.19	4.5	—
85	Lean only — 2.7 ounces	78	65	125	24	3	1	1	Trace	0	10	3.0	Trace	0.06	0.18	4.3	—
	Steak, broiled: Relatively fat, such as sirloin:																
86	Lean and fat — 3 ounces	85	44	330	20	27	13	12	1	0	9	2.5	50	0.05	0.16	4.0	—
87	Lean only — 2.0 ounces	56	59	115	18	4	2	2	Trace	0	7	2.2	10	0.05	0.14	3.6	—
	Relatively lean, such as round:																
88	Lean and fat — 3 ounces	85	55	220	24	13	6	6	Trace	0	10	3.0	20	0.07	0.19	4.8	—
89	Lean only — 2.4 ounces	68	61	130	21	4	2	2	Trace	0	9	2.5	10	0.06	0.16	4.1	—
	Beef, canned:																
90	Corned beef — 3 ounces	85	59	185	22	10	5	4	Trace	0	17	3.7	20	0.01	0.20	2.9	—
91	Corned beef hash — 3 ounces	85	67	155	7	10	5	4	Trace	9	11	1.7	—	0.01	0.08	1.8	—
92	Beef, dried or chipped — 2 ounces	57	48	115	19	4	2	2	Trace	0	11	2.9	—	0.04	0.18	2.2	—
93	Beef and vegetable stew — 1 cup	235	82	210	15	10	5	4	Trace	15	28	2.8	2,310	0.13	0.17	4.4	15
94	Beef potpie, baked, 4 1/4-inch diam., weight before baking about 8 ounces — 1 pie	227	55	560	23	33	9	20	2	43	32	4.1	1,860	0.25	0.27	4.5	7
	Chicken, cooked:																
95	Flesh only, broiled — 3 ounces	85	71	115	20	3	1	1	1	0	8	1.4	80	0.05	0.16	7.4	—
	Breast, fried, 1/2 breast:																
96	With bone — 3.3 ounces	94	58	155	25	5	1	2	1	1	9	1.3	70	0.04	0.17	11.2	—
97	Flesh and skin only — 2.7 ounces	76	58	155	25	5	1	2	1	1	9	1.3	70	0.04	0.17	11.2	—
	Drumstick, fried:																
98	With bone — 2.1 ounces	59	55	90	12	4	1	2	1	Trace	6	0.9	50	0.03	0.15	2.7	—
99	Flesh and skin only — 1.3 ounces	38	55	90	12	4	1	2	1	Trace	6	0.9	50	0.03	0.15	2.7	—
100	Chicken, canned, boneless — 3 ounces	85	65	170	18	10	3	4	2	0	18	1.3	200	0.03	0.11	3.7	3
101	Chicken potpie, baked 4 1/4-inch diam., weight before baking about 8 ounces — 1 pie	227	57	535	23	31	10	15	3	42	68	3.0	3,020	0.25	0.26	4.1	5
	Chili con carne, canned:																
102	With beans — 1 cup	250	72	335	19	15	7	7	Trace	30	80	4.2	150	0.08	0.18	3.2	—
103	Without beans — 1 cup	255	67	510	26	38	18	17	1	15	97	3.6	380	0.05	0.31	5.6	—
104	Heart, beef, lean, braised — 3 ounces	85	61	160	27	5	—	—	—	1	5	5.0	20	0.21	1.04	6.5	1
	Lamb,[3] cooked: Chop, thick, with bone, broiled — 1 chop																
105	4.8 ounces	137	47	400	25	33	18	12	1	0	10	1.5	—	0.14	0.25	5.6	—
106	Lean and fat — 4.0 ounces	112	47	400	25	33	18	12	1	0	10	1.5	—	0.14	0.25	5.6	—
107	Lean only — 2.6 ounces	74	62	140	21	6	3	2	Trace	0	9	1.5	—	0.11	0.20	4.5	—
	Leg, roasted:																
108	Lean and fat — 3 ounces	85	54	235	22	16	9	6	Trace	0	9	1.4	—	0.13	0.23	4.7	—
109	Lean only — 2.5 ounces	71	62	130	20	5	3	2	Trace	0	9	1.4	—	0.12	0.21	4.4	—
	Shoulder, roasted:																
110	Lean and fat — 3 ounces	85	50	285	18	23	13	8	1	0	9	1.0	—	0.11	0.20	4.0	—
111	Lean only — 2.3 ounces	64	61	130	17	6	3	2	Trace	0	8	1.0	—	0.10	0.18	3.7	—
112	Liver, beef, fried — 2 ounces	57	57	130	15	6	—	—	—	3	6	5.0	30,280	0.15	2.37	9.4	15

[2] Contributed largely from beta-carotene used for coloring.

[3] Outer layer of fat on the cut was removed to within approximately 1/2-inch of the lean. Deposits of fat within the cut were not removed.

Table A–1. (Cont.)

Food, Approximate Measure, and Weight (in grams)		gm	Water per cent	Food Energy calories	Protein gm	Fat gm	Fatty Acids				Carbo-hy-drate gm	Cal-cium mg	Iron mg	Vita-min A Value I.U.	Thia-mine mg	Ribo-flavin mg	Niacin mg	Ascor-bic Acid mg
							Satu-rated (total) gm	Unsaturated										
								Oleic gm	Lin-oleic gm									
	Pork, cured, cooked:																	
113	Ham, light cure, lean and fat, roasted	3 ounces	85	54	245	18	19	7	8	2	0	8	2.2	0	0.40	0.16	3.1	—
	Luncheon meat:																	
114	Boiled ham, sliced	2 ounces	57	59	135	11	10	4	4	1	0	6	1.6	0	0.25	0.09	1.5	—
115	Canned, spiced or unspiced	2 ounces	57	55	165	8	14	5	6	1	1	5	1.2	0	0.18	0.12	1.6	—
	Pork, fresh,[3] cooked:																	
116	Chop, thick, with bone	1 chop, 3.5 ounces	98	42	260	16	21	8	9	2	0	8	2.2	0	0.63	0.18	3.8	—
117	Lean and fat	2.3 ounces	66	42	260	16	21	8	9	2	0	8	2.2	0	0.63	0.18	3.8	—
118	Lean only	1.7 ounces	48	53	130	15	7	2	3	1	0	7	1.9	0	0.54	0.16	3.3	—
	Roast, oven-cooked, no liquid added:																	
119	Lean and fat	3 ounces	85	46	310	21	24	9	10	2	0	9	2.7	0	0.78	0.22	4.7	—
120	Lean only	2.4 ounces	68	55	175	20	10	3	4	1	0	9	2.6	0	0.73	0.21	4.4	—
	Cuts, simmered:																	
121	Lean and fat	3 ounces	85	46	320	20	26	9	11	2	0	8	2.5	0	0.46	0.21	4.1	—
122	Lean only	2.2 ounces	63	60	135	18	6	2	3	1	0	8	2.3	0	0.42	0.19	3.7	—
	Sausage:																	
123	Bologna, slice, 3-in diam. by 1/8 inch	2 slices	26	56	80	3	7	—	—	—	Trace	2	0.5	—	0.04	0.06	0.7	—
124	Braunschweiger, slice 2-in diam. by 1/4 inch	2 slices	20	53	65	3	5	—	—	—	Trace	2	1.2	1,310	0.03	0.29	1.6	—
125	Deviled ham, canned	1 tbsp	13	51	45	2	4	2	2	Trace	0	1	0.3	—	0.02	0.01	0.2	—
126	Frankfurter, heated (8 per lb purchased pkg)	1 frank	56	57	170	7	15	—	—	—	1	3	0.8	—	0.08	0.11	1.4	—
127	Pork links, cooked (16 links per lb raw)	2 links	26	35	125	5	11	4	5	1	Trace	2	0.6	0	0.21	0.09	1.0	—
128	Salami, dry type	1 oz	28	30	130	7	11	—	—	—	Trace	4	1.0	—	0.10	0.07	1.5	—
129	Salami, cooked	1 oz	28	51	90	5	7	—	—	—	Trace	3	0.7	—	0.07	0.07	1.2	—
130	Vienna, canned (7 sausages per 5-oz can)	1 sausage	16	63	40	2	3	—	—	—	Trace	1	0.3	—	0.01	0.02	0.4	—
	Veal, medium fat, cooked, bone removed:																	
131	Cutlet	3 oz	85	60	185	23	9	5	4	Trace	—	9	2.7	—	0.06	0.21	4.6	—
132	Roast	3 oz	85	55	230	23	14	7	6	Trace	0	10	2.9	—	0.11	0.26	6.6	—
	Fish and shellfish:																	
133	Bluefish, baked with table fat	3 oz	85	68	135	22	4	—	—	—	0	25	0.6	40	0.09	0.08	1.6	—
	Clams:																	
134	Raw, meat only	3 oz	85	82	65	11	1	—	—	—	2	59	5.2	90	0.08	0.15	1.1	8
135	Canned, solids and liquid	3 oz	85	86	45	7	1	—	—	—	2	47	3.5	—	0.01	0.09	0.9	—
136	Crabmeat, canned	3 oz	85	77	85	15	2	—	—	—	1	38	0.7	—	0.07	0.07	1.6	—
137	Fish sticks, breaded, cooked, frozen; stick 3 3/4 by 1 by 1/2 inch	10 sticks or 8 oz pkg.	227	66	400	38	20	5	4	10	15	25	0.9	—	0.09	0.16	3.6	—
138	Haddock, breaded, fried	3 oz	85	66	140	17	5	1	3	Trace	5	34	1.0	—	0.03	0.06	2.7	2
139	Ocean perch, breaded, fried	3 oz	85	59	195	16	11	—	—	—	6	28	1.1	—	0.08	0.09	1.5	—
140	Oysters, raw, meat only (13–19 med. selects)	1 cup	240	85	160	20	4	—	—	—	8	226	13.2	740	0.33	0.43	6.0	—

Mature Dry Beans and Peas, Nuts, Peanuts; Related Products

No.	Food	Measure	g	%	cal	g	g	g	g	g	g	mg	mg	I.U.	mg	mg	mg	mg
141	Salmon, pink, canned	3 oz	85	71	120	17	5	1	1	Trace	0	⁴167	0.7	60	0.03	0.16	6.8	—
142	Sardines, Atlantic, canned in oil, drained solids	3 oz	85	62	175	20	9	—	—	—	0	372	2.5	190	0.02	0.17	4.6	—
143	Shad, baked with table fat and bacon	3 oz	85	64	170	20	10	—	—	—	0	20	0.5	20	0.11	0.22	7.3	—
144	Shrimp, canned, meat	3 oz	85	70	100	21	1	—	—	—	1	98	2.6	50	0.01	0.03	1.5	—
145	Swordfish, broiled with butter or margarine	3 oz	85	65	150	24	5	—	—	—	0	23	1.1	1,750	0.03	0.04	9.3	—
146	Tuna, canned in oil, drained solids	3 oz	85	61	170	24	7	2	1	1	0	7	1.6	70	0.04	0.10	10.1	—
147	Almonds, shelled, whole kernels	1 cup	142	5	850	26	77	6	52	15	28	332	6.7	0	0.34	1.31	5.0	Trace
	Beans, dry: Common varieties as Great Northern, navy and others: Cooked, drained:																	
148	Great Northern	1 cup	180	69	210	14	1	—	—	—	38	90	4.9	0	0.25	0.13	1.3	0
149	Navy (pea)	1 cup	190	69	225	15	1	—	—	—	40	95	5.1	0	0.27	0.13	1.3	0
	Canned, solids and liquid: White with—																	
150	Frankfurters (sliced)	1 cup	255	71	365	19	18	—	—	—	32	94	4.8	330	0.18	0.15	3.3	Trace
151	Pork and tomato sauce	1 cup	255	71	310	16	7	2	3	1	49	138	4.6	330	0.20	0.08	1.5	5
152	Pork and sweet sauce	1 cup	255	66	385	16	12	4	5	1	54	161	5.9	—	0.15	0.10	1.3	—
153	Red kidney	1 cup	255	76	230	15	1	—	—	—	42	74	4.6	10	0.13	0.10	1.5	—
154	Lima, cooked, drained	1 cup	190	64	260	16	1	—	—	—	49	55	5.9	—	0.25	0.11	1.3	—
155	Cashew nuts, roasted	1 cup	140	5	785	24	64	11	45	4	41	53	5.3	140	0.60	0.35	2.5	—
	Coconut, fresh, meat only:																	
156	Pieces, approx. 2 by 2 by 1/2 inch	1 piece	45	51	155	2	16	14	1	Trace	4	6	0.8	0	0.02	0.01	0.2	1
157	Shredded or grated, firmly packed	1 cup	130	51	450	5	46	39	3	Trace	12	17	2.2	0	0.07	0.03	0.7	4
158	Cowpeas or blackeye peas, dry, cooked	1 cup	248	80	190	13	1	—	—	—	34	42	3.2	20	0.41	0.11	1.1	Trace
159	Peanuts, roasted, salted, halves	1 cup	144	2	840	37	72	16	31	21	27	107	3.0	—	0.46	0.19	24.7	0
160	Peanut butter	1 tbsp	16	2	95	4	8	2	4	2	3	9	0.3	—	0.02	0.02	2.4	0
161	Peas, split, dry, cooked	1 cup	250	70	290	20	1	—	—	—	52	28	4.2	100	0.37	0.22	2.2	—
162	Pecans, halves	1 cup	108	3	740	10	77	5	48	15	16	79	2.6	140	0.93	0.14	1.0	2
163	Walnuts, black or native, chopped	1 cup	126	3	790	26	75	4	26	36	19	Trace	7.6	380	0.28	0.14	0.9	—

Vegetables and Vegetable Products

No.	Food	Measure	g	%	cal	g	g	g	g	g	g	mg	mg	I.U.	mg	mg	mg	mg
	Asparagus, green: Cooked, drained:																	
164	Spears, 1/2-in. diam. at base	4 spears	60	94	10	1	Trace	—	—	—	2	13	0.4	540	0.10	0.11	0.8	16
165	Pieces, 1 1/2 to 2-in. lengths	1 cup	145	94	30	3	Trace	—	—	—	5	30	0.9	1,310	0.23	0.26	2.0	38
166	Canned, solids and liquid	1 cup	244	94	45	5	1	—	—	—	7	44	4.1	1,240	0.15	0.22	2.0	37

³Outer layer of fat on the cut was removed to within approximately 1/2-inch of the lean. Deposits of fat within the cut were not removed.

⁴If bones are discarded, value will be greatly reduced.

Table A–1. (Cont.)

	Food, Approximate Measure, and Weight		Water	Food Energy	Pro-tein	Fat	Fatty Acids			Carbo-hy-drate	Cal-cium	Iron	Vita-min A Value	Thia-mine	Ribo-flavin	Niacin	Ascor-bic Acid
							Satu-rated (total)	Unsaturated									
	(in grams)							Oleic	Lin-oleic								
		gm	per cent	calories	gm	gm	gm	gm	gm	gm	mg	mg	I.U.	mg	mg	mg	mg
	Beans:																
167	Lima, immature seeds, cooked, drained	1 cup	170	71	190	13	1	—	—	—	34	80	4.3	480	0.31	0.17	2.2	29
	Snap:																
	Green:																
168	Cooked, drained	1 cup	125	92	30	2	Trace	—	—	—	7	63	0.8	680	0.09	0.11	0.6	15
169	Canned, solids and liquid	1 cup	239	94	45	2	Trace	—	—	—	10	81	2.9	690	0.07	0.10	0.7	10
	Yellow or wax:																
170	Cooked, drained	1 cup	125	93	30	2	Trace	—	—	—	6	63	0.8	290	0.09	0.11	0.6	16
171	Canned, solids and liquid	1 cup	239	94	45	2	1	—	—	—	10	81	2.9	140	0.07	0.10	0.7	12
172	Sprouted mung beans, cooked, drained	1 cup	125	91	35	4	Trace	—	—	—	7	21	1.1	30	0.11	0.13	0.9	8
	Beets:																
	Cooked, drained, peeled:																
173	Whole beets, 2-in. diam.	2 beets	100	91	30	1	Trace	—	—	—	7	14	0.5	20	0.03	0.04	0.3	6
174	Diced or sliced	1 cup	170	91	55	2	Trace	—	—	—	12	24	0.9	30	0.05	0.07	0.5	10
175	Canned, solids and liquid	1 cup	246	90	85	2	Trace	—	—	—	19	34	1.5	20	0.02	0.05	0.2	7
176	Beet greens, leaves and stems, cooked, drained	1 cup	145	94	25	3	Trace	—	—	—	5	144	2.8	7,400	0.10	0.22	0.4	22
	Blackeye peas. See Cowpeas																
	Broccoli, cooked, drained:																
177	Whole stalks, medium size	1 stalk	180	91	45	6	1	—	—	—	8	158	1.4	4,500	0.16	0.36	1.4	162
178	Stalks cut into 1/2-in pieces	1 cup	155	91	40	5	1	—	—	—	7	136	1.2	3,880	0.14	0.31	1.2	140
179	Chopped, yield from 10-oz frozen pkg	1 3/8 cups	250	92	65	7	1	—	—	—	12	135	1.8	6,500	0.15	0.30	1.3	143
180	Brussels sprouts, 7–8 sprouts (1 1/4 to 1 1/2 in. diam.) per cup, cooked	1 cup	155	88	55	7	1	—	—	—	10	50	1.7	810	0.12	0.22	1.2	135
	Cabbage:																
	Common varieties:																
	Raw:																
181	Coarsely shredded or sliced	1 cup	70	92	15	1	Trace	—	—	—	4	34	0.3	90	0.04	0.04	0.2	33
182	Finely shredded or chopped	1 cup	90	92	20	1	Trace	—	—	—	5	44	0.4	120	0.05	0.05	0.3	42
183	Cooked	1 cup	145	94	30	2	Trace	—	—	—	6	64	0.4	190	0.06	0.06	0.4	48
184	Red, raw, coarsely shredded	1 cup	70	90	20	1	Trace	—	—	—	5	29	0.6	30	0.06	0.04	0.3	43
185	Savoy, raw, coarsely shredded	1 cup	70	92	15	2	Trace	—	—	—	3	47	0.6	140	0.04	0.06	0.2	39
186	Cabbage, celery or Chinese raw, cut in 1-in pieces	1 cup	75	95	10	1	Trace	—	—	—	2	32	0.5	110	0.04	0.03	0.5	19
187	Cabbage, spoon (or pakchoy), cooked	1 cup	170	95	25	2	Trace	—	—	—	4	252	1.0	5,270	0.07	0.14	1.2	26
	Carrots:																
	Raw:																
188	Whole, 5 1/2 by 1 inch, (25 thin strips)	1 carrot	50	88	20	1	Trace	—	—	—	5	18	0.4	5,500	0.03	0.03	0.3	4

No.	Food	Measure	Grams	Water (%)	Food energy	Protein	Fat				Carbohydrate	Calcium	Iron	Vitamin A	Thiamine	Riboflavin	Niacin	Ascorbic acid
189	Grated	1 cup	110	88	45	1	Trace	—	—	—	11	41	0.8	12,100	0.06	0.06	0.7	9
190	Cooked, diced	1 cup	145	91	45	1	Trace	—	—	—	10	48	0.9	15,220	0.08	0.07	0.7	9
191	Canned, strained or chopped (baby food)	1 ounce	28	92	10	Trace	Trace	—	—	—	2	7	0.1	3,690	0.01	0.01	0.1	1
192	Cauliflower, cooked, flower-buds	1 cup	120	93	25	3	Trace	—	—	—	5	25	0.8	70	0.11	0.10	0.7	66
193	Celery, raw: Stalk, large outer, 8 by about 1 1/2 inches, at root end	1 stalk	40	94	5	Trace	Trace	—	—	—	2	16	0.1	100	0.01	0.01	0.1	4
194	Pieces, diced	1 cup	100	94	15	1	Trace	—	—	—	4	39	0.3	240	0.03	0.03	0.3	9
195	Collards, cooked	1 cup	190	91	55	5	1	—	—	—	9	289	1.1	10,260	0.27	0.37	2.4	87
196	Corn sweet: Cooked, ear 5 by 1 3/4 inches[5]	1 ear	140	74	70	3	1	—	—	—	16	2	0.5	310[6]	0.09	0.08	1.0	7
197	Canned, solids and liquid	1 cup	256	81	170	5	2	—	—	—	40	10	1.0	690[6]	0.07	0.12	2.3	13
198	Cowpeas, cooked immature seeds	1 cup	160	72	175	13	1	—	—	—	29	38	3.4	560	0.49	0.18	2.3	28
199	Cucumbers, 10-ounce; 7 1/2 by about 2 inches: Raw, pared	1 cucumber	207	96	30	1	Trace	—	—	—	7	35	0.6	Trace	0.07	0.09	0.4	23
200	Raw, pared, center slice 1/8-inch thick	6 slices	50	96	5	Trace	Trace	—	—	—	2	8	0.2	Trace	0.02	0.02	0.1	6
201	Dandelion greens, cooked	1 cup	180	90	60	4	1	—	—	—	12	252	3.2	21,060	0.24	0.29	—	32
202	Endive, curly (including escarole)	2 ounces	57	93	10	1	Trace	—	—	—	2	46	1.0	1,870	0.04	0.08	0.3	6
203	Kale, leaves including stems, cooked	1 cup	110	91	30	4	1	—	—	—	4	147	1.3	8,140	—	—	—	68
204	Lettuce, raw: Butterhead, as Boston types; head, 4-inch diameter	1 head	220	95	30	3	Trace	—	—	—	6	77	4.4	2,130	0.14	0.13	0.6	18
205	Crisphead, as Iceberg; head, 4 3/4 inch diameter	1 head	454	96	60	4	Trace	—	—	—	13	91	2.3	1,500	0.29	0.27	1.3	29
206	Looseleaf, or bunching varieties, leaves	2 large	50	94	10	1	Trace	—	—	—	2	34	0.7	950	0.03	0.04	0.2	9
207	Mushrooms, canned, solids and liquid	1 cup	244	93	40	5	Trace	—	—	—	6	15	1.2	Trace	0.04	0.60	4.8	4
208	Mustard greens, cooked	1 cup	140	93	35	3	1	—	—	—	6	193	2.5	8,120	0.11	0.19	0.9	68
209	Okra, cooked, pod 3 by 5/8 inch	8 pods	85	91	25	2	Trace	—	—	—	5	78	0.4	420	0.11	0.15	0.8	17
210	Onions: Mature: Raw, onion 2 1/2-inch diameter	1 onion	110	89	40	2	Trace	—	—	—	10	30	0.6	40	0.04	0.04	0.2	11
211	Cooked	1 cup	210	92	60	3	Trace	—	—	—	14	50	0.8	80	0.06	0.06	0.4	14
212	Young green, small, without tops	6 onions	50	88	20	1	Trace	—	—	—	5	20	0.3	Trace	0.02	0.02	0.2	12
213	Parsley, raw, chopped	1 tablespoon	4	85	Trace	Trace	Trace	—	—	—	Trace	8	0.2	340	Trace	0.01	Trace	7
214	Parsnips, cooked	1 cup	155	82	100	2	1	—	—	—	23	70	0.9	50	0.11	0.12	0.2	16
215	Peas, green: Cooked	1 cup	160	82	115	9	1	—	—	—	19	37	2.9	860	0.44	0.17	3.7	33
216	Canned, solids and liquid	1 cup	249	83	165	9	1	—	—	—	31	50	4.2	1,120	0.23	0.13	2.2	22
217	Canned, strained (baby food)	1 ounce	28	86	15	1	Trace	—	—	—	3	3	0.4	140	0.02	0.02	0.4	3

[5]Measure and weight apply to entire vegetable or fruit including parts not usually eaten.

[6]Based on yellow varieties; white varieties contain only a trace of cryptoxanthin and carotenes, the pigments in corn that have biologic activity.

	Food, Approximate Measure, and Weight (in grams)		gm	Water per cent	Food Energy calories	Protein gm	Fat gm	Fatty Acids Saturated (total) gm	Unsaturated Oleic gm	Unsaturated Linoleic gm	Carbohydrate gm	Calcium mg	Iron mg	Vitamin A Value I.U.	Thiamine mg	Riboflavin mg	Niacin mg	Ascorbic Acid mg
218	Peppers, hot, red, without seeds, dried (ground chili powder, added seasonings)	1 tablespoon	15	8	50	2	2	—	—	—	8	40	2.3	9,750	0.03	0.17	1.3	2
	Peppers, sweet:																	
219	Raw, about 5 per pound: Green pod without stem and seeds	1 pod	74	93	15	1	Trace	—	—	—	4	7	0.5	310	0.06	0.06	0.4	94
220	Cooked, boiled, drained	1 pod	73	95	15	1	Trace	—	—	—	3	7	0.4	310	0.05	0.05	0.4	70
221	Potatoes, medium (about 3 per pound raw): Baked, peeled after baking	1 potato	99	75	90	3	Trace	—	—	—	21	9	0.7	Trace	0.10	0.04	1.7	20
	Boiled:																	
222	Peeled after boiling	1 potato	136	80	105	3	Trace	—	—	—	23	10	0.8	Trace	0.13	0.05	2.0	22
223	Peeled before boiling	1 potato	122	83	80	2	Trace	—	—	—	18	7	0.6	Trace	0.11	0.04	1.4	20
	French-fried, piece 2 by 1/2 by 1/2 inch:																	
224	Cooked in deep fat	10 pieces	57	45	155	2	7	2	2	4	20	9	0.7	Trace	0.07	0.04	1.8	12
225	Frozen, heated	10 pieces	57	53	125	2	5	1	1	2	19	5	1.0	Trace	0.08	0.01	1.5	12
	Mashed:																	
226	Milk added	1 cup	195	83	125	4	1	—	—	—	25	47	0.8	50	0.16	0.10	2.0	19
227	Milk and butter added	1 cup	195	80	185	4	8	4	3	Trace	24	47	0.8	330	0.16	0.10	1.9	18
228	Potato chips, medium, 2-inch diameter	10 chips	20	2	115	1	8	2	2	4	10	8	0.4	Trace	0.04	0.01	1.0	3
229	Pumpkin, canned	1 cup	228	90	75	2	1	—	—	—	18	57	0.9	14,590	0.07	0.12	1.3	12
230	Radishes, raw, small, without tops	4 radishes	40	94	5	Trace	Trace	—	—	—	1	12	0.4	Trace	0.01	0.01	0.1	10
231	Sauerkraut, canned, solids and liquid	1 cup	235	93	45	2	Trace	—	—	—	9	85	1.2	120	0.07	0.09	0.4	33
	Spinach:																	
232	Cooked	1 cup	180	92	40	5	1	—	—	—	6	167	4.0	14,580	0.13	0.25	1.0	50
233	Canned, drained solids	1 cup	180	91	45	5	1	—	—	—	6	212	4.7	14,400	0.03	0.21	0.6	24
	Squash: Cooked:																	
234	Summer, diced	1 cup	210	96	30	2	Trace	—	—	—	7	52	0.8	820	0.10	0.16	1.6	21
235	Winter, baked, mashed	1 cup	205	81	130	4	1	—	—	—	32	57	1.6	8,610	0.10	0.27	1.4	27
	Sweetpotatoes: Cooked, medium, 5 by 2 inches, weight raw about 6 ounces:																	
236	Baked, peeled after baking	1 sweetpotato	110	64	155	2	1	—	—	—	36	44	1.0	8,910	0.10	0.07	0.7	24
237	Boiled, peeled after boiling	1 sweetpotato	147	71	170	2	1	—	—	—	39	47	1.0	11,610	0.13	0.09	0.9	25
238	Candied, 3 1/2 by 2 1/4 inches	1 sweetpotato	175	60	295	2	6	2	3	1	60	65	1.6	11,030	0.10	0.08	0.8	17
239	Canned, vacuum or solid pack	1 cup	218	72	235	4	Trace	—	—	—	54	54	1.7	17,000	0.10	0.10	1.4	30
	Tomatoes:																	
240	Raw, approx. 3-in diam. 2 1/8 in high; wt., 7 oz	1 tomato	200	94	40	2	Trace	—	—	—	9	24	0.9	1,640	0.11	0.07	1.3	742
241	Canned, solids and liquid	1 cup	241	94	50	2	1	—	—	—	10	14	1.2	2,170	0.12	0.07	1.7	41

No.	Food	Measure	Grams	Water (%)	Food energy (cal.)	Protein (g)	Fat (g)	Saturated (g)	Oleic (g)	Linoleic (g)	Carbohydrate (g)	Calcium (mg)	Iron (mg)	Vitamin A (I.U.)	Thiamin (mg)	Riboflavin (mg)	Niacin (mg)	Ascorbic acid (mg)
	Tomato catsup:																	
242	Cup	1 cup	273	69	290	6	1	—	—	—	69	60	2.2	3,820	0.25	0.19	4.4	41
243	Tablespoon	1 tbsp.	15	69	15	Trace	Trace	—	—	—	4	3	0.1	210	0.01	0.01	0.2	2
	Tomato juice, canned:																	
244	Cup	1 cup	243	94	45	2	Trace	—	—	—	10	17	2.2	1,940	0.12	0.07	1.9	39[7]
245	Glass (6 fl oz)	1 glass	182	94	35	2	Trace	—	—	—	8	13	1.6	1,460	0.09	0.05	1.5	29[7]
246	Turnips, cooked, diced	1 cup	155	94	35	1	Trace	—	—	—	8	54	0.6	Trace	0.06	0.08	0.5	34
247	Turnips greens, cooked	1 cup	145	94	30	3	Trace	—	—	—	5	252	1.5	8,270	0.15	0.33	0.7	68

Fruits and Fruit Products

No.	Food	Measure	Grams	Water (%)	Food energy (cal.)	Protein (g)	Fat (g)	Saturated (g)	Oleic (g)	Linoleic (g)	Carbohydrate (g)	Calcium (mg)	Iron (mg)	Vitamin A (I.U.)	Thiamin (mg)	Riboflavin (mg)	Niacin (mg)	Ascorbic acid (mg)
248	Apples, raw (about 3 per lb)[5]	1 apple	150	85	70	Trace	Trace	—	—	—	18	8	0.4	50	0.04	0.02	0.1	3
249	Apple juice, bottled or canned	1 cup	248	88	120	Trace	Trace	—	—	—	30	15	1.5	—	0.02	0.05	0.2	2
	Applesauce, canned:																	
250	Sweetened	1 cup	255	76	230	1	Trace	—	—	—	61	10	1.3	100	0.05	0.03	0.1	3[8]
251	Unsweetened or artificially sweetened	1 cup	244	88	100	1	Trace	—	—	—	26	10	1.2	100	0.05	0.02	0.1	2[8]
	Apricots:																	
252	Raw (about 12 per lb)[5]	3 apricots	114	85	55	1	Trace	—	—	—	14	18	0.5	2,890	0.03	0.04	0.7	10
253	Canned in heavy syrup	1 cup	259	77	220	2	Trace	—	—	—	57	28	0.8	4,510	0.05	0.06	0.9	10
254	Dried, uncooked (40 halves per cup)	1 cup	150	25	390	8	1	—	—	—	100	100	8.2	16,350	0.02	0.23	4.9	19
255	Cooked, unsweetened, fruit and liquid	1 cup	285	76	240	5	1	—	—	—	62	63	5.1	8,550	0.01	0.13	2.8	8
256	Apricot nectar, canned	1 cup	251	85	140	1	Trace	—	—	—	37	23	0.5	2,380	0.03	0.03	0.5	8
257	Avocados, whole fruit, raw:[5] California (mid- and late-winter; diam. 3 1/8 in)	1 avocado	284	74	370	5	37	7	17	5	13	22	1.3	630	0.24	0.43	3.5	30
258	Florida (late summer, fall; diam. 3 5/8 in)	1 avocado	454	78	390	4	33	7	15	4	27	30	1.8	880	0.33	0.61	4.9	43
259	Bananas, raw, medium size[5]	1 banana	175	76	100	1	Trace	—	—	—	26	10	0.8	230	0.06	0.07	0.8	12
260	Banana flakes	1 cup	100	3	340	4	1	—	—	—	89	32	2.8	760	0.18	0.24	2.8	7
261	Blackberries, raw	1 cup	144	84	85	2	1	—	—	—	19	46	1.3	290	0.05	0.06	0.5	30
262	Blueberries, raw	1 cup	140	83	85	1	1	—	—	—	21	21	1.4	140	0.04	0.08	0.6	20
263	Cantaloups, raw; medium, 5-inch diameter about 1 2/3 pounds[5]	1/2 melon	385	91	60	1	Trace	—	—	—	14	27	0.8	6,540[9]	0.08	0.06	1.2	63
264	Cherries, canned, red, sour, pitted, water pack	1 cup	244	88	105	2	Trace	—	—	—	26	37	0.7	1,660	0.07	0.05	0.5	12
265	Cranberry juice cocktail, canned	1 cup	250	83	165	Trace	Trace	—	—	—	42	13	0.8	Trace	0.03	0.03	0.1	40[10]
266	Cranberry sauce, sweetened, canned, strained	1 cup	277	62	405	Trace	1	—	—	—	104	17	0.6	60	0.03	0.03	0.1	6
267	Dates, pitted, cut	1 cup	178	22	490	4	1	—	—	—	130	105	5.3	90	0.16	0.17	3.9	0
268	Figs, dried, large, 2 by 1 in	1 fig	21	23	60	Trace	Trace	—	—	—	15	26	0.6	20	0.02	0.02	0.1	0
269	Fruit cocktail, canned, in heavy syrup	1 cup	256	80	195	1	Trace	—	—	—	50	23	1.0	360	0.05	0.03	1.3	5
	Grapefruit: Raw, medium, 3 3/4-in diam.[5]																	
270	White	1/2 grapefruit	241	89	45	1	Trace	—	—	—	12	19	0.5	10	0.05	0.02	0.2	44
271	Pink or red	1/2 grapefruit	241	89	50	1	Trace	—	—	—	13	20	0.5	540	0.05	0.02	0.2	44
272	Canned, syrup pack	1 cup	254	81	180	2	Trace	—	—	—	45	33	0.8	30	0.08	0.05	0.5	76

[5] Measure and weight apply to entire vegetable or fruit including parts not usually eaten.

[7] Year-round average. Samples marketed from November through May, average 20 milligrams per 200-gram tomato; from June through October, around 52 milligrams.

[8] This is the amount from the fruit. Additional ascorbic acid may be added by the manufacturer. Refer to the label for this information.

[9] Value for varieties with orange-colored flesh; value for varieties with green flesh would be about 540 I.U.

[10] Value listed is based on products with label stating 30 mg per 6-fl-oz serving.

#	Food, Approximate Measure, and Weight (in grams)		Water per cent	Food Energy calories	Pro-tein gm	Fat gm	Fatty Acids Satu-rated (total) gm	Unsaturated Oleic gm	Lin-oleic gm	Carbo-hy-drate gm	Cal-cium mg	Iron mg	Vita-min A Value I.U.	Thia-mine mg	Ribo-flavin mg	Niacin mg	Ascor-bic Acid mg
		gm															
	Grapefruit juice:																
273	Fresh	1 cup	246	90	95	1	Trace	—	—	—	23	22	0.5	(11)	0.09	0.04	0.4	92
	Canned, white:																
274	Unsweetened	1 cup	247	89	100	1	Trace	—	—	—	24	20	1.0	20	0.07	0.04	0.4	84
275	Sweetened	1 cup	250	86	130	1	Trace	—	—	—	32	20	1.0	20	0.07	0.04	0.4	78
	Frozen concentrate, unsweetened:																
276	Undiluted, can, 6 fluid ounces	1 can	207	62	300	4	1	—	—	—	72	70	0.8	60	0.29	0.12	1.4	286
277	Diluted with 3 parts water, by volume	1 cup	247	89	100	1	Trace	—	—	—	24	25	0.2	20	0.10	0.04	0.5	96
278	Dehydrated crystals	4 oz	113	1	410	6	1	—	—	—	102	100	1.2	80	0.40	0.20	2.0	396
279	Prepared with water (1 pound yields about 1 gallon)	1 cup	247	90	100	1	Trace	—	—	—	24	22	0.2	20	0.10	0.05	0.5	91
	Grapes, raw:5																
280	American type (slip skin)	1 cup	153	82	65	1	1	—	—	—	15	15	0.4	100	0.05	0.03	0.2	3
281	European type (adherent skin)	1 cup	160	81	95	1	Trace	—	—	—	25	17	0.6	140	0.07	0.04	0.4	6
	Grapejuice:																
282	Canned or bottled	1 cup	253	83	165	1	Trace	—	—	—	42	28	0.8	—	0.10	0.05	0.5	Trace
	Frozen concentrate, sweetened:																
283	Undiluted, can, 6 fluid ounces	1 can	216	53	395	1	Trace	—	—	—	100	22	0.9	40	0.13	0.22	1.5	(12)
284	Diluted with 3 parts water, by volume	1 cup	250	86	135	1	Trace	—	—	—	33	8	0.3	10	0.05	0.08	0.5	(12)
285	Grapejuice drink, canned	1 cup	250	86	135	Trace	Trace	—	—	—	35	8	0.3	—	0.03	0.03	0.3	(12)
286	Lemons, raw, 2 1/8-in diam., size 165.5 Used for juice	1 lemon	110	90	20	1	Trace	—	—	—	6	19	0.4	10	0.03	0.01	0.1	39
287	Lemon juice, raw	1 cup	244	91	60	1	Trace	—	—	—	20	17	0.5	50	0.07	0.02	0.2	112
	Lemonade concentrate:																
288	Frozen, 6 fl oz per can	1 can	219	48	430	Trace	Trace	—	—	—	112	9	0.4	40	0.04	0.07	0.7	66
289	Diluted with 4 1/3 parts water, by volume	1 cup	248	88	110	Trace	Trace	—	—	—	28	2	Trace	Trace	Trace	0.02	0.2	17
	Lime juice:																
290	Fresh	1 cup	246	90	65	1	Trace	—	—	—	22	22	0.5	20	0.05	0.02	0.2	79
291	Canned, unsweetened	1 cup	246	90	65	1	Trace	—	—	—	22	22	0.5	20	0.05	0.02	0.2	52
	Limeade concentrate, frozen:																
292	Undiluted, can, 6 fluid ounces	1 can	218	50	410	Trace	Trace	—	—	—	108	11	0.2	Trace	0.02	0.02	0.2	26
293	Diluted with 4 1/3 parts water, by volume	1 cup	247	90	100	Trace	Trace	—	—	—	27	2	Trace	Trace	Trace	Trace	Trace	5
294	Oranges, raw, 2 5/8-in diam., all commercial varieties5	1 orange	180	86	65	1	Trace	—	—	—	16	54	0.5	260	0.13	0.05	0.5	66
295	Orange juice, fresh, all varieties	1 cup	248	88	110	2	1	—	—	—	26	27	0.5	500	0.22	0.07	1.0	124
296	Canned, unsweetened	1 cup	249	87	120	2	Trace	—	—	—	28	25	1.0	500	0.17	0.05	0.7	100
	Orange juice concentrate:																
297	Undiluted, can, 6 fluid ounces	1 can	213	55	360	5	Trace	—	—	—	87	75	0.9	1,620	0.68	0.11	2.8	360

Item No.	Food, approximate measure	Weight (g)	Water (%)	Food energy (cal)	Protein (g)	Fat (g)	Saturated (g)	Oleic (g)	Linoleic (g)	Carbohydrate (g)	Calcium (mg)	Iron (mg)	Vitamin A (I.U.)	Thiamin (mg)	Riboflavin (mg)	Niacin (mg)	Ascorbic acid (mg)
298	Diluted with 3 parts water, by volume — 1 cup	249	87	120	2	Trace	—	—	—	29	25	0.2	550	0.22	0.02	1.0	120
299	Dehydrated crystals — 4 oz	113	1	430	6	2	—	—	—	100	95	1.9	1,900	0.76	0.24	3.3	408
300	Prepared with water (1 pound yields about 1 gallon) — 1 cup	248	88	115	2	1	—	—	—	27	25	0.5	500	0.20	0.07	1.0	109
301	Orange-apricot juice drink — 1 cup	249	87	125	1	Trace	—	—	—	32	12	0.2	1,440	0.05	0.02	0.5	40[10]
	Orange and grapefruit juice: Frozen concentrate:																
302	Undiluted, can, 6 fluid ounces — 1 can	210	59	330	4	1	—	—	—	78	61	0.8	800	0.48	0.06	2.3	302
303	Diluted with 3 parts water, by volume — 1 cup	248	88	110	1	Trace	—	—	—	26	20	0.2	270	0.16	0.02	0.8	102
304	Papayas, raw, 1/2-inch cubes — 1 cup	182	89	70	1	Trace	—	—	—	18	36	0.5	3,190	0.07	0.08	0.5	102
	Peaches: Raw:																
305	Whole, medium, 2-inch diameter, about 4 per pound[5] — 1 peach	114	89	35	1	Trace	—	—	—	10	9	0.5	1,320[13]	0.02	0.05	1.0	7
306	Sliced — 1 cup	168	89	65	1	Trace	—	—	—	16	15	0.8	2,230[13]	0.03	0.08	1.6	12
	Canned, yellow-fleshed, solids and liquid: Syrup pack, heavy:																
307	Halves or slices — 1 cup	257	79	200	1	Trace	—	—	—	52	10	0.8	1,100	0.02	0.06	1.4	7
308	Water pack — 1 cup	245	91	75	1	Trace	—	—	—	20	10	0.7	1,100	0.02	0.06	1.4	7
309	Dried, uncooked — 1 cup	160	25	420	5	1	—	—	—	109	77	9.6	6,240	0.02	0.31	8.5	28
310	Cooked, unsweetened, 10–12 halves and juice — 1 cup	270	77	220	3	1	—	—	—	58	41	5.1	3,290	0.01	0.15	4.2	6
	Frozen:																
311	Carton, 12 ounces, not thawed — 1 carton	340	76	300	1	Trace	—	—	—	77	14	1.7	2,210	0.03	0.14	2.4	135[14]
	Pears:																
312	Raw, 3 by 2 1/2-inch diameter[5] — 1 pear	182	83	100	1	1	—	—	—	25	13	0.5	30	0.04	0.07	0.2	7
	Canned, solids, and liquid: Syrup pack, heavy:																
313	Halves or slices — 1 cup	255	80	195	1	1	—	—	—	50	13	0.5	Trace	0.03	0.05	0.3	4
	Pineapple:																
314	Raw, diced — 1 cup	140	85	75	1	Trace	—	—	—	19	24	0.7	100	0.12	0.04	0.3	24
	Canned, heavy syrup pack, solids and liquids:																
315	Crushed — 1 cup	260	80	195	1	Trace	—	—	—	50	29	0.8	120	0.20	0.06	0.5	17
316	Sliced, slices and juice — 2 small or 1 large	122	80	90	Trace	Trace	—	—	—	24	13	0.4	50	0.09	0.03	0.2	8
317	Pineapple juice, canned — 1 cup	249	86	135	1	Trace	—	—	—	34	37	0.7	120	0.12	0.04	0.5	22[8]
	Plums, all except prunes:																
318	Raw, 2-inch diameter, about 2 ounces[5] — 1 plum	60	87	25	Trace	Trace	—	—	—	7	7	0.3	140	0.02	0.02	0.3	3
	Canned, syrup pack (Italian prunes):																
319	Plums (with pits) and juice[5] — 1 cup	256	77	205	1	Trace	—	—	—	53	22	2.2	2,970	0.05	0.05	0.9	4

5 Measure and weight apply to entire vegetable or fruit including parts not usually eaten.

8 This is the amount from the fruit. Additional ascorbic acid may be added by the manufacturer. Refer to the label for this information.

10 Value listed is based on product with label stating 30 milligrams per 6-fl-oz serving.

11 For white-fleshed varieties value is about 20 I.U. per cup; for red-fleshed varieties, 1,080 I.U. per cup.

12 Present only if added by the manufacturer. Refer to the label for this information.

13 Based on yellow-fleshed varieties; for white-fleshed varieties value is about 50 I.U. per 114-gm peach and 80 I.U. per cup of sliced peaches.

14 This value includes ascorbic acid added by manufacturer.

Table A–1. (Cont.)

	Food, Approximate Measure, and Weight (in grams)		Water per cent	Food Energy calories	Protein gm	Fat gm	Fatty Acids			Carbohydrate gm	Calcium mg	Iron mg	Vitamin A Value I.U.	Thiamine mg	Riboflavin mg	Niacin mg	Ascorbic Acid mg
							Saturated (total) gm	Unsaturated									
		gm						Oleic gm	Linoleic gm								
	Prunes, dried, "softenized," medium:																
320	Uncooked[5] 4 prunes	32	28	70	1	Trace	—	—	—	18	14	1.1	440	0.02	0.04	0.4	1
321	Cooked, unsweetened, 17–18 prunes and 1/3 cup liquid[5] 1 cup	270	66	295	2	1	—	—	—	78	60	4.5	1,860	0.08	0.18	1.7	2
322	Prune juice, canned or bottled 1 cup	256	80	200	1	Trace	—	—	—	49	36	10.5	—	0.03	0.03	1.0	85
	Raisins, seedless:																
323	Packaged, 1/2 oz or 1 1/2 tbsp per pkg. 1 pkg	14	18	40	Trace	Trace	—	—	—	11	9	0.5	Trace	0.02	0.01	0.1	Trace
324	Cup, pressed down 1 cup	165	18	480	4	Trace	—	—	—	128	102	5.8	30	0.18	0.13	0.8	2
	Raspberries, red:																
325	Raw 1 cup	123	84	70	1	1	—	—	—	17	27	1.1	160	0.04	0.11	1.1	31
326	Frozen, 10-ounce carton, not thawed 1 carton	284	74	275	2	1	—	—	—	70	37	1.7	200	0.06	0.17	1.7	59
327	Rhubarb, cooked, sugar added 1 cup	272	63	385	1	Trace	—	—	—	98	212	1.6	220	0.06	0.15	0.7	17
	Strawberries:																
328	Raw, capped 1 cup	149	90	55	1	1	—	—	—	13	31	1.5	90	0.04	0.10	1.0	88
329	Frozen, 10-ounce carton, not thawed 1 carton	284	71	310	1	1	—	—	—	79	40	2.0	90	0.06	0.17	1.5	150
330	Tangerines, raw, medium, 2 3/8-in diam., size 176[5] 1 tangerine	116	87	40	1	Trace	—	—	—	10	34	0.3	360	0.05	0.02	0.1	27
331	Tangerine juice, canned, sweetened 1 cup	249	87	125	1	1	—	—	—	30	45	0.5	1,050	0.15	0.05	0.2	55
332	Watermelon, raw, wedge, 4 by 8 inches (1/16 of 10 by 16-inch melon, about 2 pounds with rind)[5] 1 wedge	925	93	115	2	1	—	—	—	27	30	2.1	2,510	0.13	0.13	0.7	30
	Grain Products																
	Bagel, 3-in diam.:																
333	Egg 1 bagel	55	32	165	6	2	—	—	—	28	9	1.2	30	0.14	0.10	1.2	0
334	Water 1 bagel	55	29	165	6	2	—	—	—	30	8	1.2	0	0.15	0.11	1.4	0
335	Barley, pearled, light, uncooked 1 cup	200	11	700	16	2	Trace	1	1	158	32	4.0	0	0.24	0.10	6.2	0
336	Biscuits, baking powder from home recipe with enriched flour, 2-in diam. 1 biscuit	28	27	105	2	5	1	2	1	13	34	0.4	Trace	0.06	0.06	0.1	Trace
337	Biscuits, baking powder from mix, 2-in diam. 1 biscuit	28	28	90	2	3	1	1	1	15	19	0.6	Trace	0.08	0.07	0.6	Trace
338	Bran flakes (40% bran), added thiamine and iron 1 cup	35	3	105	4	1	—	—	—	28	25	12.3	0	0.14	0.06	2.2	0
339	Bran flakes with raisins, added thiamine and iron 1 cup	50	7	145	4	1	—	—	—	40	28	13.5	Trace	0.16	0.07	2.7	0
	Breads:																
340	Boston brown bread, slice 3 by 3/4 in 1 slice	48	45	100	3	1	—	—	—	22	43	0.9	0	0.05	0.03	0.6	0
	Cracked-wheat bread:																
341	Loaf, 1 lb 1 loaf	454	35	1,190	40	10	2	5	2	236	399	5.0	Trace	0.53	0.41	5.9	Trace
342	Slice, 18 slices per loaf 1 slice	25	35	65	2	1	—	—	—	13	22	0.3	Trace	0.03	0.02	0.3	Trace

No.	Food	Measure	Grams	Water (%)	Food energy (cal)	Protein (g)	Fat (g)	Saturated (g)	Oleic (g)	Linoleic (g)	Carbohydrate (g)	Calcium (mg)	Iron (mg)	Vitamin A (IU)	Thiamine (mg)	Riboflavin (mg)	Niacin (mg)	Ascorbic acid (mg)
	French or Vienna bread:																	
343	Enriched, 1-lb loaf	1 loaf	454	31	1,315	41	14	3	8	2	251	195	10.0	Trace	1.27	1.00	11.3	Trace
344	Unenriched, 1-lb loaf	1 loaf	454	31	1,315	41	14	3	8	2	251	195	3.2	Trace	0.36	0.36	3.6	Trace
	Italian bread:																	
345	Enriched, 1-lb loaf	1 loaf	454	32	1,250	41	4	1	1	2	256	77	10.0	0	1.32	0.91	11.8	0
346	Unenriched, 1-lb loaf	1 loaf	454	32	1,250	41	4	1	1	2	256	77	3.2	0	0.41	0.27	3.6	0
	Raisin bread:																	
347	Loaf, 1 lb	1 loaf	454	35	1,190	30	13	3	8	2	243	322	5.9	Trace	0.23	0.41	3.2	Trace
348	Slice, 18 slices per loaf	1 slice	25	35	65	2	1	—	—	—	13	18	0.3	Trace	0.01	0.02	0.2	Trace
	Rye bread:																	
	American, light (1/3 rye, 2/3 wheat):																	
349	Loaf, 1 lb	1 loaf	454	36	1,100	41	5	—	—	—	236	340	7.3	0	0.82	0.32	6.4	0
350	Slice, 18 slices per loaf	1 slice	25	36	60	2	Trace	—	—	—	13	19	0.4	0	0.05	0.02	0.4	0
351	Pumpernickel, loaf, 1 lb	1 loaf	454	34	1,115	41	5	—	—	—	241	381	10.9	0	1.04	0.64	5.4	0
	White bread, enriched:[15]																	
	Soft-crumb type																	
352	Loaf, 1 lb	1 loaf	454	36	1,225	39	15	3	8	2	229	381	11.3	Trace	1.13	0.95	10.9	Trace
353	Slice, 18 slices per loaf	1 slice	25	36	70	2	1	—	—	—	13	21	0.6	Trace	0.06	0.05	0.6	Trace
354	Slice, toasted	1 slice	22	25	70	2	1	—	—	—	13	21	0.6	Trace	0.05	0.05	0.6	Trace
355	Slice, 22 slices per loaf	1 slice	20	36	55	2	1	—	—	—	10	17	0.5	Trace	0.05	0.04	0.5	Trace
356	Slice, toasted	1 slice	17	25	55	2	1	—	—	—	10	17	0.5	Trace	0.05	0.04	0.5	Trace
357	Loaf, 1 1/2 lb	1 loaf	680	36	1,835	59	22	5	12	3	343	571	17.0	Trace	1.70	1.43	16.3	Trace
358	Slice, 24 slices per loaf	1 slice	28	36	75	2	1	—	—	—	14	24	0.7	Trace	0.07	0.06	0.7	Trace
359	Slice, toasted	1 slice	24	25	75	2	1	—	—	—	14	24	0.7	Trace	0.07	0.06	0.7	Trace
360	Slice, 28 slices per loaf	1 slice	24	36	65	2	1	—	—	—	12	20	0.6	Trace	0.06	0.05	0.6	Trace
361	Slice, toasted	1 slice	21	25	65	2	1	—	—	—	12	20	0.6	Trace	0.06	0.05	0.6	Trace
	Firm-crumb type:																	
362	Loaf, 1 lb	1 loaf	454	35	1,245	41	17	4	10	2	228	435	11.3	Trace	1.22	0.91	10.9	Trace
363	Slice, 20 slices per loaf	1 slice	23	35	65	2	1	—	—	—	12	22	0.6	Trace	0.06	0.05	0.6	Trace
364	Slice, toasted	1 slice	20	24	65	2	1	—	—	—	12	22	0.6	Trace	0.06	0.05	0.6	Trace
365	Loaf, 2 lb	1 loaf	907	35	2,495	82	34	8	20	4	455	871	22.7	Trace	2.45	1.81	21.8	Trace
366	Slice, 34 slices per loaf	1 slice	27	35	75	2	1	—	—	—	14	26	0.7	Trace	0.07	0.05	0.6	Trace
367	Slice, toasted	1 slice	23	25	75	2	1	—	—	—	14	26	0.7	Trace	0.07	0.05	0.6	Trace
	Whole-wheat bread, soft-crumb type:																	
368	Loaf, 1 lb	1 loaf	454	36	1,095	41	12	2	6	2	224	381	13.6	Trace	1.36	0.45	12.7	Trace
369	Slice, 16 slices per loaf	1 slice	28	36	65	3	1	—	—	—	14	24	0.8	Trace	0.09	0.03	0.8	Trace
370	Slice, toasted	1 slice	24	24	65	3	1	—	—	—	14	24	0.8	Trace	0.09	0.03	0.8	Trace
	Whole-wheat bread, firm-crumb type:																	
371	Loaf, 1 lb	1 loaf	454	36	1,100	48	14	3	6	3	216	449	13.6	Trace	1.18	0.54	12.7	Trace
372	Slice, 18 slices per loaf	1 slice	25	36	60	3	1	—	—	—	12	25	0.8	Trace	0.06	0.03	0.7	Trace
373	Slice, toasted	1 slice	21	24	60	3	1	—	—	—	12	25	0.8	Trace	0.06	0.03	0.7	Trace
374	Breadcrumbs, dry, grated	1 cup	100	6	390	13	5	1	2	1	73	122	3.6	Trace	0.22	0.30	3.5	Trace
375	Buckwheat flour, light, sifted	1 cup	98	12	340	6	1	—	—	—	78	11	1.0	0	0.08	0.04	0.4	0
376	Bulgur, canned, seasoned	1 cup	135	56	245	8	4	—	—	—	44	27	1.9	0	0.08	0.05	4.1	0
	Cakes made from cake mixes:																	
	Angel food:																	
377	Whole cake	1 cake	635	34	1,645	36	1	—	—	—	377	603	1.9	0	0.03	0.70	0.6	0
378	Piece, 1/12 of 10-in diam. cake	1 piece	53	34	135	3	Trace	—	—	—	32	50	0.2	0	Trace	0.06	0.1	0

[5]Measure and weight apply to entire vegetable or fruit including parts not usually eaten.

[8]This is the amount from the fruit. Additionl ascorbic acid may be added by the manufacturer. Refer to the label for this information.

[15]Values for iron, thiamine, riboflavin, and niacin per pound of unenriched white bread would be as follows:

	Iron (mg)	Thiamine (mg)	Riboflavin (mg)	Niacin (mg)
Soft crumb	3.2	.31	.39	5.0
Firm crumb	3.2	.32	.59	4.1

	Food, Approximate Measure, and Weight (in grams)		gm	Water per cent	Food Energy calories	Protein gm	Fat gm	Fatty Acids			Carbohydrate gm	Calcium mg	Iron mg	Vitamin A Value I.U.	Thiamine mg	Riboflavin mg	Niacin mg	Ascorbic Acid mg
								Saturated (total) gm	Unsaturated									
									Oleic gm	Linoleic gm								
	Cakes made from cake mixes (cont.)																	
	Cupcakes, small, 2 1/2 in diam.:																	
379	Without icing	1 cupcake	25	26	90	1	3	1	1	1	14	40	0.1	40	0.01	0.03	0.1	Trace
380	With chocolate icing	1 cupcake	36	22	130	2	5	2	2	1	21	47	0.3	60	0.01	0.04	0.1	Trace
	Devil's food, 2-layer, with chocolate icing:																	
381	Whole cake	1 cake	1,107	24	3,755	49	136	54	58	16	645	653	8.9	1,660	0.33	0.89	3.3	1
382	Piece, 1/16 of 9-in diam. cake	1 piece	69	24	235	3	9	3	4	1	40	41	0.6	100	0.02	0.06	0.2	Trace
383	Cupcake, small, 2 1/2-in diam	1 cupcake	35	24	120	2	4	1	2	Trace	20	21	0.3	50	0.01	0.03	0.1	Trace
	Gingerbread:																	
384	Whole cake	1 cake	570	37	1,575	18	39	10	19	9	291	513	9.1	Trace	0.17	0.51	4.6	2
385	Piece, 1/9 of 8-in square cake	1 piece	63	37	175	2	4	1	2	1	32	57	1.0	Trace	0.02	0.06	0.5	Trace
	White, 2-layer, with chocolate icing:																	
386	Whole cake	1 cake	1,140	21	4,000	45	122	45	54	17	716	1,129	5.7	680	0.23	0.91	2.3	2
387	Piece, 1/16 of 9-in diam. cake	1 piece	71	21	250	3	8	3	3	1	45	70	0.4	40	0.01	0.06	0.1	Trace
	Cakes made from home recipes:[16]																	
388	Boston cream pie; piece 1/12 of 8-in. diam.	1 piece	69	35	210	4	6	2	3	1	34	46	0.3	140	0.02	0.08	0.1	Trace
	Fruitcake, dark, made with enriched flour:																	
389	Loaf, 1 lb	1 loaf	454	18	1,720	22	69	15	37	13	271	327	11.8	540	0.59	0.64	3.6	2
390	Slice, 1/30 of 8-in loaf	1 slice	15	18	55	1	2	Trace	1	Trace	9	11	0.4	20	0.02	0.02	0.1	Trace
	Plain sheet cake:																	
	Without icing:																	
391	Whole cake	1 cake	777	25	2,830	35	108	30	52	21	434	497	3.1	1,320	0.16	0.70	1.6	2
392	Piece, 1/9 of 9-in square cake	1 piece	86	25	315	4	12	3	6	2	48	55	0.3	150	0.02	0.08	0.2	Trace
393	With boiled white icing, piece, 1/9 of 9-in square cake	1 piece	114	23	400	4	12	3	6	2	71	56	0.3	150	0.02	0.08	0.2	Trace
	Pound:																	
394	Loaf, 8 1/2 by 3 1/2 by 3 in	1 loaf	514	17	2,430	29	152	34	68	17	242	108	4.1	1,440	0.15	0.46	1.0	0
395	Slice, 1/2-in thick	1 slice	30	17	140	2	9	2	4	1	14	6	0.2	80	0.01	0.03	0.1	0
	Sponge:																	
396	Whole cake	1 cake	790	32	2,345	60	45	14	20	4	427	237	9.5	3,560	0.40	1.11	1.6	Trace
397	Piece, 1/12 of 10-in diam. cake	1 piece	66	32	195	5	4	1	2	Trace	36	20	0.8	300	0.03	0.09	0.1	Trace
	Yellow, 2 layer, without icing:																	
398	Whole cake	1 cake	870	24	3,160	39	111	31	53	22	506	618	3.5	1,310	0.17	0.70	1.7	2
399	Piece, 1/16 of 9-in diam. cake	1 piece	54	24	200	2	7	2	3	1	32	39	0.2	80	0.01	0.04	0.1	Trace
	Yellow, 2-layer, with chocolate icing:																	
400	Whole cake	1 cake	1,203	21	4,390	51	156	55	69	23	727	818	7.2	1,920	0.24	0.96	2.4	Trace
401	Piece, 1/16 of 9-in diam. cake	1 piece	75	21	275	3	10	3	4	1	45	51	0.5	120	0.02	0.06	0.2	Trace
	Cake icings. See Sugars, Sweets																	

No.	Food	Measure	Weight (g)	Water (%)	Food energy	Protein (g)	Fat (g)	Saturated (g)	Oleic (g)	Linoleic (g)	Carbohydrate (g)	Calcium (mg)	Iron (mg)	Vitamin A (IU)	Thiamine (mg)	Riboflavin (mg)	Niacin (mg)	Ascorbic acid (mg)
	Cookies:																	
	Brownies with nuts:																	
402	Made from home recipe with enriched flour	1 brownie	20	10	95	1	6	1	3	1	10	8	0.4	40	0.04	0.02	0.1	Trace
403	Made from mix	1 brownie	20	11	85	1	4	1	2	1	13	9	0.4	20	0.03	0.02	0.1	Trace
	Chocolate chip:																	
404	Made from home recipe with enriched flour	1 cookie	10	3	50	1	3	1	1	1	6	4	0.2	10	0.01	0.01	0.1	Trace
405	Commercial	1 cookie	10	3	50	1	2	1	1	Trace	7	4	0.2	10	Trace	Trace	Trace	Trace
406	Fig bars, commercial	1 cookie	14	14	50	1	1	—	—	—	11	11	0.2	20	Trace	0.01	0.1	Trace
407	Sandwich, chocolate or vanilla, commercial	1 cookie	10	2	50	1	2	1	1	Trace	7	2	0.1	0	Trace	Trace	0.1	0
	Corn flakes, added nutrients:																	
408	Plain	1 cup	25	4	100	2	Trace	—	—	—	21	4	0.4	0	0.11	0.02	0.5	0
409	Sugar-covered	1 cup	40	2	155	2	Trace	—	—	—	36	5	0.4	0	0.16	0.02	0.8	0
	Corn (hominy) grits, degermed, cooked:																	
410	Enriched	1 cup	245	87	125	3	Trace	—	—	—	27	2	0.7	[17]150	0.10	0.07	1.0	0
411	Unenriched	1 cup	245	87	125	3	Trace	—	—	—	27	2	0.2	[17]150	0.05	0.02	0.5	0
	Cornmeal:																	
412	Whole-ground, unbolted, dry	1 cup	122	12	435	11	5	1	2	2	90	24	2.9	[17]620	0.46	0.13	2.4	0
413	Bolted (nearly whole-grain) dry	1 cup	122	12	440	11	4	Trace	1	2	91	21	2.2	[17]590	0.37	0.10	2.3	0
	Degermed, enriched:																	
414	Dry form	1 cup	138	12	500	11	2	—	—	—	108	8	4.0	[17]610	0.61	0.36	4.8	0
415	Cooked	1 cup	240	88	120	3	1	—	—	—	26	2	1.0	[17]140	0.14	0.10	1.2	0
	Degermed, unenriched:																	
416	Dry form	1 cup	138	12	500	11	2	—	—	—	108	8	1.5	[17]610	0.19	0.07	1.4	0
417	Cooked	1 cup	240	88	120	3	1	—	—	—	26	2	0.5	[17]140	0.05	0.02	0.2	0
418	Corn muffins, made with enriched degermed cornmeal and enriched flour; muffin 2 3/8-in diam.	1 muffin	40	33	125	3	4	2	2	Trace	19	42	0.7	[17]120	0.08	0.09	0.6	Trace
419	Corn muffins, made with mix, egg, and milk; muffin 2 3/8-in diam.	1 muffin	40	30	130	3	4	1	2	1	20	96	0.6	100	0.07	0.08	0.6	Trace
420	Corn, puffed, presweetened, added nutrients	1 cup	30	2	115	1	Trace	—	—	—	27	3	0.5	0	0.13	0.05	0.6	0
421	Corn, shredded, added nutrients	1 cup	25	3	100	2	Trace	—	—	—	22	1	0.6	0	0.11	0.05	0.5	0
	Crackers:																	
422	Graham, 2 1/2-in square	4 crackers	28	6	110	2	3	—	—	—	21	11	0.4	0	0.01	0.06	0.4	0
423	Saltines	4 crackers	11	4	50	1	1	—	—	—	8	2	0.1	0	Trace	Trace	0.1	0
	Danish pastry, plain (without fruit or nuts):																	
424	Packaged ring, 12 ounces	1 ring	340	22	1,435	25	80	24	37	15	155	170	3.1	1,050	0.24	0.51	2.7	Trace
425	Round piece, approx. 4 1/4-in diam. by 1 in	1 pastry	65	22	275	5	15	5	7	3	30	33	0.6	200	0.05	0.10	0.5	Trace
426	Ounce	1 oz	28	22	120	2	7	2	3	1	13	14	0.3	90	0.02	0.04	0.2	Trace
427	Doughnuts, cake type	1 doughnut	32	24	125	1	6	1	4	Trace	16	13	[18]0.4	30	[18]0.05	[18]0.05	[18]0.4	Trace
428	Farina, quick-cooking, enriched, cooked	1 cup	245	89	105	3	Trace	—	—	—	22	147	[19]0.7	0	[19]0.12	[19]0.07	[19]1.0	0

[16] Unenriched cake flour used unless otherwise specified.

[17] This value is based on product made from yellow varieties of corn; white varieties contain only a trace.

[18] Based on product made with enriched flour. With unenriched flour, approximate values per doughnut are: iron, 0.2 mg; thiamine, 0.01 mg; riboflavin, 0.03 mg; niacin, 0.2 mg.

[19] Iron, thiamine, riboflavin, and niacin are based on the minimum levels of enrichment specified in standards of identity promulgated under the Federal Food, Drug, and Cosmetic Act.

661

| | Food, Approximate Measure, and Weight | | Water per cent | Food Energy calories | Pro-tein gm | Fat gm | Fatty Acids | | | Carbo-hy-drate gm | Cal-cium mg | Iron mg | Vita-min A Value I.U. | Thia-mine mg | Ribo-flavin mg | Niacin mg | Ascor-bic Acid mg |
| | | | | | | | Satu-rated (total) gm | Unsaturated | | | | | | | | | |
	(in grams)	gm	per cent	calories	gm	gm	gm	Oleic gm	Lin-oleic gm	gm	mg	mg	I.U.	mg	mg	mg	mg
	Macaroni, cooked: Enriched:																
429	Cooked, firm stage (undergoes additional cooking in a food mixture)	1 cup, 130	64	190	6	1	—	—	—	39	14	[19]1.4	0	[19]0.23	[19]0.14	[19]1.8	0
430	Cooked until tender	1 cup, 140	72	155	5	1	—	—	—	32	8	[19]1.3	0	[19]0.20	[19]0.11	[19]1.5	0
	Unenriched:																
431	Cooked, firm stage (undergoes additional cooking in a food mixture)	1 cup, 130	64	190	6	1	—	—	—	39	14	0.7	0	0.03	0.03	0.5	0
432	Cooked until tender	1 cup, 140	72	155	5	1	—			32	11	0.6	0	0.01	0.01	0.4	0
433	Macaroni (enriched) and cheese, baked	1 cup, 200	58	430	17	22	10	9	2	40	362	1.8	860	0.20	0.40	1.8	Trace
434	Canned	1 cup, 240	80	230	9	10	4	3	1	26	199	1.0	260	0.12	0.24	1.0	Trace
435	Muffins, with enriched white flour; muffin, 3-inch diam.	1 muffin, 40	38	120	3	4	1	2	1	17	42	0.6	40	0.07	0.09	0.6	Trace
	Noodles (egg noodles), cooked:																
436	Enriched	1 cup, 160	70	200	7	2	1	1	Trace	37	16	[19]1.0	110	[19]0.22	[19]0.13	[19]1.9	0
437	Unenriched	1 cup, 160	70	200	7	2	1	1	Trace	37	16	1.0	110	0.05	0.03	0.6	0
438	Oats (with or without corn) puffed, added nutrients	1 cup, 25	3	100	3	1	—	—	1	19	44	1.2	0	0.24	0.04	0.5	0
439	Oatmeal or rolled oats, cooked	1 cup, 240	87	130	5	2	—	—	1	23	22	1.4	0	0.19	0.05	0.2	0
	Pancakes, 4-inch diam.:																
440	Wheat, enriched flour (home recipe)	1 cake, 27	50	60	2	2	Trace	1	Trace	9	27	0.4	30	0.05	0.06	0.4	Trace
441	Buckwheat (made from mix with egg and milk)	1 cake, 27	58	55	2	2	1	1	Trace	6	59	0.4	60	0.03	0.04	0.2	Trace
442	Plain or buttermilk (made from mix with egg and milk)	1 cake, 27	51	60	2	2	1	1	Trace	9	58	0.3	70	0.04	0.06	0.2	Trace
	Pie (piecrust made with unenriched flour): Sector, 4-in, 1/7 of 9-in-diam. pie:																
443	Apple (2-crust)	1 sector, 135	48	350	3	15	4	7	3	51	11	0.4	40	0.03	0.03	0.5	1
444	Butterscotch (1-crust)	1 sector, 130	45	350	6	14	5	6	2	50	98	1.2	340	0.04	0.13	0.3	Trace
445	Cherry (2-crust)	1 sector, 135	47	350	4	15	4	7	3	52	19	0.4	590	0.03	0.03	0.7	Trace
446	Custard (1-crust)	1 sector, 130	58	285	8	14	5	6	2	30	125	0.8	300	0.07	0.21	0.4	0
447	Lemon meringue (1-crust)	1 sector, 120	47	305	4	12	4	6	2	45	17	0.6	200	0.04	0.10	0.2	4
448	Mince (2-crust)	1 sector, 135	43	365	3	16	4	8	3	56	38	1.4	Trace	0.09	0.05	0.5	1
449	Pecan (1-crust)	1 sector, 118	20	490	6	27	4	16	5	60	55	3.3	190	0.19	0.08	0.4	Trace
450	Pineapple chiffon (1-crust)	1 sector, 93	41	265	6	11	3	5	2	36	22	0.8	320	0.04	0.08	0.4	1
451	Pumpkin (1-crust)	1 sector, 130	59	275	5	15	5	6	2	32	66	0.7	3,210	0.04	0.13	0.7	Trace
	Piecrust, baked shell for pie made with:																
452	Enriched flour	1 shell, 180	15	900	11	60	16	28	12	79	25	3.1	0	0.36	0.25	3.2	0
453	Unenriched flour	1 shell, 180	15	900	11	60	16	28	12	79	25	0.9	0	0.05	0.05	0.9	0

No.	Food, approximate measure, and weight	Measure	Grams	Water (%)	Food energy (cal.)	Protein (g)	Fat (g)	Saturated (g)	Oleic (g)	Linoleic (g)	Carbohydrate (g)	Calcium (mg)	Iron (mg)	Vitamin A (I.U.)	Thiamine (mg)	Riboflavin (mg)	Niacin (mg)	Ascorbic acid (mg)
454	Piecrust mix including stick form: Package, 10 oz, for double crust; 1/8 of 14-in diam. pie	1 pkg.	284	9	1,480	20	93	23	46	21	141	131	1.4	0	0.11	0.11	2.0	0
455	Pizza (cheese) 5 1/2-in sector; 1/8 of 14-in diam. pie	1 sector	75	45	185	7	6	2	3	Trace	27	107	0.7	290	0.04	0.12	0.7	4
	Popcorn, popped:																	
456	Plain, large kernel	1 cup	6	4	25	1	Trace	—	—	—	5	1	0.2	—	—	0.01	0.1	0
457	With oil and salt	1 cup	9	3	40	1	2	Trace	1	—	5	1	0.2	—	—	0.01	0.2	0
458	Sugar coated	1 cup	35	4	135	2	1	Trace	1	—	30	2	0.5	—	—	0.02	0.4	0
	Pretzels:																	
459	Dutch, twisted	1 pretzel	16	5	60	2	1	—	—	—	12	4	0.2	0	Trace	Trace	0.1	0
460	Thin, twisted	1 pretzel	6	5	25	1	Trace	—	—	—	5	1	0.1	0	Trace	Trace	Trace	0
461	Sticks, small 2 1/4 inches	10 sticks	3	5	10	Trace	Trace	—	—	—	2	1	Trace	0	Trace	Trace	Trace	0
462	Stick, regular, 3 1/8 inches	5 sticks	3	5	10	Trace	Trace	—	—	—	2	1	Trace	0	Trace	Trace	Trace	0
	Rice, white:																	
	Enriched:																		
463	Raw	1 cup	185	12	670	12	1	—	—	—	149	44	[20]5.4	0	[20]0.81	[20]0.06	[20]6.5	0
464	Cooked	1 cup	205	73	225	4	Trace	—	—	—	50	21	[20]1.8	0	[20]0.23	[20]0.02	[20]2.1	0
465	Instant, ready to serve	1 cup	165	73	180	4	Trace	—	—	—	40	5	[20]1.3	0	[20]0.21	—	[20]1.7	0
466	Unenriched, cooked	1 cup	205	73	225	4	Trace	—	—	—	50	21	0.4	0	0.02	0.02	0.8	0
467	Parboiled, cooked	1 cup	175	73	185	4	Trace	—	—	—	41	33	[20]1.4	0	[20]0.19	[20]0.02	[20]2.1	0
468	Rice, puffed, added nutrients	1 cup	15	4	60	1	Trace	—	—	—	13	3	0.3	0	0.07	0.01	0.7	0
	Rolls, enriched:																		
	Cloverleaf or pan:																		
469	Home recipe	1 roll	35	26	120	3	3	1	1	1	20	16	0.7	30	0.09	0.09	0.8	Trace
470	Commercial	1 roll	28	31	85	2	2	Trace	1	Trace	15	21	0.5	Trace	0.08	0.05	0.6	Trace
471	Frankfurter or hamburger	1 roll	40	31	120	3	2	1	1	1	21	30	0.8	Trace	0.11	0.07	0.9	Trace
472	Hard, round or rectangular	1 roll	50	25	155	5	2	Trace	1	Trace	30	24	1.2	Trace	0.13	0.12	1.4	Trace
473	Rye wafers, whole-grain, 1 7/8 by 3 1/2 inches	2 wafers	13	6	45	2	Trace	—	—	—	10	7	0.5	0	0.04	0.03	0.2	0
474	Spaghetti, cooked, tender stage, enriched	1 cup	140	72	155	5	1	—	—	—	32	11	[19]1.3	0	[19]0.20	[19]0.11	[19]1.5	0
	Spaghetti with meat balls, and tomato sauce:																		
475	Home recipe	1 cup	248	70	330	19	12	4	6	1	39	124	3.7	1,590	0.25	0.30	4.0	22
476	Canned	1 cup	250	78	260	12	10	2	3	1	28	53	3.3	1,000	0.15	0.18	2.3	5
	Spaghetti in tomato sauce with cheese:																		
477	Home recipe	1 cup	250	77	260	9	9	2	5	1	37	80	2.3	1,080	0.25	0.18	2.3	13
478	Canned	1 cup	250	80	190	6	2	1	1	1	38	40	2.8	930	0.35	0.28	4.5	10
479	Waffles, with enriched flour, 7-in diam.	1 waffle	75	41	210	7	7	2	4	1	28	85	1.3	250	0.13	0.19	1.0	Trace
480	Waffles, made from mix, enriched, egg and milk added, 7-in diam.	1 waffle	75	42	205	7	8	3	3	1	27	179	1.0	170	0.11	0.17	0.7	Trace
481	Wheat, puffed, added nutrients	1 cup	15	3	55	2	Trace	—	—	—	12	4	0.6	0	0.08	0.03	1.2	0
482	Wheat, shredded, plain	1 biscuit	25	7	90	2	1	—	—	—	20	11	0.9	0	0.06	0.03	1.1	0
483	Wheat flakes, added nutrients	1 cup	30	4	105	3	Trace	—	—	—	24	12	1.3	0	0.19	0.04	1.5	0
	Wheat flours:																		
484	Whole wheat, from hard wheats, stirred	1 cup	120	12	400	16	2	Trace	1	1	85	49	4.0	0	0.66	0.14	5.2	0

[19] Iron, thiamine, riboflavin, and niacin are based on the minimum levels of enrichment specified in standards of identity promulgated under the Federal Food, Drug, and Cosmetic Act.

[20] Iron, thiamine, and niacin are based on the minimum levels of enrichment specified in standards of identity promulgated under the Federal Food, Drug, and Cosmetic Act. Riboflavin is based on unenriched rice. When the minimum level of enrichment specified in the standards of identity becomes effective the value will be 0.12 mg per cup of parboiled rice and of white rice.

Table A–1. (Cont.)

No.	Food, Approximate Measure, and Weight		Water per cent	Food Energy calories	Pro-tein gm	Fat gm	Fatty Acids Satu-rated (total) gm	Unsaturated Oleic gm	Lin-oleic gm	Carbo-hy-drate gm	Cal-cium mg	Iron mg	Vita-min A Value I.U.	Thia-mine mg	Ribo-flavin mg	Niacin mg	Ascor-bic Acid mg
		gm															
	Wheat flours (cont.)																
	All-purpose or family flour, enriched:																
485	Sifted 1 cup	115	12	420	12	1	—	—	—	88	18	3.3[19]	0	0.51[19]	0.30[19]	4.0[19]	0
486	Unsifted 1 cup	125	12	455	13	1	—	—	—	95	20	3.6[19]	0	0.55[19]	0.33[19]	4.4[19]	0
487	Self-rising, enriched 1 cup	125	12	440	12	1	—	—	—	93	331	3.6[19]	0	0.55[19]	0.33[19]	4.4[19]	0
488	Cake or pastry flour, sifted 1 cup	96	12	350	7	1	—	—	—	76	16	0.5	0	0.03	0.03	0.7	0
	Fats, Oils																
	Butter:																
	Regular, 4 sticks per pound:																
489	Stick 1/2 cup	113	16	810	1	92	51	30	3	1	23	0	3,750[21]	—	—	—	0
490	Tablespoon (approx. 1/8 stick) 1 tbsp.	14	16	100	Trace	12	6	4	Trace	Trace	3	0	470[21]	—	—	—	0
491	Pat (1-in sq, 1/3-in high; 90 per lb) 1 pat	5	16	35	Trace	4	2	1	Trace	Trace	1	0	170[21]	—	—	—	0
	Whipped, 6 sticks or 2, 8-oz containers per pound:																
492	Stick 1/2 cup	76	16	540	1	61	34	20	2	Trace	15	0	2,500[21]	—	—	—	0
493	Tablespoon (approx. 1/8 stick) 1 tbsp.	9	16	65	Trace	8	4	3	Trace	Trace	2	0	310[21]	—	—	—	0
494	Pat (1 1/4-in sq 1/3-in high; 120 per lb) 1 pat	4	16	25	Trace	3	2	1	Trace	Trace	1	0	130[21]	—	—	—	0
	Fats, cooking:																
495	Lard 1 cup	205	0	1,850	0	205	78	94	20	0	0	0	0	0	0	0	0
496	1 tbsp	13	0	115	0	13	5	6	1	0	0	0	0	0	0	0	0
497	Vegetable fats 1 cup	200	0	1,770	0	200	50	100	44	0	0	0	—	0	0	0	0
498	1 tbsp	13	0	110	0	13	3	6	3	0	0	0	—	0	0	0	0
	Margarine:																
	Regular, 4 sticks per pound:																
499	Stick 1/2 cup	113	16	815	1	92	17	46	25	1	23	0	3,750[22]	—	—	—	0
500	Tablespoon (approx. 1/8 stick) 1 tbsp	14	16	100	Trace	12	2	6	3	Trace	3	0	470[22]	—	—	—	0
501	Pat (1-in sq 1/3-in high; 90 per lb) 1 pat	5	16	35	Trace	4	1	2	1	Trace	1	0	170[22]	—	—	—	0
	Whipped, 6 sticks per pound:																
502	Stick 1/2 cup	76	16	545	1	61	11	31	17	Trace	15	0	2,500[22]	—	—	—	0
	Soft, 2 8-oz tubs per pound:																
503	Tub 1 tub	227	16	1,635	1	184	34	68	68	1	45	0	7,500[22]	—	—	—	0
504	Tablespoon 1 tbsp	14	16	100	Trace	11	2	4	4	Trace	3	0	470[22]	—	—	—	0
	Oils, salad or cooking:																
505	Corn 1 cup	220	0	1,945	0	220	22	62	117	0	0	0	—	0	0	0	0
506	1 tbsp	14	0	125	0	14	1	4	7	0	0	0	—	0	0	0	0
507	Cottonseed 1 cup	220	0	1,945	0	220	55	46	110	0	0	0	—	0	0	0	0
508	1 tbsp	14	0	125	0	14	4	3	7	0	0	0	—	0	0	0	0
509	Olive 1 cup	220	0	1,945	0	220	24	167	15	0	0	0	—	0	0	0	0
510	1 tbsp	14	0	125	0	14	2	11	1	0	0	0	—	0	0	0	0
511	Peanut 1 cup	220	0	1,945	0	220	40	103	64	0	0	0	—	0	0	0	0
512	1 tbsp	14	0	125	0	14	3	7	4	0	0	0	—	0	0	0	0

No.	Food	Measure	Grams	Water (%)	Food energy (cal)	Protein (g)	Fat (g)	Saturated (g)	Oleic (g)	Linoleic (g)	Carbohydrate (g)	Calcium (mg)	Iron (mg)	Vitamin A (IU)	Thiamine (mg)	Riboflavin (mg)	Niacin (mg)	Ascorbic acid (mg)
513	Safflower	1 cup	220	0	1,945	0	220	18	37	165	0	0	0	—	0	0	0	0
514		1 tbsp	14	0	125	0	14	2	2	10	0	0	0	—	0	0	0	0
515	Soybean	1 cup	220	0	1,945	0	220	33	44	114	0	0	0	—	0	0	0	0
516		1 tbsp	14	0	125	0	14	2	3	7	0	0	0	—	0	0	0	0
	Salad dressing:																	
517	Blue cheese	1 tbsp	15	32	75	1	8	2	2	4	1	12	Trace	30	Trace	0.02	Trace	Trace
	Commercial, mayonnaise type:																	
518	Regular	1 tbsp	15	41	65	Trace	6	1	1	3	2	2	Trace	30	Trace	Trace	Trace	—
519	Special dietary, low calorie	1 tbsp	16	81	20	Trace	2	Trace	Trace	1	2	3	Trace	40	Trace	Trace	Trace	—
	French:																	
520	Regular	1 tbsp	16	39	65	Trace	6	1	1	3	3	2	0.1	—	—	—	—	—
521	Special dietary, low fat with artificial sweeteners	1 tbsp	15	95	Trace	Trace	Trace	—	—	—	Trace	2	0.1	—	—	—	—	—
522	Home cooked, boiled	1 tbsp	16	68	25	1	2	Trace	1	Trace	2	14	0.1	80	0.01	0.03	Trace	Trace
523	Mayonnaise	1 tbsp	14	15	100	Trace	11	2	2	6	Trace	3	0.1	40	Trace	0.01	Trace	Trace
524	Thousand island	1 tbsp	16	32	80	Trace	8	2	2	4	3	2	0.1	50	Trace	Trace	Trace	Trace

Sugars, Sweets

No.	Food	Measure	Grams	Water (%)	Food energy (cal)	Protein (g)	Fat (g)	Saturated (g)	Oleic (g)	Linoleic (g)	Carbohydrate (g)	Calcium (mg)	Iron (mg)	Vitamin A (IU)	Thiamine (mg)	Riboflavin (mg)	Niacin (mg)	Ascorbic acid (mg)
	Cake icings:																	
525	Chocolate made with milk and table fat	1 cup	275	14	1,035	9	38	21	14	1	185	165	3.3	580	0.06	0.28	0.6	1
526	Coconut (with boiled icing)	1 cup	166	15	605	3	13	11	1	Trace	124	10	0.8	0	0.02	0.07	0.3	0
527	Creamy fudge from mix with water only	1 cup	245	15	830	7	16	5	8	3	183	96	2.7	Trace	0.05	0.20	0.7	Trace
528	White, boiled	1 cup	94	18	300	1	0	—	—	—	76	2	Trace	0	Trace	0.03	Trace	0
	Candy:																	
529	Carmels, plain or chocolate	1 oz	28	8	115	1	3	2	1	Trace	22	42	0.4	Trace	0.01	0.05	0.1	Trace
530	Chocolate, milk, plain	1 oz	28	1	145	2	9	5	3	Trace	16	65	0.3	80	0.02	0.10	0.1	Trace
531	Chocolate-coated peanuts	1 oz	28	1	160	5	12	3	6	2	11	33	0.4	Trace	0.10	0.05	2.1	Trace
532	Fondant; mints, uncoated; candy corn	1 oz	28	8	105	Trace	1	—	—	—	25	4	0.3	0	Trace	Trace	Trace	0
533	Fudge, plain	1 oz	28	8	115	1	4	2	1	Trace	21	22	0.3	Trace	0.01	0.03	0.1	Trace
534	Gum drops	1 oz	28	12	100	Trace	Trace	—	—	—	25	2	0.1	0	0	0	Trace	0
535	Hard	1 oz	28	1	110	0	Trace	—	—	—	28	6	0.5	0	0	Trace	0	0
536	Marshmallows	1 oz	28	17	90	1	Trace	—	—	—	23	5	0.5	0	0	Trace	Trace	0
	Chocolate-flavored syrup or topping:																	
537	Thin type	1 fl oz	38	32	90	1	1	Trace	Trace	Trace	24	6	0.6	Trace	0.01	0.03	0.2	0
538	Fudge type	1 fl oz	38	25	125	2	5	3	2	Trace	20	48	0.5	60	0.02	0.08	0.2	Trace
	Chocolate-flavored beverage powder (approx. 4 heaping teaspoons per oz):																	
539	With nonfat dry milk	1 oz	28	2	100	5	1	Trace	Trace	Trace	20	167	0.5	10	0.04	0.21	0.2	1
540	Without nonfat dry milk	1 oz	28	1	100	Trace	1	Trace	Trace	Trace	25	9	0.6	—	0.01	0.03	0.1	0
541	Honey, strained or extracted	1 tbsp	21	17	65	Trace	0	—	—	—	17	1	0.1	0	Trace	0.01	0.1	Trace
542	Jams and preserves	1 tbsp	20	29	55	Trace	Trace	—	—	—	14	4	0.2	Trace	Trace	0.01	Trace	Trace
543	Jellies	1 tbsp	18	29	50	Trace	Trace	—	—	—	13	4	0.3	Trace	Trace	0.01	Trace	1
	Molasses, cane:																	
544	Light (first extraction)	1 tbsp	20	24	50	—	—	—	—	—	13	33	0.9	—	0.01	0.01	Trace	—
545	Blackstrap (third extraction)	1 tbsp	20	24	45	—	—	—	—	—	11	137	3.2	—	0.02	0.04	0.4	—
	Syrups:																	
546	Sorghum	1 tbsp	21	23	55	—	—	—	—	—	14	35	2.6	—	0.02	Trace	Trace	—

[19]Iron, thiamine, riboflavin, and niacin are based on the minimum levels of enrichment specified in standards of identity promulgated under the Federal Food, Drug, and Cosmetic Act.

[21]Year-round average.

[22]Based on the average vitamin A content of fortified margarine. Federal specifications for fortified margarine require a minimum of 15,000 I.U. of vitamin A per pound.

Table A–1. (Cont.)

| | Food, Approximate Measure, and Weight (in grams) | | Water per cent | Food Energy calories | Protein gm | Fat gm | Fatty Acids | | | Carbo-hydrate gm | Cal-cium mg | Iron mg | Vita-min A Value I.U. | Thia-mine mg | Ribo-flavin mg | Niacin mg | Ascor-bic Acid mg |
| | | gm | | | | | Satu-rated (total) gm | Unsaturated | | | | | | | | | |
								Oleic gm	Lin-oleic gm								
	Syrups (cont.)																
547	Table blends, chiefly corn, light and dark	1 tbsp	21	24	60	0	0	—	—	—	15	9	0.8	0	0	0	0	0
	Sugars:																	
548	Brown, firm packed	1 cup	220	2	820	0	0	—	—	—	212	187	7.5	0	0.02	0.07	0.4	0
	White:																	
549	Granulated	1 cup	200	Trace	770	0	0	—	—	—	199	0	0.2	0	0	0	0	0
550		1 tbsp	11	Trace	40	0	0	—	—	—	11	0	Trace	0	0	0	0	0
551	Powdered, stirred before measuring	1 cup	120	Trace	460	0	0	—	—	—	119	0	0.1	0	0	0	0	0
	Miscellaneous Items																	
552	Barbecue sauce	1 cup	250	81	230	4	17	2	5	9	20	53	2.0	900	0.03	0.03	0.8	13
	Beverages, alcoholic:																	
553	Beer	12 fl oz	360	92	150	1	0	—	—	—	14	18	Trace	—	0.01	0.11	2.2	—
	Gin, rum, vodka, whiskey:																	
554	80 proof	1 1/2 fl oz jigger	42	67	100	—	—	—	—	—	Trace	—	—	—	—	—	—	—
555	86 proof	1 1/2 fl oz jigger	42	64	105	—	—	—	—	—	Trace	—	—	—	—	—	—	—
556	90 proof	1 1/2 fl oz jigger	42	62	110	—	—	—	—	—	Trace	—	—	—	—	—	—	—
557	94 proof	1 1/2 fl oz jigger	42	60	115	—	—	—	—	—	Trace	—	—	—	—	—	—	—
558	100 proof	1 1/2 fl oz jigger	42	58	125	—	—	—	—	—	Trace	—	—	—	—	—	—	—
	Wines:																	
559	Dessert	3 1/2 fl oz glass	103	77	140	Trace	0	—	—	—	8	8	—	—	0.01	0.02	0.2	—
560	Table	3 1/2 fl oz glass	102	86	85	Trace	0	—	—	—	4	9	0.4	—	Trace	0.01	0.1	—
	Beverages, carbonated, sweetened, nonalcoholic:																	
561	Carbonated water	12 fl oz	366	92	115	0	0	—	—	—	29	—	—	0	0	0	0	0
562	Cola type	12 fl oz	369	90	145	0	0	—	—	—	37	—	—	0	0	0	0	0
563	Fruit-flavored sodas and Tom Collins mixes	12 fl oz	372	88	170	0	0	—	—	—	45	—	—	0	0	0	0	0
564	Ginger ale	12 fl oz	366	92	115	0	0	—	—	—	29	—	—	0	0	0	0	0
565	Root beer	12 fl oz	370	90	150	0	0	—	—	—	39	—	—	0	0	0	0	0
566	Bouillon cubes, approx. 1/2 in	1 cube	4	4	5	1	Trace	—	—	—	Trace	—	—	—	—	—	—	—
	Chocolate:																	
567	Bitter or baking	1 oz	28	2	145	3	15	8	6	Trace	8	22	1.9	20	0.01	0.07	0.4	0
568	Semisweet, small pieces	1 cup	170	1	860	7	61	34	22	1	97	51	4.4	30	0.02	0.14	0.9	0
	Gelatin:																	
569	Plain, dry powder in envelope	1 envelope	7	13	25	6	Trace	—	—	—	0	—	—	—	—	—	—	—
570	Dessert powder, 3-oz package	1 pkg	85	2	315	8	0	—	—	—	75	—	—	—	—	—	—	—
571	Gelatin dessert, prepared with water	1 cup	240	84	140	4	0	—	—	—	34	—	—	—	—	—	—	—

No.	Food, approximate measure, and description	Measure	Grams	Water (%)	Food energy (cal)	Protein (g)	Fat (g)	Saturated fat (g)	Oleic (g)	Linoleic (g)	Carbohydrate (g)	Calcium (mg)	Iron (mg)	Vitamin A (IU)	Thiamin (mg)	Riboflavin (mg)	Niacin (mg)	Ascorbic acid (mg)
572	Olives, pickled: Green	4 medium or 3 extra large or 2 giant	16	78	15	Trace	2	Trace	2	Trace	Trace	8	0.2	40	—	—	—	—
573	Ripe: Mission	3 small or 2 large	10	73	15	Trace	2	Trace	2	Trace	Trace	9	0.1	10	Trace	Trace	—	—
574	Pickles, cucumber: Dill, medium, whole, 3 3/4 in long, 1 1/4 in diam.	1 pickle	65	93	10	1	Trace	—	—	—	1	17	0.7	70	Trace	0.01	Trace	4
575	Fresh, sliced, 1 1/2 in diam., 1/4 in thick	2 slices	15	79	10	Trace	Trace	—	—	—	3	5	0.3	20	Trace	Trace	Trace	1
576	Sweet, gherkin, small, whole, approx. 2 1/2 in long, 3/4 in diam.	1 pickle	15	61	20	Trace	Trace	—	—	—	5	2	0.2	10	Trace	Trace	Trace	1
577	Relish, finely chopped, sweet	1 tbsp	15	63	20	Trace	Trace	—	—	—	5	3	0.1	—	—	—	—	—
	Popcorn. See Grain Products																	
578	Popsicle, 3-fl oz size	1 popsicle	95	80	70	0	0	—	—	—	18	0	Trace	0	0	0	0	0
	Pudding, home recipe with starch base:																	
579	Chocolate	1 cup	260	66	385	8	12	7	4	Trace	67	250	1.3	390	0.05	0.36	0.3	1
580	Vanilla (blancmange)	1 cup	255	76	285	9	10	5	3	Trace	41	298	Trace	410	0.08	0.41	0.3	2
581	Pudding mix, dry form, 4-oz package	1 pkg	113	2	410	3	2	1	1	Trace	103	23	1.8	Trace	0.02	0.08	0.5	0
582	Sherbet	1 cup	193	67	260	2	2	—	—	—	59	31	Trace	120	0.02	0.06	Trace	4
	Soups: Canned, condensed, ready-to-serve: Prepared with an equal volume of milk:																	
583	Cream of chicken	1 cup	245	85	180	7	10	3	3	3	15	172	0.5	610	0.05	0.27	0.7	2
584	Cream of mushroom	1 cup	245	83	215	7	14	4	4	5	16	191	0.5	250	0.05	0.34	0.7	1
585	Tomato	1 cup	250	84	175	7	7	3	2	1	23	168	0.8	1,200	0.10	0.25	1.3	15
	Prepared with an equal volume of water:																	
586	Bean with pork	1 cup	250	84	170	8	6	1	2	2	22	63	2.3	650	0.13	0.08	1.0	3
587	Beef broth, bouillon consommé	1 cup	240	96	30	5	0	—	—	—	3	Trace	0.5	Trace	Trace	0.02	1.2	—
588	Beef noodle	1 cup	240	93	70	4	3	1	1	1	7	7	1.0	50	0.05	0.07	1.0	Trace
589	Clam chowder, Manhattan type (with tomatoes, without milk)	1 cup	245	92	80	2	3	—	—	—	12	34	1.0	880	0.02	0.02	1.0	—
590	Cream of chicken	1 cup	240	92	95	3	6	1	2	3	8	24	0.5	410	0.02	0.05	0.5	Trace
591	Cream of mushroom	1 cup	240	90	135	2	10	1	3	5	10	41	0.5	70	0.02	0.12	0.7	Trace
592	Minestrone	1 cup	245	90	105	5	3	—	—	—	14	37	1.0	2,350	0.07	0.05	1.0	1
593	Split pea	1 cup	245	85	145	9	3	1	1	1	21	29	1.5	440	0.25	0.15	1.5	—
594	Tomato	1 cup	245	90	90	2	3	Trace	1	1	16	15	0.7	1,000	0.05	0.05	1.2	12
595	Vegetable beef	1 cup	245	92	80	5	2	—	—	—	10	12	0.7	2,700	0.05	0.05	1.0	—
596	Vegetarian	1 cup	245	92	80	2	2	—	—	—	13	20	1.0	2,940	0.05	0.05	1.0	—
	Dehydrated, dry form:																	
597	Chicken noodle (2-oz package)	1 pkg	57	6	220	8	6	2	3	1	33	34	1.4	190	0.30	0.15	2.4	3
598	Onion mix (1 1/2-oz package)	1 pkg	43	3	150	6	5	1	2	1	23	42	0.6	30	0.05	0.03	0.3	6
599	Tomato vegetable with noodles (2 1/2-oz pkg)	1 pkg	71	4	245	6	6	2	3	1	45	33	1.4	1,700	0.21	0.13	1.8	18
	Frozen, condensed: Clam chowder, New England type (with milk, without tomatoes):																	
600	Prepared with equal volume of milk	1 cup	245	83	210	9	12	—	—	—	16	240	1.0	250	0.07	0.29	0.5	Trace

| | Food. Approximate Measure, and Weight (in grams) | | Water per cent | Food Energy calories | Pro-tein gm | Fat gm | Fatty Acids | | | Carbo-hy-drate gm | Cal-cium mg | Iron mg | Vita-min A Value I.U. | Thia-mine mg | Ribo-flavin mg | Niacin mg | Ascor-bic Acid mg |
| | | | | | | | Satu-rated (total) gm | Unsaturated | | | | | | | | | |
		gm						Oleic gm	Lin-oleic gm								
	Soups, frozen (cont.)																
	Clam chowder, New England type																
601	Prepared with equal volume of water	1 cup	240	89	130	4	8	—	—	—	11	91	1.0	50	0.05	0.10	0.5	—
	Cream of potato:																
602	Prepared with equal volume of milk	1 cup	245	83	185	8	10	5	3	Trace	18	208	1.0	590	0.10	0.27	0.5	Trace
603	Prepared with equal volume of water	1 cup	240	90	105	3	5	3	2	Trace	12	58	1.0	410	0.05	0.05	0.5	—
	Cream of shrimp:																
604	Prepared with equal volume of milk	1 cup	245	82	245	9	16	—	—	—	15	189	0.5	290	0.07	0.27	0.5	Trace
605	Prepared with equal volume of water	1 cup	240	88	160	5	12	—	—	—	8	38	0.5	120	0.05	0.05	0.5	—
	Oyster stew:																
606	Prepared with equal volume of milk	1 cup	240	83	200	10	12	—	—	—	14	305	1.4	410	0.12	0.41	0.5	Trace
607	Prepared with equal volume of water	1 cup	240	90	120	6	8	—	—	—	8	158	1.4	240	0.07	0.19	0.5	—
608	Tapioca, dry, quick cooking	1 cup	152	13	535	1	Trace	—	—	—	131	15	0.6	0	0	0	0	0
	Tapioca desserts:																
609	Apple	1 cup	250	70	295	1	Trace	—	—	—	74	8	0.5	30	Trace	Trace	Trace	Trace
610	Cream pudding	1 cup	165	72	220	8	8	4	3	Trace	28	173	0.7	480	0.07	0.30	0.2	2
611	Tartar sauce	1 tbsp	14	34	75	Trace	8	1	1	4	1	3	0.1	30	Trace	Trace	Trace	Trace
612	Vinegar	1 tbsp	15	94	Trace	Trace	0	—	—	—	1	1	0.1	—	—	—	—	—
613	White sauce, medium	1 cup	250	73	405	10	31	10	10	1	22	288	0.5	1,150	0.10	0.43	0.5	2
	Yeast:																
614	Bakers', dry, active	1 pkg	7	5	20	3	Trace	—	—	—	3	3	1.1	Trace	0.16	0.38	2.6	Trace
615	Brewers', dry	1 tbsp	8	5	25	3	Trace	—	—	—	3	17	1.4	Trace	1.25	0.34	3.0	Trace
	Yogurt. See Milk, Cheese, Cream, Imitation Cream																

Table A–2. Mineral and Vitamin Content of Foods

Explanatory notes. The data in this table are intended to provide assistance in the planning of diets modified for sodium and potassium, and to give information on food composition for nutrients listed in the table of Recommended Dietary Allowances (1968) for the first time. The data are derived from a number of sources listed below. For these nutrients many of the values must be regarded as tentative inasmuch as only a few determinations have been made on many kinds of foods. No recent data are available for folacin, and there is a paucity of data for vitamin E.

In some instances, the sources do not indicate whether the product analyzed was raw or cooked; it has been assumed that the values are for the raw product unless specifically stated. Cooking procedures would reduce the values somewhat.

Sodium. The values for sodium apply to foods as they are purchased in the retail market. Further additions for salt and leavening agents are accounted for in home-prepared products for which recipes state an exact measure.

Foods to which salt and other sodium compounds have ordinarily been added include canned vegetables, regular pack, assuming 0.6 per cent salt concentration; canned meats, fish, poultry, soups; cured meats; cheeses; baked products including bread, quick breads, rolls, cakes, cookies, pies; ready-to-eat and cooked breakfast cereals; salad dressings; butter, margarine.

The amount of salt added to some foods is so highly variable that the values listed in this table pertain to the unsalted product. Included are cooked fresh and frozen vegetables; cooked fresh meats, fish, and poultry; cooked legumes; cooked macaroni, spaghetti, noodles.

SOURCES OF DATA

Bunnell, R. H., *et al.:* "Alpha-Tocopherol Content of Foods," *Am. J. Clin. Nutr.,* **17**:1–10, 1965.

Composition of Foods—Raw, Processed, Prepared, Handbook No. 8. U.S. Department of Agriculture, Washington, D.C., 1963. (All values for mineral elements)

Hardinge, M. G., and Crooks, H.: "Lesser Known Vitamins in Foods," *J. Am. Diet. Assoc.,* **38**:240–45, 1961. (Folacin)

Meyer, B. H., *et al.:* "Pantothenic Acid and Vitamin B_6 in Beef," *J. Am. Diet. Assoc.,* **54**: 122–25, 1969.

Orr, M. L.: *Pantothenic Acid, Vitamin B_6, and Vitamin B_{12} in Foods,* Home Economics Research Report No. 36, Agricultural Research Service. U.S. Department of Agriculture, Washington, D.C., 1969.

Polansky, M. M.: "Vitamin B_6 Components in Fresh and Dried Vegetables," *J. Am. Diet. Assoc.,* **54**:118–21, 1969.

Toepfer, E. W., *et al.:* *Folic Acid Content of Foods,* Handbook No. 29. U.S. Department of Agriculture, Washington, D.C., 1951.

Table A–2. Mineral and Vitamin Content of Foods: Sodium, Potassium, Phosphorus, and Magnesium; Folacin, Pantothenic Acid, Vitamin B₆, Vitamin B₁₂, and Vitamin E

(Values for 100 gm edible portion)

Item No.	Food	Sodium mg	Potassium mg	Phosphorus mg	Magnesium mg	Folacin mcg	Pantothenic Acid mcg	Vitamin B$_6$ mcg	Vitamin B$_{12}$ mcg	Vitamin E mg
1	Almonds, dried	4	773	504	270	45	470	100	0	
2	Roasted, salted	198	773	504	—[1]		250	95	0	
3	Apples, raw, not peeled	1	110	10	8	2	105	30	0	0.31
4	Apple brown Betty	153	100	22	—	Trace	—		0	
5	Apple juice, bottled	1	101	9	4			30	0	
6	Applesauce, sweetened	2	65	5	5		85	30	0	
7	Apricots, raw	1	281	23	12	3	240	70	0	
8	Canned	1	234	15	7	1	92	54	0	
9	Dried, sulfured, uncooked	26	979	108	62	5[2]	753[2]	169[2]	0	
10	Cooked, sweetened	7	278	31	20					
11	Apricot nectar	Trace	151	12	—					
12	Asparagus, green, cooked	1	183	50	20 (raw)	109				
13	Canned, regular pack	236	166	53	—	27	195	55	0	
14	Low sodium	3	166	53	—					
15	Frozen, spears, cooked	1	238	67	14	109	410	155	0	
16	Avocado	4	604	42	45	30	1070	420	0	
17	Bacon, cooked, drained	1021	236	224	25	—	330 (raw)	125 (raw)	0.70 (raw)	0.53
18	Canadian, cooked	2555	432	218	24					
	Baking powder, home use:									
19	Sodium aluminum sulfate	10,953	150	2904						
20	Straight phosphate	8220	170	9438						
21	Tartrate	7300	3800	0						
22	Low sodium, commercial	6	10,948							
23	Low sodium, noncommercial formula		20,729							
24	Banana	1	370	26	33	10	260	510	0	0.22
25	Barley, pearled, light	3	160	189	37		503	224	0	
26	Bass, sea, raw	68	256	—	—		512	—	—	
	Beans, common, mature:									
27	White, dry	19	1196	425	170	125	725	560	0	0.47
28	Cooked	7	416	148	—		92	—	—	
29	Canned with pork and tomato sauce	463	210	92	37					

No.	Food									
30	Red, dry	10	984	406	163	180[1]	500	441	0	
31	Cooked	3	340	140	—	34			0	
	Beans, Lima, immature:									
32	Cooked	1	422	121	67 (raw)	13			0	
33	Canned, regular pack	236	222	70	—	34	130	90	0	
34	Low sodium	4	222	70	—					
35	Frozen, Fordhook, cooked	101	426	90	48 (raw)	34	240	150	0	
36	Mature seeds, dry	4	1529	385	180	103	975	580	0	
37	Cooked	2	612	154	—	128				
38	Beans, Mung, sprouts, cooked	4	156	48	—	145	190	80 (raw)	0	
39	Beans, snap, green, cooked	4	151	37	32 (raw)	28				
40	Canned, regular pack	236	95	25	14	12	75 (raw)	40	0	0.03
41	Low sodium	2	95	25	—					
42	Frozen, cooked	1	152	32	21 (raw)	28	135	70	0	0.11
43	Yellow, cooked	3	151	37	—	32	250 (raw)	— (raw)	0	
44	Canned, regular pack	236	95	25	—		—	42 (raw)	0	
45	Low sodium	2	95	25	—					
	Beef:									
46	All cuts, lean, broiled or roasted, average	60	370	246	29	11	620 (raw)	435 (raw)	1.8 (raw)	0.13
47	Simmered, average	60	370	194	18					
48	Hamburger, regular, cooked	47	450	194	21	7				0.37
49	Beef, canned, roast beef	—	259	116	—					
50	Beef, corned, cooked	1740	150	93	—			75 (with potato)	1.84 (canned)	
51	Hash, canned	540	200	67	—					
52	Beef, dried	4300	200	404	—					1.84
53	Beef potpie, commercial	366	93	48	—					
54	Home recipe	284	159	71	—					
55	Beef and vegetable stew, canned	411	174	45	—					0.65
56	Home recipe	37	250	75	—					

[1]Dashes denote lack of reliable data for a constituent believed to be present in measurable amounts.

[2]Source of data does not indicate whether raw or cooked; it is assumed that the values are for the raw food.

Table A–2. (Cont.)

Item No.	Food	Sodium mg	Potassium mg	Phosphorus mg	Magnesium mg	Folacin mcg	Pantothenic Acid mcg	Vitamin B6 mcg	Vitamin B12 mcg	Vitamin E mg
57	Beets, cooked	43	208	23	25 (raw)	14	150 (raw)	55 (raw)	0	
58	Canned, regular pack	236	167	18	15	3	100	50	0	
59	Low sodium	46	167	18	—					
60	Beet greens, cooked	76	332	25	106 (raw)	60	250 (raw)	100 (raw)	0	
	Beverages, alcoholic									
61	Beer	7	25	30			80	60	0	
62	Gin	1	2							
63	Wine, table	5	92	10	10		30	40	0	
	Biscuits, baking powder:									
64	Enriched	626	117	175	—					
65	Self-rising flour	660[3]	64	317[3]	—					
66	Biscuit dough, commercial in cans	868	65	497	—					
67	Blackberries, raw	1	170	19	30	14	240	50	0	
68	Blueberries, raw	1	81	13	6	8	156	67	0	
69	Frozen, sweetened	1	66	11	4	8	121	54	0	
70	Bluefish, baked or broiled, prepared with butter	104	—	287	—					
71	Bouillon cube	24,000	100	—	—					
72	Bran, with sugar and malt extract	1060	1070	1176	—					
73	Bran flakes (40 per cent bran)	925	—	495	—		875	384	0	
74	Bran flakes with raisins	800		396	—					
75	Brazil nuts	1	715	693	225	5	231	170	0	
	Breads:									
76	Boston brown	251	292	160	—		607	92		
77	Cracked wheat	529	134	128	35	25	378	53	0	
78	French or Vienna	580	90	85	22	9			0	
79	Italian	585	74	77	—	—				
80	Raisin	365	233	87	24					
81	Rye, American	557	145	147	42	16	450	100	0	
82	Pumpernickel	569	454	229	71		500	160	0	
83	White, 3–4 per cent nonfat milk solids	507	105	97	22	15	430	40	Trace	0.10
84	Whole-wheat bread, 2 per cent nonfat milk solids	527	273	228	78	30	760	180	0	0.45

No.	Food									
85	Broccoli spears, cooked	10	267	62	24 (raw)	54	525	170	0	1.00
86	Frozen, cooked	12	220	58	21	54	420 (frozen)	175 (frozen)	0	
87	Brownies with nuts	251	190	148	—	49				
88	Brussels sprouts, cooked	10	273	72	29 (raw)					
89	Butter, salted	987	23	16	2	—	—	3 (frozen)	Trace	
90	Unsalted	Under 10								
91	Buttermilk	130	140	95	14	11	307	36	0.22	
92	Cabbage, raw	20	233	29	13	32[2]	205	160	0	
93	Cooked, small amount of water	14	163	20	—					
94	Cabbage, celery or Chinese	23	253	40	14					
	Cakes (home recipe)[4]:									
95	Angel food	283	88	22	—			—	—	
96	Chocolate with icing	235	154	131	—		200 (commercial)		—	
97	Fruitcake, dark	158	496	113	—					
98	Gingerbread	237	454	65	—					
99	Plain with icing	229	114	104	—					
100	Plain without icing	300	79	102	—		—	40[5]	—	1.10
101	Poundcake, old fashioned	110	60	79	—					
102	Sponge	167	87	112	—					
	Candy:									
103	Caramels	226	192	122	—					
104	Chocolate, milk, plain	94	384	231	58					1.10
105	Fudge, plain	190	147	84	—					
106	Hard	32	4	7	Trace					
107	Marshmallows	39	6	6	—					
108	Peanut brittle	31	151	95	—					
109	Cantaloupe	12	251	16	16	7	250	86	0	0.14
110	Carrots, raw	47	341	36	23	8	280	150	0	0.11[2]
111	Cooked	33	222	31	—					
112	Canned, regular pack	236	120	22	—	3	130	30	0	0.11
113	Low sodium	39	120	22	—					
114	Cashew nuts, unsalted	15	464	373	267	—	1300	—	0	

[2] Source of data does not indicate whether raw or cooked; it is assumed that the values are for the raw food.

[3] Based on use of self-rising flour containing anhydrous monocalcium phosphate.

[4] Based on calculations using sodium aluminum sulfate baking powder with monocalcium phosphate monohydrate.

[5] Nature of samples not clearly defined.

Table A–2. (Cont.)

Item No.	Food	Sodium mg	Potassium mg	Phosphorus mg	Magnesium mg	Folacin mcg	Pantothenic Acid mcg	Vitamin B6 mcg	Vitamin B12 mcg	Vitamin E mg
115	Cauliflower, raw	13	295	56	24	22[2]	1000	210	0	
116	Cooked	9	206	42	—	—	540	190	0	
117	Frozen, cooked	10	207	38	13 (raw)	—		—		0.38
118	Celery, raw	126	341	28	22 (raw)	7	429	60	0	
119	Cooked	88	239	22	—					
120	Chard, Swiss, cooked	86	321	24	65 (raw)	42	172 (raw)	—	0	
	Cheese:									
121	Cheddar or American	700	82	478	45	16	500	80	1	
122	Cheddar, process	1136[6]	80	771[6]	—	11	400	80	0.80	
123	Cottage, creamed	229	85	152	—	31	220	40	1	
124	Uncreamed	290	72	175	—					
125	Cream	250	74	95	—		270	55	0.22	
126	Parmesan	734	149	781	48		530	96	—	
127	Swiss	710	104	563	14		370	75	1.80	
128	Cherries, raw, sweet	2	191	19	14	6	261	32	0	
129	Canned, syrup pack	1	124	12	9	3	—	30	0	
130	Frozen, sweetened	2	130	15	8		83	58	0	
	Chicken, broiled:									
131	Light without skin	64	411	265	19	3	800	683	0.45	0.37
132	Dark without skin	86	321	229	—	3	1000	325	0.40	
133	Chicken, canned, boneless	—	138	247	—		850	300	0.79	
134	Chicken potpie, frozen, commercial	411	153	50	—					
135	Chicory	7	182	21	13	28	—	45	0	
136	Chili con carne, canned with beans	531	233	126	169		140	103	—	
137	Chili powder with seasonings	1574	1000	204	292					
138	Chocolate, bitter	4	830	384	63		190	35	0	
139	Chocolate syrup, thin	52	282	92	—					
140	Clams, raw, soft, meat only	36	235	183	—		300	80	98	
141	Hard, round, meat only	205	311	151	—					
142	Canned	—	140	137	—	2	—	83	—	
143	Cocoa, breakfast, dry powder	6	1522	648	420					
144	Processed with alkali	717	651	648	—					
145	Coconut, fresh, shredded	23	256	95	46	28	200	44	0	

No.	Food									
146	Dried, sweetened	—	353	112	77		400	32	0	0.05
147	Coffee, instant, dry powder	72	3256	383	456		4	Trace	0	
148	Beverage	1	36	4					0	
149	Collards, cooked	25	234	39	57 (raw)	102	450 (frozen)	195 (frozen)	0	
150	Cookies, plain and assorted	365	67	163	15					
151	Fig bars	252	198	60						
152	Corn, sweet, cooked	Trace	165	89	48 (raw)	28[2]	540 (raw)	161 (raw)	0	
153	Canned, whole kernel, regular pack	236	97	49	19	8	220	200	0	
154	Low-sodium pack	2	97	49						
	Corn cereals, ready to eat:									
155	Cornflakes	1005	120	45	16	6	185	65	0	0.12
156	Cornflakes, sugar coated	775	—	24			288	—		
157	Corn, puffed	1060	—	90					0	
158	Corn, shredded	988	—	39						
159	Corn, rice, and wheat flakes	950	—	120						
160	Corn grits, dry	1	80	73	20		—	147	0	0.31
161	Cooked	—	11	10	3					
162	Cornbread, southern style, degermed cornmeal	591	157	156						
	Cornmeal, white or yellow, dry:									
163	Whole ground	(1)	(284)	256	106	7	580[5]	250[5]	0	0.64[5]
164	Degermed, dry	1	120	99	47	9				
165	Cooked	—	16	14	7					
166	Cowpeas, immature, cooked	1	379	146	55	41		95 (frozen)		
167	Canned, regular pack	236	352	112		26	162	53	0	
168	Cowpeas, dry seeds, cooked	8	229	95	230	439	1050	562	0	
169	Crabmeat, canned	1000	110	182	34	Trace	600	300	10	
170	Crackers, graham, plain	670	384	149	51		—			
171	Saltines	(1100)	(120)	90			—	68	0	
172	Soda	1100	120	89	29					
173	Cranberry juice	1	10	3						
174	Cranberry sauce	1	30	4	2			22	0	

[2]Source of data does not indicate whether raw or cooked; it is assumed that the values are for the raw food.

[5]Nature of samples not clearly defined.

[6]Values for phosphorus and sodium are based on use of 1.5 per cent anhydrous disodium phosphate as the emulsifying agent. If the emulsifying agent does not contain either phosphorus or sodium, the content of these nutrients per 100 gm is sodium, 650 mg; phosphorus, 444 mg.

Table A–2. (Cont.)

Item No.	Food	Sodium	Potassium	Phosphorus	Magnesium	Folacin	Pantothenic Acid	Vitamin B6	Vitamin B12	Vitamin E
		mg	mg	mg	mg	mcg	mcg	mcg	mcg	mg
175	Cream, half-and-half	46	129	85	—					
176	Light, coffee	43	122	80	11		321	33	0.25	
177	Whipping, light	36	102	67	9		—	29	0.20	
178	Cream substitute (cream, skim milk, lactose)	575	—	—	—					
179	Cucumbers, not peeled	6	160	27	11	7	250[5]	42[5]	0	
180	Custard, baked	79	146	117	—					
181	Dandelion greens, cooked	44	232	42	36 (raw)					
182	Dates, domestic	1	648	63	58	25	780	153	0	
183	Doughnuts, cake type	501	90	190	—		387[5]	—		
184	Duck, flesh only, raw	74	285	(203)					—	
185	Eggplant, cooked	1	150	21	16 (raw)	10	220 (raw)	81 (raw)	0	
186	Eggs, whole	122	129	205	11 (raw)	5	1600 (raw)	110 (raw)	2.0 (raw)	0.46 (cooked)
187	White	146	139	15	9	1	200 (raw)	2 (raw)	0.10 (raw)	
188	Yolk	52	98	569	16	13	4400 (raw)	300 (raw)	6 (raw)	
189	Endive, curly	14	294	54	10	47	90 (canned)	20 (canned)	0	
190	Farina, regular, dry	2	83	107	25	13	515	67	0	
191	Cooked, salted	144	9	12	3					
192	Instant cooking, cooked	188	13	60	4					
193	Fats, vegetable	0	0	0	0					
194	Figs, raw	2	194	22	20	14	300	113	0	
195	Canned	2	149	13	—		69	—	0	
196	Dried, uncooked	34	640	77	71	32	435	175	0	
197	Flounder, raw	78	342	195			850	170	1.2	
198	Fruit cocktail	5	161	12	7			33		
199	Gelatin, dry	—	—	—	33		—	7	—	
200	Sweetened, ready to eat	51	—	—						
201	Goose, flesh only, raw	86	420	203						
202	Grapefruit, raw	1	135	16	12	3	283	34	0	
203	Canned, sweetened	1	135	14	11		120	20	0	

No.	Food								
204	Grapefruit juice, canned	1	162	14	—	2	130	11	0	0.04
205	Frozen, diluted	1	170	17	9	1	162	14	0	
206	Grapes, American	3	158	12	13	5	75[5]	80[5]	0	
207	European	3	173	20	6					
208	Grape juice, bottled	2	116	12	12					
209	Haddock, raw	61	304	197	24		130	180	1.3	0.60 (broiled)
210	Fried (dipped in egg, milk, bread crumbs)	177	348	247	24					
211	Heart, beef, lean, raw	86	193	195	18		2500	250	11	
212	Cooked, braised	104	232	181	—					
213	Herring, raw, Pacific	74	420	225	—		—	—	2	
214	Smoked, hard	6231	157	—			500	200	7	
215	Honey, strained	5	51	6	3	3	200	20	0	
216	Honeydew melon	12	251	16	14	5	207	56	0	
217	Ice cream, no added salt, approximately 12% fat	40	112	99			492	—	—	0.06
218	Ice milk, no added salt	68	195	124	—		—	25	0	
219	Jams and preserves	12	88	9	5				0	
220	Jellies	17	75	7	4					
221	Kale, cooked, leaves with stems	43	221	46	37 (raw)	70	376 (frozen)	185 (frozen)		
222	Lamb, average of lean cuts, cooked	70	290	223	21	3	550 (raw)	275 (raw)	2.15 (raw)	0.16
223	Lard	0	0	0	0					
224	Lemon juice, fresh	1	141	10	8	1	103	20	0	
225	Lemonade, frozen, diluted	Trace	16	1	1		11	46	0	
226	Lettuce, butterhead	9	264	26	11	25		5		
227	Crisphead	9	175	22	—	21[5]	200[5]	55[5]	0	0.06
228	Looseleaf	9	264	25	—	44				
229	Lime juice, fresh or canned	1	104	11			314 (sweet)	— (sweet)	0	
230	Limeade, frozen, diluted	Trace	13	1						
	Liver, cooked, fried:									
231	Beef	184	380	476	18	294 (raw)	7700 (raw)	840 (raw)	80 (raw)	0.63 (broiled)
232	Calf	118	453	537	26		8000 (raw)	670 (raw)	60 (raw)	
233	Pork	111	395	539	24	221	6400 (raw)	650 (raw)	32 (raw)	

[5]Nature of samples not clearly defined.

Table A–2. (Cont.)

Item No.	Food	Sodium mg	Potassium mg	Phosphorus mg	Magnesium mg	Folacin mcg	Pantothenic Acid mcg	Vitamin B6 mcg	Vitamin B12 mcg	Vitamin E mg
234	Lobster, canned or cooked	210	180	192	22 (raw)		1500 (raw)	— (raw)	0.5 (raw)	0.04
235	Macaroni, dry	2	197	162	48		—	64	0	
236	Cooked, firm state	1	79	65	20					
237	Tender	1	61	50	18					
238	Macaroni and cheese, baked	543	120	161	—					
239	Margarine, salted	987	23	16		—				
240	Unsalted	Under 10								
241	Milk, whole	50	144	93	13	1	340	40	0.4	
242	Skim	52	145	95	14	Trace	370	42	0.4	
243	Dry, nonfat, instant	526	1725	1005	143		3600	380	3.2	
244	Evaporated, undiluted	118	303	205	25	1	640	50	0.16	
245	Milk, goat's	34	180	106	17		320	45	0.08	
246	Milk, human	16	51	14	4		220	10	0.04	
	Milk beverages:									
247	Chocolate flavored, with skim milk	46	142	91	—					
248	Malted, with whole milk	91	200	122	—					
249	Molasses, light	15	917	45	46	10[5]	350[5]	200[5]	0[5]	
250	Blackstrap	96	2927	84	258					
251	Muffins, corn, enriched degermed cornmeal	481	135	169	—					
252	Plain	441	125	151	—					
253	Mushrooms, raw	15	414	116		24	2200	125	0	
254	Canned	400	197	68	8	4	1000	60	0	
255	Mustard, prepared, yellow	1252	130	73	48					1.75
256	Mustard greens, cooked	18	220	32	27	60	164 (frozen)	133 (frozen)	0 (frozen)	1.75
257	Nectarine	6	294	24	13 (raw)	20				(raw)
258	Noodles, enriched, dry	5	136	183			—	17	0	
259	Cooked	2	44	59	—		—	88	Trace	
260	Oatmeal, dry	2	352	405	144	30	1500	140	0	2.27[2]
261	Cooked, salted	218	61	57	21	33				
262	Oil, vegetable	0	0	0	0	—				36.0 (corn)[7]

No.	Food									Vit. E
263	Okra, cooked	2	174	41	41 (raw)	24	215 (frozen)	45 (frozen)	0 (frozen)	
264	Olives, green	2400	55	17	22	1	18	14	0	
265	Ripe	813	34	16	—	11	15	130	0	
266	Onions, mature, raw	10	157	36	12	10	130	—	0	
267	Cooked	7	110	29	—	14	144	60		
268	Onions, young green	5	231	39	—	5	250	40	0	
269	Oranges, peeled	1	200	20	11	2	190	35	0	
270	Orange juice, fresh	1	200	17	11	2	150	28	0	
271	Canned	1	199	18	—	2	164	50	0	
272	Frozen, diluted	1	186	16	10	11	250		0	
273	Oysters, eastern, raw	73	121	143	32	(canned)			18	0.04
274	Pancakes, buckwheat, from mix	464	245	337	—					
275	Wheat, home recipe	425	123	139	—					
276	Papayas, raw	3	234	16	—	38	218	—	0	
277	Parsley	45	727	63	41	23	300	164	0[2]	
278	Parsnips, cooked	8	379	62	32		600[2]	90[2]	0[2]	
279	Peaches, raw	1	202	19	10 (raw)	4	170	24	0	
280	Canned	2	130	12	6	1	50	19	0[2]	
281	Dried, sulfured, uncooked	16	950	117	48	5	—[2]	100[2]	0[2]	
282	Cooked with sugar	4	261	32	15				0	
283	Frozen	2	124	13	6	4	132	18	0	
284	Peach nectar	1	78	11	—				0	
285	Peanuts, roasted	5	701	407	175	57	2100	400	0	7.70 (dry)
286	Salted	418	674	401	175	57			0	
287	Peanut butter	607	670	407	173	2	—	330	0	
288	Pears, raw	2	130	11	7		70	17	0	
289	Canned	1	84	7	5		22	14	0	
290	Pear nectar	1	39	5	—	25			0	
291	Peas, green, cooked	1	196	99	35 (raw)		150		0	0.55
292	Canned, regular pack	236	96	76	20	10		50	0	
293	Low-sodium pack	3	96	76	—				0	0.02

[2] Source of data does not indicate whether raw or cooked; it is assumed that the values are for the raw food.

[5] Nature of samples not clearly defined.

[7] Vitamin E in other oils as follows: cottonseed, 60.5; olive, 67.0; peanut, 61.0; safflower, 90.0; and soybean, 21.0 mg per 100 gm.

Table A-2. (Cont.)

Item No.	Food	Sodium mg	Potassium mg	Phosphorus mg	Magnesium mg	Folacin mcg	Pantothenic Acid mcg	Vitamin B6 mcg	Vitamin B12 mcg	Vitamin E mg
294	Frozen, not thawed[8]	129[8]	150	90	24	25	315	130	0	0.25
295	Peas, dry, split, raw	40	895	268	180	51[2]	2000	130	0	
296	Cooked	13	296	89	—		220 (canned)	20 (canned)	0 (canned)	
297	Pecans	Trace	603	289	142	27	1707	183	0	
298	Peppers, sweet, green, raw	13	213	22	18	7	230	260	0	
299	Perch, ocean, Atlantic, raw	79	269	207	—					
300	Persimmons, Japanese	6	174	26	8					
301	Pickles, dill	1428	200	21	12		—[5]	7[5]	0[5]	
302	Relish, sweet	712	—	14						
	Pies, home recipe:									
303	Apple	301	80	22	—		110	—	0	2.50
304	Cherry	304	105	25	—					
305	Custard	287	137	113	—		946	—	0	
306	Lemon meringue	282	50	49	—					
307	Mince	448	178	38	—					
308	Pumpkin	214	160	69	—		519	—	—	
309	Piecrust, baked	611	50	50	—					
310	Pike, walleye, raw	51	319	214	—					
311	Pineapple, raw	1	146	8	13	6	160	115	—	
312	Canned	1	96	5	8	1	100	88	0	
313	Pineapple juice, canned	1	149	9	12	1	100	74	0	
314	Pizza, cheese, home recipe	702	130	195	—			96	0	
315	Plums, raw	2	299	17	9		186	52	0	
316	Canned, purple	1	142	10	5	1	72	27	0	
317	Popcorn, salted	1940	—	216	—		—	204	0	
	Pork, fresh:									
318	Ham, lean, roasted	65	390	308	29	2 (loin)	790 (raw)	450 (raw)	0.70 (raw)	0.16 (chops, fried)
319	Picnic ham, lean, simmered	65	390	176	18					
	Pork cured:									
320	Ham, light cure, lean, cooked	930	326	200	20	11	675 (raw)	400 (raw)	0.60 (raw)	0.28 (fried)

321	Canned, spiced or unspiced	(1100)	(340)	156	—		—	360	—	
322	Potatoes, baked	4	503	65	22 (raw)	7		233[5]		0.03
323	Boiled, unsalted	2	285	42	—			174	0	0.04
324	French fried	6	853	111	—		540 (frozen)	180		0.28
325	Mashed, with milk, table fat, salted	331	250	48	—					
326	Potato chips	Variable to 1000	1130	139	—		—	180	0	6.40
327	Pretzels	1680[9]	130	131	40	5	540	19	Trace	0.15
328	Prunes, dried, uncooked	118	694	79	20			240[2]	0[2]	
329	Cooked, without sugar	4	327	37	10		460[2]			
330	Prune juice, canned	2	235	20						
	Pudding, home recipe:									
331	Bread with raisins	201	215	114						
332	Chocolate	56	171	98						
333	Cornstarch (blanc mange)	65	138	91						
334	Rennin, using mix	46	128	92						
335	Rice with raisins	71	177	94						
336	Tapioca cream	156	135	109						
337	Pumpkin, canned, unsalted	2	240	26	12 (raw)	8	400	56	0	
338	Radishes, raw	18	322	31	15	7	184	75	0	
339	Raisins, dried	27	763	101	35	10	45	240	0	
340	Raspberries, red, raw	1	168	22	20	5	240	60	0	
341	Frozen	1	100	17	—	5	270 (frozen)	38	0	
342	Rhubarb, cooked	2	203	15	13	4[5]	70	25	0	
343	Rice, white, dry	5	92	94	28			170	0	0.18
344	Cooked, salted	374	28	28	8	16	550			
	Rice cereals:									
345	Flakes	987	180	132	—	8	340	125	0	0.04
346	Puffed, without salt	2	100	92	—		378	75	0	
347	Rolls, commercial, plain	506	95	85	—		310	35		—
348	Sweet	389	124	107	—					
349	Whole wheat	564	292	281	—				—	

[2]Source of data does not indicate whether raw or cooked; it is assumed that the values are for the raw food.

[5]Nature of samples not clearly defined.

[8]Average weighted in accordance with commercial practices in freezing vegetables.

[9]Sodium content is variable. For example, very thin pretzel sticks contain about twice the average amount listed.

Table A–2. (Cont.)

Item No.	Food	Sodium mg	Potassium mg	Phosphorus mg	Magnesium mg	Folacin mcg	Pantothenic Acid mcg	Vitamin B6 mcg	Vitamin B12 mcg	Vitamin E mg
350	Rutabagas, cooked	4	167	31	15 (raw)	5	160[2]	100[2]	0[2]	
351	Rye flour, light	1	156	185	73	16	720	90	0	
352	Rye wafers	882	600	388	—					
	Salad dressings:[10]									
353	Blue cheese	1094	37	74						
354	Commercial, mayonnaise type	586	9	26						
355	French	1370	79	14	10					
356	Home cooked	728	116	93						
357	Mayonnaise	597	34	28	2					
358	Thousand island	700	113	17						
359	Salmon, pink, raw	64	306	—	—		300	700	4	1.35 (broiled)
360	Canned	387[11]	361	286	30	1	550	300	6.89	
361	Sardines, Pacific, canned in tomato sauce	400	320	478	24	1	700	160	10	
362	Sauerkraut	747[12]	140	18	—		93	130	0	
	Sausage:									
363	Bologna	1300	230	128	—	—	—	100	—	0.06
364	Frankfurters, raw	1100	220	133	—	—	430	140	1.30	
365	Pork links, cooked	958	269	162	16	12	682	165	0.54	0.16 (fried)
366	Scallops, bay steamed	265	476	338	—		132 (raw)	—	1.20 (raw)	0.60 (frozen, deep fried)
367	Shad, raw	54	330	260	—					
368	Baked, with butter or margarine	79	377	313	—		608	—	—	
369	Sherbet, orange	10	22	13	—					
370	Shrimp, raw	140	220	166	42		280	100	0.90	0.60 (fried)
371	Canned, dry pack	—	122	263	51	2	210	60	—	
	Soup, canned, diluted with equal part water:									
372	Bean with pork	403	158	51	—					
373	Beef bouillon	326	54	13	—					

682

No.	Food									
374	Beef noodle	382	32	20	—					
375	Chicken noodle	408	23	15	—					
376	Clam chowder, Manhattan type	383	75	19	—					
377	Cream soup (mushroom), prepared with milk	424	114	69	—					
378	Minestrone	406	128	24	—					
379	Pea, green	367	80	46	—					
380	Tomato	396	94	14	9					
381	Vegetable with beef broth	345	98	16	—		140	—	0	
382	Spaghetti, dry	2	197	162	—		—	64	0	
383	Cooked, tender	1	61	50	—					
384	Spaghetti with meatballs, canned	488	98	45	—					
385	Spaghetti in tomato sauce with cheese, home recipe	(382)	163	54	—					
386	Spinach, raw	71	470	51	88	77	300	280	0	
387	Cooked	50	324	38	—	75	75 (frozen)	130 (frozen)	0	
388	Canned, regular pack	236	250	26	63	49	65	70 (frozen)	0	0.02
389	Low sodium	32	250	26	—		(frozen)	(frozen)		
390	Squash, summer, cooked	1	141	25	16	11	173 (frozen)	63 (frozen)	0	
391	Winter, cooked	1	258	32	17 (raw)	12	282 (frozen)	91 (frozen)	0	
392	Strawberries, raw	1	164	21	12	9	340	55 (frozen)	0	0.13
393	Frozen	1	112	17	9	9	135	43	0	0.21
394	Sugar, brown	30	344	19	—					
395	Granulated	1	3	0	Trace					
396	Sweet potatoes, baked	12	300	58	31 (raw)	12[5]	820 (raw)	218 (raw)	0	
397	Boiled	10	243	47	—					
398	Candied	42	190	43	—					
399	Syrup, table blend	68	4	16	—					
400	Tangerines, raw	2	126	18	—	7	200	67	0	
401	Tangerine juice, canned	1	178	14	—	—	—	32	0	
402	Tapioca, dry	3	18	18	3	6				

[2] Source of data does not indicate whether raw or cooked; it is assumed that the values are for the raw food.

[5] Nature of samples not clearly defined.

[10] For salad dressings without salt, sodium content is low, ranging from less than 10 mg to 50 mg per 100 gm; the amount is usually indicated on the label.

[11] If canned without salt, the sodium value is about the same as for raw salmon.

[12] Based on salt content of 1.9 per cent; may vary significantly from this level.

Table A–2. (Cont.)

Item No.	Food	Sodium mg	Potassium mg	Phosphorus mg	Magnesium mg	Folacin mcg	Pantothenic Acid mcg	Vitamin B6 mcg	Vitamin B12 mcg	Vitamin E mg
403	Tea, instant, dry powder	—	4530	—	395					
404	Beverage	—	25		22					
405	Tomatoes, raw	3	244	27	14	8	330	100	0	0.40
406	Canned, regular pack	130	217	19	12	4	230	90	0	
407	Low sodium	3	217	19	—					
408	Tomato catsup, regular pack	1042	363	50	21		—			0.22
409	Tomato juice, canned, regular pack	200	227	18	10	7	250	107	0	
410	Canned, low sodium	3	227	18	—			192	0	
411	Tongue, beef, braised	61	164	117	16					
412	Tuna, canned, in oil, solids and liquid	800	301	294	28 (raw)	2	320	425	2.20	
413	Turkey, light, roasted	82	411	(251)	—	8[5]	591	—	—	
414	Dark, roasted	99	398	(251)	20		1128		0	
415	Turnips, cooked, diced	34	188	24	—	4	200 (raw)	90 (raw)		
416	Turnip greens, canned, regular pack	236	243	30	58 (raw)	42	68	— (raw)	0	
417	Frozen, not thawed	23	188	41	—		140	100	0	
418	Veal, lean, stewed	80	500	140	— (raw)	5	1060 (raw)	400 (raw)	1.75 (raw)	
419	Roasted	80	500	235	19					0.05 (fried)
420	Vinegar, cider	1	100	9	1				0	
421	Waffles, home recipe	475	145	173	—		650	1[5]	—	
422	Walnuts, black	3	460	570	190	77		—		
423	English	2	450	380	131		900	730	0	
424	Watermelon	1	100	10	8	1	300	68	0	
425	Wheat bran, crude	9	1121	1276	490	195				
	Wheat cereals, cooked:									
426	Wheat and malted barley, dry	1	—	350	168	33				
427	Cooked	72	Trace	59	31					
428	Wheat, rolled, cooked	Trace	84	76	—	49				0.61[2]
	Wheat cereals, ready to eat:									
429	Wheat flakes	1032	—	309	—	47	469	292	0	
430	Wheat, puffed, without salt	4	340	322	—		—	170	0	

No.									
431	Wheat, shredded, plain	3	348	388	133	55	706	244	0
	Wheat flours:								
432	All purpose or family	2	95	87	25	8	465	60	0
433	Cake	2	95	73		5	320	45	0
434	Self-rising	1079	90[13]	466	—				
435	Whole wheat	3	370	372	113	38	1100	340	0
436	Wheat germ	3	827	1118	336	305	1200	1150	0
437	White sauce, medium	379	139	93	—				
	Yeast, bakers':								
438	Compressed	16	610	394	59		3500	600	0
439	Dry active	(52)	(1998)	(1291)	—		11,000	2000	0
440	Brewers', dry	121	1894	1753	231	2022	12,000	2500	0
441	Yogurt, made from partially skimmed milk	51	143	94	—		313	46	0.11

[2] Source of data does not indicate whether raw or cooked; it is assumed that the values are for the raw food.

[5] Nature of samples not clearly defined.

[13] Ninety milligrams potassium per 100 gm contributed by flour. Small quantities of additional potassium may be contributed by other ingredients.

Table A–3 Nutritive Values of Baby Foods*
(Per 100 gm Edible Portion—About 7 Tablespoons)

Food	Energy cal	Protein gm	Fat gm	Carbo-hydrate gm	Calcium mg	Iron mg	Vitamin A Value I.U.	Thiamine mg	Riboflavin mg	Niacin mg	Ascorbic Acid mg
Cereals, Precooked, Dry and Other											
Cereal Products											
Barley, added nutrients	348	13.4	1.2	73.6	736	53.2	(0)	3.71	1.20	32.2	(0)
High protein, added nutrients	357	35.2	3.7	48.1	815	63.1	—	3.67	1.15	24.0	(0)
Mixed, added nutrients	368	15.2	2.9	70.6	820	56.4	—	3.15	1.35	22.3	(0)
Oatmeal, added nutrients	375	16.5	5.5	66.0	757	48.2	(0)	2.58	1.05	21.3	(0)
Rice, added nutrients	371	6.6	1.6	80.0	858	50.2	(0)	2.56	1.24	19.7	(0)
Dinners, Canned											
Cereal, vegetable, meat mixtures (approx. 2%–4% protein):											
Beef noodle dinner	48	2.8	1.1	6.8	12	0.5	620	0.02	0.05	0.5	2
Cereal, egg yolk, and bacon	82	2.9	4.9	6.6	29	0.8	520	0.05	0.06	0.4	—
Chicken noodle dinner	49	2.1	1.3	7.2	27	0.3	800	0.03	0.06	0.4	1
Macaroni, tomatoes, meat, and cereal	67	2.6	2.0	9.6	21	0.5	500	0.14	0.12	1.0	1
Split peas, vegetables, and ham or bacon	80	4.0	2.1	11.2	29	0.7	600	0.08	0.05	0.5	1
Vegetables and bacon, with cereal	68	1.7	2.9	8.7	17	0.6	2200	0.07	0.05	0.6	1
Vegetables and beef, with cereal	56	2.7	1.6	7.6	17	0.8	2800	0.03	0.04	0.9	1
Vegetables and chicken, with cereal	52	2.1	1.4	7.7	33	0.4	1000	0.03	0.04	0.5	Trace
Vegetables and ham, with cereal	64	2.8	2.2	8.3	25	0.3	1000	0.08	0.05	0.5	3
Vegetables and lamb, with cereal	58	2.2	2.0	7.7	23	0.7	2200	0.03	0.05	0.7	1
Vegetables and liver, with cereal	47	3.1	.4	7.8	17	2.7	4700	0.04	0.37	1.6	3
Vegetables and liver, with bacon and cereal	57	2.4	1.9	7.5	11	2.6	4600	0.03	0.33	1.3	2
Vegetables and turkey, with cereal	44	2.1	0.8	7.2	22	0.3	400	0.01	0.03	0.4	1
Meat or poultry (approx. 6%–8% protein)											
Beef with vegetables	87	7.4	3.7	6.0	13	1.2	1100	0.07	0.17	1.6	2
Chicken with vegetables	100	7.4	4.6	7.2	22	0.9	1000	0.09	0.15	1.6	2
Turkey with vegetables	86	6.7	3.2	7.6	38	0.6	1000	0.13	0.13	1.8	2
Veal with vegetables	63	7.1	1.6	5.1	11	0.8	800	0.08	0.15	2.0	2
Fruits and Fruit Products with or Without Thickening, Canned											
Applesauce	72	0.2	0.2	18.6	4	0.4	40	0.01	0.02	0.1	Trace
Applesauce and apricots	86	0.3	0.1	22.6	4	0.3	600	0.01	0.02	0.1	2

Meats, Poultry, and Eggs; Canned and *Vegetables, Canned*

Food											
Bananas (with tapioca or cornstarch, added ascorbic acid) strained	84	0.4	0.2	21.6	13	0.2	70	0.02	0.02	0.2	35
Bananas and pineapple (with tapioca or cornstarch)	80	0.4	0.1	20.7	20	0.2	30	0.01	0.01	0.1	2
Fruit dessert with tapioca (apricot, pineapple and/or orange)	84	0.3	0.3	21.5	15	0.4	450	0.02	0.01	0.2	4
Peaches	81	0.6	0.2	20.7	6	0.3	500	0.01	0.02	0.7	3
Pears	66	0.3	0.1	17.1	7	0.2	30	0.02	0.02	0.2	2
Pears and pineapple	69	0.4	0.2	17.6	7	0.2	20	0.03	0.02	0.2	2
Plums with tapioca, strained	94	0.4	0.2	24.3	5	0.4	250	0.01	0.02	0.2	2
Prunes with tapioca	86	0.3	0.2	22.4	7	0.9	400	0.02	0.06	0.4	4
Meats, Poultry, and Eggs; Canned											
Beef:											
Strained	99	14.7	4.0	(0)	8	2.0	—	0.01	0.16	3.5	0
Junior	118	19.3	3.9	(0)	8	2.5	—	0.02	0.20	4.3	0
Chicken	127	13.7	7.6	(0)	—	1.9	—	0.02	0.16	3.5	0
Egg yolks, strained	210	10.0	18.4	.2	81	3.0	1900	0.12	0.12	Trace	Trace
Lamb:											
Strained	107	14.6	4.9	(0)	9	2.1	—	0.02	0.17	3.3	—
Junior	121	17.5	5.1	(0)	13	2.7	—	0.02	0.21	4.1	—
Liver, strained	97	14.1	3.4	1.5	6	5.6	24,000	0.05	2.00	7.6	10
Liver and bacon, strained	123	13.7	6.6	1.3	6	4.2	22,000	0.05	1.99	7.8	7
Pork:											
Strained	118	15.4	5.8	(0)	8	1.5	—	0.19	0.20	2.7	—
Junior	134	18.6	6.0	(0)	8	1.2	—	0.23	0.23	2.8	—
Veal:											
Strained	91	15.5	2.7	(0)	10	1.7	—	0.03	0.20	4.3	—
Junior	107	18.8	3.0	(0)	8	1.6	—	0.03	0.22	6.0	—
Vegetables, Canned											
Beans, green	22	1.4	0.1	5.1	33	1.1	400	0.02	0.06	0.3	3
Beets, strained	37	1.4	0.1	8.3	18	0.7	20	0.02	0.03	0.1	3
Carrots	29	0.7	0.1	6.8	23	0.5	13,000	0.02	0.03	0.4	3
Mixed vegetables, including vegetable soup	37	1.6	0.3	8.5	22	0.9	4700	0.05	0.04	0.6	2
Peas, strained	54	4.2	0.2	9.3	11	1.2	500	0.08	0.09	1.2	10
Spinach, creamed	43	2.3	0.7	7.5	64	0.6	5000	0.02	0.13	0.3	6
Squash	25	0.7	0.1	6.2	24	0.4	2400	0.02	0.04	0.3	8
Sweetpotatoes	67	1.0	0.2	15.5	16	0.4	4900	0.04	0.03	0.4	8
Tomato soup, strained	54	1.9	0.1	13.5	24	0.4	1000	0.05	0.12	0.7	3

*Items selected from Table 1 in *Composition of Foods—Raw, Processed, Prepared*, by B. K. Watt and A. L. Merrill, Handbook No. 8, Consumer and Food Economics Research Division, U.S. Department of Agriculture, Washington, D.C., 1963.

Table A-4. Food Exchange Lists for Calculating Diets*

(Foods are divided into six groups, according to their composition)

Food Exchange	Quantity for One Exchange Measure	Weight gm	Carbo-hydrate gm	Protein gm	Fat gm	Calories
Milk	8 ounces	240	12	8	10	170
Vegetables—A	As desired	—	—	—	—	—
Vegetables—B	1/2 cup	100	7	2	—	35
Fruit	Varies	—	10	—	—	40
Bread	Varies	—	15	2	—	70
Meat	1 ounce	30	—	7	5	75
Fat	1 teaspoon	5	—	—	5	45

*Caso, E. K.: "Calculation of Diabetic Diets," *J. Am. Diet. Assoc.,* **26**: 575, 1950.

List 1—Milk Exchanges
Per exchange: carbohydrate, 12 gm; protein, 8 gm; fat, 10 gm

	Measure	Weight
Milk, whole (plain or homogenized)	1 cup (8 ounces)	240
Milk, skim, liquid†	1 cup	240
Milk, evaporated	1/2 cup	120
Milk, powdered whole	3–5 tablespoons‡	35
Milk, nonfat dry†	3–5 tablespoons‡	35
Buttermilk (from whole milk)	1 cup	240
Buttermilk (from skim milk)†	1 cup	240

†Since these forms of milk contain no fat, two fat exchanges may be added to the diet when they are used; or one exchange of these forms of milk may be calculated as carbohydrate, 12; protein, 8; and fat, 0.

‡The amount of milk powder to use depends upon the brand used; read package directions for the equivalent for 1 cup liquid milk.

List 2—Vegetable Exchanges
Group A vegetables—negligible carbohydrate, protein, and fat if 1 cup (200 gm) or less is used. Count each additional cup as one exchange of group B vegetable.

Asparagus
Beans, string, young
Broccoli§
Brussels sprouts
Cabbage
Cauliflower
Celery
Chicory§
Cucumbers
Escarole§

Eggplant
Greens§
  beet greens
  chard, Swiss
  collard
  dandelion
  kale
  mustard
  spinach
  turnip greens

Lettuce
Mushrooms
Okra
Pepper§
Radish
Sauerkraut
Squash, summer
Tomatoes§
Watercress§

Group B vegetables—per exchange: carbohydrate, 7 gm; protein, 2 gm; fat, negligible. One exchange = 1/2 cup = 100 gm.

Beets
Carrots§
Onion

Peas, green
Pumpkin§
Rutabaga

Squash, winter§
Turnip

§These vegetables have high vitamin A value. At least one serving should be included in the diet each day.

List 3—Fruit Exchanges
Per exchange: carbohydrate, 10 gm; protein, and fat, negligible
Fruits may be used fresh, cooked, canned or frozen, unsweetened

	Measure	Weight
		gm
Apple	1 small, 2-in. diameter	80
Applesauce	1/2 cup	100
Apricots, dried	4 halves	20
Apricots, fresh	2 medium	100
Banana	1/2 small	50
Blackberries	1 cup	150
Blueberries	2/3 cup	100
Cantaloupe‖	1/4, 6-inch diameter	200
Cherries	10 large	75
Dates	2	15
Figs, dried	1 small	15
Figs, fresh	2 large	50
Grapefruit‖	1/2 small	125
Grapefruit juice‖	1/2 cup	100
Grape juice	1/4 cup	60
Grapes	12	75
Honeydew melon‖	1/8, 7-inch diameter	150
Mango	1/2 small	70
Nectarines	1 medium	80
Orange‖	1 small	100
Orange juice‖	1/2 cup	100
Papaya	1/3 medium	100
Peach	1 medium	100
Pear	1 small	100
Pineapple	1/2 cup cubed	80
Pineapple juice	1/3 cup	80
Plums	2 medium	100
Prunes, dried or fresh	2 medium	25
Raisins	2 tablespoons	15
Raspberries	1 cup	150
Strawberries‖	1 cup	150
Tangerine	1 large	100
Watermelon	1 cup diced	175

‖These fruits are rich sources of ascorbic acid. At least one exchange should be included in the diet each day.

List 4—Bread Exchanges
Per exchange: carbohydrate, 15 gm; protein, 2 gm; fat, negligible

	Measure	Weight gm
Bread	1 slice	25
biscuit, roll (2 inch diameter)	1	30
muffin	1 medium	35
cornbread	1 1/2-inch cube	35
Cereal, cooked	1/2 cup	100
Cereal, dry	3/4 cup	20
Crackers, graham	2	20
oyster	20 (1/2 cup)	20
saltines (2 inches square)	5	20
soda (2 1/2 inches square)	3	20
round, thin (1 1/2 inch diameter)	6–8	20
Flour	2 1/2 tablespoons	30
Grits	1/2 cup cooked	100
Ice cream, vanilla (omit two fat exchanges)	1/2 cup	70
Macaroni	1/2 cup cooked	100
Matzoth	1/2 (6 1/2 inch square)	20
Noodles	1/2 cup cooked	100
Rice	1/2 cup cooked	100
Spaghetti	1/2 cup cooked	100
Sponge cake, no icing	1 1/2-inch cube	25
Vegetables		
beans, baked; no pork	1/4 cup	50
beans and peas, dried (includes kidney, Lima, navy beans, blackeyed, split, and cowpeas, etc.)	1/2 cup cooked	100
beans, Lima, fresh	1/2 cup	100
corn, popped	1 cup	20
corn, fresh	1/3 cup or 1/2 small ear	80
parsnips	2/3 cup	125
potatoes, white	1 small (2-inch diameter)	100
potatoes, white, mashed	1/2 cup	100
potatoes, sweet or yam	1/4 cup	50

List 5—Meat Exchanges
Per exchange: carbohydrate, negligible; protein, 7 gm; fat 5 gm
Measures and weights are for cooked meat

	Measure	Weight
		gm
Meat and poultry (medium fat)	1 ounce	30
(beef, lamb, pork, veal, liver, chicken, turkey, etc.)		
cold cuts (bologna, liver sausage, luncheon loaf, boiled ham, salami, etc.)	1 slice, 4 1/2 inches square, 1/8 inch thick	45
frankfurt (9 per pound)	1	50
Fish		
cod, haddock, halibut, herring, etc.	1 ounce	30
crab, lobster, salmon, tuna	1/4 cup	30
clams, oysters, shrimp	5 small	45
sardines	3 medium	30
Cheese, Cheddar	1 ounce	30
cottage	1/4 cup	45
Egg	1	50
Peanut butter#	2 tablespoons	30

\#Limit to one exchange daily or adjust for carbohydrate. Deduct 5 gm carbohydrate for each additional exchange.

List 6—Fat Exchanges
Per exchange: fat, 5 gm; protein and carbohydrate, negligible

	Measure	Weight
		gm
Butter or margarine	1 teaspoon	5
Bacon, crisp	1 slice	10
Cream, light, 20 per cent	2 tablespoons	30
Cream, heavy, 35–40 per cent	1 tablespoon	15
Cream cheese	1 tablespoon	15
French dressing	1 tablespoon	15
Mayonnaise	1 teapsoon	5
Nuts	6 small	10
Oil or cooking fat	1 teaspoon	5
Olives	5 small	50
Avocado	1/8, 4-inch diameter	25

Foods Allowed As Desired
Protein, fat, and carbohydrate negligible

Coffee
Tea
Clear broth
Bouillon
  (fat free)
Herbs (see list, page 569)

Gelatin, unsweetened
Rennet tablets
Saccharin
Spices (see list, page 569)

Vinegar
Cranberries, unsweetened
Lemon
Mustard, dry
Pickle, dill, unsweetened
Rhubarb, unsweetened

Table A–5. Amino Acid Content of Selected Foods*

(per 100 gm food, edible portion)

Food	Protein gm	Tryptophan gm	Threonine gm	Isoleucine gm	Leucine gm	Lysine gm	Sulfur Containing Methionine gm	Sulfur Containing Cystine gm	Phenylalanine gm	Tyrosine gm	Valine gm	Arginine gm	Histidine gm
Milk													
Cow:													
Fluid, whole and nonfat	3.5	0.049	0.161	0.223	0.344	0.272	0.086	0.031	0.170	0.178	0.240	0.128	0.092
Canned:													
unsweetened	7.0	0.099	0.323	0.447	0.688	0.545	0.171	0.063	0.340	0.357	0.481	0.256	0.185
Condensed, sweetened	8.1	0.114	0.374	0.518	0.796	0.631	0.198	0.072	0.393	0.413	0.557	0.296	0.214
Dried													
Whole	25.8	0.364	1.191	1.648	2.535	2.009	0.632	0.231	1.251	1.316	1.774	0.944	0.680
Nonfat	35.6	0.502	1.641	2.271	3.493	2.768	0.870	0.318	1.724	1.814	2.444	1.300	0.937
Goat	3.3	0.039	0.217	0.087	0.278	0.312	0.065	—	0.121	—	0.139	0.174	0.068
Human	1.4	0.023	0.062	0.075	0.124	0.090	0.028	0.027	0.060	0.071	0.086	0.055	0.030
Milk Products													
Buttermilk	3.5	0.038	0.165	0.219	0.348	0.291	0.082	0.032	0.186	0.137	0.262	0.168	0.099
Casein	100.0	1.335	4.227	6.550	10.048	8.013	3.084	0.382	5.389	5.819	7.393	4.070	3.021
Cheese													
Blue mold	21.5	0.293	0.799	1.449	2.096	1.577	0.559	0.121	1.153	1.028	1.543	0.785	0.701
Camembert	17.5	0.239	0.650	1.179	1.706	1.284	0.455	0.099	0.938	0.837	1.256	0.639	0.571
Cheddar	25.0	0.341	0.929	1.685	2.437	1.834	0.650	0.141	1.340	1.195	1.794	0.913	0.815
Cheddar processed	23.2	0.316	0.862	1.563	2.262	1.702	0.604	0.131	1.244	1.109	1.665	0.847	0.756
Cottage	17.0	0.179	0.794	0.989	1.826	1.428	0.469	0.147	0.917	0.917	0.978	0.802	0.549
Cream cheese	9.0	0.080	0.408	0.519	0.923	0.721	0.229	0.085	0.547	0.408	0.538	0.313	0.278
Swiss	27.5	0.375	1.021	1.853	2.681	2.017	0.715	0.155	1.474	1.315	1.974	1.004	0.896
Swiss processed	26.4	0.360	0.981	1.779	2.574	1.937	0.687	0.149	1.415	1.262	1.895	0.964	0.861
Eggs													
Whole	12.8	0.211	0.637	0.850	1.126	0.819	0.401	0.299	0.739	0.551	0.950	0.840	0.307
Whites	10.8	0.164	0.477	0.698	0.950	0.648	0.420	0.263	0.689	0.449	0.842	0.634	0.233
Yolks	16.3	0.235	0.827	0.996	1.372	1.074	0.417	0.274	0.717	0.756	1.121	1.132	0.368
Meat and Poultry													
Beef cuts, medium fat													
Chuck	18.6	0.217	0.821	0.973	1.524	1.625	0.461	0.235	0.765	0.631	1.033	1.199	0.646
Hamburger	16.0	0.187	0.707	0.837	1.311	1.398	0.397	0.202	0.658	0.543	0.888	1.032	0.556
Porterhouse	16.4	0.192	0.724	0.858	1.343	1.433	0.407	0.207	0.674	0.556	0.911	1.057	0.569
Rib roast	17.4	0.203	0.768	0.910	1.425	1.520	0.432	0.220	0.715	0.590	0.966	1.122	0.604
Round	19.5	0.228	0.861	1.020	1.597	1.704	0.484	0.246	0.802	0.661	1.083	1.257	0.677
Rump	16.2	0.189	0.715	0.848	1.327	1.415	0.402	0.205	0.666	0.550	0.899	1.045	0.562
Sirloin	17.3	0.202	0.764	0.905	1.417	1.511	0.429	0.219	0.711	0.587	0.960	1.116	0.601
Beef, dried or chipped	34.3	0.401	1.515	1.795	2.810	2.996	0.851	0.434	1.410	1.163	1.904	2.212	1.191
Lamb cuts, medium fat													
Leg	18.0	0.233	0.824	0.933	1.394	1.457	0.432	0.236	0.732	0.625	0.887	1.172	0.501
Rib	14.9	0.193	0.682	0.772	1.154	1.206	0.358	0.195	0.606	0.517	0.734	0.970	0.415
Shoulder	15.6	0.202	0.714	0.809	1.208	1.263	0.374	0.205	0.634	0.542	0.769	1.016	0.434

Pork cuts, medium fat, fresh													
Ham	15.2	0.197	0.705	0.781	1.119	1.248	0.379	0.178	0.598	0.542	0.790	0.931	0.525
Loin	16.4	0.213	0.761	0.842	1.207	1.346	0.409	0.192	0.646	0.585	0.853	1.005	0.567
Miscellaneous lean cuts	14.5	0.188	0.673	0.745	1.067	1.190	0.362	0.169	0.571	0.517	0.754	0.889	0.501
Pork, cured													
Bacon, medium fat	9.1	0.095	0.306	0.399	0.728	0.587	0.141	0.106	0.434	0.234	0.434	0.622	0.246
Fat back or salt pork	3.9	0.006	0.141	0.110	0.367	0.317	0.055	0.043	0.157	0.052	0.168	0.379	0.035
Ham	16.9	0.162	0.692	0.841	1.306	1.420	0.411	0.273	0.646	0.652	0.879	1.068	0.544
Luncheon meat	22.8	0.219	0.934	1.135	1.762	1.915	0.554	0.368	0.872	0.879	1.186	1.441	0.733
Canned, spiced	14.9	0.143	0.610	0.741	1.151	1.252	0.362	0.241	0.570	0.575	0.775	0.942	0.479
Veal cuts, medium fat													
Round	19.5	0.256	0.846	1.030	1.429	1.629	0.446	0.231	0.792	0.702	1.008	1.270	0.627
Shoulder	19.4	0.255	0.841	1.024	1.422	1.620	0.444	0.230	0.788	0.698	1.003	1.263	0.624
Stew meat	18.3	0.240	0.793	0.966	1.341	1.528	0.419	0.217	0.744	0.659	0.946	1.192	0.589
Chicken, flesh only													
Broilers or fryers	20.6	0.250	0.877	1.088	1.490	1.810	0.537	0.277	0.811	0.725	1.012	1.302	0.593
Hens	21.3	0.259	0.907	1.125	1.540	1.871	0.556	0.286	0.838	0.750	1.046	1.346	0.613
Fish and Shellfish													
Blue fish	20.5	0.203	0.889	1.040	1.548	1.797	0.597	0.276	0.761	0.554	1.092	1.155	—
Cod, fresh	16.5	0.164	0.715	0.837	1.246	1.447	0.480	0.222	0.612	0.446	0.879	0.929	—
dried	81.8	0.811	3.547	4.149	6.178	7.172	2.382	1.099	3.036	2.212	4.358	4.607	—
Flounder	14.9	0.148	0.646	0.756	1.125	1.306	0.434	0.200	0.553	0.403	0.794	0.839	—
Haddock	18.2	0.181	0.789	0.923	1.374	1.596	0.530	0.245	0.676	0.492	0.970	1.025	—
Halibut	18.6	0.185	0.806	0.943	1.405	1.631	0.542	0.250	0.690	0.503	0.991	1.048	—
Herring, Atlantic	18.3	0.182	0.793	0.928	1.382	1.605	0.533	0.246	0.679	0.495	0.975	1.031	—
Mackerel, raw, common Atlantic	18.7	0.186	0.811	0.948	1.412	1.640	0.545	0.251	0.694	0.506	0.996	1.053	—
Salmon, raw, Pacific	17.4	0.173	0.754	0.883	1.314	1.526	0.507	0.234	0.646	0.470	0.927	0.980	—
canned, red, solids and liquid	20.2	0.200	0.876	1.025	1.526	1.771	0.588	0.271	0.750	0.546	1.076	1.138	—
Sardines, canned, solids and liquid, Atlantic	21.1	0.209	0.915	1.070	1.593	1.850	0.614	0.284	0.783	0.571	1.124	1.188	—
Shrimp, canned, solids and liquid	18.7	0.186	0.811	0.948	1.412	1.640	0.545	0.251	0.694	0.506	0.996	1.053	—
Products from Meat, Poultry, and Fish													
Fish flour	76.0	0.754	4.378	4.232	6.189	7.381	2.019	—	2.845	—	3.916	5.204	1.289
Gelatin	85.6	0.006	1.912	1.357	2.930	4.226	0.787	0.077	2.036	0.401	2.421	7.866	0.771
Liver, beef or pork	19.7	0.296	0.936	1.031	1.819	1.475	0.463	0.243	0.993	0.738	1.239	1.201	0.523
Sausage													
Bologna	14.8	0.126	0.606	0.718	1.061	1.191	0.313	0.185	0.540	0.481	0.744	1.028	0.398
Frankfurters	14.2	0.120	0.582	0.688	1.018	1.143	0.300	0.177	0.518	0.461	0.713	0.986	0.382
Liverwurst	16.7	0.187	0.724	0.818	1.400	1.301	0.347	0.203	0.759	0.510	1.037	1.034	0.497
Pork, links or bulk, raw	10.8	0.092	0.442	0.524	0.774	0.869	0.228	0.135	0.394	0.351	0.543	0.750	0.290
Pork, bulk, canned	15.4	0.131	0.631	0.747	1.104	1.239	0.325	0.192	0.562	0.500	0.774	1.069	0.414
Salami	23.9	0.203	0.979	1.159	1.713	1.923	0.505	0.298	0.872	0.776	1.201	1.660	0.642
Tongue, beef	16.4	0.197	0.708	0.792	1.286	1.364	0.357	0.207	0.661	0.548	0.840	1.065	0.412

*Items selected from *Amino Acid Content of Foods,* by M. L. Orr and B. K. Watt, Home Economics Research Rep. No. 4, Agricultural Research Service, U.S. Department of Agriculture, Washington, 1957.

Table A–5. (Cont.)

Food	Protein gm	Tryptophan gm	Threonine gm	Isoleucine gm	Leucine gm	Lysine gm	Methionine gm	Cystine gm	Phenylalanine gm	Tyrosine gm	Valine gm	Arginine gm	Histidine gm
							Sulfur Containing						
Legumes													
Beans													
Red kidney													
raw	23.1	0.214	1.002	1.312	1.985	1.715	0.233	0.229	1.275	0.891	1.401	1.390	0.658
canned, solids and liquid	5.7	0.053	0.247	0.324	0.490	0.423	0.057	0.057	0.315	0.220	0.346	0.343	0.162
Other common beans including navy, pea-bean, white marrow:													
raw	21.4	0.199	0.928	1.216	1.839	1.589	0.216	0.212	1.181	0.825	1.298	1.287	0.609
baked with pork, canned	5.8	0.057	0.274	0.291	0.486	0.354	0.059	0.018	0.333	0.165	0.312	0.251	0.186
Chickpeas	20.8	0.170	0.739	1.195	1.538	1.434	0.276	0.296	1.012	0.692	1.025	1.551	0.559
Cowpeas	22.9	0.220	0.901	1.110	1.715	1.491	0.352	0.297	1.198	0.678	1.293	1.473	0.692
Lentils, whole	25.0	0.216	0.896	1.316	1.760	1.528	0.180	0.204	1.104	0.664	1.360	1.908	0.548
Lima beans	20.7	0.195	0.980	1.199	1.722	1.378	0.331	0.311	1.222	0.543	1.298	1.315	0.669
Peanuts	26.9	0.340	0.828	1.266	1.872	1.099	0.271	0.463	1.557	1.104	1.532	3.296	0.749
Peanut flour	51.2	0.647	1.575	2.410	3.563	2.091	0.516	0.881	2.963	2.100	2.916	6.273	1.425
Peanut butter	26.1	0.330	0.803	1.228	1.816	1.066	0.263	0.449	1.510	1.071	1.487	3.198	0.727
Peas, split	24.5	0.259	0.945	1.380	2.027	1.795	0.294	0.318	1.235	0.988	1.372	2.164	0.670
Soybeans, whole	34.9	0.526	1.504	2.504	2.946	2.414	0.513	0.678	1.889	1.216	2.005	2.763	0.911
Soybean flour, flakes and grits													
Low fat	44.7	0.673	1.926	2.630	3.773	3.092	0.658	0.869	2.419	1.558	2.568	3.538	1.166
Full fat	35.9	0.541	1.547	2.112	3.030	2.483	0.528	0.698	1.943	1.251	2.062	2.842	0.937
Soybean milk	3.4	0.051	0.176	0.175	0.305	0.269	0.054	0.071	0.195	0.193	0.186	0.302	0.121
Nuts													
Almonds	18.6	0.176	0.610	0.873	1.454	0.582	0.259	0.377	1.146	0.618	1.124	2.729	0.517
Brazil nuts	14.4	0.187	0.422	0.593	1.129	0.443	0.941	0.504	0.617	0.483	0.823	2.247	0.367
Cashews	18.5	0.471	0.737	1.222	1.522	0.792	0.353	0.527	0.946	0.712	1.592	2.098	0.415
Coconut	3.4	0.033	0.129	0.180	0.269	0.152	0.071	0.062	0.174	0.101	0.212	0.486	0.069
Pecans	9.4	0.138	0.389	0.553	0.773	0.435	0.153	0.216	0.564	0.316	0.525	1.185	0.273
Walnuts (English or Persian)	15.0	0.175	0.589	0.767	1.228	0.441	0.306	0.320	0.767	0.583	0.974	2.287	0.405
Other Seeds													
Cottonseed flour and meal	42.3	0.591	1.764	1.884	2.945	2.139	0.686	0.814	2.610	1.365	2.458	5.603	1.325
Safflower seed meal	42.1	0.675	1.462	1.914	2.740	1.525	0.731	—	2.605	—	2.446	4.623	0.985
Sesame seed	19.3	0.331	0.707	0.951	1.679	0.583	0.637	0.495	1.457	0.951	0.885	1.992	0.441
Meal	33.4	0.573	1.223	1.645	2.905	1.008	1.103	0.857	2.521	1.645	1.531	3.447	0.763
Sunflower meal	39.5	0.589	1.565	2.191	2.981	1.491	0.760	0.797	2.094	1.110	2.325	4.069	1.006
Grains and Their Products													
Barley	12.8	0.160	0.433	0.545	0.889	0.433	0.184	0.257	0.661	0.466	0.643	0.659	0.239
Bread, white (4% nonfat dry milk, flour basis)	8.5	0.091	0.282	0.429	0.668	0.225	0.142	0.200	0.465	0.243	0.435	0.340	0.192

Food													
Cereal combinations													
Corn and soy grits	18.0	0.161	0.792	0.841	1.656	0.772	0.271	0.311	0.832	0.562	1.054	0.982	0.472
Infant food, precooked, mixed cereals with nonfat dry milk and yeast	19.4	0.118	—	—	—	0.273	0.310	0.137	0.543	0.447	—	0.447	0.233
Oat-corn-rye mixture, puffed	14.5	0.172	0.545	0.841	1.368	0.343	0.388	0.234	0.933	0.622	0.900	0.776	0.326
Corn grits	8.7	0.053	0.347	0.402	1.128	0.251	0.161	0.113	0.395	0.532	0.444	0.306	0.180
Cornmeal, degermed	7.9	0.048	0.315	0.365	1.024	0.228	0.147	0.102	0.359	0.483	0.403	0.278	0.163
Corn flakes	8.1	0.052	0.275	0.306	1.057	0.154	0.135	0.152	0.354	0.283	0.386	0.231	0.226
Oatmeal	14.2	0.183	0.470	0.733	1.065	0.521	0.209	0.309	0.758	0.524	0.845	0.935	0.261
Rice flakes or puffed	5.9	0.046	—	—	—	0.056	—	0.044	0.286	0.124	—	0.137	0.137
Rice, white and converted	7.6	0.082	0.298	0.356	0.655	0.300	0.137	0.103	0.382	0.347	0.531	0.438	0.128
Rye flour, medium	11.4	0.129	0.422	0.485	0.766	0.465	0.180	0.227	0.538	0.368	0.594	0.557	0.260
Wheat flour													
Whole grain	13.3	0.164	0.383	0.577	0.892	0.365	0.203	0.292	0.657	0.497	0.616	0.636	0.271
White	10.5	0.129	0.302	0.483	0.809	0.239	0.138	0.210	0.577	0.359	0.453	0.466	0.210
Wheat products													
Bran	12.0	0.196	0.342	0.485	0.717	0.491	0.145	0.270	0.434	0.259	0.552	0.742	0.280
Burghul	12.4	0.070	—	—	—	0.430	0.300	0.319	0.579	—	—	0.424	0.268
Farina	10.9	0.124	0.356	0.496	0.891	0.199	0.143	0.184	0.478	0.447	0.572	0.559	0.231
Flakes	10.8	0.121	—	—	—	0.360	0.127	0.191	0.311	—	—	—	—
Germ	25.2	0.265	1.343	1.177	1.708	1.544	0.404	0.287	0.908	0.882	1.364	1.825	0.687
Macaroni or spaghetti	12.8	0.150	0.499	0.642	0.849	0.413	0.193	0.243	0.669	0.422	0.728	0.582	0.303
Noodles, containing egg solids	12.6	0.133	0.533	0.621	0.834	0.411	0.212	0.245	0.610	0.312	0.745	0.621	0.301
Shredded wheat	10.1	0.085	0.405	0.449	0.684	0.331	0.139	0.204	0.481	0.236	0.577	0.523	0.236
Whole wheat with added germ	12.8	0.136	—	—	—	0.466	—	0.246	0.755	0.481	0.742	0.742	0.371
Fruit													
Bananas, ripe	1.2	0.018	0.061	0.074	0.077	0.055	0.011	—	0.063	0.031	0.094	0.049	0.049
Dates	2.2	0.061	—	—	—	0.065	0.027	—	—	0.050	—	—	—
Grapefruit	0.5	0.001	—	—	—	0.006	0.000	—	—	—	—	—	—
Guavas, common	1.0	0.010	—	—	—	0.030	0.010	—	—	—	—	—	—
Limes	0.8	0.003	—	—	—	0.015	0.002	—	—	—	—	—	—
Mangos	0.7	0.014	—	—	—	0.093	0.008	—	—	—	—	—	—
Muskmelons	0.6	0.001	—	—	—	0.015	0.002	—	—	—	—	—	—
Oranges	0.9	0.003	—	—	—	0.024	0.003	—	—	—	—	—	—
Papayas	0.6	0.012	—	—	—	0.038	0.002	—	—	—	—	—	—
Pineapple	0.4	0.005	—	—	—	0.009	0.001	—	—	—	—	—	—
Vegetables													
Asparagus, raw	2.2	0.027	0.066	0.080	0.096	0.103	0.032	—	0.069	—	0.106	0.123	0.036
Beans, snap	2.4	0.033	0.091	0.109	0.139	0.126	0.035	0.024	0.057	0.050	0.115	0.101	0.045
Beet greens	2.0	0.024	0.076	0.084	0.129	0.108	0.034	—	0.116	—	0.101	0.083	0.026
Beets	1.6	0.014	0.034	0.051	0.055	0.086	0.006	—	0.027	—	0.049	0.028	0.022
Broccoli	3.3	0.037	0.122	0.126	0.163	0.147	0.050	—	0.119	—	0.170	0.192	0.063
Brussels sprouts	4.4	0.044	0.153	0.186	0.194	0.197	0.046	—	0.148	—	0.193	0.279	0.106
Cabbage	1.4	0.011	0.039	0.040	0.057	0.066	0.013	0.028	0.030	0.030	0.043	0.105	0.025
Carrots	1.2	0.010	0.043	0.046	0.065	0.052	0.010	0.029	0.042	0.020	0.056	0.041	0.017
Cauliflower	2.4	0.033	0.102	0.104	0.162	0.134	0.047	—	0.075	0.034	0.144	0.110	0.048

Table A–5. (Cont.)

Food	Protein gm	Tryptophan gm	Threonine gm	Iso-leucine gm	Leucine gm	Lysine gm	Sulfur Containing		Phenylalanine gm	Tyrosine gm	Valine gm	Arginine gm	Histidine gm
							Methionine gm	Cystine gm					
Celery	1.3	0.012	—	—	—	0.021	0.015	0.006	—	0.016	—	—	—
Chard	1.4	0.014	0.058	0.060	0.076	0.055	0.004	—	0.046	—	0.055	0.035	0.018
Chicory	1.6	0.024	—	—	—	0.052	0.016	0.006	—	0.040	—	—	0.024
Corn, sweet	3.7	0.023	0.151	0.137	0.407	0.137	0.072	0.062	0.207	0.124	0.231	0.174	0.095
Cowpeas	9.4	0.099	0.353	0.465	0.653	0.617	0.131	—	0.523	—	0.513	0.615	0.310
Cucumbers	0.7	0.005	0.019	0.022	0.030	0.031	0.007	—	0.016	—	0.024	0.053	0.001
Eggplant	1.1	0.010	0.038	0.056	0.068	0.030	0.006	—	0.048	—	0.065	0.037	0.019
Kale	3.9	0.042	0.139	0.133	0.252	0.121	0.035	0.036	0.158	—	0.184	0.202	0.062
Lettuce	1.2	0.012	—	—	—	0.070	0.004	—	—	—	—	—	—
Lima beans	7.5	0.097	0.338	0.460	0.605	0.474	0.080	0.083	0.389	0.259	0.485	0.454	0.247
Mustard greens	2.3	0.037	0.060	0.075	0.062	0.111	0.024	0.035	0.074	0.121	0.108	0.167	0.041
Onions, mature	1.4	0.021	0.022	0.021	0.037	0.064	0.013	—	0.039	0.046	0.031	0.180	0.014
Peas	6.7	0.056	0.245	0.308	0.418	0.316	0.054	0.073	0.257	0.163	0.274	0.595	0.109
Peppers	1.2	0.009	0.050	0.046	0.046	0.051	0.016	—	0.055	—	0.033	0.024	0.014
Potatoes, raw	2.0	0.021	0.079	0.088	0.100	0.107	0.025	0.019	0.088	0.036	0.107	0.099	0.029
Spinach	2.3	0.037	0.102	0.107	0.176	0.142	0.039	0.046	0.099	0.073	0.126	0.116	0.049
Squash, summer	0.6	0.005	0.014	0.019	0.027	0.023	0.008	—	0.016	—	0.022	0.027	0.009
Sweetpotatoes, raw	1.8	0.031	0.085	0.087	0.103	0.085	0.033	0.029	0.100	0.081	0.135	0.094	0.036
Tomatoes	1.0	0.009	0.033	0.029	0.041	0.042	0.007	—	0.028	0.014	0.028	0.029	0.015
Turnips	1.1	—	—	0.020	—	0.057	0.012	—	0.020	0.029	—	—	—
Turnip greens	2.9	0.045	0.125	0.107	0.207	0.129	0.052	0.045	0.146	0.105	0.149	0.167	0.051
Miscellaneous Food Items													
Yeast													
Bakers', compressed	10.6†	0.122	0.655	0.655	1.151	0.914	0.248	0.120	0.607	0.580	0.840	0.536	0.353
Brewers', dried	36.9†	0.710	2.353	2.398	3.226	3.300	0.836	0.548	1.902	1.902	2.723	2.250	1.251
Primary, dried													
Saccharomyces cerevisiae	36.9†	0.636	2.353	2.708	3.300	3.337	0.851	0.444	1.813	2.472	2.553	1.931	1.103
Torulopsis utilis	36.9†	0.636	2.331	3.323	3.707	3.648	0.710	0.422	2.361	2.464	2.901	3.337	1.251

†Assumes 4/5 of total nitrogen is protein.

Table A–6. Cholesterol Content of the Edible Portion of Food*

Food	Cholesterol mg per 100 gm food	Food	Cholesterol mg per 100 gm food
Beef, raw	70	Ice cream	45
Brains, raw	>2000	Kidney, raw	375
Butter	250	Larnb, raw	70
Caviar or fish roe	>300	Lard and other animal fat	95
Cheese:		Liver, raw	300
Cheddar	100	Lobster	200
Cottage, creamed	15	Margarine:	
Cream	120	All vegetable fat	0
Other (25% to 35% fat)	85	Two-thirds animal fat, one-third	
Cheese spread	65	vegetable fat	65
Chicken, flesh only, raw	60	Milk:	
Crab	125	Fluid, whole	11
Egg, whole	550	Dried, whole	85
Egg, white	0	Fluid, skim	3
Egg, yolk:		Mutton	65
Fresh	1500	Oysters	>200
Frozen	1280	Pork	70
Dried	2950	Shrimps	125
Fish, steak or fillet	70	Sweetbreads (thymus)	250
Heart, raw	150	Veal	90

*Adapted from Table 4 in *Composition of Foods—Raw, Processed, Prepared*. Handbook No. 8, U.S. Department of Agriculture, Washington, D.C., 1963, p. 146.

Except as noted, the following foods contain no cholesterol:
Breads, crackers, and rolls (small amounts of cholesterol if made with egg and/or whole milk)
Cereals: breakfast; macaroni, sphaghetti, etc; rice
Cottage cheese made with skim milk
Fats: vegetable oils and shortenings; margarine made with vegetable fat
Fruits
Nonfat milk
Sugars and sweets
Vegetables (not seasoned with butter or whole milk)

Table A–7. Composition of Some Alcoholic Beverages

Beverage	Approximate Measure	Weight gm	Energy calories*	Alcohol gm	Carbohydrate gm
Ale, American	1 glass	250	150	15	11
Beer	1 glass	250	110	10	10
Brandy	1 cordial glass	20	50	7	
Cocktails†					
Daiquiri (1 1/2 jiggers rum)	1 cocktail glass	90	180	22	5
Manhattan (1 1/2 jiggers whiskey)	1 cocktail glass	90	200	28	1
Martini (1 1/2 jiggers gin)	1 cocktail glass	90	220	31	1
Creme de menthe	1 cordial glass	20	75	7	6
Gin—90 proof	1 jigger	45	126	18	
Rum—80 proof	1 jigger	45	105	15	
Vermouth, dry	1 jigger	45	47	7	1
Vermouth, sweet	1 jigger	45	75	8	5
Vodka—100 proof	1 jigger	45	135	19	
Whiskey—86 proof	1 jigger	45	112	16	
Wine					
Champagne, dry	1 champagne glass	135	105	13	3
Champagne, sweet	1 champagne glass	135	160	13	17
California, red	1 claret glass	120	100	12	4
white	1 claret glass	120	95	11	4
Port	1 sherry glass	30	50	5	4
Sherry	1 sherry glass	30	45	5	2

*Alcohol yields 7 calories per gram. The percentage of alcohol varies widely in different preparations.

†Recipes from Rombauer's *Joy of Cooking* used in these calculations and based upon the proof of the liquor listed in the above table. Calories and alcohol content of cocktails will vary widely depending upon the recipes used.

Table A–8. Average Weight-for-Height Table*

(For boys from birth to school age)

Height	Age (Months)											
(Inches)	1	3	6	9	12	18	24	30	36	48	60	72
20	8											
21	9	10										
22	10	11										
23	11	12	13									
24	12	13	14									
25	13	14	15	16								
26		15	17	17	18							
27		16	18	18	19							
28			19	19	20	20						
29			20	21	21	21						
30			22	22	22	22	22					
31				23	23	23	23	24				
32				24	24	25	25	25				
33					26	26	26	26	26			
34						27	27	27	27			
35						29	29	29	29	29		
36							30	31	31	31		
37							32	32	32	32	32	
38								33	33	33	34	
39								35	35	35	35	
40									36	36	36	36
41										38	38	38
42										39	39	39
43										41	41	41
44											43	43
45											45	45
46												48
47												50
48												52
49												55

*Used by the courtesy of the American Child Health Association. Prepared by Robert M. Woodbury.

Table A–9. Average Weight-for-Height Table*

(*For boys from 5 to 19 years*)

Height (Inches)	5	6	7	8	9	10	11	12	13	14	15	16	17	18	19
									Age (Years)						
38	34	34													
39	35	35													
40	36	36													
41	38	38	38												
42	39	39	39	39											
43	41	41	41	41											
44	44	44	44	44											
45	46	46	46	46	46										
46	47	48	48	48	48										
47	49	50	50	50	50	50									
48		52	53	53	53	53									
49		55	55	55	55	55	55								
50		57	58	58	58	58	58	58							
51			61	61	61	61	61	61							
52			63	64	64	64	64	64	64						
53			66	67	67	67	67	68	68						
54				70	70	70	70	71	71	72					
55				72	72	73	73	74	74	74					
56				75	76	77	77	77	78	78	80				
57					79	80	81	81	82	83	83				
58					83	84	84	85	85	86	87				
59						87	88	89	89	90	90	90			
60						91	92	92	93	94	95	96			
61							95	96	97	99	100	103	106		
62							100	101	102	103	104	107	111	116	
63							105	106	107	108	110	113	118	123	127
64								109	111	113	115	117	121	126	130
65								114	117	118	120	122	127	131	134
66									119	122	125	128	132	136	139
67									124	128	130	134	136	139	142
68										134	134	137	141	143	147
69										137	139	143	146	149	152
70										143	144	145	148	151	155
71										148	150	151	152	154	159
72											153	155	156	158	163
73											157	160	162	164	167
74											160	164	168	170	171

*Used by the courtesy of the American Child Health Association. Prepared by Bird T. Baldwin and Thomas D. Wood.

Table A–10. Average Weight-for-Height Table*

(For girls from birth to school age)

Height (Inches)	Age (Months)											
	1	3	6	9	12	18	24	30	36	48	60	72
20	8											
21	9	10										
22	10	11										
23	11	12	13									
24	12	13	14	14								
25	13	14	15	15								
26		15	16	17	17							
27		16	17	18	18							
28			19	19	19	19						
29			19	20	20	20						
30			21	21	21	21	21					
31				22	22	23	23	23				
32					23	24	24	24	25			
33						25	25	25	26			
34						26	26	26	27			
35						29	29	29	29	29		
36							30	30	30	30	31	
37							31	31	31	31	32	
38								33	33	33	33	
39								34	34	34	34	34
40									35	36	36	36
41										37	37	37
42										39	39	39
43										40	41	41
44											42	42
45												45
46												47
47												50
48												52

*Used by the courtesy of the American Child Health Association. Prepared by Robert M. Woodbury.

Table A–11. Average Weight-for-Height Table*

(For girls from 5 to 18 years)

Height	Age (Years)													
(Inches)	5	6	7	8	9	10	11	12	13	14	15	16	17	18
38	33	33												
39	34	34												
40	36	36	36											
41	37	37	37											
42	39	39	39											
43	41	41	41	41										
44	42	42	42	42										
45	45	45	45	45	45									
46	47	47	47	48	48									
47	49	50	50	50	50	50								
48		52	52	52	52	53	53							
49		54	54	55	55	56	56							
50		56	56	57	58	59	61	62						
51			59	60	61	61	63	65						
52			63	64	64	64	65	67						
53			66	67	67	68	68	69	71					
54				69	70	70	71	71	73					
55				72	74	74	74	75	77	78				
56					76	78	78	79	81	83				
57					80	82	82	82	84	88	92			
58						84	86	86	88	93	96	101		
59						87	90	90	92	96	100	103	104	
60						91	95	95	97	101	105	108	109	111
61							99	100	101	105	108	112	113	116
62							104	105	106	109	113	115	117	118
63								110	110	112	116	117	119	120
64								114	115	117	119	120	122	123
65								118	120	121	122	123	125	126
66									124	124	125	128	129	130
67									128	130	131	133	133	135
68									131	133	135	136	138	138
69										135	137	138	140	142
70										136	138	140	142	144
71										138	140	142	144	145

*Used by the courtesy of the American Child Health Association. Prepared by Bird T. Baldwin and Thomas D. Wood.

Table A–12. Desirable Weights for Men of Ages 25 and Over*

Weight in Pounds According to Frame (Indoor Clothing)

Height (with shoes on) 1-inch heels		Small Frame	Medium Frame	Large Frame
Feet	Inches			
5	2	112–120	118–129	126–141
5	3	115–123	121–133	129–144
5	4	118–126	124–136	132–148
5	5	121–129	127–139	135–152
5	6	124–133	130–143	138–156
5	7	128–137	134–147	142–161
5	8	132–141	138–152	147–166
5	9	136–145	142–156	151–170
5	10	140–150	146–160	155–174
5	11	144–154	150–165	159–179
6	0	148–158	154–170	164–184
6	1	152–162	158–175	168–189
6	2	156–167	162–180	173–194
6	3	160–171	167–185	178–199
6	4	164–175	172–190	182–204

*Metropolitan Life Insurance Company, New York.

Table A–13. Desirable Weights for Women of Ages 25 and Over*†

Weight in Pounds According to Frame (In Indoor Clothing)

Height (with shoes on) 2-inch heels		Small Frame	Medium Frame	Large Frame
Feet	Inches			
4	10	92– 98	96–107	104–119
4	11	94–101	98–110	106–122
5	0	96–104	101–113	109–125
5	1	99–107	104–116	112–128
5	2	102–110	107–119	115–131
5	3	105–113	110–122	118–134
5	4	108–116	113–126	121–138
5	5	111–119	116–130	125–142
5	6	114–123	120–135	129–146
5	7	118–127	124–139	133–150
5	8	122–131	128–143	137–154
5	9	126–135	132–147	141–158
5	10	130–140	136–151	145–163
5	11	134–144	140–155	149–168
6	0	138–148	144–159	153–173

*Metropolitan Life Insurance Company, New York.
†For girls between 18 and 25, subtract 1 pound for each year under 25.

Table A–14. Normal Constituents of the Blood in the Adult

Physical Measurements

Specific gravity		1.025–1.029
Viscosity (water as unity)		4.5
Bleeding time (capillary)	min	1–3
Prothrombin time (plasma) (Quick)	sec	10–20
Sedimentation rate (Wintrobe method)		
Men	mm in 1 hr	0–9
Women	mm in 1 hr	0–20

Hematologic Studies

Cell volume	per cent	39–50
Red blood cells	million per cu mm	4.25–5.25
White blood cells	per cu mm	5000–9000
Lymphocytes	per cent	25–30
Neutrophils	per cent	60–65
Monocytes	per cent	4–8
Eosinophils	per cent	0.5–4
Basophils	per cent	0–1.5
Platelets	per cu mm	125,000–300,000

Proteins

Total protein (serum)	gm per 100 ml	6.5–7.5
Albumin (serum)	gm per 100 ml	4.5–5.5
Globulin (serum)	gm per 100 ml	1.5–2.5
Albumin: globulin ratio		1.8–2.5
Fibrinogen (plasma)	gm per 100 ml	0.2–0.5
Hemoglobin		
Males	gm per 100 ml	14–17
Females	gm per 100 ml	13–16

Nitrogen Constituents

Nonprotein N (serum)	mg per 100 ml	20–36
(Whole blood)	mg per 100 ml	25–40
Urea (whole blood)	mg per 100 ml	18–38
Urea N (whole blood)	mg per 100 ml	8–18
Creatinine (whole blood)	mg per 100 ml	1–2
Uric acid (whole blood)	mg per 100 ml	2.5–5.0
Amino acid N (whole blood)	mg per 100 ml	3–6

Blood Gases

CO_2 content (serum)	volumes per cent	55–75
	mM per liter	(24.5–33.5)
CO_2 content (whole blood)	volumes per cent	40–60
	mM per liter	(18.0–27.0)
Oxygen capacity (whole blood)		
Males	volumes per cent	18.7–22.7
Females	volumes per cent	17.0–21.0
Oxygen saturation		
Arterial blood	per cent	94–96
Venous blood	per cent	60–85

Carbohydrates and Lipids

Glucose (whole blood)	mg per 100 ml	70–90
Ketones—as acetone (whole blood)	mg per 100 ml	1.5–2
Fats (total lipids) (serum)	mg per 100 ml	570–820
Cholesterol (serum)	mg per 100 ml	100–230
Bilirubin (serum)	mg per 100 ml	0.1–0.25
Icteric index (serum)	units	4–6

Acid-Base Constituents

Base, total fixed (serum)	mEq per liter	142–150
Sodium (serum)	mg per 100 ml	320–335
	mEq per liter	(139–146)
Potassium (serum)	mg per 100 ml	16–22
	mEq per liter	(4.1–5.6)
Calcium (serum)	mg per 100 ml	9.0–11.5
	mEq per liter	(4.5–5.8)
Magnesium (serum)	mg per 100 ml	1.0–3.0
	mEq per liter	(1.0–2.5)
Phosphorus, inorganic (serum)	mg per 100 ml	3.0–5.0
	mEq per liter	(1.0–1.6)
Chlorides, expressed as Cl (serum)	mg per 100 ml	352–383
	mEq per liter	(99–108)
As NaCl (serum)	mg per 100 ml	580–630
	mEq per liter	(99–108)
Sulfates, inorganic as SO_4 (serum)	mg per 100 ml	2.5–5.0
	mEq per liter	(0.5–1.0)
Lactic acid (venous blood)	mg per 100 ml	10–20
	mEq per liter	(1.1–2.2)
Serum protein base binding power	mEq per liter	(15.5–18.0)
Base bicarbonate HCO_3 (serum)	mEq per liter	(19–30)
pH (blood or plasma at 38° C)		7.3–7.45

Miscellaneous

Phosphatase (serum)	Bodansky units per 100 ml	5
Iron (whole blood)	mg per 100 ml	46–55
Ascorbic acid (whole blood)	mg per 100 ml	0.75–1.50
Carotene (serum)	mcg per 100 ml	75–125

---

ml = milliliters
mg = milligrams
mcg = micrograms
mEq = milliequivalents

gm = grams
cu mm = cubic millimeters

$$\text{mEq per liter} = \frac{\text{mg per liter}}{\text{equivalent weight}}$$

$$\text{equivalent weight} = \frac{\text{atomic weight}}{\text{valence of element}}$$

$$\text{mM (millimoles) per liter} = \frac{\text{mg per liter}}{\text{molecular weight}}$$

$$\text{volumes per cent} = \text{mM per liter} \times 2.24$$

Table A–15. Normal Constituents of the Urine of the Adult

Specific gravity		1.010–1.025
Reaction	pH	5.5–8.0
Volume	ml per 24 hr	800–1600
		gm per 24 hr
Total solids		*55–70*
Nitrogenous constituents		
Total nitrogen		10–17
Ammonia		0.5–1.0
Amino acid N		0.4–1
Creatine		None
Creatinine		1–1.5
Protein		None
Purine bases		0.016–0.060
Urea		20–35
Uric acid		0.5–0.7
Acetone bodies		0.003–0.015
Bile		None
Calcium		0.2–0.4
Chloride (as NaCl)		10–15
Glucose		None
Indican		0–0.030
Iron		0.001–0.005
Magnesium (as MgO)		0.15–0.30
Phosphate, total (as phosphoric acid)		2.5–3.5
Potassium (as K_2O)		2.0–3.0
Sodium (as Na_2O)		4.0–5.0
Sulfates, total (as sulfuric acid)		1.5–3.0

General References

Normal and Therapeutic Nutrition

Anderson, L., and Browe, J. H.: *Nutrition and Family Health Services*. W. B. Saunders Company, Philadelphia, 1960.

Beaton, G. H., and McHenry, E. W., eds.: *Nutrition. A Comprehensive Treatise. Vol. I. Macronutrients and Nutrient Elements, 1964. Vol. II. Vitamins, Nutrient Requirements and Food Selections, 1964. Vol. III. Nutritional Status: Assessment and Applications, 1966.* Academic Press, New York.

Bogert, L. J., Bridges, G. M., and Calloway, D. H.: *Nutrition and Physical Fitness,* 8th ed. W. B. Saunders Company, Philadelphia, 1966.

Bourne, G. H., ed.: *World Review of Nutrition and Dietetics.* Annual. Hafner Publishing Co., New York.

Burton, B. T.: *The Heinz Handbook of Nutrition,* 2nd ed. McGraw-Hill Publishing Company, New York, 1965.

Chaney, M. S. and Ross, M. L.: *Nutrition,* 7th ed. Houghton Mifflin Company, Boston, 1966.

Davidson, S., and Passmore, R.: *Human Nutrition and Dietetics,* 4th ed. The Williams and Wilkins Company, Baltimore, 1969.

Department of Nutrition: *Recent Advances in Therapeutic Diets.* Iowa State University Press, Ames, 1970.

Duncan, G. G., ed.: *Diseases of Metabolism,* 5th ed. W. B. Saunders Company, Philadelphia, 1964.

Eppright, E., Pattison, M., and Barbour, H.: *Teaching Nutrition,* 2nd ed. Iowa State University Press, Ames, Iowa, 1963.

Fleck, H.: *Introduction to Nutrition,* 2nd ed. The Macmillan Company, New York, 1971.

Francis, D. E. M., and Dixon, D. J. W.: *Diets for Sick Children,* 2nd ed. F. A. Davis Company, Philadelphia, 1969.

Goldsmith, G. A.: *Nutritional Diagnosis.* Charles C Thomas Company, Springfield, Ill., 1959.

Guthrie, H. A.: *Introductory Nutrition,* 2nd ed. The C. V. Mosby Company, St. Louis, 1971.

Jolliffe, N., *et al.: Clinical Nutrition,* 2nd ed. Harper & Row, New York, 1962.

Krause, M. V.: *Nutrition and Diet Therapy.* 4th ed. W. B. Saunders Company, Philadelphia, 1966.

Lowenberg, M. E., Todhunter, E. N., Wilson, E. D., Feeney, M. C. and Savage, J. P.: *Food and Man.* John Wiley & Sons, Inc., New York, 1968.

Martin, E. A.: *Roberts' Nutrition Work with Children.* University of Chicago Press, Chicago, 1954.

Mitchell, H. H.: *Comparative Nutrition of Man and Domestic Animals.* 2 vols. Academic Press, New York, 1962, 1964.

Mitchell, H. S., Rynbergen, H. J., Anderson, L., and Dibble, M. V.: *Cooper's Nutrition in Health and Disease,* 15th ed. J. B. Lippincott Company, Philadelphia, 1968.

Pike, R. L., and Brown, M. L.: *Nutrition: An Integrated Approach.* John Wiley & Sons, Inc., New York, 1967.

Present Knowledge of Nutrition, 3rd ed. The Nutrition Foundation, Inc., New York, 1967.

Pyke, M.: *Food and Society.* John Murray, London, 1968.

Taylor, C. M., and Pye, O. F.: *Foundations of Nutrition,* 6th ed. The Macmillan Company, New York, 1966.

Turner, D. F.: *Handbook of Diet Therapy,* 5th ed. University of Chicago Press, Chicago, 1970.

Wayler, T. J., and Klein, R. S.: *Applied Nutrition.* The Macmillan Company, New York, 1965.

Williams, S. R.: *Nutrition and Diet Therapy.* C. V. Mosby Company, St. Louis, 1969.

Wilson, E. D., Fisher, K. H., and Fuqua, M. E.: *Principles of Nutrition,* 2nd ed. John Wiley & Sons, Inc., New York, 1965.

Wohl, M. G., and Goodhart, R. S.: *Modern Nutrition in Health and Disease,* 4th ed. Lea & Febiger, Philadelphia, 1968.

Nutrition Books for Lay Readers

Howe, P. S.: *Nutrition for Practical Nurses,* 4th ed. W. B. Saunders Company, Philadelphia, 1967.

Leverton, R. M.: *Food Becomes You,* 3rd ed. Iowa State University Press, Ames, Iowa, 1965.

McHenry, E. W.: *Foods Without Fads.* J. B. Lippincott Company, Philadelphia, 1960.

Martin, E. A.: *Nutrition in Action,* 3rd ed. Holt, Rinehart, and Winston, New York, 1971.

Mickelson, O.: *Nutrition Science and You.* National Science Teachers Association, Inc., Washington, D.C., 1964.

Mowry, L., and Williams, S. R.: *Basic Nutrition and Diet Therapy for Practical Nurses,* 4th ed. The C. V. Mosby Company, St. Louis, 1969.

Robinson, C. H.: *Basic Nutrition and Diet Therapy,* 2nd ed. The Macmillan Company, New York, 1970.

Shackelton, A. D.: *Practical Nurse Nutrition Education.* W. B. Saunders Company, Philadelphia, 1966.

Stare, F. J.: *Eating for Good Health.* Doubleday, New York, 1964.

U.S. Department of Agriculture:
Consumers All. Yearbook of Agriculture, 1965.
Food for Us All. Yearbook of Agriculture, 1969.
Food, the Yearbook of Agriculture, 1959.

White, P. L.: *Let's Talk About Food.* American Medical Association, Chicago, 1967.

Tables of Food Composition

Amino Acid Content of Foods and Biological Data on Proteins. FAO Nutritional Studies No. 24, Food and Agriculture Organization, Rome, 1970.

Aykroyd, W. R., et al.: *The Nutritive Value of Indian Foods and the Planning of Satisfactory Diets.* Indian Council Med. Res. Bull. 23, 1956.

Bocobo, D. L., et al.: *Food Composition Tables Recommended for Use in the Philippines.* Handbook No. 1, Institute for Nutrition, Department of Health, Manila, 1951.

Chatfield, C.: *Food Composition Tables for International Use.* Nutritional Studies No. 3, Food and Agriculture Organization, Rome, 1949.

————: *Food Composition Tables—Minerals and Vitamins—for International Use.* Nutritional Studies No. 11, Food and Agriculture Organization, Rome, 1954.

Church, C. F., and Church, H. N.: *Food Values of Portions Commonly Used,* 11th ed. J. B. Lippincott Company, Philadelphia, 1970.

Consumer and Food Economics Research Division, Agricultural Research Service: *Nutritive Value of Foods,* HG 72, U.S. Department of Agriculture, Washington, D.C. 1970.

————: *Pantothenic Acid, Vitamin B_6 and Vitamin B_{12} in Foods.* U.S. Department of Agriculture, Washington, D.C., 1969.

Leung, W. T. W., *et al.*: *Composition of Foods Used in Far Eastern Countries.* Handbook No 34, U.S. Department of Agriculture, Washington, D.C., 1952.

Leung, W. T. W.: *Food Composition Table for Use in Latin America.* Interdepartmental Committee on Nutrition for National Defense, National Institutes of Health, Bethesda, Maryland, 1961.

McCance, R. A., and Widdowson, E. M.: *The Composition of Foods,* 3rd ed. Spec. Rep. Series No. 297, Medical Research Council, London, 1960.

Orr, M. L., and Watt, B. K.: *Amino Acid Content of Foods.* Home Econ. Res. Rep., No. 4, U.S. Department of Agriculture, Washington, D.C., 1957.

Platt, B. S.: *Tables of Representative Values of Foods Commonly Used in Tropical Countries.* Special Rep. Series No. 302, Med. Research Council, London: H.M. Stationery Office, 1962.

Watt, B. K., and Merrill, A. L.: *Composition of Foods—Raw, Processed, Prepared.* Handbook No. 8, U.S. Department of Agriculture, Washington, D.C., 1963.

FOODS AND FOOD PREPARATION

Handbook of Food Preparation. American Home Economics Association, Washington, D.C., 1970.

Heseltine, M., and Dow, U. M.: *The New Basic Cook Book.* Houghton Mifflin Company, Boston, 1957.

Hughes, O, and Bennion, M.: *Introductory Foods,* 5th ed. The Macmillan Company, New York, 1970.

McWilliams, M.: *Food Fundamentals.* John Wiley & Sons, Inc., New York, 1966.

Peckham, G. C.: *Foundations of Food Preparation,* 2nd ed. The Macmillan Company, New York, 1969.

Rombauer, I. S., and Becker, M. R.: *Joy of Cooking.* Bobbs-Merrill Company, Inc., Indianapolis, 1962.

Vail, G. E., Griswold, R. M., Justin, M. M., and Rust, L. O.: *Foods,* 5th ed. Houghton Mifflin Company, Boston, 1967.

MEDICAL SCIENCES

Beland, I. L.: *Clinical Nursing,* 2nd ed. The Macmillan Company, 1970.

Beeson, P. B., and McDermott, W.: *Cecil and Loeb's Textbook of Medicine.* W. B. Saunders Company, Philadelphia, 1967.

Best, C. H., and Taylor, N. B.: *The Physiological Basis of Medical Practice,* 8th ed. The Williams & Wilkins Company, Baltimore, 1966.

Cantarow, A., and Schepartz, B.: *Biochemistry,* 4th ed. W. B. Saunders Company, Philadelphia, 1967.

Goodman, L. S., and Gilman, A.: *The Pharmacological Basis of Therapeutics,* 4th ed. The Macmillan Company, New York, 1970.

Grollman, S.: *The Human Body: Its Structure and Function,* 2nd ed. The Macmillan Company, New York, 1969.

Guyton, A. C.: *Textbook of Medical Physiology,* 3rd ed. W. B. Saunders Company, Philadelphia, 1966.

Hanlon, J. J.: *Principles of Public Health Administration,* 5th ed. The C. V. Mosby Company, St. Louis, 1969.

Harrison, T. R., *et al.: Principles of Internal Medicine,* 5th ed. Blakiston McGraw-Hill, New York, 1966.

McCammon, R. W.: *Human Growth and Development.* Charles C Thomas, Springfield, Ill., 1970.

Miller, M. A., and Leavell, L. C.: *Kimber-Gray-Stackpole's Anatomy and Physiology,* 16th ed. The Macmillan Company, New York, 1972.

Nelson, W. E.: *Textbook of Pediatrics,* 9th ed. W. B. Saunders Company, Philadelphia, 1970.

West, E. S., Todd, W. R., Mason, H. W., and Van Bruggen, J. T.: *Textbook of Biochemistry,* 4th ed. The Macmillan Company, New York 1966.

JOURNALS

American Journal of Clinical Nutrition
American Journal of Digestive Diseases
American Journal of Diseases of Children
American Journal of Nursing
American Journal of Obstetrics and Gynecology
American Journal of Public Health
Annals of Internal Medicine
Annual Review of Biochemistry
Archives of Internal Medicine
Borden's Review of Nutrition Research
British Journal of Nutrition
Chemical Abstracts—Nutrition Division
Diabetes
Federation Proceedings
Food Science
Food Technology
Geriatrics
Journal of the American Dietetic Association
Journal of the American Medical Association

Journal of Biological Chemistry
Journal of Clinical Investigation
Journal of Geriatrics
Journal of Gerontology
Journal of Home Economics
Journal of Nutrition
Journal of Pediatrics
Lancet
Metabolism
New England Journal of Medicine
Nursing Outlook
Nutrition Abstracts and Reviews
Nutrition Today
Pediatrics
Physiological Reviews
Public Health Nursing
Public Health Reports
Science
Today's Health

SOURCES OF NUTRITION EDUCATION MATERIALS

American Can Company. 730 Park Avenue, New York, New York 10017.

American Diabetes Association. 18 East 48th Street, New York, New York 10017.

American Dietetic Association. 620 North Michigan Avenue, Chicago, Illinois 60611.

American Heart Association. 44 East 23rd Street, New York, New York 10010.

American Home Economics Association. 1600 Twentieth Street, N.W., Washington, D.C. 20009.

American Institute of Baking. Consumer Service Department, 400 East Ontario Street, Chicago, Illinois 60611

American Public Health Association. 1790 Broadway, New York, New York 10019.

American School Food Service Association. P.O. Box 10095, Denver, Colorado 80210.

The Borden Company. 350 Madison Avenue, New York, New York 10017.

Home Economics Department, The Campbell Soup Company. 385 Memorial Avenue, Camden, New Jersey 08101.

Cereal Institute, Inc., Educational Director. 135 South LaSalle Street, Chicago, Illinois 60603.

Chicago Dietetic Supply House, Inc. 1750 West Van Buren Street, Chicago, Illinois 60612.

Children's Bureau. Department of Health, Education, and Welfare. Washington, D.C. 20201.

Council on Foods and Nutrition. American Medical Association. 535 North Dearborn Street, Chicago, Illinois 60610.

Evaporated Milk Association. 228 North LaSalle Street, Chicago, Illinois 60601.

Food and Drug Administration. Department of Health, Education, and Welfare. Washington, D.C. 20204.

Food and Nutrition Board, National Research Council. 2101 Constitution Avenue, Washington, D.C. 20418.

General Foods Corporation. 250 North Street, White Plains, New York 10602.

Public Relations Department. General Mills, Inc. 9200 Wayzata Boulevard, Minneapolis, Minnesota 55426.

Gerber Products. Department of Nutrition. Fremont, Michigan 49412.

John Hancock Life Insurance Company. 200 Berkeley Street, Boston, Massachusetts 02117.

Department of Home Economics Services. Kellogg Company. 215 Porter Street, Battle Creek, Michigan 49016.

Metropolitan Life Insurance Company. Health and Welfare Division. One Madison Avenue, New York, New York 10010.

National Dairy Council. 111 North Canal Street, Chicago, Illinois 60606.

National Live Stock and Meat Board, Home Economics Department. 36 South Wabash Avenue, Chicago, Illinois 60603.

The Nutrition Foundation, Inc. 99 Park Avenue, New York, New York 10016.

Poultry and Egg National Board. 250 West 57th Street, New York, New York 10019.

School Lunch Branch, Food Distribution Division, Agricultural Marketing Service, U.S. Department of Agriculture, Washington, D.C. 20250.

Superintendent of Documents, U.S. Government Printing Office, Washington, D.C. 20402.

Office of Information, U.S. Department of Agriculture, Washington, D.C. 20250.

Common Abbreviations

AcCoa: acetyl coenzyme A
ACTH: adrenocorticotropic hormone
ADH: antidiuretic hormone
ADP: adenosine-5'-diphosphate
AMP: adenosine-5'-phosphate
ATP: adenosine-5'-triphosphate

BMR: basal metabolic rate

cal: calorie
CoA, CoASH: coenzyme A

DNA: deoxyribonucleic acid

EAA: essential amino acids
EFA: essential fatty acids

FAD: flavin adenine dinucleotide, oxidized form
FADH: flavin adenine dinucleotide, reduced form
FAO: Food and Agriculture Organization
FDA: Food and Drug Administration
FFA: free fatty acids
FMN: flavin mononucleotide
FSH: follicle-stimulating hormone

GFR: glomerular filtration rate
gm: gram(s)

Hb: hemoglobin
HbO_2: oxyhemoglobin
HMP shunt: hexose monophosphate shunt

I.U.: international unit

J: joule

kcal: kilocalorie
kg: kilogram
kJ: kilojoule

L: liter
lb: pound
LCT: long-chain triglycerides

mcg: microgram(s)
MCT: medium-chain triglyceride
mEq: milliequivalent(s)
mg: milligram(s)

NAD: nicotinamide adenine dinucleotide
NADP: nicotinamide adenine dinucleotide phosphate
NRC: National Research Council

PABA: para-amino benzoic acid
PBI: protein-bound iodine
pH: hydrogen ion concentration
PKU: phenylketonuria

RDA: Recommended Dietary Allowances
RNA: ribonucleic acid

SH: sulfhydryl

TCA: tricarboxylic acid cycle
TPP: thiamine pyrophosphate
TSH: thyroid-stimulating hormone

UNESCO: United Nations Educational, Scientific, and Cultural Organization
UNICEF: United Nations Children's Fund
USDA: United States Department of Agriculture
USP: United States Pharmacopeia

WHO: World Health Organization

Glossary

absorption (ab-sorp′shun): the transfer of nutrients across cell membranes; following digestion, nutrients are transferred from the intestinal lumen across the mucosa and into the blood and lymph circulation

acetoacetic acid (as′et-o-as-e′tik): a 4-carbon keto-acid; one of the acetone bodies in diabetic urine

acetone (as′et-ōn): dimethyl ketone; accumulates in the blood and excretions when fats are incompletely oxidized as in diabetes mellitus; gives fruity odor to the breath

acetyl coenzyme A (as′et-il co-en′zīm): condensation product of acetic acid and coenzyme A; form by which 2-carbon fragment enters the tricarboxylic acid cycle

achlorhydria (a-klor-hi′dri-ah): absence of hydrochloric acid in gastric juice

acids: see individual names

acidosis (as-ĭd-o′sis): condition caused by accumulation of an excess of acids (anions) in the body, or by excessive loss of base (mineral cations) from the body

acrolein (ak-ro′le-in): an irritating volatile decomposition product of glycerol that results from overheating fat

adenine (ad′en-in): one of the purines (bases) that are constituents of nucleic acid

adenosine triphosphate (ad-en′o-sin tri-fos′fāt): a compound consisting of 1 molecule each of adenine and ribose and 3 molecules of phosphoric acid; two of the phosphate groups are held by high-energy bonds; ATP

adipose (ad′ip-ōs): fat; fatty

aerobic (a-er-o′bik): growing in presence of air

agar (ah′gar): an indigestible polysaccharide prepared from moss and seaweed; has property of holding water and is often used to relieve constipation

alanine (al′an-in): a nonessential amino acid occurring widely in foods

albumin (al-bu′min): a protein in tissues and body fluids soluble in water and coagulated by heat; principal protein in blood regulating osmotic pressure; lactalbumin of milk

aldehyde (al′de-hīd): any of a large group of compounds containing the grouping -CHO

aldohexose (al-dō-hex′ōs): a 6-carbon sugar containing a -CHO grouping; glucose, galactose

aldosterone (al-dos′ter-ōn): a steroid hormone produced by the adrenal cortex; increases sodium retention and potassium loss

alkalosis (al-kah-lo′sis): increased alkali reserve (blood bicarbonate) of the blood and other body fluids; caused by excessive ingestion of sodium bicarbonate, persistent vomiting, or hyperventilation; pH of blood is usually increased

allergen (al′ler-jen): substance (usually protein) capable of producing altered response of cell, resulting in manifestation of allergy

amino acid (am′in-o as′id): an organic acid containing an amino (NH_2) group; the building blocks of protein molecules

amylase (am′i-lās): salivary or pancreatic enzyme that hydrolyzes starch; ptyalin, amylopsin

amylopectin (am′il-o-pek′tin): polysaccharide found in starch consisting of branched chains of glucose

amylose (am′il-ōs): polysaccharide of starch consisting of unbranched chains of glucose

anabolism (an-ab′oh-lizm): processes for building complex substances from simple substances

anaerobic (an-aer-oh′bik): living in the absence of air

androgen (an′dro-jen): a substance such as testosterone that produces male sex characteristics

anemia (an-e′me-ah): deficiency in the circulating hemoglobin, red blood cells, or packed cell volume

anion (an′i-on): an ion that contains a negative charge of electricity and therefore goes to a positively charged anode

anorexia (an-o-rek′se-ah): loss of appetite

antagonist (an-tag′on-ist): a substance that opposes or neutralizes the action of another substance, e.g., a vitamin antagonist

anthropometry (an-thro-pom′et-re): branch of anthropology dealing with comparative measurements of the parts of the human body.

anti-: a prefix meaning against or opposing; e.g., antiscorbutic means preventing scurvy

antibiotic (an'ti-bi-ot'ik): a substance that inhibits the growth of bacteria

antibody (an'te-bod-e): a protein substance produced in an organism as a response to the presence of an antigen

antigen (an'ti-jen): any substance such as bacteria or foreign protein that, as a result of contact with tissues of the animal body, produces an immune response; an increased reaction such as hypersensitivity may result

antiketogenesis (an-ti-ke-tō-jen'es-is): the prevention of ketosis by stimulating the tricarboxylic acid cycle and thus bringing about oxidation of the ketone bodies

antioxidant (an-te-ok'sid-ant): a substance that prevents deterioration by hindering oxidation, e.g., tocopherols prevent oxidation and rancidity of fats

anuria (an-u're-ah): lack of urinary secretion

apathy (ap'ath-e): indifference; lack of interest or concern

apatite (ap'ah-tīt): complex calcium phosphate salt giving strength to bones

apoenzyme (ap-o-en'zīm): the protein part of an enzyme

arachidonic acid (ar-ak-id-on'ik): a 20-carbon fatty acid with four double bonds; the physiologically functioning essenial fatty acid

arginase (ar'jin-ās): enzyme that splits arginine to urea and ornithine

arginine (ar'jin-in): a diamino acid; required for growth but not required by adults

arteriosclerosis (ar-te-re-o-skle-ro'sis): thickening and hardening of the inner walls of the arteries

ascites (a-si'tēz): accumulation of fluid in the abdominal cavity

ascorbic acid (a-skor'bik): water-soluble vitamin required for collagenous intercellular substance; prevents scurvy; also known as vitamin C

aspartic acid (as-par'tik): a nonessential dibasic amino acid

asymptomatic (a-sim-tō-mat'ik): without symptoms

ataxia (a-tak'se-ah): loss of ability of muscular coordination

atherosclerosis (ath-er-o-skle-ro'sis): thickening of the walls of blood vessels by deposits of fatty materials, including cholesterol

atony (at'o-ne): lack of normal tone or strength

atrophy (at'ro-fe): a wasting away of cell, tissue, or organ

autosome (aw'tō-sōm): any chromosome other than a sex chromosome

avidin (av'id-in): protein substance in raw egg white which binds biotin and prevents its absorption from the digestive tract

azotemia (a-zo-te'me-ah): elevated levels of nitrogenous constituents in the blood; uremia

basal metabolism (ba'zal me-tab'o-lizm): energy expenditure of the body at rest in the postabsorptive state

base (bās): substance that combines with an acid to form a salt; any molecule or ion that will add on a hydrogen ion

benign (bi-nīn'): mild nature of an illness; with reference to a neoplasm, not malignant

beriberi (ber'ē-ber'ē): a deficiency disease caused by lack of thiamine and characterized by extreme weakness, polyneuritis, emaciation, edema, and cardiac failure

beta-hydroxybutyric acid (ba-tah-hi-drox'e-bu-tir'-ik): a 4-carbon intermediate in oxidation of fatty acids; one of the acetone bodies excreted in the urine in uncontrolled diabetes

bio- (bi-o-): prefix denoting life

bioassay (bi'-o-as-say): testing of activity or potency, as of a vitamin or hormone, on an animal or microorganism

biopsy (bi'op-sē): examination of a piece of tissue removed from a living subject

biotin (bi'o-tin): a vitamin of the B complex; participates in fixation of carbon dioxide in fatty acid synthesis

Bitot's spots (be'tōz): gray, shiny spots on the conjunctiva resulting from malnutriiton, especially vitamin A deficiency

botulism (bot'u-lizm): frequently fatal poisoning caused by toxin produced in inadequately sterilized canned food by the *Clostridium botulinum*

buffer (buf'er): a mixture of an acid and its conjugate base that is capable of neutralizing either an acid or a base without appreciably changing the original acidity or alkalinity, e.g., $H_2CO_3/HCO_3{}^-$

calciferol (kal-sif'er-ol): vitamin D_2; fat-soluble vitamin of plant origin formed by irradiation of ergosterol; prevents rickets

calcification (kal-sif-ik-a'shun): hardening of tissue by a deposit of calcium and also magnesium salts

calculus (kal'ku-lus): an abnormal concretion occurring in any part of the body; usually consists of mineral salts around an organic nucleus

calorie (kal'o-rē): a unit of heat measurement; in nutrition, the kilocalorie is the amount of heat required to raise the temperature of 1 kg water 1° C

calorimetry (kal-or-im′et-rē): measurement of heat produced by the body, or from a food; *direct:* measure of heat produced by a subject in a closed chamber; *indirect:* measurement of heat by determining consumption of oxygen and sometimes carbon dioxide and calculating the amount of heat produced

carbonic acid (kar-bon′ik): the acid formed when carbon dioxide is dissolved in water; H_2CO_3

carboxylase (kar-bok′sil-ās): a thiamine-containing enzyme that catalyzes the removal of the carboxyl group of alpha keto acids, e.g., decarboxylation of pyruvic acid

carboxypeptidase (kar-box-e-pep′tid-ās): an intestinal enzyme which catalyzes the splitting of peptides

carotene (kar′o-tēn): precursor of vitamin A; yellow plant pigments occurring abundantly in dark-green leafy and deep-yellow vegetables

casein (ka′se-in): principal protein in milk; a phosphoprotein

catabolism (kat-ab′o-lizm): process for breaking down complex substances to simpler substances; usually yields energy

catalyst (kat′ah-list): a substance which in minute amounts initiates or modifies the speed of a chemical or physical change without itself being changed

cation (kat′i-on): an ion that carries a positive charge and migrates to the negatively charged pole

cellulose (sel′u-lōs): the structural fibers of plants; an indigestible polysaccharide

cephalin (sef′al-in): a phospholipid in brain and nervous tissue

ceruloplasmin (ser-ul′o-plaz-min): copper-containing protein in blood plasma

cheilosis (ki-lo′sis): lesions of the lips and the angles of the mouth; characteristic of riboflavin deficiency

chelation (ke-la′shun): formation of a bond between a metal ion and two or more polar groupings of a single molecule

cholecalciferol (ko-le-kal-sif′er-ol): vitamin D_3 formed from 7-dehydrocholesterol

cholecystitis (ko-le-sis-ti′tis): inflammation of the gallbladder

cholecystokinin (ko-le-sis-tō-kin′in): hormone produced in duodenum in presence of fat; stimulates contraction of gallbladder and release of bile

cholelithiasis (ko-le-lith-i′a-sis): gallstones in the gallbladder

cholesterol (ko-les′ter-ol): the commonest member of the sterol group; found in animal foods and made within the body; a constituent of gallstones and of atheroma

choline (ko′lēn): a nitrogenous base that donates methyl groups; a component of lecithin and acetylcholine; sometimes classed as a B complex vitamin

chondroitin sulfate (kon-droi′tin): a mucopolysaccharide widely distributed in skin and cartilage

chylomicrons (ki′lo-mi′krons): large molecules of fat occurring in lymph and plasma after a fat-rich meal; consist of triglycerides attached to a small amount of protein

chymotrypsin (ki-mo-trip′sin): enzyme produced in pancreas for the hydrolysis of protein

citric acid (sit′rik): an organic acid containing three carboxyl groups; one of compounds in the Krebs or citric acid cycle; a constituent of citrus fruits

citrovorum factor (sit-ro-vor′um): folinic acid, the active form of folic acid

citrulline (sit-rul′in): an amino acid formed from ornithine in the urea cycle

Clostridium (klos-trid′i-um): a genus of bacteria, chiefly anaerobic, found in soils and in the intestinal tract, e.g., *botulinum, perfringens*

coagulation (ko-ag-u-la′shun): process of changing into a clot, as in heating of an egg, curdling of milk

cobalamine (ko-bal′ah-min): compound containing cobalt grouping found in vitamin B_{12}

cocarboxylase (ko-kar-box′il-ās): thiamine-containing coenzyme of carboxylase

coenzyme (ko-en′zīm): the prosthetic group of an enzyme; a substance, for example, a vitamin, that conjugates with a protein molecule to form an active enzyme

coenzyme A: a complex nucleotide containing pantothenic acid; combines with acetyl groups to yield active acetate which can enter the Krebs cycle; involved in fatty acid oxidation and synthesis and cholesterol synthesis

coenzyme Q: involved in transfer of electrons in cytochrome chain

colitis (ko-li′tis): inflammation of the colon

collagen (kol′aj-in): widely distributed protein that makes up the matrix of bone, cartilage, and connective tissue

colloid (kol′oid): matter dispersed through another medium; particles are larger than crystalline molecules but not large enough to settle out; do not pass through an animal membrane

colostrum (ko-los′trum): milk secreted during the first few days after the birth of a baby

coma (ko′mah): state of unconsciousness

congenital (kon-jen′it-al): existing at or before

birth with reference to certain physical or mental traits

coronary (kor′o-na-re): like a crown; related to blood vessels supplied to the heart muscle

cortex (kor′tex): outer layers of an organ, e.g., adrenal cortex

cortisone (kor′ti-sōn): hormone of the adrenal cortex; influences carbohydrate metabolism

creatine (kre′at-in): a nitrogenous constituent of muscle; phosphorylated form essential for muscle contraction

creatinine (kre-at′in-in): a nitrogen-containing substance derived from catabolism of creatine and present in the urine

cryptoxanthine (kript-o-zan′thin): a yellow pigment present in some foods; precursor of vitamin A

cystine (sis′tin): sulfur-containing nonessential amino acid

cytochrome (si′tō-krōm): a respiratory enzyme; consists of a number of hemochromogens; undergoes alternate reduction and oxidation

cytology (si-tol′oh-je): the anatomy, chemistry, physiology, and pathology of the cell

cytoplasm (si′to-plazm): substance within the cell exclusive of the nucleus

cytosine (si′tō-sin): one of the nitrogenous bases in nucleic acid

deamination, deaminization (de-am-in-a′shun): removal of the amino (NH₂) group from an amino acid

debility (de-bil′i-te): weakness

dehydrocholesterol, 7- (de-hi-dro-ko-les′ter-ol): cholesterol derivative in the skin that is converted to vitamin D

dehydrogenases (de-hi-dro′jen-ās-es): enzymes that catalyze oxidation by transferring hydrogen to a hydrogen acceptor

denaturation (de-na-tur-a′shun): to use chemical or physical means to alter the natural properties of a substance; e.g., heat coagulation of protein

deoxypyridoxine (de-ok′se-pir-id-oks′in): a compound similar in structure to pyridoxine that is antagonistic to the action of pyridoxine

deoxyribonucleic acid (DNA) (de-ok′se-ri-bo-nu-kla′ik): giant molecule in cell nucleus which determines hereditary traits; consists of four bases attached to ribose and phosphate

dermatitis (der-mat-i′tis): inflammation of the surface of the skin

dextrin (dex′trin): intermediate product in breakdown of starches; a polysaccharide

dicoumarin (di-koo′mah-rin): antiprothrombin; anticlotting factor first isolated from sweet clover

diffuse (dif-ūs′): not localized

digestion (di-jes′chun): the hydrolysis of foods in the digestive tract to simpler substances so they can be used by the body

diglyceride (di-glis′er-id): a fat containing 2 fatty acid molecules

disaccharidase (di-sak′ar-id-ās): enzyme which hydrolyzes disaccharides

disaccharide (di-sak′ar-id): a carbohydrate that yields two simple sugars upon hydrolysis; sucrose, maltose, lactose

distal (dis′tal): part of structure farthest from the point of attachment

diuresis (di-u-re′sis): increased secretion of urine

duodenum (du-o-de′num): first portion of the small intestine, extending from the pylorus to the jejunum

dyspepsia (dis-pep′se-ah): indigestion or upset stomach

dysphagia (dis-fa′je-ah): difficulty in swallowing

dyspnea (disp′ne-ah): difficulty or distress in breathing

eclampsia (ĕ-klamp′se-ah): convulsions occurring during pregnancy and associated with edema, hypertension, and proteinuria

edema (ĕ-de′mah): presence of abnormal amounts of fluid in intercellular spaces

elastin (ĕ-las′tin): insoluble yellow elastic protein in connective tissue

electrolyte (el-ek′tro-līt): any substance which dissociates into ions when dissolved and thus conducts an electric current

emaciation (e-ma-se-a′shun): wasting of the body; excessive leanness

emulsion (e-mul′shun): a system of two immiscible liquids in which one is finely divided and held in suspension by another

endemic (en-dem′ik): prevalence of a disease in a given region

endo-: prefix meaning inner or within

endocrine (en′do-krin): pertaining to glands that secrete substances into the blood for control of metabolic processes

endogenous (en-doj′en-us): originating in the cells or tissues of the body

endoplasmic reticulum (en′do-plaz-mik ret-ic′u-lum): the system of membranes within the cell that permits communication between cellular, nuclear, and extracellular environment

endosperm (en′do-sperm): reserve food material of the plant; the starchy center of the cereal grain

enter-: combining term denoting intestine

enteritis (en-ter-i′tis): inflammation of the intestine

enterocrinin (en-ter-o-krī′nin): hormone of small intestine that stimulates secretion of intestinal juice

enterogastrone (en-ter-o-gas′trōn): hormone secreted by duodenal mucosa upon stimulation by fat; inhibits secretion of gastric juice and reduces motility

enterokinase (en-ter-o-kīn′ās): enzyme of intestinal juice that converts trypsinogen to trypsin

enteropathy (en-ter-op′ath-e): any disease of the intestine

enzyme (en′zīm): an organic compound of protein nature produced by living tissue to accelerate metabolic reactions; hydrolases, oxidases, transferases, dehydrogenases, peptidases, and others

epinephrine (ep-in-ef′rin): secretion of the medulla of the adrenal gland that stimulates energy metabolism; adrenaline

epithelium (ep-ith-e′le-um): the covering layer of the skin and mucous membranes

ergosterol (er-gos′ter-ol): a sterol found chiefly in plants; when exposed to ultraviolet light becomes vitamin D

erythrocyte (er-ith′ro-sīt): mature red blood cell

erythropoieses (er-ith-ro-po-e′sis): formation of red blood cells

essential amino acid: an amino acid that must be supplied in the diet to provide the body's need for it

essential fatty acid: a fatty acid that must be present in the diet and that prevents certain deficiencies of the skin and blood capillaries; linoleic acid, arachidonic acid

estrogen (es′tro-jen): hormone secreted by the ovary

etiology (e-te-ol′o-je): cause of a disease

exacerbation (ex-as-er-ba′shun): increase in severity of symptoms

exogenous (ex-oj′en-us): originating or produced from the outside

extracellular (extra-sel′u-lar): situated or occurring outside the cells

extrinsic factor (ex-trin′sik): vitamin B_{12}; term used by Castle prior to identification of the nature of the compound

exudate (ex′u-dāt): a fluid discharged into the tissues or any cavity

familial (fam-il′e-al): common to a family

fatty acids (fat′e): open-chain monocarboxylic acids containing only carbon, hydrogen, and oxygen

favism (fa′vism): condition caused by eating certain species of beans, e.g., *Vicia faba*; symptoms include fever, abdominal pain, headache, anemia, coma

febrile (feb′ril): feverish; having a fever

ferritin (fer′it-in): an iron-protein complex containing up to 23 per cent iron and formed by combining iron with apoferritin

fetor hepaticus (fe′tor hep-at′ik-us): offensive odor to the breath present in persons with severe liver disease

fibrosis (fi-bro′sis): formation of fibrous tissue in repair processes

fistula (fis′tu-lah): a tubelike ulcer leading from an abscess cavity or organ to the surface, or from one abscess cavity to another

flatulence (flat′u-lens): distention of stomach or intestines with gases

flavin adenine dinucleotide, FAD (fla′vin ad′en-in di-nu′kle-o-tīd): a coenzyme consisting of riboflavin and adenosine diphosphate required for the action of various dehydrogenases

flavin mononucleotide, FMN (fla′vin mon-o-nu′kle-o-tīd): a riboflavin-containing coenzyme involved in the action of dehydrogenases

flavoprotein (fla-vo-pro′te-in): a conjugated protein that contains a flavin and is involved in tissue respiration

fluoridation (floo-or-id-a′shun): the use of fluorine, as in water, to reduce the incidence of tooth decay

folacin (fo′lah-sin): folic acid, a vitamin of the B complex

folic acid (fo′lik): a vitamin of the B complex necessary for the maturation of red blood cells and synthesis of nucleoproteins; also known as folacin and pteroylglutamic acid

folinic acid (fo-lin′ik): the active form of folacin; citrovorum factor

follicle (fol′ikl): small excretory sac or gland, e.g., hair follicle, ovarian follicle

fortification (for-ti-fik-a′shun): the addition of one or more nutrients to a food to make it richer than the unprocessed food, e.g., vitamin D milk

fructose (fruk′tōs): a 6-carbon sugar found in fruits and honey; also obtained from the hydrolysis of sucrose; fruit sugar, levulose

galactose (gal-ak′tōs): a single sugar resulting from the hydrolysis of lactose

galactosemia (gal-ak′tō-se′me-ah): accumulation of galactose in the blood owing to a hereditary lack of an enzyme to convert galactose to glucose; accompanied by severe mental retardation

gastrectomy (gas-trek′tō-me): surgical removal of part or all of the stomach

gastrin (gas′trin): hormone secreted by pyloric mucosa that stimulates secretion of hydrochloric acid by parietal cells

genetic (jen-et′ik): congenital or inherited

gingivitis (jin-jĭ-vi′tis): inflammation of the gums

gliadin (gli′ad-in): a protein fraction of wheat gluten

globulin (glob′u-lin): a class of proteins insoluble in water and alcohol; serum globulin, lactoglobulin, myosin

glomerulus (glom-er′u-lus): the tuft of capillaries at the beginning of each tubule in the kidney

glossitis (glos-i′tis): inflammation of the tongue

glucagon (gloo′kag-on): hormone produced by the alpha cells of the islands of Langerhans; raises blood sugar by increasing glycogen breakdown

glucocorticoid (glu′ko-kor-tĭ-koid): hormone produced by the adrenal cortex that influences glucose metabolism

glucogenic (glu-ko-jen′ik): glucose forming

gluconeogenesis (glu′ko-ne-o-jen′e-sis): formation of glucose from noncarbohydrate sources, namely certain amino acids and the glycerol fraction of fats

glucose (glu′kōs): a single sugar occurring in fruits and honey; also obtained by the hydrolysis of starch, sucrose, maltose, and lactose; the sugar found in the blood; dextrose, grape sugar

glutamic acid (glu-tam′ik): a dibasic nonessential amino acid widely distributed in proteins

glutathione (glu-ta-thi′ōn): a tripeptide of glycine, glutamic acid, and cystine; can act as hydrogen acceptor and hydrogen donor

gluten (glu′ten): protein in wheat and other cereals that gives elastic quality to a dough

glyceride (glis′er-id): organic ester of glycerol; fats are esters of fatty acids and glycerol

glycerol (glis′er-ol): a 3-carbon alcohol derived from the hydrolysis of fats

glycine (gli′sin): aminoacetic acid; a nonessential amino acid

glycogen (gli′ko-jen): polysaccharide produced from glucose by the liver or the muscle; "animal" starch

glycogenesis (gli′ko-jen′ĭ-sis): formation of glycogen from glucose by the liver or muscle

glycogenolysis (gli-ko-jen-ol′ĭ-sis): enzymatic breakdown of glycogen to glucose

glycolysis (gli-kol′ĭ-sis): the anaerobic conversion of glucose to lactose, an energy-yielding process

glycosuria (gli-ko-su′re-ah): presence of sugar in the urine

goiter (goi′tèr): enlargement of the thyroid gland

goitrogen (goi′tro-jen): a substance that leads to goiter

guanine (gwan′in): one of the nitrogenous bases in nucleic acids

hematocrit (he-mat′o-krit): separation of red cells from the plasma

hematuria (he-mat-u′re-ah): condition in which urine contains blood

heme (hēm): deep red pigment consisting of ferrous iron linked to protoporphyrin

hemicellulose (hem-i-sel′u-lōs): a class of indigestible polysaccharides that form the cell wall of plants

hemochromatosis (hem-o-kro-ma-to′sis): a condition in which excessive iron absorption leads to skin pigmentation and deposits of hemosiderin in the liver and other organs

hemoglobin (he-mo-glo′bin): the iron-protein pigment in the red blood cells; carries oxygen to the tissues

hemolytic (he-mo-lit′ik): causing separation of hemoglobin from the red blood cells

hemopoietic, hematopoietic (he-mo-poi-et′ik): concerned with the formation of blood

hemorrhage (hem′or-ej): loss of blood from the vessels; bleeding

hemosiderin (he′mo-sid′er-in): iron-containing pigment in liver and other organs in disorders of iron metabolism, including excessive iron absorption or excessive blood destruction

heparin (hep′ar-in): a mucopolysaccharide that prevents clotting of blood

hepatic (hep-at′ik): pertaining to the liver

hepatomegaly (hep-at-o-meg′ah-le): enlargement of the liver

heterozygous (het-er-o-zi′gus): possessing dissimilar pairs of genes for any hereditary trait

hexose (heks′ōs): a 6-carbon sugar; glucose, fructose, galactose

histidine (his′tid-in): a basic amino acid essential for growing children but not for adults

homeostasis (ho-me-o-sta′sis): tendency to maintain equilibrium in normal body states

homogenize (ho-moj′en-īz): to make of uniform quality throughout

homozygous (ho-mo-zi′gus): having identical pairs of genes for any given pair of hereditary traits

hormone (hor′mōn): substance produced by an organ to produce a specific effect in another organ

hydrogenation (hi′dro-jen-a′shun): the addition of

hydrogen to a compound, such as an unsaturated fatty acid to produce a solid fat

hydrolysate (hi-drol′is-āt): the product of hydrolysis; e.g., protein hydrolysate is a mixture of the constituent amino acids when the protein molecule is split by acids, alkalies, or enzymes

hydrolysis (hi-drol′is-is): the splitting up of a product by the addition of water

hydroxyproline (hi′drok-se-pro′lin): a nonessential amino acid occurring abundantly in collagen

hyper-: a prefix meaning above, beyond, or excessive

hypercalcemia (hi-per-kal-se′me-ah): abnormally high calcium level in the blood

hypercalciuria (hi-per-kal-se-u′re-ah): abnormal calcium excretion in the urine

hyperchlorhydria (hi-per-klor-hi′dre-ah): increased hydrochloric acid secretion by stomach cells

hyperchromic (hi-per-krōm′ik): abnormally high color

hyperemia (hi-per-e′me-ah): excess of blood in any part of the body

hyperesthesia (hi-per-es-the′zĭ-ah): increased sensitivity to touch or pain

hyperglycemia (hi-per-glĭ-se′me-ah): an excess of sugar in the blood

hyperkalemia (hi-per-kah-le′me-ah): an increased level of potassium in the blood

hyperplasia (hi-per-pla′se-ah): abnormal multiplication of normal cells

hypertrophic (hi-per-tro′fik): pertaining to enlargement of an organ due to increase in size of its constituent cells

hyperuricemia (hi-per-u-ris-e′me-ah): excess of uric acid in the blood; one of the characteristics of gout

hypervitaminosis (hi-per-vi-tah-min-o′sis): condition produced by excessive ingestion of vitamins, especially vitamins A and D

hypo-: prefix meaning lack or deficiency

hypoalbuminemia (hi-po-al-bu-min-e′me-ah): low albumin level of the blood

hypochlorhydria (hi-po-klor-hid′re-ah): decreased secretion of hydrochloric acid by the cells of the stomach

hypochromic (hi-po-krom′ik): below normal color; e.g., pale red blood cells lacking hemoglobin

hypoglycemia (hi-po-gli-se′me-ah): a lower than normal level of glucose in the blood

hypokalemia (hi-po-kal-e′me-ah): decreased potassium level in the blood

hypothalamus (hi-po-thal′am-us): a group of nuclei at the base of the brain; includes centers of appetite control, cells that produce antidiuretic hormone

idiopathic (id-e-o-path′ik): pertaining to a disease of unknown origin

idiosyncrasy (id-e-o-sin′kra-se): a susceptibility to action of food or drugs that is characteristic or peculiar to an individual person

ileum (il′e-um): lower portion of the small intestine extending from the jejunum to the cecum

ileus (il′e-us): obstruction of the bowel

infarction (in-fark′shun): the formation of an area of dead tissue resulting from obstruction of blood vessels supplying the part

ingest (in-jest′): to take food into the body

inositol (in-os′it-ol): a 6-carbon alcohol found especially in cereal grains; combines with phosphate to form phytic acid

insidious (in-sid′e-us): pertaining to the progress of a disease with few if any symptoms to indicate its seriousness

insulin (in′su-lin): hormone secreted by beta cells of the islands of Langerhans of the pancreas; promotes utilization of glucose and lowers blood sugar

interstitial (in-ter-stish′al): situated in spaces between tissues

intra-: prefix meaning within

intracellular (in-trah-sel′u-lar): within the cell

intravenous (in-trah-ve′nus): into or from within a vein

intrinsic factor (in-trin′sik): mucoprotein in gastric juice which facilitates absorption of vitamin B_{12}; deficient in patients with pernicious anemia

iodopsin (i-o-dop′sin): pigment found in cones of the retina; visual violet

ion (i′on): an atom or group of atoms carrying a charge of electricity; e.g., cations, anions

ionize (i′on-īz): to separate molecules into electrically charged atoms or group of atoms; the number of negative charges exactly equals the number of positive charges

ischemia (is-ke′me-ah): a local deficiency of blood, chiefly from narrowing of the arteries

isocaloric (i-sō-kal-or′ik): containing an equal number of calories

isoleucine (i-sō-lu′sin): an essential amino acid

isotopes (i′so-tōps): atoms of the same element having the same atomic numbers and chemical properties but differing in the nuclear masses

jaundice (jon′dis): condition characterized by elevated bilirubin level of the blood and deposit of bile pigments in skin and mucous membranes

jejunum (je-joo′num): middle portion of small intestine; extends from duodenum to ileum

joule (jool): the unit of energy in the metric system; 1 calorie equals 4.184 joules (J)

keratin (ker′at-in): an insoluble sulfur-containing protein found in the skin, nails, hair

keratomalacia (ker′at-o-mal-a′shah): dryness and ulceration of the cornea resulting from vitamin A deficiency

keto-: a prefix denoting the presence of the carbonyl (CO) group

ketogenesis (ke-tō-jen′es-is): formation of ketones from fatty acids and some amino acids

α-ketoglutaric acid (ke-tō-gloo-tar′ik): one of the intermediates in the tricarboxylic acid cycle; also the product of oxidative deamination of glutamic acid

ketone (ke′tōn): any compound containing a ketone (CO) grouping; ketone bodies include acetone, beta-hydroxybutyric acid, and acetoacetic acid

ketosis (ke-tō′sis): condition resulting from incomplete oxidation of fatty acids, and the consequent accumulation of ketone bodies

kilocalorie (kil′o-ka′lo-re): the unit of heat used in nutrition; the amount of heat required to raise 1000 gm water 1° C (from 15.5 to 16.5° C); also known as the large calorie

kwashiorkor (kwash-e-or′kor): deficiency disease related principally to protein lack and seen in severely malnourished children; characterized by growth failure, edema, pigment changes in the skin

labile (la′bil): chemically unstable

lactalbumin (lak-tal-bu′min): a protein in milk

lactic acid (lak′tik): 3-carbon acid produced in milk by bacterial fermentation of lactose; also produced during muscle contraction by anaerobic glycolysis

lactose (lak′tōs): a disaccharide composed of glucose and galactose; the form of carbohydrate in milk

lamina propria (lam′in-ah pro′pre-ah): connective-tissue structure that supports the epithelial cells of the intestinal mucosa

lecithin (les′ith-in): a phospholipid occurring in nervous and organ tissues, and in egg yolk; effective emulsifier

leucine (lu′sin): an essential amino acid

linoleic acid (lin-o-le′ic): an 18-carbon fatty acid with two double bonds; essential for growth and skin health

linolenic acid (lin-o-len′ik): an 18-carbon fatty acid with three double bonds; not an essential fatty acid

lipase (lip′ās): an enzyme that hydrolyzes fat

lipid (lip′id): a term for fats including neutral fats, oils, fatty acids, phospholipids, cholesterol

lipogenesis (lip-o-jen′es-is): formation of fat

lipoic acid (lip-o′ik): thioctic acid; protogen; a factor that functions with thiamine pyrophosphate in removing the carboxyl group from alpha keto acids such as pyruvic acid

lipolysis (lip-ol′is-is): the splitting up of fat

lipoprotein (li-po-pro′te-in): a conjugated protein that incorporates lipids to facilitate transportation of the lipids in an aqueous medium

lipotropic (lip-o-trop′ik): pertaining to substances that prevent accumulation of fat in the liver

lithiasis (li-thi′a-sis): the formation of calculi of any kind

lysine (li′sēn): a diamino essential amino acid

lysosomes (li′so-sōms): structures of cell cytoplasm that contain digestive enzymes

macrocyte (mak′ro-sīt): an abnormally large red blood cell

malaise (mal-āz′): discomfort, distress, or uneasiness

malignant (mal-ig′nant): occurring in severe form, frequently fatal; in tumors refers to uncontrollable growth as in cancer

maltose (mawl′tōs): a disaccharide resulting from starch hydrolysis; yields 2 molecules glucose on further hydrolysis

marasmus (mar-az′mus): extreme protein-calorie malnutrition marked by emaciation, especially severe in young children who receive insufficient amounts of food

matrix (ma′trix): the groundwork in which something is cast; for example, protein is the bone matrix into which mineral salts are deposited

megaloblast (meg′al-o-blast): primitive red blood cell of large size with large nucleus; present in blood when there is deficiency of vitamin B_{12} and/or folic acid

menadione (men-a-di′on): synthetic compound with vitamin K activity

metabolic pool (met-ah-bol′ik): the assortment of nutrients available at any given moment of time for the metabolic activities of the body, e.g., amino acid pool, calcium pool

metabolism (me-tab′o-lism): physical and chemical changes occurring within the organism; includes synthesis of biologic materials and breakdown of substances to yield energy methionine (meth-i'o-nin): an essential sulfur-containing amino acid; supplies labile methyl groups

micelle (mis-el'): a microscopic particle of lipids and bile salts

microcyte (mi'kro-sīt): small red blood cell

microvilli (mi'kro-vil'li): minute structures visible by electron microscope, present on surface of mucosal epithelium; the "brush border"

milliequivalent, mEq (mil'lĭ-e-kwiv'ah-lent): concentration of a substance per liter of solution; obtained by dividing the milligrams per liter by the equivalent weight

mitochondria (mit-o-kon'dre-ah): rod-shaped or round structures in cell that trap energy-rich ATP.

monoglyceride (mono-glis'er-id): an ester of glycerol with one fatty acid

monosaccharide (mon-o-sak'ar-id): a single sugar not affected by hydrolysis; includes glucose, fructose, galactose

monounsaturated (mon-o-un-sat'u-ra-ted): having a single double bond as in a fatty acid, e.g., oleic acid

morbidity (mor-bid'it-e): the proportion of disease to health in a community

motility (mo-til'it-e): ability to move spontaneously

mucin (mu'sin): a substance containing mucopolysaccharides secreted by goblet cells of the intestine and other glandular cells; has a protective and lubricating action

mucopolysaccharide (mu'ko-pol-e-sak'er-id): any of a group of polysaccharides combined with other groups such as protein

mucoprotein (mu'ko-pro'te-in): a conjugated protein containing a carbohydrate group such as chondroitin sulfuric acid

mucosa (mu-ko'sah): membrane lining the gastrointestinal, respiratory, and genitourinary tracts

myocardium (mi-o-kar'de-um): the heart muscle

myoglobin (mi-o-glo'bin): an iron-protein complex in muscle that transports oxygen; somewhat similar to hemoglobin

myosin (mi'o-sin): a soluble protein in muscle; combines with actin to form actomyosin, an enzyme that catalyzes the dephosphorylation of ATP during muscle contraction

nausea (naw'se-ah): sickness at the stomach; inclination to vomit

necrosis (ne-kro'sis); death of a cell or cells or of a portion of tissue

neonatal (ne-o-na'tal): pertaining to the newborn

neoplasm (ne'o-plazm): new or abnormal, uncontrolled growth, such as a tumor

nephron (nef'ron): the functional unit of the kidney consisting of a tuft of capillaries known as the glomerulus attached to the renal tubule

neuritic (nu-rit'ik): pertaining to inflammation of a nerve

neuropathy (nu-rop'ath-e): disease of the nervous system

niacin (ni'ah-sin): one of the water-soluble B complex vitamins which functions as a coenzyme in cell respiration; antipellagra factor

niacin equivalent: the total niacin available from the diet including preformed niacin plus that derived from the metabolism of tryptophan; 60 mg tryptophan = 1 mg niacin

niacinamide (ni'ah-sin-am'id): biologically active form of niacin occurring in the tissues

nicotinamide adenine dinucleotide, NAD (nik'o-tin-am'id ad'en-in di-nu'kle-o-tid): coenzyme for a number of enzymes, chiefly dehydrogenases

nicotinic acid (nik-o-tin'ik): niacin

nocturia (nok-tu're-ah): excessive urination at night

nucleic acid (nu-kle'ik): complex organic acid containing four bases—adenine, guanine, cytosine, and thymine—attached to ribose and phosphate

nucleoprotein (nu-kle-o-pro'te-in): conjugated protein found in the nuclei of cells; yields a protein fraction and nucleic acid

nucleotide (nu'kle-o-tid): a hydrolytic product of nucleic acid; contains one purine or pyrimidine base and a sugar phosphate

nutrient (nu'tre-ent): chemical substance in foods which nourishes, e.g., amino acid, fat, calcium

nyctalopia (nik-tal-o'pe-ah): night blindness

nystagmus (nis-tag'mus): rhythmic rapid movement of the eyeball

oleic acid (o-le'ik): an 18-carbon fatty acid containing one double bond; widely distributed in foods

oliguria (ol-ig-u're-ah): scanty secretion of urine

-ology: suffix meaning science of, study of

ophthalmia (of-thal'me-ah): severe inflammation of the eye

organelles (or-gan-elz'): the various structures of the cell such as lysosomes, mitochondria

ornithine (or'nith-in): an amino acid formed from arginine when urea is split off

osmosis (oz-mo'sis): passage of a solvent from the lesser to the greater concentration when two solutions are separated by a membrane

ossification (os-if-ik-a'shun); formation of bone

osteo-: prefix meaning bone

osteomalacia (os-te-o-mal-a'se-ah): softening of the bone, chiefly in adults

osteoporosis (os-te-o-po-ro'sis): reduction of the

quantity of bone, occurring principally in women after middle age; the remaining bone is normally mineralized

oxalic acid (oks-al'ik): a dicarboxylic acid present in foods such as spinach, chard, rhubarb; forms insoluble salts with calcium

oxaloacetic acid (oks-al-o-as-e'tik): a 3-carbon ketodicarboxylic acid; an intermediate in the tricarboxylic acid cycle

oxidation (oks-id-a'shun): increase of positive charges on an atom or loss of negative charges

palmitic acid (pal-mit'ik): a 16-carbon saturated fatty acid widespread in foods

pancreozymin (pan'kre-o-zi'min): hormone produced in duodenal mucosa that stimulates secretion of pancreatic enzymes

pantothenic acid (pan-to-then'ik): one of the B complex vitamins; a constituent of coenzyme A

parenchyma (par-en'ki-mah): functional tissue of an organ or gland as distinct from its supporting framework

parenteral (par-en'ter-al): by other means than through the gastrointestinal tract; introduction of nutrients by vein or into subcutaneous tissues

paresthesia (par-es-the'zi-ah): abnormal sensation such as numbness, burning, pricking

parturition (par-tu-rish'un): giving birth to a child

path-, patho-, -pathy: combining forms meaning disease, e.g., *patho*genic, nephro*pathy*

pathology (path-ol'o-je): science dealing with disease; structural and functional changes caused by disease

pectin (pek'tin); a polysaccharide found in many fruits and having gelling properties

pellagra (pel-lah'gra): a deficiency disease of the skin, gastrointestinal tract, and nervous system caused by lack of niacin and associated with other nutritional deficiencies

pentose (pen'tōs): a simple sugar containing 5 carbon atoms; ribose, arabinose, xylose

peptide linkage (pep'tid): the CO-NH linkage of two amino acids by condensation of the amino group of one amino acid with the carboxyl group of another amino acid

peptone (pep'tone): an intermediate product of protein digestion

perinatal (per-ĭ-na'tal): pertaining to before, during, or after the time of birth

peristalsis (per-is-tal'sis): the rhythmic, wavelike movement produced by muscles of the small intestine to move food forward

phagocyte (fag'o-sīt): a cell capable of ingesting bacteria or other foreign material

phenylalanine (fen-il-al'ah-nin): an essential amino acid; consists of a phenyl group attached to alanine

phenylketonuria (fe-nil-ke-to-nu're-ah): excretion of phenylpyruvic acid and other phenyl compounds in urine because of congenital lack of an enzyme required for conversion of phenylalanine to tyrosine; characterized by mental retardation

phospholipid (fos'fo-lip'id): a fatlike compound that contains a phosphate and another group such as a nitrogen base in addition to glycerol and fatty acids, e.g., lecithin, cephalin

phosphoprotein (fos-fo-pro'te-in): a conjugated protein that contains phosphorus, e.g., nucleoprotein, casein

phosphorylate (fos-fo'ril-ate): to introduce a phosphate grouping into an organic compound, e.g., glucose monophosphate produced by action of enzyme *phosphorylase*

photosynthesis (fo-to-sin'the-sis): the process whereby the chlorophyll in green plants utilizes the energy from the sun to synthesize carbohydrate from carbon dioxide and water

phylloquinone (fil'o-kwin-ōn): vitamin K

phytic acid (fi'tik): a phosphoric acid ester of inositol found in seeds; interferes with absorption of calcium, magnesium, iron

pica (pi'kah): a hunger for substances not fit for food

pinocytosis (pin-o-si-to'sis): the taking up of droplets (for example, fat) by a cell by surrounding the liquid with part of the membrane

plaque (plak): any patch or flat area; atherosclerotic plaque in a deposit of lipid material in the blood vessel

plasma (plaz'mah): fluid portion of the blood before clotting has taken place

poly-: prefix meaning much or many

polyneuritis (pol-e-nu-ri'tis): inflammation of a number of nerves

polypeptide (pol-e-pep'tid): a compound consisting of more than three amino acids; an intermediate stage in protein digestion

polyphagia (pol-e-fa'je-ah): excessive eating

polysaccharide (pol-e-sak'ar-id): a class of carbohydrates containing many single sugars; includes starch, glycogen, dextrins, pectins, cellulose, and others

polyunsaturated fatty acid: fatty acids containing two or more double bonds; linoleic, linolenic, and arachidonic acids

porphyrin (por'fir-in): a pigmented compound containing four pyrrole nuclei joined in a ring structure; combines with iron in hemoglobin

prenatal (prē-na'tal): preceding birth

proenzyme (pro-en'zīm): inactive form of an enzyme, e.g., pepsinogen

progesterone (prō-jes'ter-ōn): hormone of corpus luteum which prepares endometrium for reception and development of the fertilized ovum

prognosis (prog-no'sis): forecast of probable result from attack of disease

proline (pro'lēn): a nonessential amino acid

prophylaxis (pro-fil-ak'sis): prevention of disease

prosthetic group (pros-thet'ik): chemical group attached to a molecule such as protein; nonprotein part of an enzyme

protease (pro'te-ās): an enzyme that digests protein

proteinuria (pro'te-in-u'ri-ah): excretion of protein in the urine

proteolytic (pro'te-o-lit'ik): effecting the hydrolysis of protein

proteose (pro'te-ōs): a derivative of protein formed during digestion

prothrombin (pro-throm'bin): factor in blood plasma for blood clotting; precursor of thrombin

protoplasm (pro'to-plazm): form of living matter in all cells

protoporphyrin (pro'tō-por'fir-in): a porphyrin combined with iron and globin forming hemoglobin

provitamin (pro-vi'tah-min): precursor of a vitamin

proximal (prok'sim-al): nearest to the head or point of attachment

pteroylglutamic acid (ter'o-il-glu-tam'ik): folic acid

puerperium (pur-pe'ri-um): the period after labor until involution of the uterus

purine (pu'rin): organic compounds containing heterocyclic nitrogen structures that are catabolized to uric acid; supplied especially by flesh foods and synthesized in the body

pyridoxal phosphate (pir-ĭ-dok'sal fos'fate): a coenzyme that contains vitamin B_6

pyridoxine (pi-ri-dox'in): one of the forms of vitamin B_6

pyruvic acid (pi-ru'vik): a 3-carbon keto acid; an intermediate in glucose metabolism

rancid (ran'sid): term that describes rank taste or smell that results from decomposition of fatty acids

regurgitation (re-gur-jit-a'shun): the backward flow of food; casting up of undigested food

relapsing (re-laps'ing): return of symptoms

remission (re-mish'un): a lessening of the severity or temporary abatement of symptoms

renal (re'nal): pertaining to the kidney

renal threshold: the level of concentration of a substance in the blood beyond which it is excreted in the urine

rennin (ren'in): enzyme in gastric juice that coagulates milk protein

repletion (rep-le'shun): plethora; to fill up; to restore

resection (re-sek'shun): removal of part of an organ

residue (rez'i-du): remainder; the contents remaining in the intestinal tract after digestion of food; includes fiber and other unabsorbed products

resorption (re-sorp'shun): a loss of substance, e.g., loss of mineral salts from bone

reticulocyte (re-tik'u-lo-sīt): a young red blood cell occurring during active blood regeneration

reticuloendothelium (re-tik'u-lo-en-dō-the'le-um): a system of macrophages concerned with phagocytosis; present in spleen, liver, bone marrow, connective tissues, and lymph nodes

retinene (ret'in-ēn): vitamin A aldehyde; intermediate step in bleaching of visual purple

retinopathy (ret-in-op'ath-e): degenerative disease of the retina

rhodopsin (ro-dop'sin): visual purple; pigment of the rods of the retina bleached by light; vitamin A required for regeneration

riboflavin (ri'bo-fla'vin): heat-stable B complex vitamin and a constituent of flavin enzymes; vitamin B_2

ribonucleic acid, RNA (ri-bo-nu-kle'ik): molecules in cytoplasm which serve for transfer of amino acid code from nucleus and the synthesis of protein

ribose (ri'bōs): 5-carbon sugar; a constituent of nucleic acid

ribosomes (ri'bo-sōms): dense particles in cell cytoplasm that are the site of protein synthesis

rickets (rik'ets): a deficiency disease of the skeletal system caused by a lack of vitamin D or calcium or both, and often resulting in bone deformities

saccharin (sak'ah-rin): a sweetening agent that is 300 to 500 times as sweet as sugar; yields no calories

Salmonella (sal-mo-nel'ah): group of bacteria causing intestinal infection; frequently contaminates foods

saponification (sap-on'if-ik-a'shun): the action of alkali on a fat to form a soap

satiety (sat-i'et-e): feeling of satisfaction following meals

saturated (sat'u-ra-ted): a state in which a substance holds the most of another substance that it can

scurvy (skur′vē): a deficiency disease caused by lack of ascorbic acid and leading to swollen bleeding gums, hemorrhages of the skin and mucous membranes, and anemia

secretin (se-kre′tin): a hormone secreted by the epithelium of the duodenum upon stimulation by the acid chyme; stimulates secretion of pancreatic juice and bile

serine (se′rin): one of the amino acids occurring in protein; nonessential

serosa (ser-o′sah): the membranes lining the peritoneal, pericardial, and pleural cavities and covering their contents

serum (se′rum): the fluid portion of the blood that separates from the blood cells after clotting

siderophilin (sid′er-o-fil′in): an iron-transferring protein

sorbitol (sor′bit-ol): a 6-carbon sugar alcohol with a sweet taste; used commercially to maintain moisture and inhibit crystal formation

sphincter (sfink′ter): a muscle surrounding and closing an orifice

sphingomyelin (sfing-go-mi′el-in): a phospholipid found in the brain, spinal cord, and kidney

stasis (sta′sis): retardation or cessation of flow of blood in the vessels; congestion

steapsin (ste-ap′sin): a hormone in pancreatic juice that hydrolyzes fat; lipase

stearic acid (ste′rik): a saturated fatty acid containing 18 carbon atoms

steatorrhea (ste-at-o-re′ah): excessive amount of fat in the feces

stenosis (sten-o′sis): narrowing of a passage

steroid (ste′roid): a group of compounds similar in structure to cholesterol; includes bile acids, sterols, sex hormones

sterol (ste′rol): an alcohol of high molecular weight; cholesterol, ergosterol

stomatitis (sto-ma-ti′tis): inflammation of the mucous membranes of the mouth

sub-: prefix denoting beneath, or less than normal

substrate (sub′strāt): substance upon which an enzyme acts

succinic acid (suk-sen′ik): a 3-carbon dicarboxylic acid that is an intermediate in the tricarboxylic acid cycle

sucrose (su′krōs): cane or beet sugar; a disaccharide that yields glucose and fructose when hydrolyzed

syn-: prefix meaning with, together

syndrome (sin′drōm): a set of symptoms occurring together

synergism (sin′er-jizm): the joint action of agents which when taken together increases each other's effectiveness

synthesis (sin′thes-is): process of building up a compound

systemic (sis-tem′ik): pertaining to the body as a whole

tachycardia (tak-e-kar′de-ah): rapid beating of the heart

testosterone (tes-tos′ter-ōn): testicular hormone responsible for male secondary sex characteristics

tetany (tet′an-e): a condition marked by intermittent muscular contraction accompanied by fibrillar tremors and muscular pains; seen in hypocalcemia, alkalosis, etc.

thiamine (thi′am-in): a B complex vitamin; with phosphate forms coenzymes of decarboxylases; essential for carbohydrate metabolism

thio-: prefix meaning sulfur containing

threonine (thre′o-nin): an essential amino acid

thrombus (throm′bus): a clot in a blood vessel formed by coagulation of blood

thymine (thi′min): one of the four nitrogenous bases in nucleic acid

thyroxine (thī-rok′sin): iodine-containing hormone produced by the thyroid gland; regulates the rate of energy metabolism

tocopherol (tok-of′er-ōl): vitamin E; antioxidant alcohol occurring in vegetable germ oils; alpha-, beta-, gamma-, delta-tocopherol

-tomy: suffix meaning to cut into, e.g., gastrectomy

tophi (to′fi): sodium urate deposits in fibrous tissues near the joints; present in gout

tox-: prefix meaning poison

toxemia of pregnancy (tok-se′me-ah): a disorder of pregnancy characterized by hypertension, edema, albuminuria

transamination (trans′am-in-a′shun): transfer of an amino group to another molecule, e.g., transfer to a keto acid, thus forming another amino acid

transferase (trans′fer-ās): an enzyme that transfers a chemical grouping from one compound to another, for example, transaminase, transphosphorylase

transferrin (trans-fer′in): iron-binding protein for transport of iron in blood; siderophilin

trauma (traw-mah): wound or injury usually inflicted suddenly

trichinosis (trik-in-o′sis): illness caused by eating raw pork that is infested by *Trichinella spiralis,* a worm

triglyceride (tri-glis′er-id): an ester of glycerol and three fatty acids

trypsin (trip′sin): a protein-digesting enzyme secreted by the pancreas and released into the small intestine

trypsinogen (trip-sin′o-jen): inactive form of trypsin

tryptophan (trip′tō-fan): an essential amino acid that contains the indole ring; a precursor of niacin

tyramine (tir′am-en): a pressor amine that has an action similar to epinephrine; produced by decarboxylation of tyrosine; found especially in cheeses and some wines

tyrosine (ti′ro-sin): semiessential amino acid; spares phenylalanine; the amino acid in thyroxine

urea (u-re′ah): chief nitrogenous constituent of the urine; formed by the liver when amino acids are deaminized

uremia (u-re′me-ah): presence of urinary constituents in the blood resulting from deficient secretion of urine

uric acid (u-rik): a nitrogenous constituent formed in the metabolism of purines; excreted in the urine; blood levels increased in gout

valine (va′lin): an essential amino acid

villus (vil′us): fingerlike projection of the intestinal mucosa

viosterol (vi-os′ter-ol): vitamin D formed by irradiation of ergosterol

visual purple: photosensitive pigment found in the rods of the retina; rhodopsin

vitamin (vi′tah-min): organic compound occurring in minute amounts in foods and essential for numerous metabolic reactions; fat-soluble A, D, E, and K; water-soluble ascorbic acid and B complex including thiamine, riboflavin, niacin, pantothenic acid, biotin, vitamin B_6, vitamin B_{12}, folacin, and others

xanthine (zan′thin): an intermediate in the metabolism of purines; related to uric acid

xanthomatosis (zan-thō-mat-o′sis): accumulation of lipids in the form of tumors in various parts of the body

xerophthalmia (zer-of-thal′me-ah): dry infected eye condition caused by lack of vitamin A

xerosis (ze-ro′sis): abnormal dryness of skin and eye

xylose (zi′lōs): a 5-carbon aldehyde sugar that is not metabolized by the body

zein (za′in): a protein of low biologic value present in corn

zymogen (zi′mo-jen): the inactive form of an enzyme

Index

Illustrations are indicated by numbers in **boldface** type.